A Curriculum for Plastic Surgery

Edward Luce

A Curriculum for Plastic Surgery

A Cognitive and Case-Based Approach

Volume I

Springer

Edward Luce
Adjunct Professor of Plastic Surgery
University of South Carolina School of Medicine
Colombia, SC, USA

ISBN 978-3-031-62086-7 ISBN 978-3-031-62087-4 (eBook)
https://doi.org/10.1007/978-3-031-62087-4

This Springer imprint is published by the registered company Springer Nature Switzerland AG
The registered company address is: Gewerbestrasse 11, 6330 Cham, Switzerland

Foreword

The field of plastic surgery stands at an intriguing crossroad. With advancements in technology and a rapidly evolving medical landscape, the demands on plastic surgeons are more complex and diverse than ever. This book, *A Curriculum for Plastic Surgery: A Cognitive and Case-Based Approach*, First Edition, by Dr. Edward Luce, aims to bridge the current gap in our educational framework by providing a comprehensive, modular curriculum designed to cultivate not only clinical excellence but also ethical, compassionate, and innovative leaders in plastic surgery.

My journey with Dr. Luce, already at that time an experienced and renowned surgeon and consummate educator, began in 1996 when I was a third-year medical student at Case Western Reserve University in Cleveland, Ohio, where he served as Chairman of the Department of Plastic Surgery. I first witnessed his visionary approach to medical education at Case. Dr. Luce's curriculum was both meticulous and inspiring, transforming our understanding of what medical training could achieve. The depth of his commitment to fostering well-rounded, highly skilled plastic surgeons left a profound impact on me, shaping the way I approached my own career. His dedication to creating a structured yet adaptable learning environment was evident in every interaction, every case, and every conference. Observing him brought home the importance of innovation in medical education—an ethos that has guided my professional journey ever since. I remain indebted to him for his commitment both to me as an individual and to the specialty as whole.

Rooted in the traditions of graduate medical education, the curriculum outlined by Dr. Luce in this book reimagines the methods of instruction and evaluation. From embracing adult learning principles to the integration of mobile technology and case-based conferences, this book sets forth a vision for what the future of plastic surgery training could—and should—be. The traditional "apprenticeship" model, while foundational, must adapt to the realities of the challenges to modern residency programs and the accreditation mandates. This book addresses those challenges head-on, offering a structure that emphasizes cognitive understanding, skill development, and practical application.

The approach within these pages prioritizes interactive learning, recognizing that the ability to diagnose, plan, and execute treatment is as much an art as a science. The text encourages a shift from passive absorption of information to active engagement in the learning process. For both faculty and residents, this book is a call to embrace a transformative model of education that meets the needs of tomorrow's plastic surgeons. The work is a comprehensive guide for residency programs aiming to foster well-rounded, proficient practitioners who are ready to lead the field into the future.

This book is organized into 12 sections, a sum totaling 110 modules/sessions, covering the breadth and depth of plastic surgery. With each meticulously developed module are integrated case studies and cognitive conferences, which lay the groundwork for a structured and adaptable curriculum that can be tailored to the unique needs of each resident. More than a roadmap—an invitation to elevate the standards of plastic surgery education and, ultimately, the quality of patient care. I saw the roots of this in action in 1996 and in a fully developed form presented here in 2024. Certainly, it couldn't be timelier, although still ahead of its time, truth be told. Dr. Luce's vision remains precocious, precedential, and impactful, and above all else, inspirational, an "educational North star."

Ohio State University Wexner Medical Center
Columbus, OH, USA

Jeffrey E. Janis

Preface

To compose a curriculum in plastic surgery is a daunting task because the specialty is truly comprehensive but also in an ongoing evolution. The content only faintly resembles that of 50 years ago, yet the concepts of reconstructive and aesthetic surgery remain the same.

What is a curriculum anyway? A variety of definitions exist including the redundant "studies prescribed for study in a school" or "a program of study." In medical education, at least in undergraduate and graduate medical education, a curriculum references those areas of medicine to be mastered as a graduate of a medical school in the instance of a medical student or to become a competent physician in the case of a resident. Viewed from the perspective of graduate medical education, a curriculum should serve both as a template and as a guide. The former in application within any institutional resident program, the latter in flexibility to modify in application to a particular residency. Of course, a surgical curriculum incorporates technical and nontechnical skills. This curriculum is designed to address the acquisition of the necessary foundation of cognitive knowledge and analytic reasoning or problem-solving capability, all to progress toward the objective of achievement of competency in the practice of plastic surgery.

This book offers a comprehensive curriculum on plastic surgery, centered on adult learning principles. The pedagogical structure includes a base of cognitive information that consists of the entire spectrum of plastic surgery; reconstructive and aesthetic; a guide for an interactive discussion of each component of the knowledge base; a set of multiple-choice questions with relevant references; and clinical cases to illustrate each element. Over 100 modules constitute the curriculum, all of which are grouped into twelve general categories. Each module includes a selected bibliography of relevant and contemporary readings that provide a base of cognitive information, a discussion guide of broad questions and answers for a faculty member to drive an interactive discussion of the module, a set of multiple choice questions to serve as a short written quiz, and 1–3 cases that are utilized in a case-based conference to discuss the practical application of cognitive knowledge to problem-solving of a clinical scenario in a broad question format about analysis and development of a treatment plan. Each clinical case is attended by a full discussion centered on the appropriate responses to the question format. The cases could equally serve as mock oral boards or for American Board of Plastic Surgery board preparation. Finally, a several page review of the particular case provides an optimal approach to diagnosis and treatment.

A Curriculum for Plastic Surgery provides an encyclopedic yet facile vehicle to deliver a comprehensive, contemporary, and interactive curriculum. The work is intended for plastic surgery faculty, residents and fellows, board candidates, and practitioners. The curriculum reflects the author's four decade long career in academic practice and teaching within this field.

The development of this curriculum would not have been possible with the unswerving support of Jack Hoopes MD and the John E. Hoopes Foundation. Thanks to the production staff of Springer Verlag. A very special thank you to Gwyneth McMahon BS for your assistance as a scribe, illustrator, and advisor in composition of this work.

Colombia, SC, USA Edward Luce

Curriculum Outline

(Master List)

(110 Sessions)

I. BASIC PRINCIPLES AND PHYSIOLOGY: 11 sessions
II. CONGENITAL ANOMALIES OF HEAD AND NECK: 13 sessions
III. SKIN CANCER: 9 sessions
IV. HEAD AND NECK TUMORS: 6 sessions
V. MAXILLOFACIAL TRAUMA: 10 sessions
VI. TRUNK, LOWER EXTREMITY, AND PERINEUM: 8 sessions
VII. BURNS: 6 sessions
VIII. HAND: 15 sessions
IX. BREAST: 13 sessions
X. AESTHETIC : 14 sessions
XI. GENDER AFFIRMATION, PERINEAL AESTHETIC SURGERY: 2 sessions
XII. PATIENT SAFETY: 2 sessions

General Precepts:

1. Patient Care 5: Consultant can be integrated into specific cases even at Level I–V, for example, V.A.1, 2; VIII A.
2. Patient Care 6: Surgical maturity and surgical care. This component of the patient care milestone can be integrated into *any* of the cases.
3. The outline is not primarily designed to assess the following competencies:
   - System-based practice 2, 3
   - Practice-based learning and improvement 1, 2
   - Professionalism 1, 2, 3
   - Interpersonal and communication skills 1, 2
   - All of the above could be assessed in case-based conferences but only indirectly and at the cost of considerable consumption of time. Assessment of the above list is probably best executed by the day-to-day clinical responsibilities of the resident.
4. Some submodules, for example, IVB1,2a, within the curriculum could be optimally assessed at milestone level 1–4 in the cognitive conference.
5. The cases represent the ability of the resident to not only analyze the dysfunction and/or deformity, develop a treatment plan, but also *describe*: so either has scrubbed, performed, or read or watched a video, so… dependent on Milestone achieved either as scrubbed, performed, or read about the particular case.
6. Assumes that performance of Level 1 would primarily be cognitive and assessed with a written exam. The notable exceptions are Patient Care 5: Consultant for V.A.1, 2 and VIII.A.
7. The assignment of milestone levels within the individual case conference discussions is clearly somewhat arbitrary.

I. General Principles (11 Sessions)

A. Wound healing 1, 2
   1. Physiology of wound healing, chronic wounds, ancillary measures: Hyperbaric oxygen, negative pressure wound care (NWPT)
      - No cases
   2. Nutrition and wound healing, impediments to wound healing by adjuvant therapy
      - Case 1:Difficult wound
      - Case 2: Subacute wound
      - Case 3: Elbow ulcer

B. Hypertrophic scar, keloids, skin grafts (Patient Care 7: Wound, Burn, Infection)
   - Case 1: Keloid
   - Case 2: Keloid

C. Local anesthetics, conscious sedation, regional anesthesia
   - No cases

D. Bone and cartilage healing, bone and cartilage grafts, osteomyelitis, bone substitutes
   - No cases

E. Flaps
   1. Classification, physiology, selection
      - No cases
   2. Design
      - No cases
   3. Tissue expansion
      - Case 1: Scalp burn alopecia

F. Microsurgery, general principles, flap failure
   - No cases

G. Biomaterials: Synthetics, skin substitutes
   - No cases

H. Lasers: Basic principles
   - No cases

II. Congenital Anomalies of the Head and Neck (Also Includes Ear Deformities) (13 Sessions)

A. Cleft lip and palate
   1. Unilateral cleft lip: General, anatomy, preoperative management, lip–nose repair
      - Case 1: Unilateral cleft lip
   2. Bilateral cleft lip: Anatomy, preoperative management, lip–nose repair
      - Case 1: Bilateral cleft lip
   3. Secondary cleft lip deformities: Late secondary deformities, cleft rhinoplasty
      - Case 1: Cleft lip deformity
      - Case 2: Cleft lip nasal deformity
   4. Cleft palate: Epidemiology and embryology, anatomy, operative repair, complications, submucous cleft palate, Pierre Robin syndrome
      - Case 1: Cleft palate
   5. Velopharyngeal insufficiency: General; anatomy and function, treatment, specific operations, complications
      - Case 1: Speech disorder

B. Craniofacial, orthognathic surgery, distraction osteogenesis
   1. Alveolar cleft, cephalometrics and orthognathic surgery, distraction osteogenesis, palatal fistulas
      - Case 1: Cleft lip; late facial deformity
      - Case 2: Palatal fistula
      - Case 3: Alveolar cleft
   2. Craniofacial anomalies: Fibrous dysplasia, Romberg's disease, neurofibromatosis, craniofacial microsomia, Treacher-Collins, other syndromes
      - Case 1: Craniofacial deformity
      - Case 2: Maxillary tumor
      - Case 3: Torticollis
   3. Overview of craniosynostosis, specific craniosynostosis, deformational plagiocephaly, orbital deformities
      - No cases

C. Cysts, sinuses
   - Case 1: Glabellar mass

D. Vascular anomalies (including non-head and neck)
   1. Hemangiomas: Pathology, natural history, clinical picture, treatment
      - Case 1: Vascular anomaly in an infant
   2. Vascular malformations of the head, neck, extremities
      - Case 1: Large mass of cheek

E. Ear deformities (1, 2), including otoplasty
   1. Anatomy, embryology, otoplasty
      - Case 1: Protruding ears
   2. Ear deformities: Microtia, other ear deformities besides protruding ears
      - Case 1: Ear deformity

III. Skin and Soft Tissue Cancer Including Reconstruction (9 Sessions)

A. Non-melanotic, skin cancer: Sunscreens, epidemiology, basal cell, squamous cell, Moh's micrographic surgery
   - Case 1: Multiple basal cell cancers

B. Non-melanotic, reconstruction, specific areas
   1. Eyelid: Anatomy, reconstruction, upper lid, lower lid
      - Case 1: Cancer of the lower eyelid
      - Case 2: Cancer of the lower eyelid
      - Case 3: Upper lid lesion
      - Case 4: Upper lid reconstruction
   2. Cheek reconstruction: Anatomy, reconstruction
      - Case 1: Skin cancer of the cheek
      - Case 2: Cancer of the face
      - Case 3: Lip cheek defect
   3. Nose: Anatomy, reconstruction
      - Case 1: Nasal lesion
      - Case 2: Nasal lesion
      - Case 3: Nasal lesion
      - Case 4: Nasal lesion
      - Case 5: Nasal lesion
      - Case 6: Nasal lesion
      - Case 7: Nasal lesion

4. Scalp, forehead: Anatomy, reconstruction
   - Case 1: Recurrent cancer of the scalp
   - Case 2: Scalp reconstruction
5. Ear reconstruction: Anatomy, reconstruction
   - Case 1: Cancer of the ear
   - Case 2: Cancer of the ear

C. Melanoma, pigmented lesions
1. Melanoma: Pathology, staging, excision, sentinel lymph node, advanced disease
   - Case 1: Melanoma
   - Case 2: Melanoma
2. Pigmented lesions: Congenital, lentigo
   - Case 1: Pigmented lesion

D. Adnexal tumors, Merkel cell carcinoma, dermatofibrosarcoma protuberans, sarcomas
- Case 1: Recurrent cancer of the scalp

IV. Head and Neck Tumors (6 Sessions)

A. Anatomy, work-up, principles of treatment, including surgery, radiation, and chemotherapy
- Case 1: Malignant neck mass

B. Lip, oral cavity, oropharynx, hypopharynx, maxilla
1. Lip: Anatomy, pathology, upper and lower lip reconstruction
   - Case 1: Tumor of the upper lip
   - Case 2: Cancer of the lower lip
   - Case 3: Basal cell cancer upper lip

2a. Mandibular reconstruction: Classification, options, virtual surgical planning
   - Case 1: Draining fistula

2b. Intraoral defect reconstruction
   - Case 1: Oral cavity lesion
   - Case 2: Cancer of the oropharynx

3. Hypopharynx, maxilla reconstruction: Anatomy, flap options
   - Case 1: Hypopharyngeal stricture
   - Case 2: Cancer of the maxilla

C. Salivary gland: Anatomy, pathology, treatment, benign disease
- Case 1: Cheek mass

V. Maxillofacial Trauma (10 Sessions)

A. General principles
1. Anatomy, airway, bleeding, radiology, clinical examination
   - Case 1: Initial care of maxillofacial trauma
   - Case 2: Initial care of maxillofacial trauma
2. Ocular injuries, operative approaches, reduction and fixation
   - Case 1: Ocular trauma

B. Soft tissue injury
1. Soft tissue injury: Parotid, eyelid, orbital adnexa
   - Case 1: Acute eyelid injury
   - Case 2: Ectropion
   - Case 3: Facial laceration
2. Gunshot wounds: Wound ballistics, reconstruction
   - Case 1: GSW to the face

3. Facial nerve (including non-traumatic)
   - Case 1: Facial paralysis
   - Case 2: Facial paralysis
   - Case 3: Facial paralysis

Note: All facial fracture modules, C–F, include anatomy, evaluation, general principles, reduction and fixation, complications

C. Upper one-third (skull, orbital roof, frontal sinus)
   - Case 1: Orbital roof
   - Case 2: Frontal sinus injury
   - Case 3: Frontal sinus fracture
   - Case 4: Cranioplasty
   - Case 5: Infected cranioplasty

D. Complex maxillary, NEO, and nasal fractures
   - Case 1: Midface fractures

E. Zygoma, orbit
   - Case 1: Facial fracture
   - Case 2: Facial fracture
   - Case 3: Orbital floor fracture

F. Mandible
   1. Mandible
      - Case 1: Mandible fracture
   2. Mandible: Condylar, pediatric fractures, complications
      - Case 1: Mandible fracture
      - Case 2: Infected mandible fracture

VI. Lower Extremity, Perineum, and Trunk (8 Sessions)

A. Lower extremity
   1. Trauma: Anatomy, limb salvage vs. amputation, management, osteomyelitis
      - Case 1: Lower extremity trauma
   2. Foot reconstruction, reconstruction of limb bony oncologic defects, specific flaps, (Session 2)
      - Case 1: Soft tissue loss, foot
   3. Complex groin wounds, extremity lymphedema (Session 3)
      - Case 1: Radiotherapy ulcer
      - Case 2: Exposure of vascular reconstruction
      - Case 3: Swollen extremity

B. Perineum
   1. Reconstruction of the vagina, congenital and acquired, perineum
      - Case 1: Persistent perineal sinus
      - Case 2: Perineal reconstruction
   2. Decubiti, others
      - Case 1: Sacral decubitus

C. Chest wall, back, abdomen
   1. Myelomeningocele, complex back wounds (Session 6)
      - Case 1: Complex back wound
      - Case 2: Myelomeningocele
      - Case 3: Back wound
   2. Abdominal wall (Session 7)
      - Case 1: Abdominal wall reconstruction
      - Case 2: Abdominal wall reconstruction

   3. Chest wall, sternum (Session 8)
      - Case 1: Chest wall ulcer
      - Case 2: Open chest wound
      - Case 3: GSW of shoulder-neck
      - Case 4: Sternal dehiscence

VII. Burns, Difficult Wounds (6 Sessions)

A. Burns: Pathophysiology, resuscitation, pulmonary complications
   - Case 1: Acute burn

B. Wound care and coverage (Session 2)
   - Case 1: Acute burn

C. Nutrition and metabolic support, electrical and chemical burn injury (Session 3)
   - Case 1: Electrical burn of scalp
   - Case 2: Electrical burns of trunk, extremities

D. Reconstruction
   1. Eyelids, ears, nose, cheek/face, neck (Session 4)
      - Case 1: Acute, late burn of the eyelids
      - Case 2: Head/neck burn reconstruction
   2. Hand/upper extremity, axilla, breast, foot, splints, and scar management (Session 5)
      - Case 1: Hand burn
      - Case 2: Burn contracture of the trunk in adolescent female

E. Soft tissue infections, difficult wounds (Session 6)
   - Case 1: Severe infection of the axillae

VIII. Hand and Upper Extremity (15 Sessions)

A. Anatomy, function, initial management of hand trauma, anesthesia
   - Case 1: Initial care of the injured hand

B. Congenital
   - Case 1: Thumb duplication
   - Case 2: Congenital anomalies of the hand
   - Case 3: Webbed fingers

C. Fingertip loss, amputations, local flaps, flap coverage including micro
   1. Fingertip loss, amputations
      - Case 1: Thumb soft tissue injury
      - Case 2: Pediatric digit soft tissue loss
      - Case 3: Thumb tip injury
   2. Regional flap coverage, thumb reconstruction
      - Case 1: Arm defect
      - Case 2: Deep burn/wound of hand
      - Case 3: Thumb reconstruction
      - Case 4: Avulsion injury of the hand

D. Fractures
   1. Metacarpal and phalangeal fractures
      - Case 1: Phalangeal fracture
      - Case 2: Multiple metacarpal fractures
      - Case 3: Metacarpal base fracture
      - Case 4: Proximal phalanx fracture

2. Dislocations and ligament injuries
   - Case 1: PIP joint dislocation
   - Case 2: Injured thumb
   - Case 3: MP joint dislocation
3. Carpal fractures and dislocations
   - No cases

E. Vascular problems, complex regional pain syndrome
   - Case 1: Ischemia of the hand
   - Case 2: SGW of forearm; late sequelae

F. Peripheral nerve
1. Nerve Injuries: Pathophysiology, repair, conduits, and grafts
   - Case 1: Pain and weakness of the hand
   - Case 2: Possible nerve injury
   - Case 3: Reconstruction of neurovascular injury of arm
   - Case 4: Peripheral nerve injury
2. Nerve compression syndromes, brachial plexus: Diagnosis
   - Case 1: Compression neuropathy

G. Flexor tendons: Acute and reconstructive
   - Case 1: Flexor tendon injury
   - Case 2: Flexor tendon injury
   - Case 3: Flexor tendon injury
   - Case 4: Failed flexor tendon repair
   - Case 5: Flexor tendon reconstruction

H. Extensor tendons: Acute and reconstructive
   - Case 1: Finger injury
   - Case 2: Finger injury
   - Case 3: Hand laceration

I. Ganglia, tumors, Dupuytren's
   - Case 1: Digital tumor
   - Case 2: Hand contracture
   - Case 3: Volar wrist mass

J. Infections, tendinopathies, rheumatoid arthritis, and other arthritides
   - Case 1: Injection injury of the finger
   - Case 2: Hand infection

K. Replantation, micro-transfers (toe to thumb, etc.)
   - No cases

IX. Breast (13 Sessions)

A. Anatomy and aesthetics
   - No cases

B. Augmentation, including silicone controversy
1. Augmentation, mammoplasty
   - Case 1: Cosmetic breast surgery
   - Case 2: Mammary hypoplasia
2. Problems, complications, ALCL, and breast implant-related illness
   - Case 1: Late complication of augmentation mammoplasty

C. Reduction mammaplasty
1. Reduction mammoplasty: Evaluation, techniques
   - Case 1: Macromastia
   - Case 2: Young patient with macromastia
   - Case 3: Gigantomastia

2. Mastopexy, explantation: Mastopexy, tuberous breast
   - Case 1: Cosmetic breast surgery

D. Post-mastectomy reconstruction
1. Oncologic principles, decision making
   - No cases
2. Nipple-sparing, oncoplastic reconstruction
   - Case 1: Lumpectomy
3. Alloplastic reconstruction (Session 8)
   - Case 1: Breast cancer
   - Case 2: Breast cancer
   - Case 3: Breast cancer
   - Case 4: Breast cancer
4. Autogenous reconstruction (Session 9)
   - Case 1: Delayed breast reconstruction
   - Case 2: Lumpectomy defect
   - Case 3: Delayed breast reconstruction
   - Case 4: Immediate post-mastectomy breast reconstruction
   - Case 5: Alternate autologous reconstruction
5. Perforator flaps (Session 10)
   - Case 1: Perforator flap reconstruction of lumpectomy defect
6. Science of fat grafting, fat grafting of the breast (Session 11)
   - No cases
7. Mastectomy skin necrosis, perfusion assessment, nipple-areola reconstruction (Session 12)
   - Case 1: Nipple reconstruction

E. Gynecomastia, Poland's, chest wall deformities including pectus
- Case 1: Gynecomastia, moderate
- Case 2: Gynecomastia, severe
- Case 3: Poland's syndrome
- Case 4: Pectus excavatum

X. Aesthetic (14 Sessions)

A. General, psychological aspects, patient selection
- No cases

B. Skin resurfacing, injectables, hair restoration
1. Skin resurfacing: Lasers, chemical peels
   - No cases
2. Facial injectables: Soft tissue fillers, Botox
   - Case 1: Facial rejuvenation
3. Hair physiology and restoration
   - No cases

C. Blepharoplasty, brow lift: Anatomy and techniques
1. Anatomy, evaluation, upper lid blepharoplasty including the Asian eyelid (Patient Care 4: Aesthetic (Level 2, 3))
   - No cases
2. Operative procedures, transconjunctival blepharoplasty, festoons
   - Case 1: Periorbital rejuvenation
   - Case 2: Upper eyelid rejuvenation
   - Case 3: "Westernization" of Asian face
3. Complications, brow lift procedures
   - No cases

D. Rhinoplasty, septoplasty, and genioplasty
   1. Anatomy, definitions, facial analysis
      - No cases
   2. Work-up, operative plan, operative approaches, complications
      - Case 1: Rhinoplasty
      - Case 2: Nasal deformity
      - Case 3: Rhinoplasty
   3. Nasal physiology, nasal airway obstruction, genioplasty
      - No cases

E. Rhytidectomy: Anatomy, pathology of aging, techniques, ancillary procedures
   1. Anatomy, aging process, evaluation
      - Case 1: Facial rejuvenation
   2. Operative principles, fat grafting, neck lifting
      - No cases

F. Suction lipectomy, body sculpting, abdominoplasty
   1. Anatomy, evaluation, operative approaches, liposuction
      - Case 1: Abdominal cosmetic surgery
      - Case 2: Liposuction
      - Case 3: Diastasis
   2. Abdominal torso, thigh reduction, brachioplasty, gluteal augmentation (Session 14)
      - Case 1: Post-bariatric surgery
      - Case 2: Massive weight loss
      - Case 3: Post-bariatric surgery

XI. Gender Affirmation: Surgery of the External Genitalia (Sessions 1, 2)

A. General principles, non-surgical treatment, top and bottom surgery
   - No cases

B. Facial feminization, labiaplasty, buried penis
   - No cases

XII. Patient Safety (Session 1)

- Case 1: Perioperative care

Cases with Milestones

I. General Principles (11 Sessions)

(No medical knowledge milestones exist for this entire module)

A. Wound healing 1, 2
   1. Physiology of wound healing, chronic wounds, ancillary measures: Hyperbaric oxygen, negative pressure wound care (NWPT) (Patient Care 7: Wound, burn, Infection Level 1–2)
      - No cases
   2. Nutrition and wound healing, impediments to wound healing by adjuvant therapy (Patient care 7: Wound, burn, Infection Level 1–3)
      - Case 1: Difficult wound (Patient Care 7: Wound, burn, Infection Level 1–2)
      - Case 2: Subacute wound (Patient Care 7: Wound, burn, Infection Level 2–3)
      - Case 3: Elbow ulcer (Patient Care 7: Wound, burn, Infection Level 3–4)

B. Hypertrophic scar, keloids, skin grafts (Patient Care 7: Wound, burn, infection)
   - Case 1: Keloid (Patient Care 7: Wound, burn, Infection Level 2–3)
   - Case 2: Keloid (Patient Care 7: Wound, burn, Infection Level 2–3)

C. Local anesthetics, conscious sedation, regional anesthesia (no comparable milestones either for patient care or medical knowledge)
   - No cases

D. Bone and cartilage healing, bone and cartilage grafts, osteomyelitis, bone substitutes (no comparable milestones either for patient care or medical knowledge)
   - No cases

E. Flaps
   1. Classification, physiology, selection (Patient Care 3: Flaps and Grafts Level 1–3)
      - No cases
   2. Design (Patient Care 3: Flaps and Grafts Level 1–3)
      - No cases
   3. Tissue expansion (Patient Care 3: Flaps and Grafts Level 1–3)
      - Case 1: Scalp burn alopecia (Patient Care 3: Flaps and Grafts Level 3–4)

F. Microsurgery, general principles, flap failure (Patient Care 2: Microsurgery Level 2–4)
   - No cases

G. Biomaterials: Synthetics, skin substitutes (Patient Care 7: Wound, burns, Infection Level 2, 3)
   - No cases

H. Lasers: Basic principles (no comparable milestones either for patient care or medical knowledge)
   - No cases

II. Congenital Anomalies of the Head and Neck (Also Includes Ear Deformities) (13 Sessions)

(No patient care milestones exist for this entire module: exceptions below)

A. Cleft lip and palate
   1. Unilateral cleft lip: General, anatomy, preoperative management, lip–nose repair (Medical Knowledge 5: Pediatric, congenital) (Level 1–4)
      - Case 1: Unilateral cleft lip (Medical Knowledge 5: Pediatric, congenital) (Level 3, 4)
   2. Bilateral cleft lip: Anatomy, preoperative management, lip–nose repair (Medical Knowledge 5: Pediatric, congenital) (Level 1–4)
      - Case 1: Bilateral cleft lip (Medical Knowledge 5: Pediatric, congenital) (Level 3, 4)
   3. Secondary cleft lip deformities: Late secondary deformities, cleft rhinoplasty (Medical Knowledge 5: Pediatric, congenital) (Level 1–4)
      - Case 1: Cleft lip deformity (Medical Knowledge 5: Pediatric, congenital) (Level 3, 4)
      - Case 2: Cleft lip nasal deformity (Medical Knowledge 5: Pediatric, congenital, Patient Care 4: Aesthetic surgery) (Level 3, 4)
   4. Cleft palate: Epidemiology and embryology, anatomy, operative repair, complications, submucous cleft palate, Pierre Robin syndrome (Medical Knowledge 5: Pediatric, congenital) (Level 1–4)
      - Case 1: Cleft palate (Medical Knowledge 5: Pediatric, congenital) (Level 2–4)
   5. Velopharyngeal insufficiency: General; anatomy and function, treatment, specific operations, complications (Medical Knowledge 5: Pediatric, congenital) (Level 1–4)
      - Case 1: Speech disorder (Medical Knowledge 5: Pediatric, congenital) (Level 2–4)

B. Craniofacial, orthognathic surgery, distraction osteogenesis
   1. Alveolar cleft, cephalometrics and orthognathic surgery, distraction osteogenesis, palatal fistulas (Medical Knowledge 5: Pediatric, congenital) (Level 1–4)
      – Case 1: Cleft lip; Late facial deformity (Medical Knowledge 5: Pediatric, congenital) (Level 2–4)
      – Case 2: Palatal fistula (Medical Knowledge 5: Pediatric, congenital) (Level 2–4)
      – Case 3: Alveolar cleft (Medical Knowledge 5: Pediatric, congenital) (Level 2–4)
   2. Craniofacial anomalies: Fibrous dysplasia, Romberg's disease, neurofibromatosis, craniofacial microsomia, Treacher-Collins, other syndromes (Medical Knowledge 5: Pediatric, congenital) (Level 1–4)
      – Case 1: Craniofacial deformity (Medical Knowledge 5: Pediatric, congenital) (Level 2–4)
      – Case 2: Maxillary tumor (Medical Knowledge 5: Pediatric, congenital) (Level 2–4)
      – Case 3: Torticollis (Medical Knowledge 5: Pediatric, congenital) (Level 2–4)
   3. Overview of craniosynostosis, specific craniosynostosis, deformational plagiocephaly, orbital deformities (Medical Knowledge 5: Pediatric, congenital) (Level 1–4)
      – No cases

C. Cysts, sinuses
   – Case 1: Glabellar mass (Medical Knowledge 5: Pediatric, congenital) (Level 2–4)

D. Vascular anomalies (including non-head and neck)
   1. Hemangiomas: Pathology, natural history, clinical picture, treatment (Medical Knowledge 5: Pediatric, congenital) (Level 1–4)
      – Case 1: Vascular anomaly in an infant (Medical Knowledge 5: Pediatric, congenital) (Level 2–4)
   2. Vascular malformations of the head, neck, extremities (Medical Knowledge 5: Pediatric, congenital) (Level 1–4)
      – Case 1: Large mass of cheek (Medical Knowledge 5: Pediatric, congenital; Patient Care 2: Microsurgery) (Level 3, 4)

E. Ear deformities (1, 2) including otoplasty
   1. Anatomy, embryology, otoplasty (Medical Knowledge 5: Pediatric, congenital) (Level 1–4)
      – Case 1: Protruding ears (Medical Knowledge 5: Pediatric, congenital; Patient Care 4: Aesthetic surgery) (Level 2, 4)
   2. Ear deformities: Microtia, other ear deformities besides protruding ears (Medical Knowledge 5: Pediatric, congenital) (Level 1–4)
      – Case 1: Ear deformity (Medical Knowledge 5: Pediatric, congenital) (Level 2–4)

III. Skin and Soft Tissue Cancer Including Reconstruction (9 Sessions)

A. Non-melanotic, skin cancer: Sunscreens, epidemiology, basal cell, squamous cell, Moh's micrographic surgery (Medical Knowledge 3: Facial soft tissue pathology) (Level 1–4)
   – Case 1: Multiple basal cell cancers (Medical Knowledge 3: Facial soft tissue pathology) (Level 1, 2)

B. Non-melanotic, reconstruction, specific areas
   1. Eyelid: Anatomy, reconstruction, upper lid, lower lid (Medical Knowledge 3: Facial soft tissue pathology; Patient Care 3: Flaps and Grafts) (Level 1–4)
      – Case 1: Cancer of the lower eyelid (Medical Knowledge 3: Facial soft tissue pathology; Patient Care 3: Flaps and grafts) (Level 3–4)
      – Case 2: Cancer of the lower eyelid (Medical Knowledge 3: Facial soft tissue pathology; Patient Care 3: Flaps and grafts) (Level 3–4)

- Case 3: Upper lid lesion (Medical Knowledge 3: Facial soft tissue pathology; Patient Care 3: Flaps and grafts) (Level 3–4)
- Case 4: Upper lid reconstruction (Medical Knowledge 3: Facial soft tissue pathology; Patient Care 3: Flaps and grafts) (Level 3–4)

2. Cheek reconstruction: Anatomy, reconstruction (Medical Knowledge 3: Facial soft tissue pathology; Patient Care 3: Flaps and grafts) (Level 1–4)
   - Case 1: Skin cancer of the cheek (Medical Knowledge 3: Facial soft tissue pathology; Patient Care 3: Flaps and grafts) (Level 2–4)
   - Case 2: Cancer of the face (Medical Knowledge 3: Facial soft tissue pathology; Patient Care 3: Flaps and grafts) (Level 3–4)
   - Case 3: Lip cheek defect (Medical Knowledge 3: Facial soft tissue pathology; Patient Care 3: Flaps and grafts) (Level 3–4)
3. Nose: Anatomy, reconstruction (Medical Knowledge 3: Facial soft tissue pathology; Patient Care 3: Flaps and grafts) (Level 1–4)
   - Case 1: Nasal lesion (Medical Knowledge 3: Facial soft tissue pathology; Patient Care 3: Flaps and grafts) (Level 2–3)
   - Case 2: Nasal lesion (Medical Knowledge 3: Facial soft tissue pathology; Patient Care 3: Flaps and grafts) (Level 3–4)
   - Case 3: Nasal lesion (Medical Knowledge 3: Facial soft tissue pathology; Patient Care 3: Flaps and grafts) (Level 2–4)
   - Case 4: Nasal lesion (Medical Knowledge 3: Facial soft tissue pathology; Patient Care 3: Flaps and grafts) (Level 2–4)
   - Case 5: Nasal lesion (Medical Knowledge 3: Facial soft tissue pathology; Patient Care 3: Flaps and grafts) (Level 2–4)
   - Case 6: Nasal lesion (Medical Knowledge 3: Facial soft tissue pathology; Patient Care 3: Flaps and grafts) (Level 2–4)
   - Case 7: Nasal lesion (Medical Knowledge 3: Facial soft tissue pathology; Patient Care 3: Flaps and grafts) (Level 2–4)
4. Scalp, forehead: Anatomy, reconstruction (Medical Knowledge 3: Facial soft tissue pathology; Patient Care 3: Flaps and grafts) (Level 1–4)
   - Case 1: Recurrent cancer of the scalp (Medical Knowledge 3: Facial soft tissue pathology; Patient Care 2: Microsurgery; Patient Care 3: Flaps and grafts) (Level 3–4)
   - Case 2: Scalp reconstruction (Medical Knowledge 3: Facial soft tissue pathology; Patient Care 3: Flaps and grafts) (Level 2–4)
5. Ear reconstruction: Anatomy, reconstruction (Medical Knowledge 3: Facial soft tissue pathology; Patient Care 3: Flaps and grafts) (Level 1–4)
   - Case 1: Cancer of the ear (Medical Knowledge 3: Facial soft tissue pathology; Patient Care 3: Flaps and grafts) (Level 2–3)
   - Case 2: Cancer of the ear (Medical Knowledge 3: Facial soft tissue pathology; Patient Care 3: Flaps and grafts) (Level 2–3)

C. Melanoma, pigmented lesions

1. Melanoma: Pathology, staging, excision, sentinel lymph node, advanced disease (Medical Knowledge 3: Facial soft tissue pathology; Patient Care 3: Flaps and grafts) (Level 1–4)
   - Case 1: Melanoma (Medical Knowledge 3: Facial soft tissue pathology; Patient Care 3: Flaps and grafts) (Level 3–4)
   - Case 2: Melanoma (Medical Knowledge 3: Facial soft tissue pathology; Medical Knowledge 4: Trunk, extremities; Patient Care 3: Flaps and grafts) (Level 3–4)
2. Pigmented lesions: Congenital, lentigo (Medical Knowledge 3: Facial soft tissue pathology; Patient Care 3: Flaps and grafts) (Level 3–4)
   - Case 1: Pigmented lesion (Medical Knowledge 3: Facial soft tissue pathology; Patient Care 3: Flaps and grafts) (Level 3–4)

D. Adnexal tumors, Merkel cell carcinoma, dermatofibrosarcoma protuberans, sarcomas (Medical Knowledge 3: Facial soft tissue pathology; Patient Care 2: Microsurgery; Patient Care 3: Flaps and grafts) (Level 3–4)
   - Case 1: Recurrent cancer of the scalp (Medical Knowledge 3: Facial soft tissue pathology; Patient Care 2: Microsurgery; Patient Care 3: Flaps and grafts) (Level 3–4)

IV. Head and Neck Tumors (6 Sessions)

(No medical knowledge milestones exist for B1, C: Exceptions below)

A. Anatomy, work-up, principles of treatment, including surgery, radiation, and chemotherapy (Patient Care 3: Flaps and grafts) (Level 1–4)
   - Case 1: Malignant neck mass (Patient Care 3: Flaps and grafts) (Level 1–3)

B. Lip, oral cavity, oropharynx, hypopharynx, maxilla
   1. Lip: Anatomy, pathology, upper and lower lip reconstruction (Patient Care 3: Flaps and grafts; Medical Knowledge 3: Facial soft tissue pathology) (Level 1–4)
      - Case 1: Tumor of the upper lip (Patient Care 3: Flaps and grafts; Medical Knowledge 3: Facial soft tissue pathology) (Level 2–3)
      - Case 2: Cancer of the lower lip (Patient Care 3: Flaps and grafts; Medical Knowledge 3: Facial soft tissue pathology) (Level 2–3)
      - Case 3: Basal cell cancer upper lip (Patient Care 3: Flaps and grafts; Medical Knowledge 3: Facial soft tissue pathology) (Level 3–4)

   2a. Mandibular reconstruction: Classification, options, virtual surgical planning (Patient Care 2: Microsurgery; Patient Care 3: Flaps and grafts) (Level 1–4)
      - Case 1: Draining fistula (Patient Care 2: Microsurgery; Patient Care 3: Flaps and grafts) (Level 3–4)

   2b. Intraoral defect reconstruction (Patient Care 2: Microsurgery; Patient Care 3: Flaps and grafts) (Level 1–4)
      - Case 1: Oral cavity lesion (Patient Care 2: Microsurgery; Patient Care 3: Flaps and grafts) (Level 3–4)
      - Case 2: Cancer of the oropharynx (Patient Care 3: Flaps and grafts) (Level 3–4)

   3. Hypopharynx, maxilla reconstruction: Anatomy, flap options (Patient Care 2: Microsurgery; Patient Care 3: Flaps and grafts) (Level 1–4)
      - Case 1: Hypopharyngeal stricture (Patient Care 2: Microsurgery; Patient Care 3: Flaps and grafts) (Level 3–4)
      - Case 2: Cancer of the maxilla (Patient Care 3: Flaps and grafts) (Level 1–4)

C. Salivary gland: Anatomy, pathology, treatment, benign disease (Medical Knowledge 3: Facial soft tissue pathology; Patient Care 2: Microsurgery; Patient Care 3: Flaps and grafts) (Level 1–4)
   - Case 1: Cheek mass (Medical Knowledge 3: Facial soft tissue pathology; Patient Care 2: Microsurgery; Patient Care 3: Flaps and grafts) (Level 3–4)

V. Maxillofacial Trauma (10 Sessions)

A. General Principles
   1. Anatomy, airway, bleeding, radiology, clinical examination (Patient Care 5: Consultant)
      - Case 1: Initial care of maxillofacial trauma (Patient Care 5: Consultant; Medical Knowledge 3: Facial soft tissue) (Level 1–4)
      - Case 2: Initial care of maxillofacial trauma (Patient Care 5: Consultant; Medical Knowledge 3: Facial soft tissue) (Level 1–4)

2. Ocular injuries, operative approaches, reduction and fixation (Patient Care 5: Consultant; Medical Knowledge 3: Facial soft tissue) (Level 1–3)
   - Case 1: Ocular trauma (Patient Care 5: Consultant; Medical Knowledge 3: Facial soft tissue) (Level 1–3)

B. Soft Tissue Injury
1. Soft tissue injury: Parotid, eyelid, orbital adnexa (Patient Care 3: Flaps and grafts; Medical Knowledge 3: Facial soft tissue) (Level 1–4)
   - Case 1: Acute eyelid injury (Patient Care 3: Flaps and grafts (Level 2–4); Medical Knowledge 3: Facial soft tissue (Level 2–4))
   - Case 2: Ectropion (Patient Care 3: Flaps and grafts (Level 2–4); Medical Knowledge 3: Facial soft tissue (Level 2–4))
   - Case 3: Facial laceration (Patient Care 3: Flaps and grafts (Level 2–4); Medical Knowledge 3: Facial soft tissue (Level 2–4))
2. Gunshot wounds: Wound ballistics, reconstruction (Patient Care 1: Fractures (Level 3, 4); Patient Care 3: Flaps and grafts (Level 3, 4); Medical Knowledge 3: Facial soft tissue (Level 2, 4))
   - Case 1: GSW to the face (Patient Care 1: Fractures (Level 3, 4); Patient Care 3: Flaps and grafts (Level 3, 4); Medical Knowledge 3: Facial soft tissue (Level 2–4))
3. Facial nerve (including non-traumatic) (Patient Care 2: Microsurgery (Level 3, 4); Patient Care 3: Flaps and grafts (Level 3, 4); Medical Knowledge 3: Facial soft tissue (Level 2–4))
   - Case 1: Facial paralysis (Patient Care 2: Microsurgery (Level 3, 4); Patient Care 3: Flaps and grafts (Level 3, 4); Medical Knowledge 3: Facial soft tissue (Level 2–4))
   - Case 2: Facial paralysis (Patient Care 2: Microsurgery (Level 3, 4); Patient Care 3: Flaps and grafts (Level 3, 4); Medical Knowledge 3: Facial soft tissue (Level 2–4))
   - Case 3: Facial paralysis (Patient Care 2: Microsurgery (Level 3, 4); Patient Care 3: Flaps and grafts (Level 3, 4); Medical Knowledge 3: Facial soft tissue (Level 2–4))

Note: All facial fracture modules, C–F, include anatomy, evaluation, general principles, reduction and fixation, complications

C. Upper one-third (skull, orbital roof, frontal sinus) (Patient Care 1: Fractures (Level 2–4); Medical Knowledge 3: Facial soft tissue (Level 2–4))
   - Case 1: Orbital roof (Patient Care 1: Fractures (Level 3, 4); Medical Knowledge 3: Facial soft tissue (Level 2– 4))
   - Case 2: Frontal sinus injury (Patient Care 1: Fractures (Level 3, 4); Medical Knowledge 3: Facial soft tissue (Level 2–4))
   - Case 3: Frontal sinus fracture (Patient Care 1: Fractures (Level 3, 4); Medical Knowledge 3: Facial soft tissue (Level 2–4))
   - Case 4: Cranioplasty (Patient Care 1: Fractures (Level 3, 4); Medical Knowledge 3: Facial soft tissue (Level 2–4))
   - Case 5: Infected cranioplasty (Patient Care 1: Fractures (Level 3, 4); Patient Care 7: Wound, burn, infection (Level 3, 4); Medical Knowledge 3: Facial soft tissue (Level 2–4))

D. Complex maxillary, NEO, and nasal fractures (Patient Care 1: Fractures (Level 3, 4); Medical Knowledge 3: Facial soft tissue (Level 3, 4))
   - Case 1: Midface fractures (Patient Care 1: Fractures (Level 3, 4); Medical Knowledge 3: Facial soft tissue (Level 3, 4))

E. Zygoma, orbit (Patient Care 1: Fractures (Level 3, 4); Medical Knowledge 3: Facial soft tissue (Level 3, 4))
   - Case 1: Facial fracture (Patient Care 1: Fractures (Level 3, 4); Medical Knowledge 3: Facial soft tissue (Level 3, 4))
   - Case 2: Facial fracture (Patient Care 1: Fractures (Level 3, 4); Medical Knowledge 3: Facial soft tissue (Level 3, 4))
   - Case 3: Orbital floor fracture (Patient Care 1: Fractures (Level 3, 4); Medical Knowledge 3: Facial soft tissue (Level 3, 4))

F. Mandible (Patient Care 1: Fractures (Level 3, 4); Medical Knowledge 3: Facial soft tissue (Level 3, 4))

1. Mandible
   - Case 1: Mandible fracture (Patient Care 1: Fractures (Level 3, 4); Medical Knowledge 3: Facial soft tissue (Level 3, 4))
2. Mandible: Condylar, pediatric fractures, complications
   - Case 1: Mandible fracture (Patient Care 1: Fractures (Level 3, 4); Medical Knowledge 3: Facial soft tissue (Level 3, 4))
   - Case 2: Infected mandible fracture (Patient Care 1: Fractures (Level 3, 4); Medical Knowledge 3: Facial soft tissue (Level 3, 4))

VI. Lower Extremity, Perineum, and Trunk (8 Sessions)

A. Lower extremity

1. Trauma: Anatomy, limb salvage vs. amputation, management, osteomyelitis (Patient Care 1: Fractures (Level 3, 4); Patient Care 2: Microsurgery (Level 3, 4); Patient Care 3: Flaps and grafts (Level 3, 4); Medical Knowledge 4: Trunk, lower extremity (Level 2–4))
   - Case 1: Lower extremity trauma (Patient Care 1: Fractures (Level 3, 4); Patient Care 2: Microsurgery (Level 3, 4); Patient Care 3: Flaps and grafts (Level 3, 4); Medical Knowledge 4: Trunk, lower extremity (Level 2–4))
2. Foot reconstruction, reconstruction of limb bony oncologic defects, specific flaps, (Session 2)
   - Case 1: Soft tissue loss, foot (Patient Care 1: Fractures (Level 3, 4); Patient Care 2: Microsurgery (Level 3, 4); Patient Care 3: Flaps and grafts (Level 3, 4); Medical Knowledge 4: Trunk, lower extremity (Level 2–4))
3. Complex groin wounds, extremity lymphedema (Session 3)
   - Case 1: Radiotherapy ulcer (Patient Care 1: Fractures (Level 3, 4); Patient Care 2: Microsurgery (Level 3, 4); Patient Care 3: Flaps and grafts (Level 3, 4); Patient Care 7: Wound, burn, infection (Level 3, 4); Medical Knowledge 4: Trunk, lower extremity (Level 2–4))
   - Case 2: Exposure of vascular reconstruction (Patient Care 1: Fractures (Level 3, 4); Patient Care 2: Microsurgery (Level 3, 4); Patient Care 3: Flaps and grafts (Level 3, 4); Patient Care 7: Wound, burn, infection (Level 3, 4); Medical Knowledge 4: Trunk, lower extremity (Level 2–4))
   - Case 3: Swollen extremity (Patient Care 2: Microsurgery (Level 3, 4); Patient Care 3: Flaps and grafts (Level 3, 4); Medical Knowledge 4: Trunk, lower extremity (Level 2–4))

B. Perineum

1. Reconstruction of the vagina, congenital and acquired, perineum (Patient Care 3: Flaps and grafts (Level 2–4); Patient Care 7: Wound, burn, infection (Level 2–4); Medical Knowledge 4: Trunk, lower extremity (Level 2–4))
   - Case 1: Persistent perineal sinus (Patient Care 3: Flaps and grafts (Level 2–4); Patient Care 7: Wound, burn, infection (Level 2–4); Medical Knowledge 4: Trunk, lower extremity (Level 2–4))
   - Case 2: Perineal reconstruction (Patient Care 3: Flaps and grafts (Level 2–4); Patient Care 7: Wound, burn, infection (Level 2–4); Medical Knowledge 4: Trunk, lower extremity (Level 2–4))

2. Decubiti, others
   - Case 1: Sacral decubitus (Patient Care 3: Flaps and grafts (Level 2–4); Patient Care 7: Wound, burn, infection (Level 2–4); Medical Knowledge 4: Trunk, lower extremity (Level 2–4))

C. Chest wall, back, abdomen
1. Myelomeningocele, complex back wounds (Session 6)
   - Case 1: Complex back wound (Patient Care 3: Flaps and grafts (Level 2–4); Patient Care 7: Wound, burn, infection (Level 2–4); Medical Knowledge 3: Facial soft tissue pathology (Level 2–4))
   - Case 2: Myelomeningocele (Patient Care 3: Flaps and grafts (Level 2–4); Patient Care 7: Wound, burn, infection (Level 2–4); Medical Knowledge 3: Facial soft tissue pathology (Level 2–4))
   - Case 3: Back wound (Patient Care 3: Flaps and grafts (Level 2–4); Patient Care 7: Wound, burn, infection (Level 2–4); Medical Knowledge 3: Facial soft tissue pathology (Level 2–4))
2. Abdominal wall (Session 7)
   - Case 1: Abdominal wall reconstruction (Patient Care 3: Flaps and grafts (Level 3, 4); Medical Knowledge 4: Trunk, extremities (Level 2–4))
   - Case 2: Abdominal wall reconstruction (Patient Care 3: Flaps and grafts (Level 3, 4); Medical Knowledge 4: Trunk, extremities (Level 2–4))
3. Chest wall, sternum (Session 8)
   - Case 1: Chest wall ulcer (Patient Care 2: Microsurgery (Level 3, 4); Patient Care 3: Flaps and grafts (Level 3, 4); Patient Care 7: Wound, burn, infection (Level 2–4); Medical Knowledge 4: Trunk, extremities (Level 2–4))
   - Case 2: Open chest wound (Patient Care 2: Microsurgery (Level 3, 4) Patient Care 3: Flaps and grafts (Level 3, 4); Patient Care 7: Wound, burn, infection (Level 2–4); Medical Knowledge 4: Trunk, extremities (Level 2–4))
   - Case 3: GSW of shoulder: Neck (Patient Care 2: Microsurgery (Level 3, 4); Patient Care 3: Flaps and grafts (Level 3, 4); Patient Care 7: Wound, burn, infection (Level 2–4); Medical Knowledge 4: Trunk, extremities (Level 2–4))
   - Case 4: Sternal dehiscence (Patient Care 2: Microsurgery (Level 3, 4); Patient Care 3: Flaps and grafts (Level 3, 4); Patient Care 7: Wound, burn, infection (Level 2–4); Medical Knowledge 4: Trunk, extremities (Level 2–4))

VII. Burns, Difficult Wounds (6 Sessions)

(No Medical Knowledge Milestones for A, B, C)

A. Burns: Pathophysiology, resuscitation, pulmonary complications
   - Case 1: Acute burn (Patient Care 7: Wound, burn, infection (Level 2–4))

B. Wound care and coverage (Session 2)
   - Case 1: Acute burn (Patient Care 3: Flaps and grafts (Level 2–4); Patient Care 7: Wound, burn, infection (Level 2–4))

C. Nutrition and metabolic support, electrical and chemical burn injury (Session 3)
   - Case 1: Electrical burn of scalp (Patient Care 2: Microsurgery (Level 2–4); Patient Care 3: Flaps and grafts (Level 3, 4); Patient Care 7: Wound, burn, infection (Level 2–4))
   - Case 2: Electrical burns of trunk, extremities (Patient Care 2: Microsurgery (Level 2–4); Patient Care 3: Flaps and grafts (Level 3, 4); Patient Care 7: Wound, burn, infection (Level 2–4))

D. Reconstruction
  1. Eyelids, ears, nose, cheek/face, neck (Session 4)
     - Case 1: Acute, late burn of the eyelids (Patient Care 3: Flaps and grafts (Level 2–4); Patient Care 7: Wound, burn, infection (Level 2–4); Medical Knowledge 3: Facial soft tissue pathology (Level 2–4))
     - Case 2: Head/neck burn reconstruction (Patient Care 3: Flaps and grafts (Level 2–4); Patient Care 7: Wound, burn, infection (Level 2–4); Medical Knowledge 3: Facial soft tissue pathology (Level 2–4))
  2. Hand/upper extremity, axilla, breast, foot, splints, and scar management (Session 5)
     - Case 1: Hand burn (Patient Care 3: Flaps and grafts (Level 2–4); Patient Care 7: Wound, burn, infection (Level 3, 4); Medical Knowledge 1: Hand (Level 2, 3); Medical Knowledge 3: Facial soft tissue pathology (Level 2–4))
     - Case 2: Burn contracture of the trunk in adolescent female (Patient Care 3: Flaps and grafts (Level 2–4); Patient Care 7: Wound, burn, infection (Level 3, 4); Medical Knowledge 1: Hand (Level 2, 3); Medical Knowledge 3: Facial soft tissue pathology (Level 2–4))

E. Soft tissue infections, difficult wounds (Session 6)
  - Case 1: Severe infection of the axillae (Patient Care 3: Flaps and grafts (Level 2–4); Patient Care 7: Wound, burn, infection (Level 2–4); Medical Knowledge 1: Hand (Level 2, 3); Medical Knowledge 4: Trunk, extremities (Level 2–4))

VIII. Hand and Upper Extremity (15 Sessions)

A. Anatomy, function, initial management of hand trauma, anesthesia
  - Case 1: Initial care of the injured hand (Patient Care 5: Consultant (Level 1–4); Medical Knowledge 1: Hand (Level 1–2))

B. Congenital
  - Case 1: Thumb duplication (Medical Knowledge 1: Hand (Level 2–4); Medical Knowledge 5: Pediatric congenital (Level 2–4))
  - Case 2: Congenital anomalies of the hand (Medical Knowledge 1: Hand (Level 2–4); Medical Knowledge 5: Pediatric congenital (Level 2–4))
  - Case 3: Webbed fingers (Medical Knowledge 1: Hand (Level 2–4); Medical Knowledge 5: Pediatric congenital (Level 2–4))

C. Fingertip loss, amputations, local flaps, flap coverage including micro
  1. Fingertip loss, amputations
     - Case 1: Thumb soft tissue injury (Patient Care 3: Flaps and grafts (Level 2–4); Medical Knowledge 1: Hand (Level 2–4))
     - Case 2: Pediatric digit soft tissue loss (Patient Care 3: Flaps and grafts (Level 2–4); Medical Knowledge 1: Hand (Level 2–4))
     - Case 3: Thumb tip injury (Patient Care 3: Flaps and grafts (Level 2–4); Medical Knowledge 1: Hand (Level 2–4))
  2. Regional flap coverage, thumb reconstruction
     - Case 1: Arm defect (Patient Care 2: Microsurgery (Level 3, 4); Patient Care 3: Flaps and grafts (Level 2–4); Medical Knowledge 1: Hand (Level 2–4))
     - Case 2: Deep burn/wound of hand (Patient Care 2: Microsurgery (Level 3, 4); Patient Care 3: Flaps and grafts (Level 2–4); Medical Knowledge 1: Hand (Level 2–4))
     - Case 3: Thumb reconstruction (Patient Care 2: Microsurgery (Level 3, 4); Patient Care 3: Flaps and grafts (Level 2–4); Medical Knowledge 1: Hand (Level 2–4))
     - Case 4: Avulsion injury of the hand (Patient Care 2: Microsurgery (Level 3, 4); Patient Care 3: Flaps and grafts (Level 2–4); Medical Knowledge 1: Hand (Level 2–4))

D. Fractures
  1. Metacarpal and phalangeal fractures
     - Case 1: Phalangeal fracture (Patient Care 1: Fractures (Level 2–4); Medical Knowledge 1: Hand (Level 2–4))
     - Case 2: Multiple metacarpal fractures (Patient Care 1: Fractures (Level 2–4); Medical Knowledge 1: Hand (Level 2–4))
     - Case 3: Metacarpal base fracture (Patient Care 1: Fractures (Level 2–4); Medical Knowledge 1: Hand (Level 2–4))
     - Case 4: Proximal phalanx fracture (Patient Care 1: Fractures (Level 2–4); Medical Knowledge 1: Hand (Level 2–4))
  2. Dislocations and ligament injuries
     - Case 1: PIP joint dislocation (Patient Care 1: Fractures (Level 2–4); Medical Knowledge 1: Hand (Level 2–4))
     - Case 2: Injured thumb (Patient Care 1: Fractures (Level 2–4); Medical Knowledge 1: Hand (Level 2–4))
     - Case 3: MP joint dislocation (Patient Care 1: Fractures (Level 2–4); Medical Knowledge 1: Hand (Level 2–4))
  3. Carpal fractures and dislocations
     - No cases

E. Vascular problems, complex regional pain syndrome
  - Case 1: Ischemia of the hand (Patient Care 2: Microsurgery (Level 3, 4); Patient Care 7: Wounds, burns, infection (Level 3, 4); Medical Knowledge 1: Hand (Level 2–4))
  - Case 2: SGW of forearm; late sequelae (Patient Care 2: Microsurgery (Level 3, 4); Patient Care 7: Wounds, burns, infection (Level 3, 4); Medical Knowledge 1: Hand (Level 2–4))

F. Peripheral nerve
  1. Nerve injuries: Pathophysiology, repair, conduits, and grafts
     - Case 1: Pain and weakness of the hand (Patient Care 2: Microsurgery (Level 2–4); Medical Knowledge 1: Hand (Level 1–4))
     - Case 2: Possible nerve injury (Patient Care 2: Microsurgery (Level 2–4); Medical Knowledge 1: Hand (Level 1–4))
     - Case 3: Reconstruction of neurovascular injury of arm (Patient Care 2: Microsurgery (Level 2–4); Medical Knowledge 1: Hand (Level 1–4))
     - Case 4: Peripheral nerve injury (Patient Care 2: Microsurgery (Level 2–4); Medical Knowledge 1: Hand (Level 1–4))
  2. Nerve compression syndromes, brachial plexus: Diagnosis
     - Case 1: Compression neuropathy (Patient Care 1: Fractures (Level 1–4))

G. Flexor tendons: Acute and reconstructive
  - Case 1: Flexor tendon injury (Medical Knowledge 1: Hand (Level 2–4))
  - Case 2: Flexor tendon injury (Medical Knowledge 1: Hand (Level 2–4))
  - Case 3: Flexor tendon injury (Medical Knowledge 1: Hand (Level 2–4))
  - Case 4: Failed flexor tendon repair (Medical Knowledge 1: Hand (Level 2–4))
  - Case 5: Flexor tendon reconstruction (Medical Knowledge 1: Hand (Level 2–4))

H. Extensor tendons: Acute and reconstructive
  - Case 1: Finger injury (Medical Knowledge 1: Hand (Level 2–4))
  - Case 2: Finger injury (Medical Knowledge 1: Hand (Level 2–4))
  - Case 3: Hand laceration (Patient Care 7: Wounds, burns, infections (Level 1, 2); Medical Knowledge 1: Hand (Level 2, 3))

I. Ganglia, tumors, Dupuytren's
  - Case 1: Digital tumor (Medical Knowledge 1: Hand (Level 2–4))
  - Case 2: Hand contracture (Medical Knowledge 1: Hand (Level 2–4))
  - Case 3: Volar wrist mass (Medical Knowledge 1: Hand (Level 2–4))

J. Infections, tendinopathies, rheumatoid arthritis, and other arthritides
  - Case 1: Injection injury of the finger (Patient Care 7: Wounds, burns, infections (Level 2–4); Medical Knowledge 1: Hand (Level 1–4))
  - Case 2: Hand infection (Patient Care 7: Wounds, burns, infections (Level 2–4); Medical Knowledge 1: Hand (Level 1–4))

K. Replantation, micro-transfers (toe to thumb, etc.)
  - No cases

IX. Breast (13 Sessions)

A. Anatomy and aesthetics (Patient Care 4: Aesthetic surgery (Level 1–3))
  - No cases

B. Augmentation, including silicone controversy
  1. Augmentation, mammoplasty
     - Case 1: Cosmetic breast surgery (Patient Care 4: Aesthetic surgery (Level 1–3); Medical Knowledge 2: Breast (Level 2–3))
     - Case 2: Mammary hypoplasia (Patient Care 4: Aesthetic surgery (Level 1–3); Medical Knowledge 2: Breast (Level 2–3))
  2. Problems, complications, ALCL, and breast implant-related illness
     - Case 1: Late complication of augmentation mammoplasty (Patient Care 4: Aesthetic surgery (Level 2–3); Medical Knowledge 2: Breast (Level 2–3))

C. Reduction mammaplasty
  1. Reduction mammoplasty: Evaluation, techniques
     - Case 1: Macromastia (Patient Care 4: Aesthetic surgery (Level 2–3); Medical Knowledge 2: Breast (Level 2–3))
     - Case 2: Young patient with macromastia (Patient Care 4: Aesthetic surgery (Level 2–3); Medical Knowledge 2: Breast (Level 2–3))
     - Case 3: Gigantomastia (Patient Care 4: Aesthetic surgery (Level 2–3); Medical Knowledge 2: Breast (Level 2–3))
  2. Mastopexy, explantation: Mastopexy, tuberous breast
     - Case 1: Cosmetic breast surgery (Patient Care 4: Aesthetic surgery (Level 2–4); Medical Knowledge 2: Breast (Level 2–3))

D. Post-mastectomy reconstruction
  1. Oncologic principles, decision making (Medical Knowledge 2: Breast (Level 2–4))
     - No cases
  2. Nipple-sparing, oncoplastic reconstruction
     - Case 1: Lumpectomy (Patient Care 3: Flaps and grafts (Level 2–4); Medical Knowledge 2: Breast (Level 2–4))
  3. Alloplastic reconstruction (Session 8)
     - Case 1: Breast Cancer (Medical Knowledge 2: Breast (Level 2–4))
     - Case 2: Breast Cancer (Medical Knowledge 2: Breast (Level 2–4))
     - Case 3: Breast Cancer (Medical Knowledge 2: Breast (Level 2–4))
     - Case 4: Breast Cancer (Medical Knowledge 2: Breast (Level 2–4))
  4. Autogenous reconstruction (Session 9)
     - Case 1: Delayed breast reconstruction (Patient Care 3: Flaps and grafts (Level 2–4); Medical Knowledge 2: Breast (Level 2–4))
     - Case 2: Lumpectomy defect (Patient Care 3: Flaps and grafts (Level 2–4); Medical Knowledge 2: Breast (Level 2–4))
     - Case 3: Delayed breast reconstruction (Patient Care 3: Flaps and grafts (Level 2–4); Medical Knowledge 2: Breast (Level 2–4))

- Case 4: Immediate post-mastectomy breast reconstruction (Patient Care 2: Microsurgery (Level 2–4); Patient Care 3: Flaps and grafts (Level 2–4); Medical Knowledge 2: Breast (Level 2–4))
- Case 5: Alternate autologous reconstruction (Patient Care 3: Flaps and grafts (Level 2–4); Medical Knowledge 2: Breast (Level 2–4))

5. Perforator flaps (Session 10)
   - Case 1: Perforator flap reconstruction of lumpectomy defect (Patient Care 3: Flaps and grafts (Level 3–4); Medical Knowledge 2: Breast (Level 3–4))
6. Science of fat grafting, fat grafting of the breast (Session 11)
   - No cases
7. Mastectomy skin necrosis, perfusion assessment, nipple-areola reconstruction (Session 12)
   - Case 1: Nipple reconstruction (Patient Care 3: Flaps and grafts (Level 2–4); Medical Knowledge 2: Breast (Level 2–4))

E. Gynecomastia, Poland's, chest wall deformities including pectus
- Case 1: Gynecomastia, moderate (Patient Care 4: Aesthetic surgery (Level 3, 4); Medical Knowledge 2: Breast (Level 2–4))
- Case 2: Gynecomastia, severe (Patient Care 4: Aesthetic surgery (Level 3, 4); Medical Knowledge 2: Breast (Level 2–4))
- Case 3: Poland's syndrome (Patient Care 4: Aesthetic surgery (Level 3, 4); Medical Knowledge 2: Breast (Level 2–4))
- Case 4: Pectus excavatum (Patient Care 4: Aesthetic surgery (Level 3, 4); Medical Knowledge 2: Breast (Level 2–4))

X. Aesthetic (14 Sessions)

A. General, psychological aspects, patient selection (Patient Care 4: Aesthetic (Level 2, 3))
- No cases

B. Skin resurfacing, injectables, hair restoration
1. Skin resurfacing: Lasers, chemical peels (Patient Care 4: Aesthetic (Level 2–4); Medical Knowledge 3: Facial soft tissue (Level 2–4))
   - No cases
2. Facial injectables: Soft tissue fillers, Botox (Patient Care 4: Aesthetic (Level 2–4); Medical Knowledge 3: Facial soft tissue (Level 2–4))
   - Case 1: Facial rejuvenation (Patient Care 4: Aesthetic (Level 2–4); Medical Knowledge 3: Facial soft tissue (Level 2–4))
3. Hair physiology and restoration (Patient Care 4: Aesthetic (Level 2–4); Medical Knowledge 3: Facial soft tissue (Level 2–4))
   - No cases

C. Blepharoplasty, brow lift: Anatomy and techniques
1. Anatomy, evaluation, upper lid blepharoplasty including the Asian eyelid (Patient Care 4: Aesthetic (Level 2, 3))
   - No cases
2. Operative procedures, transconjunctival blepharoplasty, festoons
   - Case 1: Periorbital rejuvenation (Patient Care 4: Aesthetic (Level 2–4); Medical Knowledge 3: Facial soft tissue (Level 2–4))
   - Case 2: Upper eyelid rejuvenation (Patient Care 4: Aesthetic (Level 2–4); Medical Knowledge 3: Facial soft tissue (Level 2–4))
   - Case 3: "Westernization" of Asian face (Patient Care 4: Aesthetic (Level 2–4); Medical Knowledge 3: Facial soft tissue (Level 2–4))
3. Complications, brow lift procedures (Patient Care 4: Aesthetic (Level 2–4); Medical Knowledge 3: Facial soft tissue (Level 2–4))
   - No cases

D. Rhinoplasty, septoplasty, and genioplasty
  1. Anatomy, definitions, facial analysis (Patient Care 4: Aesthetic (Level 2, 3); Medical Knowledge 3: Facial soft tissue (Level 2, 3))
     – No cases
  2. Work-up, operative plan, operative approaches, complications (Patient Care 4: Aesthetic (Level 2, 3); Medical knowledge 3: Facial soft tissue (Level 2, 3))
     – Case 1: Rhinoplasty (Patient Care 4: Aesthetic (Level 2–4); Medical Knowledge 3: Facial soft tissue (Level 2–4))
     – Case 2: Nasal deformity (Patient Care 4: Aesthetic (Level 2–4); Medical Knowledge 3: Facial soft tissue (Level 2–4))
     – Case 3: Rhinoplasty (Patient Care 4: Aesthetic (Level 2–4); Medical Knowledge 3: Facial soft tissue (Level 2–4))
  3. Nasal physiology, nasal airway obstruction, genioplasty (Patient Care 4: Aesthetic (Level 2–4); Medical Knowledge 3: Facial soft tissue (Level 2–4))
     – No cases

E. Rhytidectomy: Anatomy, pathology of aging, techniques, ancillary procedures
  1. Anatomy, aging process, evaluation (Patient Care 4: Aesthetic (Level 2–4); Medical Knowledge 3: Facial soft tissue (Level 2–4))
     – Case 1: Facial rejuvenation (Patient Care 4: Aesthetic (Level 2–4); Medical Knowledge 3: Facial soft tissue (Level 2–4))
  2. Operative principles, fat grafting, neck lifting
     – No cases

F. Suction lipectomy, body sculpting, abdominoplasty
  1. Anatomy, evaluation, operative approaches, liposuction (Patient Care 4: Aesthetic (Level 2–4). No medical knowledge milestones apply to body aesthetic surgery procedures.)
     – Case 1: Abdominal cosmetic surgery (Patient Care 4: Aesthetic (Level 2–4). No medical knowledge milestones apply to body aesthetic surgery procedures.)
     – Case 2: Liposuction (Patient Care 4: Aesthetic (Level 2–4). No medical knowledge milestones apply to body aesthetic surgery procedures.)
     – Case 3: Diastasis (Patient Care 4: Aesthetic (Level 2–4). No medical knowledge milestones apply to body aesthetic surgery procedures.)
  2. Abdominal torso, thigh reduction, brachioplasty, gluteal augmentation (Session 14)
     – Case 1: Post-bariatric surgery (Patient Care 4: Aesthetic (Level 2–4). No medical knowledge milestones apply to body aesthetic surgery procedures.)
     – Case 2: Massive weight loss (Patient Care 4: Aesthetic (Level 2–4). No medical knowledge milestones apply to body aesthetic surgery procedures.)
     – Case 3: Post-bariatric surgery (Patient Care 4: Aesthetic (Level 2–4). No medical knowledge milestones apply to body aesthetic surgery procedures.)

XI. Gender affirmation, surgery of the external genitalia (Sessions 1, 2)

A. General principles, non-surgical treatment, top and bottom surgery (Patient Care 4: Aesthetic (Level 2–4). No medical knowledge milestones apply to this module.)
  – No cases

B. Facial feminization, labiaplasty, buried penis (Patient Care 4: Aesthetic (Level 2–4). No medical knowledge milestones apply to this module.)
  – No cases

XII. Patient Safety (Session 1)

– Case 1: Perioperative care

Contents of Volume I

Contents of Volume II

Introduction

1

The future of plastic surgery, the continuing ability of the specialty to deliver high-quality care and engage in productive innovation, rests squarely on our capability to produce well-educated, well-trained, ethical, and compassionate plastic surgeons. Nevertheless, the challenges have never been as enormous to do so. If the future of plastic surgery is inextricably tied to the future of graduate medical education, the successful accomplishment and implementation of that education should be the business of all plastic surgeons, both academic and private practice. To transform our present system of resident education to one that not only addresses the current challenges but is also flexible to endure into the future requires a substantial alteration in didactics, embracing adult learning principles, universal incorporation of mobile digital technology into graduate medical education, adoption of approved tenets in teaching motor skills, and incorporation of objective methods in assessment of resident performance [1].

Where Are We Now?

The current system of surgical resident education is frequently dubbed the Halstedian system [2], and the words "apprenticeship" and "training" are used interchangeably and often in a deprecatory manner. Actually, Halsted inoculated structure into the surgical residency, dictated that clinical care would hinge on science not empiricism, and that successful completion of residency was attainment of competency (as judged by Halsted) and not time based [3]. However, the traditional or Halstedian model cannot survive the contemporary pressures on graduate surgical education, including those imposed by the limitation of work hours. The mandatory requirements of the Accreditation Council of Graduate Medical Education, ACGME, leveled in 2003 of an 80-h work week and updated in 2011, principally directed toward the first postgraduate year, resulted in some unintended consequences deleterious toward resident education [4, 5]. These unintended consequences include the necessities for hand-offs ("transitions of care"), the development of protocols and standards for the execution of hand-offs to minimize loss of continuity and errors secondary to inadequate communication [6], a burgeoning bureaucracy to ensure compliance with those protocols ("institutional compliance officer"), and the work hours limitation [7, 8]. Overlaid onto the working hours requirement is the advent of the ACGME Next Accreditation System, assessment of performance within the six competencies (as defined by the ACGME), and the accompanying milestones project. The efforts of the ACGME to emphasize outcomes rather than process and structure in accreditation should be lauded; nevertheless, the resultant documentation workload on both staff and faculty has increased dramatically [9]. To fully realize the promise of the new accreditation system will require a substantial infusion of money and resources because implementation of the initiative was essentially unfunded. An additional stress for plastic surgery faculty, a welcome stress but a stress nevertheless, is the advent of the integrated program that imposes responsibility on the plastic surgery faculty for the education and welfare of the residents from day one of their residency. As plastic surgery has shifted from the independent or fellowship model after general surgery to an integrated plan of resident education driven solely by the specialty, the responsibility for the core education has shifted as well from primarily general surgery to the plastic surgery program and faculty [10]. That responsibility is particularly acute in consideration of the educational needs of the junior, year one and two, versus the senior, year five and six, plastic surgery residents.

In all likelihood, these contemporary pressures on graduate surgical education are immutable, not subject to significant modification. Because we are unlikely to alter or impact these current influences and forces in any significant way, how can we optimally direct our energy and efforts toward a transformation of our current graduate surgical education into a system that will provide for the future? The current model or structure is based on mostly pedagogic methods of teaching that pose a betrayal of the principles of adult

E. Luce, *A Curriculum for Plastic Surgery*, https://doi.org/10.1007/978-3-031-62087-4_1

learning, by the philosophy that one learning style fits all, and significant variability in the quality of operating room teaching and instruction [1, 11]. Although not intended as a sweeping indictment of all programs, these characteristics are all too common and probably represent the majority. In summary, as educators we, our specialty, must accept the necessity for a fundamental metamorphosis of resident education, in particular, the formal or didactic component.

Two premises underlie the need for a new conceptual approach to conference didactics:

1. Didactics are driven by the mission of conference: the primary thrust is education of the resident, graduate medical education, not continued medical education of faculty.
2. With the limitations of work hour regulations, a substantial increase in clinical load of both faculty and residents has occurred over time (increased number of faculty members, increase in number of cases, and the limits of the expansion of the resident workforce by ACGME), conference time is a valuable resource not to be squandered or wasted in an imprudent manner, perhaps thought of as an inherited trust fund.

The plastic surgery conferences are the traditional foundation of the formal or didactic component of resident education [12]. Organized to be secure from scheduled clinical activity, attendance is expected of all faculty and residents. The format is most commonly one of two, either a lecture (talk) on a particular topic drawn from a developed list (the curriculum), or a conference structured around a clinical case or cases frequently accompanied by a short talk as well. Viewed from the principles of adult learning, substantial criticism can be leveled at both. Lecturing as an educational instrument suffers from the use of a pedagogic approach to teaching-learning. Pedagogy ("to lead the child") views learning in a teacher-centered ("sage of the stage") model and the learners or students as passive vessels to receive the necessary knowledge [1, 12] (Fig. 1.1). The lecture (talks given to a weekly conference either by residents or faculty are essentially lectures) is an anachronism in the literal sense of the word because lectures are derived from medieval times when books were rare and unobtainable. The low value attached to lecture-based conferences is attested to by several observations: the conference rarely starts promptly, attendance is mandated and perhaps monitored by a sign-in process, and attention lapses after 10–12 min [13] (See Fig. 1.2).

The contributions by the faculty [14] are anecdotal and cite relevant information from published sources uncommonly.

The other component of plastic surgery didactics is the case-based conference. The case-based conference, as the name implies, is centered on a recent case or cases or scheduled operations (preoperative or indications conference), heavily dependent

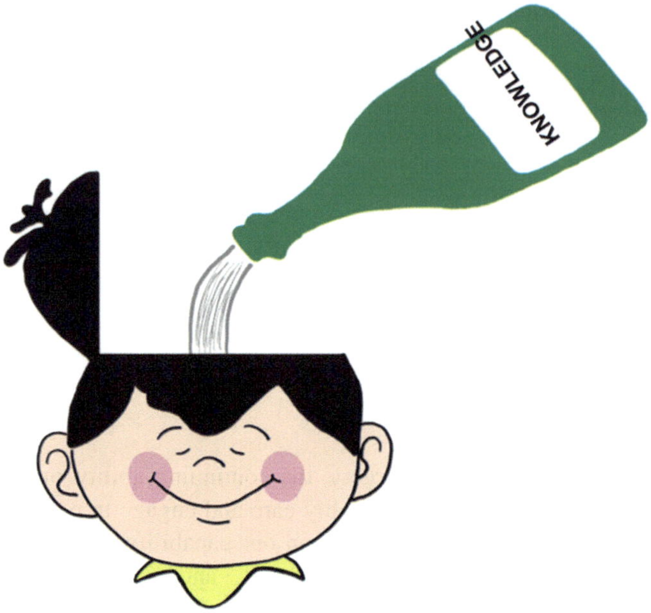

Fig. 1.1 Pedagogy

on case mix and flow. The use of case-based conferences as an educational vehicle in GME is designed to enable residents to acquire clinical knowledge and involvement by the use of a current patient case to illustrate the principles of diagnosis and treatment. The necessity for this educational vehicle is impelled by the loss of operative autonomy and diminished operative experience [15] with the advent by mandate of close attending supervision in the operating room, readily defensible, but nevertheless a mandate with a potential detrimental ripple effect on graduate medical education. The evolution or devolution of operative experience from one of the independent and autonomous surgeons to supervised operative experience has been implemented to the ultimate benefit of the patient, but has de facto increased the valence, importance, of the case-based conference as a vehicle to drive the acquisition of clinical experience.

Yet, the case conference fails to do so. The mechanics of the conference most commonly consist of presentation of the case by the resident, followed by a short summary of the relevant literature. The remainder of the discussion is conducted principally by the attendings with an occasional question by the resident, a discussion dominated by faculty with ad hoc and anecdotal information—"seems I've seen a number of these cases recently" or "In my experience…." In addition, the cases for presentation have some type of interesting dimension and are rarely mundane. As a result, two significant liabilities are imparted; first, the established educational curriculum is ignored and; second, the clinical strengths or case mix of the program is overemphasized and in parallel programmatic deficiencies in case distribution are magnified.

In summary, both the traditional talk and the case-based conference as currently structured or formatted are inadequate, woefully inadequate, educational vehicles. Yet, when

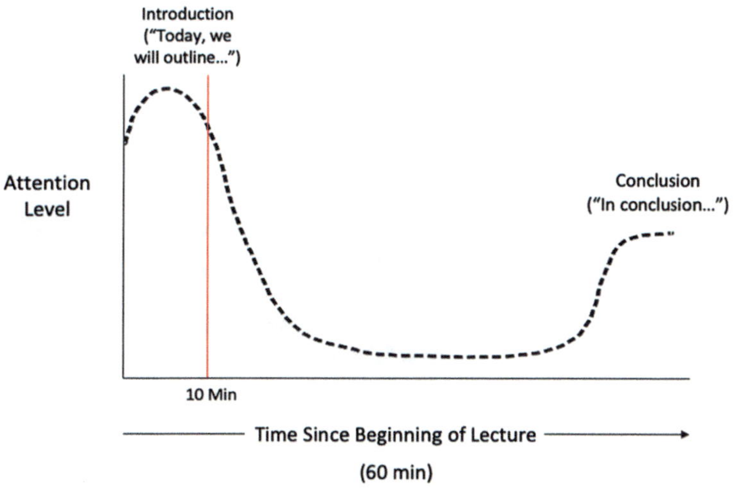

Fig. 1.2 (Redrawn from H. Niemantsverdriet and J.K. Felderhof, "Scientific Leadership" DeGruyter, Berlin 2017)

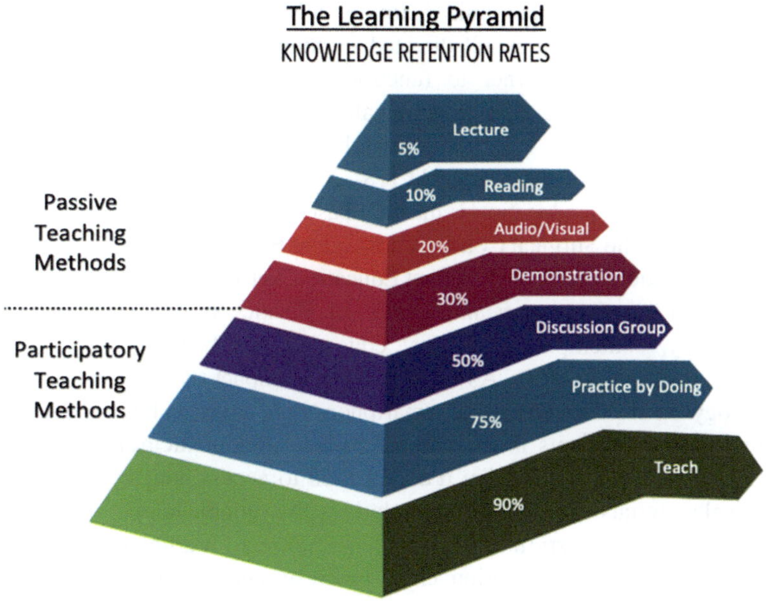

Fig. 1.3 The learning pyramid

viewed from the constraints of working hour regulations and dictates with respect to attending OR responsibilities, both have emerged as an essential element of the didactics of plastic surgery graduate medical education. As such, a radical restructuring of the conference foundation and design is mandatory to fulfill the objective of provision of the cognitive and intuitive tools of a competent plastic surgeon.

Guidance toward construction of a conference model that will achieve education goals is available. Educational research has established a hierarchy of teaching models, the rank or level achieved by learner retention rate (Fig. 1.3).

The common thread is the degree of teacher-learner interaction from the least, the talk, to the highest, the use of the information, and teaching others. Attempts to mollify the pedagogic aspects of a conference talk by post-talk discussion or prior distribution of reading material accomplishes little. The former is uniformly anecdotal, the latter rarely examined.

To sum, the properties of an optimal didactic conference are:

1. Structured and organized
2. Interactive between faculty and residents, not faculty to faculty—a proven concept of education
3. Built upon a comprehensive curriculum [16]

Where Should We Be?

If we accept the lecture or conference talk as a traditional but outmoded and ineffective teaching tool, what is the replacement, the vehicle to accomplish formal, didactic education? Some current enthusiasm exists about the use of "self-directed" learning, given a body of knowledge to master, learning initiated by the learner with minimal or no faculty

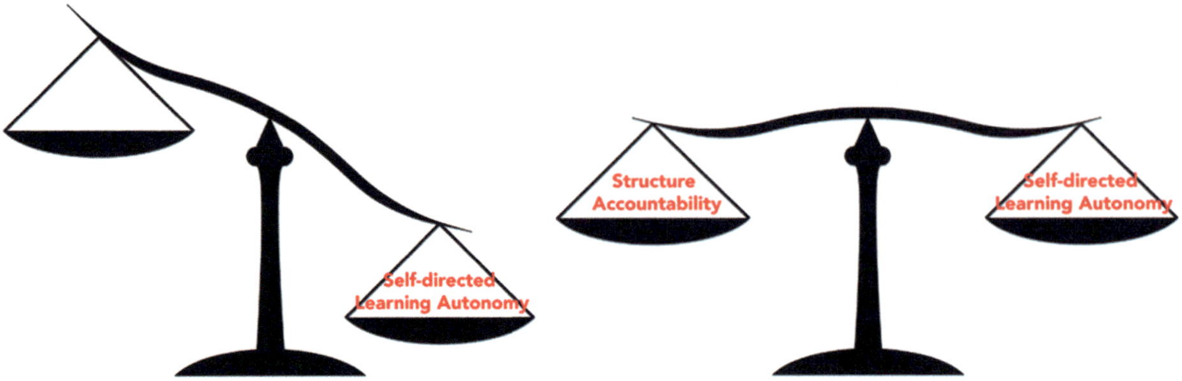

Fig. 1.4 Self-directed learning lends autotomy to the learner but no balance. (Right) An element of structure and accountability achieves a balance between autonomous self-directed learning and teacher-centered learning. (Luce EA. "The Future of Plastic Surgery Resident Education". Plast Reconstr Surg. 2016;137(3):1065. (Reprinted with permission))

involvement [17]. Electronic learning, termed e-learning, folds into the concept of self-directed learning and facilitates the ability of the learner to function autonomously. The capacity to place and store electronically (digitally) tutorials, graphics, and videos has been proven by the success of the Khan Academy in the lay world [18]. Within the arena of graduate surgical education is the web-based general surgery curriculum, the Surgical Council on Resident Education [19], and in plastic surgery, the Resident Education Network (REC) managed by the American Society of Plastic Surgeons. Certainly, contemporary resident education has benefited from digital technology. As evidence of the impact of technology on resident education, smartphones are used widely by surgical residents in the care of patients (telemedicine) [20] and tablets such as the iPad are used to access educational materials "on the fly," particularly with available applications such as *Plastic and Reconstructive Surgery* for articles or videos [21, 22]. In addition, cloud-based storage of institutional archived materials can be accomplished with minimal cost. Access to the material is available 24 hours per day, 7 days per week, and in this context, e-learning is self-directed [23]. However, evidence exists that self-directed learning is no more effective in education than the traditional lecture [24]. Self-directed learning alone provides learner autonomy but at the price of structure and accountability (Fig. 1.4).

Only when an element of interaction is introduced by the teacher ("the guide by the side") is learning, as judged by a statistically significant increase in test scores, enhanced. The power of group interactive discussion conducted with prepared learners is inestimable. A model to accomplish the integration of self-directed learning accompanied by the essential element of interactive discussion is the concept of the "flipped classroom." [25] The flipped classroom, viewed from the perspective of undergraduate or graduate studies, reverses the traditional sequence of classroom lecture followed by classwork completed on the student's own time into a sequence of the lecture available as a tutorial online,

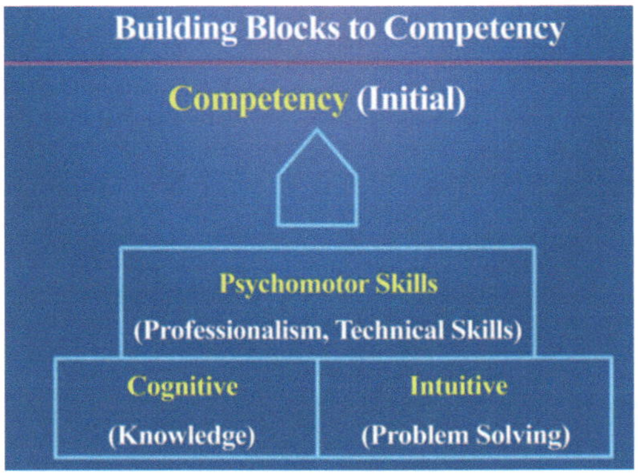

Fig. 1.5 Building blocks toward competency. (Luce EA. "Beyond Working Hours: Part II. Incentive to Improve". Plast Reconstr Surg. 2012;129(4):718e. (Reprinted with permission))

reviewed by the students on their own cognizance (homework time), and the use of the classroom for interactive discussion of the lecture material [26, 27].

Any number of didactic protocols exist to accomplish the objectives of incorporation of self-directed learning that would include an electronic vehicle and the use of a flipped classroom approach to ensure interactive discussion. A common thread of success to all is adherence to the main principles of andrology: experientially derived learning including the capacity to commit mistakes, problem-oriented rather than teacher-centered, immediate relevance and feedback, ability to apply the information shortly after learning, and participation by the learners in the establishment of their educational goals [28]. For example, one template is the American Board of Plastic Surgery certification process, a process that examines the candidate's body of cognitive knowledge (written examination), intuitive or problem-solving capabilities (Theory and Practice component of the oral examination), and operative and professional skills (Board-selected case reports), all important elements of the assessment of competency [29] (Fig. 1.5).

Another model is Miller's Pyramid. Miller's pyramid [30] classifies the development of clinical competence into four levels of ascending complexity of performance. The fundamental or Level I is medical knowledge, the second the application of that knowledge, but in a basic or fundamental way. The third is the acquisition of clinical skills and the highest or fourth level, performance in a clinical setting (Fig. 1.6).

To separate or group didactics in that manner, a single conference can be structured to focus either entirely on broad type of goals as acquisition of cognitive knowledge (Miller's Level I) *or* the application of such knowledge to problem-solving clinical situations (Miller's Levels 2 and 3). Division of conference didactics into either cognitive or case-based, conceptually and structurally, establishes a format substantially different between the two for residents and faculty. The structure of the cognitive conference requires prior (10–14 days) electronic distribution of material including tutorials, readings (review and CME articles in *Plastic and Reconstructive Surgery* are an excellent source), and videos. Conference time is directed toward an interactive discussion of the modular material, consistent with the flipped classroom concept, designed by questions directed by the faculty moderator in Socratic fashion [31, 32] toward a learner comprehension of the assigned cognitive information. The interactive component is implemented by not only questions and answers to ensure comprehension but also a discussion of the debatable elements, if any, within the readings. Thorough preparation of the faculty is imperative by the prior development of a series of discussion points (lesson plan), sufficiently specific in focus, to drill down into residents' grasp of the concepts involved. The prior preparation and utilization of a faculty discussion and study guide avoids an ad hoc approach to conference teaching and also enables attendance and conduct of the conference by one or two faculty members only. To add the component of accountability, a short, 10 min, written examination consisting of archived multiple choice questions, matched to the module, is administered the subsequent week, a mechanism that has demonstrable efficacy [33].

The intuitive conference, separate temporally and conceptually from the cognitive conference, is devoted entirely to learning clinical problem-solving skills in general and in specific scenarios. The analysis of deformity and dysfunction is an acquired skill not innate to most individuals [34]. The successful application by the resident of those acquired skills to a plastic surgery case for the development of a treatment plan is the objective of this conference. Grantcharov and Reznick [35] have emphasized the educational value of modular teaching-learning, so the clinical cases should be drawn from the same module (e.g., velopharyngeal insufficiency) assigned and discussed in the prior cognitive conference. To duplicate actual practice and virtual learning, cases are distributed 48–72 h in advance. To ensure structure, a case is assigned to a single resident and faculty member, an assignment that would include broadly defined and distributed discussion goals. Once assigned, the resident can pursue available resources, reflect on the case, and construct a diagnostic and therapeutic framework, all of which are application of adult learning principles. Experience has taught the equal importance of faculty preparation as well, independent of the assigned resident, to ensure that the relevant learning points are thoroughly reviewed in conference. Proper conduct of the intuitive conference is crucial to the desired outcome. Similar to the oral examination of the American Board of Plastic Surgery, question composition is designed to test the analytical reasoning of the resident, a definition of expected responses, and the similarity of process errors to those of a faulty board candidate performance. Different, though, is the dialogue nature and the extended time allotted

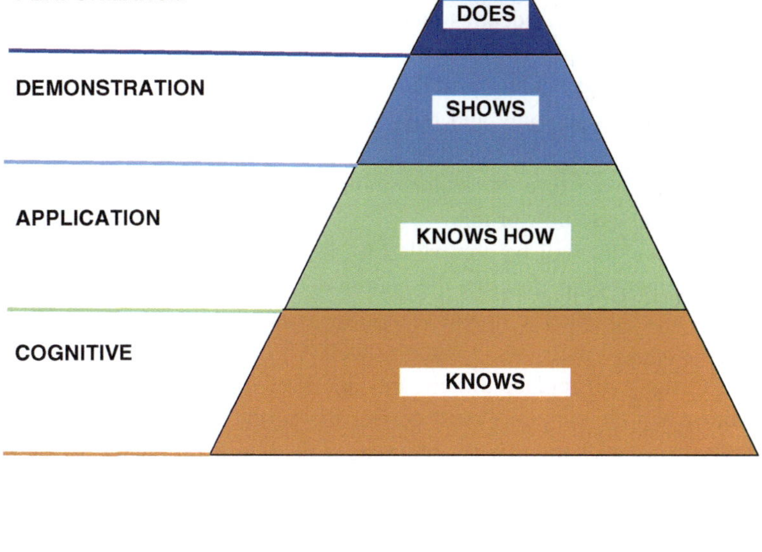

Fig. 1.6 Miller's pyramid of clinical competence

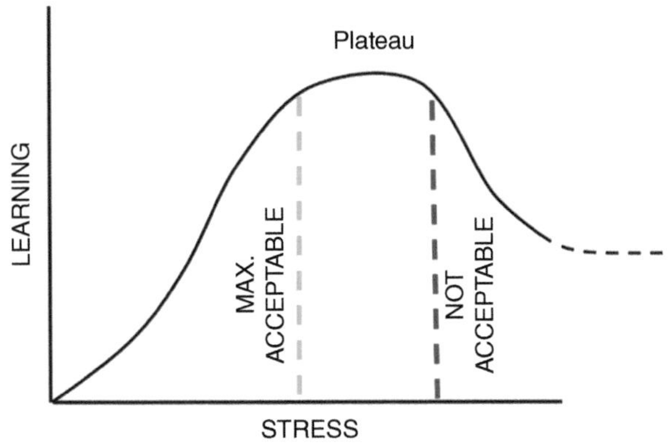

Fig. 1.7 Yerkes-Dodson Curve. The optimum balance of stress and learning; the bell-shaped curve of performance versus level of stress. (Luce EA. "The Future of Plastic Surgery Resident Education. Plast Reconstr Surg. 2016;137(3). (Reprinted with permission))

per case; a dialogue limited to the assigned faculty-resident pair. Different also is the capability of feedback, educational as well as constructive (formative) criticism. Some element of stress is unavoidable and perhaps to a degree desirable [14], but badgering and intimidation are not acceptable nor should be tolerated (Fig. 1.7).

The case conference can play an integral role in the development of the clinical skills necessary to become a competent plastic surgeon, a requisite structure that fulfills several criteria. First, the selection of cases should be tailored to and follow a comprehensive curriculum. Second, the conference structure should adhere to the principles of adult learning, be interactive in format, and duplicate virtually, clinical scenarios. Those criteria can be addressed by assignment to specific residents of cases 2–3 days in advance as well as a set of questions also distributed in advance designed to enhance an interactive dialogue between the resident and a specific assigned faculty member. Matching a specific faculty member with a subspecialty interest to the particular clinical scenario posed by the case is not necessary, given the several day hiatus for preparation.

What is necessary, though, is the case difficulty matched to the level of the resident as dictated by the ACGME milestones. For example, the level of education and expertise to address a wound healing problem is substantially different than a post-lumpectomy and radiotherapy deformity of the breast. To repeat, the intuitive or case-based conference should be linked to a curricular module, not the particular institutional case flow or mix.

The resident will be compelled to develop a diagnostic and treatment plan, describe the plan in detail, including the selection of a specific operative option in most cases, and draw proposed incisions in some as well. Of course, no virtual format will replace the circumstances of the operating room when the surgeon "must deliver the goods." Yet, residents do not wish to fail in the presence of peers and although not a reenactment or duplication of the demands inherent within the operating room, the desire to perform superbly is in part a substitute or surrogate.

Table 1.1 Recommendations

1. Replace the pedagogic (teacher-centered) educational style with adult learning principles or an educational avenue of andragogy (learner-centered)
2. Adopt the "flipped classroom" concept of conference didactics
3. Promote universal acceptance of a uniform curriculum, supplemented with faculty discussion guides
4. Establish formalized faculty training in the performance of optimal resident education

The "flipped classroom" format, besides an enhancement of the educational process, also expands the number of weekly hours devoted to education. For example, of the 3 h of actual weekly conference time, the residents in an annual survey report 4–6 h preparation for the cognitive (reading) conference and 3–4 h for the case-based conference, if a case is assigned. In addition, the rotation of faculty responsibility in this manner for conference teaching (2 h of preparation for cognitive and 3 h for the three cases in the intuitive conference) addresses, in part, the demands on faculty time described above.

What is of paramount importance is to recognize residents as both students and adults, not as apprentices or passive and dependent learners. We all learn optimally by the process of active inquiry, embodied in those principles of plastic surgery problem-solving and clinical judgment, conducted in a supportive environment that provides constructive feedback.

Thus, what does the future hold for plastic surgery resident education in the arena of conference didactics? Universal adoption of a uniform standardized curriculum, program to program, that would enable, for example, use of the same conference case transmitted electronically and used regionally in simultaneous conference(s). Actually, the media means to do so exists today but the universal uniform curriculum does not. From a personal perspective one objective of this project is to provide such a curriculum (Table 1.1).

Journal Club

Although programmatic didactics are designed to provide the resident with the pathway to competency, an important component is the inoculation of habits of the life-long learner. Certainly, in medicine in general and plastic surgery in particular, a practitioner must have a plan of continuing medical education of which a review of the current literature is certainly key. A journal club is the forum to accomplish the goals of acquisition of a critical appraisal of the published literature as well as a method to promote the practice of evidence-based medicine, EBM.

The roots appear to be with William Osler who initiated a journal club at McGill in Toronto and later at Johns Hopkins [36]. Surely, Halsted at Hopkins adopted the same in the department of surgery and currently journal clubs are universal throughout graduate surgical education. Some considerable variability exists, though, in administration and conduct [37], particularly within the constraints within the working hours mandate. Regardless, the ingredients of a successful journal club, successfully judged by the criteria of longevity, attendance, and resident favorable reviews, include a number of ingredients [37, 38]. Those ingredients listed below were experientially derived and also by a review of published observations.

The structure is defined by the educational objectives—Is the goal to review the current literature to imbue the principles of EBM *or* to teach critical appraisal skills in analysis of a scientific paper, or both? The former implies the review of 5–7 papers and a discussion centered on integration of the information into current practice. The latter requires fewer articles, 4–5, and a discussion of the methodology and limitations of the specific article. Incorporation of both can be accomplished by article selection criteria and discussion format.

The selection criteria include excellent papers such as random controlled trials with few, if any limitations, an investigation with a novel perspective of a clinical problem or issue, or an article perhaps not of pristine methodology but accompanied by an excellent discussion of the different aspects of the question under consideration. If the thrust of the objective is to review some current literature, the discussion will be driven, mostly, by faculty (attendings). In a hybrid model, developed at two institutions, the majority of the discussion is conducted by the residents with utilization of a pro-con framework, one resident presenting a brief summary and the positive aspects, the second a critique and the limitations of the study. Any resident can expect a request to discuss the pro or con side of a given article selected from the list. A previously assigned attending for each article renders a balanced summary. A moderator, preferably a mid-level attending, is necessary to move the agenda and solicit discussion. This model incorporates both the educational goals listed above and minimizes anecdotal comments by attendings, a frequent occurrence in journal clubs of other formats.

Prior distribution of a list of articles, or preferentially an electronic copy of the articles particularly if drawn from multiple journals, should be accomplished at least 2 weeks in advance. Attendance can be maximized not only by a mandatory requirement but also by the setting. Journal clubs are optimally conducted independently of conventional conference time, in the evening, with the provision of food in a setting of the home of a faculty member or a restaurant [39]. A short social time can precede the actual journal club. Even the physical arrangement of the conference can enhance interaction. A circle or round table, if logistically possible, will promote eye contact and discussion. To do so strengthens faculty-resident interaction in an informal and collegial milieu. To adhere to working hours restrictions and attention span, duration should be limited to 2 h.

Table 1.2 Characteristics of a successful Journal Club [37–39]

1. Educational objectives defined
2. Criteria of article selection developed
3. Physical layout to enhance discussion
4. Discussion format codified

Consistent with the environment of all didactic conferences, the learners must be comfortable with their limitations and the capacity to err without a threatening atmosphere. Junior residents must be permitted to pro-con discuss an article that does not hinge on the necessity of prior clinical experience. Consistent with the goals of continuous quality improvement, the results of an annual anonymous resident and faculty survey will enable the necessary modifications to ensure a successful journal club.

A final note on the temptation to implement a totally online journal club. Efforts of a virtual online journal club, when evaluated, concluded that the traditional onsite option was preferred [38] (Table 1.2).

Morbidity and Mortality Conference

Mandated by the ACGME, Morbidity and Mortality conference, M&M, is a requirement within all residency programs. The heritage of the M&M conference well predates the ACGME, however. Over a century ago, Emory Codman advocated a review of outcomes and discussion of same both as an educational process and a method for identification of issues. Because of the central and essential role of the M&M conference, a considerable volume of publications have discussed the function and mechanics. As in the preceding section "The Journal Club," the recommendations listed and discussed are the product of both experience and a literature review.

From Codman's time onward, the objectives of the M&M conference have been a yin-yang of two objectives, occasionally in conflict, education, and quality improvement [40]. Is the goal of the conference primarily education and quality improvement, QI, is a secondary consequence *or* a QI exercise with GME as a by-product? Although not a dichotomy, concise definition determines the format and who drives the discussion. With the rising prominence of offices of risk management and system error investigation, the M&M conference can be hijacked and resident education fade into the background. Not to deprecate a multidisciplinary and collaborative approach to the investigation and discussion of complications, but if root cause analysis and implementation of specific and continuous QI is the primary objective, perhaps a separate conference driven by attendings alone is justified.

Nevertheless, the execution of the components of case selection, structure, and format of the M&M conference are crucial to achievement of the educational objectives. Compilation of the list is mandatory by inclusion of either all adverse events and complications or the use of a standardized set of criteria. Both have benefits and liabilities: the former can create a burdensome list that ultimately requires a selection, the latter the potential to exclude an educational case. The use of NSQIP complication indices has been advocated by some [41] but if so should be supplemented by criteria unique to plastic surgery.

Once selected, the number of cases included hinge in part by the frequency of conference, monthly or bi-monthly, and should be limited to 4 or 5 cases for a 90-min conference. The results of this selection process should be distributed 2 weeks prior to the particular conference. Resident presentations must be succinct and concise. A useful framework is the SABR (situation, background, assessment, recommendation) [42] such that following resident presentation and analysis of the case, an open discussion is conducted. Experience has dictated an appointment of a moderator, optimally an academic mid-level attending, again similar to journal club. To foster only constructive feedback, of cardinal importance is the assurance of an environment free of the "blame and shame" or "blood in the water" tendencies of a surgical M&M conference.

The M&M conference can be explicitly linked to the ACGME six core competencies [43]. To do so implies a reflection of issues of not just the speciality-specific competencies of medical knowledge and patient care, but also the issues of practice-based learning, systems-based practice, professionalism, and communication and interpersonal skills. Finally, another educational element of an M&M conference that has not been defined in the past is the opportunity for resident observation of exemplary attending role modeling in humility and professionalism.

ACGME, the Milestones, and Entrustable Professional Activities

Although this book, the organization discussed below, is primarily focused on the structure and function of education, assessment of any educational process is a key element. The ACGME is the body primarily responsible for the approval, the accreditation council, of graduate medical education, a responsibility assigned to the ACGME by all of organized medicine.

A curriculum, at least as conceived by this book and discussed above, is a vehicle to transport the resident on the pathway to competency in the cognitive and intuitive (problem-solving) domains of plastic surgery. A periodic assessment of the progress on that pathway is an integral part of the Milestone project of the ACGME. The impetus of the project was to shift resident education and training from a time-based to a competency-based system. The journey toward achievement of competency is by a series of steps or levels termed milestones. The milestones, as the name implies, are interval points on the path or journey toward the destination of independent practice. In turn, the definition of competency has been divided into six components of which only two, medical knowledge and patient care, are unique to plastic surgery. Of those six components, the remaining four are systems-based practice, practice-based learning, professionalism, interpersonal skills and communication, and the assessment of all six in plastic surgery residents' performance is the keystone of the conceptual arch of graduate medical education, GME, as envisioned by the ACGME. Attainment of a milestone is easily discerned in, for example, a road race (where one passes a mile marker) but logarithmically more difficult to ascertain in the complex tasks of the practice of medicine. Assessment tools are a necessity to determine progress in that journey [44].

In summary, plastic surgery training programs have been tasked, an unfunded mandate, with the adoption of methods of resident assessment that are objective, consistent, and sufficiently granular to provide particular rather than global feedback to residents. Outlined below is how incorporation of this curriculum can provide a discharge of nonoperative elements of resident performance assessment.

The curriculum as constituted in the book could readily provide assessment in the two competencies of medical knowledge and patient care. The former by an interactive discussion of cognitive knowledge on the part of the resident within a specific area or topic in each of the chapters, the latter by evaluation of performance in the case-based conference dialogue. Rather than global, the evaluation should be specific with listed objectives, for example, photo analysis of deformity/dysfunction, description of pathologic anatomy and/or pathophysiology, and development of a treatment plan. The overall assessment would be judged by if the resident met (or not) the anticipated milestone. Besides medical knowledge and patient care, the competency of interpersonal skills and communication could be indirectly assessed in some cases. The competency of practice-based learning implies a sequential improvement of performance. Since each case is drawn from a submodule, evaluation is within a narrowly defined clinical area. Of course, these objective and summative assessments could be maintained in the resident's portfolio for use by the Clinical Competency Committee [45].

As a result of the perspective that the Milestones were too broad and abstract, entrustable professional activities [46], EPAs, have been developed as an effort to translate the

Milestones into a mechanism that would enable assessment in the workplace on a day-to-day, real-time basis. An EPA is a directly observed clinical behavior of resident performance in the management of a single entity as cleft palate. EPAs are designed to enable specific faculty evaluation after an observed clinical encounter.

At the time of this writing, a number of EPAs are under development by plastic surgery.

Overview of Book Structure

This book was written with a vision, provoked by a question: if a program director was to implement a plastic surgery residency *de novo*, what elements would he or she need to implement for the formal educational structure? The answer appears simple—any number of "curricula" exist, everything from a simple list of broad topics to a much more detailed compilation. Yet, those curricula whether 1 or 10 pages remain, perhaps as originally intended, a roadmap of a journey of a resident from novice to com*p*etence. The novice plastic surgery resident can read those lists on day one and yet have made no progress in that journey. This book is structured as a conveyance, somewhat complex, a vehicle for that journey. The aforementioned program director can adopt this curriculum as a "turn key" design for resident education.

The organization follows the lines established in the prior section and assumes the weekly didactics would consist of two conferences: a 1-h cognitive conference and a 1.5 or a 2-h case conference. Overall, the curriculum consists of modules, the general topics of plastic surgery. Each of the 12 modules is subdivided into, varying according to topic, of two to 15 submodules or a total of 110.

An individual cognitive conference is entirely devoted to a single submodule, for example, bilateral cleft lip. The material for the cognitive conference consists of a bibliography of selected reading, a faculty discussion guide, and a set of multiple choice questions including the relevant references. The selected readings, mostly articles, were chosen on the basis of several criteria: relevance, comprehensive, and current. Book chapters, although not excluded, compose a minority of the selections. To render the workload palatable and to minimize overlap, only sections of any given article or chapter rather than the entire article or chapter were identified and assigned (see example below of a bibliography). The bibliography as a reading assignment is distributed to resident staff and faculty member responsible for the conference 7–10 days in advance. The faculty discussion guides were developed to set the interactive discussion as sufficiently specific and granular to ensure a thorough comprehension of the material. Prior preparation of the faculty by a review of both the guide and the material is essential to the success of the conference. An example of the bibliography of a submodule within the broader module, Skin Tumors, is listed below. To minimize overlap and repetition for the reader, selected pages of each reference are listed.

Bibliography: Melanoma

Netscher, DT, Leong M, Orengo I, et al., "Cutaneous Malignancies: Melanoma and Nonmelanoma Types", *Plast. Reconstr. Surg.*, (2011); 127(3):**48e-52e ONLY.**

Dźwierzyński WW, "Managing Malignant Melanoma", *Plast. Reconstr. Surg.*, (2013); 132(3):**446e-460e (Skip 450e-455e but include Figure 7 and Table 3 on pg 451e and also include videos).**

Cochran AM, Buchanan PJ, Bueno Jr. RA, Neumeister, MW, "Subungual Melanoma: A review of Current Treatment", *Plast. Reconstr. Surg.*, (2014); 134: **259-262 (to literature review), 271-272.**

Knackstedt, T, Knackstedt R W, Couto R, Gastman Brian, " Malignant Melanoma: Diagnostic and Management Update", *Plast. Reconstr. Surg.*, (2018);(142):**202e-212e and Video 1.**

Upadhyaya S.N., Knackstedt R.W., Ko J.S., Gastman B.R.,The Use and Technique of Sentinel Node Biopsy for Skin Cancer, *Plast Reconstr Surg.*, (2022);149(5):**995e-1005e ONLY.**

Pavri SN, Clune J, Ariyan S, Narayan D, "Malignant Melanoma: Beyond the Basics", *Plast. Reconstr. Surg.*, (2016); 138(2):**330e-338e ONLY.**

Supplemental:

- Ariyan S and Berger A, Ch. 31: "Melanoma", Neligan PC, Plastic Surgery 3rd Edition (2013); 1:**748-771, 776-784 ONLY.**

Written examinations are provided for each chapter consisting of three to four multiplechoice questions based on the topic of the prior cognitive conference. Dependent on programmatic preference, the results can be distributed electronically. Experience indicates only 8–10 min are necessary for completion of the short exam.

The material for the intuitive or case conference consists of a selected case (or cases) for the particular submodule linked to the prior cognitive conference that includes representative photos, a short description and several, three to four, broad questions to frame the discussion. The problem-solving format of the questions is dictated by the "Here-There" [33] concept that compels the dialogue into an analysis of the deformity and/or dysfunction, identifies the causative mechanisms as well as the pathologic anatomy and pathophysiology and then based on those responses, develops a treatment plan. At the completion of the dialogue between resident and the selected attendings, 20 min duration in most instances, a short period is devoted to general discussion.

Assessment of resident performance in the identification of the case representation of deformity/dysfunction, the description of the pathologic anatomy and pathophysiology, and the articulation of a treatment plan is conducted in a formative and constructive manner, usually at the completion of the discussion. To determine attainment of the core competency-based milestones, an alternate faculty member with the use of a prescribed form can complete a written summative assessment, subsequently available to the Clinical Competency Committee [45]. In addition, each case has a four to six page discussion including postoperative results centered on the question format, distributed in follow-up to the particular resident as an outline of the anticipated "correct" responses. The Table of Contents have separately been linked to the ACGME milestones.

Conclusions

As educators, we must discard the current outmoded and ineffective methods of resident education and embrace a contemporary method that embodies structured learning and interactive discussion. To reiterate, the mission of the book is to fulfill the definition of a curriculum, a course of study that incorporates the "flipped classroom" format and conference structure for the acquisition of the requisite cognitive knowledge and intuitive problem-solving skills. The principal thrust of our educational efforts, integral to such a transformation, is to shift the performance expertise and professionalism curve of all residents to the right (Fig. 1.8).

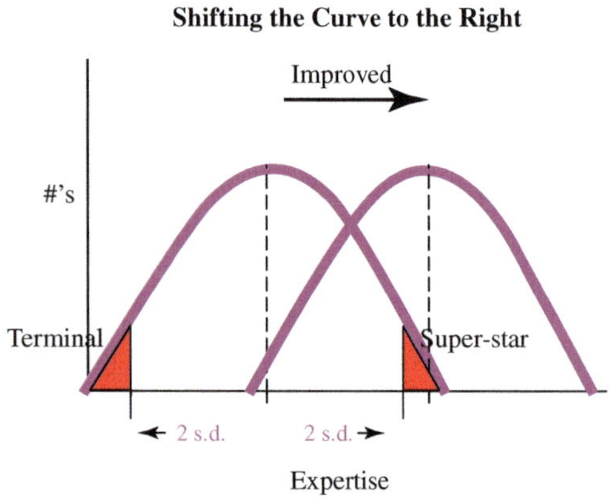

Fig. 1.8 Shifting the resident curve of performance and professionalism to the right. (Luce EA. Beyond working hours: Part II. Incentive to improve. *Plast Reconstr Surg.*, (2012);129:717e–720e. (Reprinted with permission))

References

1. Luce E.A., "The Future of Plastic Surgery Resident Education", *Plast Reconstr Surg.*, (2016);137(3):1063-1070.
2. Reznick RK, MacRae H. Teaching surgical skills: Changes in the wind. N Engl J Med. 2006;355:2664–2669.
3. Marsh JL. AOA 2014–2015 Presidential Address. "Tipping points" in surgical education: AOA critical issues. J Bone Joint Surg. 2015;97:e14.
4. Luce EA. Beyond working hours: Part I. Genesis and current difficulties. Plast Reconstr Surg. 2012;129:1015–1021.
5. Luce, E.A. Beyond Working Hours: Part II. Incentive to Improve. Plastic and Reconstr Surg. 2012;129:717e-720e.
6. Anderson CE, Nicksa GA, Stewart L. Distractions during resident handoffs: Incidence, sources, and influence on handoff quality and effectiveness. JAMA Surg. 2015;150:396–401.
7. Arrighi JA, Hebert JC. Duty hour requirements: Time for a new approach? JAMA 2014;312:2342–2344.
8. Ahmed N, Devitt KS, Keshet I, et al. A systematic review of the effects of resident duty hour restrictions in surgery: Impact on resident wellness, training, and patient outcomes. Ann Surg. 2014;259:1041–1053.
9. Williams RG, Dunnington GL, Mellinger JD, et al. Placing constraints on the use of the ACGME Milestones: A commentary on the limitations of global performance ratings. Acad Med. 2015;90:404–407.
10. Luce EA. Integrated training in plastic surgery: Concept, implementation, benefits, and liabilities. Plast Reconstr Surg. 1995;95:119–123.
11. Mellinger JD, Damewood R, Morris JB. Assessing the quality of graduate surgical training programs: Perception vs reality. J Am Coll Surg. 2015;220:785–789.
12. Luce EA. The plastic surgery teaching conference: A horse and buggy educational vehicle for supersonic times. Plast Reconstr Surg. 1996;97:1234–1237.
13. Luce EA. Discussion: Teaching plastic surgeons how to be better teachers. Plast Reconstr Surg. 2012;129:1198–1199.
14. DeRosa D. Maximally invasive teaching: Presentation to the Institute of Excellence in Education, Johns Hopkins, March 20, 2014. http://www.hopkinsmedicine.org/institute_excellence_education/. Accessed June 1, 2015.
15. Bell R.H. Why Johnny Cannot Operate. Surgery. 2009;146(4):533-42.
16. Kaufman DM. Applying educational theory in practice. BMJ 2003;326:213–216.
17. Larvin M. E-learning in surgical education and training. ANZ J Surg. 2009;79:133–137.
18. Noer M. One man, one computer, 10 million students: How Khan Academy is reinventing education. Forbes November 19, 2012:1–8.
19. Klingensmith ME, Jones AT, Smiley W, et al. Subscription to the surgical council on resident education web portal and qualifying examination performance. J Am Coll Surg. 2014;218:566–570.
20. Plant MA, Fish JS. Resident use of the Internet, e-mail, and personal electronics in the care of surgical patients. Teach Learn Med. 2015;27:215–223.
21. Al-Hadithy N, Ghosh S. Smartphones and the plastic surgeon. J Plast Reconstr Aesthet Surg. 2013;66:e155–e161.
22. Gerstle T, Hassanein AH, Eriksson E. iPad integration in plastic surgical training: Optimizing clinical efficiency, education, and compliance with the health insurance portability and accountability act. Plast Reconstr Surg. 2015;135:223e–225e.

23. Lobo MJ, Crandley EF, Rumph JS, et al. Pilot study of iPad incorporation into graduate medical education. J Grad Med Educ. 2013;5:142–144.
24. Porte MC, Xeroulis G, Reznick RK, Dubrowski A. Verbal feedback from an expert is more effective than self-accessed feedback about motion efficiency in learning new surgical skills. Am J Surg. 2007;193:105–110.
25. Deslauriers L, Schelew E, Wieman C. Improved learning in a large-enrollment physics class. Science 2011;332:862–864.
26. Prober CG, Heath C. Lecture halls without lectures: A proposal for medical education. N Engl J Med. 2012;366:1657–1659.
27. McLaughlin JE, Roth MT, Glatt DM, et al. The flipped classroom: A course redesign to foster learning and engagement in a health professions school. Acad Med. 2014;89:236–243.
28. Knowles MS, Holton EF III, Swanson RA. The Adult Learner. 7th ed. Amsterdam: Elsevier; 2011.
29. Luce EA. A survival plan. Plast Reconstr Surg. 2001;108:776–782.
30. Witheridge A., Ferns G., Scotts-Smith W. "Revisiting Miller's pyramid in Medical Education: The Gap Between Traditional Assessment and Diagnostic Reasoning", *International Journal of Medical Education* (2019) Vol 10; pg 191-192.
31. Rohrich RJ, Johns DF. The Socratic method in plastic surgery education: A lost art revisited. Plast Reconstr Surg. 2000;105:1803–1805.
32. Farnsworth, Ward. *The Socratic Method: A Practitioner's Handbook*. Godine, 2021.
33. de Virgilio C, Chan T, Kaji A, Miller K. Weekly assigned reading and examinations during residency, ABSITE performance, and improved pass rates on the American Board of Surgery Examinations. J Surg Educ. 2008;65:499–503.
34. Luce EA. Analysis of complex postextirpative deformity. Clin Plast Surg. 1995;22:1–8.
35. Grantcharov TP, Reznick RK. Training tomorrow's surgeons: What are we looking for and how can we achieve it? ANZ J Surg. 2009;79:104–107.
36. Topf JM, Sparks MA, Phelan PJ, Shah N, Lerma EV, Graham-Brown MPM, Madariaga H, Iannuzzella F, Rheault MN, Oates T, Jhaveri KD, Hiremath S. The Evolution of the Journal Club: From Osler to Twitter. Am J Kidney Dis. 2017;69(6):827-836.
37. Williams AD, Mann BD, Lipman J. Understanding the Modern Surgical Journal Club. J Surg Educ. 2019;76(3):637-643.
38. Campbell ST, Kang JR, Bishop JA. What Makes Journal Club Effective?-A Survey of Orthopaedic Residents and Faculty. J Surg Educ. 2018;75(3):722-729.
39. Gottlieb M, King A, Byyny R, Parsons M, Bailitz J. Journal Club in Residency Education: An Evidence-based Guide to Best Practices from the Council of Emergency Medicine Residency Directors. West J Emerg Med. 2018;19(4):746-755.
40. de Vos MS, Marang-van de Mheen PJ, Smith AD, Mou D, Whang EE, Hamming JF. Toward Best Practices for Surgical Morbidity and Mortality Conferences: A Mixed Methods Study. J Surg Educ. 2018;75(1):33-42.
41. Endicott KM, Zettervall SL, Rettig RL, Patel N, Buckley L, Sidawy A, Knoll S, Vaziri K. Use of Structured Presentation Formatting and NSQIP Guidelines Improves Quality of Surgical Morbidity and Mortality Conference. J Surg Res. 2019;233:118-123.
42. Sacks GD, Lawson EH, Tillou A, Hines OJ. Morbidity and Mortality Conference 2.0. Ann Surg. 2015;262(2):228-9.
43. Kravet SJ, Howell E, Wright SM. Morbidity and mortality conference, grand rounds, and the ACGME's core competencies. J Gen Intern Med. 2006;21(11):1192-4.
44. Luce, Edward A. M.D. Discussion: Competency, the NAS, and the Milestones: Sea Change or Deluge?. Plast Reconstr Surg. 2016.137(4):1334-1336.
45. Luce EA, Wallace R, Suavee E., "Use of a Case-base Conference to Assess Achievement of Milestones and Noncognitive Skills", *PRS GO*, (2016);4(6):e1156.
46. Brasel KJ, et al, "Implementation of Entrustable Professional Activities in General Surgery: Results of a National Pilot Study", *Ann Surg.*, (2023);278(4):578-586.

Part I

General Principles

Wound Healing 1: General Principles

2

Bibliography

Broughton G, Janis JE, Attinger CE, "Wound healing: An overview", *Plast. Reconstr. Surg.*, (2006); 117(7S):**1-10eS ONLY**.

Jones, C., Rothermel, A. and Mackay, D., "Evidence - Based Medicine: Wound Management"., *Plast. Reconstr. Surg.*, (2017), 140:**204e, 207e-209e ONLY**.

Anghel, E., et al., "Current Concept in Debridement: Science and Strategies.", *Plast. Reconstr. Surg.*, (2016),138:**82S-91S**.

Orgill DP and Bayer LR, "Update on negative-pressure wound therapy", *Plast. Reconstr. Surg.*, (2011); 127(1S):**107S-113S ONLY**.

Singh D, Chopra K, Sabino J, Brown E, "Practical Things You Should Know About Wound Healing and Vacuum-Assisted Closure Management", *Plast. Reconstr. Surg.*, (2020); 145(4):**839e-852e (skip laser angiography 845e-49e).**

Gompelman M., van Asten SAV., Peters EJG., "Update on the Role of Infection and Biofilms in Wound Healing: Pathophysiology and Treatment", *Plast Reconstr Surg.*, (2016);138 (Supplement):**61S-67S.**

Faculty Discussion and Study Guide

Editor's Note: Difficult wounds are also discussed in Chap. 64.

Physiology of Wound Healing

1. Describe the principal events of the first stage of wound healing. (The first stage, referred to as the cellular or inflammatory phase, consists of a brief period of vasoconstriction that lasts literally minutes, followed by active vasodilatation and the appearance of a cellular infiltrate morphologically and a variety of kinins biochemically. The initial infiltrate consists of PMNs and neutrophil cells, as well as lymphocytes slightly later. The neutrophils are the source of proteolytic enzymes that are bactericidal. At 24–48 h, macrophages appear as a bactericidal agent, cleansing the wound of acellular debris, and are also the source of multiple growth factors.)
   (a) What is the role and duration of fibronectin? (Cellular adhesion and migration; 24–48 h)
   (b) What is the primary cellular agent that initiates the inflammatory phase? (Platelets release the cytokines or platelet factors that participate in the coagulation cascade and attract the other cells that begin the first phase of wound healing such as polymorphonuclear cells (PMNs) and macrophages.)
2. Describe the principal events of the second stage, the fibroblastic or proliferative phase. (The onset is 48–72 h, and the primary events are the migration of fibroblasts along the scaffolding provided by fibrin, the formation of ground substance, and the early deposition of collagen, as well as angiogenesis or capillary neovascularization.)
   (a) What is the composition of the ground substance? (Hyaluronic acid and chondroitin sulfate)
3. What is the principal stimulus to epithelial cell migration? (Loss of contact inhibition and disruption of the basement membrane)
   (a) What are integrin receptors? (Receptors that bind to extracellular proteins to maintain intimate contact between epithelial cells)
4. What is the principal agent in the contraction of a wound? (Myofibroblasts)
5. What is the timing of and what occurs during the maturation or remodeling phase? (Although there is no net increase in collagen after a month or so after injury, both synthesis and degradation are increased, and cross-linkage begins to occur. The timing is approximately 3–4 weeks although obviously not exact.)

E. Luce, *A Curriculum for Plastic Surgery*, https://doi.org/10.1007/978-3-031-62087-4_2

(a) What are the two principal amino acids contained in collagen? (Hydroxyproline and hydroxylysine)
(b) Will a biopsy of a wound at one week and a biopsy of adjacent normal skin differ in content of collagen type? (At one week, the wound will be substantially higher in type III collagen although type I collagen will predominate overall; normal adult skin has a 4:1 ratio of type I to type III collagen.)

6. What elements are required to be present for the attachment of hydroxy moiety to proline to convert to hydroxyproline? (Fe^{++}, vitamin C or ascorbic acid, oxygen, and alpha ketoglutarate)
7. Define tensile and bursting strength. (Tensile strength is the measure of the wound strength per unit area, while bursting strength is an absolute force that is required to disrupt the wound.)
8. You have performed an abdominal wall reconstruction and placed the patient in a binder 24/7. You want the strength of the wound to be at least 30% of the normal strength before discontinuing the binder. What will that time interval be? (The curve flattens at about 80% of normal, so 30% tensile strength is about one month, 80% at three months.)
   (a) What is the biochemical explanation for the increase in wound tensile strength with time? (Progressive cross-linkage of the collagen)
9. A young calf drifts away from the herd; discovers a clump of sweet peas, which he eats daily; and suddenly dies. The autopsy reveals a ruptured aorta. What is the explanation? (Lathyrism, named after the Latin word for the plant sweet pea: the naturally occurring presence of beta-aminopropionitrile (BAPN) with the loss of the ability to cross-link collagen)
   (a) What are the other agents? (Penicillamine chelates copper in enzymatic agents and blocks the assembly of helical collagen into fibrils; colchicine acts intracellularly to prevent cleavage of hydroxy moiety to produce collagen.)
10. While discussing the adverse effects of some agents or modalities on the healing process, briefly discuss the following local effects:
    (a) Smoking (Smoking can induce an adverse effect on healing through a number of factors, but probably the most important is the vasoconstriction and thus hypoxia from a decreased arterial PO_2. An effect at the cellular level also occurs including increased blood viscosity, increased platelet aggregation, and diminished collagen deposition.)
    (b) Infection (Infection prolongs the inflammatory phase of healing, so collagen deposition is diminished because of increased collagenolytic activity, as discussed below.)
    (c) Edema (As dramatically demonstrated by the ability of the VAC to decrease local tissue edema, edema has a deleterious effect on wound healing. Edema increases tissue pressure that results in critical capillary closing pressures, relative ischemia, and the adverse effects of cellular hypoxia.)
11. Discuss the adverse effects of the following systemic factors:
    (a) Diabetes (Although in the past the microvascular occlusive disease has been regarded as the villain and ischemia from peripheral vascular disease certainly has a profound negative effect on wound healing, the adverse effects of diabetes are mediated via elevated glucose levels. Those adverse effects include glycosylation of the key enzymes and collagen that affect the proliferative phase by decreased granulation tissue formation and the maturation phase by defects in the collagen. Hyperglycemia will delay the migration of inflammatory cells and fibroblasts and deposition of matrix components and decrease ascorbic-acid transport. All of these elements lead to impaired wound healing in the presence of hyperglycemia.)
    (b) Steroids: How to counteract the effect. (Steroids impair all stages of wound healing including wound contracture. The decrease in inflammatory infiltrate includes a decrease in growth factor profile. Some evidence show that megadoses of vitamin A 25,000 IU by mouth daily for three days may reverse some deleterious effects of steroids but not the increased susceptibility to infection.)
    (c) Age (Not clear, perhaps less growth factors present. Also, the increased incidence of comorbidities with advancing age play a role.)
    (d) Mild-to-moderate anemia (None)
12. In terms of content, how do fetal wounds differ from postnatal wounds? (Substantially higher content of hyaluronic acid and type III collagen)
    (a) What appears to be the benefit? (Minimal or no scar and the absence of the inflammatory stage of healing)

Editor's Note: Nutrition as well as the effects of chemo- and radiotherapy are covered in Chap. 3.

Physiology of Chronic Wounds

Antibiotic-containing solutions are addressed in the Part VII. Skin substitutes are addressed in Chap. 11.

1. What is the significance of matrix metalloproteinases (MMPs)? (MMPs are inflammation- and infection-produced enzymes that are capable of lysis of matrix proteins including growth factors and cytokines, all important

elements of wound healing. The concentration of proteolytic enzymes in chronic wounds produces further tissue damage and diminishes crucial growth factors essential for wound healing.)

2. Define what occurs in a "stalled" or chronic wound. (Colonization with bacteria, overproduction of matrix metalloproteinases (MMP), wound debris, decreased wound oxygen, and fibrosis)
3. What is one example or evidence that an element of chronic wounds is an imbalance of synthesis/degradation of extracellular matrix? (Elevated levels of proteases or enzymatic proteolytic activity such as the production of matrix metalloproteinases and diminished levels of their inhibitors)
4. The readings reference the necessity for bacterial colonization of less than a certain number. What is the number? (Depending on the reading, 10^5 or 10^6)
   (a) The readings describe the deleterious effects of wound proteases. What proteases in particular does this refer to? (Matrix metalloproteinases are increased in chronic wounds.)
5. What is a biofilm and what is its importance? (A biofilm is the presence in a chronic colonized wound of an almost parasitic relationship of the bacteria to the host. Biofilm is a complex network of bacteria within a protective film that provides an extracellular response mechanism and a physical barrier to antibiotics and a host response. In addition, the normal healing process is inhibited.)
6. Tie the answers to the above questions into a concept of the physiology of the chronic wound. (One perspective of the chronic wound is a "steady-state" alteration of the normal synthesis/degradation ratio of the matrix elements necessary for wound healing. Degradation or lysis is the result of elevated proteases or enzymatic proteolytic activity. An additional component of the chronic wound is the development of a biofilm.)
7. What is the essential philosophy of the readings underlying treatment; and what is the mainstay of the debridement approach to wounds? (Adequate and aggressive debridement to convert the fibrotic wound to an acute one; the aggressive removal of infected, nonviable tissue removes the established proteases and decreases bacterial colonization.)
   (a) What is the specific characteristic of debridement intended to eradicate a biofilm? (The evidence is that biofilm lodges within the deeper wound tissue rather than adhering to the surface. So debridement, by definition, must be aggressive.)
8. Comment on the following: pulse lavage, lavage with antibiotic-containing solutions, and dressings with Dakin's solution. (Pulse lavage is of value in the acute wound to rid the wound of bacteria and debris. The value is substantially less in a chronic wound unless surface debris exists that can be removed with pulse lavage. The Versajet® can also be substituted for pulse lavage and has a debridement component as well, established by a vacuum around the high-pressure water stream. Adding antibiotics to lavage solutions is of no value. Dakin's solution, although bactericidal, is cytotoxic to living tissue. Hypochlorous solutions and povidone iodine can be diluted to the point of little or no cytotoxicity to the host tissue but are also of little bactericidal efficacy.)

Dressings

1. What is the one simple criterion of wound characteristics that separate wound dressing into two groups? (Magnitude of the wound exudates. Highly exudative wounds dictate a more absorptive dressing as calcium alginate. Less-exudative wounds dictate the use of dressing that maintains a moist environment as hydrogels. The use of the wound VAC has nullified many of these precepts.)
2. A dressing applied to a granulating wound should have what characteristics? (The contemporary emphasis on wound dressings is to the use of those that maintain moisture and temperature as well as serve as a bacterial barrier. These dressings tend to be more occlusive in nature and are changed less frequently than the traditional wet-to-wet gauze dressings, which are changed three to four times a day. These dressings include hydrogels and hydrocolloids. In addition, an absorptive component is beneficial.)
3. A commonly used agent in exudative wounds is alginate dressing. What are alginate dressings? (Alginates are derived from seaweed and are highly absorbent and biodegradable. Once placed into the wound, they form a gel, which can maintain a moist wound-healing environment. Alginates are often combined with the use of a silver-impregnated dressing.)
4. Comment on and give an example of a wound topical antiseptic. (Wound antiseptics such as a sustained silver dressing, Acticoat®, have a slow release of nanoparticles of silver in sufficient tissue concentrations to achieve antisepsis. More traditional antibiotic-based wound preparations are silver sulfadiazine and mafenide acetate, applicable to burns and acute wounds rather than chronic wounds.)
5. Discuss the use of tissue dye and surgical debridement. (Instillation of methylene blue topically into the wound aids in complete excision and facilitates identification of tunneling and sinus tracts.)
6. Give an example of an enzymatic debriding agent. (Collagenase is probably one of the more commonly used enzymatic debriding agents under the brand name Santyl and is used as a once- or twice-a-day dressing.)

   (a) What is Accuzyme®, and what agent is contraindicated in simultaneous use with Accuzyme®? (Accuzyme® is the brand name of an agent composed of papain and urea. Accuzyme® is inactivated in the presence of a silver-containing dressing such as Acticoat.)
7. Regranex®, recombinant platelet–derived growth factor (PDGF), is the only approved growth factor for use in wounds. What are the necessary prerequisites that need to be present? (Clean, granulating wound without a covering coagulum)
   (a) What etiology of wound does Regranex® seem to benefit? (Diabetic foot)

Ancillary Measures in Wound Healing: Hyperbaric Oxygen (HBO)

1. What is the argument for the use of HBO in wounds? (It improves oxygenation by improving the partial pressure of oxygen in serum.)
2. Does the use of hyperbaric oxygen, HBO, primarily increase the hemoglobin oxygen (Hgb–O_2) saturation or the serum PO_2? (Since Hgb–O_2 saturation is typically greater than 90%, the primary mechanism of HBO is to increase the partial pressure of O_2 dissolved in the serum.)
3. Tissue hypoxia is defined as tissue O_2 pressures less than 30 mm Hg. Even in the circumstances of normal systemic O_2 pressures, 100 mm Hg, why might a wound be hypoxic? (Anything that impairs adequate circulation like vasoconstriction, hypothermia, or ischemia may result in local tissue hypoxia. Also, chronic fibrotic wounds, by definition, are hypoxic, particularly in the interior of the wound.)
4. What wound conditions could potentially benefit from the use of HBO? (Necrotizing fasciitis, deep diabetic foot ulcers, gangrene, and radiated wounds. All are relative indications and do not replace aggressive debridement when warranted.)
5. What are the principal complications of HBO? (Otitic barotrauma or perforated ear drums and seizures)

> **Editor's Note:** With the exception of diabetic foot ulcers, the use and purported efficacy of HBO in the treatment of chronic wounds are controversial. Substantial logistical issues deter meaningful clinical trials.

Negative Pressure Wound Therapy (NPWT)

1. What is the relationship between negative pressure wound therapy (NPWT) and blood flow? (Blood flow diminishes at the immediate edge of the wound, but at a distance from the edge, blood flow increases under the influence of the negative pressure. With vacuum release, the blood flow is also increased at the wound edge, which would suggest that intermittent pressure may further increase the flow. Microdeformation may be responsible for the enhanced angiogenesis and granulation tissue formation.)
2. Outline the principal benefits of the application of VAC to a wound. (Decrease in edema, chronic drainage removed continuously, provision of a moist environment for wound healing, drawing the viable soft tissues closer together or macrodeformation, and enhancement of blood flow)
   (a) Link these benefits to the proposed efficacy of Prevena™ or the use of NPWT on a closed surgical incision. (The two significant factors are probably macrodeformation and enhanced blood flow.)
3. How much of a difference in efficacy in NPWT can be attributed to the type of wound filler? (Little. The negative pressure transmitted to the wound and the enhanced blood flow are the same. Wound contracture in larger wounds may be enhanced with polyurethane foam.)
4. The demonstrable primary benefit of NPWT is because of, among other factors, the reduction of the quantitative bacterial load. True or false? (Essentially, false. The benefit is derived from edema reduction, increased perfusion, enhanced granulation tissue formation, and wound contracture, and bacterial load may be secondarily decreased because of the effects.)
5. If the overall efficacy is the same for foam vs. gauze as a wound filler, what patient comfort factors should be considered in the choice of filler? (Since tissue ingrowth into the wound filler is considerably more in foam than gauze, pain and bleeding are increased with dressing changes with the former. If the treatment plan is VAC changes under general anesthesia, that factor becomes irrelevant but otherwise important.)
6. What other factors should be considered in the choice of wound filler? (Because of the stimulus provided by foam, more tissue ingrowth and more rapid granulation tissue formation occurs, and wound contracture is more rapid than gauze-based wound fillers. More complex-shaped and irregular wounds require considerable pre-shaping and time, and some ingenuity with the use of foam as wound filler and gauze may be more suitable.)
7. What are the factors in choosing the level of negative pressure? (Pain: The higher the negative pressure, for example, a choice between the settings of −75 mm Hg and −125 mm Hg, the greater the pain experienced by the patient. Volume of wound drainage: Highly exudative wounds may require more negative pressure, perhaps higher than −125 mm Hg. Wound ischemia: Although blood flow is increased overall with negative wound pressure therapy, blood flow in the immediate

vicinity of the wound is decreased, so high negative pressure, certainly greater than −125 mm Hg, should be avoided.)

8. What are the pressure limits, high or low, where efficacy is lost or minimal? (−40 mm Hg or less and higher than −200 mm Hg)
9. Discuss the variation of instillation and dwell. (The modification of traditional constant negative wound pressure therapy has been one of periodic instillation of a variety of solutions, which are then either immediately suctioned free or allowed to dwell for a variable period of time. Ongoing work is investigating the variables of solution, dwell time, and types of included dressings.)
10. What is the sine qua non before implementation of the wound VAC for chronic wounds? (Adequate debridement)
11. What are the contraindications to NPWT? (The presence of osteomyelitis, necrotic tissue, exposed vascular anastomosis, and wound malignancy)

In-Service Examination

1. The initial event in the first stage of wound healing is:
   (a) Cellular infiltrate of PMNS
   (b) Vasodilation
   (c) Vasoconstriction
   (d) Appearance of proteolytic enzymes
2. The principal component of ground substance is:
   (a) Fibronectin
   (b) Metalloproteinases
   (c) Chondroitin sulfate
   (d) Tetra hydroxy acid
3. The conversion of proline to hydroxyproline requires the following **EXCEPT:**
   (a) Alpha ketoglutarate
   (b) Collagenase
   (c) Iron
   (d) Oxygen

Role of Nutrition and Cancer Therapy in Wound Healing, Specific Wound Healing Problems, Dietary Supplements and Vitamins, and Principles of Radiotherapy

3

Bibliography

Janis J, Harrison B, "Wound Healing: Part II. Clinical Applications", *Plast. Reconstr. Surg.*, (2014); 133(3):**383e-86e, 388e-89e and Videos 1 and 2.**

Arnold M., Barbul A., "Nutrition and Wound Healing", *Plast Reconstr Surg.*, (2006);117 (Supplement):**42S-45S (To "Amino Acids") ONLY.**

Kavalukas SL., Barbul A., "Nutrition and Wound healing: An Update", Plast Reconstr Surg., (2011);127 (Supplement):**38S-39S 40-42S (Skip Amino Acids).**

Xue A.S., Dayan E., Rohrich R.J., "Dietary Supplements and Current Available Evidence", *Plast Reconstr Surg.*, (2020);146(4):**474e-481e.**

Borrelli M.R., Shen A.H., Lee G.K., et al., "Radiation-Induced Skin Fibrosis: Pathogenesis, Current Treatment Options, and Emerging Therapeutics", *Annals of Plastic Surgery*, (2019);83(4S):**1-7.**

Kotha VS., Rewari A., Lakhiani C., et al., "Radiation Oncology Applications in Plastic and Reconstructive Surgery: A Nonsystematic Review of Concepts and Principles", *PlastReconstrSurg.*, (2021);147(2):**314e-320e ONLY.**

Drake DB., Oishi SN., Wound Healing Considerations In Chemotherapy And Radiation Therapy", *Clinics in Plastic Surgery*, (1995);22:**31-37.**

Jacobson, L.K., Johnson M.B., Dedhia R.D., al. "Impaired wound healing after radiation therapy: A systematic review of pathogenesis and treatment", *Jpras Open*, (2017);13:**92, 93-99 ONLY.**

Faculty Discussion and Study Guide

Nutrition and Wound Healing

1. What is the effect of malnutrition on the wound-healing process? (Malnutrition is a general term applied to insufficient calories of the three elements of intermediate metabolism, carbohydrates, proteins, and fats, but, most commonly, an overall total calorie–protein deficiency. The impact of malnutrition is upon all three phases of wound healing including collagen synthesis. The detrimental effect on phagocytic activity as well as complement and antibody levels renders the wound prone to infection.)
2. Does the postoperative period ameliorate or enhance the adverse effects on wound healing? (Enhances. The postoperative period results in a state of catabolism, the severity of which is dependent on several factors including the extent and magnitude of the operation and duration of postoperative fasting, among others.)
3. Give a hierarchy of laboratory values of assessment of nutrition in the order of increasing sensitivity and short-term changes. (Albumin, prealbumin, and serum retinol–binding protein. Albumin has a half-life of about 18 days, prealbumin, 3–5 days, and serum retinol–binding protein, 3 or 4 days. Albumin and prealbumin are the most common lab values obtained.)
   (a) Categorize the severity of malnutrition based on clinical exam. (A 10%-weight loss risk of malnutrition is considered moderate. A 20%-weight loss is considered severe. Other findings such as cachexia or muscle wasting are also important.)
4. What is the importance of adequate carbohydrates in the postoperative period? (Intrinsic gluconeogenesis in the presence of inadequate carbohydrate stores will be accomplished at the expense of protein catabolism. The expense of protein catabolism is accomplished by muscle breakdown, and unfortunately, protein catabolism is the preferential metabolic route in starvation rather than depletion of fat stores.)
5. Discuss the role of deficiencies of vitamins A and C in impaired wound healing. (Vitamin C is involved in the hydroxylation of proline and lysine in collagen synthesis and cross-linking; a deficiency will lead to scurvy. Vitamin A enhances collagen synthesis and deposition by fibroblasts and can offset some of the detrimental effects of steroids on wound healing.)

E. Luce, *A Curriculum for Plastic Surgery*, https://doi.org/10.1007/978-3-031-62087-4_3

(a) Give a historical perspective or notation of the occurrence of scurvy. (Scurvy was noted in British sailors who, during long maritime trips deficient in fresh fruits, had spontaneous disruption of old healed wounds, indicative of an imbalance in collagen synthesis and breakdown.)

(b) What are the implications of water versus fat-soluble vitamins? (Vitamins B and C are water-soluble. The remainder is fat-soluble, which has implications in the total dosage or duration of therapy since toxicity is a potential in the administration of fat-soluble vitamins but not water-soluble ones.)

6. If you had to supplement a malnourished patient with a single trace element, what would that element be and why? (Zinc. Zinc is a cofactor in DNA and protein synthesis and perhaps cellular proliferation as well. Iron deficiency can also result in impaired collagen synthesis but only in severe states. Patients on long-term steroids are particularly susceptible to zinc deficiency.)

Impediments to Wound Healing by Adjuvant Therapy

1. In general, does neutropenia secondary to intra- or immediate postoperative chemotherapy affect the inflammatory phase of wound healing? Explain. (The early inflammatory phase is characterized by increased vascular permeability, fibrin deposition, and influx of neutrophils and monocytes. Neutrophils predominate in the first 48 h. Neutropenia secondary to chemotherapy generally takes 7–14 days to develop, so the inflammatory phase has generally given way to the proliferative phase by this time. but chemotherapy can adversely affect healing if initiated preoperatively within this time window.)
2. How do chemotherapeutic agents adversely affect the proliferative phase of healing? (Most cytotoxic agents interfere with cell division, protein production, or DNA or RNA production. The proliferative phase of healing, which begins at 3–5 days post-wounding and persists for up to 2 weeks, is characterized by fibroblast proliferation, neovascularization, collagen deposition, and mucopolysaccharide production. Cytotoxic agents thwart this process by reducing fibroblast and myofibroblast cellular turnover, slowing healing, and decreasing wound strength.)
3. Does chemotherapy affect the third phase of wound healing? How? (The maturation phase begins at 2 or 3 weeks and lasts for several months, characterized by deposition and resorption of collagen into the direction of wound tension. Since cytotoxic agents can interfere with collagen metabolism, they can slow or impede this phase and diminish ultimate wound strength.)
4. What class are 5-fluorouracil (5-FU) and methotrexate members of? What are their effects on wound healing? (5-FU and methotrexate are antimetabolites, pyridime analogs that have been shown in clinical studies to increase wound healing complications.)
5. How do steroids affect wound healing? What drug can counteract prednisone's effects? (Steroids exert an anti-inflammatory effect that decreases fibroblast proliferation and neovascularization, reduces collagen formation, delays healing, and impacts all three phases of wound healing. High-dose vitamin A may counteract this effect.)
6. Discuss the timing for cessation of chemotherapy preoperatively and initiation of the same postoperatively. (Chemotherapy affects wound healing only if given during the first 10–14 days following wounding. Practically, the readings recommend delaying chemotherapy until 2–4 weeks postoperatively, until the early phases of wound healing are complete.)
   (a) When should the cessation of chemotherapy be performed preoperatively? (Four weeks: Recovery from chemotherapy protocols begins between 2 and 3 weeks, and a 4-week lag between chemotherapy injections is the standard since WBC counts usually reach acceptable levels at 4 weeks.)
7. How does chemotherapy affect tissue expansion when utilized in breast reconstruction? (Tissue expansion may be continued with ongoing communication with the oncologist. If the patient becomes severely leukopenic, less than 1000 WBC, the percutaneous injection may risk infection and therefore is not advisable.)
8. What are the two mechanisms of the effects of radiation therapy on tissues that result in injury to those same tissues? (DNA disruption and loss of cell replication and production of oxygen-free radicals)
   (a) What are the clinical implications? (Ongoing process of injury. To be effective, radiotherapy needs oxygen and tissues well-vascularized.)
9. What is the measure of radiotherapy dose? (cGy = rads or Gy = 100 rads.)
10. Compare the routes of delivery of radiation therapy and the determination of depth of skin penetration. (External versus brachytherapy; energy level as in the magnitude of voltage; for example, orthovoltage versus linear accelerator or super voltage)
11. What are isodose curves? What are portals? (Portals are the anatomically defined limits of the therapeutic dose of administered radiation. Radiation portals can be discerned on the patient by the presence of small indelible marks or tattoos. Isodose curves are calculations by radiation physics of the estimated radiation dose given at that particular point.)
    (a) Define penumbra. (Diminishing or fall of the dose at the edges of the radiation beam)

12. Define tumor control–tissue complication curves. (See Fig. 3.1)
    (a) Would curves that achieved LD_{50} of tumor cells at 40 cGy be favorable or unfavorable? What about at 72 cGy?
13. What is the information about prior radiotherapy that you would need to estimate the probability of late radiotherapy damage? (Total dose and dose per fraction)
14. What are the skin findings in chronic radiotherapy damage? (Fibrosis, telangiectasia, and pigment changes)
15. The discussion of specific clinical problems can be optimally done in a preoperative conference, but what are the general principles in the management of late post-radiotherapy complications? (Ruling out recurrent cancer with a biopsy, if necessary; resection of ulcer, fistula etc.; and provision of well-vascularized tissue in closure or reconstruction)
16. What is brachytherapy? What are its advantages? (Sealed radioactive sources, usually iridium-192 seeds, within catheters are placed into a tumor site percutaneously or at the time of surgical extirpation. Molds can also be used for sinonasal, vaginal, or other sites. The radioactivity drops steeply with increasing distance from the sources, minimizing radiation toxicity to surrounding normal tissues, thus increasing the tolerated doses.)
    (a) What is the contemporary method for administration of brachytherapy? (Usually, seeds are placed into an intracavitary space such as the breast or pelvis intraoperatively, and the radiation is "loaded" onto the seeds in a protected environment postoperatively.)
17. What is a standard fractionation regimen, for example, after mastectomy? What is hyperfractionation and how does it allow a greater total dose to be administered? (180–200 cGy per day to a total dose of 5000–7000 cGy, 5 weeks for the former and 7 weeks for the latter with weekends off. Hyperfractionation reduces the dose fraction but increases the number of fractions per day, or the days remain constant but the daily dosage is increased.)
18. What tissues are primarily affected by acute radiation injury? When does this occur? (Acute injury affects rapidly proliferating tissues, like skin and mucosa, but this resolves within one month of XRT, radiotherapy.)
    (a) Late radiation injuries. (Defined as those occurring after six months and primarily involve tissues with slow cellular turnover like endothelium, bone, and cartilage.)
19. What is the tolerance dose (TD) for skin, bone, and nerves? (TD for 100 cm^2 of skin is 7000 cGy; more XRT can be given if smaller areas are treated. For the mandible, TD is 6500 cGy if one-third or less of the mandible is treated and 6000 for a larger area. Peripheral nerves

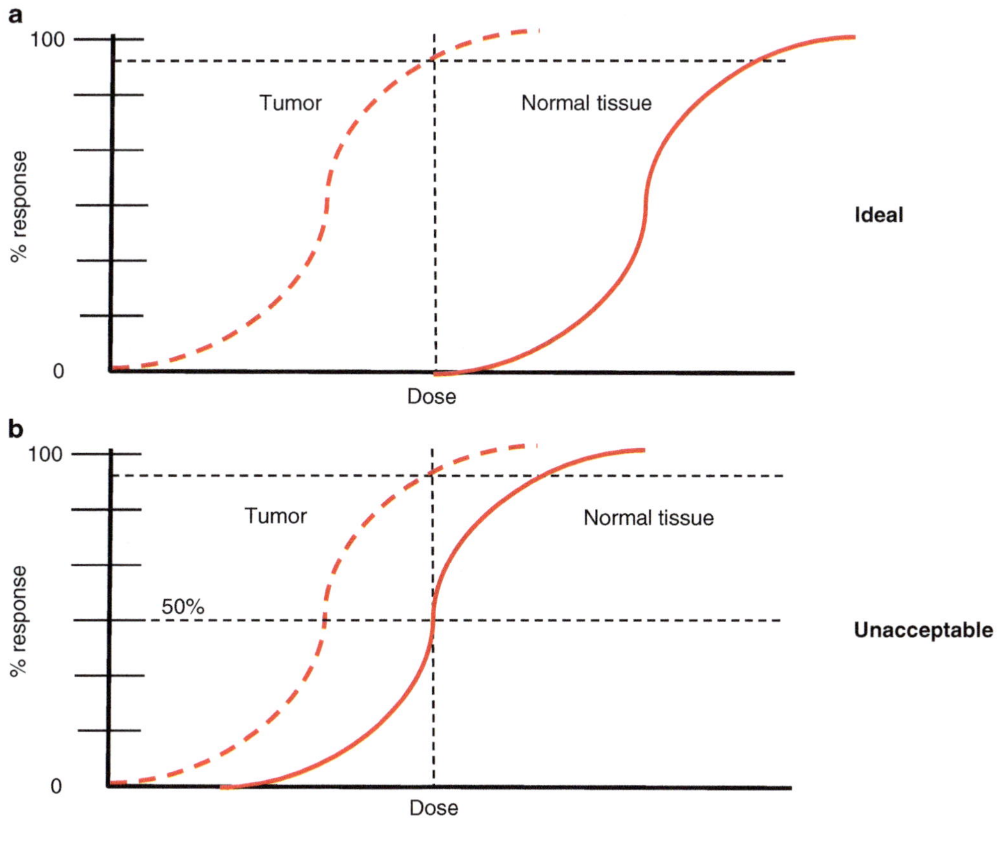

Fig. 3.1 Tumor control–tissue complication curves

tolerate high doses because they are not mitotically active and the cell bodies' nuclei are often outside the portals. Intensity-modulated radiotherapy has modified traditional radiotherapy by more accurate 3D treatment planning that increases the tumor dosage and decreases the dosage to the adjacent normal tissues.)

   (a) What are the minimum and maximum tolerable doses for skin necrosis? (Defined as 5 and 50% probability and is approximately 5500 for the former and 7000 for the latter for a 100 cm^2 portal)

20. Define chronic radiation injury pathologically. (The pertinent pathologic changes include cellular depletion, extracellular matrix, and hypoxia from microvascular damage. Cellular depletion is the result of the impairment of cellular proliferation including the fibroblast. The extracellular matrix is altered secondary to overexpression of matrix metalloproteinases. Progressive endothelial thickening leads to obliterative endarteritis.)
21. Discuss the role of hyperbaric oxygen (HBO) in chronic radiotherapy damage including the intensity and duration and the most likely diagnostic candidate. (Osteoradionecrosis of the mandible is the most likely candidate. HBO is given at 2½ atmospheres of pressure time and 30 "dives" for most radiotherapy chronic complications. Efficacy, outside of osteoradionecrosis, has not been established for chronic radiation damage.)

Dietary Supplements and Vitamins

1. The role of vitamins A, C, and D in perioperative care is discussed in the readings. Frame that discussion briefly. (All play an essential role in varying ways in wound healing and deficiencies may negatively impact postoperative wound healing and susceptibility to surgical-site infections. Yet, other than isolated reports, a paucity of studies have examined the overall benefit of supplementation. Vitamin A supplementation has the capacity to reverse the detrimental effects of steroids in wound healing. Severe sufficiency of vitamin C results in scurvy as a result of an imbalance between collagen synthesis, which is decreased, and collagen degradation. The site of action of vitamin C, ascorbic acid, is the facilitation of collagen cross-linkage.)
2. Comment on the role of vitamins B12 and E in surgical perioperative care. (Deficiency of vitamin B12 is distinctly uncommon and is signaled by the presence of anemia with a distinctive profile on CBC analysis. Vitamin E may have an adverse effect on platelet function and collagen synthesis. They should be discontinued 2 or 3 weeks preoperatively.)
3. Comment on the use and potential liabilities of arnica and bromelain. (Both are plant-derived. Arnica has been demonstrated to decrease edema and ecchymosis in aesthetic surgery, in particular rhytidectomy, blepharoplasty, and rhinoplasty, although the evidence is debatable. Bromelain has been advocated to decrease edema and inflammation, but again, similar to arnica, irrefutable proof is lacking.)
4. What are the concerns regarding the commonly used herbal supplements, echinacea, and St. John's wort? (With echinacea, the concerns are immunosuppression with chronic use and possible interactions with some medications. St John's wort alters the metabolism of a number of drugs utilized in the surgical armamentarium. Both should be discontinued 2 weeks preoperatively.)

Specific Wound Healing Problems

1. What is the specific pathology in venous stasis ulcers? (The ulcers occur because of the direct transmission of increased venous pressure, secondary to the obliteration of a portion of the deep venous system, to the subcutaneous tissues. The result is a decrease in perfusion and fibrosis and a further decrease in perfusion, ultimately resulting in ulceration.)
   (a) Treatment (Compression therapy, most commonly with bandages as the Unna boot. Surgery is reserved for recalcitrant situations and consists of excision and reconstruction.)
2. What are the specific issues with diabetic foot ulcers? (Diabetics are susceptible to the development of chronic ulceration of the plantar aspect of the foot. The pathogenesis is a combination of diabetic neuropathy and small-vessel vascular disease including microvascular occlusion. The abnormal pressure distribution and diminished sensation culminate in chronic ulceration that is recalcitrant to therapy. Prophylaxis is important for assiduous foot care. Treatment is wound care with periodic conservative debridement and dressing. The use of platelet-derived and transforming growth factors applied topically has had some success in healing.)

Case-Based Conference

Case 1: Difficult Wound

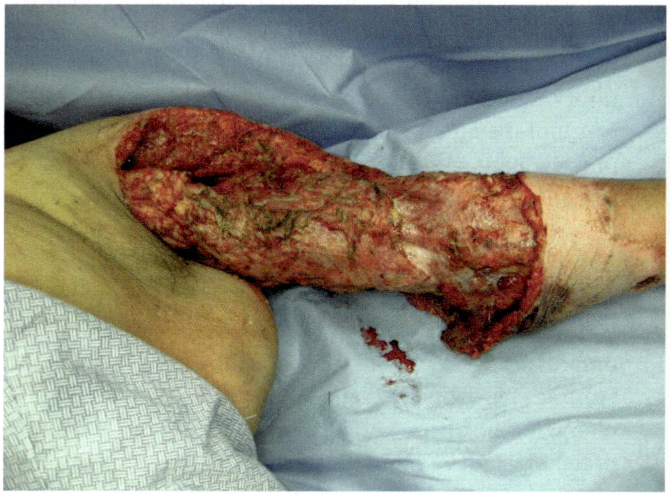
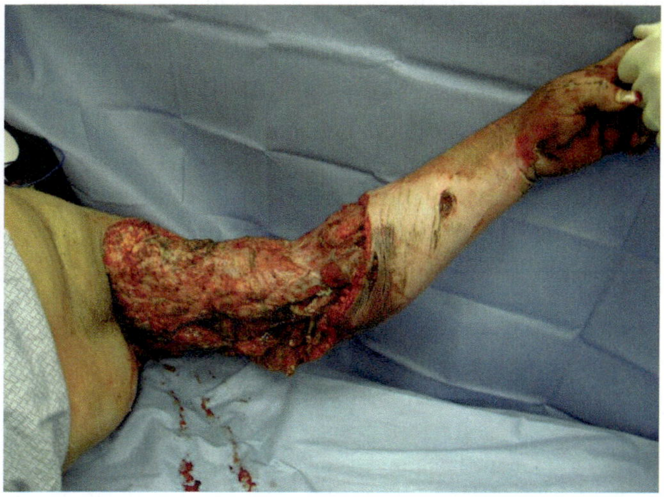

A 40-year-old injured 18 hours ago in a farming accident and required an emergency laparotomy. The patient is without fractures or dislocations. The patient was in prior excellent health. The thrust of this case is wound management.

1. Describe the findings in the slide(s). Outline a focused clinical exam.
2. Since the thrust of this case is wound management, what is the pathologic physiology of this wound, and how does that pathology impact your proposed treatment plan?
3. Outline a treatment plan. Give the milestones in that plan with the different decision points, if any, in the flow of the plan.
4. As the last step, describe definitive wound closure.

Case-Based Conference: Discussion

Case 1: Difficult Wound

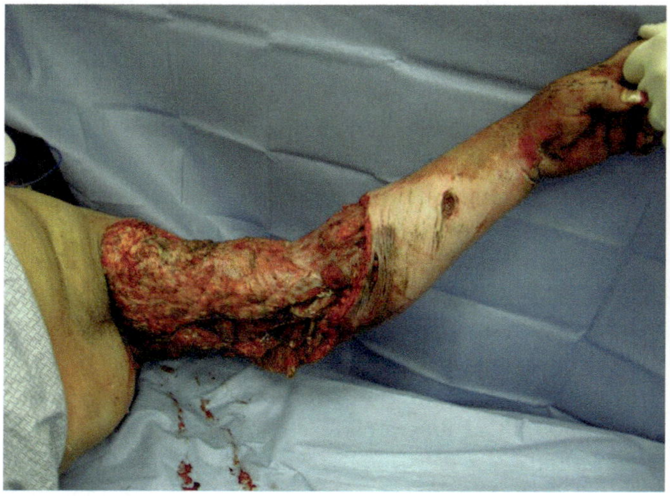
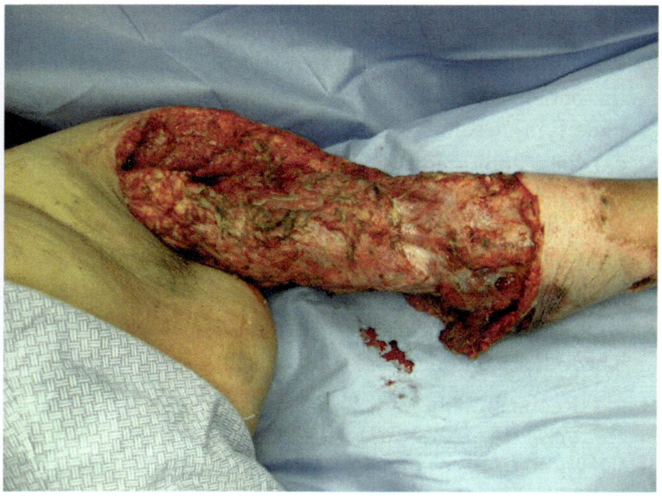

A 40-year-old injured 18 hours ago in a farming accident and required an emergency laparotomy. The patient is without fractures or dislocations. The patient is in prior excellent health. The thrust of this case is wound management and is directed toward a mid-level resident.

1. Describe the findings in the photos(s). Outline a focused clinical exam. (The first photo encompasses the entire upper extremity including the hand, shoulder, and adjacent chest wall. The area of concern is an extensive soft-tissue injury. All of the skin envelope is absent from the level of the axilla to several centimeters distal to the antecubital fossa. The level of injury appears to be subcutaneous fat although biceps fascia may be exposed distally. Dirt or foreign material is evident within the subcutaneous fat, particularly proximal and medial. On the posterior and lateral aspects of the arm, the soft tissue appears to droop with loose attachment to the medial arm. Distally, the proximal forearm skin is dark for several centimeters from radial to ulnar, and a single 1- or 2-cm skin-soft-tissue defect is present at the junction of the middle and distal one-third of the volar forearm. The palm is dirty but without evident soft-tissue injury. In summary, the volar photos demonstrate an extensive soft-tissue avulsive loss with a heavily contaminated wound. The photo also suggests a continuation of the avulsive mechanism of injury further distal and probable detachment and undermining of the volar forearm skin.

   The additional slide, restricted to the area of the axilla to the antecubital fossa, confirms the findings including an apparently intact deep brachial fascia. Again, dirt contamination and impregnation of the wound are visualized, as well as an intact fascia overlying the biceps. The loss of attachment of the distal flap the forearm skin can be visualized. However, the shoulder has been internally rotated and a disruption of muscle, possibly deltoid, is evident.

   The patient is probably immediate postoperative but some details of the accident should be ascertained from the patient and/or family. The preamble assures that no underlying fracture is present and the patient has no preexisting comorbidities. The pertinent physical exam would focus on the neurovascular status of the hand, given the potential for injury either in the axilla, arm, or volar forearm. Palpation of wrist pulses and examination for median-, ulnar-, and radial-nerve function in the hand would complete that aspect of the clinical examination. The other component would be an assessment of the degree of injury of the distal skin envelope. The slide of the volar aspect strongly suggests an undermining with devascularization and injury of a portion of the volar forearm skin.)
2. Since the thrust of this case is wound management, what is the pathologic physiology of this wound, and how does that pathology impact your proposed treatment plan? (The clinical scenario is one of an extensive, avulsive, heavily contaminated wound with circumferential skin and soft-tissue loss from axilla to elbow but probable involvement and injury of at least the volar forearm. An additional element is the delay between injury and definitive management, eighteen hours, as a result of the emergency laparotomy. Optimal interdisciplinary management would have entailed intraoperative consultation of plastic surgery at the time of the laparotomy. The delay has permitted early bacterial colonization of a heavily contaminated wound. Since the environment of injury was a farming accident, the soil contamination also raises the specter of gram-negative organisms.)
3. Outline a treatment plan. Give the milestones in that plan with the different decision points, if any, in the flow of the plan. (Assuming the neurovascular status is intact, the initial treatment step is operative debridement. Hopefully, timewise, the consult was initiated such that the same general anesthetic as the laparotomy would provide the opportunity for wound toilet. If not, then as soon as the patient appears stable postoperatively, perhaps 24 h or less, the patient would return to the operating room. Aggressive sharp debridement of grossly contaminated subcutaneous fat and excision of devitalized skin should be accomplished. Digital exploration to determine the extent of undermining, probably combined with a vertical volar forearm incision to access and expose the wound and facilitate debridement. Once accomplished, a bulky dressing is applied, combined with a splint of the hand in a functional position. The patient should be returned to the operating room for reexploration and re-debridement 24–48 h later. At that juncture, assuming the absence of evidence of wound sepsis, the application of negative pressure wound therapy will assist in the achievement of a wound suitable for closure. Early definitive wound closure is imperative in the upper extremity. To do so permits aggressive physical therapy and rehabilitation. Certainly, an intermediate step at this junction could consist of the application of allograft. Given the magnitude of autograft required, an allograft "take" would indicate that wound colonization, if any, is minimal and the bed is suitable for split-thickness skin graft.)
4. As the last step, describe definitive wound closure. (Definitive wound closure is achieved by split-thickness skin graft, either with or without an intermediate step of allograft. If an allograft is elected, the time interval should be brief, 3–5 days, prior to a definitive split-thickness skin graft. Use of negative pressure wound therapy after the application of autografts will enhance the likelihood of a successful take.)

Case-Based Conference

Case 2: Subacute Wound

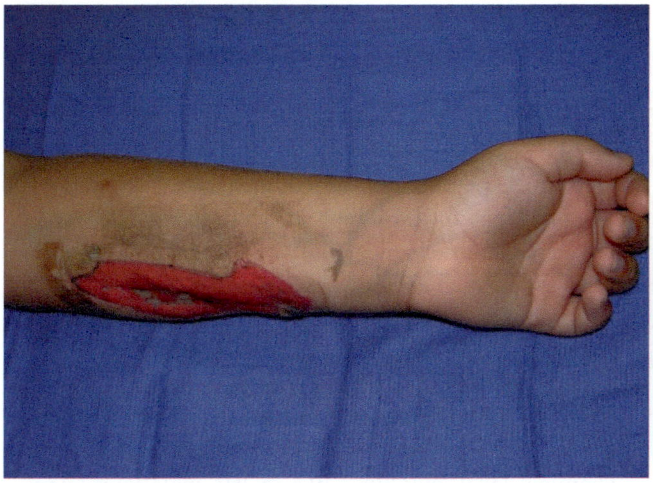

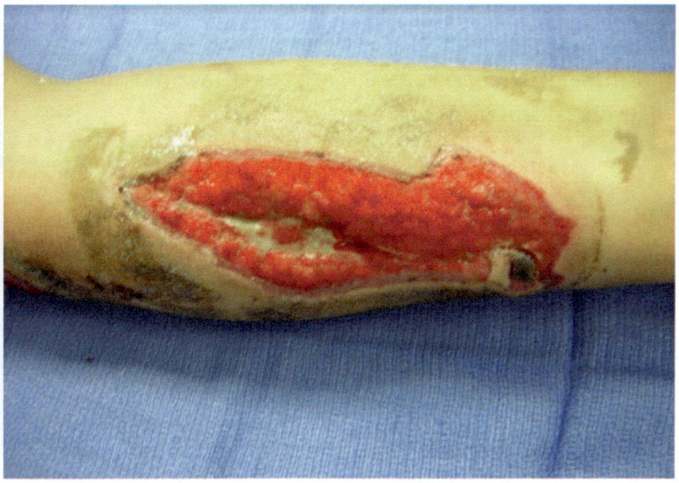

A 28-year-old male sustained an injury to his forearm in a boating accident 6 weeks ago. The wound has been managed by dressings performed by the patient. Hand function is intact.

> **Editorial Note**: The case is directed toward a mid-level resident.

1. Describe the slides and add a clinical examination.
   (a) Is any test indicated?
2. Outline the pathophysiology of the patient's wound.
3. Based on the response to question 2, what is the appropriate treatment plan?

Case-Based Conference: Discussion

Case 2: Subacute Wound

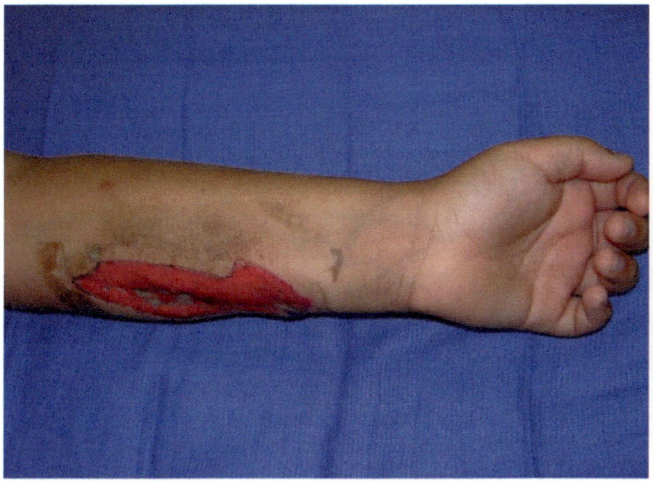

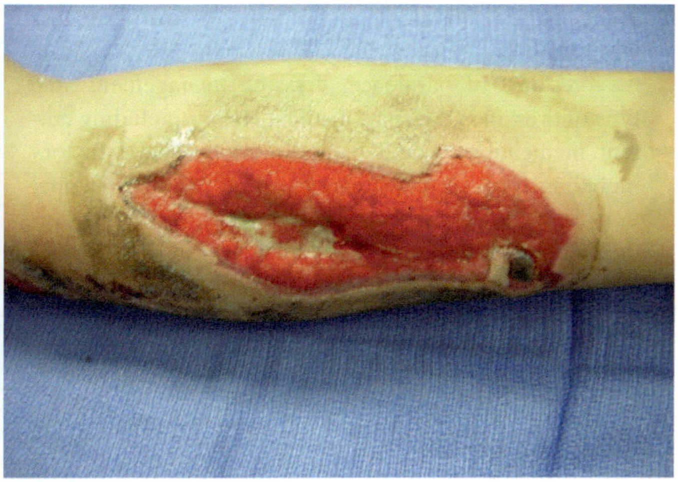

A 28-year-old male sustained an injury to his forearm in a boating accident 6 weeks ago. The wound has been managed by dressings performed by the patient. Hand function is intact.

Editorial Note: The case is directed toward a mid-level resident in Wound Care.

1. Describe the slides and add a clinical examination. (Two views are provided: the first, a hand and forearm in a supinated position demonstrating the volar–palmar aspect, and the second, a close-up of the central volar forearm only. In the first slide, the hand position and digital cascade appear normal. The predominant finding is a large open wound on the ulnar–volar aspect in the central one-half of the forearm. Dimensions appear to be approximately 15 cm in length and 5 cm in width. The surrounding intact skin is non-erythematous and appears normal except for tape marks. The visible wound is marked by the presence of red granulation tissue. The second slide is focused on the wound that confirms the presence of proliferative granulation tissue over most of the surface except for an area of 4 or 5 cm in length and approximately 2 cm in width centrally. That area, in the proximal one-third of the wound, is more depressed than the surrounding granulation tissue and, in contrast to the granulation, is gray–white in color. A thin rim, 1 or 2 mm in size, of pink tissue is present circumferentially on the wound borders.

   The hiatus would focus on a determination of the evolution of the wound and begin with the circumstances of the injury and initial management, progressing to the appearance on the first several days after injury. Crucial in the history is the element of initial skin-soft-tissue loss with the injury. History questions would also ascertain the presence of purulence, dressing management, and type of dressings. The past medical history including current medications would be followed by social history including tobacco or recreational drug use and occupation. Since hand function has been determined to be normal and wound appearance is depicted by the slides, little additional information will be elicited from the physical examination. The initial dressings should be inspected for the amount and character of the drainage.)

   (a) Is any test indicated? (Lacking any evidence of a deep-seated infection that would dictate imaging, the principal test indicated would be a quantitative wound culture. Although prior surface or qualitative wound cultures may have been performed, a determination of the degree of bacterial colonization as measured by the number of colonies per cc of tissue will assist in subsequent wound management. Although the appearance of the wound dictates the treatment plan outlined below, quantitative bacteriology will index the degree of colonization.)

2. Outline the pathophysiology of the patient's wound. (The essential pathology is a subacute-to-chronic wound. Given the duration since injury of 4 weeks, some chronicity is established that consists of fibrosis, diminished vascular supply, and an increase in bacterial colonization. Although the gross appearance of the granulation tissue appears healthy, that appearance may be deceptive and, from a microscopic and bacteriologic perspective, may not be suitable for wound closure. In addition, on a biochemical level, cytokines like matrix metalloproteinases detrimental to normal wound healing are secreted and accumulate. The wound also has an area that may represent residual necrotic tissue. In summary, the pathology is a sizable soft-tissue defect that is on the threshold of a chronically inflamed and problematic wound. At some juncture, the wound is further characterized by the development of a biofilm, an environment hostile to physiologic healing.)
3. Based on the response to question 2, what is the appropriate treatment plan? (Several therapeutic options exist, but the underlying assumption is that wound closure with a split-thickness skin graft will be necessary, an assumption further propelled if, in all likelihood, the patient's livelihood is adversely impacted by the necessities of prolonged wound care. The most expeditious management would consist of operative debridement including attention directed toward the area in the center of the wound as described above that may represent necrotic fascia as well as sharp and abrasive debridement of granulation tissue. Although probably protected by the flexor carpi ulnaris (FCU) muscle belly, care should be taken to not injure the ulnar nerve and artery. Once assured of adequate debridement, the wound is placed into negative pressure wound therapy for several days. A return to the OR would be planned for definitive closure with a skin graft and placed again into negative pressure wound therapy. As discussed above, the results of quantitative culture may not alter treatment substantially unless a particular recalcitrant organism is detected.)

Case-Based Conference

Case 3: Elbow Ulcer

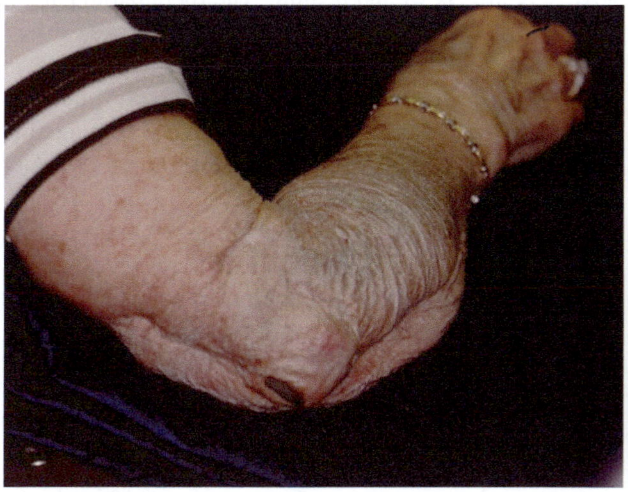

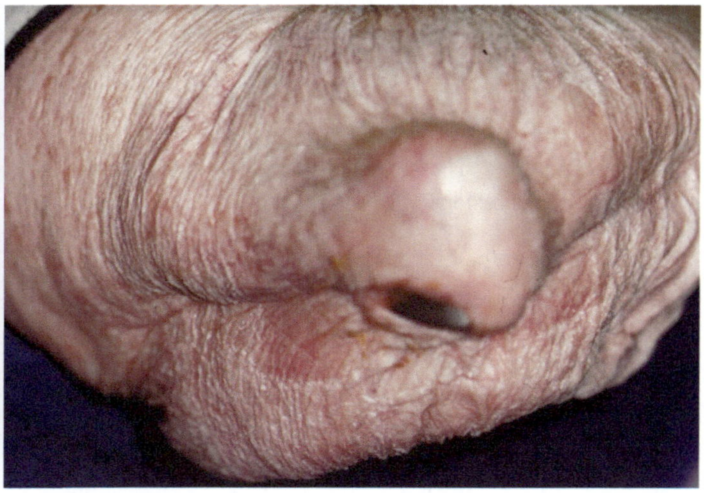

A 70-year-old woman, a rheumatoid arthritis patient on long-term steroids, had total elbow joint replacement 6 months ago, with the onset of drainage a month ago, followed by a one-week history of extrusion of the prosthesis. The orthopedist plans the removal and replacement of the joint prosthesis and desires your input and assistance.

> **Editorial Note:** The case is directed toward an advanced-level resident.

1. Describe the slides and add a clinical examination.
   (a) Is any test indicated? Justify.
2. What is the pathophysiology of the patient's clinical picture?
3. What is your treatment plan? Develop different scenarios dependent on the orthopedist's plan.

Case-Based Conference: Discussion

Case 3: Elbow Ulcer

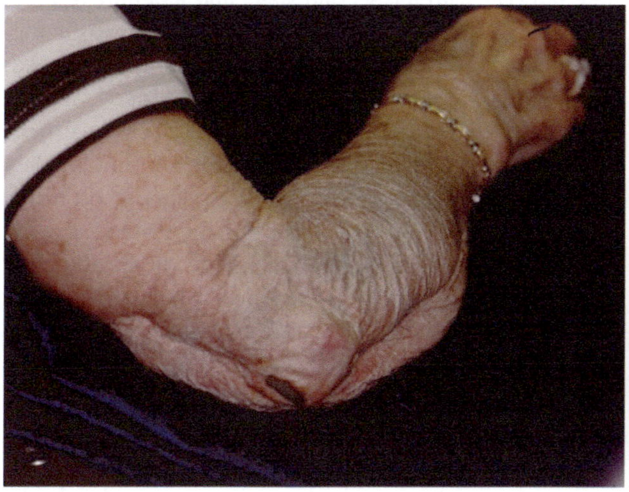

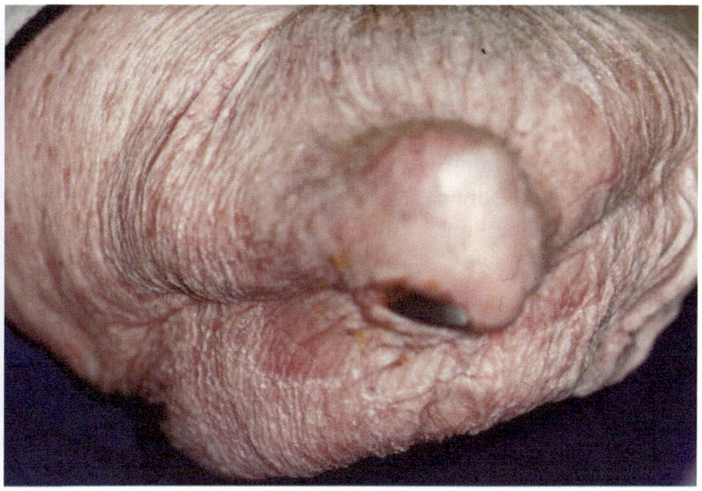

A 70-year-old woman, a rheumatoid arthritis patient on long-term steroids, had total elbow joint replacement 6 months ago, with the onset of drainage a month ago, followed by a one-week history of extrusion of the prosthesis. The orthopedist plans the removal and replacement of the joint prosthesis and desires your input and assistance.

Editorial Note: The case is directed toward an advanced-level resident.

1. Describe the slides and add a clinical examination. (Two views are provided. The first depicts the entire upper extremity of an elderly woman from the dorsal aspect, the elbow in the foreground, and the hand in the distance. The elbow is positioned at 90°. Visible at the point of the elbow in the vicinity of the olecranon, protruding from the skin, is a smooth, dark-colored object, consistent with an exposed joint prosthesis. Superior and inferior to that point is a longitudinal straight-line infolding of skin and soft tissue. The surrounding skin does not appear inflamed or swollen. The second slide is a close-up and does not provide additional information except that the longitudinal skin- and soft-tissue-infolding appears to be a well-healed surgical scar. The extruded prosthesis is again visualized, as well as some immediately adjacent, well-circumscribed 2-cm swelling.

   The history component of the clinical exam would focus on the duration of the rheumatoid arthritis, other joint involvement, and steroid dosage and duration, as well as the determination by history of upper extremity function before and after the total elbow replacement. A general assessment by history of overall functional status should be accomplished. The patient and/or medical record should be queried about other agents, particularly immune-modulating drugs. Because of the higher probability, the presence of comorbidities should be ascertained, if possible. Although not likely, systemic sepsis is ruled out by the absence of a history of fever and chills. The physical exam is primarily centered on the wound, the nature of the drainage, and current elbow function and range of motion. Some estimates by physical exam should determine the degree of frailty of the patient and the ability to undergo a reconstructive procedure.)

   (a) Is any test indicated? Justify. (If not already performed by the referring orthopedist, a CT scan would be of value to detect the presence of fluid collection or local osteomyelitis. A concomitant CT angiogram, if of sufficient resolution, could define the local vasculature.)
2. What is the pathophysiology of the patient's clinical picture? (Several factors are active in this clinical picture. First, the underlying disease process, rheumatoid arthritis, is a chronic inflammatory state of the joint synovium that may also be attended by an associated vasculitis that adversely affects wound healing. The rheumatoid patient may also be in a chronically malnourished state. More specifically, the sequence of events that culminated in joint prosthesis exposure may have begun with an incident of minor trauma, followed by bacterial colonization of the wound cavity. The history of one month of drainage suggests an established infection. The joint prosthesis, although biologically inert if colonized, can result in the formation of a biofilm. Biofilm, as the name suggests, is a film composed of noncellular elements that coat, in this instance, the surface of the prosthesis and afford protection for the polymicrobial aggregate that represents chronic infection. The biofilm permits ongoing colonization and infection by a number of mechanisms including a blunting of the local-host response, release of inflammatory cytokines, and a resistance or barrier to antibiotic penetration. If the patient has undergone multiple operative procedures (e.g., arthroplasties, curettage, and debridement), prior to total joint replacement, the overall wound bed would be scarred and fibrotic.)
3. What is your treatment plan? Develop different scenarios dependent on the orthopedist's plan. (First would be a conversation with the orthopedist to ascertain the details of the planned procedure. Of the orthopedic management of this patient's presentation are four options although, in reality, only two and possibly one is appropriate. The options are resection debridement of the infected cavity with the removal of the prosthesis, namely an arthroplasty; excisional debridement and arthrodesis; single-stage resection and replacement of the prosthesis; and a two-stage excisional debridement of the involved cavity and placement of an antibiotic spacer, followed by a variable interval with the second stage and a definitive prosthesis placement. The first two result in unsatisfactory outcomes, the first because of lack of stability and load-bearing and the second because of limitation of range of motion. Although a single-stage approach has been adopted in some instances of infected total joint replacement, several factors including an immunocompromised patient, the hiatus between onset and definitive treatment, and the probable polymicrobial nature of the infection would dictate a two-stage treatment plan. Assuming a two-stage approach is selected by the referring orthopedist; the involvement of the plastic surgeon will be driven by the anticipation of a soft-tissue deficiency. The configuration of the antibiotic spacer is either a ball or packet, placed in the area of the previous elbow-joint space. Depending on the magnitude of the excisional debridement, a skin-soft-tissue deficiency may be the outcome but not likely in this patient.

The hiatus or interval between the two stages is driven by the orthopedist, but a common duration is six weeks. Some evidence show that some of the deleterious effects of the steroids and wound healing can be, in part, ameliorated by preoperative administration of vitamin A. In the same vein, nutritional deficiency, particularly if documented objectively by diminished albumin and prealbumin levels, should be addressed in this interval between the first and second stages. However, in the second stage, with the removal of the antibiotic spacer and prosthesis insertion, the probability of uneventful healing could be enhanced by rotation and coverage of the prosthesis with well-vascularized tissue. The reconstructive ladder would dictate the selection of a local flap, in this instance, a forearm muscle. The immediately adjacent flexor carpi ulnaris is a candidate if the radial wrist flexors are intact. The vascular supply of the FCU is the posterior ulnar recurrent artery, a branch located proximally, which permits an excellent arch of rotation for the muscle. Minor branches of the ulnar artery more distal can be safely ligated. If necessary, a split-thickness skin graft can be applied to the rotated muscle, but primary closure of the native skin would be preferable.)

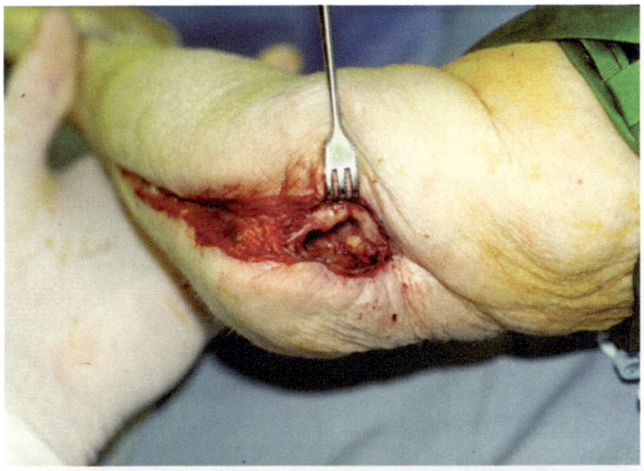

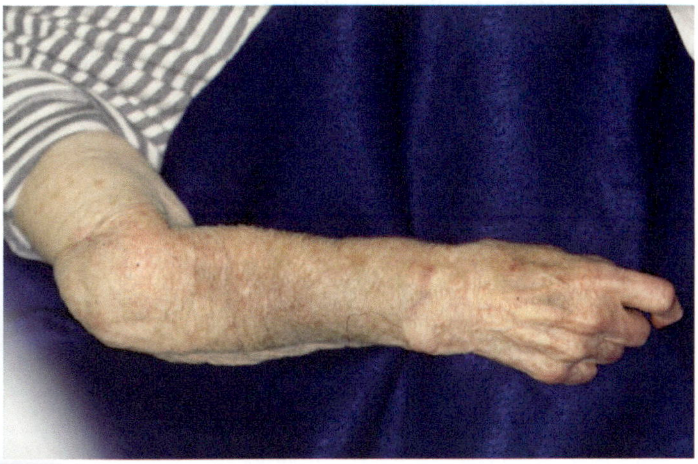

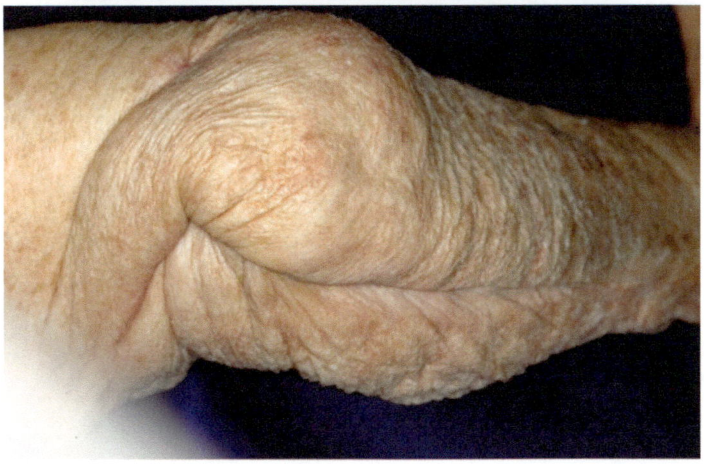

Postoperative (6 Months)

Three photos are provided: an apparent intraoperative and two postoperative photos. The intraoperative photo depicts a longitudinal surgical incision and wound on the ulnar aspect on the forearm, the proximal extent at the elbow. Exposed at the elbow is the thickened empty prosthesis capsule. There are two postoperative photos, the first of the upper extremity in a semi-extended position and the second, a close-up of the intact healed wound.

Critique

Photos of the elbow range of motion would be helpful in the assessment of the result, but the two-stage approach has achieved a healed wound and, presumably, a satisfactory functional result.

In-Service Examination

1. The role of vitamin C in wound healing is:
   (a) Hydroxylation of proline and lysine
   (b) Enhanced deposition of fibroblasts
   (c) To serve as a cofactor in the synthesis of ground substance
   (d) To increase the permeability of platelets to release cytokines
2. Steroids can adversely affect wound healing by all of the following **EXCEPT:**
   (a) Reduction of fibroblast proliferation
   (b) Creation of leukopenia
   (c) Reduction of collagen production
   (d) Decrease in neovascularization
3. The term penumbra, when applied to radiotherapy, is:
   (a) The calculated maximal dose at the center of the radiation beam
   (b) The LD_{50} of tumor cells
   (c) The LD_{50} of normal tissue
   (d) The diminished dose at the edge of the radiation beam or portal

Hypertrophic Scars, Keloids, and Skin Grafts

4

Bibliography

Loder J., Levi B., Clark A., Ch. 17 "Skin Grafting", Neligan PC, Plastic Surgery, Elsevier 5th Edition, (2023), Volume 1: pg. **206-219.**

Broughton G, Janis JE, Attinger CE, "Wound healing: An overview", *Plast. Reconstr. Surg.*, (2006); 117(7S):**17-23eS ONLY**. (Overview)

Van de Kar, A. L., et al., "The Results of Surgical Excision and Adjuvant Irradiation for Therapy-Resistant Keloids: A Prospective Clinical Outcome Study", *Plast. Reconstr. Surg.,* (2007); 119(7):**2248-2254.** Erratum in: *PRS,* (2007); 120(2):**579.**

Ogawa R, "The Most Current Algorithms for the Treatment and Prevention of Hypertrophic Scars and Keloids", *Plast. Reconstr. Surg.*, (2010); 125(2):**557-566.**

Al-Attar, A., et al., "Keloid Pathogenesis and Treatment.", *Plast. Reconstr. Surg.*, (2006); 117(1):**286-296.**

Khansa I, Harrison B, and Janis JE, "Evidence-Based Scar Management: How to Improve Results with Technique and Technology.", *Plast. Reconstr. Surg., (*2016); 138:**168S-173S (Start with "Onion Extract" and stop at "Keloids").**

Shah VV, Aldahan AS, Mlacker S, et al., "5-Fluorouracil in the Treatment of Keloids and Hypertrophic Scars: A Comprehensive Review of the Literature", *Dermatol Ther.*, (2016); 6:**178-180.**

Perez JL, Rohrich RJ, "Optimizing Post Surgical Scars: A Systematic Review on Best Practices in Preventative Scar Management", *Plast. Reconstr. Surg.,* (2017); 140(6):**789-92**.

Faculty Discussion and Study Guide

Skin Grafts

1. Where does the component or major common unit of the blood supply to the skin exist? (Subdermal arterial plexus)
   (a) Where does the skin capillary bed exist? (Papillary dermis)
2. Differentiate between musculocutaneous and direct cutaneous perforators, a topic also covered in the flaps module. (Direct cutaneous perforators run parallel to the skin just superficial to the muscle fascia; musculocutaneous perforators are the classic angiosome units of an arterial supply "perforating" the musculocutaneous fascia and then running relatively perpendicular to the skin surface to supply the subdermal arterial plexus.)
3. Define the "blush" zone. (Considering the area above the clavicles, the skin once transplanted has more of a blush component rather than a yellowish tan appearance from truncal and extremity skin.)
   (a) What are the implications? (A full-thickness skin graft harvested from this area provides a better color match for facial skin defects.)
4. Define serum imbibition. What are its practical applications? (Imbibition is the phenomenon of passage of oxygen and nutrients from the interstitial fluid of the bed into the skin graft, which is capable of sustaining mostly anaerobic metabolism for 24–48 h. Practically speaking, that phenomenon implies firm adherence to the underlying bed such that a fluid collection such as seroma, which will be inert biochemically, does not occur.)

E. Luce, *A Curriculum for Plastic Surgery*, https://doi.org/10.1007/978-3-031-62087-4_4

5. Define inosculation. What are its practical applications? (Inosculation is the term applied to revascularization of the skin graft, either by capillary connections from the underlying recipient bed into the capillaries of the skin graft or perhaps by direct angiogenic ingrowth of capillaries into the graft. Regardless, any shearing force can rupture these new fragile capillaries. The implication is that a firm compressive dressing, such as a bolster, is necessary to prevent shearing and, of course, fluid collection.)
6. Differentiate primary and secondary skin graft contracture. (Primary contracture is the contraction of the graft that occurs once the graft is harvested. The thicker the dermis, the more elastin fibers are present, and the greater the degree of primary contracture, estimated to be about 20% in a full-thickness skin graft or a flap. Secondary contracture is the phenomenon once the graft has been transplanted into the recipient bed and the healing processes are underway. Secondary contracture is probably mediated by native fibroblast in the wound bed. A contracture process occurs over time, weeks or months, similar to wound healing. The observation has been that the thicker the dermis obtained with the graft, the less secondary contracture occurs. A variety of theories have been offered to explain that observation.)
7. You plan to skin-graft a fingertip injury. From the perspective of the innervation, would you opt for a full-thickness skin graft or split-thickness skin graft? (A full-thickness skin graft experimentally permits more sensory nerve ingrowth than a split-thickness skin graft, but practically speaking, the evidence indicates that no difference is present in fingertip-grafting closure by split-thickness or full-thickness skin graft.)
8. What is the principal cell of the epidermis that is responsible for the immune functions of the skin? (Langerhans cells)
9. Compare and contrast the following features in full- vs. split-thickness skin grafts: sweating, hair growth, and pigmentation. (The ability to sweat, lubricate, and regrow hair are all features dependent on the incorporation of the appendages of skin with the harvest of the graft. A full-thickness skin graft will harvest more dermis that will have a higher probability of incorporation of skin appendages and therefore sweat, lubricate, and regrow hair. Curiously, pigmentation occurs more frequently in thin grafts than thick, perhaps due to activation of the melanosomes.)
10. What are the phases of hair follicle growth? (Anagen or proliferative phase, catagen or regressing phase, and telogen or resting phase. These are discussed more fully in the Chap. 96.)
11. Sweat glands are divided into eccrine and apocrine glands. Where are apocrine glands located? (Exclusively in the axillae and the perianal, perivulvar, scrotal, areolar, and pubic areas. These areas also parallel to the principal locations of hidradenitis, a disease of obstruction of the perifollicular apocrine glands.)

Fibroproliferative Scars

1. Differentiate clinically keloids and hypertrophic scars (HS). What do they share in common? (Keloids and hypertrophic scars are both erythematous, raised, and pruritic. Clinically, keloids extend outside the boundaries of the original wound and involve the adjacent normal tissue. Hypertrophic scars appear relatively early in the healing phase, as early as 3 or 4 weeks, while keloids tend to occur months later. Areas that are prone to hypertrophy of scars include the posterior shoulder, anterior chest, and suprapubic area. Hypertrophic scars will eventually regress with time, while keloids do not.)
   (a) Differentiate histiologically on standard H and E preparation. (As in clinical appearance, keloids will extend into the adjacent normal tissue. Collagen in keloids is more random in distribution and composed of larger and thicker bundles. Also, keloids will have abundant eosinophils, mast cells, and plasma cells.)
2. Cite a single cytokine, of the several cytokines, that is elevated in keloids. (Transforming growth factor-beta (TGF-β) and platelet-derived growth factor (PDGF))
   (a) Is there a difference in the *type* of collagen in keloids as opposed to hypertrophic and other scars? (Yes, the ratio of type I to type III collagen has decreased significantly in keloids compared to normal skin or scar from 3:1 to 2:1, but type I is still predominant.)
3. Outline a hypothesis for keloid formation. (Simplistically, the pathologic mechanism in keloids is an overproduction of collagen and a diminished breakdown of collagen. This imbalance in synthesis and degradation may be the result of inhibition of collagenase with the resultant decrease in levels of the degradative enzymes. The trigger mechanism, other than trauma, is unknown.)
4. Contrast the epidemiologic characteristics of hypertrophic scars and keloids. (Keloids occur predominantly in Black and Hispanic individuals, with a higher incidence in the teenage population. Hypertrophic scars are more common in Asians and, if all other variables are held constant, in young children. Both hypertrophic scars and keloids, particularly keloids, are rare in the elderly.)
5. What is the explanation for both keloids and hypertrophic scars being pruritic? (Both have elevated levels of mast cells, and mast cells are responsible for the release of histamine. Antihistamines can be useful as a symptomatic treatment.)

6. Comment on the value of surgical excision of keloids. (The results of surgery alone seem doomed to a high recurrence rate. A number of technical recommendations have been made including the intralesional excision with preservation of a lateral rim as well as adjunctive techniques such as steroids, pressure, and radiation, all of which are discussed below. A singular exception may be earlobe keloids, but data is lacking.)
7. What is the theoretical basis for the possible efficacy of steroids in the treatment of keloids and hypertrophic scars? (Long-acting steroids such as Kenalog® inhibit the proliferation of fibroblast and collagen synthesis and may also increase collagen degradation. From a treatment-outcome standpoint, steroids have been moderately successful in the treatment of hypertrophic scars. In the treatment of keloids, steroids are usually combined with surgical excision with highly variable outcomes. In addition, reported protocols vary from administration preoperatively, intraoperatively, and postoperatively, as well as the number of injections and total dosage.)
   (a) What are the potential side effects of steroid injections? (Of course, systemic effects are possible with higher doses, but local adverse effects can include hypopigmentation as well as dermal and subcutaneous fat atrophy and depression deformity of the skin.)
8. Describe the role, if any, of the use of radiation therapy in the treatment of keloids. (Radiation therapy has only been used postoperatively after keloid excision and is characteristically given in a relatively low dose, 12–1500 cGy, given immediately postoperatively in three fractions over 3 days.)
9. A reading has been included that gives a substantially negative view of the use of radiation therapy in post-excisional keloids. Summarize. (A small group of patients had a highly significant, 72% recurrence rate, which perhaps could be explained since their patients had failed multiple other treatment modalities. The article also discusses the high variability of methods used in other publications of ostensibly good results with radiotherapy.)
10. Outline a short list of other agents that may be efficacious in a keloid treatment but are still largely experimental. (Imiquimod or Aldara, 5-fluorouracil (5-FU), and interferon all have been described in the management of keloids and hypertrophic scars. A growing body of evidence would indicate that interferon is of little value and the injection of imiquimod has not been adequately evaluated. A substantial experience with the use of 5-FU locally has been garnered that would indicate some efficacy in the reduction of keloids, particularly when combined with steroid injections.)
11. Comment on laser therapy and prophylaxis for the management of hypertrophic scars. (Essentially, CO_2 laser does not appear to offer any advantage to sharp-knife excision of keloids in terms of recurrence. The 585-nm pulsed dye laser (PDL) may well have efficacy, but in African–American patients, the most common ethnic group with keloids, melanin is a competing chromophore. The use of PDL as prophylaxis has yielded, at best, mixed results. Some efficacy has been demonstrated in the treatment of immature hypertrophic scars. The non-ablative fractional laser may outperform the PDL in patients with darker skin, Fitzpatrick IV and higher, in the treatment of hypertrophic scars. Discussion of efficacy continues to be centered not only on the specific laser but also on the timing: prophylaxis in the early postoperative period or therapeutic, aimed toward established scars.)
12. What is the mechanism of action for the efficacy, if present, in the use of pressure garments for hypertrophic scars? (Local tissue pressures may lead to relative tissue ischemia and hypoxia, which would diminish collagen production and increase collagen degradation.)
   (a) What is the minimum pressure? (15–30 mmHg)
   (b) What are the stipulations in the use of compression garments, and what pressure is necessary? (Garments must be worn 24/7 for 9–12 months, and the pressure should be between 15 and 30 mmHg, but recently those higher pressures have been called into question. In burn patients, pressure garments are often combined with silicone conformers in an effort to derive some additional effect from silicone/coated material as a treatment for hypertrophic scars.)
13. Besides the injection of long-acting steroids and the use of compression garments, what other modalities are available for the treatment of hypertrophic scars? (Silicone gel may be useful in the treatment of hypertrophic scars. If so, the effect can be enhanced by the addition of an occlusive dressing. The mechanism of action may be hydration of the scar.)
14. A factor under the surgeon's control, in part, is the placement of incisions. Discuss. (Tension placed upon wounds triggers a number of mechanisms at the molecular level that enhance collagen production and perhaps inhibit collagen degradation. One method to take advantage of this biology is the placement of incisions, if possible, within the relaxed skin tension lines. Relaxed skin tension lines are most commonly distributed at right angles to the axis of motion of the underlying muscles. The use of Z-plasty in addressing hypertrophic scars is an example of the modulation of mechanical forces. The technique of the use of deep dermal sutures and wound closure is another example, but such sutures are usually absorbable, so the effect is probably temporary. A number of available commercial products purportedly serve to off-load the mechanical forces on incisions. See Fig. 4.1.)

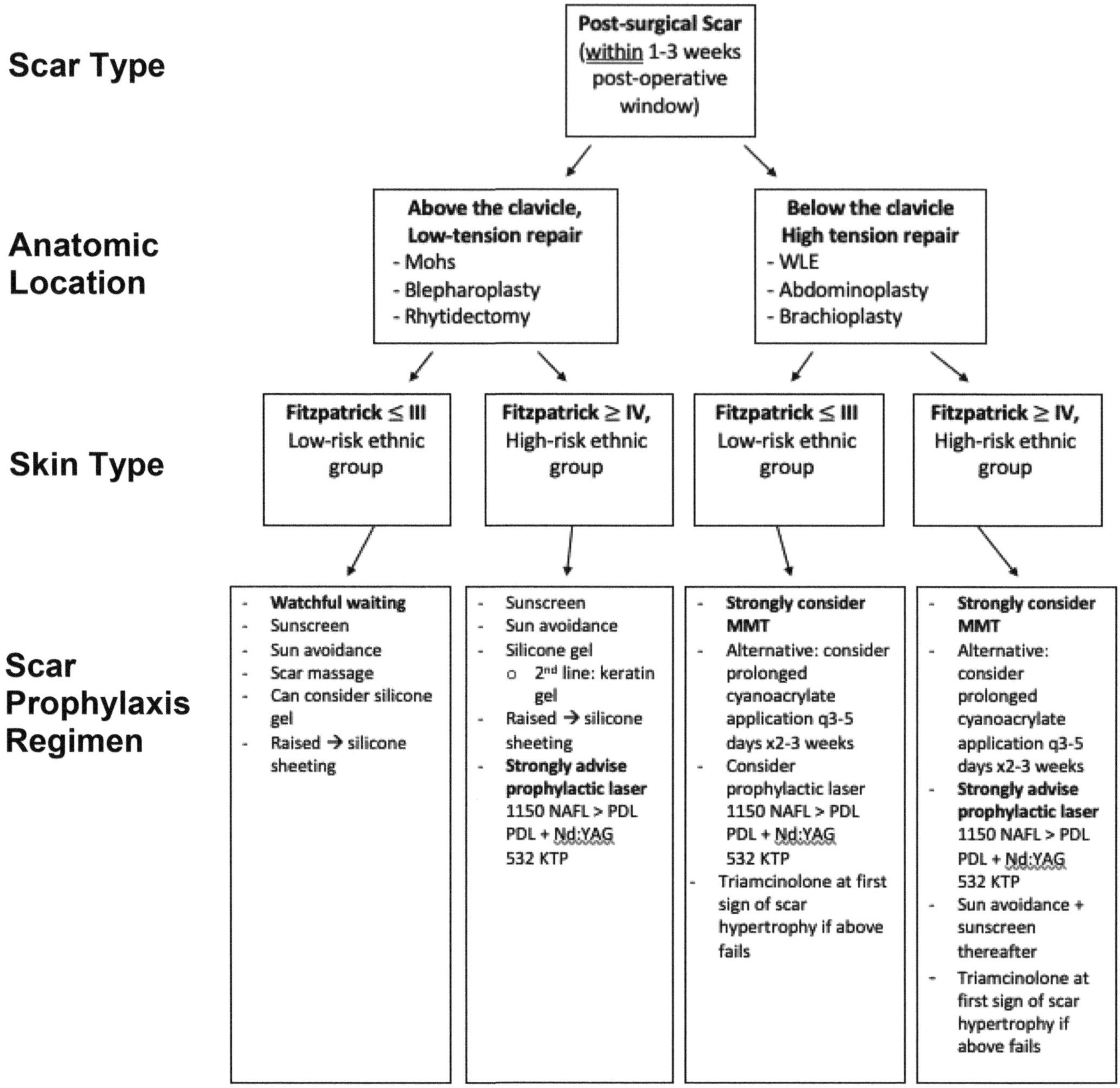

Fig. 4.1 Placement of incisions

Case-Based Conference

Case 1: Keloid

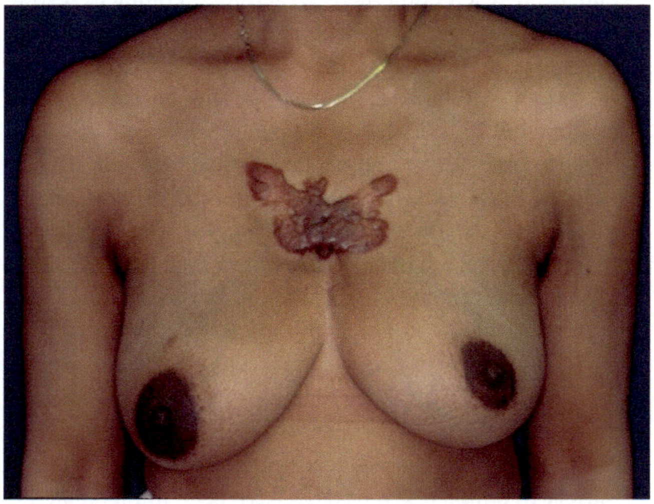

A 30-year-old woman who had "laser" removal of a tattoo with complaints of pruritus and appearance.

1. Describe the slide. Add a focused clinical examination.
   (a) Are any tests indicated? Justify. (Probably not. The clinical examination established the diagnosis.)
2. Discuss the pathophysiology of the patient's diagnosis. Explain the treatment paradox inherent to the diagnosis.
3. Outline a treatment plan. If your treatment plan is nonoperative, be prepared for an operative approach including pre-, intra-, and postoperative care as well.

Case-Based Conference: Discussion

Case 1: Keloid

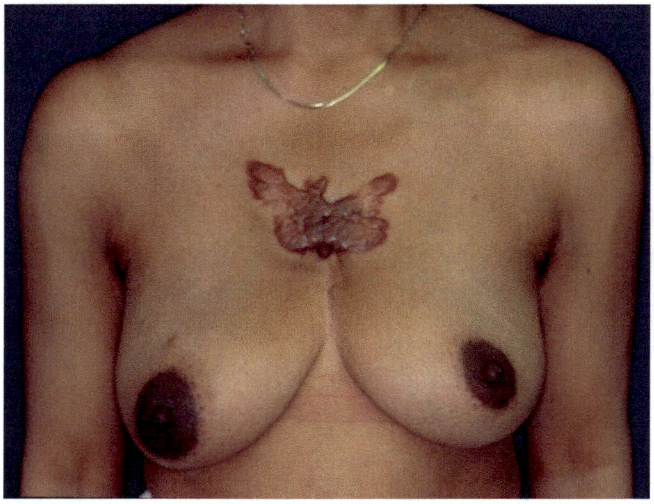

A 30-year-old woman who had "laser" removal of a tattoo with complaints of pruritus and appearance.

1. Describe the slide. Add a focused clinical examination. (A single slide depicts a frontal view of the chest of an African–American woman. The most obvious feature is a large, butterfly-shaped, raised, non-ulcerated part of the central sternum. The color is variegated, dark in some areas and lighter in others. The dimensions appear to be 5 or 6 cm in width and 3 cm in height. No other lesions are evident. The breasts are not distorted by the lesion.

   The history would establish the duration since the treatment of the tattoo, the subsequent healing process and wound appearance, as well as the growth of the lesion over time. Additional questions are posed about similar lesions elsewhere on the body. The impact of the appearance and symptoms on the activities of daily living would also be assessed. Determination of the past medical history including medications and the social history including occupation would be added. A family history of occurrence of similar lesions will complete the history component of the clinical examination. The physical examination would include, if the patient had lesions elsewhere, determining if they are similar in appearance. Examination of the lesion in question mainly consists of inspection; palpation will yield little additional information.)
   (a) Are any tests indicated? Justify. (The clinical examination established the diagnosis.)
2. Discuss the pathophysiology of the patient's diagnosis. Explain the treatment paradox inherent to the diagnosis. (The presumptive diagnosis is a keloid. The differentiation in this patient is hypertrophic scar versus keloid. Other instances with a different scenario, e.g., the occurrence of a de novo lesion without an antecedent history of trauma, could raise the possibility of an alternate diagnosis of dermatofibroma or even dermatofibrosarcoma that may mimic hypertrophic scar in appearance. The differentiation of hypertrophic scar from keloid hinges on the propensity of the latter to proliferate beyond the confines of the original wound. In addition, the surface of a keloid will be considerably irregular and the color variegated, as is the case of this patient. Hypertrophic scars appear relatively early in the healing phase, as early as 3 or 4 weeks, while keloids tend to occur months later. Hypertrophic scars will eventually regress with time, while keloids do not.

   The pathogenesis of keloid is unclear. A number of biochemical abnormalities of the normal wound-healing process have been identified, but on a cellular level, the triggering factor has not. Simplistically, the pathologic mechanisms in keloid and hypertrophic scars are overproduction and diminished breakdown of collagen. This imbalance in synthesis and degradation may be the result of inhibition of collagenase with a resultant decrease in levels of the degradative enzymes. Keloids occur predominantly in African–American and Hispanic individuals and perhaps more commonly in young patients. Fair-skinned individuals, Fitzpatrick 1, particularly those with red hair and Celtic skin are more prone to hypertrophic scars. Certain anatomical regions such as the sternum, posterior shoulder, and back are more commonly afflicted with both hypertrophic scars and keloids. Keloids can occur virtually anywhere with skin wounding including earlobes, face, and areas with chronic folliculitis like posterior scalp and suprapubic region.

The treatment paradox arises from the necessity to develop a successful treatment for a condition that is inherent to the patient with an incomplete understanding of pathophysiology. As a result, the various options, given below, are empirical in nature.)

3. Outline a treatment plan. If your treatment plan is nonoperative, be prepared for an operative approach including pre-, intra-, and postoperative care as well. (As discussed above, a number of nonoperative modalities are available, all with an established record of mixed results, and include the local intralesional injections of long-acting steroids, antimetabolites like 5-FU, and immunomodulators like imiquimod; pressure therapy; and the use of laser. The use of local agents by intralesional injection like long-acting steroids, such as riamcinolone, has a broad range of scar suppression effects; 5-FU inhibits fibroblast proliferation. The use of either appears to be enhanced when combined. Regardless, complete resolution of the keloid cannot be anticipated but rather some amelioration of the patient's symptoms and softening of the lesion. Although the use of pressure garments and/or silicone gel has yielded some benefit in the treatment of hypertrophic scars and following excision of earlobe keloids, little success has been garnered in the management of keloids in general. In a similar vein, the pulsed dye laser (PDL) has been applied to hypertrophic scars, but the mode of action is limited to penetration of 1 mm or less and would not be appropriate for this patient.

A surgical approach alone would mandate a split-thickness skin graft for wound closure and is attended by an extremely high recurrence rate and raises the additional specter of keloid occurrence at the donor site. A variety of adjunctive measures have been implemented in an effort to reduce their recurrence including injection of steroids intra-and postoperatively. Another protocol is the administration of immediate postoperative radiotherapy at the dose of 1200 cGY. Studies have dispelled concerns about carcinogenesis. The surgical option would require careful consideration by both the patient and surgeon regarding the possible outcome of a recurrence even larger than the primary lesion.)

Case-Based Conference

Case 2: Keloid

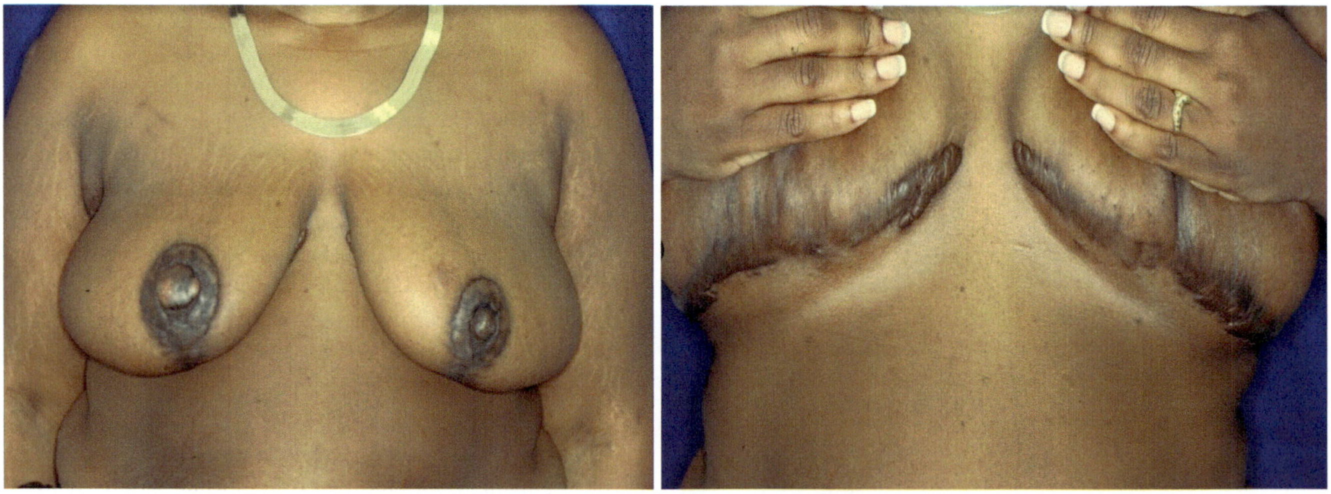

A 40-year-old woman, 1 year after breast reduction, who complains of thickened scars that are pruritic

1. Describe the slides and obtain a clinical examination. Establish a presumptive clinical diagnosis.
   (a) Are any test(s) indicated?
2. What is the pathophysiology of the clinical diagnosis?
3. Based on the response to question 2, what is your treatment plan?

Case-Based Conference: Discussion

Case 2: Keloid

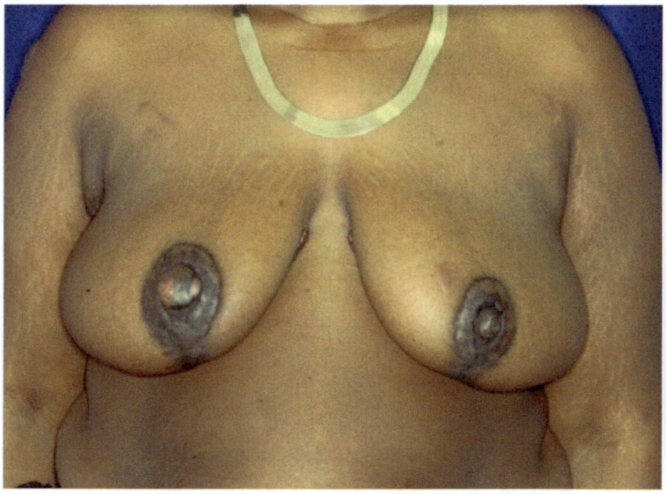

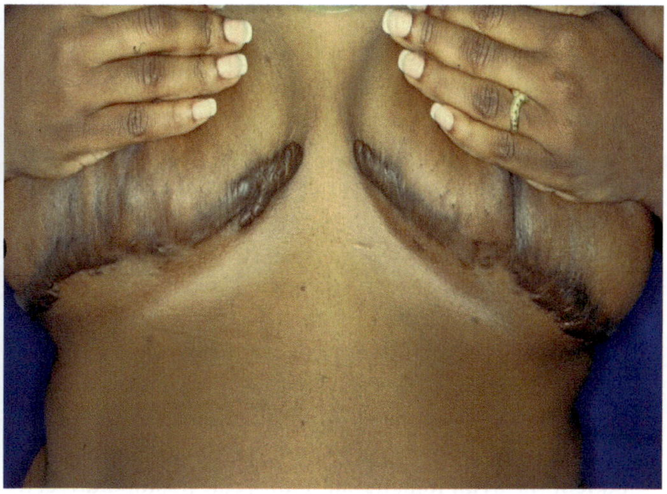

A 40-year-old woman, 1 year in both after breast reduction, who complains of thickened scars that are pruritic

1. Describe the slides and obtain a clinical examination. Establish a presumptive clinical diagnosis. (Two views are provided of a postoperative reduction-mammoplasty African–American patient. The first is a truncal view of the breast. What is evident is the presence of enlarged thickened nipples and some thickening of the circumference of the areola but not dramatically so. The most medial aspects of the inframammary scars are evident and appear thickened. The second photo provides a focused view of the post-breast-reduction inframammary crease incision scars. The view demonstrates widened and thickened scars, perhaps more remarkable medially but evident throughout the visible three-fourths of the visible inframammary fold. The scars are raised but perhaps not proliferative. Only the most inferior portion of the vertical scar is visible and, although widened, does not appear thickened similar to the crease scars. No other diagnostic clues are provided in either view.

   The presumptive clinical diagnosis of this case is postoperative hypertrophic scars, based on appearance and the dominant complaint of pruritus. The differential diagnosis is keloid. The clinical differential diagnosis hinges on the appearance: keloids are proliferative lesions, initiated by trauma, that are clinically distinguished by the propensity to invade normal tissue. The appearance of the lesions in this case should be compared to the keloids in the other case in this module.

   The clinical examination begins with the history: Did uneventful healing occur postoperatively? At what point was the thickening of the inframammary crease incisions evident? Pruritus is apparently a prominent symptom; at what time point postoperatively did the onset occur? Of course, past medical history is pursued including medications. The physical exam would include the search for other scars elsewhere, which could be inspected for a similar appearance or not to the breast scars. In addition to inspection, palpation of the scars will not probably further delineate between hypertrophic scars and keloids.)
   (a) Are any test(s) indicated? (Although a number of sophisticated tests may be of assistance in the differential diagnosis, none are indicated at this juncture.)
2. What is the pathophysiology of the clinical diagnosis? (The clinical diagnosis is postoperative hypertrophic scars (HS), and as mentioned above, the differential in this case is keloid. Certainly, in another set of clinical circumstances such as an occurrence of a de novo lesion, an alternate diagnosis of dermatofibroma or even dermatofibrosarcoma could be considered. The differentiation of HS and keloid hinges on the capacity of the latter to involve adjacent normal tissue beyond the borders of the original wound. Hypertrophic scars appear promptly after wounding, weeks later, while the time hiatus for keloids is months, perhaps years. Finally, if left untreated, HS eventually regress, but keloids do not. In many aspects, the pathophysiology of HS and keloids appear to differ principally in degree. For example, histologically, both contain an abundance of collagen, much in random orientation, although, with maturation, the collagen in HS becomes more organized and uniform. Both have an increase in fibroblast density and an imbalance between collagen production and degradation with the resultant disruption of the collagen equilibrium. Abnormalities in certain cytokines and growth factors are unique to keloids but are not of practical clinical significance. The trigger mechanism or mechanisms are not clearly understood,

but the role of wound tension has been most consistently implemented. Biologically, mechanical tension drives fibroblast proliferation and collagen synthesis and may also dictate collagen orientation. Certainly, some tension exists at the inframammary fold with wound closure of breast-reduction operations, and hypertrophic scars of that incision are not a rare occurrence. Genetically, African–American patients have a higher risk for the development of keloids, as do Asian and perhaps fair-skinned individuals, Fitzpatrick 1. Certainly, the last, fair-skinned patients, are more prone to the development of hypertrophic scars.)

3. Based on the response to Question 2, what is your treatment plan? (Given the presumptive diagnosis of hypertrophic scar, several treatment strategies are available. The first, and most conservative, is simply observation and patient reassurance. The difficulty of that option is that the time frame for resolution is uncertain and the patient is symptomatic at one year postoperatively. Other interventions include the use of silicone gel or sheets held in place with a bra. The injection of a long-acting steroid, triamcinolone, can be efficacious either as a single treatment or as a series, each three or four weeks apart. Care must be exercised to avoid overdosage in any given area because of the complication of soft-tissue atrophy and/or depigmentation. Injected agents such as 5-fluorouracil and imiquimod have had some success in the treatment of keloids, but little experience has been published in the management of hypertrophic scar. Also, the use of lasers, particularly the pulsed dye laser, has been applied to incisional scars, particularly in the early postoperative period, but since the depth of penetration is limited to 1 mm or less, little efficacy could be expected in this patient. An operative option does exist: excision and reclosure with an unknown probability of success, success judged by the lack of recurrence or at least a substantially thinner and less-prominent scar. Given the considerable thickening of the periareolar scars at this point postoperatively, one year, the patient should be counseled, if that option is under consideration, about appropriate expectations. A favorable circumstance, perhaps, is less tension with closure than the original operation.)

In-Service Examination

1. The principal difference in outcomes between a thick and thin skin graft is:
   (a) Less pigmentation and more secondary contraction in a thin skin graft
   (b) Less pigmentation and more secondary contraction in a thick skin graft
   (c) More pigmentation and less secondary contracture in a thick skin graft
   (d) Less pigmentation and less secondary contracture in a thick skin graft
2. A consideration of the relationship between types I and III collagens in keloids is:
   (a) The ratio of 1:3 is decreased compared to normal tissue
   (b) The ratio of 1:3 is increased compared to normal tissue
   (c) No difference
   (d) No difference, but the absolute amounts of both are increased
3. Skin graft survival in the initial postoperative period is dependent on:
   (a) Revascularization
   (b) Inosculation
   (c) Imbibition
   (d) Fibroblast migration

5 Local Anesthetics and Complications of General Anesthesia

Bibliography

Armstrong K, "A Primer on Local Anesthetics for Plastic Surgery", *Clin Plastic Surg.*, (2013); 40: **515-26 (Overview).**

Becker DE, Reed KL, "Local Anesthetics: Review of Pharmacological Considerations", *Anesth Prog.*, (2012); 59:**90-94 (skip local toxicity).**

Gitman M, Fettiplace MR, Weinberg GL, et al., "Local Anesthetic Systemic Toxicity: A Narrative Literature Review and Clinical Update on Prevention, Diagnosis, and Management", *Plast. Reconstr. Surg.*, (2019); 144(3): **783-790.**

Neal JM, Woodward CM, Harrison TK, "The American Society of Regional Anesthesia and Pain Medicine Checklist for Managing Local Anesthetic Systemic Toxicity 2017 Version", *Regional Anesthesia and Pain Medicine*, (2018); 43(2):**150-153.**

Mustoe TA, Buck DW, Lalonde DH, "The Safe Management of Anesthesia, Sedation and Pain in Plastic Surgery", *Plast. Reconstr. Surg.*, (2010); 126(4):**165e-167e and Video 1.**

Jo YY, Kwak HJ, "Sedation Strategies for Procedures Outside the Operating Room", *Yonsei Med J*, (2019); 60(6):**491-495.**

Gutowski KA, "Tumescent Analgesia in Plastic Surgery", *Plast. Reconstr. Surg.*, (2014); 134(4S-2):**50S-57S.**

Pace MM, Chatterjee A, Merrill DG, et al., "Local Anesthetics in Liposuction: Considerations for New Practice Advisory Guidelines to Improve Patient Safety", *Plast. Reconstr. Surg.*, (2013); 131(5):**820e-826e.**

Malik O, Kaye Ad, Kaye A, et al., "Emerging Roles of Liposomal Bupivacaine in Anesthesia Practice", *J Anesthesiol Clin Pharmacol.*, (2017); 33(2):**151-154.**

Momoh AO, Hilliard PE, Chung KC, "Regional and Neuraxial Analgesia for Plastic Surgery: Surgeon's and Anesthesiologist's Perspectives", *Plast. Reconstr. Surg.*, (2014); 134(4S-2):**60S-62S ONLY.**

Gurunluoglu R, Swanson JA, Haeck PC, "Evidence-Based Patient Safety Advisory: Malignant Hyperthermia", *Plast. Reconstr. Surg.*, (2009): 124(4S):**68S-71S, 74S-76S ONLY.**

Faculty Discussion and Study Guide

Editor's Note: Some elements of conscious sedation and general anesthesia are included in the Part XII.

Pharmacology and Toxicity of Local Anesthetics

1. Some understanding of the pharmacology of local anesthesia is necessary for its safe use. What is the hierarchy of sensitivity to local anesthetics among the autonomic, motor, proprioceptive, and pain fibers? (Autonomic, pain, proprioceptive, and motor, in that order. A wrist block of the median and ulnar nerves will render the digits anesthetic, but intrinsic function will be retained initially.)
2. Essentially, what is the mechanism of action of local anesthetics? (Although local anesthetics have a number of molecular actions, at the cellular level, local anesthetics act upon sodium channels and block the depolarization–repolarization process.)
3. In general, two classes of local anesthesia (LA) exist. List and describe their chemical differences and metabolism. (Amides and esters. Although both are quite similar in chemical structure and share a lipophilic core and hydrophilic tertiary amine, the intermediate stem or linkage is moderately different between the two; amides have an amide link. Amides are metabolized in the liver by one of the principal hepatic enzymes, P450 and esters in the plasma by cholinesterases and excreted in the urine. See Fig. 5.1)

E. Luce, *A Curriculum for Plastic Surgery*, https://doi.org/10.1007/978-3-031-62087-4_5

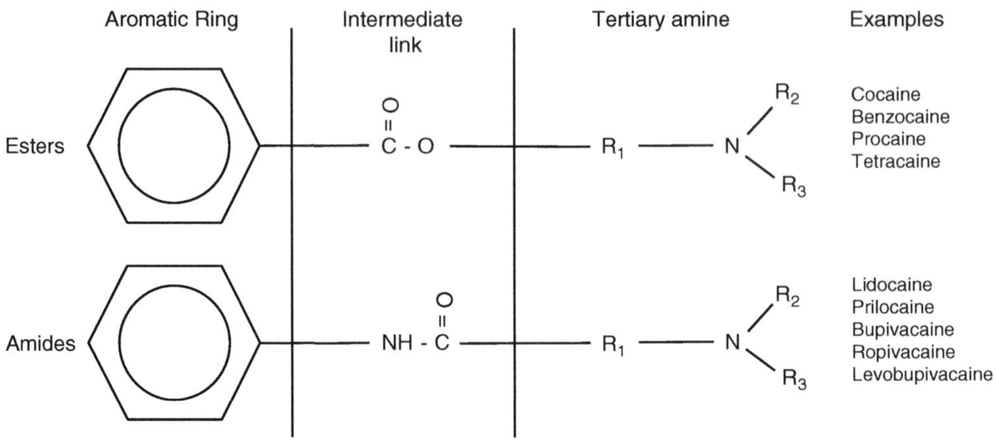

Fig. 5.1 Local anesthesia

4. What is the biochemical explanation for the difference in potency from agent to agent? (The difference in potency is mostly the result of a difference in lipid solubility. High lipophilic agents can diffuse more readily through lipid-rich nerve sheaths and cellular membranes. Of course, a higher concentration of any given agent in solution enhances potency as well as a number of factors including the characteristics of the local environment and the pKa of the agent. Potency can be defined as the completeness of anesthesia.)
5. The family of LA has different individual rapidity of onset and duration of action. Explain. (The principal biochemical explanation for a difference in rapidity of onset is the pKa of the agent since, without a detailed discussion of the Henderson–Hasselbalch equation, the pKa of the agent, when subject to the physiologic pH of tissues, will dictate the number of lipid-soluble molecules available to penetrate the cellular membrane. The *duration* of action is primarily due to their affinity or not to be bound by serum proteins. A high protein-binding property prolongs the duration of action. For example, bupivacaine is initially 95% protein-bound in plasma and has a long duration of neural blockade. Another factor is the inherent vasodilatory action of the local anesthetic agent, which varies from drug to drug. As a result, epinephrine is usually added to produce local vasoconstriction and delay systemic absorption.)
6. True or false: the probability of local anesthetic systemic toxicity is directly correlated with serum levels? (True. Although any number of factors can directly or indirectly affect serum levels, the probability of toxicity is directly proportional to serum levels. For example, prodromal signs and symptoms may be present at 4–5 μg/mL, CNS convulsions at 10–12 μg/mL, and cardiovascular collapse and respiratory arrest at 20 μg/mL, all expressed as the concentration of lidocaine in this instance. See Fig. 5.2)
7. What are the prodromal signs and symptoms of local anesthetic systemic toxicity (LAST)? (The most common are tinnitus, perioral numbness, metallic taste, and dysarthria although all may be absent prior to the onset of major manifestations. See Table 5.1.)

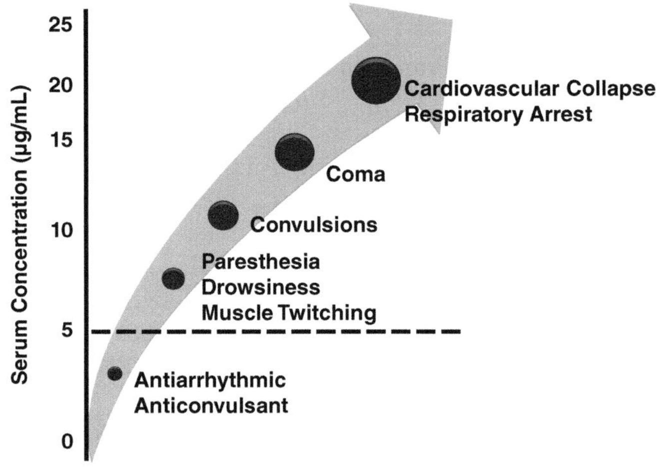

Fig. 5.2 Classes of local anesthesia. (Becker DE, Reed KL, "Local Anesthetics: Review of Pharmacological Considerations," *Anesth Prog.*, (2012); 59:93. (Reprinted with permission))

8. What are the major CNS presentations and explanations of LAST? (Excitability and convulsions, presumably due to selective depression of central inhibitory tracts, followed by coma with an increased serum concentration.)
9. What are the cardiovascular presentations of LAST? (The same sodium channel blockade on nerves that is responsible for the desired therapeutic effect can also produce a detrimental depression of conduction in the heart. The initial signs may be tachycardia and hypertension that is replaced by arrhythmias, bradycardia, and hypotension. The EKG expressions of the conduction abnormalities consist of the prolongation of QRS and ST intervals.)
10. What is the principal difference between a shorter-acting agent such as lidocaine and a longer-acting agent such as bupivacaine in cardiac toxicity? (The adverse cardiac effects of both are the result of the conduction system

Table 5.1 Clinical picture of local anesthetic systemic toxicity (LAST)

Prodrome
Perioral numbness
Tinnitus
Confusion
Dysarthria
Dysphoria
Dizziness
Drowsiness
Dysgeusia
Neurologic
Agitation
Loss of consciousness
Seizure
Cardiovascular
Arrhythmias (bradycardia, tachycardia, ventricular ectopy/tachycardia/fibrillation)
Hypotension or hypertension
Conduction disturbances (e.g., widened QRS complex)
Cardiac arrest (asystole, pulseless electrical activity)

blockade discussed above, but the toxicity of bupivacaine is substantially more severe. The greater lipophilic nature of bupivacaine has a higher tissue-binding capacity, creating a cardiac depression that is much more refractory to resuscitation.)

11. What are the risk factors in the production of local anesthetic systemic toxicity (LAST)? (The principal patient-independent risk factor is the rate of administration; the most obvious example is inadvertent intravenous administration that can produce toxic serum levels. Differences between the sites of injection, mucosa vs. skin-soft tissue, for equivalent doses result in an enhanced uptake in the former. Patient risk factors include the extremes of age, infancy and elderly; congestive heart failure; and/or preexistent arrhythmias and hepatic dysfunction. The patient risk factor for obesity is not well-defined. Observed systemic toxic reactions may be a reflection that the calculated maximum safe dosage limits, mg/kg, may not be linear in the obese and may predispose to overdosage.)
12. What is the clinical picture or threshold that signals the initiation of treatment for possible local anesthetic systemic toxicity (LAST)? (Certainly, any of the cardiovascular signs, arrhythmias or hyper- or hypotension, as well as CNS manifestations such as excitability and confusion. Prodromal signs and symptoms may require, in addition to cessation of injections, if relevant, the initiation of the first steps of a protocol for the treatment of potential LAST.)
13. Describe the protocol for the treatment of LAST. (In addition to cessation of injections, if any, the patient should be oxygenated and CNS toxicity treated with benzodiazepines intravenously. The 2017 recommendations of the American Society of Regional Anesthesia and Pain Medicine are an infusion of lipid emulsion, a fixed dose of 100 cc bolus of 20% rapidly administered over 2–3 min for patients of 70 kg or greater, followed by 200–250 cc over the subsequent 15–20 min. Patients less than 70 kg are given a weight-based infusion of 1.5 mL/kg, also over 2–3 min, followed by 0.5 cc/kg/min. Cardiac arrest protocols should not include epinephrine, calcium channels, or beta blockers (Table 5.2).
14. Explain the benefit of the addition of epinephrine to the composition of LA. (Simply stated, epinephrine, by vasoconstriction of the vessels in the local environment, decreases the rate of systemic uptake of the LA and raises the maximum tolerable dose. See below.)

Table 5.2 Treatment checklist

<table>
<tr><td colspan="2">Checklist for the treatment of local anesthetic systemic toxicity (LAST)[a]</td></tr>
<tr><td colspan="2">The pharmacologic treatment for LAST is different from other cardiac arrest scenarios</td></tr>
<tr><td colspan="2">– Reduce individual epinephrine boluses to ≤1 mcg/kg
– Avoid vasopressin, calcium channel blockers, beta blockers, or other local anesthetics
– Stop injecting local anesthetics
– Get help
  – Consider lipid emulsion therapy at the first sign of a serious LAST event
  – Call for the LAST Rescue Kit
  – Alert the nearest cardiopulmonary bypass team; resuscitation may be prolonged
– Airway management
  – Ventilate with 100% oxygen/avoid hyperventilation/advanced airway device if necessary
– Control seizures
  – Benzodiazepines preferred
  – Avoid large doses of propofol, especially in hemodynamically unstable patients
– Treat hypotension and bradycardia If pulseless, start CPR
– Continue monitoring
  – At least 4–6 h after a cardiovascular event
  – At least 2 h after a limited CNS event
– Do not exceed 12 mL/kg lipid emulsion (particularly important in the small adult or child)
  – Much smaller doses are typically needed for LAST treatment</td></tr>
<tr><td colspan="2">Lipid emulsion 20% (Precise volume and flow rate are not crucial)</td></tr>
<tr><td>Greater-than-70-kg patient</td><td>Less-than-70-kg patient</td></tr>
<tr><td>Bolus 100 mL lipid emulsion 20%
Rapidly over 2–3 min
– Lipid emulsion infusion 200–250 mL over 15–20 min</td><td>Bolus 1.5 mL/kg lipid emulsion 20%
Rapidly over 2–3 min
– Lipid emulsion infusion ~0.25 mL/kg/min (ideal body weight)</td></tr>
<tr><td colspan="2">If the patient remains unstable:
– Re-bolus once or twice at the same dose and double infusion rate; be aware of the dosing limit (12 mL/kg)
– Total volume of lipid emulsion can approach 1 L in a prolonged resuscitation (e.g., >30 min)</td></tr>
</table>

[a] Modified from the ASRA Checklist for Treatment of Local Anesthetic Systemic Toxicity (LAST)

Clinical Use

1. List the recommended doses for the following agents with and without epinephrine: lidocaine, bupivacaine, and mepivacaine. (Although rarely administered without the addition of epinephrine, the maximum dosage of plain lidocaine is 3 mg/kg, and with epinephrine 7 mg/kg or a total dosage of 500 mg in a 70-kg patient. Also, as discussed above, extrapolation of the total dosage in a linear fashion for heavier patients should be done with caution. The maximum tolerable dose of bupivacaine is 2 mg/kg and mepivacaine is 5 mg/kg. Evidence indicates that neither the duration nor the dosage is extended appreciably by the addition of epinephrine in bupivacaine or mepivacaine.)
2. Discuss the variables of concentration and total permissible dosage of epinephrine. (The effect of vasoconstriction is not enhanced in concentrations greater than 1:200,000. The recommended total dosage is 0.07 mg/kg. A 50-cc vial of lidocaine with a 1:200,000 concentration of epinephrine contains a total of 0.25 mg of epinephrine. Total-dosage concerns are mostly limited to tumescent anesthesia techniques. See below.)
3. The above recommendations of lidocaine dosage, 7 mg/kg with epinephrine, are modified in the technique of tumescent anesthesia in liposuction and other body-contouring procedures. How and why? (The infusion of large volumes of saline or Ringer's lactate that contain highly diluted lidocaine and epinephrine are essential for the performance of liposuction. A number of formulas have been adopted, but a common example is 30–50 cc of 1% lidocaine and 1 cc or 1 mg of 1:1000 epinephrine in 1000 cc of Ringer's lactate or saline, the former balanced for pH. That formula yields a dosage of 300–500 mg of lidocaine and an epinephrine concentration of 1:1,000,000. The threshold for large-volume liposuction is 5 L. Assuming a patient of 70 kg, the total lidocaine dosage in that set of circumstances would be 21 mg/kg if 30 cc at 1% lidocaine per liter is utilized or 35 mg/kg if 50 cc of 1% lidocaine per liter is used)
4. Liposomal bupivacaine has emerged as a potential local postoperative pain-control measure administered either as a continuous infusion via catheters or as a fascial block placed in the operative site. Discuss in terms of toxicity, not efficacy. (The concept of liposomal bupivacaine is a slow release of the agent from encapsulation with particles composed of a liposomal platform. To do so prolongs the duration of action and, possibly, enhances safety. The recommended maximum dosage is 265 mg.)

Conscious Sedation

1. What is the hierarchy of sedation from least to most in the clinical criteria? (In moderate or conscious sedation, the patient, although sedated, is capable of purposeful response to verbal or tactile stimuli as well as spontaneous ventilation and maintenance of the airway. In deep sedation, the patient is purposely responsive to painful stimulation, but ventilation may be inadequate, and airway intervention may be required. Both have specific monitoring requirements. See Table 5.3.)
2. List and briefly describe the agents employed for sedation. (Benzodiazepines such as diazepam, valium, and midazolam or Versed®, as well as short-acting opioids such as fentanyl. Other drugs that may result in deep sedation include ketamine, a dissociative agent, and propofol, a hypnotic, administered intravenously and not related to the above class of drugs.)
   (a) What are the antagonists? (For benzodiazepines, flumazenil is given at 0.2 mg incremental doses to a maximum of 1 mg. For opioids, naloxone is administered at 0.1–0.2 mg doses until reversal of toxic effects.)

Table 5.3 Statement on Continuum of Depth of Sedation: Definition of General Anesthesia and Levels of Sedation/Analgesia, American Society of Anesthesiologists, 2019 is reprinted with permission of the American Society of Anesthesiologists, 1061 American Lane, Schaumburg, Illinois 60173-4973

	Minimal sedation (anxiolysis)	Moderate sedation/analgesia (conscious sedation)	Deep sedation/analgesia	General anesthesia
Responsiveness[a]	Normal response to verbal stimulation	Purposeful response to verbal or tactile stimulation	Purposeful response following repeated or painful stimulation	Unarousable even with painful stimulus
Airway	Unaffected	No intervention required	Intervention may be required	Intervention often required
Spontaneous ventilation	Unaffected	Adequate	May be inadequate	Frequently inadequate
Cardiovascular function	Unaffected	Usually maintained	Usually maintained	May be required

Source: http://www.asahq.org

[a] Reflex withdrawal from a painful stimulus is not considered a purposeful response

Regional Anesthesia

1. A paravertebral block can be utilized for breast and abdominal surgery. Briefly explain what are the techniques and drawbacks. (A spinal needle is inserted into the paravertebral space dorsal to the transverse process but ventral or anterior to the vertebral body and also accesses the epidural space. The complications include pneumothorax, epidural spread with hypopnea, and hypoxia. As a result, paravertebral block is not widely used.)
2. The transversus abdominis plane block (TAP) has been increasingly utilized in abdominal procedures including abdominal-based breast reconstruction. Describe the anatomy and technique. (TAP block is accomplished by deposition of a long-acting anesthetic in the fascial plane of the sensory component of a segmental intercostal nerve or nerves. Typically, thoracic 10 through lumbar 1 are the branches targeted by a TAP block. The block can be placed preoperatively with ultrasound guidance or by intraoperative exposure. The block is injected into the plane between the transversus and the internal oblique muscle, posteriorly, lateral to the latissimus dorsi. Continuous anesthesia postoperatively is possible by placement of an infusion catheter. Complications are possible with the use of bilateral blocks by violation of toxic dose limits.)
3. What is the anatomy of an axillary block? (An axillary block is accompanied with the aid of ultrasound to achieve a block of the radial nerve, posterior to the artery, median nerve, anterior and superior to the artery, and ulnar nerve, anterior and inferior to the artery. Frequently, the musculocutaneous exits the sheath proximal to the point of injection. Since the musculocutaneous conducts the eventual medial and lateral antebrachial sensory nerves, additional injection of local anesthetic should be instilled into the coracobrachialis. Some institutions utilize infraclavicular and supraclavicular blocks instead of axillary blocks.)

In-Service Examination

1. What are the nerve fibers that are the most sensitive to the least sensitive to local anesthetic?
   (a) Pain, autonomic, proprioceptive, motor
   (b) Proprioceptive, autonomic, pain, motor
   (c) Pain, proprioceptive, autonomic, motor
   (d) Autonomic, pain, proprioceptive, motor
   (e) Autonomic, proprioceptive, pain, motor
2. The physiological mechanism of the action of local anesthetic is:
   (a) Releasing acetylcholine from the nerve fibers
   (b) Delaying the release of acetylcholine
   (c) Blocking the sodium channels and suspending the depolarization–repolarization process
   (d) Enhancing the rate of Ca^{++} loss from the nerve fibers
3. A 70-kg patient will have liposuction. What is the maximal dose of epinephrine plus lidocaine per kg of body weight?
   (a) 7 mg
   (b) 35 mg
   (c) 140 mg
   (d) 280 mg

Bone Healing, Bone and Cartilage Grafts, and Bone Substitutes

6

Bibliography

Buck DW and Dumanian GA, "Bone Biology and Physiology: Part I. The Fundamentals", *Plast. Reconstr. Surg.*, (2012); 129(6):**1316-1319 ONLY.**

Buck DW and Dumanian GA, "Bone Biology and Physiology: Part II. Clinical correlates", *Plast. Reconstr. Surg.*, (2012); 129(6):**950e-955e ONLY.**

Lipschitz MD, A. H. and Kenkel MD, J. M., "Implantation: Bone, Cartilage, and Alloplasts". *Selected Readings in Plastic Surgery*, (2004), 10(2):**15-18 ONLY (Cartilage) (Overview).**

Liu W and Cao Y, Chapter 20: "Repair, grafting, and engineering of cartilage", Neligan PC, Plastic Surgery 3rd Edition, Elsevier, (2013); 1:**397-399, 404-408.**

Campana V, Milano G, Pagano E, Barba M, Cicione C, Salonna G, Lattanzi W,

Logroscino G, "Bone Substitutes in Orthopaedic Surgery: From Basic Science to

Clinical Practice", *J Mater Sci Mater Med.*, (2014);25(10):**2445-47, 2452-55 ONLY.**

Gosain AK, Chim H, Arneja JS, "Application-Specific Selection of Biomaterials for Pediatric Craniofacial Reconstruction: Developing a Rational Approach to Guide Clinical Use", *Plast. Reconstr. Surg.*, (2009); 123(1):**319-330 (Skip Results).**

Cierny G, "Surgical treatment of osteomyelitis", *Plast. Reconstr. Surg.*, (2011); 127(1S):**190S-204S.**

Faculty Discussion and Study Guide

Bone Healing and Bone Grafts

1. What is the primary functional unit of cortical bone? (The osteon. Concentric layers of lamella of bone surround an individual central canal, the haversian canal, that contains a vascular network.)
2. Briefly describe the components of the vascular supply to the bone and rank those components in the order of importance. (The three components are the nutrient artery within the medullary cavity, the metaphyseal and epiphyseal blood vessels in the region of the joint that supply cortical and cancellous bone at the terminal portions of long bones, and blood flow within the fine vascular network of the periosteum, both outer and inner, or the lining of the medullary cavity. Although somewhat arbitrary, the diaphyseal nutrient vessels traveling the length of the bone are perhaps most important since they are the vascular supply to the medullary cavity as well as the inner two-thirds of the cortical bone. Fractures, of course, would disrupt this source of vascular supply.)
3. From the standpoint of vascularization and blood supply alone, why might a spiral fracture of the tibia be more likely to heal than a segmental displaced fracture of the same bone? (Of the three principal routes of blood supply to a long bone listed above, the metaphyseal vessels, the periosteal vessels, and the principal nutrient artery and vein course throughout endosteum and marrow cavity and would be severely disrupted in any segmental fracture but likely would remain intact in a spiral fracture.)
4. List and briefly describe the three constituents of bone. (Cellular: the various stages of cellular function of the osteocytes, osteoblasts, or osteoclasts; organic matrix: collagen and ground substance; and inorganic matrix: hydroxyapatite)
5. Give the stages of bone healing and the approximate time frame. (The three stages are similar to that of soft tissue healing and are inflammatory, reparative, and remodeling. The inflammatory stage, again similar to soft tissue, peaks at approximately 48 h and may last several days. The reparative phase commences about 3–4 days after fracture or injury and fades into the remodeling phase, which, theoretically, can last several months to years.)

E. Luce, *A Curriculum for Plastic Surgery*, https://doi.org/10.1007/978-3-031-62087-4_6

6. In distraction osteogenesis, does bone healing occur by a process similar to primary or secondary bone healing? (Primary bone healing. No cartilaginous or intermediate phase is apparent during the healing process, but rather membranous ossification occurs, so the intermediate or cartilaginous phase is minimal or absent, at least theoretically.)
   (a) What are the three phases of distraction osteogenesis; and what is the predominant form of ossification? (Osteotomies create a bone gap and latent phase similar to fracture healing, subsequently placed under tension and will produce the distraction phase when tension forces are applied to the early formative callus; and the consolidation phase during which mineral deposition and remodeling occurs. The ossification is principally intramembranous.)
7. Describe the basic features of primary and secondary bone repair or healing, both in terms of the principles underlying primary bone healing and the histologic characteristics. (Primary bone healing refers to healing by direct deposition of embryonic woven bone without an intervening or intermediate cartilaginous component, which is characteristic of *membranous* bone formation. Primary bone healing occurs when the bone is compressed and rigidly fixed and is also a feature of facial and calvarial bone healing. Secondary bone healing is the model that follows the stages of wound healing listed above, namely, an inflammatory stage characterized by inflammatory cells including macrophages that act to eradicate necrotic bone and other material, followed by the deposition of a cartilage framework as the intermediate stage, and last, bone deposition with remodeling, which is characteristic of *endochondral* or long bone healing. Recent evidence indicates that in addition to the embryonic origin of the healing bone, the other factor in membranous vs. endochondral type bone healing, is the local wound oxygen tension and the type of stress load placed on the graft. For example, a lower oxygen tension in the wound environment can lead to chondrocyte differentiation of the host cells and the formation of the intermediate cartilaginous callus.)
   (a) Why is primary bone healing often referred to as similar to membranous ossification? (The process in primary bone healing is similar to that seen in the healing of the membranous bones of the face such as the zygoma.)
8. What factor or factors explain enhanced healing of bone in the pediatric vs. adult population? (The active cellular layer of the periosteum and the innermost layer of the enveloping bone, the cambium, becomes much thinner and disappears with skeletal maturity.)
9. You are in the process of providing soft tissue coverage for a 2-week-old healing tibial fracture and encounter callus. What would a biopsy of that callus demonstrate? (Cartilage, minimal amounts of woven bone, and osteoid, as well as collagen and capillaries)
10. Differentiate the terms osteoconductive and osteoinductive. (Osteoconductive refers to the structure of the bone graft, namely, a scaffold of the appropriate pore size or aperture that will permit the ingrowth of capillaries and osteoprogenitor cells as well as the provision of the appropriate three-dimensional structure. Bone substitutes such as calcium hydroxyapatite should have a structure with pore size similar to that of native bone. Osteoinductive refers to the presence of bone morphogenetic proteins (BMPs) or other extracellular proteins that are substances that stimulate the recruitment and differentiation of mesenchymal stem cells into osteoblasts. Osteogenesis simply refers to the potential to synthesize new bone.)
11. You perform a non-vascularized bone graft to a segmental defect in two different patients, one with cancellous and cortical bones and the other with only cortical. Describe the process of "take" with both forms of graft, and which of the two will heal more rapidly, and why? (Non-vascularized bone graft "take" is characterized by invasion of the bone graft by inflammatory cells and blood vessels with neovascularization. Resorption of necrotic bone graft occurs as a result of activity by osteoclasts. That resorption is followed by the deposition of new bone by osteoblasts, a process known as "creeping substitution." The take of cancellous bone as opposed to cortical bone is enhanced because of the trabecular structure, greater surface area, and more rapid vascularization for the formation of new bone. Cancellous bone is both osteoconductive and osteoinductive. Cortical bone is only osteoconductive.)
    (a) More specifically, contrast the advantages and disadvantages and efficacy of a bone graft to the mandible between cancellous bone in a titanium tray and a block of cortical bone. (The block of cortical bone will lend some degree of mechanical stability and rigidity during the early post-graft period. Yet, within 6–8 weeks, with bone absorption, 60% or more of the mechanical strength will be lost. In contrast, cancellous bone in the titanium tray lends little or no mechanical rigidity but does permit more rapid revascularization and new bone deposition. On balance, most commonly, smaller segmental defects of the mandible are grafted with non-vascularized cortical bone. The physiologic process, though, provides the basis for the necessity of external rigid fixation until bone healing is sufficiently complete to withstand masticatory forces. Frequently, fixation

may be necessary for as long as 6 months depending on the size of the defect. Larger defects, 6 cm or greater, require vascularized bone grafts.)

12. True or false: the use of freshly harvested iliac cancellous bone graft for alveolar bone grafting in a cleft-lip patient does not contain viable osteoblasts but rather is dependent on host osteoblasts for new bone formation? (False. Although only a small percentage, about 15%, of the osteoblasts within the iliac cancellous bone graft survive, this is sufficient to provide new bone.)
13. Does a difference exist in the fate of two grafts: a bone graft placed for a mandibular defect and a graft placed on the zygoma for cheek enhancement? (Inlay bone grafts are subject to mechanical stress and are more likely to be incorporated and survive. Onlay bone grafts used to address contour deformities are not subjected to such stresses and are more likely to resorb.)
    (a) What is the eponym applied to this principle? (Wolff's law)
14. To summarize, what are the factors that influence the success of graft incorporation or "take?" (Autogenous over allogeneic, bone type such as cancellous or cortical, donor site such as calvarial over iliac or rib, a surrogate for membranous over endochondral, periosteum over the absence of periosteum, rigid fixation over less rigidity, inlay or onlay, and vascularized recipient bed over less-vascularized)
    (a) List some factors that adversely affect bone incorporation. (Prior radiotherapy, systemic factors such as diabetes, smoking, steroids, possibly NSAIDs, and macromotion at the fracture site)
15. A well-established clinical fact is that conventional, non-vascularized bone grafting of tibial defects greater than 5–6 cm is doomed to failure, and defects of that magnitude require vascularized free fibula bone grafts. What is the physiological explanation for this clinical fact? (Segmental bone defects grafted with non-vascularized bone require healing by "creeping substitution," namely, bone deposition initially at the graft recipient interface so that the bone deposition occurs transversely in parallel to the long axis of the graft. Because of the slow rate of old bone resorption and new bone deposition, at a critical point in time, the central cavity is replaced by fibrous tissue. In the case of the tibia, this critical size appears to be about 6 cm, probably the same for the mandible.)
    (a) What is the reconstructive approach to this dilemma, and why? (Vascularized bone transferred by microsurgical techniques such as the fibula graft. The graft is viable from the onset, so no creeping substitution is necessary although the two interfaces with native bone must still fuse by the normal process of fracture healing.)
16. In musculoskeletal oncologic surgery, segmental resection of an extremity bone may be replaced by allograft cortical bone. What complication would you anticipate would be the most common? (Late stress fracture) Why? (Allograft bone may elicit an immunogenic response that inhibits normal bone reparative processes. In addition, concerns exist about disease transmission, so tissue processing must address both of these issues. The processing consists of deep-freezing or freeze-drying and may include the addition of ethylene oxide or irradiation, all of which have adverse effects on structural strength and osteoinductive capability. As a result, although initial structural stability exists, the host tissue response to the presence of an allograft will lead to weakening and, perhaps, stress fracture. Also, size limitations exist consistent with all non-vascularized grafts.)

Cartilage Healing and Cartilage Grafts

1. List the three types of cartilage and a typical location for each. (Hyaline: ribs and joint services; fibrous: intervertebral discs; and elastic: pinna and larynx)
2. How do the metabolism and nutrition of cartilage differ from that of bone? (Cartilage, with the exception of the perichondrium on the surface, is nonvascular and must rely upon diffusion for oxygen and nutrients. Cartilage is a unique tissue with a low metabolic rate. Water is an essential component of cartilage. A corollary is that cartilage can survive substantially longer than bone prior to implantation.)
3. Do hyaline and fibrous cartilage differ in terms of collagen composition? (Type II collagen predominates in hyaline cartilage, while type I is the principal collagen component in fibrous collagen. Elastin is a component of elastic cartilage.)
4. How does cartilage heal? Is it by generation of de novo cartilage similar to bone? (No. Cartilage does not heal similarly to bone but rather heals by substitution of fibrous tissue alone. So, in the harvesting of a costochondral graft, the donor site will heal with fibrous or essentially scar tissue.)
    (a) Explain the principle underpinning the abrasion of ear cartilage in otoplasty. (Some controversy exists, but historical research by Gibson demonstrated that injured cartilage because of an alteration in tensile forces tends to heal in the opposite direction of the injury. So, in otoplasty *anterior* abrasion or the Stenström otoplasty?, the cartilage will tend to warp or heal in the reverse or posterior direction. Of course, modern otoplasty combines other methods, such as the use of Mustardé sutures?)

5. In the process of performing a facial reconstruction, you consider the use of cadaver cartilage from the tissue bank. Discuss. (Allogenic or alloplastic cartilage?, whether preserved or processed or not, has little current clinical utility because of resorption and/or warping over extended periods of time. Even though alloplastic cartilage is not highly antigenic, a sufficient immune response is mobilized by the host to yield undesirable long-term outcomes.)
6. What are the two practical applications of addressing the problem of warping of cartilage in clinical use? (The phenomenon of warping of cartilage is perhaps related to stress forces on altered cartilage such as carving. That phenomenon of stress forces is utilized in otoplasty, for example, when cartilage will bend in the opposite direction of the abrasion. So, anterior cartilage abrasion will warp the ear cartilage posteriorly. The application in nasal dorsum cartilage grafts is the necessity to symmetrically carve the implant. The second phenomenon is that warping will occur within the first 15–30 min, so a time interval prior to implantation after carving is recommended.)

Osteomyelitis

1. What are the types of osteomyelitis? (The Cierny classification is: type I is only medullary, usually a complication of an intramedullary nail or acute hematogenous; type II is only cortical as in a decubitus; type III is a cortical infection that has penetrated and involved the medullary canal such as chronic infection of an old tibial fracture, but the bone is stable; and type IV is type III plus loss of stability, either because of the diffuse nature and/or debridement.)
   (a) Add a host classification. (A: healthy; B: either local and/or systemic factors unfavorable or bone healing; and C: uncorrectable and not able to tolerate therapy)
2. What is the appropriate diagnosis of osteomyelitis? (Bone biopsy is the gold standard. Culture of soft tissue sinus tracts will not necessarily reveal the causative organism. Imaging modalities include plain X-rays, WBC labeled bone scans, and MRI.)
   (a) Discuss the sensitivity and specificity of the following imaging: plain films, CT scans, WBC labeled indium-111 scans, and MRI. (Plain films and CT scans are specific, particularly with respect to the capability of CT to determine the degree of bone involvement. Neither are particularly sensitive although CT is more sensitive than X-ray. Labeled bone scans are quite sensitive but not specific. MRI is the most accurate in sensitivity and specificity.)
3. Briefly outline the treatment for the following:
   (a) Tibial shaft fracture, managed with an intramedullary nail, complicated by intramedullary infection three weeks later. (Removal of the nail, drainage of any soft tissue infection by reaming of the medullary canal, and application of external fixation)
   (b) A tibial shaft fracture, managed with plates and screws, complicated by wound infection three weeks later. The bone is stable. (The key element is the stability of the hardware and bone. Drainage of the soft tissue infection, intravenous antibiotics, and possibly application of negative pressure wound therapy)
   (c) The same scenario as B, but the time hiatus is six weeks and debridement reveals a non-vascularized, infected sequestrum of bone. (Removal of sequestrum, removal of plates and screws, bone and soft tissue debridement, application of external fixation, and IV antibiotics. The resultant dead space can be addressed with an antibiotic bead packet. After a short hiatus, provision of soft tissue coverage)

Bone Substitutes

Editor's Note: Platelet-rich plasma is discussed in Chap. 11.

1. What are the three groups of biomaterials for use in craniofacial bone surgery? (Bone cement/paste, biomaterials designed to be replaced by bone, and prefabricated polymers)
   (a) Give an example of each. (Hydroxyapatite used as bone paste, demineralized bone as an allograft designed to be replaced by bone, and Medpor® or porous polyethylene)
2. What is the essential recommendation for the reconstruction of bone defects in the craniofacial region in a growing child? (The recommendation after the age of two when the osteogenic capability of the craniofacial skeleton is sharply reduced is the use of autogenous bone. Perhaps, as an inlay, a bioactive material such as a demineralized bone strut could be used although one could question the advisability in a load-bearing situation as the mandible.)
3. Although surgeons would prefer to use autogenous bone for most instances of bony skeletal reconstruction, in what situation would biomaterials be preferred, and why? (Non-load-bearing onlay. Resorption of autogenous bone is high in the absence of load-bearing. An example is a contour defect of the frontal bone.)

4. A commonly employed implant in orbital floor reconstruction is Medpor®. Does the implant become bone? (Probably not. Experimental investigations have determined that a lip of bone develops at the implant edges, and a limited osseous penetration occurs, but the pores of the substance are incorporated in mostly a fibrovascular process.)
5. In the discussion of the structure and components of bone, you request for repair of a bone defect a commercially available hydroxyapatite. Which component of bone would this product reconstitute? (Hydroxyapatite is the mineral crystal of calcium and phosphorus that constitutes the inorganic portion of bone.)
   (a) Alternatively, you request a demineralized bone matrix (DBM). What component of bone does the DBM represent, and what are its limitations? (As the name implies, DBM is cortical bone, processed to remove the calcium and phosphate but retaining the organic matrix including the osteoinductive extracellular proteins and eradicating hopefully the cellular component, osteocytes. DBM, which is commercially available, is highly variable in terms of the processing and final formulation. Few objective studies have been published about the efficacy, and the material is an allograft with the inherent limitations of an allograft. DBM can be combined with autograft but lacks any structural strength. Both hydroxyapatite and DBM are examples of osteoconductive materials, and DBM may also be weakly osteoinductive.)
6. Describe the subsequent biologic process after the implantation of a bone substitute constructed of $CaPO_4$ or $CaCO_2$. (To be successful, the implant must be resorbed and, in parallel fashion, replaced by native bone. By osteoconduction, the crucial cellular elements are introduced into the architecture of the implant-graft by vascular ingrowth, with resorption by osteoclasts and inorganic and matrix deposition by osteoblasts. Ultimately and ideally, the graft is replaced by a stable native bone.)
   (a) What are the limitations of that use? (Any significant bone ingrowth, particularly in larger pieces, is limited, and thus, service as a bone replacement is also limited. These substances are commercially known as Bone Source® by Stryker or Norian® by Synthes. The definition of a critical defect size in the skull is not concise but is approximately 5 cm.)
7. Discuss the properties, use, and limitations of commercially available bone morphogenetic proteins (BMPs). (Off the shelf, BMP is an allograft material by definition. In clinical application, BMP is intended to simulate native BMP's osteoinductive characteristics: stimulate the migration and differentiation of bone progenitor cells as well as angiogenesis. The powder when reconstructed is a paste, so it alone has no structural strength and is most commonly used as an adjunct or bone filler. The principal limitations are the high cost and the inevitable inflammatory response to an allogenic protein. The development of recombinant BMP may partially alleviate this disadvantage.)
8. What is the basic principle underlying the use of a bone substitute in cranioplasty such as Norian®? (Norian® and the competing product Bone Source® are composed of hydroxyapatite paste and as such are osteoconductive and are commonly used in combination with BMP. Since they do not provide any inherent osteoblastic activity, the bone replacement process is by "creeping substitution." The clinical evidence is that cranial defects larger than 4 or 5 cm will be incompletely ossified.)
   (a) Define osseointegration. (Osseointegration is the unification between the native bone and an implanted foreign body by the process of bone deposition, similar to that of primary bone healing. A number of characteristics must be present in the implanted material for the process of osseointegration to occur.)
9. The readings discuss several alloplastic materials for the reconstruction of the cranial vault. Describe the advantages and disadvantages of porous and nonporous implants. What are they? (Nonporous implants do not allow for tissue ingrowth and may have less resistance to infection, particularly if in contact with paranasal sinuses or the nose. Porous implants allow for tissue ingrowth and have a higher resistance to infection.)
   (a) Give an example of a porous and a nonporous implant. (A porous implant is Medpor® (see below) and hydroxyapatite. A nonporous implant is methyl methacrylate.)
   (b) What are the issues with the use of methyl methacrylate for cranioplasty?(Excellent soft tissue is the sine qua non for primary cranioplasty in an adult, but the use of methyl methacrylate is debatable, and a propensity for the development of a biofilm infection and eventual extrusion exists. The use has been largely supplanted by porous polymers.)

In-Service Examination

1. The phases of bone healing and distraction osteogenesis include the following **EXCEPT:**
   (a) Consolidation
   (b) Latency
   (c) Imbibition
   (d) Distraction

2. Wolff's law states that bone incorporation and survival of bone are dependent on:
   (a) Cancellous bone
   (b) Load or stress
   (c) Vascularity
   (d) The necessary presence of BMP

3. Vascularized bone grafts are preferable to non-vascularized ones because of the enhanced:
   (a) Osteogenesis
   (b) Endochondral ossification
   (c) Osteoconduction
   (d) Osteoinduction

Flaps: Physiology, Classification, and Selection

7

Bibliography

Morris SF., Taylor GI., Chapter 2 "Vascular Territories of the Integument", Blondeel, P. N., *Perforator flaps: anatomy, technique, and clinical applications.* Second Edition. (2013), **pgs 31-43.**

Hong J.P., Neligan P.C., Chapter 24: "Flap Physiology, Classification, and Applications", Neligan PC, Plastic Surgery, Elsevier 5th Edition, (2023), Volume 1: pg. **346-413 (this chapter is to be utilized in both Chaps. 7 and 8)**

Saint-Cyr M, Wong C, Schaverien M, et al., "The Perforasome Theory: Vascular Anatomy and Clinical Implications", *Plast. Reconstr. Surg.,* (2009):124(5):**1529-1544.**

Wang W. Z., Baynosa R. G., Zamboni W. A. "Update on Ischemia-Reperfusion Injury for the Plastic Surgeon", *Plast Reconstr Surg.*, (2011); 128: 685e-687e ONLY.

Ghali S. Butler PEM., Tepper OM., et al., "Vascular Delay Revisited", *Plast Reconstr Surg.*, (2007);119(6):**1735-1742.**

The references below have material, particularly videos, that you could reference when either a case arises or when we read that particular module.

Hollock GG and Morris SF, "Skin Grafts and Local Flaps", *PRS*, (2011); 127(1):**5e-22e.**

Saint-Cyr, M., et al., "Perforator Flaps: History, Controversies, Physiology, Anatomy, and Use in Reconstruction", *Plast. Reconstr. Surg.,* (2009); 123(4): **132e-145e.**

Saint-Cyr M, Wong C, Buchel EW, et al., "Free Tissue Transfers and Replantation", *Plast. Reconstr. Surg.*, (2012); 130(6): **858e-878e (Brief description of the major free flaps).**

Faculty Study and Discussion Guide

Classification and Anatomy

1. Describe the basic components of blood supply to the skin including the various plexuses. (The first and deepest plexus encountered is the subdermal plexus lying beneath or within the deepest portion of the dermis, vessels that course through the dermis that are derived from this plexus, some arteriovenous anastomoses that lie within the more superficial dermis, and finally the subepidermal plexus, or papillary plexus, that can be found in the most superficial portion of the papillary dermis. The fascial–subfascial plexus is termed the fascial plexus and lies on the surface of, or deep to, the deep fascia.)
2. Differentiate the following in terms of the anatomy of the blood supply: septocutaneous, musculocutaneous perforator, axial or direct cutaneous vessels, and random flaps. (The paper on perforator flaps attempts to simplify nomenclature. Other than direct vs. indirect, another view is the source of the blood supply. So, musculocutaneous are those perforators that arise from a blood supply to a muscle, course through the muscle, and perforate the fascia to then ramify within the fat and skin. See below. Classification systems have been derived to define whether the blood supply is or not, is initially to the intervening muscle. Septocutaneous vessels arise from the source artery and course through the intermuscular septum to provide perforating vessels into the fat and skin. Classification systems (see below) have also been derived that define further categories of these septocutaneous vessels. Perforator flaps have a specific arterial vessel incorporated into the pedicle, identified by Doppler and/or imaging. Axial or direct cutaneous are those vessels that course directly into the fat and skin without an origin from either muscle or septum. Random flaps have a blood supply that is primarily driven through the subdermal plexus and have no discernible vessel in the base either by Doppler or imaging.)
   (a) Give an example of each. (Musculocutaneous: latissimus; septocutaneous: radial forearm; axial or direct cutaneous: deltopectoral or forehead flap; and random: Z-plasty or simple transposition flap)
3. The "myocutaneous revolution" refers to the description and elucidation of the myocutaneous principle. Describe

E. Luce, *A Curriculum for Plastic Surgery*, https://doi.org/10.1007/978-3-031-62087-4_7

the myocutaneous principle and explain its clinical importance. (The myocutaneous principle, defined, enlarged, and given clinical application by the Emory group in the early and mid-1970s, described that a block of soft tissue including skin, fat, fascia, and muscle could be transferred on the axial blood supply to that muscle alone. The revolution in reconstruction was now possible because of the variety of flaps that could be utilized throughout the body, either pedicled, island, or free, massively expanding the versatility of flap reconstruction. Of course, the next step in the evolution of flap design was the harvest and sacrifice of only a portion of the muscle by dissection of a flap perforator on the skin to the source vessel—a perforator flap.)

4. Draw in cross section the following flaps: random, myocutaneous, and "direct" cutaneous. (The drawing of a random flap should include perforators, regardless of the source, that perfuse the dermal–subdermal plexus, with a drawing illustrating the progressive sacrifice of the perforators as the flap is raised. A myocutaneous illustration should be one that includes skin, muscle, and then, of course, vascular supply, with the perforators traveling through the muscle and emerging from the deep fascia. Finally, a "direct" cutaneous flap would have the main vascular supply in the subcutaneous fat or directly on the deep fascia.)
5. Describe the five types of vascular supply to myocutaneous flaps according to Mathes and Nahai. Give an example of each. (I. Single dominant pedicle: tensor fascia lata and medial gastrocnemius; II. Single dominant and a minor pedicle: gracilis; III. Two dominant pedicles: gluteus max and rectus abdominis; IV. Segmental: sartorius; and V. A dominant pedicle and several secondary pedicled latissimus. See Fig. 7.1.)
   (a) What are the disadvantages of musculocutaneous flaps? (A deformity or dysfunction may exist because of the loss of the particular muscle incorporated in the flap. Also, the bulk of the flap may be excessive in certain reconstructive circumstances.)
6. Cormack and Lamberty describe four types of fasciocutaneous flaps. Describe each and give an example. (A: multiple perforators; sural. B: single large perforators; DIEP. C: multiple perforators along the course of the vessel; fibula, anterolateral thigh flap, and radial forearm. D: includes bone; fibula. Editor's note: The actual anatomy is more important than the classification. A fasciocutaneous flap is nourished by perforators from the subfascial or suprafascial source vessel that requires elevation of the fascia with the flap.)
   (a) What are the disadvantages of fasciocutaneous flaps? (The converse the musculocutaneous flaps, namely, lack of bulk in certain circumstances where dead space exists. In some instances, technically, the harvest of the flap may be difficult. Although a classification has been derived for the vascular supply to the bone and viscera, the classification has no clinical relevance.)

Editor's Note: The discussion about the superiority of myocutaneous versus fasciocutaneous in their ability to decrease bacterial concentration is still unsettled. The variables are the bulk of the flap as well as oxygen or perfusion of the flap under consideration.

Physiology

1. Define and describe the angiosome concept. (An angiosome is a definition of the safe anatomical boundary of tissue that can be transferred safely. The angiosome concept as elucidated by Taylor dictates that the body is composed of three-dimensional blocks of tissue, perhaps 40 in all, that are fed by a single artery and drained by a

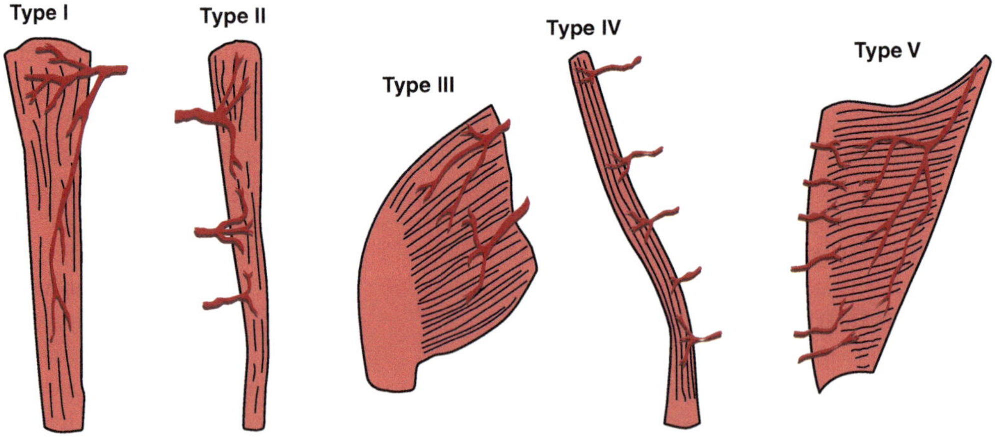

Fig. 7.1 Classification of the Vascular Supply to Muscle. (Buchanan PJ, Kung TA, Cederna PS, "Evidence-Based Medicine: Wound Closure," *Plast. Reconstr. Surg.*, (2014); 134(6):1397. (Reprinted with Permission))

vein. A block may be a composite of muscle, nerve, connective tissue, bone, and the overlying skin. Each block is connected by either a true arterial system or an anastomosis through "choke vessels.")

(a) Define "choke vessels." (Choke vessels lie in the junctional zone between adjacent angiosomes and with a stimulus, delay, for example, have the potential to enlarge and increase in flow. Choke vessels lie principally in the subdermal plexus but may exist in the peri-fascial plexus as well.)

(b) Discuss the argument, pro and con, that zone I of a superior pedicle TRAM is a random flap. (Pro is namely that zone I of a superior pedicle TRAM is a random flap since the vascular anatomy of that area is directly perfused by perforators from the deep *inferior* epigastric artery and that a *superior*-based pedicle TRAM perfusion is through a set of choke vessels. The con of the argument is what constitutes "random." Does one set of choke vessels constitute a random extension?)

(c) A basic principle is that the survival of the tip of any flap is a function of adequate vascular perfusion. Using the angiosome concept, detail how the surviving length of a flap can be increased, and give an example using any flap currently in clinical usage. (An *effective* "delay" of a flap by, presumably, the production of ischemia will open the choke vessels until the adjacent angiosome that will be transferred with the flap is adequately perfused. With the enhancement of flow through the choke vessels into the adjacent angiosome, the probability of survival of the tip of the designed flap is also enhanced. A classic example would be the TRAM flap since zone 1 is the angiosome, and the recruitment of additional tissue from either the adjacent zone 3 or across the midline to zone 2 requires patent choke vessels.)

(d) Define the random component of a groin flap and apply the angiosome concept to the improvement of the probability of survival of that random component. (The random portion is that portion beyond the watershed area of the superficial circumflex iliac artery, an area usually regarded as lateral to the anterior superior iliac spine. An *effective* delay can open the choke vessels into the adjacent angiosome, the lateral hip soft tissue, to improve the probability of survival once transferred as an extension of the standard groin flap. Conceptually, one should visualize the adjacent collateral supply that will require interruption. For example, the elongation of the groin flap will require interruption of the anterolateral extension of the intercostal vessels.)

2. Define effective delay. (The definition of effective can be viewed either technically or functionally. Technically, an effective delay is one that divides all of the collateral circulation to the particular area of tissue to be transferred, except for the major nutrient artery. This procedure usually requires not only incisions along the periphery but also undermining. Functionally, an effective delay is one that produces the maximal amount of ischemia as the inciting phenomenon without, of course, the production of tissue necrosis.)
3. What is the probable explanation of the efficacy of delay? (It is not entirely clear but probably a combination of both morphologic and biochemical changes including reorientation and increase in the size of the blood vessels, the opening of the "choke" vessels a sympathectomy that protects the flap from the effects of sympathetic stimulation, and the metabolic adaptability of the tissue on a cellular level to tolerate a decrease in the blood flow.)
4. Balancing your knowledge of the timelines between the vascular events of the inset of the pedicle flap and the timelines in the delay phenomenon, what seems to be the optimal duration of delay for a flap? (7 days)
   (a) Explain. (Viewed from one perspective, the efficacy of delay is a balance between the beneficial effects on the flap itself and the increase with time of vascular connections between the flap and the recipient bed, which is potentially detrimental once the flap is raised and transferred, as well as the progressive increase in scar fibrosis with time.)
5. What are the principal events that occur in time between an inset of a flap and the recipient bed? (Marked decrease in circulation immediately in the flap, which persists for approximately 12 h; congestive edema evident at 24 h; little change in circulation but increase in number and reorientation of the vessels at 3 days; increase in circulation by day 7; functionally significant vascular connections between the flap and recipient bed are evident by day 7; circulatory function that stays greater than normal for 2–3 weeks; and further development and maturation of vascular connections)
   (a) If true, one should be able to divide the pedicle in 3 weeks. Give a clinical scenario where this conclusion might not be the case. (If the bed is relatively ischemic, such as a chronic radiation wound, or fibrotic. Some evidence exists that <u>less</u> ischemic flaps such as well-vascularized free flaps or myocutaneous flaps may not engender a similar prompt angiogenic response from the recipient bed, and the time for safe division of the pedicle may be prolonged and indeterminate.)
6. The term "perforasome" is the next step in the definition beyond the term "angiosome." How? (The angiosome is

the determination of a major, usually named, arterial supply. The perforator is the terminal branch that will perfuse a block of soft tissue. The imaging of perforasomes beyond angiosomes requires the development of dynamic vascular imaging with CT angiogram, whereas the angiosomes are imaged with radiographic whole-body static imaging.)

7. What are two principles of the perforasome theory? (Each unit of perfusion or perforasome is linked with direct and indirect linking vessels. Direct linking vessels are larger and communicate directly from one perforator to the next and perhaps permit the capture of an adjacent perforasome. Direct linking vessels appear to lie within the subcutaneous fat superficial to the fascia and, as such, could be considered a suprafascial plexus. Indirect vessels communicate by recurrent flow through the subdermal plexus. A second principle is that perforator flaps should be oriented with the long axis in the direction of linking vessels, longitudinal on the extremities and perpendicular to the midline in the trunk. Examples include the lateral arm and ALT, anterolateral thigh, flaps on the extremities, and the internal mammary artery perforator flap on the trunk.)
8. What is the essential underlying mechanism that permits, according to the theory, the recruitment of adjacent perforasomes? (According to the readings, hyperperfusion increases the pressure/flow through the perforator and then, by the direct and indirect linking vessels, perfuses an adjacent perforasome. The occurrence of hyperperfusion is explained by the ligation of all other vessels except for the direct perforating vessel. The inevitable question arises: does the experimental injection reproduce what occurs clinically?)
9. You draw several options for flap reconstruction of a skin defect of the abdomen. Your attending demands that you respect in your selection options a 2:1 length-to-width ratio. Your response is: (The skin territory of any given flap is directly dependent on the vascular anatomy incorporated in the base. So, on the abdomen, if you have incorporated one or more perforators in the base of your flap and you have not crossed the midline, the length can be substantially longer than a 2:1 ratio. The principle is not a length-to-width ratio but rather the vascular anatomy.)
10. The readings compare and discuss surviving lengths of different types of flaps as defined by the flaps' vascular design. Compare the anticipated survival length among three theoretical flaps: a direct flap that contains two perforators at the base, each of X caliber; a myocutaneous flap that has two myocutaneous perforators, each of X caliber; and a direct flap that contains four perforators, each of X/2-caliber. (The first two flaps should be equal in surviving length, the third according to the law that defines flow as to the fourth power of radius theoretically should dictate that arterial inflow considered alone will be but a fraction of the first two, that is 1/16.)
11. The readings describe the systemic and local effects on circulation within a flap. Briefly list the same. (Systemic includes sympathetic regulation through alpha-adrenergic receptors that lead to vasoconstriction and through beta-adrenergic receptors that produce vasodilatation. Humoral and inflammatory mediators that, depending on the agent, can do either. Local effects are a decrease or increase in temperature, pH, or oxygen tension.)
12. What is the probable explanation for the success of the reverse radial forearm and sural flap despite the lack of incorporation of a named venous drainage? (A valveless system in the venae comitantes, which permits retrograde flow)

The Failing Flap

1. Differentiate clinically the findings in arterial and venous insufficiency. (The three clinical characteristics that may be of value in an arterial insufficient flap are that the flap is not firm, bleeds little when pinpricked, and has extremely slow or absent capillary refill. The venous insufficient flap is tense and swollen; bleeds dark red blood profusely; and has rapid, even too rapid, capillary refill.)
2. What is the scientific basis for leech therapy? (Hirudin that is secreted by the leech is an anticoagulant that blocks fibrinogen conversion to fibrin. Also, the leech secretes hyaluronidase. The efficacy is primarily in the use of flaps that suffer venous insufficiency.)
   (a) What are the bacteria at risk derived from the leech GI tract? (Aeromonas hydrophila)
3. With the exception of fluorescein, which essentially is not an all or none type differentiation, what is the inherent difficulty in objective monitoring of pedicle flaps?(The problem is that the gradient or threshold is established for irreversible ischemia. If the flow to skin under normal thermic and resting conditions is about 100 cc per unit of tissue, reduction of that flow can occur down to nearly 4 cc without tissue loss. The safe margin then is lost, and as little as an additional 1-cc reduction in flow can result in tissue necrosis. Currently, we have no consistent, reliable measure that provides information about the discreteness of that gradient.)
4. What is the "no-reflow" phenomenon in free and pedicled tissue transfer? (At about ≥8 h of warm ischemia, irreversible swelling of the endothelial cells with thrombus formation and stagnant blood flow occurs. At the molecular level, vasoactive cytokines and oxygen-derived free radicals are responsible.)

Flaps: Design

8

Bibliography

Jackson IT., Chapter 1 "General Considerations", Jackson IT., *Local Flaps in Head and Neck Reconstruction*, 2nd Edition, (2007), **pgs 8-31.**

Maciel-Miranda, Alejandro, MD, et al., "Local flaps, including pedicled perforator flaps: anatomy, technique, and applications", *Plast. Reconstr. Surg.*, (2013):131:pgs 896-911. **896e-908e ONLY (Including videos 2-4).**

Hundeshagen G, ZApata-Sirvent R, Goverman J, et al, "Tissue Rearrangements The Power of the Z-Plasty", *Clin Plastic Surg*, (2017) 44:pgs 805-812. **805-807 ONLY.**

Mohan AT, Rammos CK, Akhavan AA, et al., "Evolving Concepts of Keystone Perforator Island Flaps (KPIF): Principles of Perforator Anatomy, Design Modifications, and Extended Clinical Applications", *Plast Reconstr Surg.*, (2016);137(6): **1909, 1917-1920, Video 1, 2 ONLY.**

Mohan AT, Sur YJ, Zhu L, et al., "The Concepts of Propeller, Perforator, Keystone, and Other Local Flaps and Their Role in the Evolution of Reconstruction", *Plast Reconstr Surg.*, (2016);138(4):**710e-715e Videos 1, 2 and SDC ONLY.**

Hong JP, Chapter 22: "Flap Classification and Applications", Neligan PC, Plastic Surgery: Volume 1: Principles, 4th Edition, (2017), 22, **366, 393-396 "Flap applications" ONLY.**

Hudson, D.A., "Some Thoughts on Choosing a Z-Plasty: The Z Made Simple", *Plastic and Reconstructive Surgery*, (2000);106(3):**665-668 ONLY.**

Faculty Study and Discussion Guide

Flap Design

1. A conceptual approach to wound closure is the reconstructive ladder. Explain. (The reconstructive ladder is a stepwise logic framework applied to the selection process for options in the reconstruction of wounds. The lowest rung is direct closure, proceeding through skin grafts and local and distant flaps. Since the original description, additional rungs have been added for negative wound pressure therapy (NWPT), dermal matrices, tissue expansion, etc.)
2. A modification of the reconstructive ladder is the reconstructive triangle. Explain. (The reconstructive triangle incorporates microsurgery and tissue expansion. Another expression is the reconstructive elevator, a concept that states that the most efficacious reconstruction may be free tissue transfer. Efficacy is defined as the most likely choice to restore form and function to as close to normal or premorbid as possible with the maximum degree of patient safety. In reality, the most efficacious reconstructive procedure selected should fulfill all of the above criteria.)
3. Flap design and rotation: Discuss and draw the necessary length of a pedicled flap to close a defect 6 x 9 units. (See Figs. 8.1 and 8.2.)
   (a) 30° to the long axis of the defect
   (b) Perpendicular or 90° to the long axis of the defect
   (c) 180°

   (The flap at right angles or perpendicular to the defect will necessarily be considerably longer than the rotation of, for example, 30° because the arc of rotation is greater and length is consumed with the rotation of the flap through a greater arc. Rotation of a pedicled flap of 180° would not be performed with this magnitude of rotation although obviously a propeller-type perforator flap frequently is rotated 180°.)

   (a) Flap Design

   Principles
   - Flap width = 6 × 1.25 for primary flap shrinkage of 20% equals 7.5
   - Flap length = tip to maximum tension point; length necessary to ensure B to B′ without tension
   - Flap base = incorporates a perforator "X"

E. Luce, *A Curriculum for Plastic Surgery*, https://doi.org/10.1007/978-3-031-62087-4_8

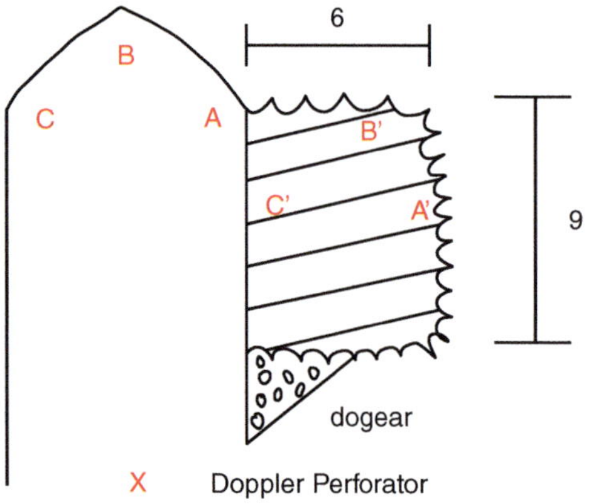

Fig. 8.1 Maximum point of tension

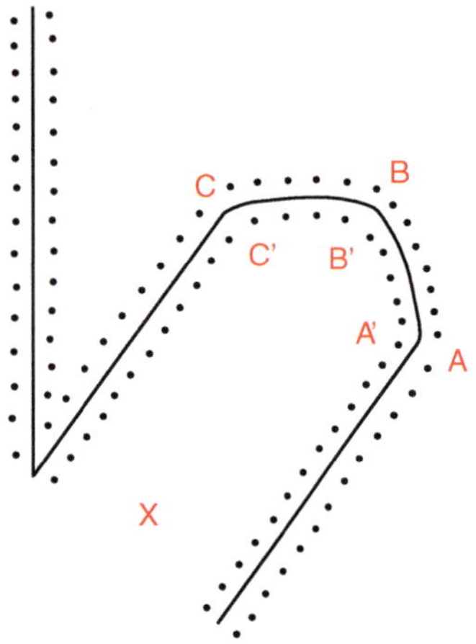

Fig. 8.2 Primary closure donor defect

- Flap rotation angle = minimum necessary to fulfill 1, 2, and 3

(b) Flap Rotated: Primary Closure Donor Defect
Axis of rotation = 37°
Excision of dog-ear

4. Define XYZ axes and points P + O in the description of flap and pedicle design in a perforator flap. (The X, Y, and Z are the three axes in the classic three dimensions of a graph. Y is the axis of blood flow of the flap, X is the transverse diameter at right angles to Y, and Z is the thickness or third dimension of the flap. Point O is the Doppler signal from the perforator of the pedicle while P is the pedicle location itself. Points P to O is the pedicle length.)
5. The design of a Z-plasty consists of two opposing triangles of equal angles. What is the outcome of transposition? (The central limb that joins the two triangles is lengthened and rearranged, theoretically, 90°. In reality, the rearrangement result of the central limb is usually slightly more acute.)
   (a) Give the theoretic elongation of the central limb with triangles of 45° and 60°. (50 and 75%, respectively. A four-flap Z-plasty with flap angles of 45° will produce 100% elongation.)
6. As described in Chap. 7, the incorporation of a perforator in the base or pedicle of the flap is more crucial than the determination of length and width ratio. What are some methods that can assist in the assurance of that incorporation? (Most importantly, a thorough and profound knowledge of the vascular anatomy of the specific region of the body. The use of a handheld Doppler can detect specific perforators based on this anatomic knowledge. CT angiogram can be useful in ambiguous situations but does require the use of IV contrast and high resolution.)
7. What is the framework of perforator flaps? Compare and contrast with musculocutaneous flaps. (A perforator flap is developed on a source vessel, a named anatomic artery, a cutaneous perforator of sufficient caliber to be demonstrable on CTA and/or Doppler exam. In turn, the perforator is dissected retrograde to the principal vessel, the source artery. The flap, now an island on that vessel, is rotated into the defect or harvested as a free flap in preparation for microvascular anastomosis. So, for example, adapted to a myocutaneous flap would be the use of a perforator exiting from the deep fascia of the muscle. The contrast is that instead of incorporating the muscle into the flap, the vessels are dissected through the muscle to be pedicled on the principal blood supply to that muscle, and the muscle is preserved.)
   (a) What are some general guidelines in the axiality of perforator flaps for different regions of the body? (In general, linking vessels from perforator to perforator, a perforasome, are parallel to the long axis of the extremities and perpendicular to the midline of the trunk.)
   (b) What is the adoption of these principles clinically? (The skin paddle should be designed parallel to the anticipated axiality of the incorporated perforator. For example, longitudinal in the extremity, the ALT perforator flap. An example on the trunk is the DIEP flap.)
8. Define "propeller" flaps. (A propeller-type flap is a perforator flap that attains the recipient site by axial rotation about the perforator.)
   (a) What is the principal potential complication? (Venous insufficiency because of the inevitable element of some twisting of the pedicle to accomplish the necessary rotation. The greater the axis of rotation, the greater the potential for compromise of venous drainage. For example, the rotation of propeller flaps 180° mandates the release of any deep fascia surrounding the vascular pedicle and, in some instances, the harvest of a small cuff of muscle.)

9. Define "keystone" flaps. (Keystone flaps are another variation of perforator flaps but differ in a design approach that does not dissect a single perforator but rather incorporates a number of identified vessels, usually with a Doppler, and a block of tissue immediately adjacent to a defect to be reconstructed. Several variations are possible, but probably the most commonly employed is a flap of elliptical design with two parallel incisions, drawn with the concavity oriented on the edge of the defect, a curvilinear trapezoid. Some discussion exists about defect-flap proportions, but a flap larger than 1:1 seems most common. See Fig. 8.3.)
   (a) Briefly describe the sequence of steps in raising a keystone flap. (Again, variations exist, but the width of the flap will hinge on, in addition to the size of the defect, the laxity of the adjacent skin. The immediately adjacent skin is incised, followed by incision of the outer limb skin and deep fascia. Undermining will permit the advancement of the flap. Undermining can be performed, but clearly preservation of the perforators is of paramount importance. Essentially, the keystone design is a bipedicle advancement flap.)
10. Describe and draw a bilobed flap. (A bilobed flap is actually two transposition flaps, the first slightly smaller in width than the defect and the second slightly smaller than the first. The design is the arch of a half-circle, the two flaps lying within the 180° extent, the furthest point of the defect, and the tip of the second flap defining 0° and 180°, respectively. The area of skin laxity adjacent to the defect determines the flap orientation. See Fig. 8.4.)
    Principles:
    - Flap width of 1 is 6 × 0.75.
    - Flap width of 2 is the width of flap 1 × 0.75.

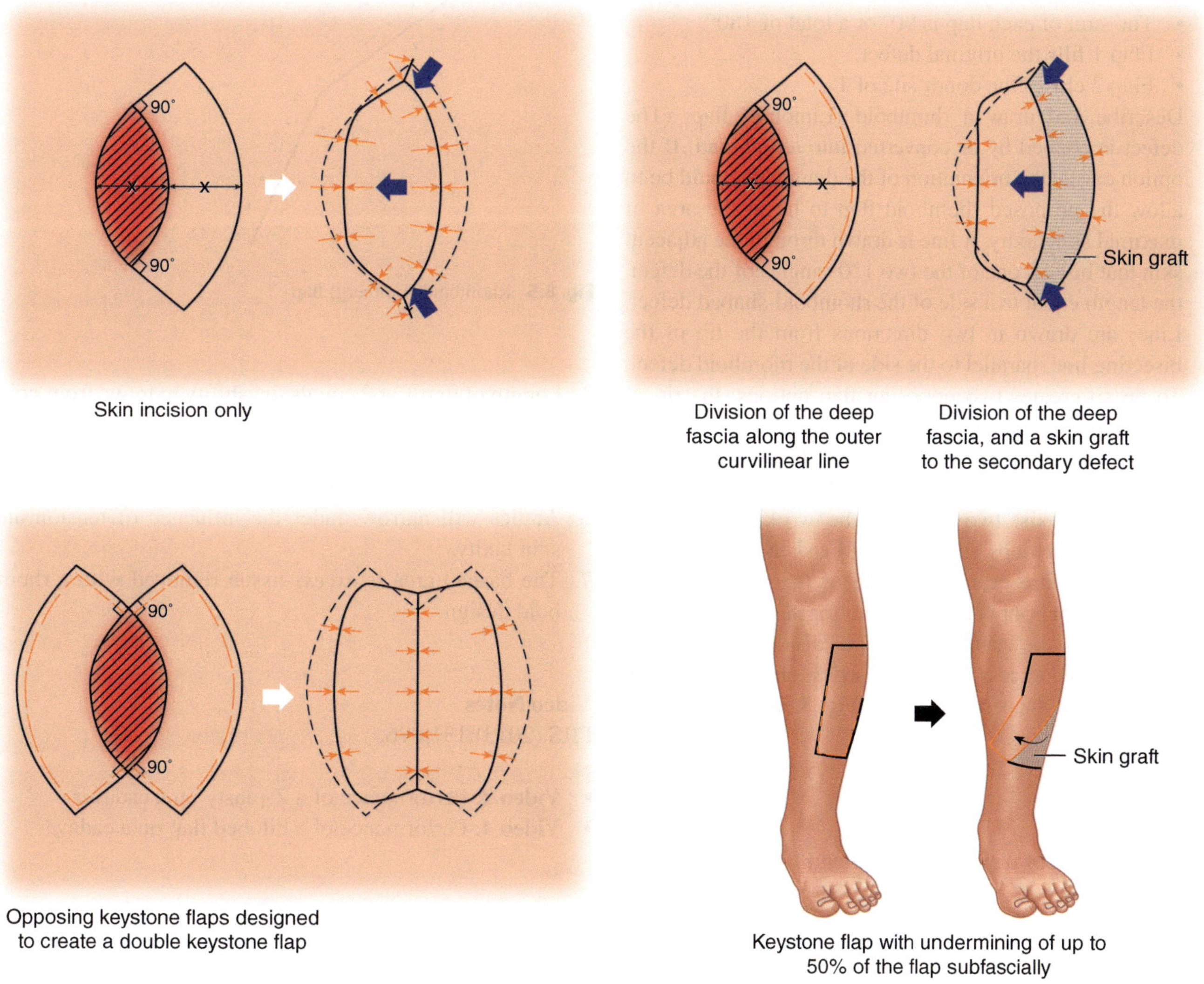

Fig. 8.3 Traditional classification of keystone island perforator flaps

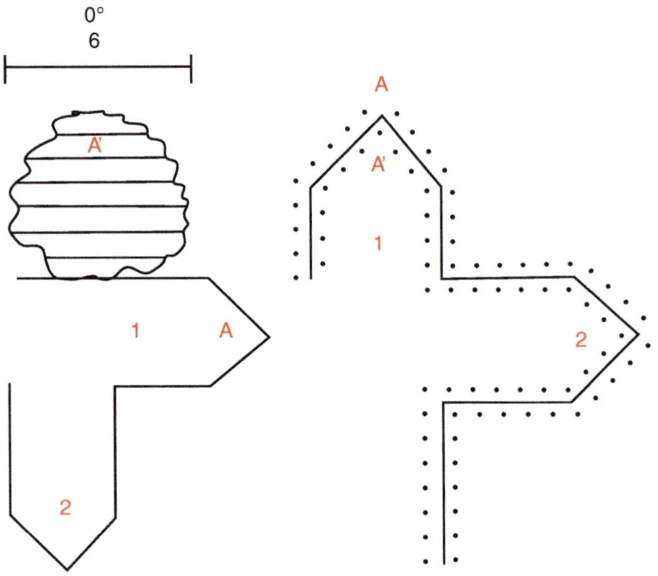

Fig. 8.4 Bilobed flap

- The sum of each flap is 90° or a total of 180°.
- Flap 1 fills the original defect.
- Flap 2 closes the donor site of 1.

11. Describe and draw a rhomboid (Limberg) flap. (The defect is created by or converted into a diamond. If the option exists, the orientation of the diamond should be to allow the proposed rhomboid flap to lie in the area of maximal skin laxity. A line is drawn through the adjacent skin that bisects one of the two 120° angles of the defect, the length equal to a side of the rhomboid-shaped defect. Lines are drawn in two directions from the tip of the bisecting line, parallel to the side of the rhomboid defect. To do so creates two opposing flap options, the tip of each formed by the initial bisecting line. After rotation of the rhomboid flap into the defect, the donor site is closed primarily. For any given rhomboid-shaped defect, four flap options exist, two at each of the two 120° angles.

    Rhomboid flaps should be utilized in areas of skin laxity to ensure primary closure of the donor site. An example of a poor anatomical site for the use of a rhomboid flap is the scalp. A potential disadvantage of the design is the excess tissue excised at either extreme of the diamond-shaped defect. See Fig. 8.5.)

A–B = 6

1. X–Y = 6.
2. A–B or width of flap equals less than 6.

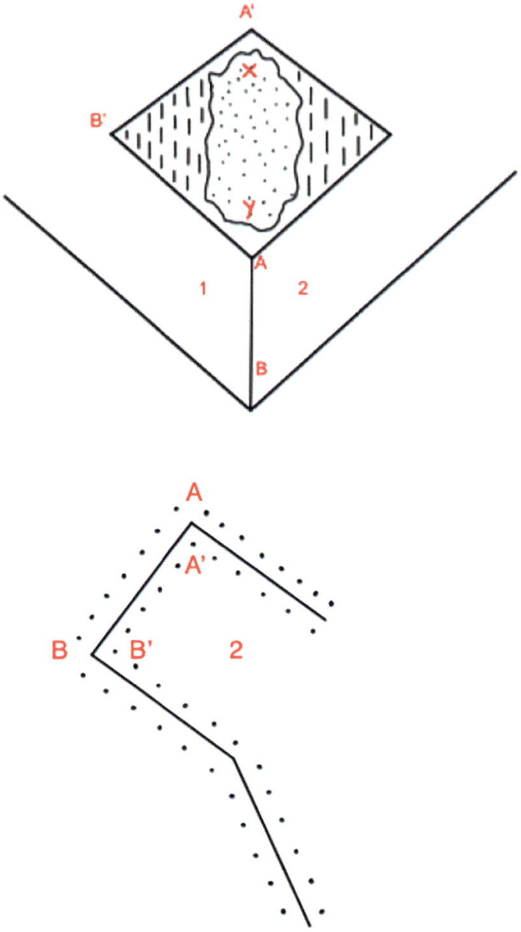

Fig. 8.5 Rhomboid (Limberg) flap

3. Length of flap 1 or 2 equals the ability to move from point A to A' without tension.
4. Width of 1 or 2 = less than 6.
5. Similar two flaps can be designed at the point X'.
6. Angles will narrow under the influence of tension and skin laxity.
7. The hashed area is *excess* tissue removed with a rhomboid design.

Video Notes

PRS (2013);131:896.

- **Video 2**: Performance of a Z-plasty on a cadaver
- **Video 4**: Performance of a bilobed flap on a cadaver

PRS (2016);137:1909

- **Video 1, 2**: Design of a large keystone flap for an anterior proximal thigh defect from sarcoma
- The principle of the technique including division of the deep fascia

PRS (2016);138:710e

- **Video 1**: Propeller flap to close a distal one-third defect of the medial tibia; good demonstration of the principals of adequate proximal dissection of the base to avoid kinking
- **Video 2**: Keystone flap; slide presentation of the principles of cases

In-Service Examination

1. An example of a type I flap according to Mathes–Nahai classification is:
   (a) Gracilis
   (b) Latissimus dorsi
   (c) Sartorius
   (d) Tensor fascia lata
   (e) Gluteus maximus
2. Normal capillary pressure is:
   (a) 6 mmHg
   (b) 12 mmHg
   (c) 24 mmHg
   (d) 36 mmHg
3. The optimal explanation for the efficacy of flap delay is:
   (a) Induction of inflammatory cytokines
   (b) Release of platelet-derived cytokines
   (c) Induction of ischemia
   (d) Induction of the coagulation cascade
4. A planned Z-plasty has flaps of 45°. The estimated increase in length of the central limb is:
   (a) 25°
   (b) 50°
   (c) 75°
   (d) 100°

Flaps: Tissue Expansion

9

Bibliography

Kuehlmann B.A, Brix E., Prantl L.M., Chapter 26: "Tissue Expansion", Neligan PC, Plastic Surgery, Elsevier 5th Edition, (2023), Volume 1: pg. **442.**

Bauer MD, B. S., et al. "The Role of Tissue Expansion in the Management of Large Congenital Pigmented Nevi of the Forehead in the Pediatric Patient", *Plast. Reconstr. Surg.*, (2001), 107(3):**669-675.**

Hallock MD, G. G., "Safety of Clinical Overinflation of Tissue Expanders", *Plast. Reconstr. Surg.*, (1995), 96(1):**153-157.**

Zide MD, B. M. and Karp MD, N. S., "Maximizing Gain from Rectangular Tissue Expanders", *Plast. Reconstr. Surg.*, (1992), 90(3):**500-504.**

Duits, Erwin H.A. M.Sc., et al. "The Modeling of Skin Expanders", *Plast. Reconstr. Surg.*, (1989), 83(2):**364-365 ONLY.**

Austad MD, E. D., Discussion: "The Modeling of Skin Expanders", *Plast. Reconstr. Surg.*, (1989), 83(2):**366-367**.

Van Rappard JH, Molenaar J, Van Doorn K, et al., "Surface-Area Increase in Tissue Expansion", *Plast. Reconstr. Surg.*, (1998); 82(5):**833-837.**

Shively R, Discussion: "Surface-Area Increase in Tissue Expansion", *Plast. Reconstr. Surg.*, (1998); 82(5):**838-839.**

Huang, X, Qu, X, and Li, Q., "Risk Factors for Complications of Tissue Expansion: A 20-Year Systematic Review and Meta-Analysis", *Plast. Reconstr. Surg.,* (2011);**792-797.**

Faculty Discussion and Study Guide

General Principles

1. What are the essential changes with respect to alteration in the dermis and epidermis of skin during the expansion process? (Although one reading was succinct, other readings were less so about the principal changes, but an acceptable response would be an increase in the thickness of the epidermis and thinning of the dermis. Thickening of the epidermis appears to be the result of increased mitosis. The thinning of the dermis may persist.)
   (a) What explains the thinning of scalp hair with the expansion process? (The hair follicles do not undergo expansion with the expansion process, but rather the intervening skin-soft tissue between follicles is expanded. As a result, gross thinning of the scalp hair can occur and frequently does and may or may not recover.)
2. Describe the effect of expansion including thickness on the following:
   (a) Bone (Thinning with normal density with periosteal reaction at the periphery; cranial affected greater than long bones; correction occurs after removal.)
   (b) What is the expansion effect on muscle, for example, the pectoralis during breast reconstruction? (Substantial thinning and atrophy and perhaps even a growth process with an increase in sarcomeres. After the removal of the expander muscle, the mass returns to normal.)
3. Increased vascularity of expanded skin is a well-accepted clinical tenet. Discuss the source of this increased vascularity. (Angiogenesis occurs as a result probably of ischemia of the expanded tissues and skin. Flaps established in expanded skin and soft tissue have significantly greater survival areas when compared with acutely raised and even delayed flaps.)
   (a) In what layer of the capsule is the increase in vascularity found in expanded skin? (The immediate subcapsular layer has increased vascularity. The practical point is with capsulotomies; careful dissection should be just deep to the capsule.)
4. In general, what are the source(s) of the increased surface area obtained with tissue expansion? (Essentially, there are three sources: first is stretching of the existent skin directly overlying the expander; second, the recruitment

E. Luce, *A Curriculum for Plastic Surgery*, https://doi.org/10.1007/978-3-031-62087-4_9

of adjacent skin by pulling that skin into the expanded area; and third, increased mitosis so additional epidermis is generated.)

5. Outline some general principles in the selection and placement of a tissue expander including access incision for placement, type of tissue expander, timing of initiation of expansion, and protocol for repeated expansion. (Generally, the incisions are best placed at the interface between the desired expanded skin and the lesion to be excised or addressed. As the readings emphasize, careful preoperative planning is necessary, which should include the design of the expanded flap to be utilized and the incisions necessary to do so. The expander pocket should be slightly larger than the expander itself so that little in the way of prosthesis folds will occur. The choice between integrated and remote ports leans toward remote ports in non-breast tissue expansion and integrated ports in most cases of breast reconstruction. External ports carry the risk of colonization and possibly infection and, in general, are not utilized. As indicated by one of the papers, a rectangular expander yields size for size and volume for volume a greater amount of expanded skin. A variety of formulas were offered for overall size and volume, but as indicated by two of the papers, the size of the base plate of the expander should be at least two to three times that of the lesion to be addressed. For larger areas, that is not a particularly practical guide; for example, a 100 cm^2 lesion would require a tissue expander of a rectangular design of 16 × 16 cm or 18 × 18 cm, not readily available.

   The readings describe the injection of at least part of the volume of the expander at the time of placement in order to smooth out the expander and fill the pocket. One approach is to place a minimal volume, 30–40 cc, only to smooth out the expander somewhat and to prevent any tension on the suture line created by higher fill volumes that may produce dehiscence and exposure. Expansion is initiated at 10–14 days and the expansion protocol (the number of expansion procedures, volume, and frequency) is dictated by patient pain and ischemia of the overlying skin. If possible, overinflation of the expander should be accomplished. After the design and elevation of the expanded flap, probably a transposition flap, further rotation advancement can be obtained by a release of the capsule at the juncture of the dome and the base since some degree of fibrous contraction or capsular contracture occurs at that point. This release must be done carefully since the blood supply lies just deep to the capsule.)
6. If expansion of a myocutaneous flap is planned, where should the expander be placed? (The potentially random portion of the distal flap would benefit the most from angiogenesis.)
   (a) What are some clinical examples of the use of this concept of expansion of an already-established flap? (One of the most frequently utilized is in extensive resurfacing of head and neck burn scar and contracture, such as the expansion of a supraclavicular flap transferred for resurfacing of the neck and lower face or expansion of a parascapular flap for similar purposes. Of course, expansion of the supraclavicular area and harvest as a free full-thickness graft can also be accomplished.)

Overexpansion and Flap Design

1. The readings were quite candid about complications in the safety of overinflation tissue expanders. Interestingly, the complication rate appears to be lower in the overexpanded than in the under-expanded group. What is the essential point? (The safety of overexpansion, and that overexpansion may allow for more flexibility in the selection of the size and volume of the tissue expander.)
2. From the readings, how much overinflation of tissue expanders can be accomplished? (It is not entirely clear. *Ex vivo* studies indicate that the expanders do not rupture until an expansion volume is 15–80 times the recommended volume of the expander, but that data does not translate to clinical utility. In the reading provided, the largest ratio described was that of 3.5 times the recommended maximal volume, but the mean overexpansion appeared to be approximately 1.5.)
3. What are the three objective parameters or constants in tissue expansion that can be used to calculate the surface area recruited with expansion? (Size, volume, and shape of expanders)
4. What are the variables in tissue expansion described by the readings? (Elastic properties of the particular skin involved, design of the expanded flap, element of primary contracture, and "stretch-back," or the phenomenon also known as stress relaxation or rebound contracture. Also, some expansion occurs inward except over bone.)
5. Now judge the usefulness of a formula or formulas. (The variables overwhelm the mathematics. The elastic properties of skin from individual to individual and on different parts of the body within the same individual, the increase of volume inward rather than outward toward the skin, and the phenomenon of "stretch-back" all invalidate formulas. In addition, one must consider tension/pressure that could rise with an increase in injected volume but no change in the configuration of the expander or the overlying skin, such as could occur with severe capsular contracture.)
6. The readings describe a porcine model to apply the formula derived in vivo. What happened? (In essence, what was determined was some factor multipled by the base of the particular expander base was necessary to recruit the

anticipated skin. The numbers as listed were those of factors of 6, 3.75, and 4.5 in the case of round-, rectangular-, and crescentic-shaped expanders. These numbers were derived by the use of advancement flaps.

At least, those numbers confirm clinical practice that rectangular expanders provide more recruited skin, volume for volume and size for size, than round or crescentic expanders. The multiplication factor of an expander 2.5–3 times that of the defect may not be completely off base if one uses an advancement rather than a transposition flap since the advancement "loses" more because of the double dog-ears, so that method is not the most efficient utilization of expanded skin. See below.)

7. If one does not wish to overexpand, what other options exist to complete the reconstruction? (Successive expansions, namely, the completion of a skin expansion, operative use of the expanded skin to excise a portion of the lesion, and reinsertion of the tissue expander into the pocket with yet another course of expansion. The cumulative complication rate increases with the number of serial expansions.)
8. What is a criterion for appropriate injection volume with an individual inflation or expansion procedure: intraluminal pressure, pain, or color changes in the skin? (All have been used and none are exact. Probably the best clinical guide is ischemic or blanching of the skin as a sign of overexpansion. Patient's pain certainly may be the determinant factor but is, of course, highly subjective and variable.)
9. The readings described three different designs for the use of expanded skin. Describe and comment. (The principal value of the readings was to outline three different methods of using the expanded skin for the reconstruction needed. The papers offered the opinion that the "over-the-top" advancement flap gave "much more tissue gain," but a cursory review of his drawing would indicate that, in actuality, more tissue is discarded and, as termed, is an advancement flap. A more efficient design that utilizes virtually all of the expanded tissue is a rotation flap. The back-cut is a key element. The back-cut enables the design of transposition and additional flap rotation and length obtained up to the point, of course, of vascular embarrassment. Since the vascularity is enhanced in the expanded skin, a narrower pedicle can be tolerated than drawn in Figs. 9.1 and 9.2.)

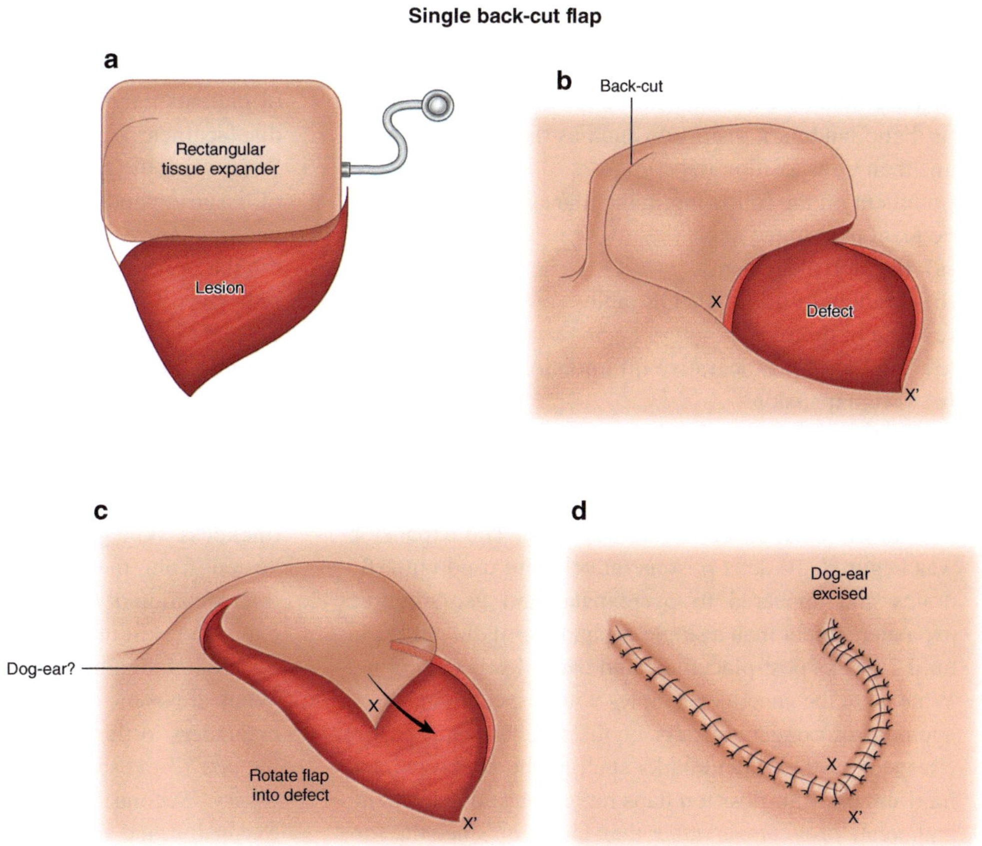

Fig. 9.1 Single backcut flap (**a**, **b**) incisions for flap (**c**, **d**) flap rotated into defect

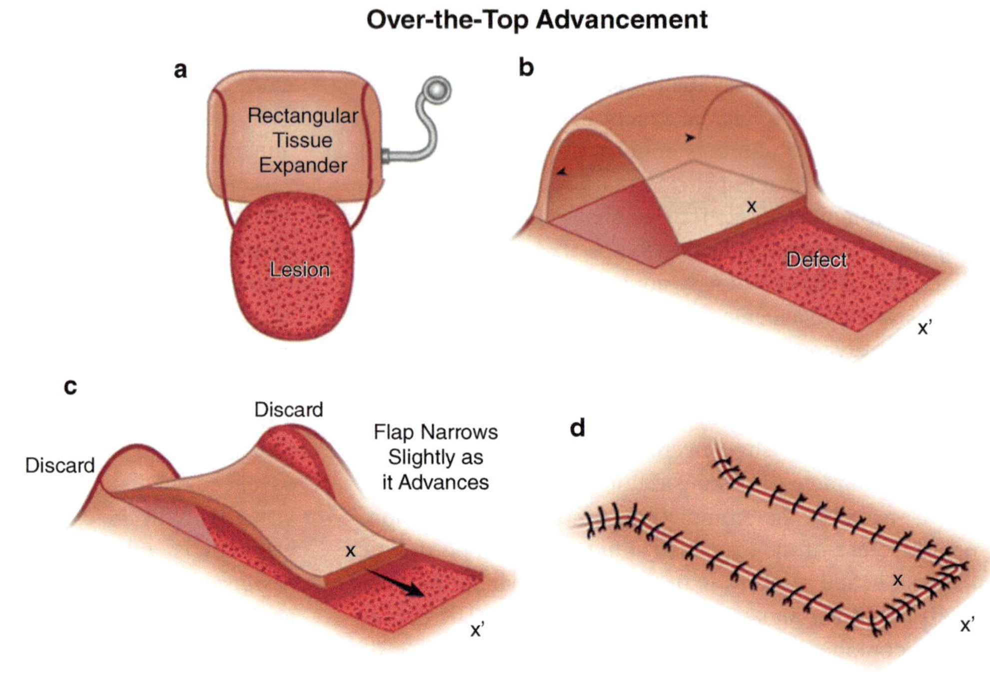

Fig. 9.2 Advancement

Specific Areas and Complications

1. The readings outline the use of tissue expansion in address of large pigmented nevi of the forehead in children. The readings outlined an approach that favored transposition over advancement flaps. Why? (The advancement of expanded skin appeared to create more aesthetic landmark distortion such as the brow and hairline than transposition flaps.)
2. Comment on the following in the management of pediatric giant pigmented nevi:
   (a) Incision placement
   (b) Amount of fill on the OR table
   (c) Use of drains
   (d) Timing of postoperative fill initiation
   (e) Overexpansion

   (From the photographs, the surgeons appeared to place the incisions at the border of the lesions and added a "comfortable intraoperative fill" to smooth the expander and fill the dead space on the OR table. The expansion was begun 7–10 days postoperatively and used butterfly drains and appeared to overexpand and use multiple expanders rather than a single expander. Fill did not begin until 2 weeks post-placement and overfill was common.)
3. What were the general principles with respect to the management of congenital nevi of the forehead and scalp? (Respect aesthetic landmarks such as the eyebrows and hairline; use transposition flaps rather than advancement; and create brow ptosis rather than elevation since the former is much more readily corrected.)
4. Give an overview or your interpretation of the complications incurred with the use of tissue expansion in the lower face and anterior neck in pediatric burn patients. (The incidence of loss of the tissue expander and the reconstruction from either infection dehiscence or flap necrosis appears to be about 10%. An additional 5–10% of patients may require reoperation for expander or port displacement.)
5. What were the general principles with respect to the use of tissue expanders in the face and neck of pediatric burn patients? (A. Advancement of cervical skin over the mandibular border frequently resulted in widening of the inset scar over time. B. Caudal or inferior rotation of the expanded cheek skin seemed superior for mandibular border scars. C. The readings thought that perhaps alternate methods such as an expanded full-thickness skin graft or an expanded cervicofacial/cervicopectoral flap might be more acceptable. Other authors, such as Feldman, have described the use of both expanded full-thickness skin grafts and expanded regional flaps harvested from the neck and upper chest. A reasonable interpretation of these conclusions is that advancement of expanded skin may be the culprit with "stretch back" and resultant widening of the scars.)
6. What are some general principles in the use of tissue expanders in the scalp of children? (First, depending on the size of the scalp lesion, serial expansion may be necessary. Second, the hair follicles are less dense with expansion and may result in thinning of the scalp hair, which may correct over time. Third, some depression of

the skull may be apparent radiographically and even clinically but apparently will resolve with the removal of the expander.)

7. Rank the major anatomical areas of the head and neck, trunk, upper extremity, and lower extremity based on the probability of complications with tissue expansion. (Using the odds ratio, the highest probability is in the lower extremity, followed by the head and neck, upper extremity, and finally the trunk. The difference in odds ratio between the lower extremity and head and neck is quite substantial, which reflects the difficulty with tissue expansion in the lower extremity, particularly below the knee.)
8. What *overall* complication rate would you quote to a potential expansion patient? (15–17%, of which infection, hematoma, exposure, and malposition account for the most.)

Case-Based Conference

Case 1: Scalp Burn Alopecia

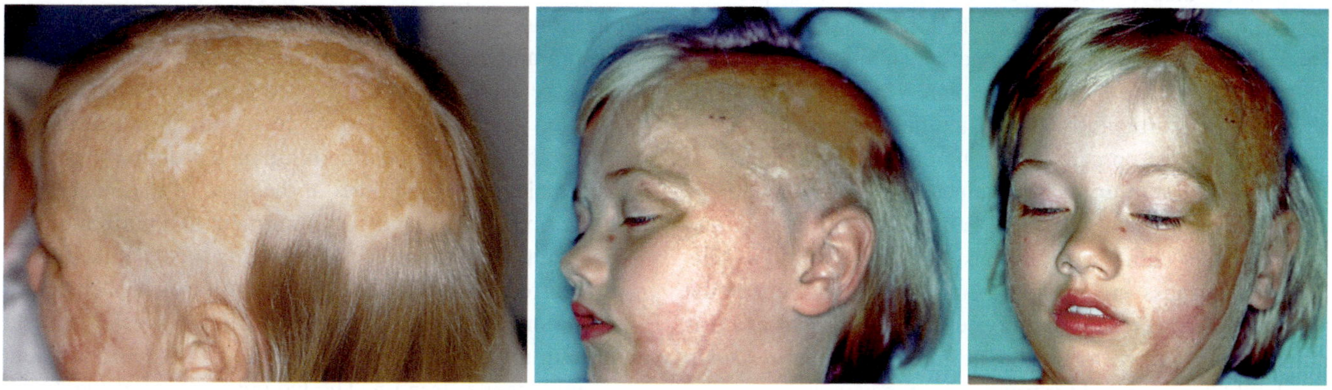

A 5-year-old one-year status-post burns with skin grafting of the scalp

1. Review slides A–C and add a focused clinical examination.
2. Assuming that you select tissue expansion for reconstruction, describe the following:
   (a) Number of expanders, if more than one
   (b) Size and volume of expander(s)
   (c) Configuration of the expanders
3. Describe your access incision(s), postoperative care, and expansion protocol. How would you counsel the parents with respect to complications including the frequency of the same?
4. In image D, draw your incisions for utilization of the expanded skin for reconstruction of the burn alopecia.

Case-Based Conference: Discussion

Case 1: Scalp Burn Alopecia

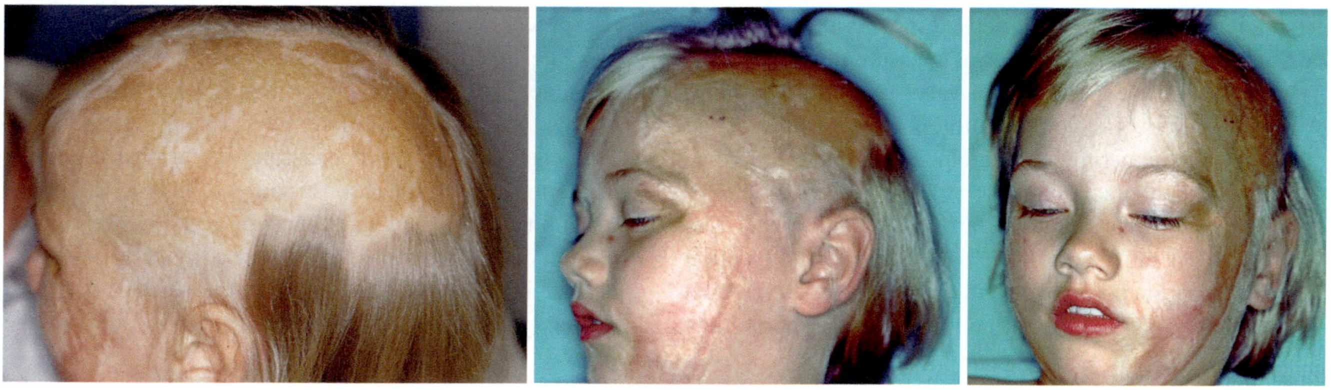

A 5-year-old one-year s/p burns with skin grafting of the scalp

1. Review slides A–C and add a focused clinical examination. (The slides provide three views: left frontal, left lateral, and left oblique. The frontal view is the only depiction of the status of the right scalp and, judged by the hair-bearing area, appears unscarred. Some well-healed, non-hypertrophic burn scars are present on the right cheek. The lateral view demonstrates the left frontal temporoparietal and cranial–occipital scalp, all of which are marked by healed skin grafts, perhaps meshed without ulceration. The remaining hair-bearing scalp in the postauricular and inferior occipital areas is seen in a monkish distribution. No areas of ulceration are present. The oblique view adds little. The left ear is intact.

   The history will probably not glean much information that will impact the treatment plan. The details of hospitalization, particularly any difficulties with general anesthesia or post-op care should be elicited. Particularly, if an inhalation injury was sustained, questions about exercise tolerance will provide a guide to cardiovascular and pulmonary fitness. Questions about the child's self-consciousness are probably superfluous but reflect the surgeon's awareness and concern. The physical exam is relatively straightforward. The intact hair-bearing scalp should be inspected for traumatic or incisional scars. The details about the size and proportion of intact-to-skin-grafted scalp are discussed below.)
2. Assuming that you select tissue expansion for reconstruction, describe the following:
   (a) Number of expanders, if more than one
   (b) Size and volume of expander(s)
   (c) Configuration of the expanders

   (The process of determination of expander selection and location is crucial for a successful outcome for this patient. The elements of that process include planned location or locations, the specifics of size and volume, and the configuration of the expanders. The attendant slides do not provide the exact dimensions of the intact scalp available for recruitment, but the principles in tissue expansion are the same. Once the potential locations are selected, the width and length of the donor site are measured to calculate and select the tissue expander. Curiously, for any given set of measurements, the volumes of tissue expanders will vary substantially among manufacturers. The configuration is of some importance as well since experimental work indicates that rectangular-shaped expanders, volume for volume, will yield greater surface area than round- or crescent-shaped ones. The other preoperative decision is the type, size, and location of the injection ports. In general, remote ports are favored in children, particularly in the scalp. Remote ports must be placed at a distance from the expander cavity and secured with sutures to avoid postoperative inversion. A low-profile and small port will exert less tension on the skin.)
3. Describe your access incision(s), postoperative care, and expansion protocol. How would you counsel the parents with respect to complications including the frequency of the same? (Once the location, number, and size of expanders are established, the access incisions are planned. To do so requires an analysis that incorporates the design of the final excisions for the harvest of the recruited skin from the expansion, followed by the selection of the initial access incisions. Experience has demonstrated that the second-stage design should be the use of transposition or rotation flaps rather than flap advancement by parallel incisions. Although the latter is considerably simpler in design and execution, advancement only fails to advantage the recruited and expanded skin to the degree that rotation flaps afford. Two access options are available, one within the hair-bearing scalp on a proposed flap rotation incision and the other at the edge of the defect. The limitation of the first is a commitment to a portion of flap design; the limitation of the second is access at the border of scarred tissue. If the second option is the choice, a minimum postoperative interval of two weeks prior to initiation of expansion is necessary to ensure sufficient wound tensile strength. The wound consists of the development of the expander cavity by subgaleal dissection slightly larger than the expander dimensions to avoid wrinkling or folds in the expander. Intraoperatively, a low initial volume of 25–50 cc of saline is placed. Drain placement should be short-term, 3 days, and as described, expansion is deferred for 2 weeks. The wound is closed in layers. Although expansion protocols differ widely, the volume of each weekly injection should be limited to 25–50 cc or 10% of the expander volume. One option is, after one or two postoperative visits, the implementation of home injections by the parents. Telemedicine offers the opportunity for healthcare provider supervision during the process. The end point is established by a dwindling injection volume possible because of increased tissue tension.

   The family should be counseled about the postoperative process of possible complications. The risk of early and late infections, expander exposure, and loss of the expander in the scalp is approximately 10%. Management in these scenarios is a different discussion.)
4. In image D, draw your incisions for utilization of the expanded skin for the reconstruction of the burn alopecia. (Planning the second-stage incision requires the consideration of two elements: first, the maximal address of the defect, i.e., the use of the expanded skin in the most advantageous rotation, and second, the location of the

base of the flap. The anterior expander flap should be based or the pedicle posterolaterally on the intact scalp to reconstruct the anterior defect and hairline. Two options exist for the posterior expander, one based posterolaterally on the right or posterolaterally on the left. The former would recruit unexpanded skin at the tip of the flap. The latter would not provide the most advantageous design for the expanded skin.)

Intraoperative

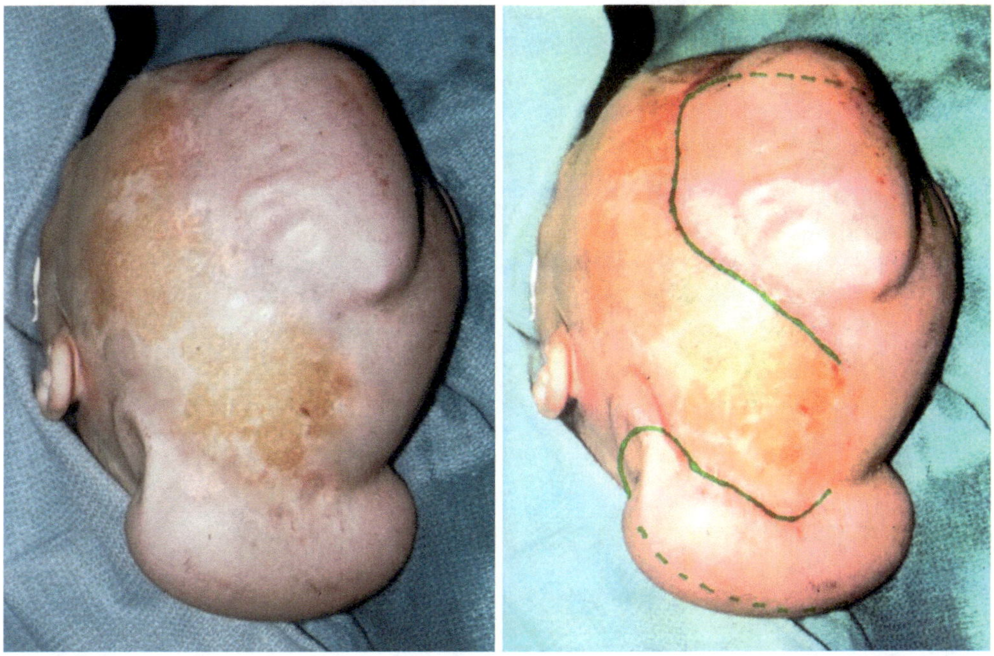

Two rectangular tissue expanders have been employed, frontal and occipital and fully expanded. The initial incisions for the creation of the rotation flaps are drawn.

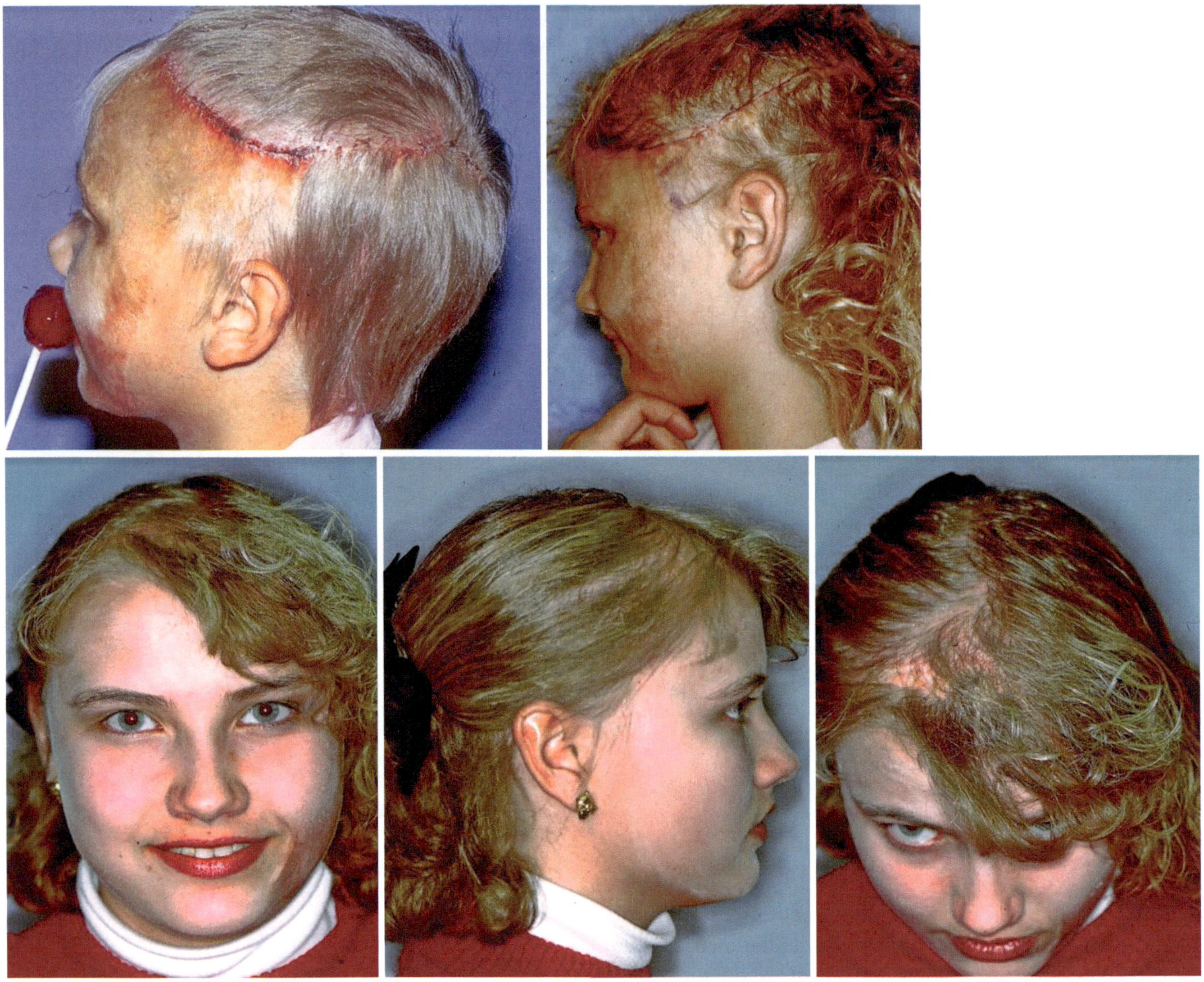

Postoperative

A series of slides demonstrates some of the steps in the expansion and flap utilization process, followed by photos of the late results.

The slides include an AP and oblique that demonstrate an expander in place, followed by a lateral view of an intermediate stage, immediately postoperative, and finally, also in lateral view, the completed reconstruction. The late follow-up, the patient as a young adult, illustrates a full head of hair and faded, flap facial burn scars. The last photo with the neck flexed reveals a hairless area that begins behind the frontal hairline on the right, triangular shaped and apex directed posteriorly that measures 2 × 3 cm. The area appears to be a scar.

Critique

If the patient desires treatment, the adjacent scalp should be assessed for mobility. The two options are hair transplantation by the follicular unit technique or excision of the alopecic element. Repeated multiple expansions of the same area of the scalp can result in alopecia as perhaps a manifestation of some relative ischemia-tension without overt tissue loss. Those small areas of alopecia can be receptive to hair transplantation. Overt scarring would be more optimally managed with excision, undermining, and closure.

In-Service Examination

1. The principal changes of the skin in tissue expansion are:
   (a) Thickening of the epidermis and dermis
   (b) Thinning of the epidermis and dermis
   (c) Thickening of the epidermis and thinning of the dermis
   (d) Thinning of the epidermis and thickening of the dermis

2. In an estimation of the surface area recruited in tissue expansion, the independent variables include the following **EXCEPT:**
   (a) Thickness of the prosthesis envelope
   (b) Size of the prosthesis
   (c) Volume of the prosthesis
   (d) Shape of the prosthesis
   (e) Elastic property of skin
3. The optimal location for placement of a scalp tissue expander is:
   (a) Subperiosteal
   (b) Subgaleal
   (c) Subcutaneous
   (d) Superficial to the frontalis

10 Microsurgery

Bibliography

Wei F.C., Lintay S.K., Deek M.F., Chapter 25: "Principles and Practice of Microvascular Surgery", Neligan PC, Plastic Surgery, Elsevier 5th Edition, (2023), Volume 1; pg. **414.**

Fan JL, Patel KM, Mardini S, et al., "Evidence to support controversy in microsurgery", *Plast. Reconstr. Surg.*, (2015); 135(3):**595e-603e.**

Wilson, J. L., et al., Chapter 12: "Avoiding complications." Wei, Fu-Chan and Mardini, S., Flaps and Reconstructive Surgery, Saunders Elsevier, (2009), **pp 117-124.**

Smit JM, Zeebregts CJ, Acosta R, Werker PM, "Advancement in free flap monitoring in the last decade: A critical review", *Plast. Reconstr. Surg.*, (2010); 125(1):**177-185.**

Davison SP, Kessler CM, Al-Attar A, "Microvascular free flap failure caused by unrecognized hypercoagulability", *Plast. Reconstr. Surg.*, (2009); 124(2):**490-495.**

Pannucci CJ, Kovach SJ, Cuker A, "Microsurgery and the Hypercoagulable State: A Hematologist's Perspective", *Plast. Reconstr. Surg.*, (2015); 136(4): **545e-552e.**

Haeck PC, Swanson JA, Schechter LS, et al., "Evidence-Based Patient Safety Advisory: Blood Dyscrasias", *Plast. Reconstr. Surg.*, (2009); 124(4S):**82S-95S.**

Sezgin B, Ayhan S, Tuncer S, et al., "Hypercoagulability in Microvascular Breast Reconstruction: An Algorithmic Approach for an Underestimated Situation", *J Reconstr Microsurg*, (2012);28:**515-519.**

Schoenbrunner A., Hackenberger P.N., DeSanto M., Chetta M., "Cost-Effectiveness of Vioptix versus Clinical Examination for Flap Monitoring of Autologous Free Tissue Breast Reconstruction", *Plast Reconstr Surg.*, (2021);148(2):**185e-86e, 187e-88 (Skip Methods and Results).**

Seruya M and Baker SB, "CME Article: Venous Thromboembolism Prophylaxis in Plastic Surgery Patients", *Plast. Reconstr. Surg.*, (2008); 122(3):**2, 4 ONLY.**

For Lab

- Chang DS, Janis JE, and Garvey PB, Chapter 8: "Basics of Microsurgery", Essentials of Plastic Surgery, Second Edition, St. Louis, Quality Medical Publishing, (2014); **pgs. 75-86.**

Wang W, Chang TS, Yi-Lu S, Chapter 3: "Basic Techniques and Operative Methods in Microsurgery", Principles, Techniques and Applications in Microsurgery, Chang TS, World Scientific Publishing, (1986); **pgs. 16-34.**

Shen-Xiu Z, Chapter 9: "Common Causes of Failure in Tissue Transplant and the Preventive Measures", Principles, Techniques and Applications in Microsurgery, Chang TS, World Scientific Publishing, (1986); **pgs. 70-75.**

Supplemental

- Saint-Cyr, M., Wong, C., Buchel, E. W., Colohan, S., Pederson, W. C. "Free tissue transfers and replantation", *Plastic and reconstructive surgery*, (2012); 130(6):**858e-878e (Brief description of major flaps).**

Faculty Discussion and Study Guide

Editor's Note: A considerable proportion of the readings for the Microsurgery module are technique-oriented. This faculty discussion and study guide focuses on the cognitive aspects of microsurgery.

Technology and Design

1. Discuss the pros and cons of the two magnification systems in microsurgery: microscope vs. loupes. (A series has been published of free flap transfer with the use of 3.5–4.5 loupes only with a 98–99% success rate.

E. Luce, *A Curriculum for Plastic Surgery*, https://doi.org/10.1007/978-3-031-62087-4_10

Although loupes offer the advantage of more mobility of the surgeon, the microscope offers the advantage of variable magnification, a quality particularly valuable in smaller-vessel anastomoses 1.5 mm or less and microvascular surgery in children.)

2. A loupe salesman comes by and offers a cheaper type of loupe. What types of loupes are available, and what are their characteristics? (Two types of surgical loupes exist: compound or Galilean and prismatic or Keplerian, invented by Galileo and Kepler, respectively. The former is much more common and employs a set of two lenses. The latter has multiple lenses incorporated into higher magnification. Prismatic loupes have better optical quality with improved magnification and a wider and longer depth of field or working distance, particularly at magnification of greater than 2.5×. Routine loop use, not microvascular use, can be accomplished with compound optics at a lower cost. The principal disadvantages are cost and more weight, particularly with increased magnification.)
   (a) What other factors need to be considered in the selection of loupes besides magnification? (The actual design, namely, through the lens of eyeglasses or, in contrast, flip-up, working angle, and focal length.)
3. Discuss the use of a coupling device for anastomosis including contraindications and efficacy. (The principal contraindications for the use of a microsurgery coupling device are the presence of prior irradiation damage with thickening, atherosclerotic calcification, and small microvessels, perhaps less than 1.0–1.5 mm in diameter. The efficacy in experienced hands is a patency rate equal to handsewn anastomosis although predominantly used for the venous side.)
4. Essentially, what are the difficulties in the adaptation of tissue adhesives to microvascular surgery? (The cyanoacrylates, used for skin closure, are quite tissue-toxic. Similar concerns arise from the use of fibrin glue with possible allergic reaction or intraluminal seepage of the glue.)
5. Discuss the role of imaging of recipient and/or donor vessels. (The topic is not readily summarized within this question because of the variability of the individual patient circumstances. In brief, imaging techniques available include the color duplex sonography, CT or MRI angiography, and conventional angiography. CT angiography requires the use of contrast, whereas MRI does not, but resolution may not be as optimal, and the efficacy of color duplex sonography is highly user-dependent. Conventional angiography requires a femoral puncture and the use of contrast with possible nephrotoxicity.)
6. Define the following: chimeric flaps, supermicrosurgery, and prefabricated and prelaminated flaps. (Chimeric flaps are multiple flaps harvested on the same pedicle. An example would be serratus anterior and latissimus dorsi muscle flaps harvested as two separate entities on the same thoracodorsal pedicle. Supermicrosurgery is the term applied to the harvest and performance of vessels less than a millimeter in diameter such as suprafascial perforator flaps. Prefabricated refers to the implantation of a vascular pedicle only into the soft tissue with a necessary hiatus and ultimate harvest of the resultant flap. Finally, prelaminated refers to the process of placement of tissues within the flap to eventually be harvested. An example would be the placement of ear cartilage on the forehead as a preliminary procedure in preparation for transfer for nasal reconstruction.)
7. Discuss the timing and sequence of flap inset vs. vessel anastomosis. (Intuitively, reestablishment of blood flow and perfusion of the flap would assume primacy over the flap inset, but mechanical factors may dictate the flap inset first. After circulation is restored, the flap swells and obviously will bleed from the edges and can render the inset of the flap difficult, particularly in the head and neck. In some instances such as free flap breast reconstruction, the anastomosis will be sufficiently deep that the anastomosis will need to be completed first.)
8. What are the indications for vein grafts in microvascular surgery? (The indications are obvious: tension at the arterial anastomosis, a short pedicle on the harvested flap, and the necessity of an anastomosis to recipient vessels outside of either an irradiated, scarred, or traumatically damaged field.)
   (a) What are the disadvantages? (The evidence would indicate that the overall success rate when vein grafts are deemed necessary is lower than primary anastomosis, probably a reflection of the operative circumstances and two anastomoses.)
9. Discuss the impact of the following on the risk of microvascular complications: age, obesity, smoking, and prior radiation therapy. (If one uses the strict definition of microvascular complications, only prior radiation therapy in the head and neck increases the incidence of microvascular complications. If the definition is expanded to all complications, obesity and smoking both increase the frequency of complications. A number of papers have been written that would indicate that age alone should not be used as a contraindication to the performance of microvascular surgery. In summary, limiting the definition of complications to the anastomosis alone is of little value in surgical decision-making.)
10. Discuss the patency outcome between end-to-end and end-to-side anastomosis. (If all other variables are equal, no difference exists in the patency rates between the two types of repair.)

Intraoperative

1. What mechanical factors can contribute to vasospasm, and what is the treatment? (Certainly, the systemic factors of hypothermia and hypovolemia can play a role, but mechanical factors are usually the etiology of vasospasm. The treatment is adventitial stripping, which is essentially a local sympathectomy of the vessel.)
   (a) List the topical agents that may be used to treat vasospasm. (The most common agents are 2–4% lidocaine, papaverine, and a calcium channel blocker such as nifedipine.)
2. What is the recommendation if the free flap is raised under tourniquet control? (The readings suggest 0.5 mg/kg of unfractionated heparin intravenous.)
3. Comment on the use of anticoagulation postoperatively. (Little has been accomplished in the way of a carefully controlled study, but once-a-day aspirin is equivalent to subcutaneous heparin in terms of efficacy with less complications. While widely practiced, the use of a postoperative anticoagulant, with a single exception of one publication to lower the incidence of anastomotic thrombosis, lacks evidence-based efficacy. The exception is the 1998 Khouri publication that prospectively demonstrated value in the use of subcutaneous heparin postoperatively.)
4. What period of time is the use of unfractionated heparin locally efficacious for? (The half-life of unfractionated heparin is about 5 h.)
5. With respect to Dextran 40, what are the potential complications? (Volume overload, severe allergic reactions, even anaphylaxis, and in severe instances, acute renal failure. Dextran is uncommonly utilized in microvascular surgery because of the complication profile.)
6. Describe the characteristics of arterial pulsation that may indicate partial or total thrombosis. (A longitudinal pulsation of the arterial vessel may indicate partial or total thrombosis. In contrast, a transverse, horizontal, or bulging pulsation is a normal finding.)
7. Describe a test of venous patency. (Probably the most commonly employed test is the stripping maneuver, which consists of the placement of two vascular clamps in close approximation on the distal vein and then stripping the vein proximally and ascertaining filling. This is a maneuver that should be done carefully because intimal damage can occur with repeated stripping.)
8. Leeches have been utilized in venous insufficiency. What are some of the potential side effects and complications? (Blood loss can be substantial, particularly with larger blocks of tissue such as a flap, and may require multiple transfusions. Blood loss in instances like fingertips and ears is less. The second potential problem is infection by the predominant organism in the enteric tract of leeches, *Aeromonas hydrophilia*.)
   (a) What is the recommended antibiotic? (Bactrim or a fourth-generation cephalosporin)
9. Besides clinical monitoring, other technology available includes an implantable Doppler, color duplex sonography, near-infrared spectroscopy, the laser Doppler, and microdialysis. Briefly describe each with the pros and cons. (The implantable Doppler is the cheapest and, perhaps, is equivalent to the other three methods in efficacy. Reading the monitoring system is relatively simple, and the expense, compared to the other three, is low. The principal disadvantage is the accurate placement and retention of the cuff on the anastomosis and the necessity to retain the cuff within the wound after the removal of the probe. This method is probably the best choice for buried flaps. Color duplex, as described in an earlier question, is highly user-dependent, time-consuming, and relatively expensive. Near-infrared spectroscopy is as accurate as any of the systems described, but in the early postoperative period when a slight decrease in oxygen saturation can exist as a normal response of free flaps, the readings may not be as reliable. The laser Doppler is probably the most widely utilized of the three monitoring systems and is as economical as the implantable Doppler. Some experience is necessary since trends rather than absolute readings may be more indicative of flap failure. Microdialysis is a more recent technique that samples the biochemistry of the flap through small double-lumen catheters. The pro is perhaps a detection of vascular compromise before clinical signs are evident. The con is the lag time, 30 min, to obtain readings; yet, it may have a value in buried or intraoral flaps. Limited experience has been published to date. Finally, a cutaneous perforator can be located intraoperatively with a hand-held pencil Doppler and marked for postoperative monitoring, also with the Doppler. See Table 10.1.)
   (a) Is the cuff of the implantable Doppler placed on the artery or the vein? Why? (On the vein. Arterial flow may persist for several hours after the thrombosis of the vein.)
10. What is the gold standard in free flap monitoring? (The gold standard in the monitoring of any flap, free or pedicled, is a frequent, skilled clinical examination. The thrust and argument for flap monitoring technology is the potential for much less or perhaps no postoperative ICU placement, but the evidence still favors clinical examination as the most cost-effective monitoring mechanism.)

Table 10.1 Different monitoring methods compared with the criteria of Creech and Miller

Monitoring technique	Positive predictive value	Negative predictive value	Continuous	Invasive	Direct	Easy to interpret	Simple technique	Applicable to all types of flaps	Costs
Conventional methods			–	–	+/–	–	+	–	
Implantable Doppler system	81–93%	100%	+	+	+	+	+	+	$3100 (monitoring box) $412 (disposable probe)
Color duplex sonography	100%	100%	–	–	+	–	–	+	$30,000–$225,000
Near-infrared spectroscopy	100%	100%	+	–	+	+	+/–	–	$16,500 (monitoring box) $150 (disposable sensor)
Microdialysis	90%	100%	–	+	–	–	–	+	$52,000 (analyzer) $570 (catheters, reagents, and consumables)
Laser Doppler flowmetry	94–100%	100%	+	–	+	+/–	+/–	–	$5460 (laser Doppler flowmeter) $1015 (probe, per ten cases)

Smit J.M., Zeebregts C.J., Acosta R., Werker P., "Advancements in Free Flap Monitoring in the Last Decade: A Critical Review", *Plast Reconstr Surg.*, 125(1):p 177-185. (Reprinted with Permission)

Flap Re-exploration

1. Define ischemia–reperfusion injury. (Prolonged periods of ischemia, particularly warm ischemia time, will create a phenomenon known as "no-reflow." The pathophysiology is ischemic tissue injury, particularly to the intima, with the release of cytokines including reactive oxygen species that in turn produce an inflammatory response and cellular swelling, platelet aggregation, and thrombosis in the small vessels of the flap. The duration of ischemia necessary to produce this injury varies from tissue to tissue.)
2. Given no other variables, what percent would you quote the microvascular consultation patient for re-exploration in flap failure? (An estimated 8–10% probability of return to the operating room for exploration and an overall 2–4% incidence of flap failure)
3. When do most flap failures occur? (0–24 h and only 10% after 72 h)
   (a) What might be the more likely etiology, rather than anastomosis failure, for a flap failure at 48 h? (More likely, an external compression source such as dressings or possibly a hematoma beneath the flap)
4. What are some of the technical recommendations for the re-exploration of a flap, which, upon milking of the vessels, reveals patency? (Open the anastomosis to inspect for thrombi and probably do a ring resection of the anastomosis with the assumption that some intimal injury has occurred.)
   (a) If milking reveals no patency (Open anastomosis for a probable thrombus; redo the anastomosis.)
5. What is the general recommendation for the use of mini-Fogarty catheters in instances of re-exploration? (Pass the vessels through the recipient vessels only.)
   (a) What is the role of r-TPA? (The use needs to be carefully considered because of potential systemic absorption and bleeding. Infusion of a bolus of recombinant TPA into a flap may lyse small vessel thrombosis. When given through the venous side the vessel, should be left open to allow efflux of the TPA.)
6. Hypercoagulable states secondary to genetic disorders are an important concern for the microvascular surgeon. Give three examples. (Factor V-Leiden, antiphospholipid syndrome, and increased homocysteine)
7. What are the medical history findings suggested by the presence of a hypercoagulable state? (Family history, history of bleeding after dental procedures, severe menometrorrhagia, and multiple miscarriages. See Fig. 10.1.)
8. List some intraoperative findings that may indicate a hypercoagulable state. (Prompt re-occlusion after an anastomotic revision, recipient vessels remain flaccid, and administration of local anti-vasospastic and thrombolytic agents are of no value)
9. What is the recommended panel of tests if suspicions, either on history or prior microvascular failure, exist? (Test for the presence of factor V or Leiden mutation, proteins C and S deficiency, antithrombin III deficiency, and increased homocysteine levels.)

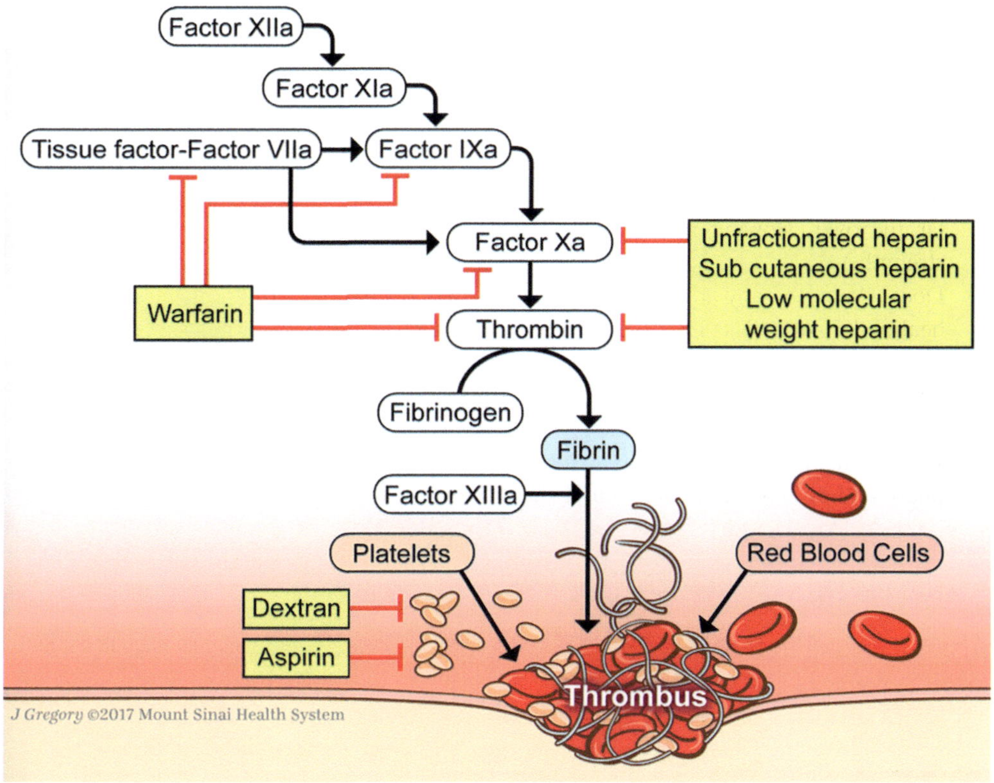

Fig. 10.1 The Coagulation cascade (Abraham et al. Thromboprophylaxis in Head and Neck Microvascular Reconstruction. *Craniomaxillofac Trauma Reconstruction*, (2018);11:92. Reprinted with permission from ©Mount Sinai Health System)

10. In the absence of a positive history, what is a reasonable panel blood test, reasonable from the aspect of cost and positive yield? (Activated partial thromboplastin time, INR, platelet count, and perhaps homocysteine levels)

In-Service Examination

1. Arterial thrombosis of a microvascular anastomosis is most likely to occur in:
   (a) 0–24 h
   (b) 24–36 h
   (c) 36–48 h
   (d) 48–72 h
   (e) Greater than 72 h
2. The principal value of the use of a venous coupler for venous anastomosis is:
   (a) Decreased time for accomplishment of the anastomosis
   (b) Ease of use
   (c) Decreased incidence of thrombosis
   (d) Decreased twisting or kinking
3. A patient has a documented family history of Leiden disorder. The pathophysiology of Leiden disorder is:
   (a) Intrinsic platelet dysfunction
   (b) Elevated plasminogen levels
   (c) Protein S deficiency
   (d) Increased resistance to activated protein

Biomaterials

11

Bibliography

Sivaray D., et al., Chapter 31: "Implants and Biomaterials", Neligan PC, Plastic Surgery, Elsevier 5th Edition, (2023), Volume 1: pg. **544.**

Jones I, Currie L, Martin R, "A guide to biological skin substitutes", *British Journal of Plastic Surgery*, (2002); 55:**185-91 ONLY.**

Nyame TT, Chiang HA, Leavitt T, et al, "Tissue-Engineered Skin Substitutes", *Plast. Reconstr. Surg.,* (2015); 136(6): **1379, 1383-87 ONLY.**

Panayi AC, Orgill DP, " Current Use of Biological Scaffolds in Plastic Surgery", *Plast. Reconstr. Surg.*, (2019); 142(1): **209e-217e ONLY.**

Yannas IV, Orgill DP, Burke JF, "Template for skin regeneration", *Plast. Reconstr. Surg.*, (2011); 127(1S):**60S-64S.**

Jordan SW, Fligor JE, Janes LE, et al, "Implant Porosity and the Foriegn Body Response", *Plast. Reconstr. Surg.*, (2018); 141(1): **103e-109e ("Absorbable Foreign Body") ONLY.**

Davis Jr. SS and Freitas AM, Ch. 6 "Tissue biologics in abdominal wall reconstruction", Loskin A and Janis JE, Advances in Abdominal Wall Reconstruction, Quality Medical Publishing, (2012); **pp. 99-115.**

Grant SA, Ramshaw B, Ch 5. "Synthetic Mesh in Abdominal Wall Reconstruction", Loskin A and Janis JE, Advances in Abdominal Wall Reconstruction, Quality Medical Publishing, (2012);**79-85 ONLY.**

Faculty Discussion and Study Guide

Editor's Note: Biomaterials are also included in Chaps. 6, 56, 60, and 95.

Synthetics

1. Understanding the application of biomaterials to skin requires knowledge of the composition of the skin. What is the composition of the dermis? (Collagen, glycosaminoglycans or ground substance, and elastin)
2. The readings make a valid point about the difference between alloplastic, allografts, and xenografts. What is the biological response to each? (Loosely, alloplastic materials are synthetics that are, or should be, biologically inert but are encapsulated by the body. Allografts are biomaterials from the human species and, as covered in a later section, contain, if not processed, antigenic cellular material that in time will be recognized by the body as foreign. Xenografts are from a different species and are immediately recognized as foreign material and provoke an inflammatory response.)
3. Characterize the different types of foreign body response. (Integration as in certain skin substitutes, see below; fibrous encapsulation as in breast implants; and ongoing inflammation and possibly dissolution as in biodegradable implants, also see below)

E. Luce, *A Curriculum for Plastic Surgery*, https://doi.org/10.1007/978-3-031-62087-4_11

4. Polytetrafluoroethylene (PTFE) or Teflon when expanded is expanded PTFE (e-PTFE) or Gore-Tex®, used extensively in vascular and, until recently, abdominal surgery. What are the physical and biologic characteristics of polytetrafluoroethylene? (PTFE is a modification of the polyethylene compound by fluoridation or the addition of fluorocarbons and is extremely stable and not biodegradable. The pore size, 10 mm, in the non-expanded variety, is quite small, which allows little in the way of tissue ingrowth. Expanded PTFE (e-PTFE) allows some limited tissue ingrowth with the larger pore sizes, 30 mm, but practically behaves similarly to PTFE.)
   (a) Some surgeons use Gore-Tex® sutures in areola insets in a mastopexy. What are the potential advantages and disadvantages? (Gore-Tex® does not resorb, which presumably could provide longer-lasting tensile strength and avoid scar-widening, but the drawback is limited tissue ingrowth, potential of extrusion, especially the knots, and fracture.)
5. What is the principal difference between Prolene® and Gore-Tex® mesh in the reconstruction of the abdominal wall? (Prolene® is polypropylene, which has sufficient pore size to allow significant tissue ingrowth into the implant. Gore-Tex®, as discussed above, has a much smaller pore size with much more limited tissue ingrowth. The bottom line is a high incidence of seroma with the use of Gore-Tex® in abdominal wall reconstruction, but in comparison, tissue ingrowth by the serosa of the bowel can lead to infection of Prolene® and even bowel fistula.)
   (a) What is Marlex mesh®? (A stiffer mesh than Prolene® and also composed of polypropyl ethylene)
6. The readings discuss aliphatic resorbable polyesters used in resorbable sutures such as Vicryl® and Monocryl®, as well as biodegradable maxillofacial plates and screws. What is the process of resorption, and what might be an anticipated complication of the process of resorption? (Some combinations of polyesters and lactone rings, known as lactide glycolide, are the constituents of every resorbable device available. The resorption is a two-phase process, the initial one of which is biochemical breakage of the ester linkages and a cellular response with macrophages and fibrovascular ingrowth. Clearly, the second phase could culminate in an inflammatory response with a sterile abscess, which is the leading drawback with resorbable devices such as plates and screws.)
7. During the closure of a breast reduction, the surgical intern offers to close the wounds with Dermabond® while you drink a cup of coffee. What is your response? (Be certain to suture and close the dermal layer and ensure that the skin edges are opposed before application of the glue. The tissue adhesives or glues can provoke an adverse tissue reaction from the byproducts and, if used, should only be applied to the skin and still require a dermal suture layer for closure. The final vote is still out on the advisability of tissue adhesives for elective wound closure.)
8. Since you do a substantial number of facial fracture cases, the CEO of the hospital calls you with a proposal for the substitution of your current plate and screw system with a much more economical system with plates and screws composed of stainless steel. What is your response? (Actually, the composition of the first plate and screw system used in maxillofacial surgery was a stainless-steel alloy, namely, iron plus nickel plus chromium plating, and was tissue reactive. Stainless steel elicits an inflammatory response when implanted in tissue. Titanium is the most biocompatible of the metals, is relatively pure, and stimulates the least reaction. This characteristic allows for osteointegration, which is the lack of a fibrous interface between the bone and implant, and presumably better and long-lasting fixation. Because of its low density, titanium does not create the "starburst" effect on CT scans.)
9. Silicone-based alloplasts are the only non-carbon-chain-polymer alloplastic materials. What determines whether the silicone implant is gel or solid? (Progressive cross-linkage of the monomers of the silicone determines the physical form, so extensive cross-linkage will produce a silicone rubber implant, a process known as vulcanization. The length of the polymer chains will also affect the ultimate form. The gel form incorporated in breast implants is produced by a change in the side chains. The catalyst is platinum; the cross-linkage occurs to produce the gel form.)
   (a) Although the topic is also included in Chap. 82, what is the argument for the biologic safety of gel breast implants? (A number of epidemiological studies including a comprehensive report by the Institute of Medicine have determined that systemic conditions are not more common in women with breast implants, basic science has not linked silicone and disease, and medical-grade silicone is ubiquitous in medical products including syringes and IV tubing.)
   (b) What is the behavior of silicone gel in soft tissues, and what is the difference in tissue reaction between the shell of a breast implant and the gel? (Silicone gel tends to migrate, particularly with gravity, and elicits a fibroblastic and perhaps a chronic inflammatory and granulomatous response. The series of events does not occur with the solid silicone of an implant shell. The difference may be secondary to the increase in the biological inertness because of the increased number of hydrophilic bonds in solid silicone.)

Skin Substitutes

1. The essence of skin replacement is captured by the difference in the management of partial and full-thickness burns. Summarize. (The partial-thickness burn is the loss of the epidermis that has the capability to regenerate. A full-thickness burn is the loss of the dermis, which is not capable of regeneration. Any skin substitute must provide for dermal replacement.)
2. What is Apligraf®, and what is the mode of action of Apligraf®? (A dermal equivalent of bovine collagen matrix composed from neonatal foreskin fibroblast. The epidermis is composed of neonatal keratinocytes. The mode of action is probably by growth factors as well as extracellular matrix components with fibrovascular ingrowth.)
   (a) What is its immunogenicity? (None apparently. No elicitable response to HLA antigens or bovine collagen)
   (b) What are its disadvantages? (Short shelf life, expense, and inconsistent clinical results)
3. What is Dermagraft®? (Composed of neonatal foreskin fibroblast and cultured onto bioresorbable glycolic acid scaffold)
   (a) What is its mode of action? (Similar to that of Apligraf®)
   (b) What is its immunogenicity? (None, similar to Apligraf®)
   (c) What are its disadvantages? (Must be kept at −75 °C, shipped frozen; expensive; and inconsistent clinically)
4. Define Biobrane®. (Biobrane® is a bilaminar of nylon and silicone that is not incorporated into the body but rather seals the wound and permits the healing process, particularly in partial-thickness wounds. No inherent bacteriostatic capability exists, so colonized wounds rapidly become infected.)
5. Define Alloderm®. (Alloderm®, although allogeneic, is processed human dermis that is created from native human skin that has been processed so that the basement membrane and cellular matrix remain intact while the cellular components that cause rejection and infection are removed. Most tissue ingrowth occurs as host tissue ingrowth; cellular repopulation and revascularization occur within Alloderm® as a result of the regenerative process. The point of emphasis is that the dermis is acellular and so serves as a *scaffold*.)
6. If you place an unaltered allograft onto a wound, what specifically triggers the immune response from the host? (The cells: epidermal, fibroblast, and endothelial cells in the dermis)
7. To repeat an earlier question, although Alloderm® has been processed to remove the cellular components responsible for the immunological response and what remains is a scaffold, what else has to occur for a successful outcome, and what is responsible for that process? (Again, the host tissue ingrowth and cellular repopulation including revascularization must occur including host fibroblasts. The unknown provocative agent or agents must be retained within the Alloderm®. Because this represents proprietary information, the company, Life-Cell®, does not release what agent might be responsible.)
8. The junior resident questions your use of Alloderm® on a wound by a challenge that it will simply be replaced by a scar. What will be your rebuttal evidence? (Evidence of the persistence of an intact basement membrane and the presence of elastin and organized neocollagen)
   (a) Why is the presence of an intact basement membrane important, and what is the clinical situation to support that point? (Cultured epithelial autografts, CTA, or split-thickness skin graft.)
9. Even though Alloderm® is non-immunogenic, what is required for a "take"? (Alloderm should be regarded as a matrix scaffold that will allow, since no inflammatory reaction has been provoked, infiltration by fibroblasts and capillaries and perhaps, eventually, epithelization.)
10. What is the composition of Integra®? (Integra®, a composition of processed xenograft bovine collagen and shark extracellular matrix, namely, chondroitin sulfate, must be replaced by host collagen and presumably host ground or extracellular substance and covered by the temporary epidermis of silicone to prevent moisture loss.)
11. What are the essential steps in the use of Integra®? (The first stage involves the application of meshing of Integra®, followed perhaps by the use of the "Vacuum Assisted Closure" (VAC) in the postoperative period. The second stage is done at 2–4 weeks and consists of the removal of the silicone outer layer, Versajet-cleansing of Integra®, and the application of a skin graft.)
12. What is the principal advantage of using the VAC? (The material can be successfully placed on exposed bone, tendons, and joints with successful skin grafting at a mean of 7.5 days compared to the usual 2–4 weeks. The incorporation of Integra® hinges on vascularization as well as colonization of fibroblasts because then, increasing adherence to the underlying bed occurs.)
    (a) What mechanisms might explain the enhanced results? (The physiologic mechanisms and the use of the VAC are those of increased bacterial clearance, decreased edema, and enhanced perfusion.)
13. What are the disadvantages of cultural epithelial autografts? (This process is different from *allogeneic* keratinocytes and requires a small piece of skin harvested from the eventual recipient, cultured process, and the

production of thin sheets of CEA. The principal disadvantages are several and include the hiatus between culture and the availability of the CEA, the absence of dermis, so little resistance to shear, low capability for substitute adherence, and cost.)

14. What is the timing of delayed application of a split-thickness skin graft to Integra®, and why? (The use varies, but the usual hiatus is two weeks, the suitability for a graft heralded by color change in Integra®. The color changes are a result of neovascularization by the host. The original timing in the initial study was a hiatus of 4–6 weeks but has been shortened clinically by the immediate application of the VAC and perhaps by fenestration of Integra®.)
15. The readings outline the four stages of integration of acellular dermal matrix examined histologically that parallel the take of a skin graft. Describe. (Imbibition, fibroblast migration, neovascularization, and remodeling)
16. What is the essential difference, other than composition, between the integration of Alloderm® and that of Integra®? (As described above, Alloderm® has infiltration of the host cellular elements, fibroblasts, and endothelial cells. Integra®, a composition of processed xenograft bovine collagen and shark extracellular matrix, namely, chondroitin sulfate, must be replaced by host collagen and presumably host ground or extracellular substance.)
    (a) What is similar between the two, Alloderm® and Integra®, in the integration process? (Host cellular infiltration of fibroblasts and endothelial cells)
17. After debridement of an acute traumatic wound of the leg, you want to close the wound temporarily and determine the suitability for a delayed autograft. You request an allograft, and the circulating nurse brings Apligraf® into the OR. What do you do? (The appropriate temporary coverage in this situation is cadaver skin or allograft. Apligraf® is not intended as a temporary dressing and is much too expensive in this setting.)
18. Give a hierarchy of cost for the above: Apligraf®, Dermagraft®, Biobrane®, Integra®, and Alloderm®. (The hierarchy from most expensive to least expensive would be Apligraf®, Dermagraf®, Alloderm®, Integra®, and finally, the cheapest by far, is Biobrane®.)

In-Service Examination

1. Compare? polytetrafluoroethylene and polypropylene:
    (a) Both have maximal tissue ingrowth.
    (b) Both have minimal tissue ingrowth.
    (c) Polytetrafluoroethylene has minimal tissue ingrowth, and polypropylene has maximal tissue ingrowth.
    (d) Polytetrafluoroethylene has maximal tissue ingrowth, and polypropylene has minimal tissue ingrowth.
2. The process of biodegradation of absorbable plates and screws involves:
    (a) Encapsulation
    (b) Fibroblastic dissolution
    (c) Macrophage destruction
    (d) TGF-alpha activation
3. In the selection of a particular bioprosthetic rather than an alloplastic material, based on the host response in the reconstruction of the abdominal wall, an important property is:
    (a) Imbibition
    (b) Encapsulation
    (c) Revascularization
    (d) Inosculation
    (e) Rigidity

12 Laser Principles

Bibliography

Burns MD, J. L., "Lasers in Plastic Surgery", *Selected Readings in Plastic Surgery*, (2008), 10:**1-23.**

Brightman MD, L. A., et al., "Ablative and Fractional Ablative Lasers", *Dermatologic Clinics*, (2009), 27(4):**479-489.**

Narurkar MD, V. A., "Nonablative Fractional Laser Resurfacing", *Dermatologic Clinics*, (2009), 27(4):**473-78.**

Riggs MD, K., et al., "Ablative laser resurfacing: high-energy pulsed carbon dioxide and erbium:yttrium-aluminum-garnet", *Clinics in Dermatology,* (2007), 25:**462-73.**

Tannous MD, Z., "Fractional Resurfacing", *Clinics in Dermatology,* (2007) 25:**480-86.**

Janik MD, J. P., et al., "Laser Resurfacing", Hollier MD, L. H., *Lasers in Plastic Surgery.* (2007), 21(3):**139-146.**

Some of this material will be repeated in Module XB1Aesthetic surgery – Skin resurfacing

Faculty Discussion and Study Guide

> **Editor's Note:** Laser principles are also included in Chap. 94.

1. Define and characterize the electromagnetic spectrum. (The electromagnetic represents all of light of which only a very narrow band of the spectrum is visible light. The spectrum is from low-frequency long wavelengths such as radio waves to the other pole of the spectrum that consists of extremely high-frequency short wavelengths such as gamma rays. Visible light falls between 385 and 760 nm with the main colors consisting of red with the longest wavelength and violet with the shortest wavelength.)
   (a) Infrared and ultraviolet light have the capability to produce DNA damage. (Ultraviolet light certainly does have that capability but infrared light does not.)
2. What are the characteristics of laser light compared to visible light other than location on the EM spectrum? (Three characteristics including monochromatic meaning one color, coherent in that the bands of emitted light are in phase with respect to cycle and lastly collimated which means the laser wave travels in the same direction at the same time.)
3. Tissue effects from the light emitted by lasers occur through what? (Essentially, the relative proportion of scatter to absorption, i.e., less absorption and more scatter equates to more tissue effect.)
4. The depth of tissue penetration by a laser beam is directly proportional to what? (The wavelength. The longer wavelengths in the infrared portion of the spectrum penetrate more deeply than laser light emitted in the shorter wavelength such as the ultraviolet portion of the spectrum.)
   (a) What is the difference between the two in terms of tissue action? (Shorter wavelengths produce controlled tissue damage like ionizing radiation while lasers that emit light in the infrared or visible light spectrum exert tissue effect by thermal or photoacoustic mechanisms.)
5. What are the four variables for the degree of clinical effect of a laser? (Wavelength in nanometers, power in watts or joules/sec, spot size in cm^2, and duration of action.)
   (a) Define power density and fluence (power density = power × spot size while fluence = power density × duration or time.)
6. What is the concept of skin cooling? (Cooling essentially eliminates heat in the epidermis as well as the dermis which in turn enables higher energy directed toward the particular target chromophore with less risk of skin burning.)

> **Editor's Note:** Is tissue damage (thermolysis) determined by scatter or absorption?

E. Luce, *A Curriculum for Plastic Surgery*, https://doi.org/10.1007/978-3-031-62087-4_12

7. What is thermal relaxation time? (The duration that tissues will dissipate the heat energy applied by a particular laser without damage. The actual number is 51% of the energy absorbed and is the same as the cooling time.)
8. The au relates the four classifications of lasers as medical devices by the US government. What are they? (Class I which are medical diagnostic lasers and do not require hazard warning, class II lasers are low powered such as a laser pointer and are safe for momentary viewing, class III and IV lasers are medical lasers and can cause fires, skin burns, and other injuries.)
9. The readings described that ocular injury by lasers can occur by two different mechanisms. What are they? (Direct burn of the cornea or sclera by CO_2 laser or lasers that are capable of transmitting light through clear fluids and striking the retina. Eye protection requires the proper use of protective goggles or glasses.)
10. You plan CO_2 laser facial skin rejuvenation and the circulating nurse places on the patient's eyes a set of clear scleral protective lenses. You argue that opaque blue lenses are necessary. Who is correct? (The nurse. For a CO_2 laser clear plastic scleral lenses are sufficient. Other lasers require opaque scleral lenses.)
11. What are chromophores? (Tissue elements that have an affinity for laser light at particular wavelengths.)
    (a) What are the clinically important tissue chromophores? (Water, hemoglobin, and melanin)

Editor's Note: Material on specific lasers is not included in this module.

Skin Resurfacing

1. What is the structural difference between chronologic and photoaging? (Chronological aging essentially is thinning of the dermis with a decrease in cellular content and blood vessels. Photoaging is also known as solar elastosis when sun-damaged skin demonstrates poor organization of the collagen fibers with lumps of elastin material evident.)
    (a) What and where is the grenz zone? (A thin layer of dermis just deep to the epidermis which is thought to be a reparative process of normal dermis.)
2. With the use of a thermal burn analogy, describe the zones of injury in lasers. (The most superficial is the zone of vaporization, a deeper layer with probable irreversible injury is a zone of coagulation, and the deeper and perhaps broader zone is a zone of reversible thermal damage.)
3. Essentially, what is the goal in skin resurfacing with CO_2 or the erb-YAG lasers? (CO_2 penetrates into the superficial and mid level of the dermis in order to create a zone of injury that will then heal with a collagen reorganization and two effects, elimination of the solar elastosis as well as "tightening" of the skin by collagen contraction with the healing process. Of course, as in the case with thermal burns, the treatment plan must sail between the rock of sufficient depth to achieve a noticeable and significant improvement and the hard place of damage to the point of scarring.)
    (a) What is the point of multiple "passes" for facial skin rejuvenation? (The first pass essentially vaporizes the epidermis to expose the dermis. Additional passes are designed to oblate deeper layers of dermis until the goal as outlined in the above question is accomplished.)
    (b) What are the side effects? (Necessity for reepithelialization and post-treatment erythema which can persist for months.)
4. From what portion of the electromagnetic spectrum are non-ablative lasers active? (Both the infrared and the adjacent visible bands of the spectrum.)
    (a) Name some non-ablative lasers. (Pulsed dye, cool-touch YAG, Q-switched Nd: YAG)
    (b) The au outlines the use of non-ablative procedures and lists several lasers that qualify. How do these lasers differ from the CO_2 laser? (A shorter wavelength for non-ablative lasers drawn from the infrared and visible portions of the electromagnetic light spectrum. Tissue penetration and energy delivered are less so recovery time is shorter. Yet, the overall effect is less and several treatments may be necessary.)
5. Give the Fitzpatrick skin type classification. (I: Pale white always burns, never tans, II: White, usually burns, tans with difficulty, III: White and tans average, IV: Medium brown skin which rarely burns and tans with ease, V: Dark brown does not burn, tans with ease, VI: Black)
6. List the appropriate laser for the following clinical situations:
    (a) Tattoos (the Q-switched Nd:YAG laser)
    (b) Pigmented lesions (Q-switched ruby laser)
    (c) Hair removal (Nd:YAG laser)
    (d) Burn excision (CO_2 laser)
7. What is the energy threshold for vaporization or human skin? (about 5 J per cm^2 with a CO_2 laser.)
    (a) What is the thermal relaxation time of skin? (1 ms)
8. What is the principal difference between Erbium:YAG laser compared to CO_2? (Shorter wavelength with an increased water absorption coefficient.)
9. What is the Fraxel laser? (Fractional photothermolysis which essentially is a more superficial laser with alternate microzones of thermal damage surrounded by zones of normal tissue. Patients require a number of sessions several weeks apart. The Fraxel laser is the newest and highly popular technology.)

Part II

Congenital Anomalies of Head and Neck

Unilateral Cleft Lip

13

Bibliography

Xue AS, Buchanan EP, Hollier LH, "Update in Unilateral Cleft Lip Surgery", *Plast. Reconstr. Surg.*, (2021); 148(2):**262e-272e ONLY, Videos 1 and 2 (Overview).**

Grayson BH and Garfinkle JS, Chapter 64: "Nasoalveolar molding and columellar elongation in preparation for the primary repair of unilateral and bilateral cleft lip and palate", Losee, J. E. and Kirschner, R. E. Comprehensive Cleft Care Second Edition, The McGraw-Hill Co. (2016); pgs.1223-1251. **1223-46 ONLY.**

Fisher DM and Sommerlad BC, "Cleft Lip, Cleft Palate, and Velopharyngeal Insufficiency", *Plast. Reconstr. Surg.*, (2011); 128(4):342e-360e. **342e-351e, (Skip 343e-45e Cleft Palate) Fig. 2, and Videos 1, 3 ONLY.**

(The material on Cleft Palate and VPI is in a later module.)

Chong DK, Swanson JW, "The Essential Anatomical Subunit Approximation Unilateral Cleft Lip Repair", *Plast Reconstr Surg.*, (2016); 138(1):**91e-94e.**

Marcus, Jeffrey, R., M.D., et al., "Principles of cleft lip repair: conventions, commonalities, and controversies", *Plast. Reconstr. Surg.*, (2017); 139:**764e-778e Videos 1, 2.**

Monson LA, Kirschner RE, Losee JE, "Primary Repair of Cleft Lip and Nasal Deformity", *Plast Reconstr Surg.*, (2013); 132(6):**1040e Videos 1, 2.**

Van Beek MD, A. L., et al., "Cleft Rhinoplasty", *Plast. Reconstr. Surg.*, (2004); 114:**61e-65e.**

Henry C, Samson T, Mackay D, "Evidence-Based Medicine: The Cleft Lip Nasal Deformity", *Plast. Reconstr. Surg.*, (2014); 133(5):**1276, Table 1, Videos 1, 2 ONLY.**

Supplemental for a Pre-op Conference

Tse R, "Unilateral cleft lip: Principles and practice of surgical management", *Seminars in plastic surgery,* (2012)26(4):**145-155.**

Faculty Discussion and Study Guide

General, Epidemiology

1. The parents of a three-year-old isolated cleft palate child are pregnant and want counseling with respect to the odds of a "hare lip" baby. (1 to 1000 or the same as the normal population. Isolated cleft palate and cleft lip/palate are genetically separate.)
   (a) If the first child had a cleft lip? (4% chance of the in utero baby having a cleft lip.)
   (b) The risk in the current child if the father has a cleft lip? (4%.)
   (c) If the first two children had cleft lips? (9%.)
   (d) Risk in the current child if the father and first child have a cleft lip? (16%.)
2. What are maternal risk factors for the occurrence of cleft lip/palate? (Smoking, alcohol, Dilantin, Accutane, and steroids.)
3. Give an approximation of the probability of a syndromic diagnosis in cleft lip/cleft palate and isolated cleft palate. (Approximately 1/3 of cleft lip patients have an associated syndrome, about 1/2 of isolated cleft palates are regarded as syndromic. A considerable portion of the latter is the Robin sequence.)
   (a) The significance of lower lip pits in a cleft lip baby? (Presence of Vander Woude syndrome, an autosomal dominant disorder.)
4. Rank in terms of frequency the occurrence of cleft lip in the following ethnic groups: Ameri-Indian, Asian, Caucasian, and African American. (In the order as written.)
   (a) Ratio of male vs. female? (2:1.)
5. At what point in utero does lip formation occur? Palate? (A variety of milestones have been offered, but for written test purposes the lip at 5–7 weeks, palate at 9–11 weeks.)

E. Luce, *A Curriculum for Plastic Surgery*, https://doi.org/10.1007/978-3-031-62087-4_13

6. Give a brief overview of the milestones and a team approach to the management of cleft lip/palate child. (A pediatric evaluation is necessary at birth including addressing any feeding difficulties. As soon as possible, nasoalveolar molding (NAM) is instituted. Lip repair is performed at 3–4 months and the palate at 9 months to a year. ENT screening for middle ear disease is instituted in infancy. Speech evaluation is instituted at age 2.5–3 years with the view toward early diagnosis of velopharyngeal insufficiency (VPI). Alveolar bone grafting is somewhat controversial but a conventional approach is at the age of eruption of the canine or 7–9 years with institution of orthodontics. The remaining milestones are dependent on any individual patient. Lip-nose revision in the more obvious deformities may be necessary in childhood or adolescence with continuance of orthodontic therapy. Orthognathic surgery is reserved for the fully grown patient.)
7. Describe a classification of clefts such as Kernahan. (The Kernahan classification uses the incisive foramen as the border between the primary and secondary palate. Then right and left primary palate clefts are drawn such that the final configuration is a Y. One to three is a right unilateral to the incisive foramen, 4–6 is left, and 7–9 is the secondary palate. The Veau classification is from 1–4 beginning with a partial soft palate, I; complete soft and hard palate, II; complete cleft of unilateral lip and palate, III; bilateral complete lip and palate, IV.)

Anatomy

1. Describe anatomically the osseous deformity in a baby with a complete cleft lip. (The alveolar deformity consists of the premaxillary or greater segment rotated anteriorly and superiorly. The lesser maxillary segment is retropositioned and collapsed lingually. Some posterior displacement and perhaps hypoplasia of the maxillary component of the bony aspect of the pyriform aperture may also exist. See Fig. 13.1.)

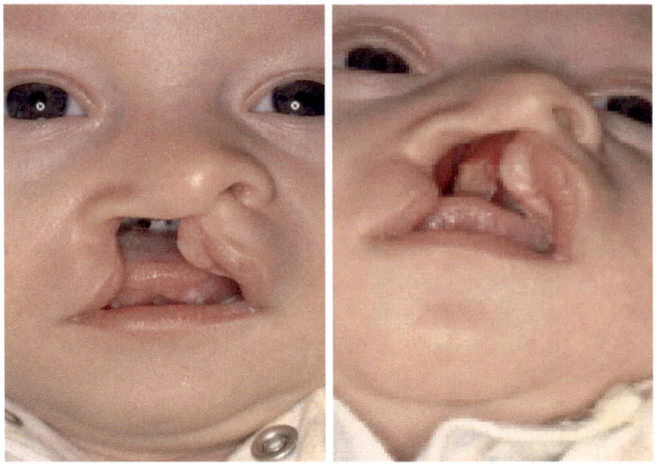

Fig. 13.1 Osseous deformity

2. Name and discuss the components of the orbicularis oris and compare and contrast their function. (Superficial or pars peripheralis and deep or pars marginalis. The deep portion is located primarily in the vermilion while the superficial portion lies beneath the skin of the upper lip, divided into the upper and lower bundles and inserts into the philtral columns. The pars marginalis appears to function mostly as an oral sphincter while the superficial, both upper and lower bundles have a principal role in facial expression and as an oral retractor.)
3. What is the configuration of the superficial component of the orbicularis in the cleft patient on the cleft side? (The lower bundle is misdirected superiorly and attaches to the inferior alar base and lateral pyriform aperture; the upper bundle is attached to the lateral aspect of the ala.)
   (a) The non-cleft side? (Abnormal insertion into the anterior nasal spine and medial crural footplates. This abnormal unopposed insertion and pull is partially responsible for the anterior and contralateral displacement of the base of the columella.)
   (b) The pars marginalis on the cleft side? (Not displaced, interrupted by the cleft, and hypoplastic in the prolabial segment.)
   (c) What pathologic changes occur in the cleft vermilion? (The vermilion is markedly deficient in the tissue adjacent to cleft in both bulk and width, probably absent mucous glands as well as the white roll.)
4. What is Noordhoff's point and the significance of the same? (Noordhoff's point is the proposed peak of Cupid's bow on the *lateral* segment of the cleft and, similar to the medial peak of Cupid's bow, is the point of adequate vermilion and white roll that is transposed. Inadvertent marking that point further medial will diminish the quality of both incorporated into the repair. Movement laterally will shorten the ultimate transverse length of the lip on the cleft side.)
5. List 8–10 components of the unilateral cleft lip nasal deformity. (1. The columella is shorter on the cleft side with an alar cartilage foot plate displaced and tethered inferiorly, 2. The base of the columella is deviated to the non-cleft side, 3. The medial crus of the alar cartilage is short and the lateral crus longer displaced laterally and flattened into a S-shaped fold and concave rather than convexity resulting in an obtuse angle of the dome rather than acute, 4. The alar cartilage is displaced in a posterior and inferior plane, 5. The medial crus-dome of the alar cartilage is drawn posteriorly and inferiorly, 6. The nasal tip is displaced to the cleft side, asymmetric, and wid-

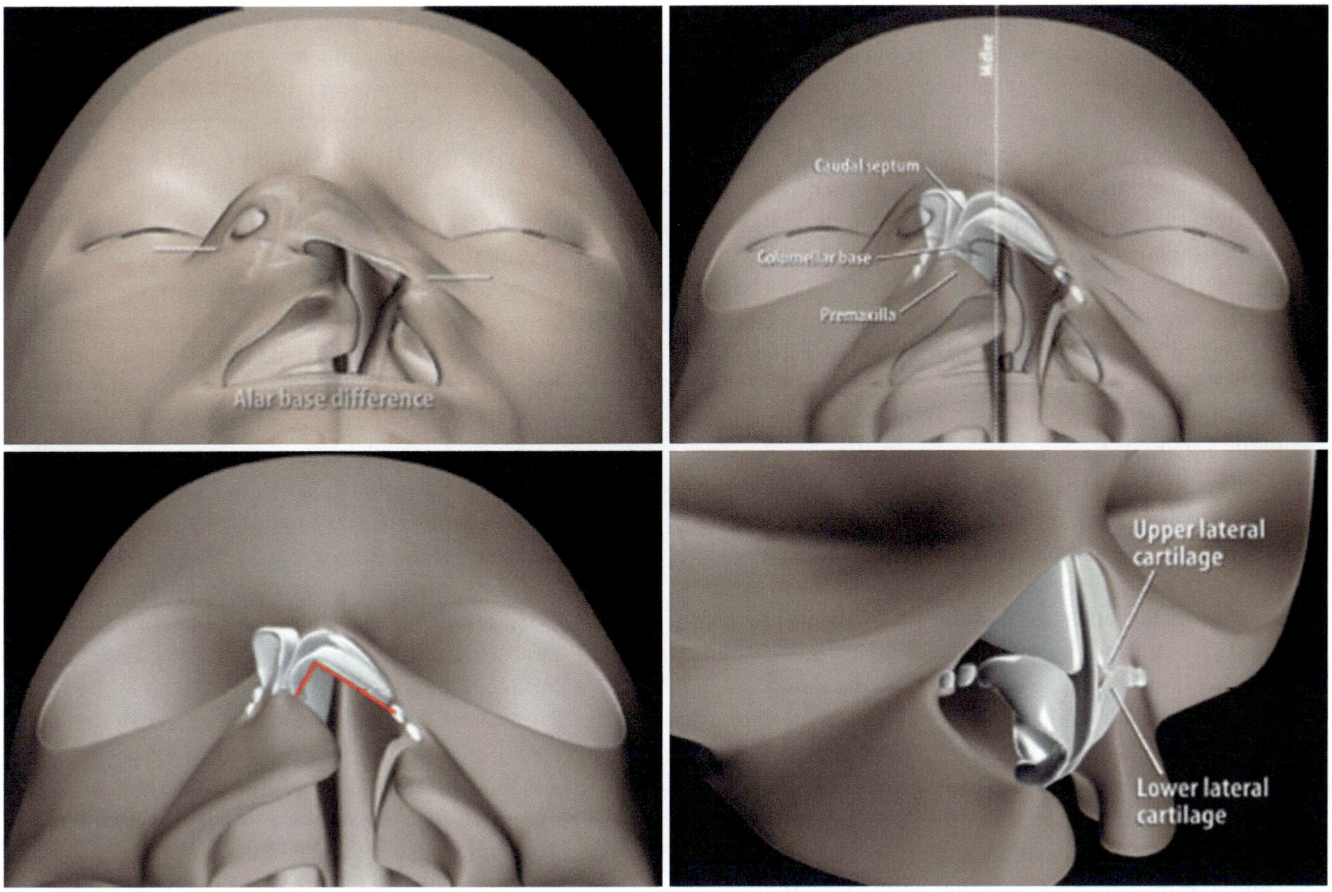

Fig. 13.2 Fisher DM and Sommerlad BC, "Cleft Lip, Cleft Palate, and Velopharyngeal Insufficiency" *Plast. Reconstr. Surg.*, (2011); 128:344e. (Reprinted with Permission)

ened, 7. The flattened alar cartilage results in a horizontal orientation of the nostril, 8. The base of the ala is displaced posteriorly, inferiorly, and laterally tethered to the underlying periosteum of the pyriform aperture, 9. The caudal septum is out of the vomerine groove and displaced to the opposite side, 10. The lateral aspect of the pyriform aperture is hypoplastic and located more posterior. See Fig. 13.2.)

6. Define Simonart's band. (In a subtotal incomplete cleft lip, a remnant of skin and soft tissue at the most superior portion of the cleft is termed Simonart's band.)

Preoperative Management

1. If you had but *one* single measurement that would express the severity of the lip cleft, what would that measurement be? (The vertical distance between the Cupid's bow on the cleft side and the base of the columella. That measurement compared to the normal side reveals the extent of deficiency or viewed differently, the necessary length of rotation. For example, in a mildly incomplete cleft, the vertical distance will be greater or the deficiency less than a wide unilateral cleft.)
2. Other than the timing of lip repair, what are the other options in terms of management of the nose and the maxillary arches or the alveolar defect? (The advisability, or not, of primary rhinoplasty for the nasal deformity, the use or not of presurgical orthopedics, and the advisability or not, of early gingivoperiosteoplasty [GPP].)
3. What are the indications, benefits, and potential liabilities of preoperative maxillary orthopedics, disregarding the nose? (Selected cases dependent on the size of the bony cleft, the maxillary arch deformity, and/or the disparity of soft tissue lip segments. Also, even in the presence of a small cleft of the alveolus, such management is indicated when gingivoperiosteoplasty is considered at the time of lip repair. Summary: According to the readings, whenever the surgeons might think a lip adhesion would be helpful then maxillary orthopedics is appropriate instead. Preoperative maxillary orthopedics can accomplish improvement in arch configuration and, if nasal alveolar molding is incorporated, improve nasal

aesthetics and achieve some ease of lip repair. The other side of the discussion is any concerns about maxillary growth restrictions.)

4. When performed, what are the treatment objectives in preoperative maxillary orthopedics? (Buccal rotation and expansion of the lateral or lesser segment; posterior, inferior, and medial rotation of the premaxillary or greater segment and closure of, to some extent, the alveolar cleft.)
5. The readings discuss the use of combined soft tissue taping and an obturator of the palate. What would occur if the palate was not obturated in the presence of lip or soft tissue taping and what is the function of the palatal obturator? (If the lateral or posterior maxillary arch is not obturated in proper position, under the posterior pressure of soft tissue taping the arch or the lesser segment will collapse further medially or lingually.)
6. Contrast the preoperative maxillary orthopedics of Latham to the other techniques described in the readings. (The Latham appliance is active in the sense that the position of the segments is manipulated by an indwelling screw, turned on a regular basis that repositions the acrylic on the anterior end of greater maxillary segments. The other methods described in the readings are more passive in the sense they are designed to prevent further *collapse* of the segments during external compression and to avoid lingual thrust. The controversy exists about whether this degree of surgical intervention of the Latham appliance restricts eventual maxillary growth and of course the operation necessary for placement.)
7. When should preoperative maxillary orthopedics be initiated and why? What is the duration of therapy? (The initiation of therapy should occur as early in the neonatal period as possible because of the beneficial effect of circulating maternal estrogens then may enhance the pliability of the segments. The duration is two to three months prior to lip repair, which is a long treatment course for *active* movement of the greater or premaxillary segment. Perhaps the traction device actually functions as a "restraining mechanism" to preclude further untethered forward and lateral growth.)
8. Briefly outline the philosophy and design aspects of nasoalveolar molding (Nasoalveolar molding (NAM)is an address principally of the underlying skeletal framework, the nasal cartilage deformity, and perhaps to a lesser degree soft tissue of the lip position. The acrylic plates are fashioned from impressions that will mold both the lesser or posterior segment and the greater or anterior segment to prevent lingual collapse of the posterior segment and to facilitate posterior and lateral and hopefully inferior rotation of the anterior or cleft segment. A spring-loaded attached outrigger holds the nasal dome into a more normal position. The compressive forces on the alveolar segments are generated by taping either connected or not to a rubber band on the appliance. Taping is used to mold the lip soft tissues into a position to facilitate surgical repair and to narrow the alveolar cleft.)
   (a) What are some practical considerations? (The surgeon may not see the patient in referral before 4–6 weeks of age and some advantage of the circulating maternal estrogen has receded; the parents must comply with the travel necessity for frequent revisions during the infant's growth perhaps weekly, and third, compliance may be a problem with parents maintaining the appliance in place. Intraoral ulcers from the acrylic edges are frequent and skin irritation from taping can be a complication.)
   (b) What are the steps? (Impressions are made, a stone cast created, and an acrylic obturator is fabricated. Frequent modifications are necessary.)
   (c) Further use of the NAM appliance is recommended for a period of 2–4 weeks postoperative.
9. Discuss the limitations of a preliminary lip adhesion. (The goals of lip adhesion are to achieve narrowing of the alveolar cleft by presence of the now intact lip and so facilitate the definitive lip repair. Lip adhesion requires the discard of soft tissue at the time of definitive lip repair, does not allow definitive address with a primary nasal repair, will require a second operation, and may have a significant dehiscence rate. Probably the principal criticism is that by the time of definitive lip repair, 8–9 months, the nasal cartilage and soft tissues are less responsive to primary nasal repair.)
10. Describe the principal advantages of gingivoperiosteoplasty (GPP)? (Close the alveolar cleft, avoid oral-nasal fistulas, avoid malpositioning of the alveolar segments. Gingivoperiosteoplasty is the closure of the alveolar and to some degree, the floor of the nose, with a flap of soft tissue, including periosteum taken from the gingiva and sutured to the other side of the cleft, performed simultaneously with lip repair. The advocacy of performance of a GPP is the potential of avoidance of secondary alveolar bone grafting. Most commonly, the procedure implies the use of preoperative NAM to improve alignment of the alveolar segment, narrow the alveolar gap, and thus shorten the length of the osteoflap required for the GPP. Considerable controversy exists about the osteogenic capability of the tissue and the possible long-term adverse effect on facial growth.)

Lip-Nose Repair

1. What are the key basic points to be marked for a Millard cleft lip repair? (On the non-cleft side the apex of Cupid's bow and the alar base as well as the base of the columella. On the medial aspect of the cleft the apex of Cupid's bow and base of columella as well as the midpoint of Cupid's bow. On the lateral lip segment, the alar base. A measurement is taken of the distance from the apex of Cupid's bow on the normal side to the alar base, namely, the height of the philtral column and that measurement is transposed to the medial side of the cleft as the length of the rotation incision. The inferior extent of the rotation incision is at the vermilion border at the Cupid's bow apex on the cleft or medial side and the length of the proposed incision is a measurement equal to the height of the non-cleft philtral column. That same measurement is then transposed to the lateral lip segment and an incision outlined parallel to and superior to the vermilion border from the alar base laterally to the Cupid's bow apex, Noordhoff's point, on the lateral lip segment. The junction of the alar base to the nasal sill and columellar base is marked on the non-cleft side and repeated on the cleft side. Many surgeons also add markings at either oral commissure or the midline of the tip of the nose.)
2. What are major steps in the dissection, prior to suturing, in cleft lip repair? (The markings as outlined above, a rotation incision with a separate dissection of the vermilion to allow inset of a vermilion flap; an advancement incision equivalent to length of the rotation incision, again with a separate dissection of the vermilion to inset as a flap into the medial vermilion; a short transverse incision at the alar base without extension as a perialar incision, complete release of the alar base from the underlying fibrous attachments, dissection of separate orbicularis muscle bundles including superficial and deep, dissection of a superiorly based septal flap for nasal floor, dissection of a lateral or vestibular flap with a separate intercartilaginous incision to be sutured to the septal flap, dissection of the skin from the lateral crus of the alar cartilage. Release of footplate and medial crura from fibrous attachments is important as well.)
3. What are the major steps in suturing? (First, repair the muscle, superficial separate from deep, place the key buried suture from the tip of the advancement flap to the apex of the rotation incision, placement of the key suture through the Cupid's bow point on both the lateral and medial lip segments as previously marked, repair the nasal floor by advancement of the lateral vestibular flap into the leading edge of the superiorly based septal flap, skin closure, and a Z-plasty of the vermilion-adjacent mucosa. See below for nasal repair.)
4. What is the most common technical error, a vertically short or long repaired lip? (Vertically short due to either inadequate rotation and/or too short of an advancement flap.)
5. What is the Fisher repair and, briefly, the conceptual approach? (The Fisher repair, dubbed the anatomic subunit approximation, is in essence, a design that incorporates a transverse triangle harvested from the lateral lip segment to address the deficiency in vertical height of the medial cleft. An estimation of the deficiency is calculated, similar to the Millard repair, by the difference between the height of the philtral column on the non-cleft and cleft sides. The difference dictates the width of the base of the triangle, the tip located approximately 1 mm superior to the vermilion, the height always 1 mm. The vertical incision on the cleft side incorporates a short, 1 mm, transverse incision at the corresponding point on the lip to permit inset of the triangular flap. See Fig. 13.3.)

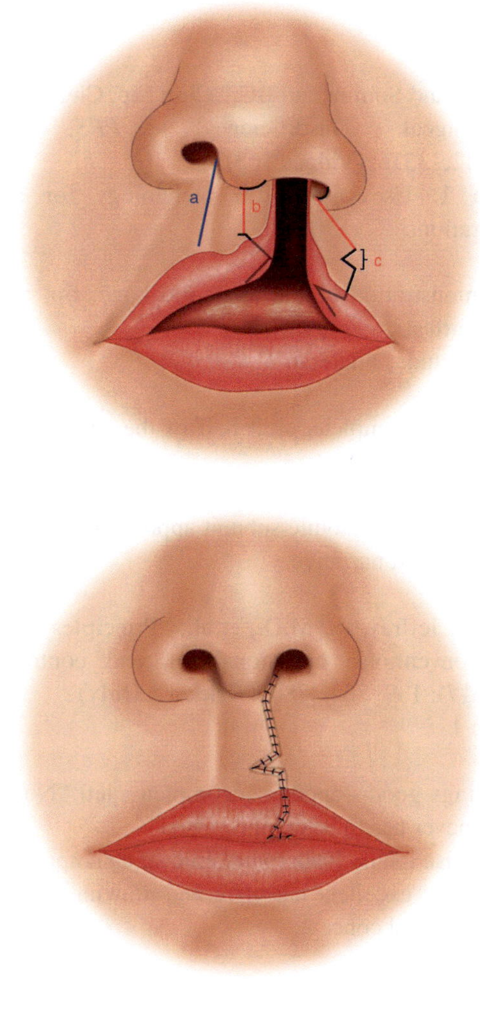

Fig. 13.3 Fisher repair

6. Describe the key elements of primary nasal repair in cleft lip as well as the underlying controversy. (The controversy about primary cleft rhinoplasty is that extensive dissection, suturing, manipulation, and incisions can set the stage for late deformity as a result of interference with normal growth. On the other hand, the first opportunity, as so often in plastic surgery, affords the best chance for a definitive repair. Virtually all cleft surgeons utilize the elements of nasal repair as described under the previous lip repair section, namely alar base advancement, septal and lateral nasal wall flaps for closure of the nasal floor, lengthening of the hemi columella and, for most, mobilization of the nasal soft tissue from the lateral crus. A more extensive approach is the use of a rim incision for dissection and direct suturing of the medial crus. Placement of key sutures over bolsters can assist in maintenance of the medial crus and dome to the opposite dome and/or upper lateral cartilage. Additional sutures and bolsters are placed through and through the lateral crus to prevent recurrence of the deformity. Long-term outcomes are conspicuously absent from the literature.)

Video Notes

Fisher DM and Sommerlad BC, "Cleft Lip, Cleft Palate, and Velopharyngeal Insufficiency", *PRS*, (2011); 128(4):342e-351e. **(Videos 1, 3)**

Video 1: Use of SMILE technology for animated demonstration.

1. A demonstration of the anatomic bone, lip, and nasal deformities.
2. *Also*, includes bilateral.

Video 3: Incomplete, cleft half of the vertical height of the lip.

1. Markings of "anatomic subunit approximation" with reasonably good narrative.

Marcus, Jeffrey, R., M.D., et al., "Principles of cleft lip repair: conventions, commonalities, and controversies", *PRS*, (2017); 139: 764e-780e. **(Video 1 Only)**

Video 1

1. Markings good—another incomplete cleft "Noordhoff's point never has to be compromised".
2. Otherwise totally Fisher anatomic subunit approximation technique; excellent narrative and drawings to illustrate markings and concept.

Monson LA, Kirschner RE, Losee JE, "Primary Repair of Cleft Lip and Nasal Deformity", *Plast Reconstr Surg.*, (2013); 132(6):**1040e Videos 1, 2.**

Video 1

1. Excellent narrative of Millard repair of 14 min in length.

Video 2

1. Closure and suturing—5.5 min also excellent narrative and videos

Xue AS, Buchanan EP, Hollier LH, "Update in Unilateral Cleft Lip Surgery", *Plast. Reconstr. Surg.*, (2021); 148(2):**262e-272e ONLY, Videos 1 and 2 (Overview).**

Video 1, 2: Millard repair with good narrative and video.

Case-Based Conference

Case 1: Unilateral Cleft Lip

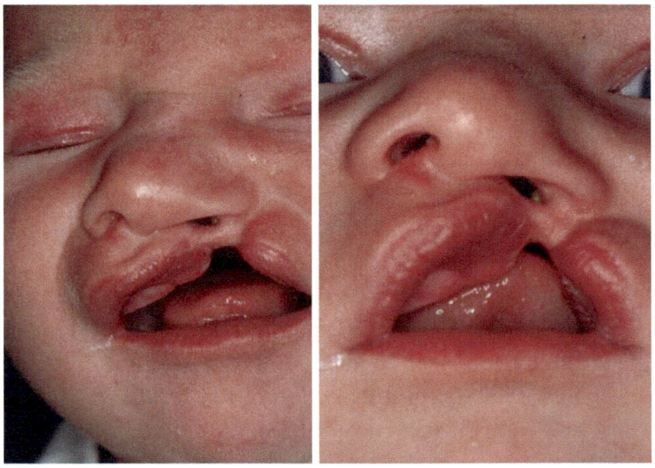

1. Describe the slide(s) and outline a brief physical examination.
   (a) Any test(s) indicated? Justify
2. Describe the pathologic anatomy. Specifically, outline the components of the osseous, soft tissue, and nasal deformity.
3. Any nonsurgical modalities indicated? If so, justify and describe.
   (a) While marking the patient the plastic surgery resident asks about the advisability of "a lip adhesion" and "gingivoperiosteoplasty". Comment. (Or perform if you believe indicated.)
4. List two repairs and select one for Qestion 4. *Briefly*, describe the other. Begin by listing the major steps in your plan of repair and then once the list is complete, draw the repair.

Case-Based Conference: Discussion

Case 1: Unilateral Cleft Lip

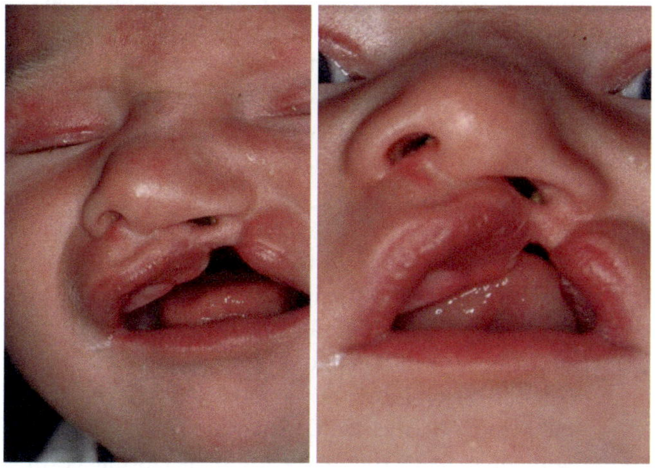

1. Describe the slide(s) and outline a brief physical examination. (Two slides are provided: one, a full frontal view, and a second an incomplete submental vertex (SMV) view. The frontal view depicts an infant with a left and subtotal unilateral cleft of the lip that appears wide. The medial edge of the alveolus or greater segment is visualized, the medial edge of the lesser segment is not. The alveolar cleft appears, though, to be 1–1.5 cm in magnitude. The associated cleft lip nasal deformity is described in the response to Question 2. No other facial deformities are evident. The SMV slide provides no additional information about an associated complete cleft of the palate. Again, the lesser palatal segment is not visualized, lending credence to the supposition of a substantial alveolar cleft. A thin band of skin is present at the nasal sill, a Simonart's band.

   The clinical exam would include a focused history to ascertain the attainment of growth and development milestones and the presence, if any, of feeding difficulties. A family history is obtained as well. In addition to an intraoral exam the remainder of the infant is examined.)

   (a) Any test(s) indicated? Justify. (In the absence of any clinical findings other than an isolated cleft lip-palate, no.)
2. Describe the pathologic anatomy. (The deformity is one of a subtotal cleft of the primary palate, namely the soft tissues of the lip, the alveolar ridge, and the palate at least to the incisive foramen and probably beyond. A subtotal cleft of the secondary palate may be present as well. On the cleft or medial side, the lip and the soft tissues of the lip are vertically oriented. The vermilion and the mucosa become sharply attenuated in the most superior aspect of the cleft. Internally, the orbicularis muscle is a haphazard arrangement with hypoplasia of the pars marginalis component within the lip and vermilion. The superficial or pars peripheralis, normally inserted into the philtral columns, are abnormally attached to the lateral alar base and the lateral aspect of the pyriform aperture. The vermilion is markedly deficient in the tissue adjacent to the cleft laterally and medially in both bulk and width. The alveolar deformity consists of the premaxillary or greater medial segment rotated anteriorly and superiorly, the lesser lateral maxillary segment is retropositioned and collapsed lingually. Some posterior displacement or perhaps hypoplasia of the maxillary component of the lateral aspect of the pyriform aperture may exist as well. Finally, the nasal deformity consists of the following: Septum deviated with the inferior edge displaced out of the vomerine groove and into the floor of opposite or normal nostril; decreased height of the ipsilateral hemi columella; a lateral flare of the alar base with posterior displacement of the lateral aspect of the pyriform aperture; the genu of the lower lateral cartilage is flattened with an obtuse angle; the alar dome on the involved side depressed inferiorly and anteriorly; the medial footplate of the alar cartilage is depressed inferiorly.)

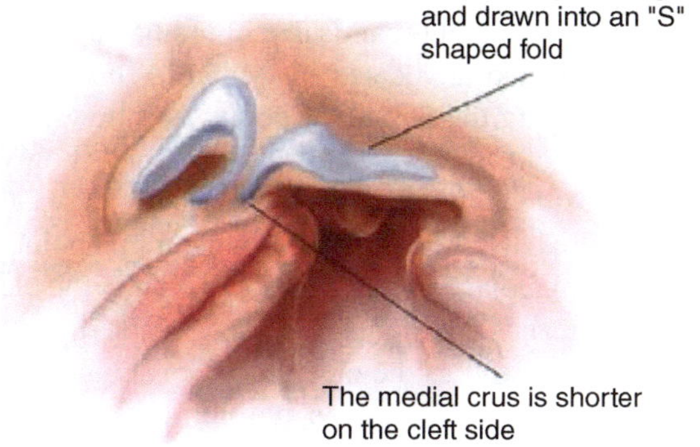

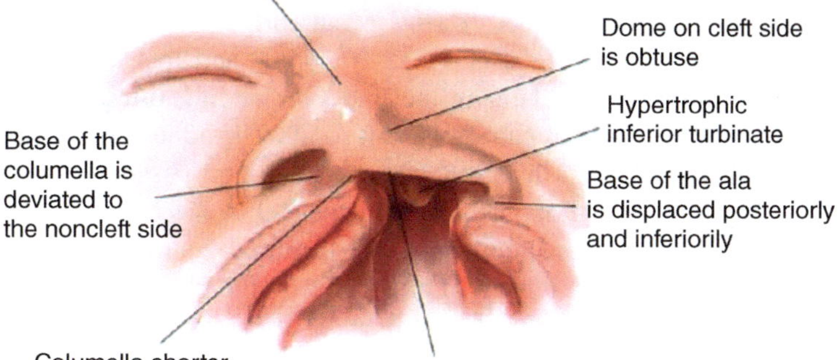

3. Any nonsurgical modalities indicated? If so, justify and describe. (This question essentially asks about the advisability of preoperative maxillary orthopedics. Preoperative maxillary orthopedics consists of either an active or passive device. Active devices are implanted onto the premaxilla and maxilla and with the aid of retaining pins and a jack screw that is turned periodically attempt to rotate the alveolar segments into a more favorable position. Specifically, the lesser segment is rotated laterally or buccal and anterior, the greater segment is posterior, inferior, and medially or lingually positioned. In doing so, the soft tissues of the cleft become less widely disparate and perhaps set the stage more favorably for lip repair. Passive devices utilize straps, tape, etc. to place pressure on the soft tissues and underlying alveolar segments in order to mold them into a more optimal position. The argument against use of passive compression is that often the tissues become inflamed or even ulcerated. Active preoperative maxillary orthopedics requires a preliminary operation for placement of the device. The devices also require parental compliance to perform the periodic manipulation of the jack screw to ensure the desired movement of the palatal segments. Nasoalveolar molding (NAM) actually can be accomplished with the use of an acrylic device and nasal outrigger to elevate into a more normal position the columella and lower lateral cartilage. The use of passive splints mandates a number of refittings over the course of treatment, usually 3 months, often on a weekly basis because of the facial growth of the infant, and may present travel and economic constraints in some patients. Some consider that the blockage of the constant movement of the tongue into the cleft may play a role in addressing the alveolar deformity.)
   (a) While marking the patient the plastic surgery resident asks about the advisability of "a lip adhesion" and "gingivoperiosteoplasty". Comment or perform if you believe indicated. (Another argument in the management of infants with wide clefts is to employ a preliminary lip adhesion rather than preoperative maxillary orthopedics.) This approach has been adopted in a number of centers and consists of a lip adhesion performed at age 2–3 months and then a definitive repair later in the first year of life, often combined with repair of the soft palate. Lip adhesion also avoids the disadvantages of active and passive molding listed above. The principal rebuttal to this argument is that although to do so facilitates lip repair and aids in attainment of a more favorable positioning of the dentoalveolar segments, the price may be the loss of an early opportunity to address the associated nasal deformity. The disadvantages also include the obvious necessity for a second operation and the possible additional scarring.

      Regardless, if maxillary orthopedics is to be instituted preoperatively, such must be accomplished as early in life as possible. The probable physiological explanation for the short "window" for institution of preoperative orthopedics is the presence of circulating maternal estrogens, diminished markedly by 6 weeks of age, in the neonate that enhances the pliability of cartilage.

      The second item of discussion is that of the advisability, or not, of the performance of a gingivoperiosteoplasty (GPP). Gingivoperiosteoplasty is the closure of the alveolar and to some degree, the floor of the nose, with a flap of soft tissue, including periosteum taken from the gingiva and sutured to the other side of the cleft, performed simultaneously with lip repair. The advocacy of performance of a GPP is the potential of avoidance of secondary alveolar bone grafting. Most commonly, the procedure implies the use of preoperative NAM to improve alignment of the alveolar segment, narrow the alveolar gap, and thus shorten the length of the periosteal flap required for the GPP. Considerable controversy exists about the osteogenic capability of the tissue and the possible long-term adverse effect on facial growth.)
4. List two repairs and select one for Question 4. *Briefly*, describe the other. (Millard and Fisher. The Millard repair will be described in the question below. The Fisher repair, dubbed the anatomic subunit approximation is, in essence, a design that incorporates a transversely oriented triangle harvested from the lateral lip segment to address the deficiency in vertical height of the medial cleft. An estimation of the deficiency is calculated, similar to the Millard repair, by the difference between the height of the philtral column on the non-cleft and cleft sides. The difference dictates the width of the base of the triangle, the tip located approximately 1 mm superior to the white roll, the height always 1 mm. The vertical incision on the cleft side incorporates a short, 1 mm, transverse incision at the corresponding point on the medial lip to permit inset of the triangular flap. Probably the most popular method of repair is that of rotation advancement described and advocated by Millard. Those steps consist of marking the key basic points as follows: The base or middle of Cupid's bow, the tip of Cupid's bow on the non-cleft side and a measurement, usually with calipers, of an equal distance from the trough or mid point of Cupid's bow to a planned Cupid's bow point on the cleft side. The alar and columellar bases are marked on the non-cleft side as well as the cleft side. The height of the philtral column is measured on the non-cleft side and

transposed to the cleft side as the length of the rotation incision. The inferior extent of the rotation incision is at the vermilion border at the Cupid's bow and the length of the rotation incision, as stated above, is equal to the height of the philtral column on the normal side. The same measurement is then transposed to the lateral lip segment and an incision is outlined parallel to and a one-half mm superior to the vermilion border from the alar base laterally. The lateral extent of that incision will ultimately contribute to the apex of Cupid's bow and is known as "Noordhoff's point". The major steps are completion of the rotation incision, a paring of the mucosa from the advancement incision and inset of the superior tip of the advancement flap into the apex of the rotation incision. Prior to suturing, a separate dissection of the vermilion to inset as a flap into the medial vermilion, a short transverse incision at the alar base with complete release of the alar base from the underlying fibrous attachments, dissection of separate orbicularis muscle bundles, including superficial and deep, dissection of a superiorly based septal flap in conjunction with dissection of a lateral or vestibular flap for repair of the nasal floor and then the dissection for a primary rhinoplasty as discussed below.

The major steps in lip suturing are to repair the muscle, superficial separate from deep, placement of the key buried suture from the tip of the advancement flap to the apex of the rotation incision, placement of the key suture through the Cupid's bow on both lateral and medial lip segments as previously marked, repair of the nasal floor by advancement of the vestibular flap into the tip of the septal flap, skin closure, and a Z-plasty of the vermilion and adjacent lip mucosa.

A more complete and diagrammatic discussion of lip repair can be found in various plastic surgical atlases and includes, among others, the Mohler and anatomic subunit approximation repairs.

Address of the cleft lip nasal deformity at the time of lip repair has become increasingly accepted and currently is performed by most, if not all, cleft surgeons. Salyer, Mulliken, and Cutting have all published technical approaches to the cleft lip nose. Complete release of the alar base, dissection of septal and lateral nasal wall flaps for closure of the nostril floor, nasal submucosal dissection with scissor spreading along the affected lower lateral cartilage with access from the alar base, placement of domal sutures from the affected lower lateral cartilage to the opposite upper lateral cartilage, a trans-cartilage suture or sutures through both foot plates, and the use of internal and external bolsters all are components of the primary rhinoplasty. Adding a rim incision for direct access to the medial crus of the affected lower lateral cartilage is another maneuver but not universally accepted.)

Postoperative (Age 4 Years)

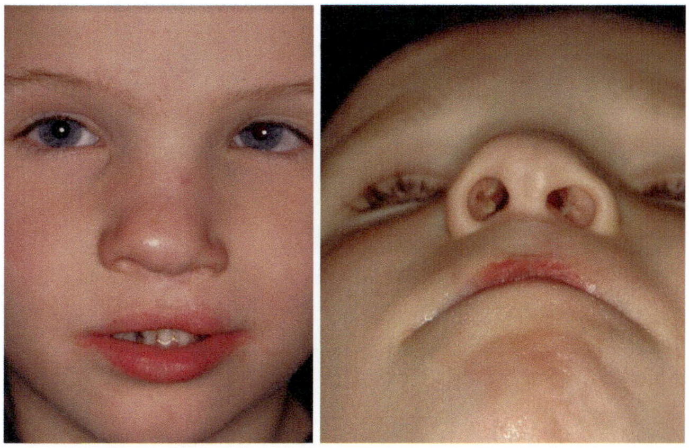

Two photos, a full face frontal and a submental vertex depict the lip repair with excellent Cupid's bow, symmetry, and mucosal fullness. The repair scar is perceptible but indistinct. The lip height is good and little transverse shortening of the left lateral lip is evident. Nasal alar bases are symmetrical and the tip is not bifid. On the submental vertex the left alar base is laterally displaced, not severely, and as a result some rounding of the nostril is evident.

In-Service Examination

1. If both father and first child have a cleft lip, what is the increased risk of cleft lip in a subsequent child?
   (a) 2%
   (b) 4%
   (c) 8%
   (d) 16%
2. If the first child has a cleft palate, what is the increased risk of a cleft lip in a subsequent child?
   (a) 0%
   (b) 2%
   (c) 4%
   (d) 8%
3. A neonate has a cleft lip and lower lip pits. What is the diagnosis?
   (a) Stickler syndrome
   (b) Van der Woude syndrome
   (c) Cri De Cault
   (d) Coute syndrome
   (e) Charcot-Tooth syndrome
4. The following are features of cleft lip nasal deformities **EXCEPT:**
   (a) The base of the columella is displaced to the non-cleft side
   (b) The alar cartilage is displaced posteriorly and superiorly
   (c) The nasal tip is displaced toward the cleft side
   (d) The caudal septum is displaced to the cleft side

Bilateral Cleft Lip

14

Bibliography

Zhang, Jacques, X., M.D., et al., "Evidence-based medicine: the bilateral cleft lip repair", *Plast. Reconstr. Surg.*, (2017); 140: **154e-161e, (Overview).**

Grayson BH and Garfinkle JS, Chapter 64: "Nasoalveolar Molding and Columella Elongation in Preparation for the Primary Repair of Unilateral and Bilateral Cleft Lip and Palate", Losee, J. E. and Kirschner, R. E. Comprehensive Cleft Care, The McGraw-Hill Co. (2016); pgs. **1223-46. (Repeat of II.A.1. reading - pg. 1241 pertinent to II.A.2.)**

Marcus JR, Allori AC, Santiago PE, "Principles of Cleft Lip Repair: Conventions, Commonalities, and Controversies", *Plast Reconstr Surg.*, 2017; 139:**764e; 769e-751e ONLY.**

Mulliken, J.B. "Primary Repair of Bilateral Cleft Lip and Nasal Deformity", *Plast. Reconstr. Surg.,* (2001); 108:**184-189 ONLY.**

Monson LA, Kirschner RE, Losee JE, "Primary repair of cleft lip and nasal deformity", *Plast. Reconstr. Surg.*, (2013); 132(6):**1047e-1051e (ONLY).**

Denadai R, Pai BCJ, Sato N, et al., "Bilateral Complete Cleft Lip Repair: A Step-by-Step Video Series", *Plast. Reconstr. Surg.*, (2020); 146(6):**1352-1356, Videos 1-4, SDC 1-3.**

Fisher DM and Sommerlad BC, "Cleft Lip, Cleft Palate, and Velopharyngeal Insufficiency", *Plast. Reconstr. Surg.*, (2011); 128(4):**342e; Video 4 ONLY.**

(The material on Cleft Palate and VPI is in a later module.)

Henry, C., Samson, T., Mackay, D., "Evidence-based medicine: the cleft lip nasal deformity", *Plast. Reconstr. Surg.*, (2014); 133:**1283-86, Table 1, and Video 1.**

Faculty Discussion and Study Guide

Anatomy, Preoperative, Background

1. What are the principal issues in bilateral cleft lip repair? (The role of premaxillary orthopedics and nasal alveolar molding (NAM); role of lip adhesion and two-stage repair; management of the asymmetric defect; the address of deficient prolabium vermilion; primary rhinoplasty.)
2. Describe the lip and soft-tissue deformity. (In both incomplete and complete clefts, the prolabial segment is of varying size. Not uncommonly in the *incomplete* bilateral cleft, the prolabial segment may be quite small while in a complete cleft of substantially larger size presumably due to the stress of the abnormally positioned premaxilla. As in a unilateral complete cleft, the lateral lip segment is attenuated superiorly as is the most superior portion of the medial lip segment. The orbicularis muscle is in the lateral segments only. The vermilion in the prolabial segment is deficient and dry with only a vestige of a white roll. The sulcus is almost nonexistent.)
3. Describe the bilateral cleft lip nasal deformity. (The short, almost absent columella; broad, almost bifid nasal tip, bilateral flared nostrils, oriented transversely, laterally displaced alar bases, webbed lateral vestibule, buckled alar rims with attenuation of the lower lateral cartilage and inferior and lateral rotation of the genu and lateral crus as well as elongation and flattening with inferior and anterior displacement of the dome. In the incomplete deformity, depending on the degree of cleft, the premaxilla may be in a more normal position lying between the tips of the maxillary segments. The alar bases are displaced laterally and posteriorly.)
4. Describe the bony or alveolar deformity. (In a complete bilateral cleft, the premaxillary segment is anteriorly and superiorly tilted. In the most severe cases, the reference is to a "fly-away premaxilla" indicative of the severity of the deformity. The lateral or posterior maxillary segments are collapsed lingually.)
5. Comment on the following in the management of bilateral cleft lip deformity: Premaxillary resection, preliminary lip adhesion. (A preliminary lip adhesion has not proved to be beneficial over that of a lip repair, including muscle and is prone to dehiscence and creates additional scar. Premaxillary complete resection is only to be con-

E. Luce, *A Curriculum for Plastic Surgery*, https://doi.org/10.1007/978-3-031-62087-4_14

demned and will result in severe class III occlusion and a dish face deformity in later childhood. Prevomerine resection and premaxillary setback are rarely employed as the readings cite.)

6. What are the specific anatomic goals of pre-surgical maxillary orthopedics in bilateral cleft lip? (Correction of the major bony deformities, including retro positioning of the premaxilla into a more posterior and inferior location, the buccal expansion of the collapsed posterior maxillary segments, and improvement of the soft-tissue relationships. In particular, the retro positioning of the premaxilla will place the lateral and prolabial lip segments in closer apposition for repair. In addition, the institution of nasal alveolar molding (NAM) as in the unilateral lip will elevate the bilateral nostril domes into a better position, similar to unilateral. Address of the lingual collapse of the maxillary segments, combined with retro positioning of the premaxilla, will permit gingivoperiosteoplasty [GPP], if so selected.)
   (a) What is the difference and the pros and cons of active vs. passive pre-surgical maxillary orthopedics? (Passive as explained in the unilateral cleft lip section, implies external traction of some type such as a band or adhesive tape and an intraoral appliance to simply maintain position of the maxillary segments. Active methods, such as the Latham appliance, actively manipulate and reposition the premaxilla and maxillary segments. The principal disadvantage of passive methods is that they are frequently inadequate and may produce soft-tissue abrasions and do nothing to expand the maxillary segments unless frequent, perhaps weekly, new appliances are fabricated. The disadvantage of the active methods is potential erosion of the intraoral soft tissues and the necessity for excellent parental compliance and of course the operation for placement. Some observers have raised concerns about the long-term effect on maxillary growth.)
   (b) Advantages of either? (Facilitates repair, possibly decrease in oral-nasal fistula, improvement in nasal aesthetics.)
7. The readings state, quite correctly, that we labored under two misconceptions about bilateral cleft lip and the repair of the same. What are they? (The two misconceptions, borrowing from the concept of unilateral lip repair, tissue had to be introduced from the lateral segment into the deficient prolabium to increase height *and* the short columella had to await secondary procedures—lengthening by the addition of flaps harvested from the lip or nasal sill.)
   (a) Comment on the alteration with time of the prolabial segment after lip repair. (An important observation is that the prolabial segment will progressively widen and lengthen with time and growth of the underlying skeletal framework. As a result, a philtral segment that is constructed too wide or even of a normal width in infancy will progressively abnormally widen with growth. Similarly, a philtrum that is constructed of adequate length with repair may become abnormally long with time.)
   (b) If the above is true, then what is the criticism of straight-line repair that would in fact produce vertical elongation of the central or philtral segment? (The segment is abnormally wide even at the time of repair and continues to widen with the inevitable tissue tension of the underlying protuberant premaxilla as well as growth.)
8. What are the methods, mostly of historical interest, of lengthening the columella? Describe? (The Cronin procedure rotated bi-pedicled flaps from the nasal floor into the columella and the forked-flap Millard procedure rotated lip skin and soft tissue into the columella as superiorly based flaps.)
   (a) What is the criticism? (The Millard forked-flap procedure produced multiple scars both in the lip and the base of the nose; lengthening accomplished with the Cronin procedure fades with time because of the lateral alar base tension on the flaps.)
   (b) Discuss "banked" forked flaps. (Millard and Mulliken both experimented with the use of the excess lateral prolabial skin-soft tissue as potential future forked flaps by banking the same in the nostril sill. The flaps contracted and given the intrinsic criticisms of the fork flap procedure, the procedure has fallen into disuse.)

Operative Plan

1. What are the principles in contemporary bilateral cleft lip repair? (Symmetry, reconstitution of the orbicularis muscle, appropriate philtral size, formation of a median tubercle, white roll, and vermilion from lateral lip elements, primary positioning of alar cartilages to construct the tip and columella; discard of the deficient prolabial white roll and vermilion; use of prolabial mucosa to line the anterior aspect of the premaxilla.)
2. What are the key elements of Mulliken's bilateral cleft lip repair? (Narrow the prolabial segment, release-excise deficient prolabial mucosa, use of laterally based vermilion-white roll labial flaps to reconstitute prolabial vermilion, white roll, and sulcus, use of prolabial mucosa to reconstitute the premaxillary labial sulcus, mobilization and repair of orbicularis muscle end to end over the bony premaxilla, open primary nasal repair with rim inci-

sions, i.e., columella is in the nose not the lip; interdomal sutures and excision of redundant alar rims.)

(a) Expand on Mulliken's philosophy about the deformity in bilateral cleft lip nose and how that sets the stage for his primary rhinoplasty repair. (Mulliken and others are of the opinion that the "columella is in the nose" meaning that the shortening of the columella is due to a lateral splay of the underlying medial crus, footplates, and dome of the lower lateral nasal cartilages and that an open repair of all those structures including open realignment and suturing of the cartilages as well a V-Y advancement of the columellar skin and soft tissues are necessary for elongation.)

3. Outline the key markings and the steps in Mulliken's bilateral cleft lip repair. (The philtral incisions are outlined first which are 6–8 mm in vertical length, 3–4 mm wide at the Cupid's bow level, and about 2 mm wide at the base of the columella. The 8 mm horizontal dimension at the base of the philtrum allows placement of the proposed bilateral Cupid's bow points and then incisions of similar length, 6–8 mm are drawn on the lateral lip segments as the advancement flap with the lateral extent of those flaps on the vermilion border tattooed as the adjoining point on the prolabial segment for the proposed peak of the Cupid's bow on that side and repeated on the opposite side. The key steps are skin incisions on the philtral segment with deepithelialization for a couple of mm laterally to add bulk to the suture line, incisions on the lateral lip segments above the white roll or vermilion border, excision of the deficient prolabial mucosa with advancement of the remaining prolabial mucosa superiorly and posteriorly to create a labial sulcus and advancement of the lateral lip segments containing the vermilion and white roll into the prolabium, muscle repair, and suturing of the lip incisions. Some other repairs are somewhat less radical in narrowing the prolabia; a width of 4 mm at Cupid's bow and 3 mm at the base of the columella. See Fig. 14.1.)

(a) Additional considerations for the nasal floor and alveolar clefts? (The nasal floors are closed bilaterally with septal and alar mucosa. If gingivoperiosteoplasty (GPP) is selected, those flaps are raised and opposed. See Fig. 14.2.)

4. Discuss the nasal repair. (Bilateral nasal rim incisions and perhaps a midline nasal tip incision, interdomal mattress sutures to oppose the genu and domes of the lower lateral cartilage, advancement and cinching of the alar base into the septum, excision of redundant soft tissue in the soft triangle and interdomal space via the rim incisions. See Fig. 14.3.)

Video Notes

Denadai R, Pai BCJ, Sato N, et al., "Bilateral Complete Cleft Lip Repair: A Step-by-Step Video Series", *Plast. Reconstr. Surg.*, (2020); 146(6):1352.

Three videos and supplemental digital content of diagrams; reasonably good with a total time of 10–11 min.

1. Millard-type repair with Noordhoff modifications.
2. Principal criticism is creation of a "nasal turbinate" flap with buccal mucosal flaps, because of the excessive mucosa and the nostrils appear stenotic at the end of the procedure.
3. **Video 4**: The authors used a Tajima incision for access for the nose repair.

Fisher DM and Sommerlad BC, "Cleft Lip, Cleft Palate, and Velopharyngeal Insufficiency", *Plast. Reconstr. Surg.*, (2011); 128(4):351e.

1. Markings: Good, excellent, and all of the 5 min devoted to preoperative markings. *No* intraoperative dissection.

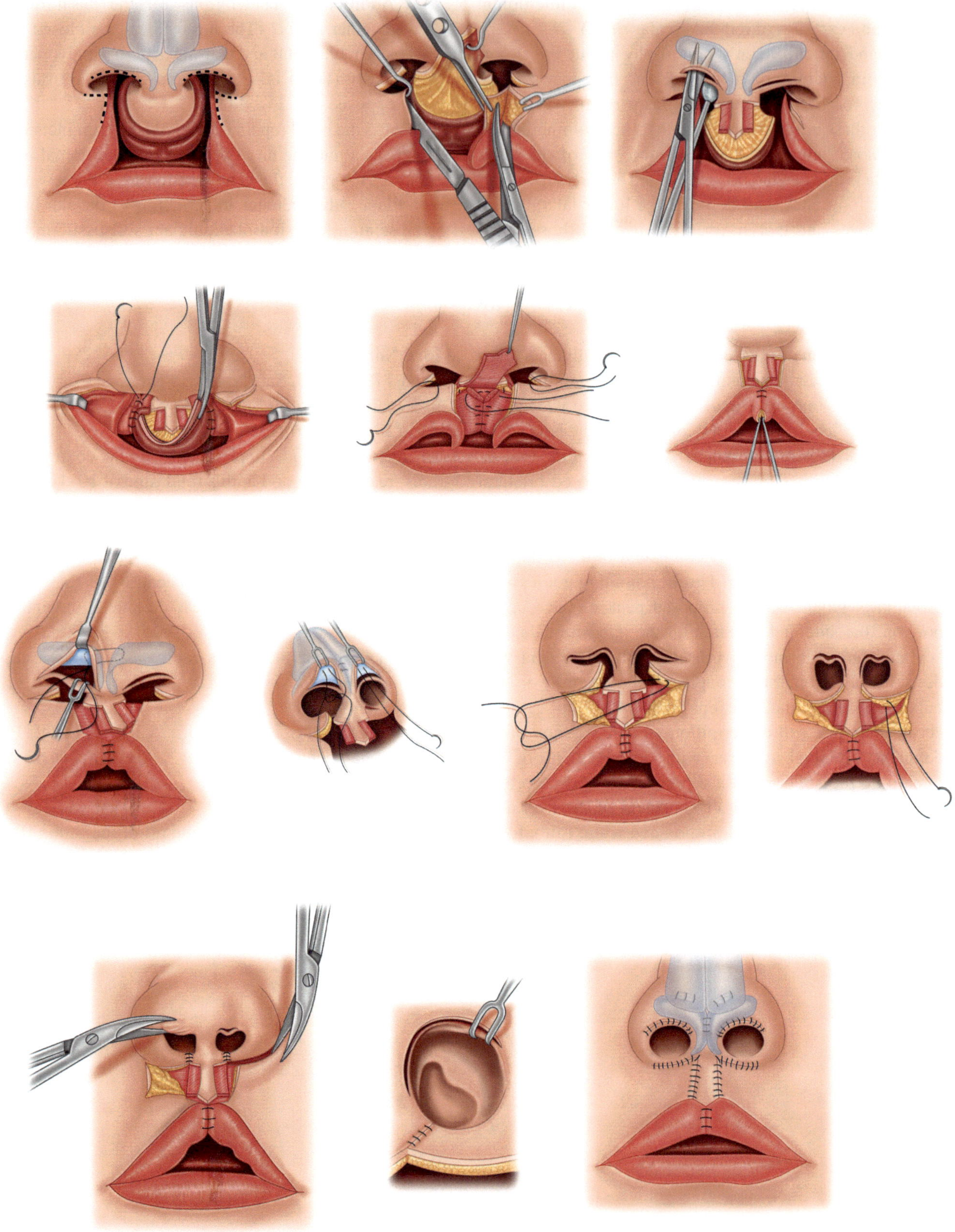

Fig. 14.1 Mulliken's bilateral cleft lip repair

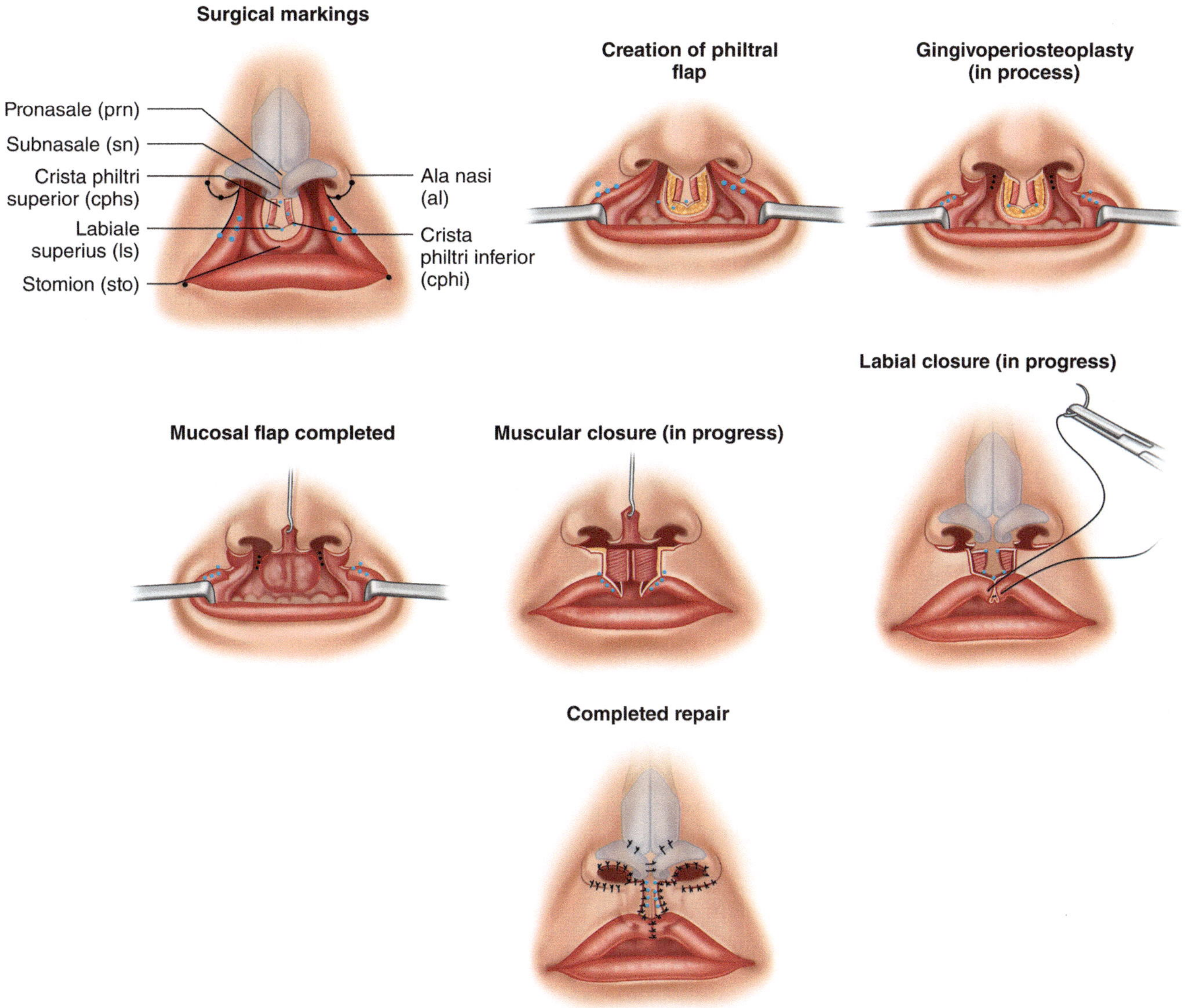

Fig. 14.2 A Detailed Description of Bilateral Cleft Lip Repair. (Marcus JR, Allori AC, and Santiago PE, "Principles of Cleft Lip Repair: Conventions, Commonalities, and Controversies", *Plas. Reconstr. Surg.*, (2017); 139: 776e. (Reprinted with Permission))

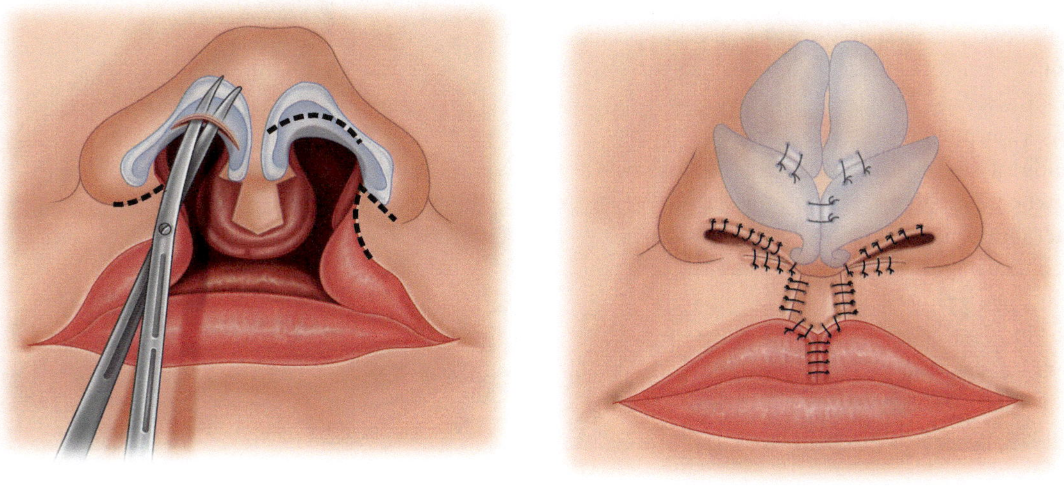

Fig. 14.3 Nasal repair

Case-Based Conference

Case 1: Bilateral Cleft Lip

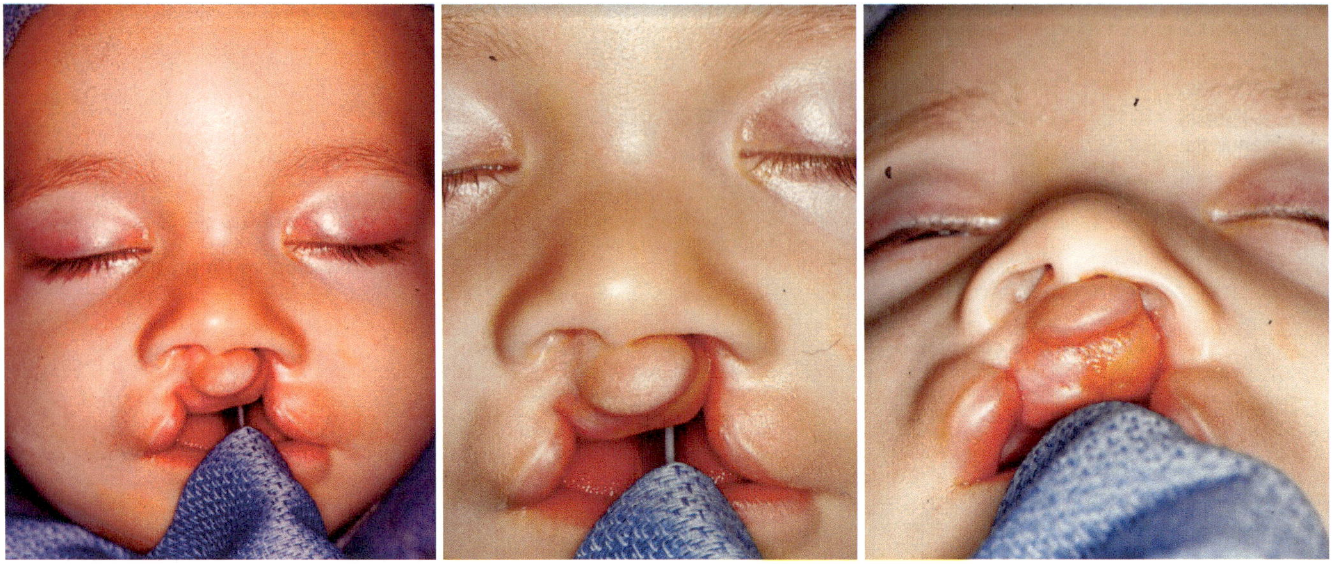

A 3-month-old infant, otherwise healthy with normal growth and development milestones.

1. Describe the slides and add other information from the clinical exam.
   (a) Any test(s) indicated? Justify.
2. Describe the deformity. What are the important variables in bilateral cleft lip that impact your treatment plan?
3. How would your treatment plan differ (or not) if you saw the patient initially as a neonate?
4. Outline the treatment plan. Draw your repair.

Case-Based Conference: Discussion

Case 1: Bilateral Cleft Lip

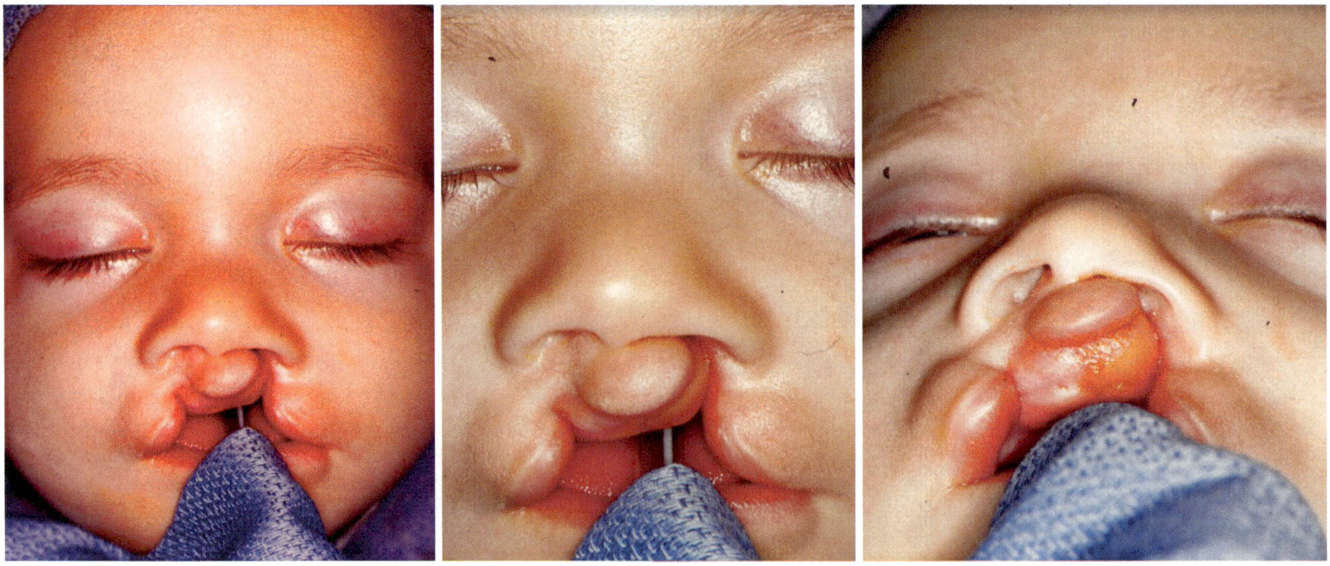

A 3-month-old infant otherwise healthy with normal growth and development milestones.

1. Describe the slides and add other information from the clinical exam. (Three views are provided: a full-face frontal, a closeup of the central one-third of the face, and a submental-vertex view. In the full-face view, an intubated infant is pictured, eyes closed, and a bilateral cleft of the lip is evident. The cleft is complete on the left side, the right side is incomplete, the cleft extending almost one-half of the height of the lip. The nose bears all the stigmata of a bilateral cleft lip nasal deformity. These findings include a short, nearly absent columella; a broad tip although perhaps not bifid as often seen in a complete bilateral cleft. The alar bases are laterally displaced with the resultant horizontally oriented nostrils. The prolabial segment is smaller than normal but not minuscule. The prolabium is also modestly tilted to the left. Although the premaxillary alveolar segment is visible, the lateral elements are not seen in this view. The closeup confirms these findings and does not add additional information. No other facial deformities or findings are evident in either view. The submental vertex does provide some additional findings and include a depiction of some buckling of the left alar rim and webbing of the lateral nasal vestibule bilaterally. In addition, the entire premaxillary segment is rotated approximately 30° counter clockwise. Again, neither the lateral alveolar segments nor the palate are visualized.

   The clinical exam would begin with ascertainment of feeding difficulties, if any, although the preamble relates normal growth and development milestones and a family history is added. The intraoral component of the physical exam would ascertain the extent of palatal involvement by the cleft and the relative positions of the lateral alveolar segments. An examination of the remainder of the body completes the physical.)
   (a) Any test(s) indicated? Justify. (No—unless the clinical exam unearths an area of concern.)
2. Describe the deformity. What are the important variables in bilateral cleft lip that impact your treatment plan? (The findings as outlined in the slide analysis include a bilateral cleft lip with a complete cleft at the left and an incomplete of the right lip. The premaxillary segment is rotated to the left or the side of the complete cleft. Although a lateral view is not available, as judged by the submental vertex, some anterior and superior displacement of the premaxillary segment is evident. In all likelihood the lateral alveolar-palatal segments are collapsed somewhat lingually. The prolabium is shortened, the vermilion is deficient and the sulcus is nearly nonexistent. The associated nasal deformity is well-characterized in the slide analysis. The nasal deformity is the result of attenuation of the lower lateral cartilage as well as lateral and inferior rotation of the genu, more severe on the left than right.

   The important variables that may impact the management of this patient are several: the magnitude of the anterior displacement of the premaxilla, the degree of lingual collapse of the lateral palatal segments, particularly if they impinge or are positioned to prevent favorable retrodisplacement of the premaxilla with the postoperative tension exerted by lip repair. The last component is not patient but rather surgeon-dependent and confident in accomplishing a single stage of repair.)
3. How would your treatment plan differ (or not) if you saw the patient initially as a neonate? (If the patient is seen as a neonate or shortly afterward, the opportunity is afforded to initiate preoperative maxillary orthopedics, directed toward expansion of the lateral palatal segments and retrodisplacement of the premaxilla. The two options in preoperative maxillary orthopedics are active and passive. Active maxillary orthopedics is implemented by the operative placement of an acrylic appliance that postoperatively by means of a jack screw turned periodically expands the elements of the appliance and translates into pressure on the malleable palate and premaxilla. Coincident with movement of the alveolar segments, an effort is also available to improve soft-tissue relationships, most particularly the nasal configuration by attachment of an outrigger to the appliance with a nostril component that maintains the nose in a more normal configuration. The passive option is a similar appliance but static and requires frequent, even weekly, repeat impressions and construction of a new appliance. Each option has advantages and disadvantages. The active appliance requires operative placement and familial compliance. The passive option mandates segmented outpatient visits for consultation and refitting of a new appliance.

   Although scenario presents a patient of 3 months of age, preoperative premaxillary orthopedics may still be of value, determined by the degree of lingual collapse of the lateral segments. In all likelihood, at least as judged by the photos, initiation of nasal-alveolar molding at this juncture would be of limited value and would only delay lip repair.)
4. Outline the treatment plan. Draw your repair. (Several different techniques address bilateral cleft lip repairs. Perhaps the most widely employed is the procedure adopted by Mulliken that centers on design of a narrow philtrum, construction of the medial or a central tubercle from the lateral lip elements including the white roll and vermilion, and reposition of the splayed lower lateral cartilages centrally to lengthen the columella. The conceptual approach is based on the observation that the philtral segment will inevitably widen with time, the pro-

labial vermilion and mucosa are deficient, and the shortened columella is secondary to the lateral splay of the underlying medial crus, dome, and foot plates. The essential markings and steps in the Mulliken repair: the philtral incisions are outlined first which are 6–8 mm in length, 3–4 mm wide at the Cupid's bow level, and about 2 mm wide at the base of the columella. The 8 mm horizontal dimension at the base of the philtrum allows placement of the proposed bilateral Cupid's bow points and then incisions of similar length, 6–8 mm are drawn on the lateral lip segments as the advancement flaps. The lateral extent of those flaps on the vermilion border is tattooed as well as the adjoining point on the prolabial segment for the proposed peak of the Cupid's bow on that side and repeated on the opposite side. The key steps are skin incisions on the philtral segment with deepithelialization for a couple of mm laterally to add bulk to the suture line, incisions on the lateral lip segments above the white roll or vermilion border, excision of the deficient prolabial mucosa and advancement of the lateral lip segments containing the vermilion and white roll into the prolabium, muscle repair, and suturing of the lip incisions.

Primary nasal repair consists of bilateral nasal rim incisions and perhaps a midline nasal tip incision, interdomal mattress sutures to oppose the genu and domes of the lower lateral cartilage, advancement and cinching of the alar base into the septum, excision of redundant soft tissue in the soft triangle and interdomal space.)

Postoperative (Age 3 Years)

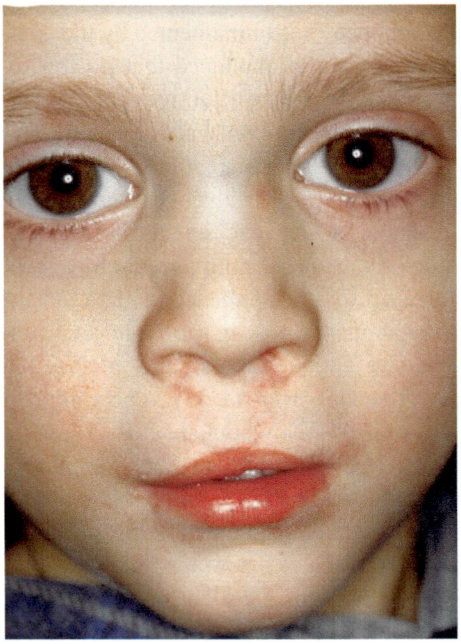

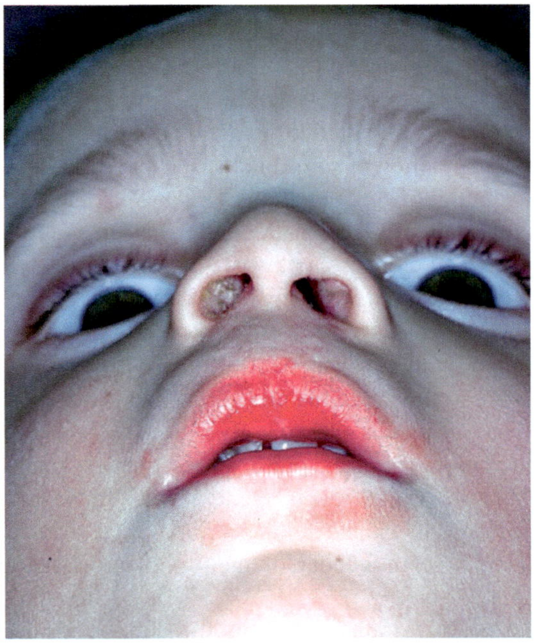

The lip lacks a defined Cupid's bow and has a slight vermilion step-off on the left. A glimpse of the maxillary incisors despite lip closure demonstrates a suggestion of a "whistle-tip" mucosal deficiency centrally. The repair scars, although visible, are not reddened and hypertrophic, and lip height is adequate. The alar bases are symmetrical and the nasal tip architecture is normal, but the nasal sills appear somewhat widened. The submental vertex depicts some lateral displacement of the left alar base and some consequent inferior displacement and asymmetry of the alar rim.

Critique

A revision, perhaps with a Tajima-type superior alar rim combined with an alar base incision would address both.

In-Service Examination

1. Objectives in nasal-alveolar molding (NAM) of the bilateral cleft lip patient include:
   (a) Lateral or buccal expansion of the posterior segments

(b) Medial movement of the lateral lip segments
(c) Lengthening of the columella
(d) Inferior displacement of the caudal septum

2. The occurrence of bilateral cleft lip is because of what elements embryologically that fail to fuse
(a) Medial nasal prominences
(b) Medial nasal and maxillary prominences
(c) Lateral nasal prominences
(d) Medial and lateral palatine prominences

3. The most likely affected tooth bilaterally in bilateral cleft lip is:
(a) Lateral incisor
(b) Medial incisor
(c) Canine
(d) First premolar

Secondary Lip Deformities, Cleft Rhinoplasty

15

Bibliography

Stal MD, S. and Hollier MD, L., "Correction of Secondary Cleft Lip Deformities", *Plast. Reconstr. Surg.*, (2002); 109:**1672-1681.**

Monsoon LA, Buchanan EP, Hollier LH, "Chapter 55: Correction of Secondary Bilateral Cleft Lip and Nose Deformities", Losee, J. E. and Kirschner, R. E. *Comprehensive Cleft Care,* The McGraw-Hill Co., (2016);**1051-60**.

Burget GC, Chapter 56: "Definitive Rhinoplasty for Adult Cleft Lip Nasal Deformity", Losee, J. E. and Kirschner, R. E. Comprehensive Cleft Care Second Edition, The McGraw-Hill Co. (2016);**1066-75.**

Allori, A.C., Mulliken J.B., "Evidence-based medicine: secondary correction of cleft lip nasal deformity", *Plast. Reconstr. Surg.*, (2017); 140: **166e-175e**.

Guyuron, B., "MOC-PS(SM) CME article: late cleft lip nasal deformity", *Plast. Reconstr. Surg.*, (2008); 121: **1-11**.

Rohrich RJ, Benkler M, Avashia YJ, Savetsky IL, "Secondary Rhinoplasty for Unilateral Cleft Nasal Deformity", *Plast Reconstr Surg.*, (2021); 148:**133-43; Videos 2-4 ONLY**.

Supplemental

Burget GC, Chapter 56: "Definitive Rhinoplasty for Adult Cleft Lip Nasal Deformity", Losee, J. E. and Kirschner, R. E. Comprehensive Cleft Care Second Edition, The McGraw-Hill Co. (2016);1075-1090 (Case Examples).

Faculty Discussion and Study Guide

Late Secondary Deformities

1. What are the essential elements of the evaluation of the patient who presents for possible cleft lip revision? (Assessment of the lip scar, status of the orbicularis, orientation of the vermilion, while roll and Cupid's bow, and excessive fullness or deficiency of the mucosa. The nasal deformity should be examined for nostril and alar base asymmetry and shape, as well as tip malpositioning. The presence of skeletal or maxillary hypoplasia should be documented.)
2. In terms of deformity of a short vertical dimension of the repaired lip, what are some guidelines to determine the method of correction? (The magnitude or degree of the shortening. A mm or less can probably be addressed with a diamond-shaped excision of scar at the white roll-vermilion junction or perhaps as Z-plasty. Deficiencies greater than 3 mm probably require a complete re-repair of the lip. Intermediate deficiencies will dictate an individual approach.)
3. Describe management of a 1.5 mm malalignment of the vermilion/white roll evident at 6 months after primary lip repair. (Nothing at this juncture, observation is warranted for at least a year.)
   (a) Evident at two years after repair? (A Z-plasty correction diagrammed in the readings, is usually successful in correction of malalignment.)
4. A 4-year-old with a prior complete unilateral cleft lip repair presents with a notching defect limited to the mucosa/vermilion only. The white lip is satisfactory. How would you analyze and manage? (One must determine whether the deficiency is simply insufficient soft tissue or does scar tethering further adds to the problem. If the notch is mild and more the result of lateral mucosa lip fullness a horizontal or transverse excision of mucosa and soft tissue hidden in the posterior labial mucosa would suffice. Moderate-sized defects can be addressed with a Y-V advancement with the apex of the V closure oriented posterior. More severe deformities may require a Z-plasty with the anterior scar placed on dry vermilion. The important aspect of the analysis is to eliminate inadequate rotation as a contributing problem.)
5. A 5-year-old presents after a prior repair of a complete unilateral cleft with a long lip. What is the most likely repair method and methods of secondary correction?

E. Luce, *A Curriculum for Plastic Surgery*, https://doi.org/10.1007/978-3-031-62087-4_15

(Most likely the repair was some type of triangular or quadrangular flap repair such as Tennison or Hagedorn or perhaps Fisher. A long cleft lip is extremely difficult to repair successfully. Probably the optimal opportunity for success is a takedown of the lip and repair both vertically and transversely.)

6. A 3-year-old with a previous bilateral cleft lip repair presents to your office with a 1 mm shortening of the lip on the right and 4 mm on the left. What is your management? (Diamond excision on the right, take down and re-rotation on the left.)
7. A 4-year-old with prior complete bilateral cleft lip repair presents with a "whistle-tip" deformity. Give your analysis and correction. ("Whistle-tip" refers to central or prolabial deficiency of mucosa. A variety of techniques have been advocated for vermilion/mucosa deficiencies in the prolabial segment. Analysis must include if a concomitant deficiency exists in the white roll and skin-soft tissue as well. Assuming not, one approach is to advance mucosal flaps from either lateral lip segment which are often quite full. More severe deficiencies will require Abbe cross-lip transfer, usually combined with columellar lengthening, and use of the deficient white lip to accomplish same. Analysis must also assess if the orbicularis muscle has been properly placed into the prolabial segment. If the child will pursue his lips, inadequate muscle advancement will be evident by a muscle bulge in the lateral lip segments.)
8. A 4-year-old with an aesthetically acceptable bilateral cleft lip repair but tight. What is the analysis and address? (The analysis should include orbicularis function and scar width. If both are satisfactory, the first consideration is treatment with fat grafting.)

Secondary Cleft Rhinoplasty

1. What are the components of the secondary *unilateral* cleft nasal deformity? (The severity of the deformity will be determined by the magnitude of the original cleft, the degree of correction obtained with primary repair, and the effect of facial growth. Please see Chap. 13. As a child or adult, the deformity to some degree will mirror the deformity encountered in the infant: the dome of the lower lateral cartilage is displaced inferior and lateral and as a result the interdomal angle is obtuse or at least less acute and the tip is wide and bifid. The skeletal component of the lateral pyriform aperture is deficient and posteriorly and laterally displaced. Similarly, the alar base is laterally displaced and wide. The nostril configuration is much more transverse than oblique. The lateral crus of the lower lateral cartilage is flattened and the alar rim may be drawn inferiorly. The hemi columella on the cleft side is shortened. The anterior nasal spine and caudal septum are deflected into the non-cleft medial nostril, and the posterior septum and ethmoid are deviated into the cleft side. The inferior turbinate may be enlarged on the non-cleft side. The dorsum is widened and deviated to the non-cleft side. In profile, the tip lacks projection, the midface may be concave.)
2. What are the components of the secondary *bilateral* cleft nose deformity? (In a sense the secondary bilateral deformity is a duplication of the unilateral on the non-cleft side. The dorsum is widened and without deviation and the tip is quite flat with uniform shortening of the columella. The alar bases are bilaterally displaced with transversely oriented nostrils. The degree of septal deviation is variable. The overall configuration of the midface is hypoplasia with malar flattening and lack of facial projection with a probable Class III malocclusion. See Table 15.1.).
3. What are the important aspects, besides nasal and facial aesthetic analysis, of the clinical examination? (The history in addition to the evaluation consistent with that performed in all potential aesthetic surgery candidates, would focus on the presence and severity of nasal obstruction and would include a nasal speculum exam and Cottle maneuvers. The dental occlusion is assessed and the prospects of any planned orthognathic surgery are explored.)
   (a) What effect, if any, does the occurrence and timing of orthognathic surgery have on planned cleft rhinoplasty surgery? (If limited to the mandible and if performed in concert with mandibular orthognathic surgery, probably none. Maxillary advancement, for example, a more likely occurrence, in correction of Class III malocclusion will alter nasal aesthetics substantially and, although in some practices, a cleft rhinoplasty is performed in the same operative setting, a more conservative approach is deferral.)
4. What is the approximate timing for secondary cleft rhinoplasty? (Essentially, two schools of thought, an intermediate correction performed in early childhood, followed by a definitive rhinoplasty in the mid-or late teens. The other is deferral of any rhinoplasty until adulthood, adulthood defined as mid-teens. To some degree, the decision hinges on the residual deformity following primary rhinoplasty performed at the time of lip repair. Regardless, as discussed below, intermediate rhinoplasty tends to be confined to manipulation of the tip cartilages, associated soft tissue, and the caudal septum. Definitive rhinoplasty incorporates dorsal osteotomies and infracture, harvest of the septum for cartilage grafts, including spreader, columellar, and extensive tip cartilage grafting. Also, see below.)

Editorial Note: This submodule optimally would follow mastery of Chaps. 99 and 100.

Table 15.1 Secondary cleft lip nasal deformity (CLND)

Anatomy	Unilateral CLND	Bilateral CLND
Upper two-thirds		
Nasal root	Minor widening and deviation	Moderate widening and deviation
Dorsum	Deviated toward noncleft side	Midline
Lower one-third		
Alar root	Inferiorly/posteriorly displaced on cleft side	Inferiorly/posteriorly displaced, bilaterally
Alar base	Wide on cleft side	Wide bilaterally
Nasal tip	Asymmetric, with relatively more projection and definition on noncleft side and "effacement" on cleft side	Flat, broad, weak tip projection
Columella	Short hemicolumella on cleft side; base deviated toward noncleft side	Short bilaterally
Alar lobule and rim	Flattened nostril on cleft side, with or without recurvatum	Flattened nostrils, with or without recurvatum
Nostril shape	Obliquely oriented on cleft side; contralateral side usually vertically oriented in Caucasians; may be variably round or obliquely oriented in other ethnicities	Obliquely oriented, bilaterally
Intranasal		
Vestibule	Vestibular web on cleft side	Vestibular webs, bilaterally
Septum	Anterocaudal septum and anterior nasal spine deviated to noncleft side; posterior septum deviated to cleft side	Midline anterocaudal septum; variable posterior deviation
Turbinates	Hypertrophied on noncleft side	Hypertrophy variably present
Facial		
Maxilla	Ipsilateral malar flattening and maxillary hypoplasia/retrusion (class III malocclusion)	Bilateral malar flattening and maxillary hypoplasia/retrusion (class III malocclusion)

5. Outline the elements of correction in an *intermediate* cleft rhinoplasty. (Centralization of the caudal edge of septum, repositioning of the alar base, correction and advancement of the lower lateral cartilage to the medial portion of the opposite upper lateral cartilage, chondro mucosal medial advancement of the lateral crus of the lower lateral cartilage. If bilateral, an open-tip incisional approach to centralization of the medial lower lateral cartilages, mimicking Mulliken's primary repair can be incorporated. In instances of severe shortening of the columella, Cronin nasal floor rotation combined with alar base advancement can also be employed to lengthen the columella.)
6. Describe the important elements of late cleft rhinoplasty. (The analysis will differ between a unilateral and a bilateral cleft lip patient. Regardless, the analysis begins with the deformity. In a unilateral cleft lip deformity the alar cartilage on the affected side duplicates to some degree the deformity seen in the unrepaired cleft. Attention must be directed toward reestablishment of normal dome height, correction of bifidity, provision of columellar support with cartilage graft, and repositioning of the skin envelope. All of these principles dictate an open rhinoplasty approach. The late bilateral cleft rhinoplasty requires address of broad and flat tip, dramatically short columella, and under projected tip as well as overall midface hypoplasia. The late rhinoplasty in the bilateral cleft patient will incorporate the above procedural components as well as perhaps dorsal cantilever bone graft. The consideration of orthognathic surgery is beyond the scope of this submodule. See Chap. 18.)
   (a) List the major steps in the late or adult cleft rhinoplasty? (Nasal dorsal reduction, osteotomy and infracture, septal resection, and spreader grafts of the upper and middle one-third. The tip requires caudal septal centralization, elevation, and advancement of the ipsilateral lower lateral cartilage with interdomal and spanning sutures to the columellar strut graft, perhaps also suture of the lower lateral to the opposite upper lateral cartilage, possible tip shield graft, alar batten graft, alar base repositioning. See Fig. 15.1.)

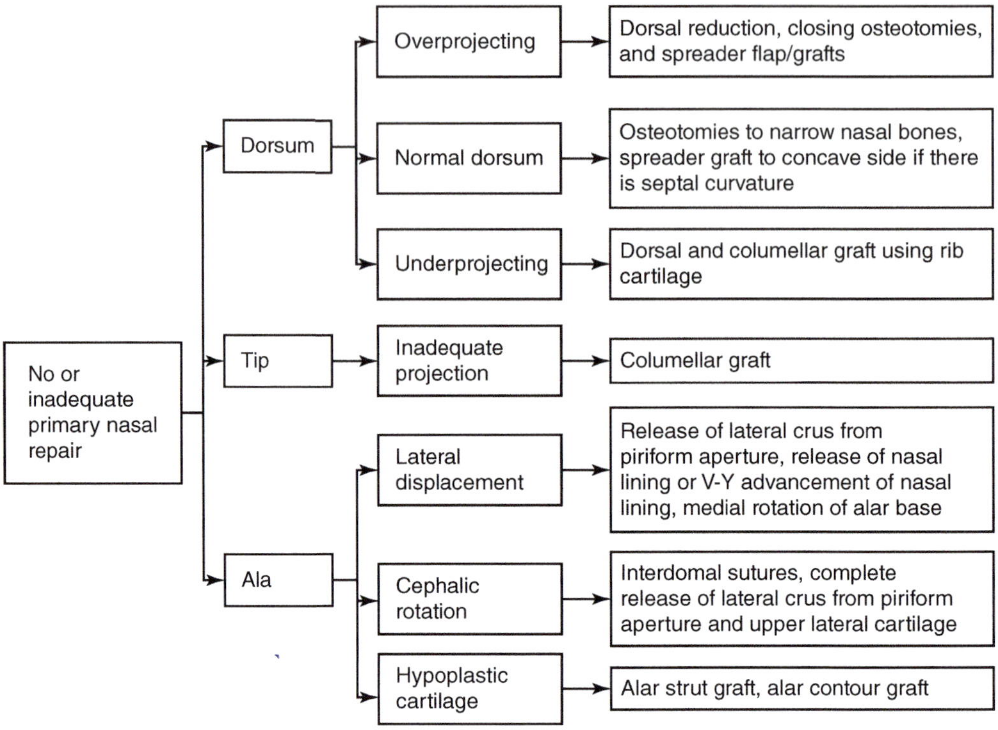

Fig. 15.1 Adult cleft rhinoplasty. (Byrd, SH, El-Musa KA, Yazdani A, Chapter 63 "Rhinoplasty in the Cleft Lip Nasal Deformity", Gunter JP, Rohrich RJ and Adams WP, Dallas Rhinoplasty Nasal Surgery by the Masters, Quality Medical Publishing, Inc., (2007);1265. (Reprinted with permission))

Case-Based Conference

Case 1: Cleft Lip Deformity

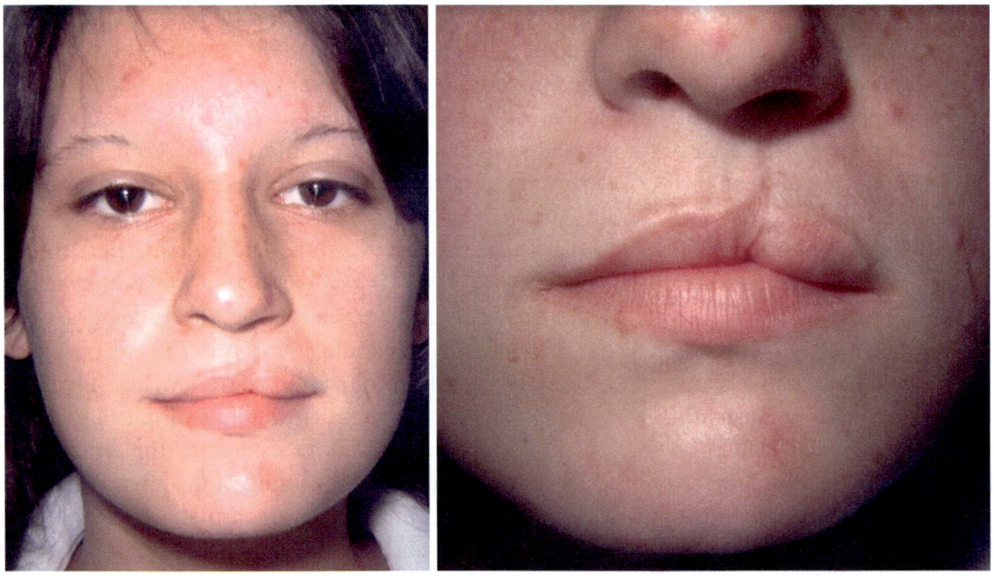

A 20-year-old woman, who had repair of a left cleft lip in infancy.

1. Describe the slide(s) and add a clinical examination.
   (a) Any tests indicated? Justify.
2. Describe the pathologic anatomy.
3. Outline a treatment plan. Include a short description of any operative procedures and nonoperative measures, if any.

Case-Based Conference: Discussion

Case 1: Cleft Lip Deformity

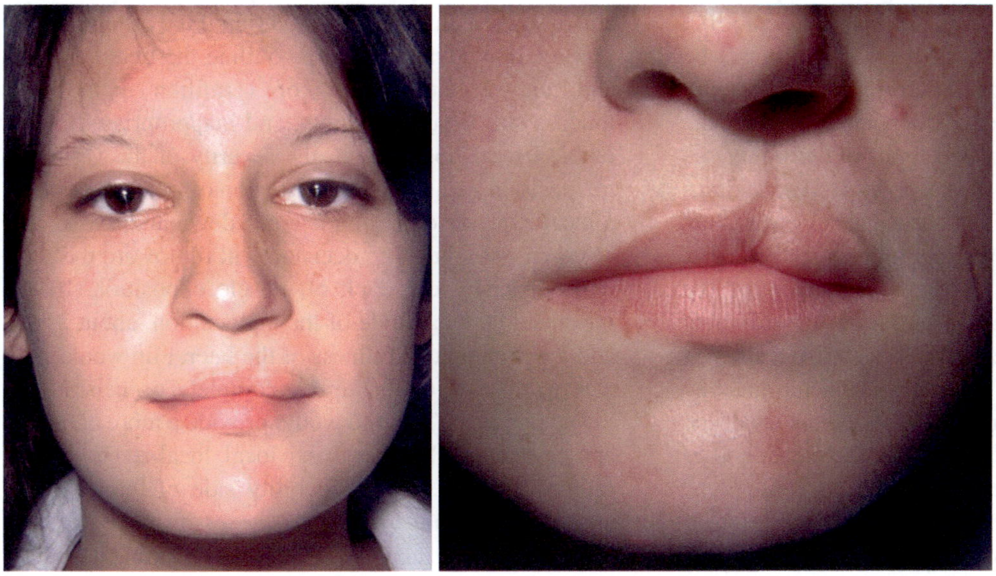

A 20-year-old woman, who had repair of a left cleft lip in infancy.

1. Describe the slide(s) and add a clinical examination. (Two photos are provided, a full frontal of the face and a close-up view of the lips and nasal tip, also frontal. The first, the full face view, represents a woman with no facial animation, the lips closed and the mouth in repose or neutral. The most evident finding depicted is an irregularity of the left upper lip, principally in the vermilion border. The irregularity occurs at the point of the normal location of Cupid's bow point on the left and consists of malposition of the lip, including the white roll common vermilion, and dry mucosa. The lip medial to the irregularity is tilted superiorly. Lateral to the break in the continuity of the vermilion, the white lip is directed inferiorly and inappropriately into dry mucosa. A fine line vertical scar is present, occupying the normal location of the philtral column. No other remarkable findings are evident. Some suggestion of inferior displacement of the left alar rim is present and only a single tip defining point is seen, on the right. Alar bases are symmetrical, the dorsum is somewhat, but not dramatically, broad. The photo was probably not taken in "portrait" mode but rather at a shorter focal length. A few scattered, small erythematous facial blemishes are evident. The close-up view adds additional information. The finding of malposition of the vermilion border is confirmed. The white roll is attenuated for several mm on either aspect, medial and lateral, of the scar disruption of the vermilion. Some deficiency of mucosa-soft tissue of the free edge of the lip is present at the same point, although the severity cannot be determined since lips are in repose. The entire dry mucosa of the upper lip from white roll to free edge is substantially fuller on the lateral lip than in comparison to the right side. The repair scar is nearly imperceptible. The nasal tip is more clearly depicted in the close-up photo and the alar rim is more inferior in position compared to the right. No other findings are evident and no suggestion of maxillary deformity, recession, or tight lip is apparent in either view, although would be optimally assessed in full lateral.

   The clinical examination would begin with ascertainment and specificity of the patient's concerns and then establish, if possible, the nature of the operative procedures accomplished in childhood. Other questions, hinging on the nature of the concerns articulated by the patient—see question two—would determine the presence of any nasal respiratory complaints. Current medications including over-the-counter and a social history, complete the overall history component of the clinical examination. The physical exam consists of observation of the lip as the patient responds during the history and then specifically when directed toward precise actions as puckering to determine muscular, orbicularis, continuity. Absence of continuity will be manifested in puckering as a bunching of the muscle in the lateral segment. The nose should be inspected for the stigmata of the cleft lip nose as well as a speculum exam of the septum, if indicated. The intraoral examination consists of detection of any persistent alveolar cleft, evaluation of the dentition, and an overall speech assessment is added.)

(a) Any tests indicated? Justify. (Barring any unanticipated detection of comorbidity or cleft-associated morbidity, no testing or imaging is indicated. To more fully evaluate this patient, although the emphasis of the case is the lip deformity, photos that depict the lateral and submental vertex perspective would be necessary to assess the nasal deformities.)

2. Describe the pathologic anatomy. (Stepping away from the issue of a possible associated cleft lip-nasal deformity, the principal pathology is the soft tissue of the lip. The findings of malposition of the vermilion border of approximately 3 mm or more and an inappropriate fullness of the lateral upper lip segment suggest incomplete rotation of the medial or cleft lip, combined with lack of sufficient advancement of the lateral segment. An associated absence of adequate muscle repair, if any, cannot be determined by the provided photos and would hinge on the results of the physical exam. As described previously, the scenario does not establish the status of the nose or alveolus.)
3. Outline a treatment plan. Include a short description of any operative procedures and nonoperative measures, if any. (A number of modalities have been described to address secondary cleft lip deformities, including fat grafting, laser therapy, and soft tissue rearrangement as well as cleft rhinoplasty and orthodontic-orthognathic surgery. Certainly, rhinoplasty can be readily combined with a soft tissue revision procedure, although any orthognathic surgery should precede the same. This discussion will center on the address of the lip. The findings outlined above suggest an inadequate rotation if the primary repair was rotation advancement. To outline the treatment plan and address the findings of vermilion malposition, mucosa-soft tissue deformity, and inappropriate fullness of the lateral lip segment, the severity of the vermilion malposition will dictate the selection of treatment option, a local Z-plasty or a complete takedown and reassembly or repair of the lip. The decision will tilt toward the latter if the exam reveals lack of muscle opposition. In this instance, the magnitude of the malposition, about 3 mm, and the pronounced fullness of the lateral lip would indicate re-rotation of the lip by complete re-incision followed by repair. To do so would provide a more definitive and optimal result rather than a local, localized to the vermilion, Z-plasty. On the liability side of the treatment plan equation, however, is the necessity to recreate an incision scar that, at present, is highly desirable in appearance. In essence, the choice is a scar substantially more noticeable that will improve with time but a considerably more comprehensive and complete solution to the clinical problem.)

Postoperative

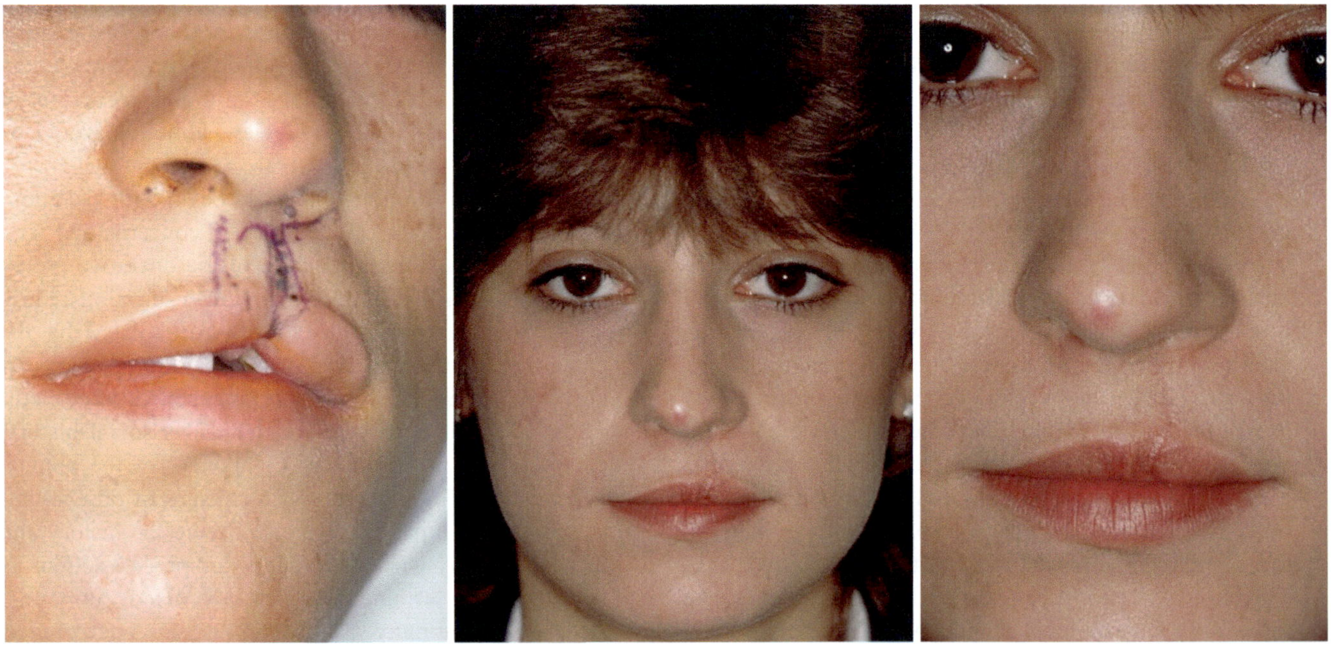

Three photos are provided: an intraoperative and two late postoperative. The intraoperative drawings demonstrate an operative plan for excision of the vertical length of the scar and some possible re-rotation and advancement. The postoperative results seen in full face and close-up reveal a mature nearly perceptible scar but some minor vermilion step off. The mucosa is full and symmetrical and the nasal configuration, tip, and alar bases, good.

Critique

The vermilion revision could be addressed with a small diamond-shaped excision.

Case-Based Conference

Case 2: Cleft Lip-Nasal Deformity

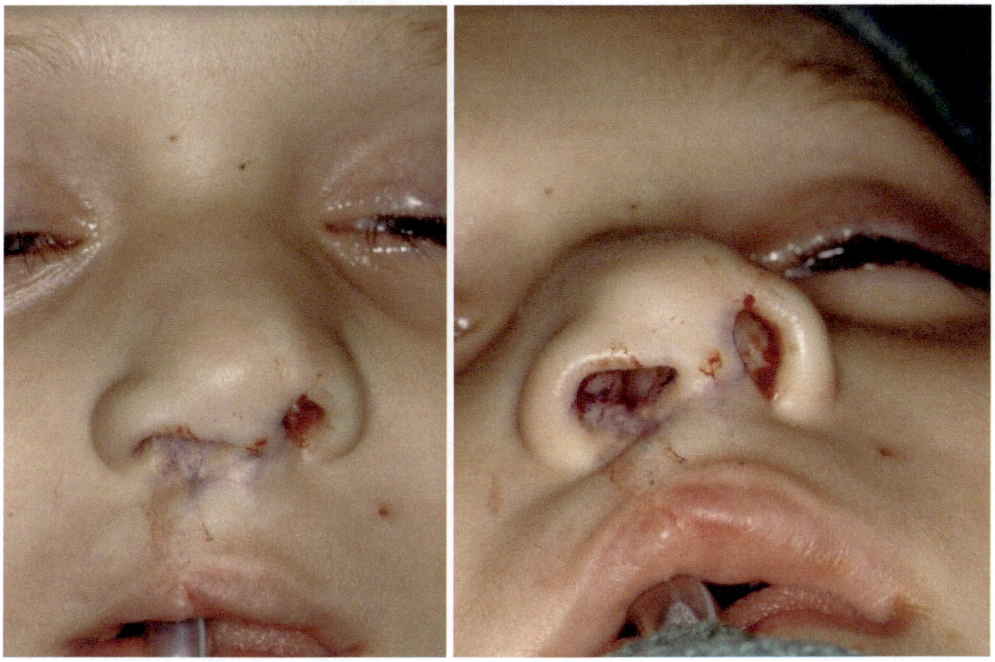

A 4-year-old who had cleft lip repair in infancy.

1. Describe the slide(s) and add a clinical examination.
   (a) Any tests or consultations indicated?
2. Describe the pathologic anatomy.
3. Outline a treatment plan. Describe the goals and essential steps for any proposed operation.

Case-Based Conference: Discussion

Case 2: Cleft Lip-Nasal Deformity

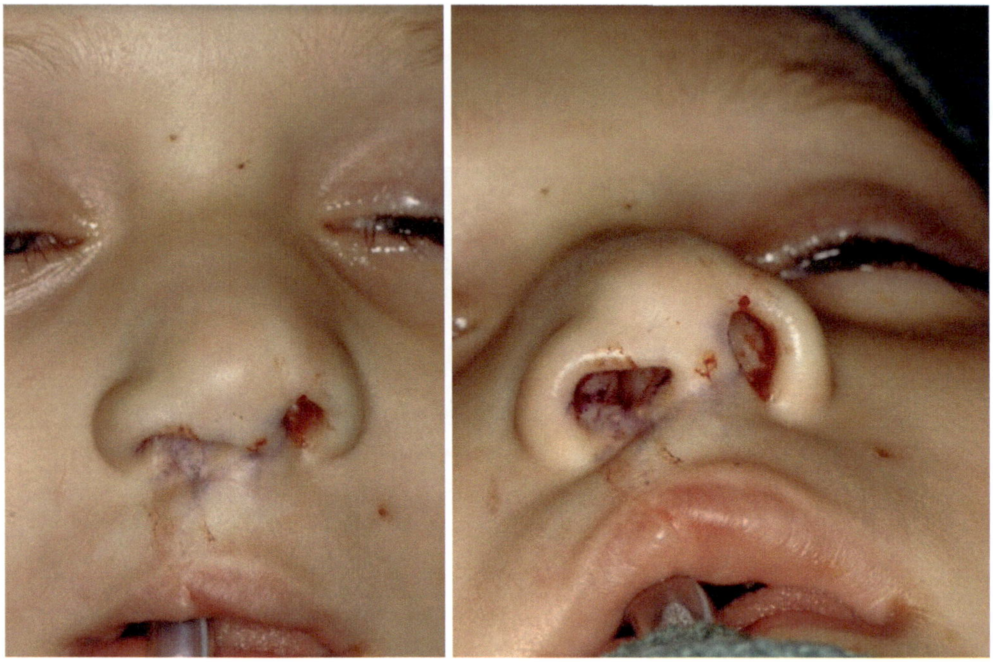

A 4-year-old who had cleft lip repair in infancy.

1. Describe the slide(s) and add a clinical examination. (The findings depicted in the two photos provided are essentially those of the cleft lip nasal deformity. The two slides are first, a central frontal midface that includes lips, nose, medial orbits, and glabella. The second is a submental vertex of approximately the same facial area. The first depicts an intubated child with remarkable findings limited to the nose and upper lip. The upper lip is symmetrical except for a minor indentation of the right dry mucosa at the point of the prior cleft repair. A fine vertical scar is present on the right, also consistent with a history of lip repair. Several nasal deformities are evident, predominately on the right, and include an alar base displaced laterally and slightly inferior and a slumped alar rim malpositioned significantly inferior. The normal convexity of the transition from the tip to lateral ala evident on the normal or left side is lost on the right and replaced by concavity and posterior collapse. The second photo or submental vertex further delineates the deformity. The findings of the nasal deformity apparent on the frontal view are confirmed. In addition, a shortened hemi columella on the right and a tilt of the columella to the non-cleft side are evident. The orientation of the nostril is transverse in contrast to the near-vertical character on the left. The alar rim on the right is inferiorly malpositioned and the nasal sill is dramatically widened. The lack of symmetry of the tip cannot be fully appreciated because the angle of the photo is slightly oblique and any potential webbing of the lateral nasal wall cannot be appreciated. No other remarkable findings are depicted.

   The history component of the clinical exam would ascertain the severity of the initial cleft, associated cleft palate repair, and the diagnosis of comorbidities, if any. The results of a recent audiologic and speech assessment would be of value as well as a review of growth and developmental milestones. Questions to determine the presence of nasal obstruction such as snoring in sleep or snorting would be important. The physical exam would establish several aspects not apparent in the photos including palpation with the examiner's thumb and forefinger at the junction of the membranous and cartilaginous portion of the columella to determine deviation of the caudal aspect of the septum, usually to the non-cleft side. If cooperative, a Q-tip is placed gently and just inside the right nostril to elevate the alar rim to define the deformity more fully. The nasal sill and vestibule should be inspected for soft tissue webbing or the existence of a nasolabial fistula. Use of a nasal speculum will probably be deferred until the OR and general anesthesia, but an intraoral exam should assess for the presence of an alveolar cleft and the status of the palate as well as again the presence of a nasolabial fistula.)

(a) Any tests or consultations indicated? (Assuming no comorbidities present, the necessity for indicated consultations would hinge off the results of the clinical exam. In particular, any suggestion of hypernasality or significant articulation errors should be further evaluated by a formal speech assessment, although the child may not have sufficient language development to assess. An appropriate consultation should be initiated in the presence of an alveolar cleft if not currently under the care of an orthodontist or pediodontist. The management of an alveolar cleft is covered in Chap. 18.)

2. Describe the pathologic anatomy. (The pathologic anatomy of the lower lateral cartilage on the cleft side, including the relationship to the ipsilateral upper lateral cartilage, the deviation of the caudal aspect of the septum and the anterior nasal spine, and the skeletal hypoplasia of the lateral aspect of the pyriform aperture also on the cleft side—all are responsible for the distortion and appearance of the tip structure. In order, those distortions consist of rotation of the columellar base, nasal spine, and caudal septum to the opposite or non-cleft side and shortening of the hemi columella on the cleft aspect, probably because of pressure created by progressive rotation of the maxillary greater segment. The lower lateral cartilage must span the cleft and have soft tissue attachments laterally to the pyriform rim. As a result, the medial footplate deviates both from the midline and its relationship to the footplate on the non-cleft side and is shortened functionally including the hemi columella. The dome of the medial crus is displaced laterally and posteriorly and the overlapping relationship of the cranial aspect of the lower lateral crus to the ipsilateral upper lateral cartilage is lost. The normal convexity of the lateral crus is flattened, splayed, lengthened, and drawn inferiorly. The normal acute angle of the dome is now obtuse. The alar base is posterior and laterally displaced that creates widening of the nostril sill. The additional pathology of the internal septum may consist of deviation of the quadrangular cartilaginous and perpendicular bony ethmoid plates into the cleft nasal airway. Finally, the severity of the associated nasal deformity is directly proportional to the severity of the cleft.)

3. Outline a treatment plan. Describe the goals and essential steps for any proposed operation. (The first issue to answer within this question is timing of any operative procedure. As discussed in Chap. 13, the extent of any nasal procedure at the time of lip repair, primary rhinoplasty, varies widely from surgeon to surgeon. A similar variance is evident in the discussion re secondary rhinoplasty. The historical perspective has been deferral until adolescence based on concerns about an adverse effect on facial and nasal growth. More contemporaneously and with the development of improved techniques, an intermediate rhinoplasty as in this 4-year-old patient limited to the tip structures and caudal septum alone has been adopted by many cleft centers. Often the correction can be combined with other operative procedures.

Access for the open rhinoplasty is through a rim incision on the cleft side. Alar base and nasal sill incisions will also be required to medially advance the alar base and narrow the nasal floor. What must be accomplished is release of the attachments of the lateral crus and soft tissue from the periosteum of the pyriform aperture, release of the footplate of the medial crus, release, and centralization of the deviated caudal septum, and cinching and narrowing of the alar base. Once dissected to correct the pathologic anatomy of the lower lateral cartilage described in question two, the dome and lateral crus should be secured to the opposite upper lateral cartilage medially supplemented by interdomal sutures. A cinch suture from the opposite alar base, passed transeptally to the cleft alar base and reversed and tied on the normal side will narrow the nasal sill and floor. An inverted "U", described and popularized by Tajima extended into the membranous septum is an operative approach and incision that will permit accomplishment of these goals. Combining a rim incision with a chondromucosal medial advancement of the lateral crus of the lower lateral cartilage can also be performed with the procedure described above.

A substantial amount of literature has been published in description of outcomes with primary and late adolescent rhinoplasty but considerably less about intermediate rhinoplasty.)

Postoperative

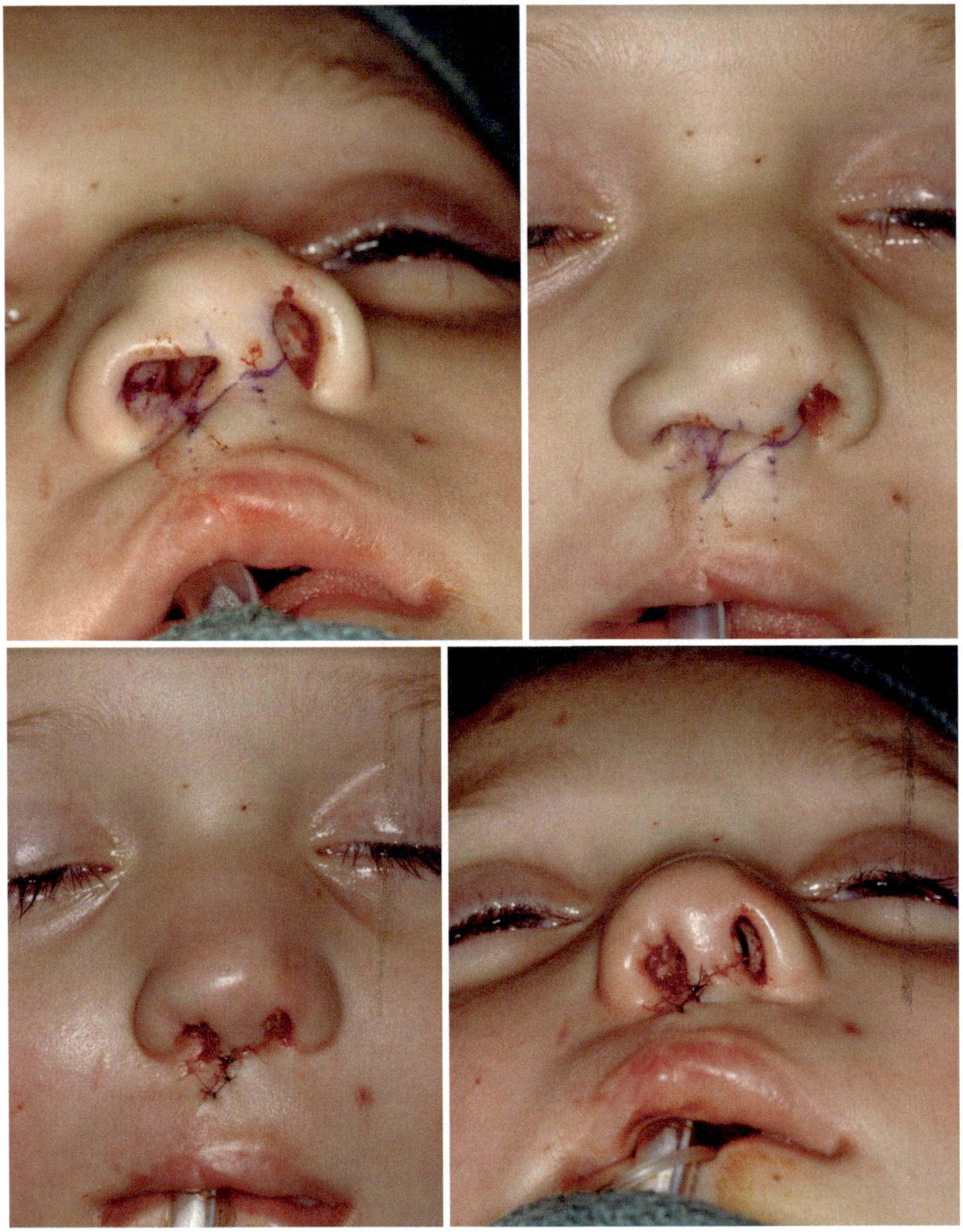

The two preoperative slides have surgical markings that depict a plan for open-tip rhinoplasty and columellar lengthening. The alar base should be advanced as well with excision of a small amount of nasal sill combined with an alar cinch stitch to the septum. The two immediate postoperative slides at the conclusion of the procedure demonstrate a lengthened columella and an alar base advancement, reorientation of the nostril into a vertical configuration, but some residual thickening of the superior nostril rim.

16 Cleft Palate

Bibliography

Applebaum, S.A., Aronson, S., Termanini, K.M., Gosain, A.K., "Evidence-Based Practices in Cleft Palate Surgery", *Plast Reconstr Surg.*, (2024);153(2):**448e-52e and Videos 1, 2, 4-6 ONLY.**

Smith DM and Losee JE, "Cleft palate repair", *Clin. Plast. Surg.*, (2014); 41:**189-205.**

Hopper RA, Tse R, Smartt J, et al., "Cleft palate repair and velopharyngeal dysfunction", *Plast. Reconstr. Surg.*, (2014); 133(6):**852e-864e (852e-856e ONLY).**

Fisher DM and Sommerlad BC, "Cleft lip, cleft palate, and velopharyngeal insufficiency", *Plast. Reconstr. Surg.*, (2011); 128(4):**342e-360e (353e-356e ONLY) Video 5, parts 1-5**.

Gosain, A.K., et al., "Submucous Cleft Palate: Diagnostic Methods and Outcomes of Surgical Treatment" *Plast. Reconstr. Surg.*, (1996); 97:**1497-1503 and summary.**

Evans KN, Sie KCY, "Pierre Robin Sequence: Assessment and Nonsurgical Management", Joseph E. Losee, Richard E. Kirschner, *Comprehensive Cleft Care*, (2016), McGraw-Hill Co.; **623-34 ONLY.**

Faculty Discussion and Study Guide

Epidemiology and Embryology

1. Rank in order of frequency the occurrence of cleft palate in the following populations: Asian, Caucasian, and African American. (Unlike cleft lip, isolated cleft palate has a similar incidence in all races: Asian, Caucasian, and African American.)
2. Syndromic cleft palate occurs in what percent of cleft palate patients? (1/3–1/2, probably closer to 1/3 if you eliminate the asymptomatic submucous cleft palate.)
   (a) List some of the most common syndromes in cleft palate patients. (Pierre Robin, Stickler, velocardiofacial, Van der Woude, Goldenhar.)
   (b) Define Pierre Robin. (Glossoptosis, upper airway obstruction, retrognathia plus cleft palate.)
   (c) Define velocardiofacial, Van der Woude, Goldenhar. (All are syndromic cleft palates. Velocardiofacial has a variety of anomalies, including Tetralogy of Fallot and ventricular septal defect, and maxillary excess with long face. Van der Woude has cleft palate plus lower lip pits, and Goldenhar has ocular colobomas and renal anomalies.)
3. What environmental factors can be causative in occurrence of cleft palate? (Steroids, retinoids, Dilantin.)
4. Outline the timing of primary and secondary palate closure in utero. (Primary palate in about four to seven weeks, the secondary palate about seven to nine weeks.)
5. Why does the association of retrognathia and cleft of the secondary palate make embryological sense? (Mandible must move anteriorly to allow the tongue to drop inferiorly which in turn would allow ascent and fusion of the palatal shelves.)
   (a) Explain the following embryologically: The increase incidence in females; clefts of the soft palate alone. (The palatine shelves fuse later in females embryologically than males and may set the stage for an increased exposure to teratogenic agents and an incidence of isolated cleft palate; clefts of the soft palate can be explained embryologically because the fusion process is from anterior to posterior.)
   (b) Name three agents that are taken during the first trimester that can increase the probability of cleft palate. (Dilantin, steroids, retinoids)
   (c) Extra Credit: Describe other head and neck anomalies that would predispose to cleft palate. (Oligohydroaminos, Klippel-Feil syndrome)
6. What is Veau's classification of palatal cleft? (A Y-shaped diagram with the stem of the Y pointing posteriorly. The left side of the Y is represented by a cleft of the left primary palate, the right arm, and a cleft of the primary palate on the right. The intersection point with the stem is the

E. Luce, *A Curriculum for Plastic Surgery*, https://doi.org/10.1007/978-3-031-62087-4_16

incisive foramen. The remaining portion of the stem represents the secondary palate.)

Anatomy

1. What is the principal blood supply to the hard palate? (Greater palatine vessels, also termed the posterior palatine vessels.)
   (a) How do those arteries enter the palatal tissue? (The arteries are a branch of the descending palatine or sphenopalatine and exit through the greater palatine foramina at the posterior aspect of the hard palate.)
2. What are the five muscles with attachment to or contained within the palate that compose the velopharyngeal mechanism? (Levator veli palatini, tensor veli palatini, superior pharyngeal constrictor, palatopharyngeus, and uvulus.)
   (a) Pick the two that are most critical in speech function. (The levator veli palatini and the superior pharyngeal constrictor.)
3. Where is the levator veli principally distributed in the velum? (The middle half of the distance as measured from the posterior nasal spine to the tip of the uvula.)
4. With respect to the palatopharyngeus, in which tonsillar pillar does the muscle lie? Discuss the anatomic relationships both medially and laterally. (The posterior tonsillar pillar. The palatopharyngeus splits in two heads in the lateral aspect of the velum and the levator crosses between those two heads. Laterally, the muscle blends with the superior pharyngeal constrictor on the lateral pharyngeal wall. The palatoglossus comprises the anterior tonsillar pillar.)
5. What is the function and distribution of the tensor levator palatini? (The muscle originates on the lateral wall and wraps laterally around the pterygoid hamulus and inserts into the palatal aponeurosis at the posterior border of the hard palate. The tensor aerates the middle ear by opening the eustachian tube orifice. The tensor veli palatini may play a role in production of tenseness of the soft palate prior to contraction of the levator sling.)
   (a) Describe the pathology in dysfunction of the tensor veli palatini. (With the abnormal course and insertion of the tensor veli palatini, the eustachian tube orifice fails to *open* and therefore the middle ear is not properly aerated. This dysfunction leads to serous otitis media followed by purulent otitis media and ultimately hearing loss. The treatment of choice is equilibration or PE tubes placed through the tympanic membrane.)
6. Discuss the function or dynamic action of the levator veli palatini. (The normal levator from the origin laterally, courses inferior, medial, and anterior. The levator on contracture moves the soft palate superior, posterior, and of course lateral. See Fig. 16.1.)

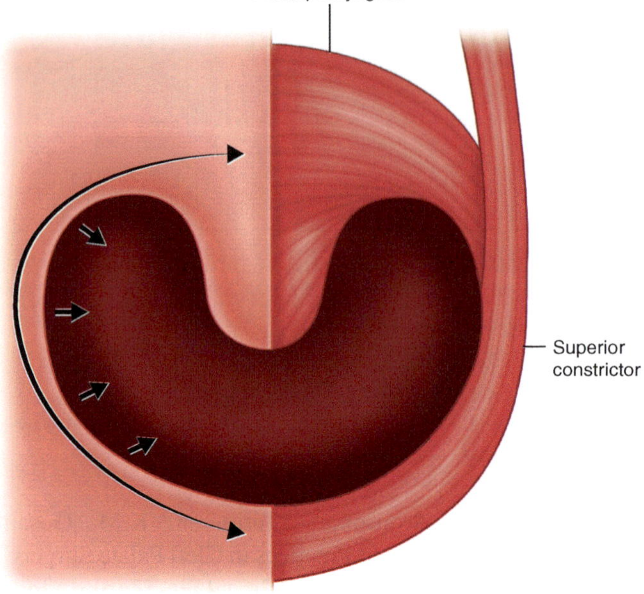

Fig. 16.1 Levator veli palatini

   (a) Discuss the same with the palatopharyngeus? (The end result is broadening or stretching of the free or nasal margin of the soft palate to increase the surface area of contact with the posterior pharyngeal wall.)
   (b) Discuss the same with the superior constrictor. (The superior pharyngeal constrictor appears to be the principal muscle for lateral pharyngeal wall movement, although the palatopharyngeus contributes in a hemi-sphincteric mechanism.)
7. Outline the degree of superior constrictor activity in the following three closure patterns: Coronal, circular, and sagittal. (Sagittal little or some, circular moderate, coronal high)
8. Describe the abnormal insertion of the levator muscles in palatal clefts. (Instead of simply ending at the edges of the cleft, the levators are usually displaced anteriorly and inserted into the posterior border of the hard palate in the region of the posterior nasal spine, palatal aponeurosis, and along the medial edges of the bony cleft. A similar malposition occurs with the distribution of the tensor veli palatini.)
9. Does a similar abnormal insertion of the levator palatini exist in the submucous cleft palate? (Yes.)
10. Discuss the following three operative procedures within the framework of these anatomic findings: Intravelar veloplasty, Furlow palatoplasty, and pharyngeal flap. (The intravelar veloplasty restores the normal muscle anatomy of the levator since pathologic anatomy in the cleft palate is an abnormal anterior insertion on the pos-

terior border of the hard palate. The Furlow repair accomplishes the same thing, but does overlap muscle in the midline, which is not a normal anatomic finding. The posterior pharyngeal flap disrupts the normal continuity on the posterior pharynx of the superior pharyngeal constrictors.)

Operative Repair

1. Outline the historical evolution of the cleft palate repair from the most simple to the most contemporary. (Simple straight-line closure of the palate, an effort at lengthening the palate, two-stage repair of cleft palate, and anatomic velopharyngeal muscle repair.)
2. In essence, what is the dilemma and argument about the appropriate timing of cleft palate repair? (The palate needs to be repaired so that an intact velopharyngeal mechanism results for correct speech, probably by the age of 9–12 months. Yet, repair of the palate at a very early age creates raw areas that must heal by secondary intention, scarring, and may have a higher probability of late maxillary deformities.)
3. The goals of palatoplasty are to achieve complete closure of the hard palate and restoration of the velopharyngeal sphincter. List the three or four components of the operation to achieve those goals. (Tension-free three-layer closure of nasal mucosa, muscle, and oral mucosa, release of the nasal layer from beneath the posterior hard palate, skeletonization of neurovascular bundle, complete release of the abnormal insertion of the levator muscle and reorientation to a transverse direction, and mattress closure of the oral layer.)
4. Describe the major points in performance of vomer flap(s) with the pros and cons. (The vomer is incised in the midline from anterior to posterior and superiorly based flaps are raised bilaterally off the vomer. These flaps are sutured end to end to the adjacent medial border of the nasal mucosa on the hard palate and as far posteriorly as possible on the anterior portion of the soft palate. The pros are the availability of a second layer of closure beneath the oral suture line in the hard palate. The cons are a possible disturbance of vomer-driven facial growth.)
5. Describe the possible long-term clinical appearance of the deleterious effect of palate repair on facial growth. (With restriction of palatal growth particularly that of maxillary anterior projection, the occlusal relationship may be a class III and a relative prognathism.)
6. What is the philosophy behind two-stage repair? (To avoid the problems outlined above. The first stage consisted of the repair of the soft palate at an early age and deferral of the hard palate closure until age 4, 5, or 6.)
   (a) The outcome in late reviews. (Evidence exists that delayed hard palate closure does not reduce the amount of dental and maxillary distortion. In addition, those patients with a two-stage repair seem to have a higher incidence of velopharyngeal insufficiency.)
7. Describe the essential or major steps in palate repair by the following techniques. (a) Von Langenbeck, (b) Wardill-Kilner or V-Y, and (c) two flaps, Bardach, repairs (Von Langenbeck consists of parallel incisions along the lateral aspect of the hard palate; the excision of the medial edge of cleft; dissection beneath periosteum to create bilateral mucoperiosteal flaps; excision of the edges of the cleft of the soft palate. The other elements are common to both types of repair and are listed below. The Wardill-Kilner or V-Y in a sense is the Von Langenbeck but incisions are completed anteriorly, leaving a triangle of mucosa intact, if cleft of the palate alone, with the tip of the triangle pointed posterior to create two posteriorly based mucoperiosteal flaps. The two-flap Bardach palatoplasty has the optimum application in a complete unilateral cleft lip and palate when essentially the two flaps posteriorly based are raised of all the hard palate oral mucosa. In any V-Y repair the flaps can be dissected from anterior to posterior and expose the vessels at the greater palatine foramina. All three repairs share the following: (1) dissection of the anterior abnormal insertion of the levator muscle from the aponeurosis and the posterior border of the hard palate; once dissected intravelar veloplasty, repairs so the two opposite muscles lie transversely across the palatal arch, midline approximation of both soft and hard palate as a two-layer closure. Variance that may or may not be included dependent on the preferred technique of the surgeon includes: (1) vomer flaps, (2) dissection of the nasal mucosa from the nasal aspect of the hard palate.)
8. What is intravelar veloplasty? (The complete dissection of the abnormally anterior insertion of the levator on the posterior border of the hard palate and repair so that the two opposite muscle bundles lie transversely across the palatal arch.)
9. In general, what is the success rate as defined by absence of velopharyngeal insufficiency in cleft palate repair? (Approximately 75–80% of patients will have good to excellent speech.)
10. You must be able to draw or design the double opposing Z-plasty velar repair. (The important keys are that on the left side of the patient, the anterior flap is a mucoperiosteal muscular flap. On the right side, the anterior flap is mucosa alone. For the posterior flaps, on the left side, the flap is nasal mucosa alone, and the right side is a musculo-mucosal flap incorporating nasal mucosa. The result is that the muscles are aligned in a transverse ori-

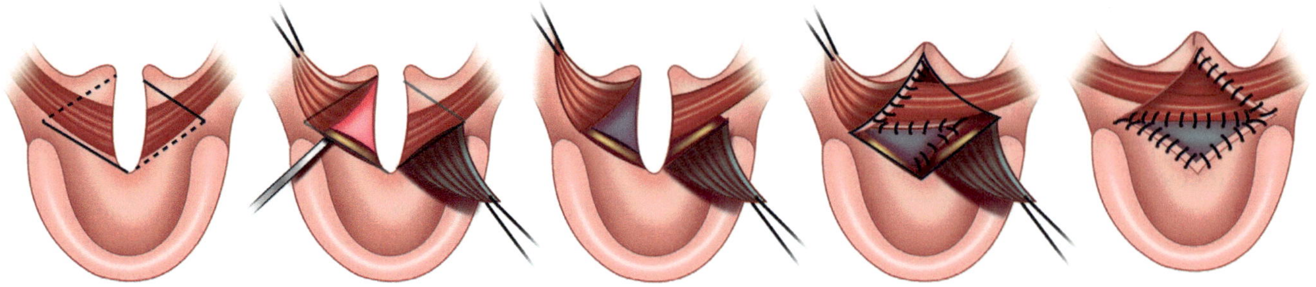

Fig. 16.2 Z-plasty velar repair

entation across the soft palate. The Z-plasty also lengthens the entire soft palate. See Fig. 16.2.)

11. What does Furlow propose for closure of the hard palate when the cleft is too wide for standard primary repair? (1. He suggests vomer flap and also suggests lateral relaxing incisions, first on the right, and then on the left if the greater palatine vessels are intact. 2. A buccinator and mucosa flap from the left side may be used. (Note: A buccal myomucosal flap performed as a primary palate repair is distinctly uncommon and not recommended as an option to the occasional cleft palate surgeon.) 3. A final option is an anterior mucoperiosteal turnover flap to close a wide cleft at the level of the alveolus.)
12. What is the recommended postoperative care for a palate patient? (A 2° silk suture transfixes the anterior portion of the tongue and is left long as a traction suture in order to control the airway in the postoperative period. Arm restraints are applied and clear liquids are begun orally as soon as tolerated by the patient. Note: Since palatal repairs are being done earlier, breastfeeding is recommended to continue if still being performed. Additionally, there are now several types of bottles and cups which are designed for postoperative palatal repair.)

Complications

1. The two principal acute complications postoperative in cleft palate repair are: (Bleeding and upper airway obstruction. Bleeding is best managed in the operating room. On most occasions may be simply a slight ooze from the suture line despite digital pressure and bleeding perceptible during observation of the baby is an operative indication. To attempt any type of control on the floor in a distressed and thrashing patient is not recommended. Sequential management of upper airway obstruction consists first of traction on the tongue suture to pull the tongue anteriorly. The next step is placement of a nasal trumpet. Some centers, particularly in Pierre Robin patients, use a nasal trumpet postoperatively as a prophylactic measure. If airway obstruction still persists, endotracheal intubation, although not desirable and distinctly uncommon, is probably the recommended course of action.)
2. Rank the following clefts in order of frequency of palatal fistulas from highest to lowest. (Bilateral cleft lip and palate, unilateral cleft lip and palate, complete cleft of the secondary palate. Remember, a definition of fistulas includes post-alveolar as well as fistulas of the hard and soft palate.)
3. Discuss possible location of postoperative palatal fistulas: (As in the above question; pre-alveolar, post-alveolar, mid-hard palate, posterior border of the hard palate at the hard palate soft palate junction, soft palate. Also discussed in Chap. 18)
   (a) What are the implications in terms of fistula location? (Pre- and post-alveolar fistulas are seen in the presence of cleft of lip and palate and particularly with a post-alveolar location may be intentional. Mid-hard palate if small may represent minor dehiscence. The posterior hard palate and soft palate fistulas carry a different implication, namely, that some dehiscence of both mucosa and muscle has occurred and the probability of the presence of velopharyngeal insufficiency is significant.)

Submucous Cleft Palate, Pierre Robin Syndrome

1. Define submucous cleft palate. (Bifid uvula, a midline blue line indicative of submucosal levator dehiscence, and a palpable notch in the posterior border of the hard palate.)
2. True or False: The presence of a triad of findings of submucosal cleft palate is an indication for operative intervention. (False, the presence of velopharyngeal insufficiency needs to be established as an operative indication. Discussion of the diagnosis and treatment of velopharyngeal insufficiency is covered in Chap. 17)
   (a) Implications in terms of timing of the repair. (Because of the difficulty in establishing the presence of velo-

pharyngeal insufficiency in children less than three years of age, the diagnosis is often established at age 5 or 6.)

3. What are the various operative options available for repair? Discuss. (Traditionally, the posterior pharyngeal flap. More currently, intravelar veloplasty with or without a posterior pharyngeal flap. The most recent description has been the use of the Furlow Z-plasty for submucous cleft palate. All have demonstrated efficacy.)
4. List the triad of Pierre Robin syndrome or sequence. (Glossoptosis, retrognathia, and upper airway obstruction. Cleft palate although a predominant finding in patients with Pierre Robin syndrome was not a component of the original descriptions.)
   (a) What is the essential anatomic abnormality? (Mandibular hypoplasia of varying extent of severity.)
   (b) Is the configuration of the cleft in Pierre Robin different from the non-Pierre Robin cleft? (Mostly yes—the cleft is more of a "wide U" than a "V" configuration.)
5. Describe the clinical presentation in the following Pierre Robin patients: Newborn vs. age 3–4 months (A neonate with Pierre Robin syndrome may present with upper airway obstruction of varying degree of severity. The most severe require intubation at birth. The moderately severe will have episodes of upper obstruction that are clinically evident during the first day or two of life. These two situations will require treatment intervention as a neonate. The less severe clinical picture, although not requiring treatment as a neonate, may present as failure to thrive with obstructive apneic episodes, but not necessarily snoring in contrast to the adult obstructive sleep apnea patient.)
   (a) The cardinal study in the 3–4 month age baby in the above scenario? (Overnight sleep study for presence of obstructive sleep apnea.)
   (b) Other considerations in the neonate with upper airway obstruction? (Posterior choanal stenosis or atresia, subglottic stenosis, tracheomalacia—all of which may dictate endoscopy.)
6. What are the treatment options for airway obstruction in the neonate with Pierre Robin syndrome? (The neonates who require intubation at birth traditionally have been managed with tracheostomy. More recently, as described in the readings, distraction osteogenesis has been performed with rapid distraction to achieve an airway. A thorough patient assessment for other possible causes of upper airway obstruction such as laryngomalacia or tracheomalacia mandates for bronchoscopy prior to initiation of distraction. Distraction can be performed with either internal or external distractors with rapid distraction and then a period of bone consolidation. Tongue-lip adhesions are still performed in some centers for those patients who have upper airway obstruction in the neonatal stage. Tongue-lip adhesion is accompanied by complications, although perhaps not as severe as tracheostomy, nevertheless those complications represent significant morbidity. Less severe cases can be managed with prone positioning, monitoring, and perhaps temporary nasopharyngeal airway.)

Video Notes

Fischer DM and Sommerlad BC, "Cleft lip, cleft palate, and velopharyngeal insufficiency", *Plast. Reconstr. Surg.*, (2011); 128(4):358e.

Video 5: Parts 1-6

Part 1: 3 min

1. Cleft to soft palate and partial of the hard palate.
2. Markings and dissection.
3. Good video (micro at low power) and narrative.

Part 2: 3 min

1. Dissected posterior aspect of the hard palate–did not expose the greater palatine vessels.
2. Exposed palatopharyngeus, oral component.

Part 3: 3 min

1. Began repair at the uvula and repaired nasal lining before dissection of the muscle.

Part 4: 8 min

1. Apparently previously dissected the oral mucosa off the underlying levator muscle.
2. Began the muscle, levator, and dissection off the *nasal* mucosa.
3. Although dissected the levator separate from the palatopharyngeus, did not appear to dissect and release the aponeurosis from the posterior hard palate.

Part 5: 4.5 min

1. Repaired muscle with interrupted sutures; narrated that he had repaired levator and palatopharyngeus incorporated in a single suture.

Part 6: 3.5 min

1. In my opinion, muscles were over-dissected and so mobile and placed posterior, but created an anterior dead space.
2. Closed oral mucosa with *vertical* mattress with a bite of nasal mucosa and a locked stitch—this writer prefers horizontal mattress sutures.

Case-Based Conference

Case 1: Cleft Palate

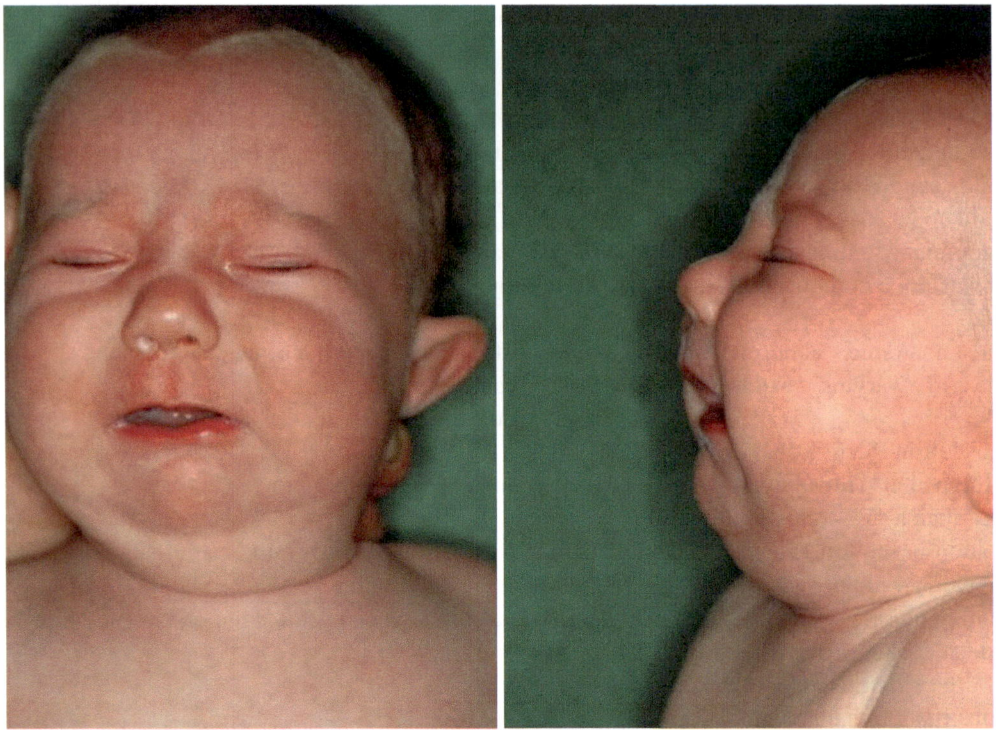

A 4-month-old cleft palate patient who has failed to gain weight and has intermittent episodes of "turning blue." He has had a normal cardiac workup.

1. What do you see on the two clinical slides? Add a pertinent clinical examination.
2. What is the pathologic anatomy in this situation?
3. What guidelines or indications will assist you in determination of the appropriate treatment options?
   (a) What is your treatment plan?

Your treatment plan has been successful and the child is now one year of age and ready for palate repair.

1. Give a menu of type(s) of repair including the pros and cons of each and your choice. Describe that procedure in detail including the steps and sequence.
2. The evening of the palate repair you are called because the infant is in respiratory distress.
   (a) Surprised?
   (b) Describe your management. Adopt a sequential or "ladder" approach.

Case-Based Conference

Case 1: Cleft Palate

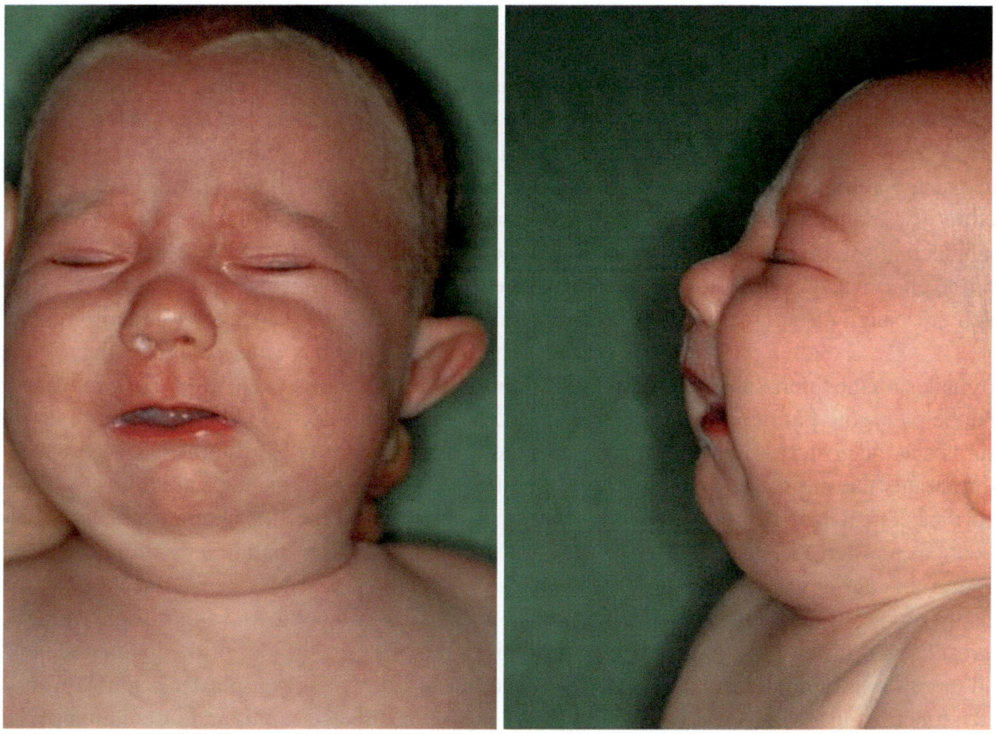

A 4-month-old cleft palate patient who has failed to gain weight and has intermittent episodes of "turning blue." He has a normal cardiac workup.

1. What is the pertinent clinical examination of this infant? (The clinical picture is consistent with the Pierre Robin syndrome of retrognathia, glossotosis, and upper airway obstruction as well as in this particular patient a cleft palate, not a component of the original description of the syndrome. Other possibilities exist in a differential diagnosis such as infantile tracheomalacia that must be ruled out, but for the purposes of this discussion, a diagnosis of Pierre Robin syndrome will be assumed. The pertinent history would further detail the failure to thrive as well as the particular details of the cyanotic episodes. Physical examination would focus on other congenital anomalies of the head and neck. Eighty percent of the patients with Pierre Robin sequence will have an associated syndrome of which the most common is Stickler and others include velocardiofacial and Nager syndromes. The cleft of the palate is usually quite wide and u-shaped which can create some difficulties in operative repair.)
2. What is the pathologic anatomy? (In normal embryologic palate formation, the tongue is positioned between the two vertically oriented palatal shelves. As the mandible grows, the tongue is permitted to move anteriorly, which in turn will permit the palatal shelves to swing into a horizontal position and fuse in the midline. The conventional hypothesis in Pierre Robin syndrome is that a retrognathic mandible interferes with tongue descent which in turn does not mechanically permit horizontal orientation of the palatal shelves. The functional pathophysiology is the infant is unable to maintain a patent upper airway because of glossoptosis. Clearly, a spectrum exists from the most severe presentation of obstruction at birth through clinical pictures such as the one given, namely, a failure to thrive later in infancy with intermittent episodes of obstruction.)
3. What are the appropriate treatment options and what will assist you in the selection of the appropriate option? (In this baby, a stepwise approach of treatment measures of an increasing interventive nature will help determine the optimal treatment. Conservative means such as a positioning of the baby prone with oxygen supplementation as is needed may suffice, although unlikely in this scenario. Pulse oximetry monitoring can also be used during sleep. Historical methods of treatment have been tongue-lip adhesion or tracheostomy. Contemporary management is mandibular distraction. Mandibular osteotomies are performed and internal distractors are placed for rapid

distraction over the following several days followed by a period of bone consolidation.)

Case 1B

The treatment plan has been successful and the child is now one year of age and ready for palate repair.

1. Outline the pertinent anatomy of the velopharynx. (The five muscles that are attached to or contained within the palate and the velopharyngeal mechanism are the levator and tensor veli palatini, superior pharyngeal constrictor, palatopharyngeus, all of which are paired structures and the midline uvulus muscle.

   The tensor veli palatini originates on the lateral wall of the pharynx and wraps around the pterygoid hamulus and inserts into the palatal aponeurosis at the posterior border of the hard palate. The tensor aerates the middle ear by opening the eustachian tube orifice. The tensor veli palatini may play a role in the production of tenseness of the soft palate prior to contraction of the levator sling. Dysfunction of the tensor palatini produced by the abnormal course and insertion will result in failure of the eustachian tube orifice to *open* and therefore the middle ear is not properly aerated. This dysfunction leads to serous otitis media followed by purulent otitis media and ultimately hearing loss. The treatment of choice is equilibration or PE tubes placed through the tympanic membrane. In cleft palates, the levator veli palatini is not in the normal anatomical configuration, namely horizontal, but rather is abnormally anteriorly inserted on the posterior and medial border of the hard palate as well as the palatal aponeurosis.

   The levator muscle is normally principally distributed in the middle half of the velum or soft palate as measured from the posterior nasal spine to the tip of the uvula. The levator functions to elevate the soft palate and move the soft palate posteriorly and superiorly to appose to the posterior pharyngeal wall during speech (see the velopharyngeal insufficiency module). The palatopharyngeus lies within the posterior tonsillar pillar and splits into two heads within the lateral aspect of the velum. The levator courses between those two heads. Laterally, the palatopharyngeus blends with the superior pharyngeal constrictor on the lateral pharyngeal wall. The superior pharyngeal constrictor appears to be the principal muscle for lateral pharyngeal wall movement, although the palatopharyngeus contributes in a hemi-sphincteric mechanism.)
2. Give a menu of types of repair including the benefits and liabilities of each. Describe the procedure in detail including the steps and sequences. (The three principal operative procedures employed for cleft palate repair are the Von Langenbeck, the V-Y, and Furlow double-Zplasty. In all likelihood, the two most common are the V-Y and Furlow palatoplasty. The dilemma about the appropriate timing of cleft palate repair is that the palate needs to be repaired so that an intact velopharyngeal mechanism is available for the development of correct speech, probably no later than the age of 9–12 months. Yet, repair of the palate at a very early age creates raw areas that must heal by secondary intention and scarring and may have a higher probability of late maxillary deformities.

   The essential or major steps in palate repair in both the Von Langenbeck and V-Y are the following: in both repairs (the V-Y repair is often referred to as the Wardill-Kilner) through lateral palatal incisions undermining of the mucoperiosteal flaps as well as freshening of the edges of the cleft is accomplished to allow for a two-layer repair. The V-Y repair differs in that the incisions are joined anteriorly to create two posteriorly based mucoperiosteal flaps. In this repair, the flaps are dissected from anterior to posterior to expose the palatine vessels at their emergence from the greater palatine foramina. Palatal repairs also share the following: (1) Dissection of the anterior abnormal insertion of the levator muscle from the aponeurosis at the posterior border of the hard palate and performance of an intravelar veloplasty, namely, a horizontal and posterior directed repair and orientation of the levator muscle fibers. (2) Many surgeons also employ vomer flaps. The vomer flaps are incised in the midline from anterior to posterior and superiorly based flaps are raised bilaterally off the vomer. These flaps are sutured end to end to the adjacent medial border of the nasal mucosa on the hard palate and sutured as far posteriorly as possible on to the anterior portion of the soft palate. The pros are the availability of a second layer of closure beneath the oral suture line in the hard palate. The cons are a possible disturbance of vomer-driven facial growth.

   The Furlow is a double opposing Z-plasty repair. For example, on the left side of the patient, the oral flap is a mucosal-periosteal muscular flap and on the right side, the oral flap is mucosa alone. For the nasal flaps, on the left side, the flap is nasal mucosa alone, and the right side is a musculo-mucosal flap incorporating nasal mucosa. The result should be the muscles are aligned in a transverse orientation across the soft palate. The Z-plasty also lengthens the entire soft palate.)
3. The evening of the palate repair, you are called because the infant is in respiratory distress. Are you surprised? Describe a management plan. (Babies with Pierre Robin sequence or syndrome have a much higher incidence of postoperative respiratory obstruction after cleft palate repair. Because of this observation, many centers prophylactically place a nasal trumpet in the operating room at the completion of the procedure. If not, the tongue suture

can be used to pull the tongue anteriorly and a nasal trumpet inserted, carefully. In most instances endotracheal intubation will not be necessary.)

In-Service Examination

1. A Passavant's ridge of mucosa consists also of what muscle?
   (a) Uvula
   (b) Superior pharyngeal constrictor
   (c) Palatoglossus
   (d) Palatopharyngeus
2. A two-flap palatoplasty involves the repair of the following muscles **EXCEPT:**
   (a) Uvulae
   (b) Palatopharyngeus
   (c) Tensor veli palatini
   (d) Levator veli palatini
3. A neonate presents with retrognathia with severe airway obstruction shortly after birth. The first step in management is:
   (a) Prone positioning
   (b) Tracheostomy
   (c) Tongue-lip adhesion
   (d) Nasotracheal intubation

17 Velopharyngeal Insufficiency

Bibliography

Kummer AW, "Speech evaluation for patients with cleft palate", *Clin. Plast. Surg.*, (2014); 41:**241–251.**

Smith B and Guyette TW, "Evaluation of cleft palate speech", *Clin. Plast. Surg.*, (2004); 31:**251–260. (Figure 2 ONLY)**

Naran S, Ford M, Losee JE, "What's New in Cleft Palate and Velopharyngeal Dysfunction Management?", *Plast. Reconstr. Surg.*, (2017); 139(6): **1343e–1353e.**

Hopper RA, Tse R, Smartt J, et al., "Cleft palate repair and velopharyngeal dysfunction", *Plast. Reconstr. Surg.*, (2014); 133(6):**861e–863e and Videos 1–4 ONLY.**

Jackson M.D., I.T, "Sphincter Pharyngoplasty", *Clin. Plast. Surg.*, (1985); 12:**712. (Table 1 ONLY)**

Marsh, J. L. MD, Chapter 42: "Sphincter Pharyngoplasty." Losee MD, J. E., and Kirschner MD, R. E., Comprehensive Cleft Care, The McGraw-Hill Co., (2009); **pp 665- 671.**

Wong KWY, Klaiman PG, Forrest CR, Chapter 59: "Posterior Pharyngeal Flaps", Losee MD, J. E., and Kirschner MD, R. E., Comprehensive Cleft Care Second Edition, The McGraw-Hill Co., (2016); **pp 1133-1151.**

Wells, M.D., Vu, T.A., Luce, E.A. "Incidence and Sequelae of Nocturnal Respiratory Obstruction Following Posterior Pharyngeal Flap Operation" *Ann. Plast. Surg.*, Lippincott Williams & Wilkins, (1999); 43(3):**252-257.**

Faculty Study and Discussion Guide

General: Anatomy and Function

1. Velopharyngeal inadequacy refers to a broad diagnosis: How can we define or classify it more specifically? (Structural, for example, a short palate; neurogenic, for example, cerebral palsy; and functional, for example, faulty learning.)
2. What is the essential definition of velopharyngeal insufficiency (VPI)? (Hypernasal speech, audible nasal emission, and weak pressure consonants are all secondary to inability because of nasopharyngeal air leakage and failure to fill the velopharyngeal "space" during speech, which is necessary to produce plosive consonants.)
   (a) What is hypernasality or hypernasal speech? (Excessive nasal resonance during vowel production and nasal emission as turbulent airflow during consonant production, the result of velopharyngeal dysfunction or insufficiency.)
3. A 6-year-old has been brought to your office because the mother has been told "he talks through his nose" by the school system. What are the first steps in the clinical evaluation? (Flesh out the history: family history of cleft palate, history in the child of oronasal regurgitation, a prior tonsillectomy and adenoidectomy, recurrent otitis media. The physical exam focuses on the function of the soft palate and the size of the tonsils. Listen to the child and then do a physical examination of soft palate function and the possible presence of tonsillar hypertrophy.)
   (a) What would be the next step? (Speech evaluation by a speech pathologist known as perceptual assessment.)
   (b) What would be the speech pathologist's role? (Determine if the velopharyngeal mechanism can be evaluated adequately or if the child needs speech therapy to correct articulation disorders and then evaluate.)
4. Define the difference between fricative and plosive consonants and give examples. (Fricative is a markedly narrowed nasal or nasopharyngeal airway with a slow release of the nasal stoppage of the airflow as in v in vowels, s in sugar, and z in zebra. Plosive is when the airway is completely stopped and then quickly released as in b in boy, t in toy, d in dog, and x in X-ray.)
   (a) What are nasal consonants? (Letters such as m, n, and ng that require in English the passage of air through the nose as well as the mouth. The production of such sounds, nasal consonants, requires an open or patulous nasopharynx for the production of nasal resonance.)

E. Luce, *A Curriculum for Plastic Surgery*, https://doi.org/10.1007/978-3-031-62087-4_17

   (b) Hold your nose while pronouncing boy and toy and then switch to m, n, and ng and note the resonance palpable in your nose with the latter.
5. What is the essence of hypernasality or hypernasal speech? Can you mimic it? (Nasal leakage during the production of fricatives and plosives that normally demand little or no nasal airflow.)
   (a) Is it correctable with speech therapy? (Although some compensatory mechanisms can be addressed, essentially an anatomical etiology for hypernasality is not correctable with speech therapy.)
   (b) What is hyponasal speech? (The opposite, namely, no nasal airflow even during the nasal consonants, for example, as present with a severe cold.)
6. A child with large tonsils and adenoids has a T and A. Postoperatively, he has hypernasal speech. Why? (The child had underlying occult hypernasality that was masked by his large adenoids that served as an obturator. Once removed, his hypernasal speech was unmasked.)
7. What are glottic stops and pharyngeal fricatives? (Both are pathological speech mechanisms. Glottic stops are the efforts of use of the false vocal cords to reduce nasal leakage, pharyngeal fricatives are the same mechanism at the level of the pharynx, and finally nasal grimacing is an effort to occlude the external nasal valve for the same reason.)
8. Describe the function, not anatomy, of the velopharyngeal mechanism. (One conceptual model of the velopharyngeal mechanism is as a sphincter: production of certain sounds requires a seal between the oropharynx and nasopharynx. The oral component of this seal is accomplished by the posterior and superior movement of the soft palate as a broad bar of muscle and soft tissue in the coronal plane at the junction of the anterior 2/3 and posterior 1/3 of the soft palate. Simultaneously, the lateral walls move medially propelled by the anterolateral distribution of the superior pharyngeal constrictor within the posterior and lateral pharyngeal walls as well as the palatopharyngeus contained in the posterior tonsillar pillar, supplemented by posterior pharyngeal movement driven anteriorly by the superior pharyngeal constrictor. Not all "normal" velopharyngeal sphincters work in this circular closure pattern. See other questions in this module.)
9. Discuss the patterns of velopharyngeal closure. (Coronal, sagittal, circular, and circular plus Passavant's ridge.)
   (a) Discuss the principal muscular components of each. (A coronal closure is achieved mostly by superior pharyngeal constrictors as well as the posterior movement and closure of the soft palate muscles, levator palatini, and tensor palatini. Sagittal closure is primarily the lateral pharyngeal walls consisting of palatopharyngeus and superior pharyngeal constrictors. Circular closure, of course, includes all of the above.)
10. Define the following as measured on lateral cephalometry: pharyngeal depth, effective palatal length, velar height, and velopharyngeal gap. (Pharyngeal depth is measured as a static transverse or horizontal measurement from a fixed point such as the posterior nasal spine to the posterior pharyngeal wall or PPW; the remaining measurements are performed on lateral cephalometric tracings taken during a sustained consonant production such as "s" and include effective palatal length or the length from a fixed point as the posterior nasal spine along the soft palate to the soft palate "knuckle" that represents the muscular bulge produced by the levator veli palatini at the contact with the posterior pharyngeal wall. Velar height is a vertical measurement from the horizontal line taken from the posterior nasal spine to the level of the soft palate "knuckle" on the posterior pharyngeal wall, vertically at a right angle to the roof of the pharynx and is not very commonly used. Finally, the velopharyngeal gap, a crucial measurement, is the space that exists between the "knuckle" of the muscular eminence of the levator veli palatini of the soft palate and the posterior pharyngeal wall during sustained production of the "s" sound, normally zero. Lateral cephalometrics have been largely replaced by cinefluoroscopy exam and endoscopy. See Fig. 17.1.)
11. Briefly outline methods of assessment of the velopharyngeal mechanism. (Essentially, two methods are available: cinefluoroscopy assessment and nasopharyngeal endoscopy. A cinefluoroscopic exam is performed principally in two views, basal or submental vertex and lateral. The tongue is usually coated with a radiopaque paste such as barium, and the child vocalizes a number of vowels and consonants. Nasopharyngeal endoscopy is

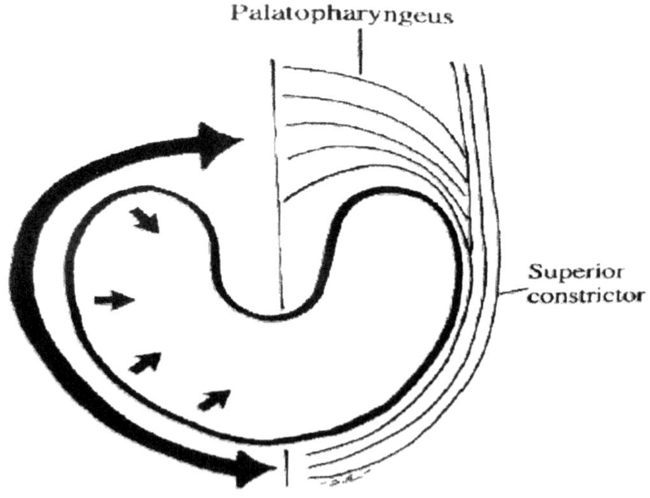

Fig. 17.1 Cinefluoroscopic examination

performed with direct visualization and usually video recording of the nasopharyngeal mechanism again during the production of certain sounds. In some sense, these two methods are complementary, but young children, under the age of 5 or 6, may not tolerate nasoendoscopy. Ancillary measures such as nasometry can be utilized even with a computerized summary of outcomes yet remain secondary in usefulness to the above two methods.)

Treatment

1. What are the options available to treat velopharyngeal insufficiency? (Speech therapy, obturator or palatal appliance, surgery by palatal lengthening, posterior pharyngeal flap (PPF), and/or pharyngoplasty.)
2. In the selection of an operative procedure, PPF, pharyngoplasty, or palatal re-repair to address velopharyngeal insufficiency, a number of variables must be considered including the severity of hypernasality, the pattern of velopharyngeal closure, the magnitude of the velar gap and velar configuration on motion assessed by cinefluoroscopy, and/or nasal endoscopy. Discuss the pattern of velopharyngeal closure specifically. (Conceptually, the selection of the two principal procedures, posterior pharyngeal flap and pharyngoplasty, is dictated in part by sparing the structure that appears to be a significant contributor to velopharyngeal closure in favor of the use of the structure that is less of a contributor. See below.)
3. With respect to the posterior pharyngeal flap (PPF), what are the structural variables? (Width, superior- or inferior-based, lined or not, the dimensions of the lateral ports, and the constructed aperture from the oropharynx to the nasopharynx, namely from the lateral edge of the PPF to the lateral pharyngeal wall.)
4. Other than the size of the lateral ports and the width of the flap, discuss the other two variables: lining and superior versus inferior based. (PPFs are best lined to avoid narrowing with contracture by healing. Logically, a superiorly based flap would be preferable and is the most widely used. The efficacy of the PPF is dependent, in part, on functional lateral ports, as defined above. Mobility of the lateral pharyngeal walls under the influence of the palatopharyngeus is desirable.)
5. In the readings' opinion the PPF is best suited to what types of velopharyngeal closure patterns? (Sagittal or circular.)
   (a) What is the role of medial movement of the lateral pharyngeal walls in outcomes with posterior pharyngeal flaps? (Some lateral pharyngeal wall motion is important to produce valving of the openings or ports on either side of the flap.)
6. What is Passavant's ridge? (A transverse bar of musculomucosal tissue seen on the posterior pharyngeal wall with velopharyngeal closure. This structure could be viewed as normal in a patient with normal speech or a pathologic finding in a patient with velopharyngeal insufficiency. Regardless, the finding is an indication of active superior pharyngeal constrictor activity.)
   (a) What is the principal muscular component of the posterior pharyngeal flap (PPF)? (The superior pharyngeal constrictor. Considerable doubt exists whether the muscular component is still actively innervated.)
7. Which patients would be poor candidates for a pharyngeal flap? (Extensive scarring because of past procedures, significant medical contraindications, and perhaps older adult patients who may have unrealistic expectations. All of the above can be managed prosthetically.)
8. Why has the operation of pharyngoplasty been attractive as a surgical alternative? (No obstruction of the nasal airway at least theoretically and the velum is not violated. Investigations, though, indicate a similar incidence of obstructive sleep apnea.)
   (a) What pattern of VP closure would lend to a pharyngoplasty? (Coronal or circular plus a Passavant's ridge. Similar to the logic employed in the selection of a PPF in the presence of a sagittal or circular pattern of velopharyngeal closure, a coronal closure would favor the use of the relatively immobile lateral pharyngeal wall as a pharyngoplasty.)
9. Consider the degree of hypernasality and describe the management:
   (a) Severe. (If the gap is small on endoscopy or cinefluoroscopy yet the hypernasality and the VPI are severe, consider a neurogenic etiology. Assess with the use of an obturator to determine if improvement is possible. If the gap is more moderate to large, it is probably a posterior pharyngeal flap.)
   (b) Moderate (Small gap is considered pharyngoplasty unless the posterior pharyngeal wall motion is poor; in other words, a pure sagittal closure then perhaps a PPF would be preferable. If the velar gap is moderate to large, a posterior pharyngeal flap would be the preferred option unless lateral pharyngeal wall motion is very poor, a pure coronal closure; then perhaps a pharyngoplasty would be preferable.)
   (c) Mild to moderate (If the gap is small, consider a palatal lengthening such as Furlow's Z-plasty palate repair. If the hypernasality is more moderate than mild, consider a PPF.)
10. What were the readings and views on palatal lengthening? (Maybe efficacious as a primary procedure but dubious as a secondary procedure, except possibly the Furlow procedure. See below.)

11. Describe the clinical setting or patients for whom a Furlow palatal repair would be efficacious. (Two. A submucous cleft palate or a prior repair, which, on assessment, appears to have residual sagittal orientation of the levator veli palatini—referred to as a 'V' deformity—*or* a small 5 mm or less of a velar gap on a cinefluoroscopy or nasal endoscopy.)
12. Although more fully discussed in Chap. 18, palatal fistulae following cleft palate repair are pertinent to a discussion of velopharyngeal insufficiency. Why? (May be responsible for nasal air leak and hypernasality.)
    (a) What are the variables in the occurrence of VPI in the presence of palatal fistulae? (The size and location, anterior versus posterior. Anterior, unless very large, tends not to cause hypernasality while posterior fistula may be indicative of an inadequate soft palate both in terms of length and function.)
    (b) How would you determine if an anterior palatal fistula was responsible for hypernasality? (Obturate with a dental appliance.)
13. Discuss posterior pharyngeal wall augmentation and prosthetic management. (Posterior pharyngeal wall augmentation with prosthetic material has fallen greatly out of favor because of migration, extrusion, etc. Some quite limited experience with autogenous fat augmentation has been reported.)
14. How can the speech therapist integrate into the care of the VPI patient? (Preoperative evaluation, possible preoperative speech therapy, and postoperative speech therapy. Preoperative evaluation, as discussed above, possible preoperative speech therapy for correction of associated articulation disorders, and postoperative speech therapy to address the compensatory mechanisms and any element of learned hypernasality.)

Specific Operations

1. What is lateral port control? (A description, originally by Hogan, of critical size of the area of the lateral ports that are created with a superiorly-based posterior pharyngeal flap. The tipping point is an area >25 mm^2 of both ports combined may allow excessive nasal airflow and conversely, a lateral port at or slightly smaller than this objective critical point would set the stage for satisfactory address of velopharyngeal insufficiency. A port smaller than these dimensions may predispose to obstructive sleep apnea. The control element is the passage of a small catheter, usually a 10 or 12F through the lateral ports either during or at the completion of construction of the posterior pharyngeal flap.)
2. Give the essential steps in the operation of PPF. (Split the soft palate in the midline, develop nasal mucosal flaps based inferiorly on the free edge of the soft palate, parallel lateral posterior pharyngeal gutter incisions and development of a bipedicled PPF, incise inferiorly to convert to a superior pedicle and cranial reflection of the flap. The raw surface of the PPF is lined with the nasal mucosal flaps, repair of the soft palate in the midline to include muscles dissected and moved medially and posteriorly so that they lie transversely, plus/minus pharyngeal donor site closure.)
3. Discuss the following technical aspects of the performance of a PPF:
    (a) Incisions in the soft palate? (Midline incision from uvula to about 1 cm posterior to the posterior border of the hard palate)
    (b) Management of the muscles? (Need to be dissected and moved medially and posteriorly so that they lie transversely)
    (c) Level of attachment or base of the PPF? (About the tubercle of the first cervical vertebra)
    (d) Management of the donor site defect? (In most cases closure of the posterior pharyngeal wall is not possible and probably not advisable)
4. You encounter some bright red blood in the posterior pharyngeal wall, what is the likely source? (The ascending pharyngeal artery-see below)
    (a) You encounter torrential arterial bleeding during the creation of a PPF. What is the problem? (Quite possibly you have performed a PPF on a patient with a velocardiofacial or 22Q11 deletion syndrome without prior imaging, MRI angiogram, of the vessel superior. These patients may have an aberrant course of the internal carotid medially well into the pharynx, and are subject to injury.)
5. Briefly describe the performance of pharyngoplasty. (Three flaps are raised: a lateral pharyngeal wall superiorly-based flap, constructed bilaterally, composed of mucosa and palatopharyngeus muscle and by anatomic definition, is located on the posterior tonsillar pillar-lateral pharyngeal wall. The third flap is a short 1–2 cm superiorly based posterior pharyngeal flap composed of mucosa and the underlying superior pharyngeal constrictor. The two lateral pharyngeal wall flaps are interdigitated in the raw area composed by construction of the superior pharyngeal wall flap. The donor sites of the lateral pharyngeal walls are closed primarily. The approach is an overall narrowing in the cross-section of the VP space.)

Complications

1. What early postoperative complication rate would you quote parents who are considering a PPF for their child's VPI? (10% assuming no syndrome present.)

2. What is the most common immediate postoperative complication? (Upper airway obstruction.)
   (a) What group of patients is at more risk? (Pierre Robin syndrome)
   (b) What measures might be considered for prophylaxis? (Nasal trumpet)
   (c) If no relief with the nasal trumpet and you consider re-intubation what are the negative aspects, besides the usual for an ET tube? (The presence of the PPF which may be disrupted by the passage of the tube)

Editor's Note: Re-intubation is rarely required and obviously the integrity of the PPF is at risk.

3. What is the frequency and type of the most common *late* complication? (Nocturnal respiratory obstruction, about 13%.)
   (a) What are the diagnostic measures that may need to be taken in the presence of a history of nocturnal respiratory obstruction (NRO) and the timing? (A sleep study after a minimum of 6–12 months; if negative, observe.)
   (b) If intervention, what are the options? (Revision plus T&A, *or* a take-down of the PPF.)
   (c) What are the considerations? (Inadequate correction of the obstruction versus recurrence of the VPI. Two of four patients who had a revision with T&A had recurrence, yet the three patients who had take-down of the PPF had resolution and none developed hypernasality.)

Case 1: Speech Disorder

Case-Based Conference

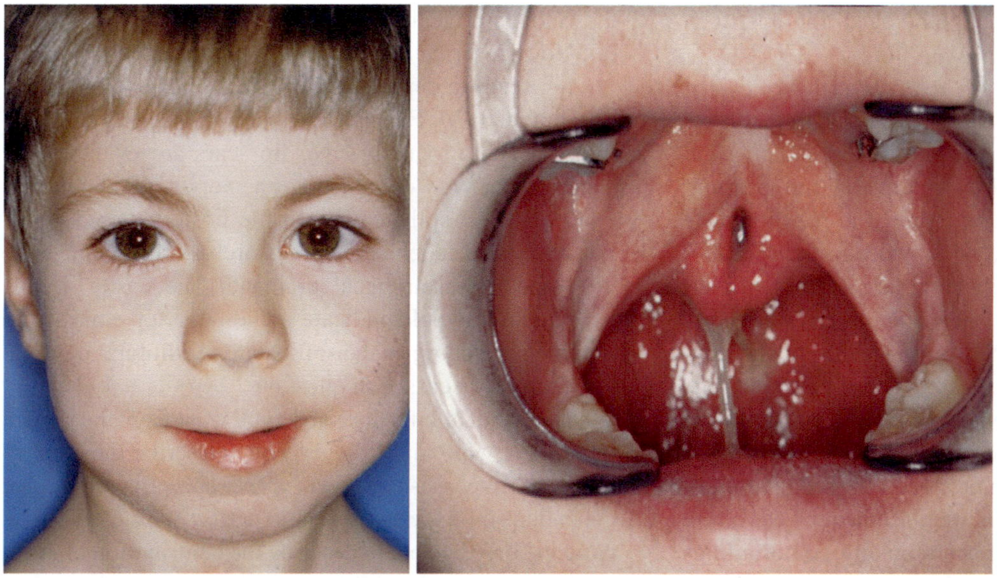

A 9-year-old who had a **cleft palate repair** at age one and has been referred by a speech pathologist for a speech disorder.

1. Prior to the description of the slides, outline your clinical examination including the pertinent history and physical exam.
   (a) Now, describe the slide(s).
2. What additional information do you want from the speech pathologist who made the referral? Describe the components of hypernasal speech.
   (a) Any additional tests indicated? Justify.
3. Describe the pathologic anatomy and pathophysiology of this patient's problem.
4. Outline a treatment plan including, if an operation is a part of that plan, your perioperative care. In the selection of an operative plan, give a menu of possible procedures and then indicate your choice and why.
5. What acute and long-term complications would you describe to the parents as part of informed consent?

Case-Based Conference: Discussion

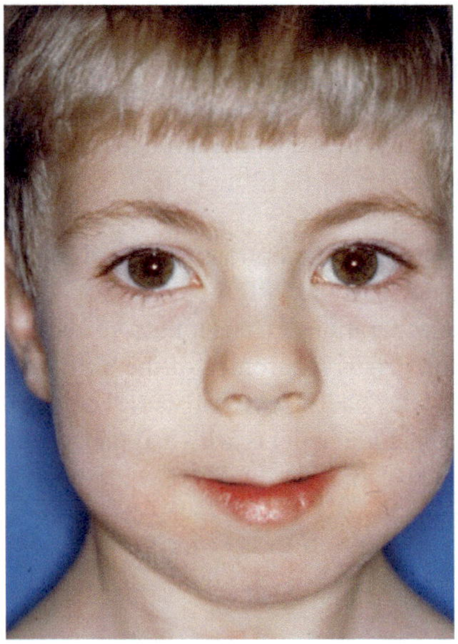
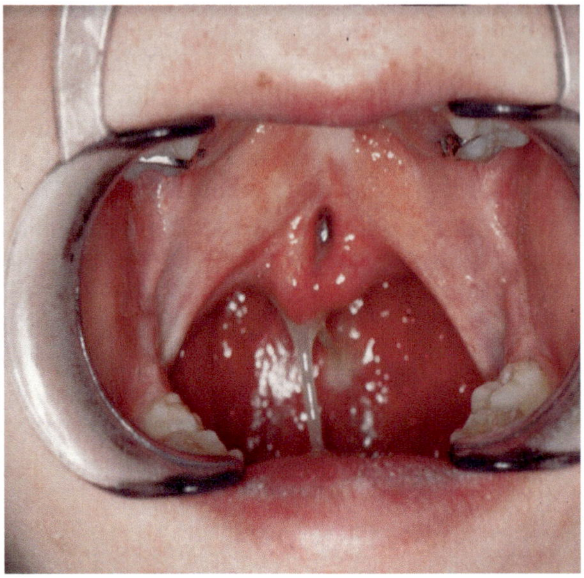

A 9-year-old who had a **cleft palate repair** at age one and has been referred by a speech pathologist for a speech disorder.

1. Prior to description of the slides, outline your clinical examination including the pertinent history and physical exam. (The preamble has already provided the information re: cleft palate repair at age one. The initial history would focus on, if possible, the knowledge the parent(s) have about the extent, namely assuming absence of cleft lip, of the palatal cleft, and if airway problems were present at birth or in infancy. Was a tonsillectomy and adenoidectomy performed recently? The history of the present illness centers on symptoms, nasal regurgitation of liquids or even solid food, intelligibility at home particularly in sustained speech or when fatigued, and treatment for ear infections including placement of ear tubes. The next tier of questions centers on any comorbidities most particularly cardiac, but also other congenital systemic anomalies or others such as asthma. The last set of questions addresses the developmental milestones—in school, special education? The subsequent physical exam would include the entire body including auscultation of the heart, but focused on the head and neck. Assessment of the facies will assist in the detection of the characteristic findings of flattened mid-face and widened nasal dorsum, all indicative of the presence of velocardiofacial or DiGeorge syndrome. Is the patient retrognathic? Intraoral exam as depicted in the slides will determine the presence of fistulas including location and dimensions. Some estimates of velar length and mobility can also be ascertained although the physical exam findings correlate poorly with function, particularly with the presence and magnitude of the velopharyngeal insufficiency (VPI).)
   (a) Now, describe the slide(s). (The full facial view does not seem to depict a child with the facies of velocardiofacial (VCF) syndrome but does suggest the presence of retrognathia. No lip scars are evident. The intraoral view demonstrates a short, scarred soft palate with a split uvula. On the posterior pharyngeal wall, the reddened adenoids are clearly visible with some nasopharyngeal drainage. The easily visible adenoids would indicate some superior contracture and shortening of the soft palate. Additional physical exam is discussed in question 2.)
2. What additional information do you want from the speech pathologist who made the referral? Describe the components of hypernasal speech. (The speech pathologist, dependent on experience and expertise with cleft palate patients, may be able to describe the contribution of articulation errors to the child's speech disorder and estimate the severity of the hypernasality.

   Hypernasality can be determined with perceptual assessment. Perceptual assessment dictates that the child engages in a number of vocalized sounds to determine the capability to seal the nasopharynx (NP) from airflow during speech. The failure to do so will permit "leakage" of air through the NP and nasal cavity. That failure is most evident during the attempted production of the plosive consonants, sounds that require the momentary increase in airway pressure such as k, x, and to some degree the vowels of e and i. While attempting to do so the child may have audible nasal emission but the cardinal characteristic of hypernasal speech is abnormal nasal resonance.

Also present in normal speech and during the production of sounds as mn, n when some NP and nasal cavity air passage occurs. Compensatory mechanisms for hypernasal speech include glottic stops, pharyngeal fricatives, and nasal grimacing. The child may have some hoarseness secondary to the first two. Glottic stops and pharyngeal fricatives are an effort on the part of the child to physically restrict airflow.)

(a) Are any additional tests indicated? Justify. (The physical exam can include a mirror placed beneath the nostril to detect abnormal nasal emission indicated by fogging of the mirror surface. An objective assessment of the presence and degree of severity of velopharyngeal insufficiency, if such is the etiology of the hypernasal speech as well as determination of the functional adequacy of the velopharyngeal mechanism can be accomplished by one or both of two methods: multi-view cineradiographic and nasoendoscopic assessment. The former utilizes dynamic lateral, anterior-posterior, and basal views during speech. A number of measurements can be determined including velar length, the magnitude of velar gap, if any, and the distance between the velar and the posterior pharyngeal wall eminence during contraction in the attempted production of plosive consonants. By utilizing the multiple views available, experienced observers can determine the pattern of closure and the relative contribution of the posterior and lateral pharyngeal walls. The other modality is directed toward visualization of the velopharyngeal mechanism by passage of an endoscope of small caliber nasally and observation during speech. All of the data described above accrued with cineradiology can be obtained with the exception of absolute measurements including perhaps most importantly, the velar gap. The critique or drawback of each is the x-ray exposure with the former which is not inconsequential with the cine technique, similar to fluoroscopic examination. The principal criticism of the latter, endoscopic observation, is the necessity for the child's cooperation which given the individual and age may be difficult.)

3. Describe the pathologic anatomy and pathophysiology of this patient's problem. (Given a diagnosis of VPI, not secondary to a hypotonic soft palate from a neurogenic cause which seems highly unlikely, the VPI in this scenario is from incomplete velopharyngeal closure at the critical moments during speech. Closure is accomplished by the five essential paired muscles of the velopharyngeal mechanism, levator veli palatini, tensor veli palatini, palatopharyngeus, superior pharyngeal constrictor, and perhaps the uvulus. The degree of participation by the palatopharyngeus and the superior pharyngeal constrictor varies somewhat, but essentially the soft palate is powered superiorly and posteriorly by the levator as well as the tensor, the latter by constriction and contraction that flattens the palate and also assists in the vector of lateral movement. Simultaneously, the lateral pharyngeal wall moves medially by the action of the palatopharyngeus residing in the posterior tonsillar pillar as well as by the anterior fibers of the superior pharyngeal constrictor which on contraction also moves the posterior pharyngeal wall anteriorly to oppose to the velar eminence at the level of C1–2. The presence of a visible transverse band of mucosa and muscle may be seen in some instances of VPI, a phenomenon known as Passavant's ridge. Patterns of velopharyngeal closure are dictated by the relative contribution of each of these components. A sagittal closure is accomplished by the lateral pharyngeal walls, coronal by the velum and posterior pharyngeal wall, and circular as the name implies by all the elements of the velopharyngeal mechanism. A pure pattern of closure, for example sagittal, is uncommon.)

4. Outline a treatment plan including, if an operation is a part of that plan, your perioperative care. In selection of an operative plan, give a menu of possible procedures and then indicate your choice and why. (To continue the assumption that the diagnosis of VPI is secondary to a scarred and shortened soft palate, the options available for address of of the dysfunctional velopharyngeal mechanism are four: posterior pharyngeal flap, palatopharyngoplasty, double-opposing Z-plasty and injection of the posterior pharyngeal wall. A posterior pharyngeal flap consists of construction of a flap of mucosa and muscle, the superior pharyngeal constrictor, usually superiorly based at the level of C1, elevated from the prevertebral fascia and inset into a midline incision in the soft palate, namely an incision from the uvula to the posterior border of the hard palate. The dimensions are approximately 5 cm in length and width of 2 cm, preserving lateral apertures to avoid complete anatomic obstruction of the NP. To minimize secondary contracture in the healing phase, the raw surface of the flap is lined with mucosa flaps harvested from the nasal aspect of the soft palate and based inferolaterally. To minimize the complication of nocturnal respiratory obstruction (NRO), [see below] the dimensions of the maintained lateral apertures should be approximately 25 cm^2 or a 12F catheter in each port. Closure of the pharyngeal donor site is advocated by some. Most commonly the width of the flap is such that complete closure is not possible but suturing the edges of the mucosa to the prevertebral fascia will facilitate secondary healing.

The second option is palatopharyngoplasty. Essentially, the superiorly-based flaps from the lateral pharyngeal wall are composed of mucosa and muscle, the palatopharyngeus, harvested from either posterior tonsillar pillar and transposed to a raw area created on the posterior pharyngeal wall by elevation of a short superior-based transverse posterior pharyngeal wall flap. The flaps are inset one superior and the other inferior, the donor sites closed primarily. Some substantial interest exists in a tailored or selection of the flap based on the pattern of velopharyngeal closure. In patients with a predominately sagittal closure, the palatopharyngeus is active but the posterior pharyngeal wall, powered by the superior pharyngeal constrictor, is less so a posterior pharyngeal flap (PPF) is optimal. The reverse would apply if the pattern was predominantly coronal, namely a palatoplasty.

The third surgical option is a double-opposing Z-plasty or Furlow palatoplasty. This operation requires a redo palatoplasty with reorientation of the muscle fibers of the levator and lengthening of the palate. A redo palatoplasty would be appropriate for the patient with a moderate velar gap, 5 mm or less, and evidence of an anteriorly abnormally displaced levator.

The last option is augmentation of the posterior pharyngeal wall by injection of a substance, alloplastic or autogenous. A variety of alloplastic substances have been injected in the past, the principal autogenous material utilized was fat and cartilage.

Each of these options have a complication profile. Posterior pharyngeal flap and palatoplasty both share a common complication concern—the production of NRO and worse, obstructive sleep apnea (OSA). Since a quiet respiratory effort consists of a combined nasal and oral airflow, particularly during sleep, total and subtotal NP obstruction has the potential for the production of NRO. The clinical picture of NRO is that of heavy snoring, perhaps attended by episodes of intermittent apnea or hypopnea. The diagnosis of obstructive sleep apnea (OSA) adds the element of daytime sleepiness as the third element of the triad. The establishment of a diagnosis of OSA requires the completion of a sleep study. A monitored sleep study will sum the frequency and duration of episodes of apnea in the calculation of an apnea index. Comparative studies have yet to determine which procedure, PPF or pharyngoplasty, is superior in this regard. Additional consideration is the possible inadequate address of a large velar gap with pharyngoplasty alone. Although conceptually a posterior pharyngeal flap would appear to provide a more comprehensive approach, little data exists to support this contention.

A Furlow Z-plasty, as mentioned above, is probably optimal for the patient with the finding of an anteriorly displaced levator and/or a moderate velar gap, 5 mm or less. Lastly, the attempted correction of VPI by posterior pharyngeal wall augmentation has yielded at best mixed results. Inferior migration and extrusion of alloplastic materials has been frequent in past reports. The injection of fat has led to incomplete correction as well as absorption. Given the appearance in this patient of a severely short and scarred soft palate, the optimal option is probably a posterior pharyngeal flap with control of the size of the lateral ports.)

5. What acute and long-term complications would you describe to the parents as part of informed consent? (The acute complications are those of bleeding and airway obstruction. Both may require a return to the operating room. The patient profile at most risk for airway obstruction is diagnosis of Pierre Robin syndrome. A risk sufficiently high that many practitioners will place a short nasal trumpet at the completion of the procedure in addition to a tongue suture and observe the patient overnight in the ICU.

   The long-term complications of the procedures of PPF and PP are the two edges of the surgical sword: incomplete correction and persistent hypernasality vs overcorrection and the production of NRO and even possibly OSA. Reputed series would indicate a 90% success rate and a 10% incidence of NRO with performance of a posterior pharyngeal flap. Of the patients with NRO a relatively small minority will require treatment. The treatment of the patient with recalcitrant NRO and OSA is transection of the PPF, a distinctly uncommon necessity. Although a concern for recurrence of VPI looms with this intervention, the limited experience would indicate that outcome is far from inevitable. Of course, fully-informed consent discusses both these possibilities, inadequate and overcorrection.)

In-Service Examination

1. The physical findings in submucous cleft palate include the following **EXCEPT**:
   (a) Class III malocclusion
   (b) Bifid uvula
   (c) Zona pellucida
   (d) Notch in posterior border of the hard palate
2. Endoscopic evaluation of a child with velopharyngeal insufficiency establishes a sagittal pattern of velopharyngeal closure. Based on those findings, what is the preferable operation?
   (a) Furlow palatoplasty
   (b) Posterior pharyngeal flap
   (c) Sphincter pharyngoplasty
   (d) A Z-flap palatoplasty and pharyngoplasty
3. An anatomical concern in the performance of a posterior pharyngeal flap in a patient with velocardiofacial syndrome is
   (a) Presence of aortic stenosis
   (b) Occult Arnold-Chiari syndrome
   (c) Medial displacement of the internal carotid arteries
   (d) Maxillary excess

18 Alveolar Clefts, Orthognathic, Palatal Fistulas

Bibliography

Murali S.P., Denadai R., Chou P., et al., "Secondary Alveolar Bone Grafting in Patients with Cleft Lip and Palate: A Step-by-Step Video Series", *Plast Reconstr Surg.*, (2022);149(6):**1176e–1179e (Videos 3 and 4) ONLY.**

Lough DM., Madsen CL., Kumar AR, Lin AY., Chapter 28 "Alveolar Cleft Surgery", Principles and Practice of Pediatric Plastic Surgery Second Edition, Quality Medical Publishing (2017);pgs. **807–15.**

Morcos SS and Patel PK, "The Vocabulary of Dentofacial Deformities", *Clinics in Plastic Surgery*, (2007); 34(3):**589–596 ONLY.**

Ferraro, J. W., Chapter 13: "Cephalometry and Cephalometric Analysis." Fundamentals of Maxillofacial Surgery, Springer-Verlag New York, Inc., (1997); **pp 236–239.**

Hurst CA, Eppley BL, Havlik RJ, and Sadove AM, "Surgical Cephalometrics: Applications and Developments", *Plast. Reconstr. Surg.*, (2007); 120(6): **92e–104e (Through 96e ONLY).**

Selber JC and Rosen HM, "Aesthetics of Facial Skeletal Surgery", *Clinics in Plastic Surgery*, (2007); 34(3):pgs. 437–445. **439, Figure 2 ONLY**.

Patel PK, Baker SB, Chapter 27 "Orthognathic Surgery in Adolescents with Dentofacial Skeletal Deformities", Principles and Practice of Pediatric Plastic Surgery, Quality Medical Publishing (2017);pgs. 949 (Surgical Phase)–954 (Postoperative Recovery), **749–754 and 784–792.**

Naran S, Steinbacher DM, D DM, et al, "Current Concepts in Orthognathic Surgery", *Plast. Reconstr. Surg.,* (2018); 141:**927e (Surgical Planning)–932e (Informed Consent) ONLY including video.**

Losee JE, Smith DM, Vecchione L, et al., Ch. 57 "Post-palatoplasty fistulae: Diagnosis, treatment, and prevention", Comprehensive Cleft Care, McGraw Hill Co., (2016); **1091–1111.**

Kalmar CL, SiuA, Alvarez E, Swanson JW, "Modified Buccal Myomucosal Flap Closure of Large Anterior Palatal oronasal Fistulas", *Plast. Reconstr. Surg.*, (2021); 147(1):**Video ONLY.**

Faculty Discussion and Study Guide

Alveolar Cleft

1. What is the essential anatomy of the unilateral bony cleft? (The bony component is a defect shaped much like a hexagon, with its base at the anterior alveolus or bony gap sloping from the anterior to posterior and from inferior to superior, a roof that consists of the nasal floor and two side walls, the medial and lateral cleft margins, the former of which is the vomer and the lateral is the pyriform margin of the maxilla. The soft tissue component has the palate as the floor and the floor of the nasal cavity as the roof. The side walls consist of nasal mucosa medially and palatal mucosa laterally. The readings established an analogy of the anatomy of the defect as a "tornado" which perhaps should be viewed as a tornado lying horizontally with the narrow end of the funnel pointed posteriorly. See Fig. 18.1.)
2. What are the goals in closure of the alveolar cleft? (To provide a bony component for eruption of the teeth, in particular the permanent canine, physical separation of the nasal and oral cavities by the construction of a stable nasal floor, and provision of a stable maxillary arch. Many cleft surgeons would add bony support of the pyriform margin as well.)
3. What are two different conceptual approaches with respect to timing of closure of the alveolar cleft? (The first conceptual approach, which could be labeled conventional, is secondary bone grafting of the alveolar cleft. The timing is between ages 8 and 11 or prior to eruption of the secondary canine, preoperative orthodontic assessment and management is necessary, as discussed below. The treatment philosophy is that earlier intervention than this age may interfere with bony growth, particularly if

E. Luce, *A Curriculum for Plastic Surgery*, https://doi.org/10.1007/978-3-031-62087-4_18

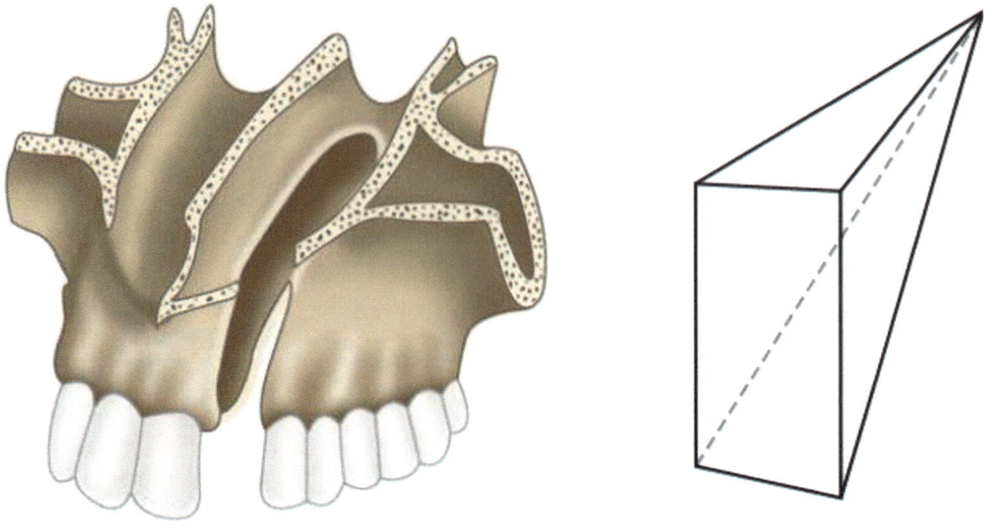

Fig. 18.1 Unilateral bony cleft

soft tissue dissection is necessary to close the soft tissue component of the cleft.

The other conceptual approach is termed primary bone grafting and is performed in infancy even at the time of lip repair. No true resolution has been accomplished of these two different treatment protocols and primary bone graft is performed by few cleft palate teams in the United States. Gingivoperiosteoplasty (GPP), performed at lip repair (see Chap. 15), does not harvest bone but the advocates believe the ultimate alveolar cleft will be substantially smaller or perhaps absent.)

4. Briefly describe the necessary preoperative orthodontic steps and goals prior to secondary alveolar bone grafting. (The process that is usually necessary consists of expansion of the maxillary arch in preparation for bone grafting. A cone or occlusal CT can construct a 3-D model of a cleft. The model can determine dental development, size of bony gap, and adjacent bony architecture. Dental impressions are necessary to ascertain the degree of maxillary collapse, occlusal relationships, and orthodontic planning. Impressions of the maxillary arch are taken and the orthodontic planning is accomplished. Preoperative orthodontic movement of the maxillary arch to accomplish an alignment is necessary and will require orthodontic bands utilizing the primary and secondary teeth. A retention appliance will be necessary postgrafting.)
5. List and discuss materials for grafting of the alveolar cleft. (The use of autogenous bone, usually harvested from the anterior iliac crest, is the most conventional and established method. Other substances have included bone substitutes such as allogeneic freeze-dried bone, recombinant bone morphogenetic protein, and BMP, with demineralized bone matrix. The search for bone substitutes has been driven by donor site morbidity including pain from the harvest of autogenous bone. The principal disadvantages of bone substitutes as BMP are several: the increase in facial edema, including the recipient site, and the lingering concern regarding the risk of malignant transformation. In addition, equivalent efficacy to autogenous bone has not been firmly established.)
6. In terms of outcomes, what is the Bergland scale? (The Bergland scale measures the interdental height of bone or bone height index that essentially measures a percentage of bone about the roots of the teeth adjacent to the alveolar cleft.)
7. An alternate technique is vertical distraction osteogenesis (VDO). Discuss including benefits and liabilities. (VDO is a conceptual extension of the procedure employed in the mandible and maxilla, most frequently in those instances of recalcitrant alveolar clefts created by repeated failed grafting. Other situations are those of extremely wide clefts and/or scarred soft tissues. The use of 3-dimensional CT scans and acrylic models assists in surgical planning. The appliance is inserted intraorally and corticotomies are completed under general anesthesia. The principal general contraindications include anticipated poor patient or familial compliance. Patients with active dental issues require optimization of oral health before surgery. Complications include infection and device failure.)

Editor's Note: The basics of distraction osteogenesis are included in module (Chap. 6).

Cephalometrics and Orthognathic Surgery

1. What is the Angle's classification of occlusion? (Class I: The mesial or most anterior buccal cusp of the first maxillary molar sits in the buccal groove of the first mandibular molar. Then, the maxillary canine sits between the mandibular canine and the first premolar. Think dentally of the maxilla sitting slightly posterior to the mandible but this is not a skeletal relationship. Class II: The mesial buccal cusp of the first maxillary molar sits mesial to the buccal groove of the first mandibular molar and the maxillary canine is mesial to the mandibular canine. Class III: In contrast, the mesial buccal cusp of the first maxillary molar sits distal or posterior to the buccal groove of the first mandibular molar, and the maxillary canine sits distal to the space or groove between the canine and first premolar of the mandible. See Fig. 18.2.)
2. Label the following points on a lateral cephalometrogram: Points A, B, S, N, Po, Or, Go, Pg. See Fig. 18.3.
3. Draw a SNA-SNB angle and give the normal in degrees. See Fig. 18.4.

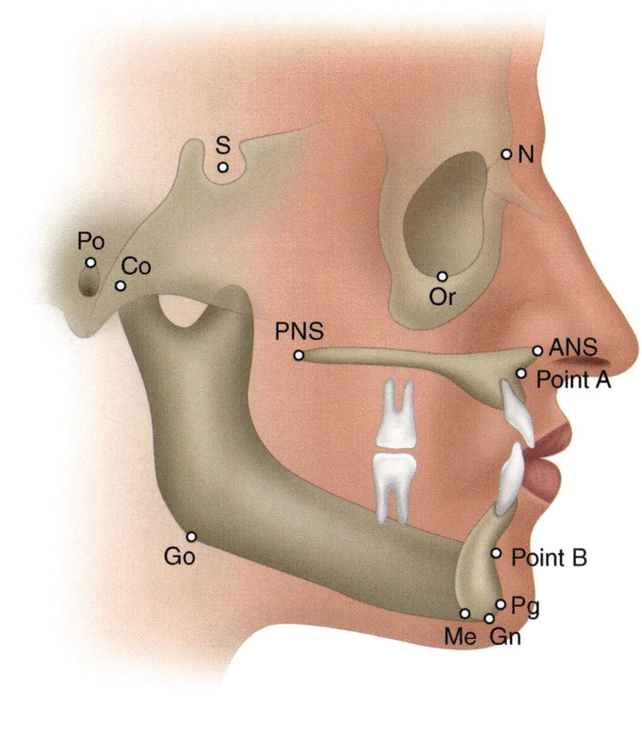

Fig. 18.3 Skeletal landmarks

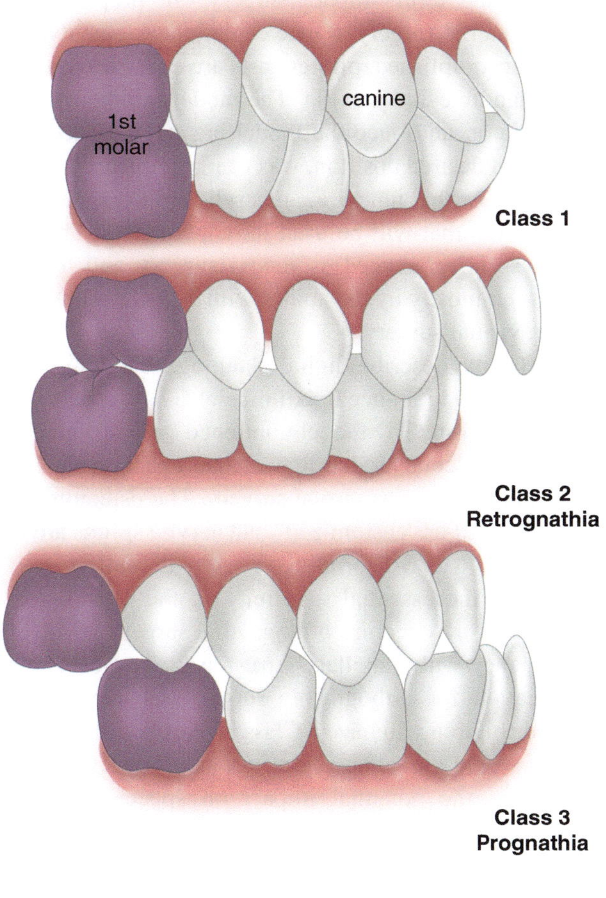

Fig. 18.2 Angle's classification of occlusion

4. Draw the Frankfort horizontal plane. See Fig. 18.5.
   (a) What is the facial plane angle? Normal value? (The facial plane angle is formed by the intersection of the Frankfort horizontal plane, a line drawn from Po to Or, and the facial plane, which is a vertical line drawn from the nasale to pogonion. The normal angle is 88° and becomes more acute in retrognathia and more obtuse and prognathism.)
5. Describe the three types of morphologic profile and the *probable* associated angle classification and SNA-SNB angles. See Fig. 18.6.
6. With dental vocabulary, define the following: distal, mesial, labial, buccal, lingual, palatal. (Distal and mesial reference the teeth more posterior, distal, or anterior, mesial in relative to the midline or sagittal plane. Buccal-labial is, as the terms infer, the outer dental surface and lingual, for the mandible, is the inner surface. Buccal is adjacent to cheek mucosa and labial is adjacent to the lip. Palatal substitutes for lingual in the maxilla. Buccal, labial, lingual, and palatal refer to specific aspect of teeth.)
7. Define the following: cross bite, open bite, overbite, over jet. (Cross bite is an abnormal relationship between maxillary and mandible teeth that reference the relationship buccal/labial and lingual/palatal; open bite is an abnormal space between the incisal surfaces of the mandibular and maxillary teeth; overbite is the distance

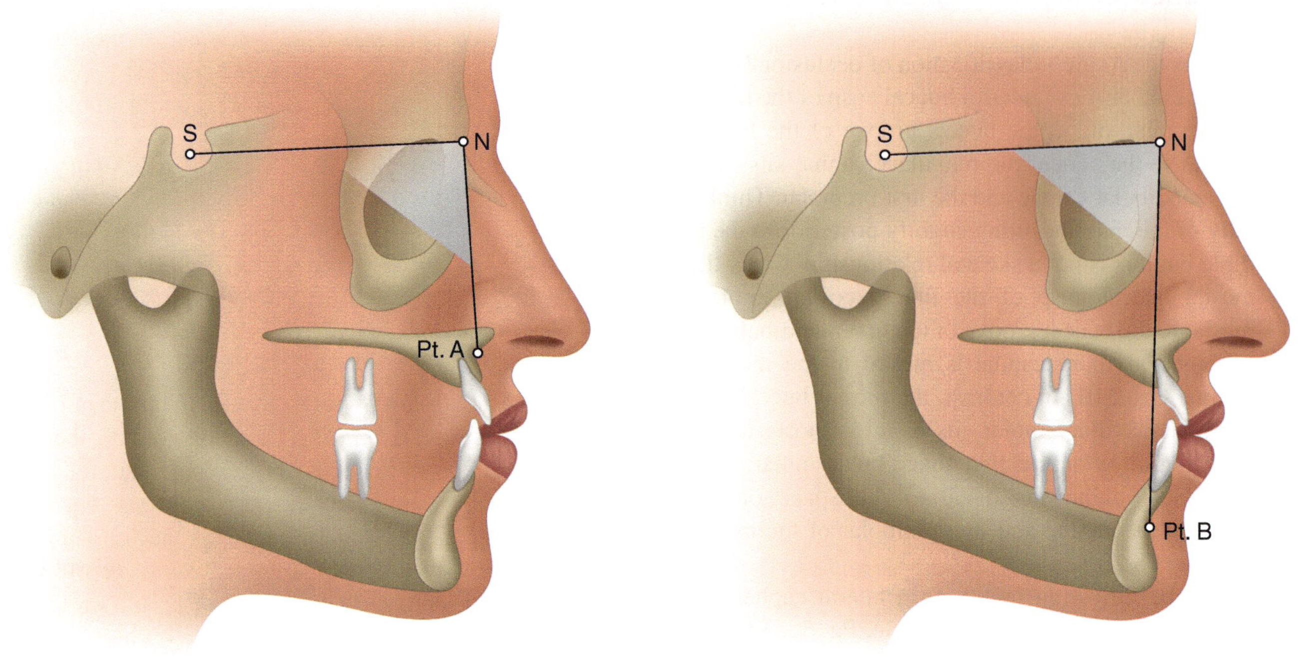

Fig. 18.4 Lateral cephalometrogram

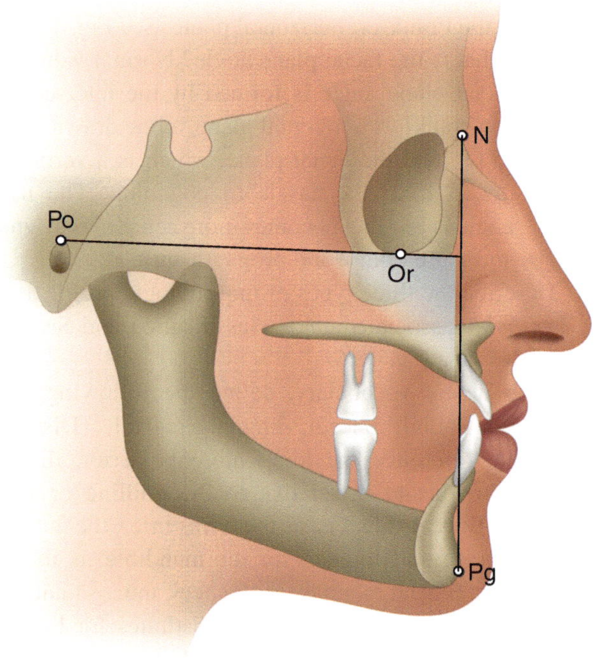

Fig. 18.5 Frankfort horizontal plane

between the maxillary and mandibular incisors when the patient is in centric occlusion. Overjet is an excessive distance between the occlusal surface of the mandible and maxillary incisor.)

8. Define the term "model surgery" in preparation for orthognathic surgery. (Once cephalometric analysis has been accomplished, plaster casts are constructed of both the mandible and maxilla. The models are placed on an articulator, and once the model has been placed in the new and desired position, wax or plaster is used to mend the gap. At that juncture, an acrylic splint is made from the model that will be used intraoperatively. The entire process is referenced as model surgery and has been replaced mostly by the ability with 3-D CT scans to perform virtual surgery.)
   (a) Briefly, describe digital planning. (The use of cone CT and thin-slice maxillofacial CT reformatted to a composite 3-D model combined with a digital scan of the dental models that enables exact surgical planning, known as virtual surgery. The osteotomies are tailored or "customized" and acrylic splints are fashioned with 3-D printing or conventionally.)
9. What is the essential deformity in the cleft lip/palate child that may require orthognathic surgery? (Maxillary deficiency with maxillary retrusion is the most frequent indication for orthognathic surgery. Characteristically, these children will have a Class III Angle malocclusion.)
10. How would you counsel the parents of a cleft lip/palate child of the potential impact on speech of planned orthognathic surgery? (Maxillary advancement may unmask an underlying borderline velopharyngeal insufficiency or move a child from normal to borderline velo-

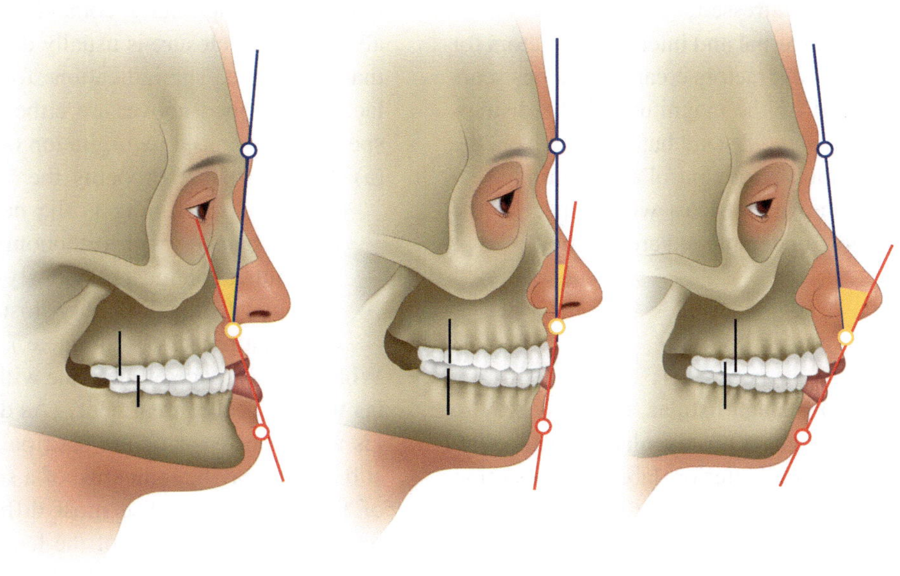

Fig. 18.6 Morphologic profile. Concave = SNA-SNB <2° and convex = SNA-SNB >2°

pharyngeal insufficiency. Preoperative assessment by a speech pathologist is essential.)

11. What group of cleft lip/palate patients would be candidates for distraction osteogenesis? (Since the degree of relapse is directly proportional, among other factors, to the severity of the maxillary retrusion and the magnitude of the necessary advancement, those children with severe maxillary retrusion, >10 mm, may be the best candidates for distraction osteogenesis at the LeFort I level.)
12. Outline the pros and cons of distraction osteogenesis for the deficient maxilla in the cleft lip/palate child. (The pros are a reduced rate of relapse and probably a lower postoperative incidence of velopharyngeal insufficiency. The cons are a two-stage procedure vs. the one-stage orthognathic surgery and the necessity in some children for additional maxillary and/or mandibular surgery.)
13. Where are the osteotomies performed for a maxillary LeFort I? (The anterior and medial maxillary walls, the lateral-posterior wall, and the pterygopalatine junction.)
    (a) Once these osteotomies are complete, the maxilla is ready for down fracture? True or false? (False) What is necessary additionally? (A osteotomy at the base of the nasal septum through the vomer.)
14. Substantial hemorrhage is encountered with a posterior-lateral wall osteotomy. What is the source? (Probably the internal maxillary artery.)
15. The most popular type of orthognathic surgery for the mandible is sagittal split osteotomy. Where is the osteotomy accomplished? (Primarily, an osteotomy in the sagittal plane of the ascending ramus of the mandible, the mandibular angle, and exiting at the buccal aspect of the posterior mandibular ramus.)
    (a) What is the principal structure at risk? (Inferior alveolar nerve.)

Distraction Osteogenesis

1. What is the essential definition of distraction osteogenesis? (The generation of new bone into a gap between bone segments in response to application of tensile stress across the gap.)
    (a) Earliest clinical application? (By Ilizarov, a Russian orthopedic surgeon, in the extremity long bones.)
2. Distraction osteogenesis has three phases: latency, distraction, and consolidation. What does the latency phase refer to? (The period between the osteotomies and the application of daily distraction, usually about 7 days.)
    (a) What type of bone is initially generated? (Membranous.)
3. If the consolidation phase is too short, fibrous instead of bony union occurs. If it is too long, bone stock is inadequate because of the absence of load-bearing. What is the

recommended duration of the consolidation phase until the new bone is loaded or stressed? (6 weeks.)

4. Compare and contrast external and internal distractors for the mandible. (External distractors create cutaneous scars and the length dictated by the magnitude of the distraction. Internal distractors avoid scars but may not have the same degree of multiple vector control and require a second procedure for removal. At least with respect to the mandible, most distractors employed are external.)

Palatal Fistulas

1. Give a classification of palatal fistulae. (An easy way to recall the system is to begin at the alveolar ridge and consider whether the fistula is anterior, labial, or posterior, lingual to the alveolar ridge. Those are type VII and VI respectively. Type V is at the incisive foramen. Type IV is anywhere in the hard palate. Type III is at the junction of the hard and soft palate. Type II is within the soft palate. Type I is a uvular fistula. See Fig. 18.7.)
2. What functional or symptomatic problems might a palatal fistula create? (The communication between the oral and nasal cavities may produce nasal regurgitation of liquids as well as sufficient nasal air escape to produce distortion and hypernasality to speech. A palatal fistula located more posteriorly, Type III or II, may indicate a submucous dehiscence of the muscular continuity at the time of cleft palate repair.)
3. What are the indications for treatment of a palatal fistula? (Type VI and VII alveolar fistulas are most commonly associated with the presence of an alveolar cleft. Since management optimally coincides with grafting of the alveolar cleft, closure is usually deferred to the timing of that procedure. The indications for more posterior fistulae, as described above, are either an adverse effect on speech and/or nasal regurgitation of liquids.)
   (a) Timing issue? (Probably the single most significant aspect of the timing is the necessity for maxillary arch expansion with orthodontics since that process may either enlarge a previously existent fistula or create a new fistula. Probably closure should be deferred until that process is complete.)
4. What is the essence of the issue with Type II and III fistulas with respect to treatment? (As described above, fistulas at the posterior or the hard palate and/or within the soft palate may be indicative of a submucous dehiscence of the prior repair. The most difficult aspect of palate repair is at the junction of the hard and soft palate. The presence of velopharyngeal insufficiency as indicated by hypernasality would dictate intervention once detected. If perceptual speech assessment has determined the presence of hypernasality, further evaluation with cinefluoroscopy and/or nasal endoscopy will assist in determination of the appropriate procedure. If those procedures determine a velar gap of >5 mm with a Type II or Ttype III fistula the velopharyngeal insufficiency should be addressed with either a pharyngoplasty or posterior pharyngeal flap combined with an intravelar veloplasty. See Chap. 17)
5. Describe an option for closure of a Type IV or mid-hard palate fistula. (Most straightforward method would be the re-creation of mucoperiosteal flaps based on the greater palatine vessels. The nasal layer can be closed with hinge flaps of the walls of the fistula based on the nasal side and the oral closure by re-apposition of the mucoperiosteal flaps.)
6. Describe the blood supply to a tongue flap used for closure of a palatal fistula. (The lingual arteries course anteriorly on the ventral surface of the tongue and give vertical branches to the dorsal tongue surface which is utilized for the tongue flap.)
7. What is an autogenous free graft option and an alloplastic option? (Chondral cartilage can be used as an adjunct between the two-layered closure and the use of acellular dermal matrix, ADM, has also been utilized as a method for closure without the use of flaps.)

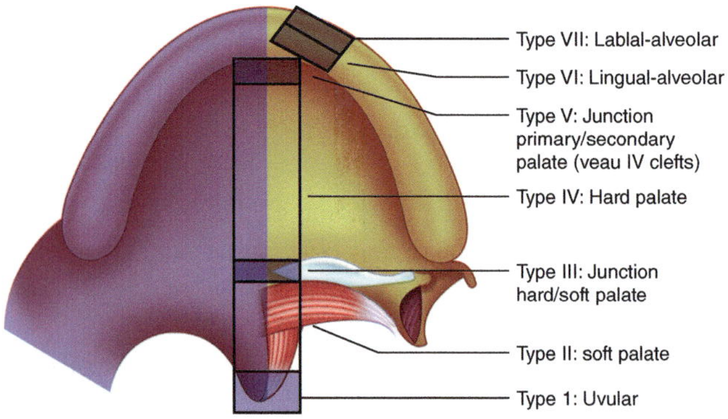

Fig. 18.7 The Pittsburg classification

Case 1: Cleft Lip Late Deformity

Case-Based Conference

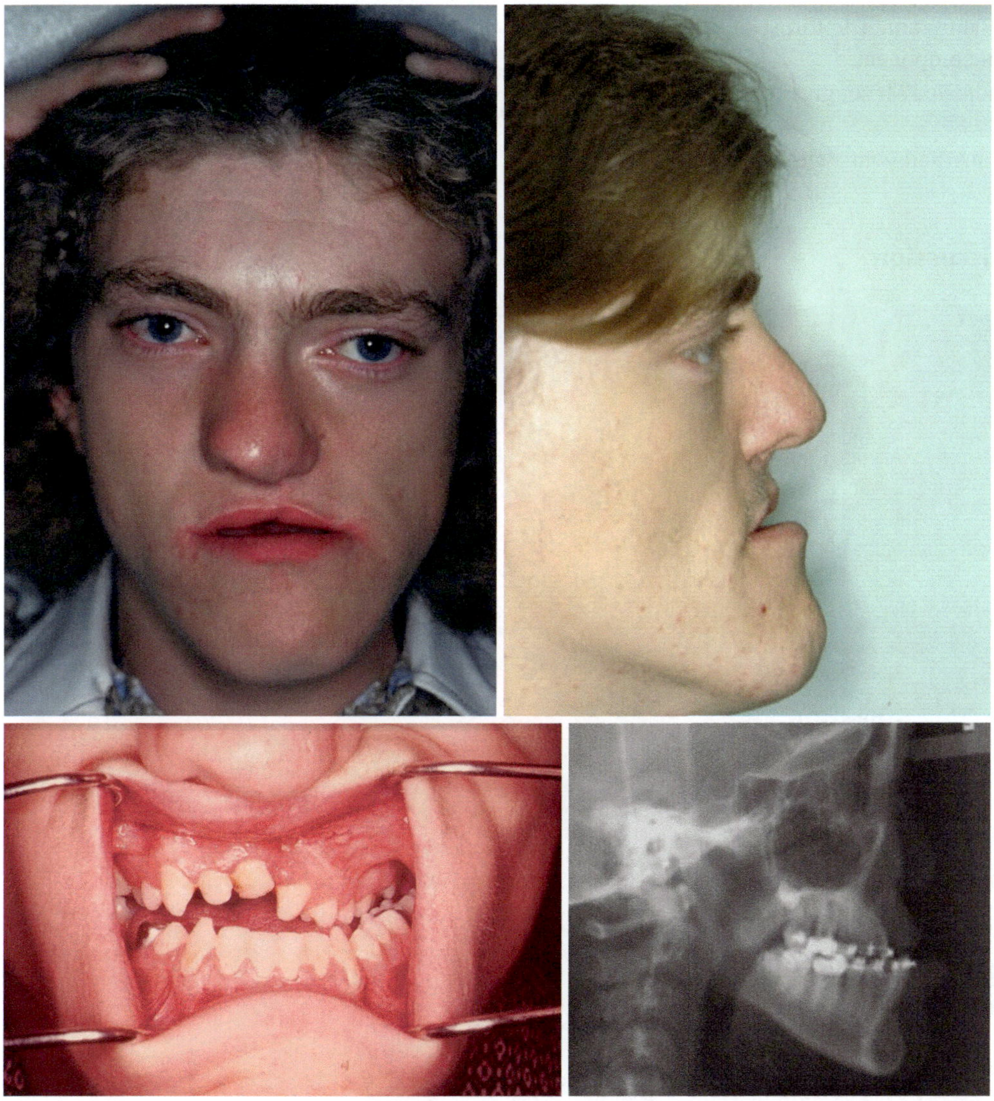

A 22 year old with a history of cleft lip/palate who desires improvement in facial appearance.

1. Describe the pertinent findings evident in the clinical slides, add information needed from the clinical exam, and then read the lateral cephalogram. The thrust of this case is the associated skeletal component.
   (a) Any diagnostic testing indicated? If so, give the anticipated results.
2. What is the pathologic anatomy and contributing factors to the same?
3. Outline a list and hierarchy of the components of a comprehensive treatment plan. Include the variables that will impact the outcomes.
4. *Briefly*, what is the type and approach of the operative component of the treatment plan?

Editor's Note: a detailed operative description is not necessary for this case conference.

Case-Based Conference: Discussion

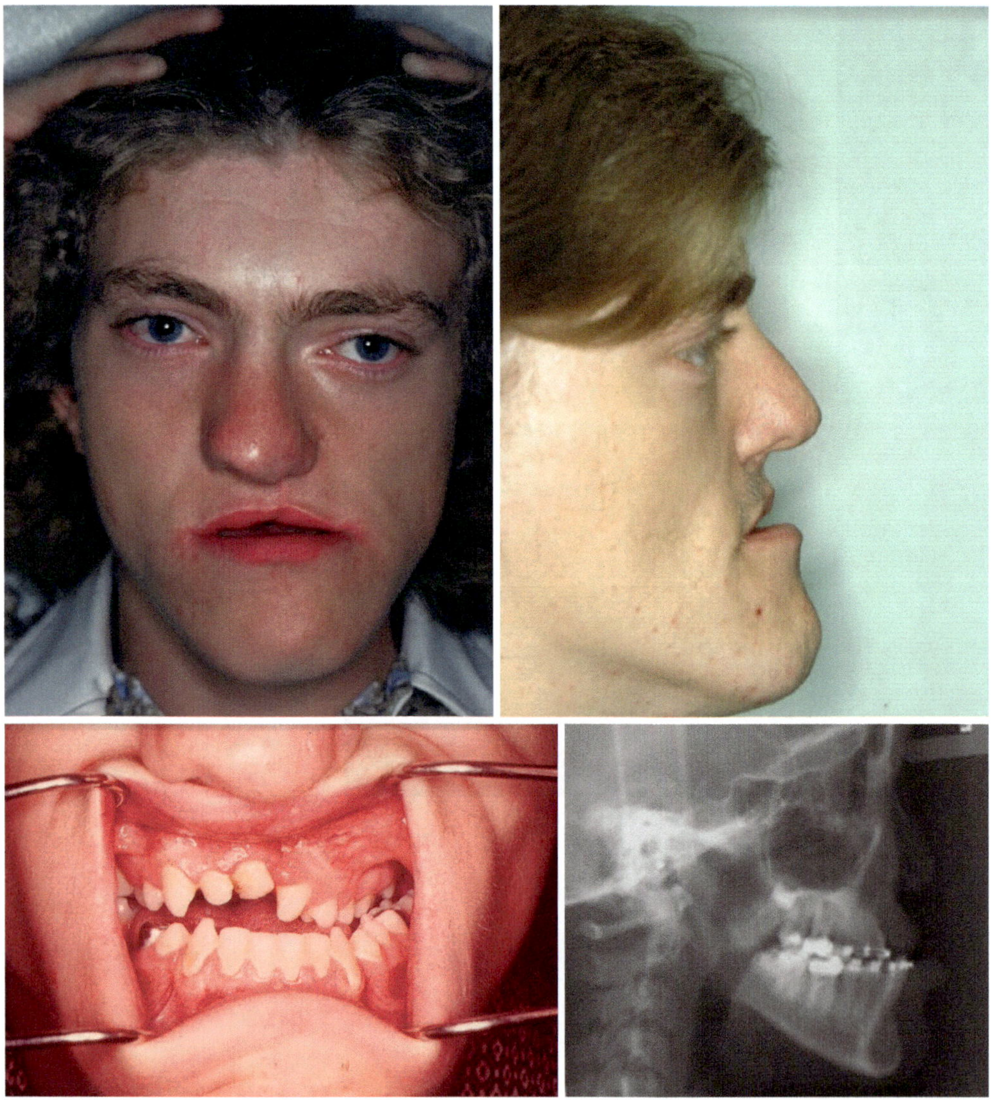

A 22 year oldwith a history of cleft lip/palate and desires improvement in facial appearance.

1. Describe the pertinent findings evident in the clinical slides, add information needed from the clinical exam, and then read the lateral cephalogram. The thrust of this case is the associated skeletal component. (Three clinical photos are provided, an anterior-posterior, lateral, and a dental or intraoral view. The full-face view demonstrates a male of stated age. The upper one-third of the face is normal. In the middle one-third, although the right side appears normal, the left eye and orbit sit lower or vertical dystopia. The transverse facial width appears equal to the right, but the malar prominence is less. The nose has the stigmata of the cleft nasal deformity with apparent depression of the tip inferiorly and medially with no tip highlight visible on the left. The upper lip is dramatically short with some vermilion malalignment and an old scar on the left that is consistent with the history of cleft lip repair. The facial proportions by divisions into transverse or horizontal thirds would indicate a middle third proportionally less than the lower one-third. The chin is disproportionately increased vertically with a disruption of the division of the normal proportion of the facial lower one-third into a superior one-third and lower two-thirds created through a transverse line through the stominon. The lower two-thirds is disproportionately greater than the superior one-third. The lateral view is from the patient's right. The upper lip is short and recessed with an obvious bony maxillary recession as well. In contrast, the chin is over projected anteriorly with the menton sitting on a vertical line dropped from the nasal tip rather than well posterior to that point. In addition to over projection anteriorly, two findings are evident: first, the inferior one-third of the face is dominated by the disproportionate chin height; second, the middle one-third of the face is disproportionately shorter than the lower one-third, confirming the impressions from the full-face view.

   The last slide demonstrates intraoral findings of disordered maxillary dentition. The malocclusion consists of a severe lingual or palatal crossbite of the left posterior dentition and an open bite of the right posterior dentition. The left maxillary central and lateral incisors, teeth 9 and 10, are absent, and teeth 7 and 8, the right maxillary incisors are canted superiorly and an anterior open bite exists as well. A mandibular premolar is missing bilaterally and root exposure is evident of both mandibular canines.

   The clinical exam would accrue historical information re: past treatment and operations particularly attempted correction of velopharyngeal insufficiency as well as other information that may indicate associated anomalies, particularly in the cardiac or renal systems. The physical exam would assess the state of dentition, most importantly the persistence of an alveolar cleft and the presence or not of an associated pre- or post-alveolar fistula. The surgeon should perform a perceptual assessment of speech, in particular, a detection of hypernasality. The posterior pharynx would be examined, if possible, for the presence of a posterior pharyngeal flap.

   The lateral cephalogram on the fourth slide depicts and illustrates a severe retrusion of the maxilla with some counter-clockwise or cephalic rotation. A more formal cephalometric analysis is discussed below.)

   (a) Any additional diagnostic testing indicated? If so, give the anticipated results. (As part of a comprehensive assessment of a cleft lip/palate patient, an audiologic exam is indicated and may determine an element of hearing loss.. Further evaluation would require lateral cephalograms as depicted in the fourth slide or, more contemporaneously, the acquisition of three-dimensional computer-generated images. The speech assessment almost certainly would determine articulation errors secondary to the patient's anterior dental configuration and, possibly, hypernasality. Cephalometrics would plot the SNA angle, determined by the angle created by the relationship of the maxilla to the cranial base, represented by a transverse line drawn from the mid-point of the sella to the nasion or the most posterior point of the junction of the nasal and frontal bones in the sagittal plane and a vertical line from the nasion to the deepest mid-point on the maxillary alveolar process, known as point A. In Caucasians, that mean angle, SNA, is 82°. A similar angle can be constructed with the S-N line intersecting with a vertical line from the nasion to a similar point on the mandible, known as point B and is the relationship of the mandible to the cranial base. The mean angle is 80° or a normal SNA-SNB of 2°. This patient would appear to have an SNA angle substantially less than normal, perhaps 70° and a SNB angle of >80°, perhaps 90°.)

2. What is the pathologic anatomy and contributing factors to the same? (The pathologic anatomy is hypoplasia and growth retardation of the maxilla, more evident on the cleft side, left than right, characterized by maxillary retrusion, cephalic rotation, and Class III malocclusion. The initial contributing cause is the cleft of the lip and palate. A major contributing cause was the repair of the palate and possibly the lip as well. The findings of a palatal crossbite on the left would indicate a constricting force combined with a palatal collapse as well as the severe lack of maxillary projection. The large and prominent chin, anterior mandible, is secondary to overgrowth. Given the cephalometrics cited above, the patient has significant maxillary recession and prognathism with a Class

III occlusion combined with anterior open bite and the previously-described crossbite.)

3. Outline a list and hierarchy of the components of a comprehensive treatment plan. Include the variables that will impact the outcomes. (Address of the patient's deformity will require two-jaw surgery, maxillary advancement, and mandibular setback. In preparation for the same, presurgical orthodontics will be mandatory, beginning with impressions, possibly isolated dental extractions, and the casting of dental stone models. The orthodontist will address and correct with palatal expansion, possibly surgically-assisted as well as correction of the compensatory anterior malocclusion. Traditionally, the stone casts created from dental compressions are placed on an articulator, re-cut and re-configured or "model surgery" to duplicate the operative procedure and prepare occlusal splints to be utilized in the OR. In two-jaw surgery, two occlusal splints will be necessary, an intermediate and a final splint that will represent the final mandibular-maxillary relationship. Contemporaneously, most of this process is completed by the use of CT technology, including 3-D models and the performance of virtual surgery. The operative procedure will be a LeFort I advancement and a bilateral mandibular setback by sagittal split osteotomies. The variables that may be critical in this patient include a past history of posterior pharyngeal flap, current borderline or overt hypernasality, the presence of residual alveolar clefts associated with pre- and post-alveolar fistulas, if any, and the magnitude of anticipated maxillary advancement. In all likelihood, determined by the patient's desires, rhinoplasty will be accomplished at some point after orthognathic surgery.)
4. *Briefly* describe the type and approach of the operative component of the treatment plan.

Editor's Note: a detailed operative description is not necessary for this case conference.

(Treatment plan:

(a) Speech and audiologic evaluation if not already accomplished
(b) Orthodontic evaluation and treatment including any tooth extraction, if necessary
(c) Orthognathic surgery or distraction osteogenesis
(d) Rhinoplasty

In a conventional LeFort I osteotomy the approach is intraoral, the maxilla is mobilized via LeFort I osteotomy lines, completed with a down-fracture, and then advanced and rotated caudally. The LeFort osteotomy for the cleft lip patient differs substantially and also differs for unilateral versus bilateral clefts. In brief, many if not most unilateral patients will require multi-segment, the greater and lesser mobilized and related separately. The cleft can be addressed with compression if necessary or bone-grafted if sufficient soft tissue exists. If inferior displacement of the maxilla is also performed, supplemental bone grafting of the osteotomy sites will be determined by the magnitude of the bone gaps.

This discussion by conventional orthognathic surgery is applicable principally to mild-moderate severity of maxillary hypoplasia. More severe, >8–10 mm of advancement anticipated as probably the instance in this patient, are plagued by a significant relapse rate. The use of distraction osteogenesis has evolved as an appropriate alternative with a proven substantially lower relapse. The mandible is retruded by bilateral osteotomies performed sagittally in the ascending raimi. The ultimate positioning is guided by the prefabricated occlusal splints.)

Case 2: Palatal Fistula

Case-Based Conference

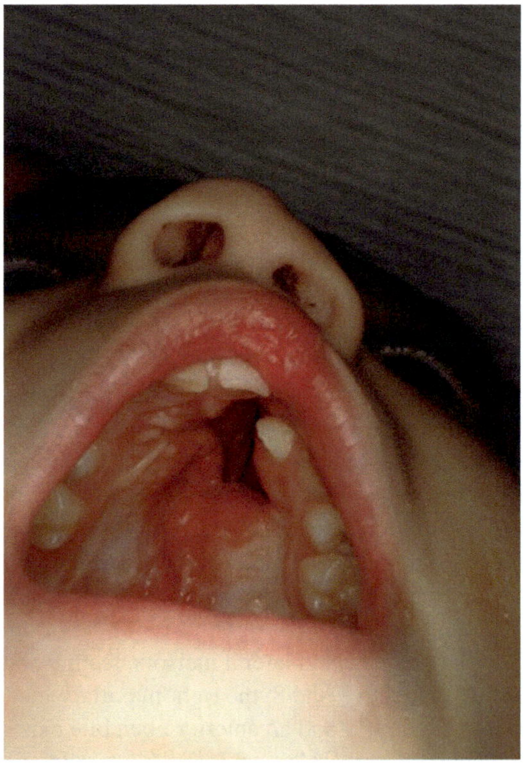

A 5-year-old who had a palate repair elsewhere. His fistula measures 2 × 1.5 cm.

1. Describe the slides, add a history, and focus physical examination.
   (a) Are any tests or consultations indicated?

2. Discuss the pathophysiology of palatal fistula including the variables of age, location, and nature of the cleft.
3. Outline your treatment plan. Begin with the goals and then a menu of operative procedure(s) (if any). Choose your preferred approach.

Case-Based Conference: Discussion

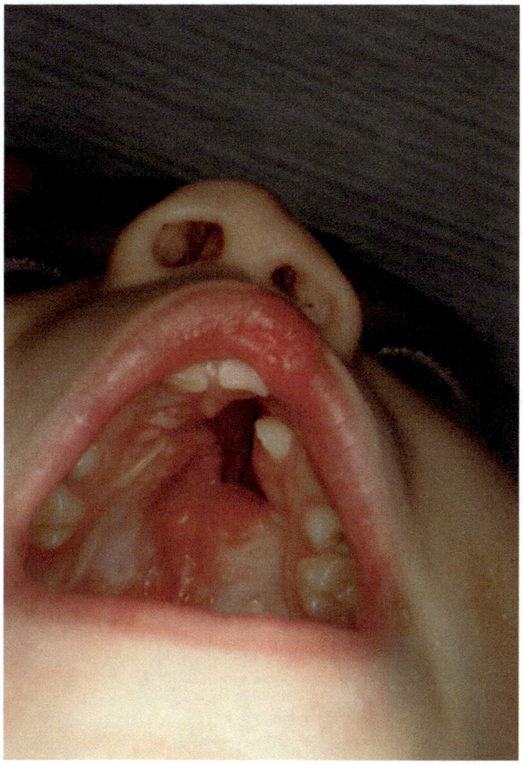

A 5 -year-old who had a palate repair elsewhere. His fistula measures 2 × 1.5 cm.

1. Describe the slides. (An intraoral photo demonstrating a large anterior hard palatal fistula that begins immediately post-alveolar. No evidence of information. The dimensions appear as stated, 2 × 1.5 cm, the remainder of the palate can not be visualized.) Add a history and physical. (The history would elicit the presence and severity of associated symptoms such as nasal regurgitation of liquids or even solids and parental opinions about affected speech as well as possible repeated middle ear infections. Whatever information can be elicited about details of the palatal repair would be of benefit as well as the timing post-operatively of the initial occurrence of nasal regurgitation of fluids. Physical exam would begin with a perceptual analysis of speech concentrating on detection of hypernasality, particularly the plosive consonants. Next, examination of the palate beyond what is depicted in the slide, detection of additional fistulae further posterior, particularly the posterior border of the hard palate and soft palate. Examination of the labial sulcus for pre-alveolar fistula should also be performed.)
   (a) Any tests or consultations indicated? (Formal speech analysis by a speech pathologist and a pediatric dentist or orthodontist if fabrication of an obturator is under consideration—see below. An endoscopy of the velopharyngeal mechanism for degree of competence may be indicated.)
2. Discuss the pathophysiology of palatal fistula including the variables of age, location, and nature of the cleft. (The location and to some degree of size of the fistula will dictate management. One system of classification, the Pittsburg classification, divides post-palatoplasty fistulas into seven categories; uvular, soft palate, posterior border of the hard palate, hard palate, junction of primary and secondary palate, post-alveolar, and pre-alveolar. That system has implications for treatment: posterior fistulae may signify excessive tension at the time of repair with dehiscence or failure to address the muscular components of the soft palate. The presence of hypernasal speech and/or repeated episodes of otitis media may also signal velopharyngeal insufficiency. Fistulae in the mid-portion of the hard palate, particularly small, may represent breakdown of the nasal closure only and not imply functional significance if not attended by the findings discussed above. Post-alveolar fistulae are seen commonly in settings of Veau III or IV palatal clefts, at least prior to alveolar bone grafting. Pre-alveolar clefts occur when inadequate attention is directed toward nasal floor closure at the time of lip repair.)
3. Outline your treatment plan. Begin with the goals and then a menu of operative procedure(s) (if any). Choose your preferred approach. (The goals of treatment of post-palatal fistula hinge on location. The occurrence of fistulae, I-III in the clinical scenario of velopharyngeal insufficiency will entail re-repair with a contemporary palate repair technique such as a two-flap or Furlow palatoplasty. Further evaluation with nasal endoscopy and/or cineradiography of the competency of the velopharyngeal mechanism will further aid in the synthesis of the treatment plan. For example, if incompetency is present with a substantial velar gap, a pharyngeal procedure as a sphincter pharyngoplasty or posterior pharyngeal flap in combination with a re-orientation of the velar muscles may be appropriate. More anterior hard palate fistulas may be closed in two layers by the use of turnover flaps based on the fistula for nasal lining and oral closure by recreation and advancement of mucoperiosteal flaps, similar to primary palate repair.

   If alveolar arch alignment requires orthodontic intervention with palatal expansion fistula closure is best deferred until those measures are accomplished. Post-alveolar fistulas, if sizable as in the case depicted, particularly in Veau IV clefts, may require the transfer of soft tissue located or recruited from the palate. The two most commonly employed regional flaps are the tongue flap and the facial artery musculomucosal flap. The tongue flap is based anteriorly on branches from the lingual artery and centered medially. Nasal closure is accomplished again with turnover flaps based on the fistula, combined with vomer flaps, if visible, and the tongue flap is used for oral closure. Recently, acellular dermal matrix has been incorporated as a third intermediate layer. Some evidence is available to indicate the use of acellular dermal matrix may be of value to permit complete healing in those instances of minor suture line breakdown and dehiscence. In young children, short-term intermaxillary fixation may be necessary with dental brackets and wires or elastics for short-term fixation. A second stage for division and definitive inset of the tongue flap is necessary. The facial artery musculo-mucosal flap, as the name implies, when based anteriorly is perfused by the facial artery. The dissection is more complex than a tongue flap and may be indicated more for large hard palatal fistulas but does not require a second stage. A third option is a buccal myomucosal flap based on the buccal artery, a branch of the internal maxillary. A peripalatal pathway is necessary for inset. Free flap reconstruction of the palate has been described but usually in an oncologic setting.

Obturator is possible for symptomatic patients if the surgery must be deferred for whatever reason. Obturation may be a satisfactory temporizing measure until the age of alveolar bone grafting is reached.)

Postoperative

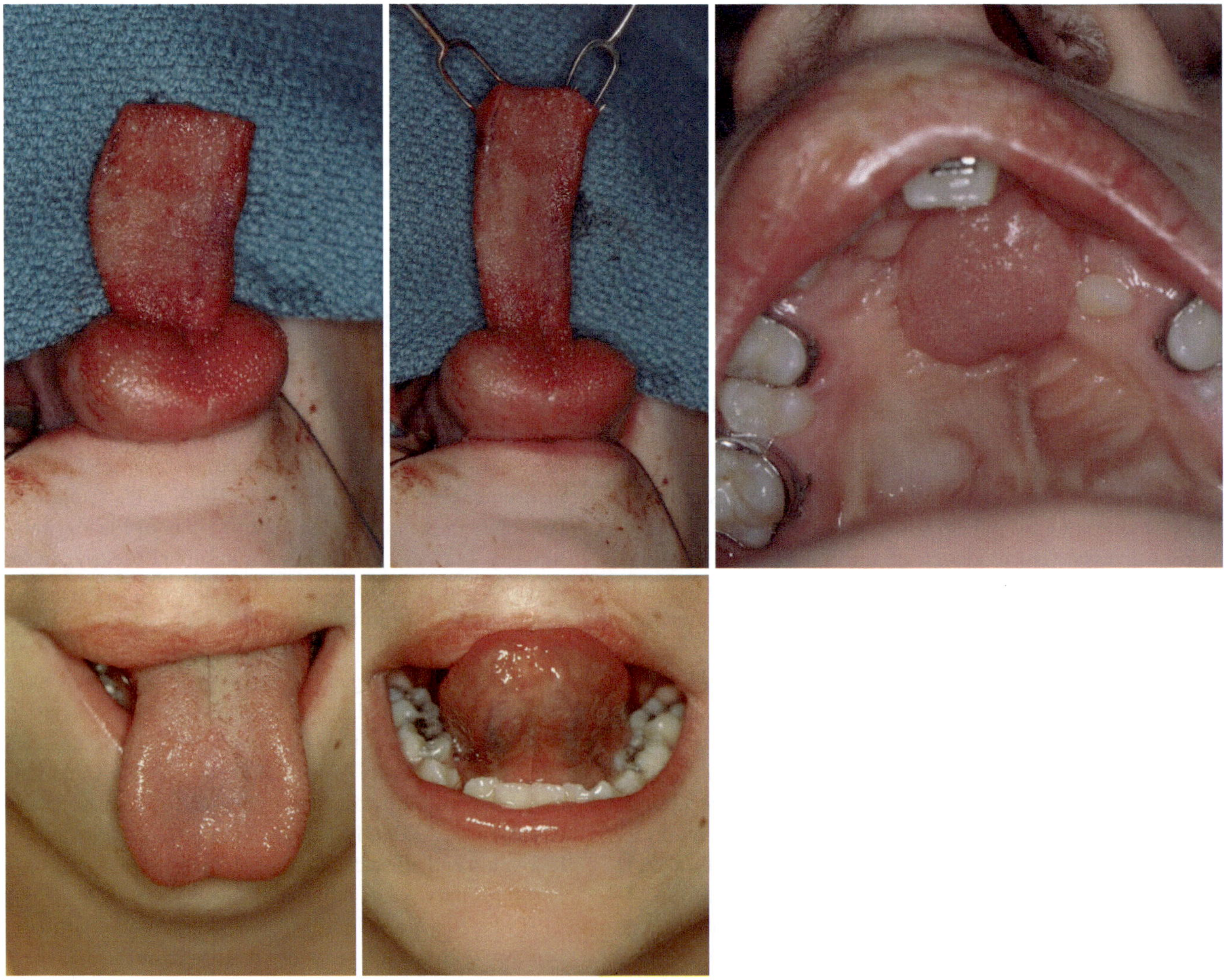

Closure of the fistula was accomplished with a tongue flap. Nasal lining was provided by turnover flaps based on the fistula. The orthodontic bands were used for immediate postoperative intermaxillary fixation, and the flap was transected and inset at 2 weeks. The postoperative tongue mobility and architecture are preserved.

Case 3: Alveolar Cleft

Case-Based Conference

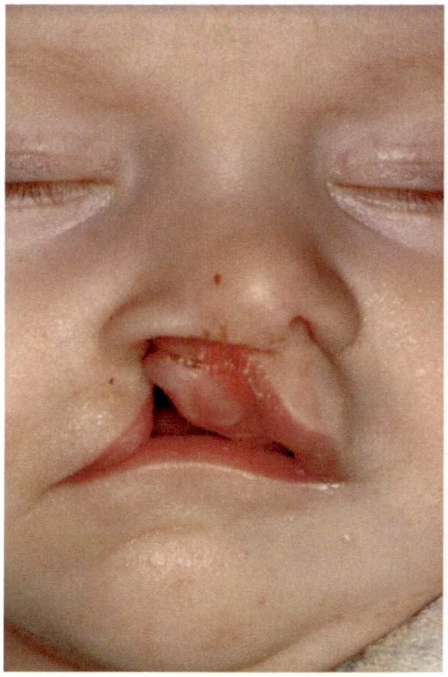

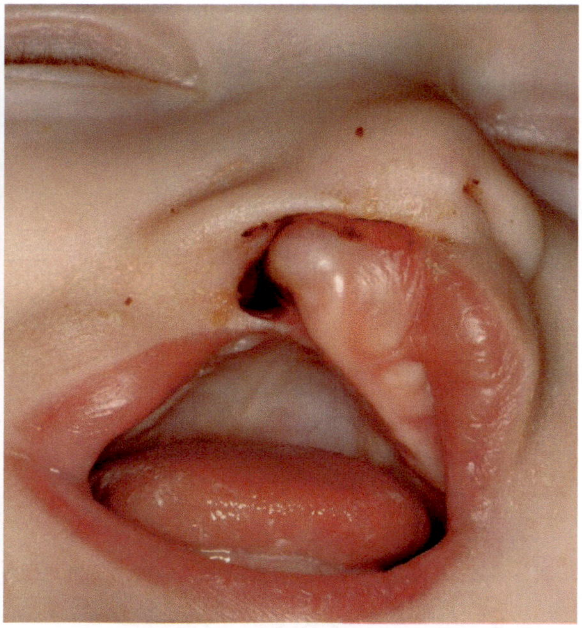

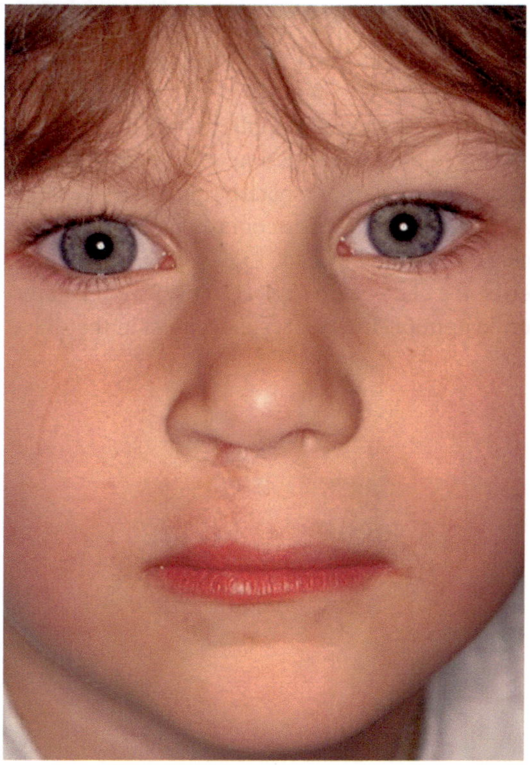

A patient who had a complete unilateral cleft repaired in infancy (first two slides) and now is 5 years of age.

A. The first portion of this case applies to the management, if any, of the alveolar cleft at the time of lip repair.
   1. Describe the slides with respect to the alveolus only.
   2. Describe options, if any, in management at this stage.

B. The child is 5 years of age. The third slide depicts operative management of the alveolar cleft (not necessarily performed at this age).
   1. Describe the slide and the anticipated alveolar findings.
   2. Outline the pathologic anatomy of the alveolar cleft.
   3. List the pertinent goals in management of the alveolar cleft.
   4. What is the conceptual approach with respect to timing?
   5. Outline your approach and describe in detail.

Case-Based Conference: Discussion

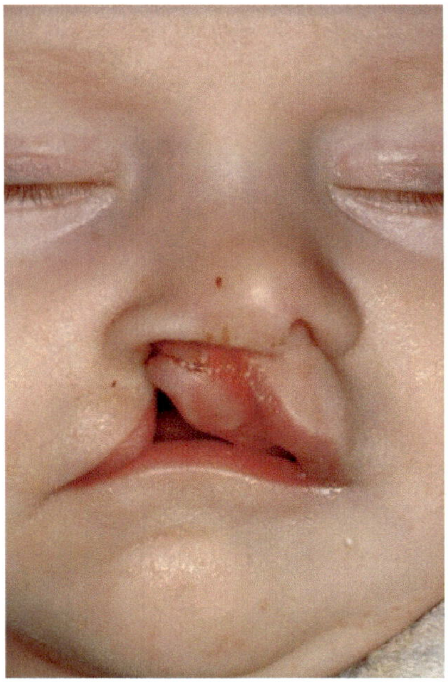

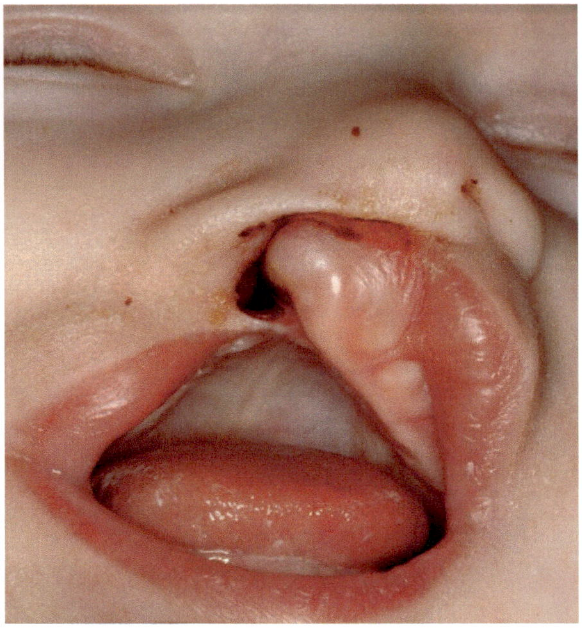

A patient who had a complete unilateral cleft repaired in infancy (first two slides) and now is 5 years of age.

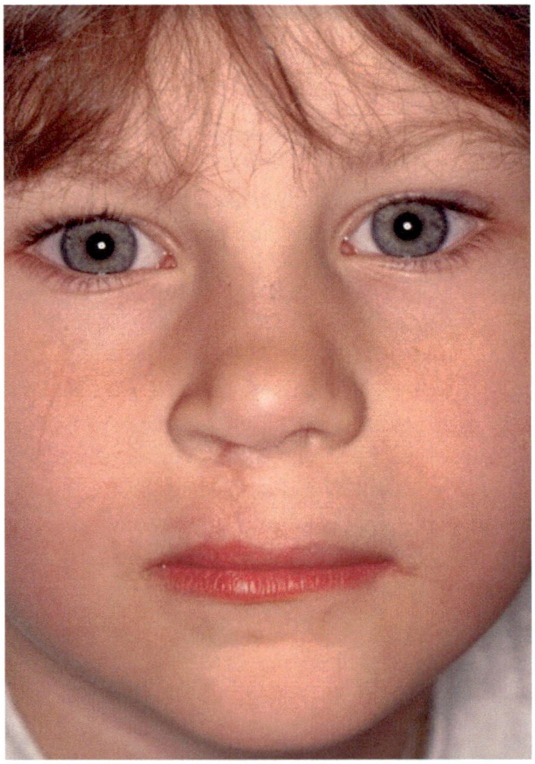

A. The first portion of this case applies to management, if any, of the alveolar cleft at the time of lip repair. (Please refer to the discussion of preoperative maxillary orthopedics, NAM, and gingivoperiosteoplasty and preoperative conference discussion in Chap. 13)
   1. Describe the slides with respect to the alveolus only.
   2. Describe options, if any, in management at this stage.

B. The child is 5 years of age. The third slide depicts operative management of the alveolar cleft (not necessarily performed at this age).

1. Describe the slide and the anticipated alveolar findings. (A single frontal view of the face is provided that includes chin, mid-face, eyes, and lower forehead. As best can be estimated, the facial proportions appear normal. The soft tissue esthetics of the lip repair are good with a well-defined cupid's bow and symmetry. The lip scars are satisfactory except for some prominence at the nasal sill and some minor blurring of the scar-vermillion interface. The nose is reflective of some of the residual stigmata of the cleft, namely, alar base inferior displacement, and a slump and hypoplasia of the alar rim. A submental-vertex view is not available that would provide additional information regarding the underlying skeletal support at the pyriform aperture and the degree of nasal floor collapse secondary to the alveolar-nasal bony defect. Further discussion of the probable associated nasal deformity is included in Chap. 15. The intraoral examination would ascertain the magnitude of the alveolar cleft and, if any, the relative relationship of the greater and lesser segments. The anticipated alveolar deformity, if present, is lingual collapse of the lesser maxillary segment and an associated posterior crossbite. The other dental abnormalities may include rotation, ectopic eruption, or absence of the lateral incisor on the cleft side. Of course, the palate should be carefully examined for associated palatal fistulas other than the adjacent anterior palate contiguous with the alveolar cleft.)
2. Outline the pathologic anatomy of the alveolar cleft. (The bony component is a defect shaped much like a hexagon with the base at the anterior alveolus or bony gap sloping from the anterior to posterior direction from inferior to superior, a roof that consists for the nasal floor and two side walls that consists of the medial and lateral cleft margins, the former of which is the vomer and the lateral of which is the pyriform margin. The soft tissue component has the palate as the floor and the floor of the nasal cavity as the roof. The side walls consist of nasal mucosa medially and palatal mucosa laterally. An analogy of the anatomy of the defect could be viewed as a pyramid lying horizontally with the apex of the pyramid pointed posteriorly.)
3. List the pertinent goals in management of the alveolar cleft. (To provide a bony component for eruption of the teeth in particular the permanent canine, physical separation of the nasal and oral cavities by construction of a stable nasal floor, and provision of a stable maxillary arch. Many cleft surgeons would add bony support of the pyriform margin as well.)
4. What is the conceptual approach with respect to timing? (The first conceptual approach, which could be labeled conventional, is secondary bone grafting of the alveolar cleft. The timing is between ages 8 and 11 or prior to eruption of the secondary canine, preoperative orthodontic assessment and management is necessary, as discussed below. The treatment philosophy is that earlier intervention may interfere with bony growth, particularly if soft tissue dissection is necessary to close the soft tissue component of the cleft.

   The other conceptual approach is termed primary bone grafting and is performed in infancy even at the time of lip repair. No true resolution has been accomplished of these two different treatment protocols. And primary bone graft is performed by few cleft palate teams in the United States. Early secondary bone grafting is performed prior to canine eruption to provide bone stock for the eruption into the now-grafted cleft.)
5. Outline your approach and describe it in detail. (The process that is usually necessary consists of expansion of the maxillary arch in preparation for bone grafting. A cone or occlusal CT can construct a 3-D model of a cleft. The model can determine dental development, the size of bony gap, and adjacent bony architecture. Dental impressions are necessary to ascertain the degree of maxillary collapse, occlusal relationships, and orthodontic planning. Impressions of the maxillary arch are taken and the orthodontic planning is accomplished. Preoperative orthodontic movement of the maxillary arch to accomplish an alignment is necessary and will require orthodontic bands utilizing the primary and secondary teeth. A retention appliance will be necessary postgrafting. The use of autogenous bone, usually harvested from the anterior iliac crest, is the most conventional and established method. Other substances have included bone substitutes as allogeneic freeze-dried bone, recombinant bone morphogenetic protein (BMP) with demineralized bone matrix. The search for bone substitutes has been driven by donor site morbidity including pain from the harvest of autogenous bone. The principal disadvantages of bone substitutes as BMP are several: the increase in facial edema including the recipient site and the lingering concern regarding the risk of malignant transformation. In addition, equivalent efficacy to autogenous bone has not been firmly established.)

In-Service Examination

1. What is the Bergland's scale?
   (a) The magnitude of a posterior cross bite
   (b) The interdental bone height in alveolar bone grafts
   (c) The degree of anterior displacement of the premaxillary segment in bilateral cleft lip
   (d) The magnitude of velar gap in velopharyngeal insufficiency
2. In a patient with SNA-SNB of −2°, one would anticipate what angle class?
   (a) Class 3
   (b) Class 2
   (c) Class 1
   (d) Equal distribution of Class 1 and 3
3. A phase in staging and distraction osteogenesis is:
   (a) Mutagen
   (b) Telogen
   (c) Consolidation
   (d) Collagen crosslinking

19 Craniofacial Anomalies

Bibliography

Hunt, Jeremy A. FRACS, and Hobar, P. Craig MD. "Common Craniofacial Anomalies: Conditions of Craniofacial Atrophy/Hypoplasia and Neoplasia", *Plast. Reconstr. Surg.*, (2003); 111:**1497–1505 ONLY.**

Birgfeld C.B., Bartlett S.P., Ch. 26 "Craniofacial Microsomia", Neligan PC, Plastic Surgery, Elsevier 5th Edition, (2023), Volume 3: **pg. 859–886.**

Mathijssen I., "Treacher – Collins Syndrome", Neligan PC, Plastic Surgery, Elsevier 5th Edition, (2023), Volume 3: pg. **923–934.**

Veienti L, Soresina M, Menozzi A, "Parascapular free flap and fat grafts: Combined surgical methods in morphological restoration of hemifacial progressive atrophy", *Plast. Reconstr. Surg.*, (2005); 116(3):**699–709 ONLY.**

Buchanan EP, Xue AS, and Hollier LH, "Craniofacial syndromes", *Plast. Reconstr. Surg.*, (2014); 134(1):**128e, 146e–148e ONLY including videos.**

Latham K, Buchanan EP, Suver D, Gruss JS, "Neurofibromatosis of the head and neck: Classification and surgical management", *Plast. Reconstr. Surg.*, (2015); 135(3):**845–855 ONLY.** (See Figures 1 in the supplemental digital content).

Patel PK, Kawamoto H, "Ch. 26 Atypical Craniofacial Clefts", *Pediatric Plastic Surgery, Second Edition, Vol. 1*, (2017); **682–683 ONLY.**

Faculty Discussion and Study Guide

Fibrous Dysplasia, Romberg's Disease, Neurofibromatosis

1. Describe the two forms of fibrous dysplasia including the characteristics of each. (Fibrous dysplasia, a tumor seen in childhood, adolescence, and early adulthood, consists of two forms: monostotic, involving a single bone, and the polyostotic, which may be associated with premature sexual development, hyperthyroidism, and other findings of the Albright syndrome. Monostotic is much more common—4 times more frequent than polyostotic and 30 times more frequent than the Albright syndrome.)
   (a) What are the most common facial bones involved in the monostotic form? (The frontal, sphenoid, and maxilla. The word monostotic is liberally applied to craniofacial fibrous dysplasia because involvement may consist of more than one facial bone such as the sphenoid, frontal, and maxilla together.)
   (b) Outside of the head and neck where else can the monostotic form occur? (Ribs, lower extremity.)
   (c) Discuss the type of bone seen and potential for malignant conversion. (Woven bone is the typical pattern seen in fibrous dysplasia. Woven bone is an intermediate stage in bone healing in route to the deposition of lamellar bone. The potential for malignant conversion is quite low about 0.5–1% and characteristically is an osteosarcoma. Malignant conversion is more common in the polyostotic form).
2. What are some absolute and relative indications for surgical intervention in fibrous dysplasia? (The principal absolute indications center on optic nerve compression by progressive sphenoid bone involvement with fibrous dysplasia. Certainly, gradual worsening vision as well as an acute loss of vision, within 1 week, are absolute indications for excision-decompression. More relative indications have to do with progressive deformity of the maxilla, exophthalmos, patterns of malocclusion, frontal bone deformities, and prophylactic decompression of pediatric patients with imaging evidence of increased impingement of the nerve.)
   (a) Most likely area of impingement-compression? (The lesser sphenoid bone component of the optic canal posterior to and at the optic foramen.)
   (b) What is the likely mechanism of vision loss? (Venous compression, engorgement, arterial occlusion.)
3. In addition to the absolute and relative indications, what are the other precepts in surgery for fibrous dysplasia?

E. Luce, *A Curriculum for Plastic Surgery*, https://doi.org/10.1007/978-3-031-62087-4_19

(Total excision of fronto-orbital, upper maxilla, and zygomatic involvement if anatomically possible, but more conservative in the tooth-bearing and central cranial base areas. The mainstay is complete or near-complete resection with reconstruction with autogenous bone.)
   (a) What is the role of radiotherapy? (None. Possibly incites malignant transformations.)
4. Romberg's disease is also known as: (Progressive facial hemiatrophy).
   (a) Characteristics? (Onset in childhood, early childhood in the case of osseous involvement; almost always unilateral. The onset is usually localized and progresses within one or more dermatomes of the divisions of the trigeminal nerve.)
   (b) What is the coup de sabre and what is the significance of same? (The localized area of soft tissue atrophy usually in the lateral mid-facial area consistent with a saber cut scar. The coup de sabre represents linear scleroderma. The differentiating point from Romberg's is the age of onset, typically adolescence rather than childhood, limited to the forehead, and no bone involvement.)
5. What is the timing of intervention in Romberg's disease? (The progressive atrophy must stabilize for a minimum of a year as judged by periodic photographic assessment. The disease is self-limiting.)
6. What are some general precepts in the operative management of Romberg's disease? (The soft-tissue deficiency is optimally addressed with free tissue transfer rather than pedicled flaps, so skin replacement is rarely necessary. Flaps composed of dermis and fat tend to be stable and not undergo the degree of atrophy characteristic of muscle flaps. Optimally, the most consistent flap cited in the literature is the scapular or parascapular flap, deepithelialized for the bulk necessary. Certainly, deepithelialized microvascular skin flaps as the groin and the ALT are suitable alternatives. The one reading describes the use of combined scapular flap and fat grafting. Fat grafting of Romberg's disease is yet to be established as an alternate treatment method, but a growing enthusiasm has emerged recently for fat grafting in mild and moderate disease. In addition, fat grafting certainly would be an option for localized scleroderma.)
   (a) What are the positive attributes of the scapular flap for this condition? (Lengthy pedicle, ample soft tissue, no major donor site drawback.)
7. Discuss neurofibromatosis from the following aspects: inheritance, tissues involved, predisposition to malignant degeneration. (Neurofibromatosis Type I is autosomal dominant with involvement of skin, soft tissue, and bone and is known as Von Recklinghausen disease. The predisposition to premalignant degeneration is low, perhaps 10% lifetime risk. The malignancy is fibrosarcoma. Type 2 is much less common and manifests as bilateral acoustic neurofibromas.)
8. Describe the typical appearance for cranial-orbital neurofibromatosis. (As illustrated in the reading, massive deformity with excess skin and soft tissue, often a blind eye, and some element of pulsation. The pathologic anatomy is loss of the sphenoid bone with migration and herniation of the brain into the orbit. Facial involvement can affect all three branches of the trigeminal nerve.)
9. A general classification of neurofibromatosis of the head and neck would include: (Cranio-orbital, facial, parotid-auricular, neck.)
   (a) Outside of the head and neck? (Plexiform neurofibromas are multiple, soft tissue tumors that occur in one-fourth to one-third of the patients with neurofibromatosis and can be present without any head or neck involvement. The overlying skin can be thickened and hyperpigmented, cafe-au-lait spots.)
   (b) Quasimoto disease? (Severe form of neurofibromatosis with development of elephantiasis-type deformity of all soft tissue structures and bone.)

Craniofacial Microsomia, Treacher-Collins, and Other Syndromes

1. Contrast the embryologic origin of the inner ear with the middle ear and also the bones of the middle ear. (The inner ear is derived from the otic capsule, while the middle ear is derived from the first and second branchial arch. In particular, the incus and malleus are derived from the first branchial arch and the stapes from the second.)
   (a) What is the embryologic origin of the zygoma, maxilla, and mandible? (The cartilage of the first branchial arch, Meckel's cartilage, contributes to the zygoma, maxilla, and palate as the maxillary process and the mandible as the mandibular process. Further discussion of the embryologic origins of the external ear is in the ear module.)
2. What is Tessier's craniofacial classification? (Tessier outlined a classification system consisting of number 0–14 proceeding from the midline laterally and dividing the orbit into two hemispheres, upper craniofacial and lower maxillofacial. His system also divided soft tissue separate from that of the osseous clefts. See Fig. 19.1.)
3. Describe the typical facial appearance of a unilateral craniofacial microsomia. (In the fully-expressed syndrome, the ear is microtia or severely deformed, the mandible hypoplastic as described above, the maxilla and zygoma underdeveloped with an occlusal cant superior, posterior, and medial on the affected side as well as deviation of the chin to the affected side, a decreased

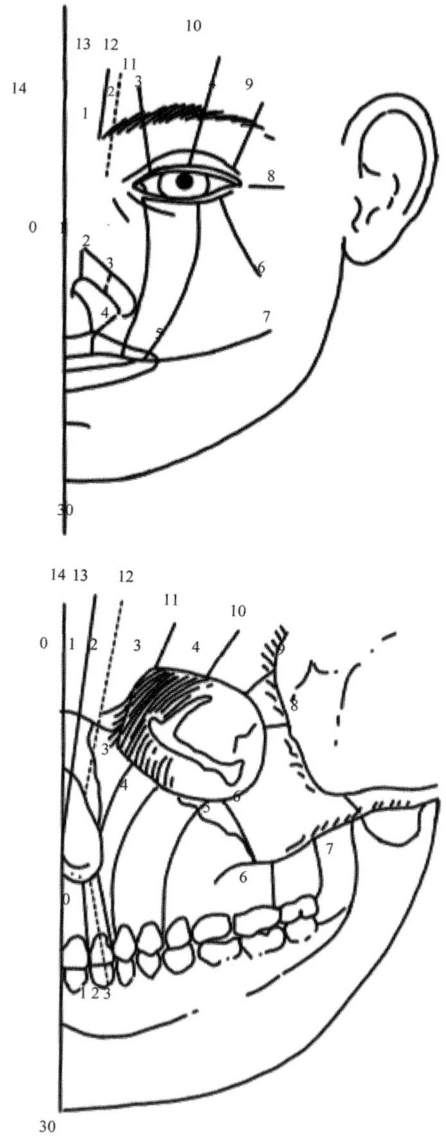

Fig. 19.1 Tessier's craniofacial classification

malar prominence, diminished facial expression and eye closure because of facial nerve absence or involvement, and quite possibly but much less common, involvement of the orbit with vertical dystopia and reduced dimensions.)

(a) What classification system addresses the overall deformity and what are the components? (OMENS)

(b) Briefly describe the OMENS system. (The OMENS system utilizes the affected orbit, mandible, ear, facial nerve, and soft tissue.)

OMENS:

O 1–3: size → position → both size and position

M 1–3:

1. small and short but normal shape

2a. glenoid fossa—temporomandibular joint (TMJ) hypoplastic but normal position

2b. TMJ inferior, medial, and anterior displaced

3. complete absence of TMJ, fossa, condyle, and vertical ramus

E 1–3: mild hypoplasia—cupping → no external auditory canal hypoplastic concha → microtia

N 1–3: temporal—zygomatic branches → lower branches → all

S 1–3: minimal deficiency → moderate → severe including muscles

4. Describe the continuum of mandibular deformity in craniofacial microsomia and the effect on the occlusal plane. Utilize a classification system in description. (The Pruzansky classification modified by Mulliken, describes a type I as all components are present and normal in shape but hypoplastic to some degree. In Type II A, the components are present and hypoplastic but also abnormal in shape, yet the fossa-condyle relationship is maintained and the temporomandibular joint (TMJ) is functional. In Type II B, the mandibular ramus is hypoplastic, markedly abnormal, abnormally located, and the relationship with the fossa is not maintained and the TMJ is not functional. The hypoplastic condyle is medial and anterior without any articulation with the temporal bone. Finally, in Type III, the mandibular ramus, condyle, and joint are absent. The occlusal plane is progressively canted further superior and posterior in this hierarchy of mandibular deformity. Of course, an associated hypoplasia and deficiency of the masseter and medial and lateral pterygoid muscles is present which accentuates the dysfunction in the mandibular opening.)
5. True or false: The degree of impairment of hearing function can be directly predicted by the magnitude of the external ear deformity. (False. The hearing loss and dysfunction can only be determined by audiometric and imaging evaluation.)
6. What is the controversy with respect to the timing of treatment of the skeletal deformity in hemifacial microsomia and outline recent developments that may bypass the controversy? (The essence of the question is whether the bony deformity, mandible, and maxilla as well as zygoma, worsen with facial growth or remain stable. Secondly, does intervention in childhood achieve an ultimately improved result over deferral of surgery until facial growth is complete?

   The development of distraction techniques has allowed for intervention in childhood but may not necessarily preclude facial skeleton reconstruction procedures subsequently.)

Editor's Note: Discussion of the clinical and physiologic particulars of distraction osteogenesis is in Chap. 6.

7. In addition to distraction osteogenesis, what two other more conventional methods are available to address the mandibular hypoplasia/deformity? (The traditional method, prior to the development of distraction osteogenesis, has been the use of rib or iliac bone. Cartilage can be harvested with the rib to simulate a condyle. Rigid skeletal fixation is necessary with intermaxillary fixation for 6–8 weeks. The microvascular technique is the use of the fibula-free flap. Of course, orthognathic surgery can be performed on the mature maxilla and/or mandible as well with or without autogenous bone grafts.)
8. Modalities available and timing for correction of the soft tissue deficiency? (Timing is probably optimal after the skeletal issues have been addressed. Like Romberg's, a microvascular free flap is the choice to augment deficient soft tissue of the cheek and preauricular areas, possibly complemented with autogenous fat grafting. Again, like Romberg's, a de-epithelialized parascapular flap has been the most frequent choice of donor tissue.)
9. Outline a series of interventions that may be necessary from neonate through adolescence. (Most likely intervention as a neonate or infant is addressed either acutely or subacutely for upper airway obstruction including sleep apnea. Early mandibular distraction can avoid the necessity for tracheostomy. Gastrostomy may be indicated.

   As discussed, in early childhood autogenous nonvascularized bone grafting of the hypoplastic mandible can be performed. A role, common to all the time phases of growth from infancy to adulthood, is that of distraction.

   Later in childhood, the involvement of orthodontics is crucial to encourage descent of the maxillary component of the occlusal plane on the involved side.

   In adolescence and adulthood distraction, orthognathic surgery, or a combination of those two may be most appropriate.)
10. What are the typical features of Treacher-Collins syndrome? (A bilateral congenital deformity that consists of an inferior obliquity and slant of the lateral canthus in combination with the colobomas of the lateral lower eyelids; hypoplasia of the zygoma and absence of the zygomatic arch; a high and narrow palate; hypoplasia of the mandible with Class II malocclusion with an anterior open bite; hypoplasia of the mandible including production of a vertical or oblique occlusal plane; microtia or other deformity of the external ear. The hallmark is the universal occurrence of bilaterality and the malar hypoplasia.)
    (a) What Tessier cleft? (6–8.)
    (b) What is the genetic pattern, if any? (Autosomal dominant.)
11. In the treatment of Treacher-Collins, outline the stages. (Intervention may be necessary as a newborn because of upper respiratory obstruction that may call for initiation of distraction and/or tracheostomy. The next phase is in early childhood, characteristically about 3 or 4 years of age, and consists of reconstruction of the zygomaticomaxillary area with autogenous bone grafts. The increase in the height of the ascending ramus and address of the anterior open bite is performed with mandibular distraction at age 5 or 6. Later in childhood, perhaps at age 7–10, the distraction of the previously bone-grafted zygomaticomaxillary complex can be performed. Additional procedures may be necessary such as orthognathic surgery once full facial growth is obtained as well as secondary soft tissue deficiency treated with autologous fat grafting.)

Editor's Note: Microtia is discussed in the Chap. 25.

12. Basically, describe the correction of the colobomas of the lower eyelid. (All three lamellae of the lid are affected. Reconstruction requires restoration of conjunctival lining together with tarsal support and correction of the vertical skin deficiency. The posterior lamella deficit can be corrected with free palatal mucoperiosteal grafts combined with advancement of the orbicularis and z-plasty and/or a Trippier laterally-based flap from the upper eyelid. In less severe cases a simple vertical wedge of the conjunctiva and tarsus may be appropriate.)
13. Describe the physical characteristics of the Binder syndrome. (Lateral view: short nose with lack of tip projection and a short columella in combination with midface recession including the radix of the nose and diminished dorsal projection. Basal view: short columella, horizontally oriented nostril, and flat nasal tip.)
14. Differentiate the following:
    (a) Unilateral craniofacial microsomia from Romberg's disease (Romberg's has an onset in childhood or adolescence, commonly involving the forehead.)
    (b) Bilateral craniofacial microsomia from Treacher-Collins (Treacher-Collins has involvement of the lower eyelid frequently with colobomas and has a very strong familial component.)
    (c) Goldenhar's syndrome (May be bilateral in one-third of the cases with epibulbar deformities of the lower eyelid and frequent vertebral anomalies.)
    (d) Nager's syndrome (Treacher-Collins plus upper lip and hand deformities, usually radial aplasia or hypoplasia.)
    (e) Mobius (Bilateral facial nerve and abducens, cranial nerve VI, palsies with a "mask facies".)

Case 1: Craniofacial Deformity

Case-Based Conference

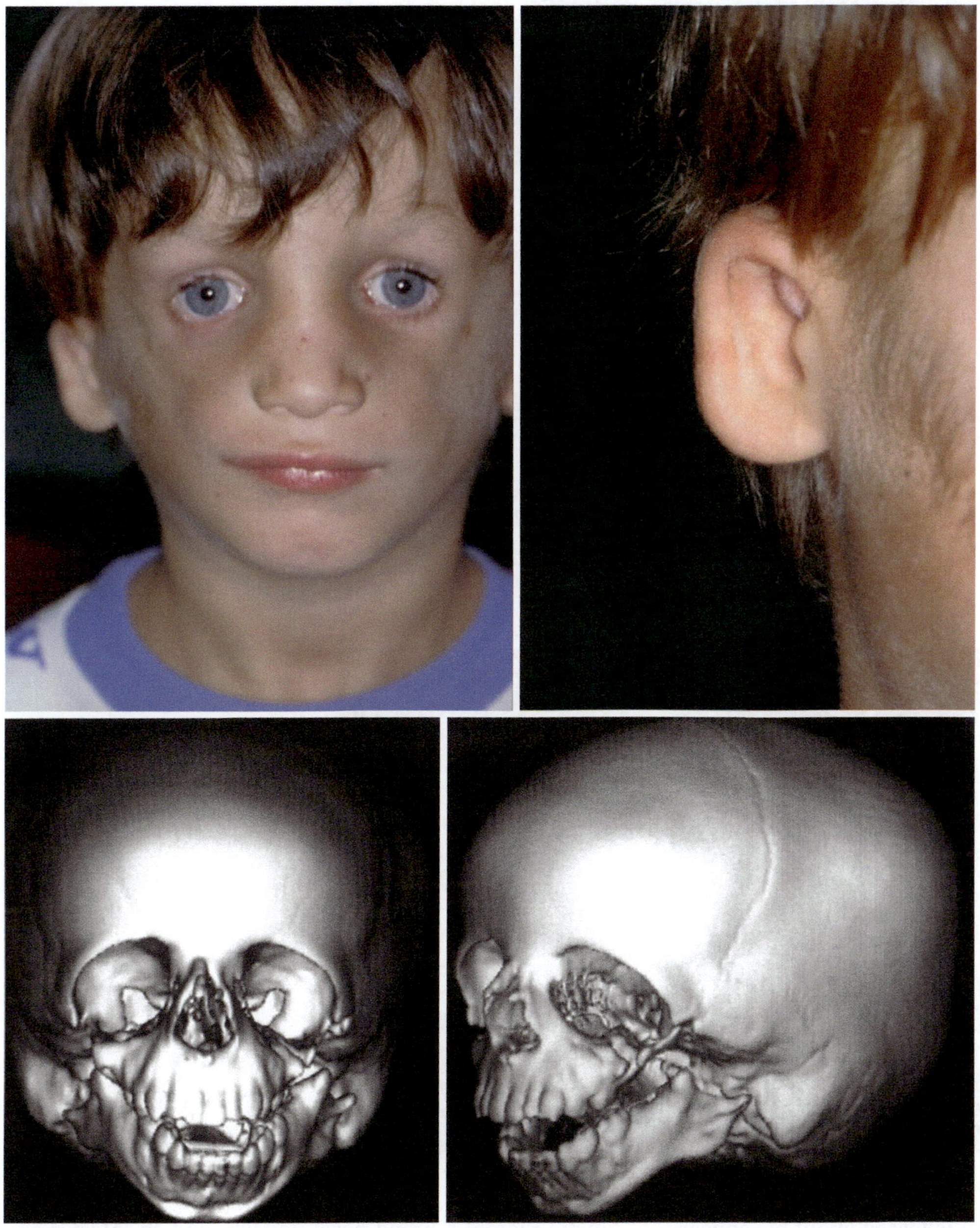

The patient is an 8-year-old who is teased about his appearance. Focus on the facial deformities rather than the ear.

1. Describe in detail what is seen on the slides (and the absence of what you do not see). Assign a name to this condition. Outline any additional information that you would desire on history and physical examination. Interpret the CT scan.
   (a) Outline any additional tests indicated. Justify.
2. Describe the pathologic anatomy of this condition.
3. Describe a treatment plan including a description of an overall list of procedures (if any) sequence and timeline. Then return to the first of your procedures and describe it in detail. Do the same for the remainder of the treatment plan.
4. A similar patient, a 6-month-old infant, presents with failure to thrive and episodes of "turning blue." What is the treatment indicated?

Case-Based Conference: Discussion

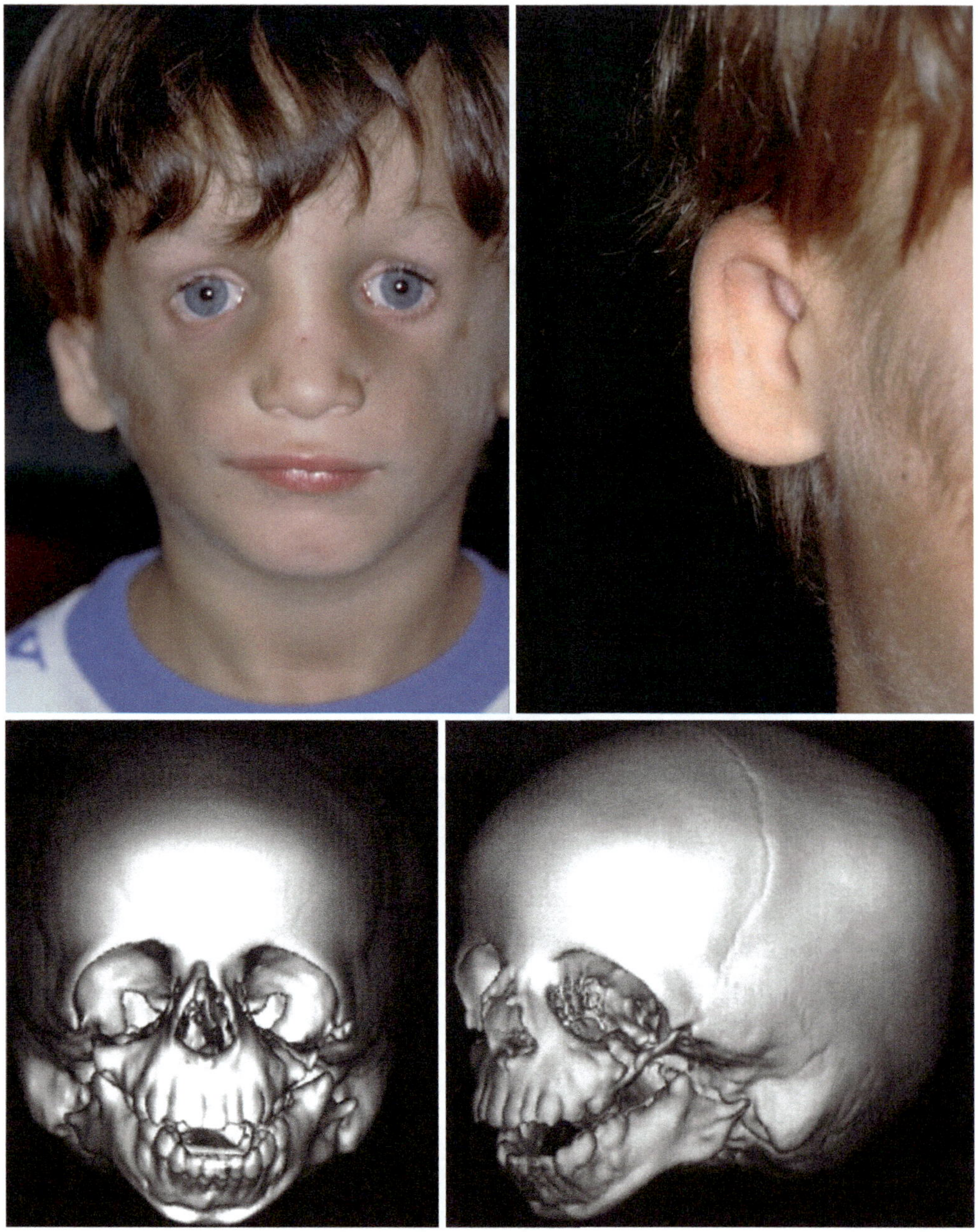

The patient is an 8-year-old who is teased about his appearance. Focus on the facial deformities rather than the ear.

1. Describe in detail what is seen on the slides (and absence of what you do not see). Assign a name to this condition. Outline any additional information that you would desire on history and physical examination. Interpret the CT scan. (A single frontal or anterior-posterior view of the patient of the head and neck area is provided. The patient has abundant hair and the contour and shape of the skull are not perceptible. The midface area is marked by several findings: the lack of prominence of the orbitozygomatic region, a broad nasal dorsum, and an inferior and lateral obliquity of the lateral lower lid, worse on the right than the left. The eyelids are further characterized by rudimentary eyelashes in the lower lids. No notching of either lid is seen. A mild vertical dystopia of the lateral canthus is suggested by a horizontal rather than a superior 2 mm relationship between medial and lateral canthi. No notching of the upper lid is evident and the mouth appears of normal configuration without macrostomia. Other findings not clearly evident on the frontal view is hair growth preauricular and extending inferiorly over the lateral cheek area. The inferior one-third suggests a defi-

ciency of vertical height of the mandible, yet measurements would indicate a related short height to the relationship of the subnasale to stomion as a one-third portion of the total height of the facial lower one-third. The right ear is not distinctly seen but appears reduced in vertical height and cupped in appearance. No other findings are evident.

The photographic depiction of the patient would have been enhanced by a lateral view. The lateral view would have illustrated the nature of the maxillo-mandibular relationship and particularly the presence, if any, of retrognathia. The lateral view will also characterize the degree of loss of facial convexity in the middle one-third. Properly staged, perhaps the skull contour and shape could have been visualized. Finally, the left ear is not seen on the frontal view. The photograph would appear to depict a patient with Treacher-Collins syndrome.

The history and physical would elicit information from the family regarding past treatment or surgery. Additional history of value including speech, hearing, or learning difficulties. Specific questions need to be directed toward the detection of obstructive sleep apnea and would consist of the standard queries regarding loud snoring, apneic episodes, and daytime sleepiness. A family history in light of the genetic pattern of Treacher-Collins syndrome would complete the history. The head and neck component of the physical exam includes the observations listed in the first segment of this question as well as an intraoral exam to determine occlusion and the status of the palate. An otoscopic exam will ascertain the presence of atresia or stenosis of the external auditory canal. A routine examination of the remainder of the body completes the clinical assessment.

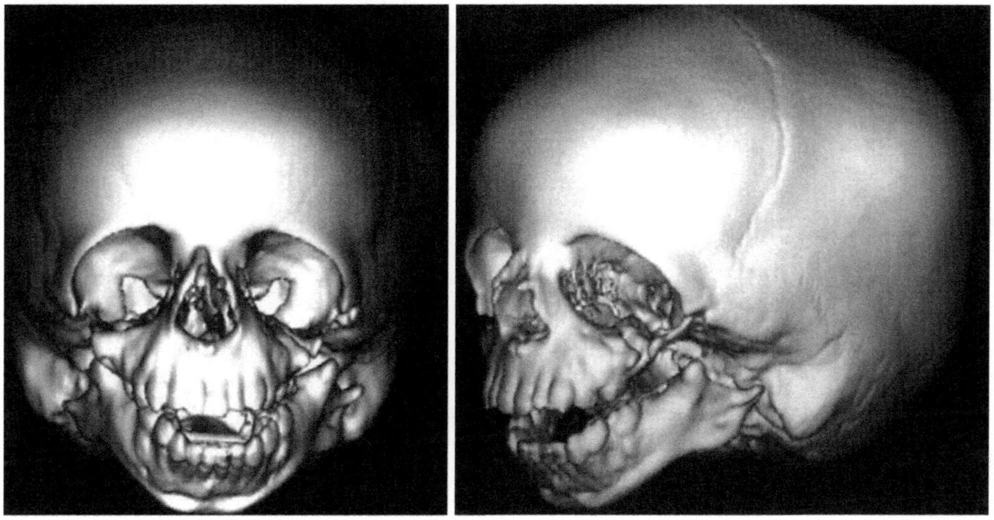

Two 3-D reconstruction CT scans are provided: an anterior-posterior and an oblique view. Several findings are evident: one, near absence of the zygoma with only a rudimentary arch, an absence of the inferior and lateral orbital wall; second, the inferior orbital rim appears depressed inferiorly and the maxilla short vertically and rotated cranially; third, the ascending ramus of the mandible is nearly absent beyond the angles; fourth, a significant open bite and probable Class II relationship is present; fifth, the mastoid is absent and an external auditory canal is not evident.)

(a) Outline any additional tests indicated. Justify. (The optimal care of the Treacher-Collins patient is multidisciplinary. Assessment of obstructive sleep apnea, if suspected, is a sleep study. Endoscopic evaluation of the upper airway may be indicated and an audiologic given the high incidence of auditory canal and middle ear involvement. An orthodontist will inevitably be employed in the management of the patient.)

2. Describe the pathologic anatomy of this condition. (The diagnosis is Treacher-Collins, an autosomal dominant genetically transmitted with a variable phenotype expressivity. Embryologically, structures affected bilaterally are derived from the first and second branchial arches, the mandibular, and the hyoid. The associated pathologic anatomy thus affected is the facial skeleton of the mandible, maxilla, and zygoma and the soft tissues of the eyelids, ear, and palate. The associated clinical findings are zygomatico-orbital hypoplasia with loss of malar prominence, absent lateral orbital floor and adjacent inferior lateral orbital wall, retrognathia, an open bite, micrognathia more severely affecting the ascending ramus and condyle, arched or cleft palate, colobomas of the eyelids and auricular malformations including microtia. The

developmental hypoplasia of the ear may also include the auditory canal and the middle ear.)

3. Describe a treatment plan including a description of an overall list of procedures (if any) sequence and timeline. Then return to the first of your procedures and describe it in detail. Do the same for the remainder of the treatment plan. (The management of the developmental anomalies is quite complex and the limitations of this discussion do not permit extensive detail. This patient's immediate needs are to address any significant hearing loss with bone conduction hearing aids, although that occurrence seems unlikely given the relatively mild degree of auricular deformity. At the patient's given age, the mandibular hypoplasia could be addressed with bi-directional distraction osteogenesis. If significant obstructive sleep apnea exists, hyoid advancement coincident with the initial performance of corticotomies could be considered. Cranio-harvested bone graft augmentation of the malar prominence combined with bone graft reconstruction of the orbit and supplemented with autologous fat grafting would be appropriate at this age. Address of the soft tissue deformities of the eyelid including colobomas are managed with a laterally-based upper eyelid, Trippier, flap combined with a lateral canthopexy. The type of ear reconstruction is dictated by the severity of the malformation, in this instance a single procedure. The timing of eyelid and ear reconstructive procedures is appropriate at this age and could coincide, procedure-wise, with operations directed toward the facial skeleton.

   At skeletal maturity, correction of residual maxillo-mandibular abnormalities will require orthognathic surgery, perhaps combined with autologous fat grafting. Rhinoplasty, if necessary, should be performed in late adolescence.)

4. A similar patient, a 6-month-old infant, presents with failure to thrive and episodes of "turning blue." What is the treatment indicated? (The patient presents with intermittent upper airway obstruction of not sufficient severity to mandate management as a neonate but nevertheless life-threatening at this stage, 6 months of life. A thorough evaluation is necessary including endoscopy of the upper airway. If the clinical picture is the result of severe micro- and retrognathia, the appropriate procedure is mandibular distraction.)

Case 2: Maxillary Tumor

Case-Based Conference

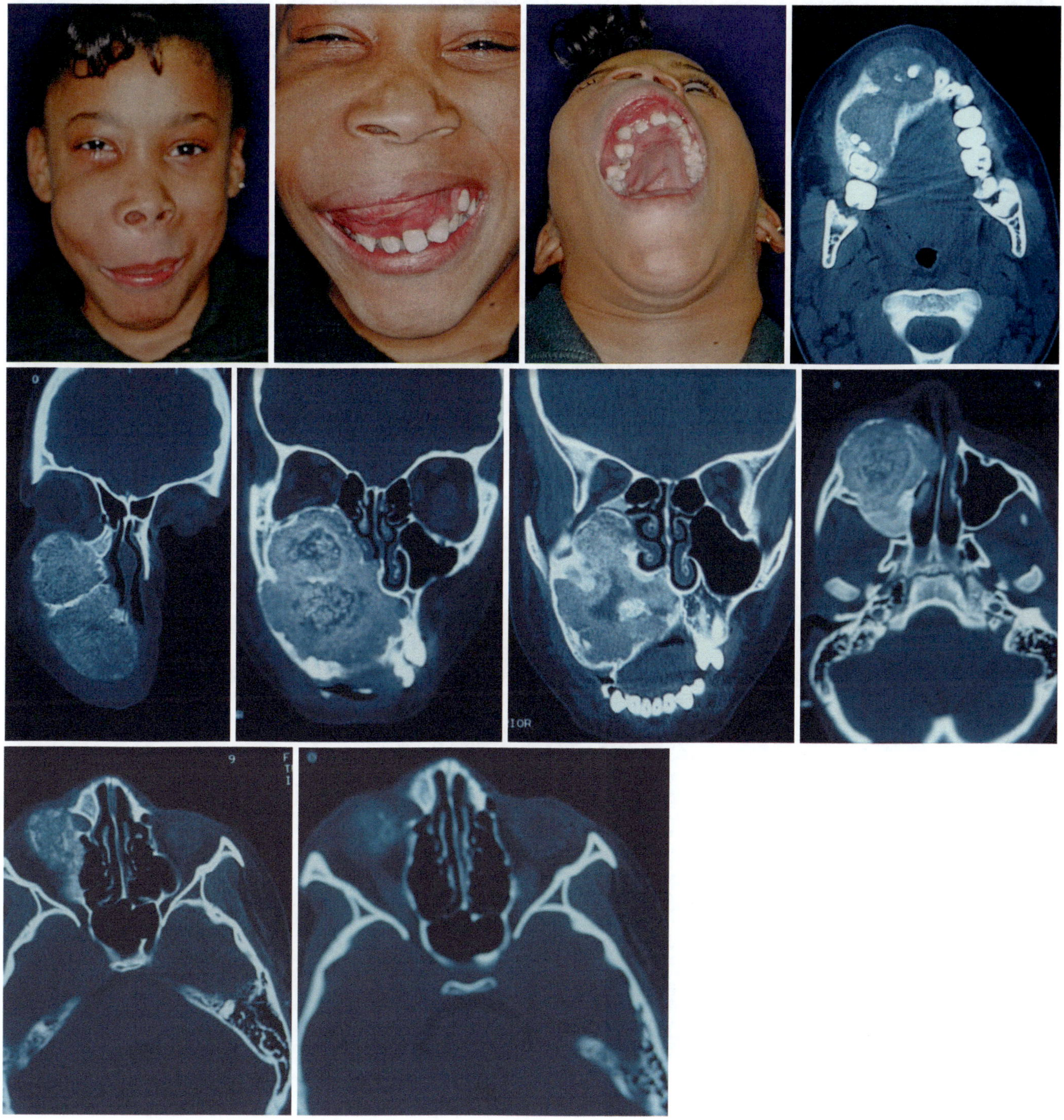

A 10-year-old with a history of progressive deformity over the past 18 months. The diagnosis is fibrous dysplasia.

1. Review the slide(s) and describe. Add a focused clinical exam.
   (a) Any tests in addition to the CT scan?
2. Then interpret the CT scan findings and outline the pathologic anatomy.
   (a) Any additional cuts in the CT necessary?
3. Describe the pathologic anatomy.
4. Outline a treatment plan including operative procedure(s), if any, begin with objectives.

Case-Based Conference: Discussion

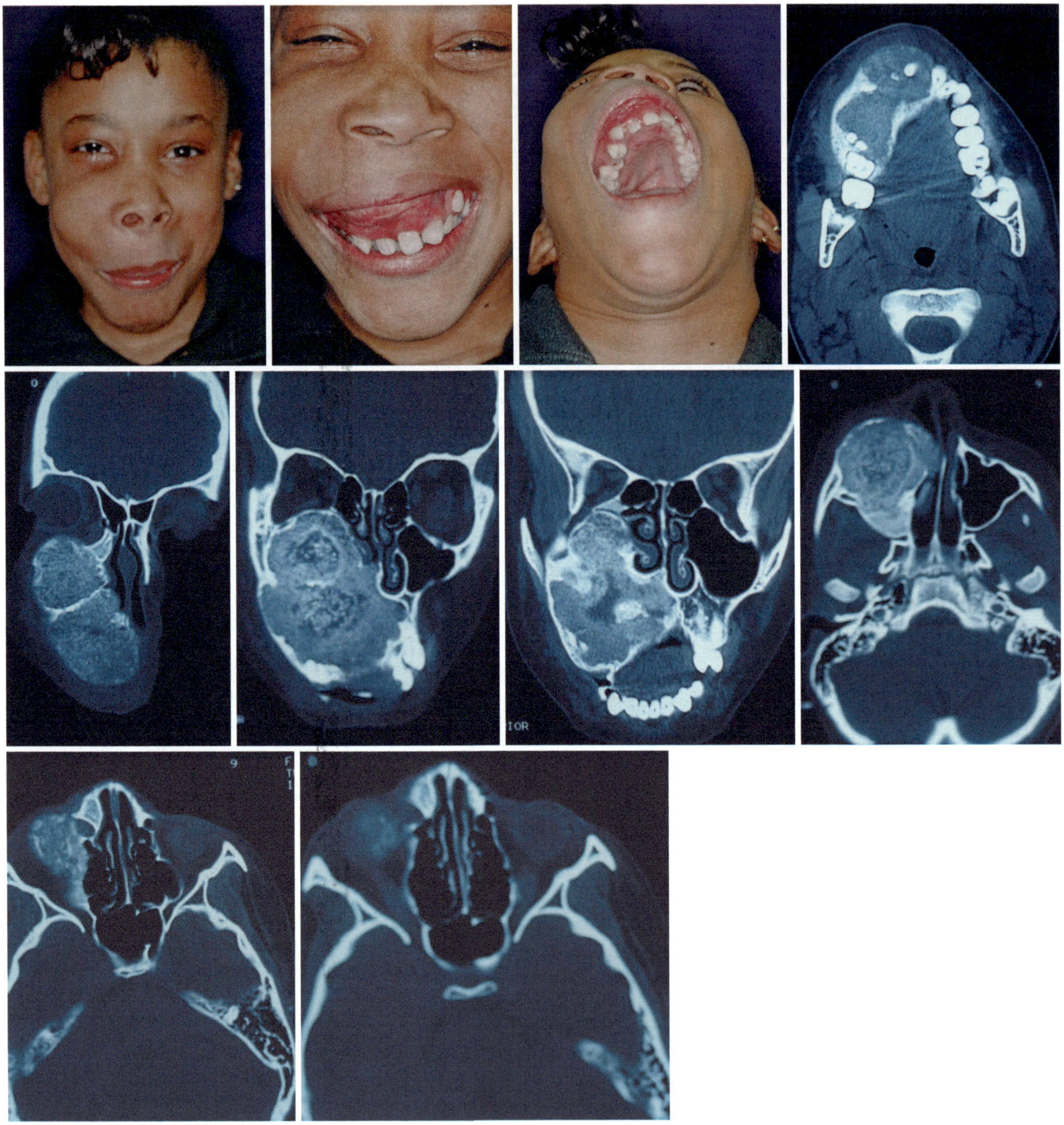

A10-year-old with a history of progressive deformity over the past 18 months. The diagnosis is fibrous dysplasia.

1. Describe the slide(s). (Young girl with swelling and deformity of the cheek with inferior and lateral displacement of the right alar base and upper lip. The right palpebral fissure appears narrowed and the orbit and/or globe appears elevated or vertical dystopia. The submental vertex or worm's eye view with the mouth open demonstrates bulging of the right hard palate and malalignment of the teeth with intact palatal mucosa. The deformity of the cheek is also evident. The close-up anterior-posterior view illustrates the inferior displacement of the entire right and the anterior portion of the left maxillary occlusal plane. The anterior and right alveolar ridge is distorted by a bulging fullness. Again, the alveolar mucosa is intact.)

   Add a focused clinical exam. (Further details should be elicited by the history re: status of the face 18 months ago, presence of facial pain, difficulty with vision in the right eye, epiphora, headaches, and/or medical problems. Does the patient have pigmented lesions on the body, bony swelling of the hips or ribs, or early menarche? The physical exam would focus on vision intact to confrontation, pupil reactivity, a nasal speculum exam for obstruction of the right nasal passageway, and stability of the maxillary teeth. Mobility of the overlying cheek skin is accessed. The trunk and extremities are examined for cafe-au-lait lesions or areas of bony prominence.)
2. Then interpret the CT scan findings and outline the pathologic anatomy.
   (a) Any additional cuts in the CT necessary? (Additional cuts would further define the findings as outlined in this question.)
3. Interpret the CT scan, suggest additional cuts and give a presumptive diagnosis. (The available axial views depict a large mass of the maxilla with a ground glass appearance with islands of radiodensity. On the two cuts available, the teeth on the left maxilla are visible but only the mass is apparent on the right on that particular cut. The other view demonstrates a mass of the floor of the right orbit and an enlarged right nasomaxillary bone. The three coronal views demonstrate a massive maxillary tumor mass but with intact cortices. The three coronal cuts are at the level of the anterior globe, the annulus of Zenn, and the most posterior orbit. The floor is intact on the latter two cuts but displaced superiorly by the large tumor mass that appears to extend to the posterior maxillary sinus wall. No evidence exists of sphenoid involvement including the lesser wing. The appearance is consistent with fibrous dysplasia.)
4. Describe the pathologic anatomy. (The pathologic anatomy is involved in the 4, possibly 5, walls of the maxillary sinus. Clinically and CT scan-wise, the patient has the involvement of the anterior and antero-lateral wall, the floor or bony palate and adjacent alveolar ridge, the medial wall or lateral wall of the nasal cavity and the roof or floor of the orbit.)
5. Outline a treatment plan including operative procedure(s), if any. Begin with objectives. (The objectives in this scenario is reconstruction after subtotal excision of fibrous dysplasia of the maxilla and adjacent zygoma, necessitating a subtotal maxillectomy. The reconstruction would provide bony support for the orbital contents, restoration of bony support of soft tissue to restore facial height and width and reconstitution of the bony palate and alveolar ridge to provide the foundation for prosthesis or integrated dental implants. The indications for intervention are those of a progressive deformity with involvement of alveolar ridge and palatine bone as well as an obvious worsening aesthetic appearance. A subtotal excision should be the essence of the operative plan which would consist of a Weber-Ferguson incision combined with a palatal mucoperiosteal flap for the maxillary and alveolar ridge resection with preservation of soft tissue and mucosa. The excision of maxilla will extend to and include infraorbital rim and the inferior medial wall as well as the anterolateral maxillary walls, nasal process of the maxilla, and the anterior orbital floor. Reconstruction can be accomplished with vascularized free tissue transfer or nonvascularized bone or combined as a free fibula with the appropriate osteotomies with additional nonvascularized autogenous bone. The infraorbital rim and orbital floor can be totally reconstructed with nonvascularized autogenous bone followed later after bone integration with dental implants.

   The components of the reconstruction would consist of: a, orbital floor and medial wall; b, the inferior orbital rim and adjacent zygoma; c, the maxilla including the palatine bone; d, the alveolar process with the ultimate need for dental implants.

   The controversial element in fibrous dysplasia is that of optic nerve compression and blindness. The controversy is the necessity or not to perform decompression of the optic nerve within the optic canal due to progressive encasement by fibrous dysplasia involvement of the lesser wing of the sphenoid. The other contrasting element of the argument is deferment of operative intervention when and if visual compromise is evident since operative decompression requires an anterior craniotomy. A decision about operative intervention cannot be undertaken lightly. Unfortunately, the loss of vision can be unpredictable and patient compliance with periodic and frequent follow-up is not always possible. This patient has no evidence of involvement of the lateral orbital wall or orbital apex. The lesser and greater wing of the sphenoid appear normal on the CT cuts available.

The choices of vascularized bone are several: fibula, iliac, scapular, radial forearm. Radial forearm does not supply sufficient bone stock for osseointegrated implants and the soft tissue reconstructive needs in this case are not great. The lateral osteocutaneous scapular flap could provide sufficient bone and can be harvested with the parascapular cutaneous component but again the soft tissue requirements are minimal and flap harvest requires a change in operative position twice. The scapular flap does offer the advantage of a separate segment of bone medially that could be utilized for the orbit. Probably on balance the scapular flap is not the ideal choice. The iliac is ideal for combining alveolar and maxillary bone as a single segment and if a small amount of soft tissue was desired, a small portion of the inferior oblique muscle included. The iliac provides the most bone stock of any of these four choices. The principal disadvantage is the more complex harvest and potentially a short pedicle. The fibula, the workhorse of vascularized osseous reconstruction, offers several advantages: excellent bone stock, the capability of separate bony segments to address both the orbit and the alveolar ridge-bony palate. Another option with the fibula, necessary with the use with the iliac bone, is utilization of nonvascularized bone to reconstruct the infraorbital rim and orbital floor.)

Intraoperative

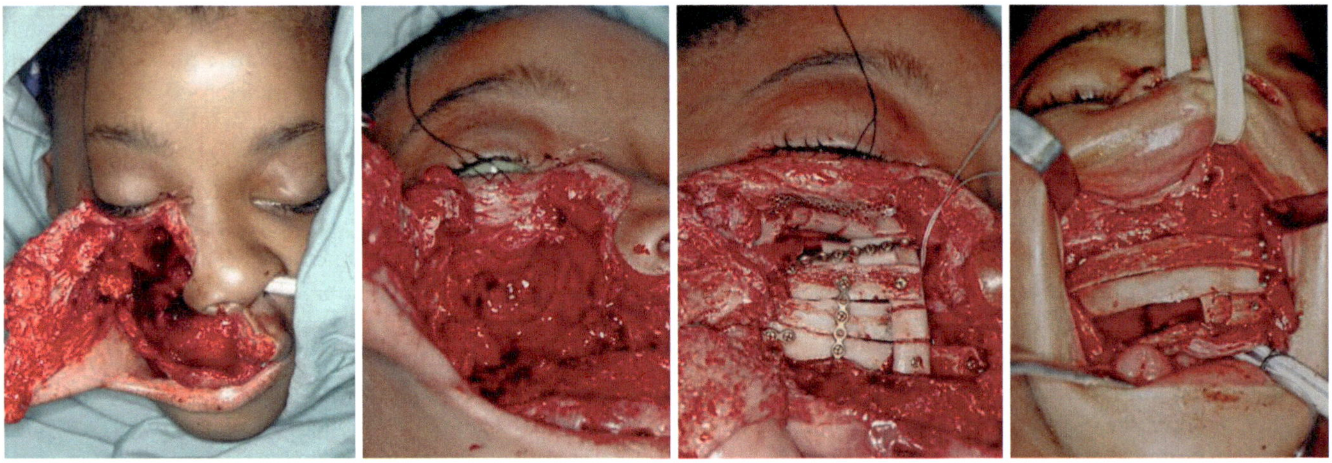

The first four slides demonstrate a Weber-Ferguson incision, the specimen, and autogenous split-rib grafts and titanium mesh to orbital floor, rim, and suprapalatal maxilla. The last slide, 1 year later illustrates resection of the alveolar ridge and palate with preservation of the palatal mucosa. Access was via a facial degloving and reconstruction with additional split-rib grafts.

Postoperative (18 Months)

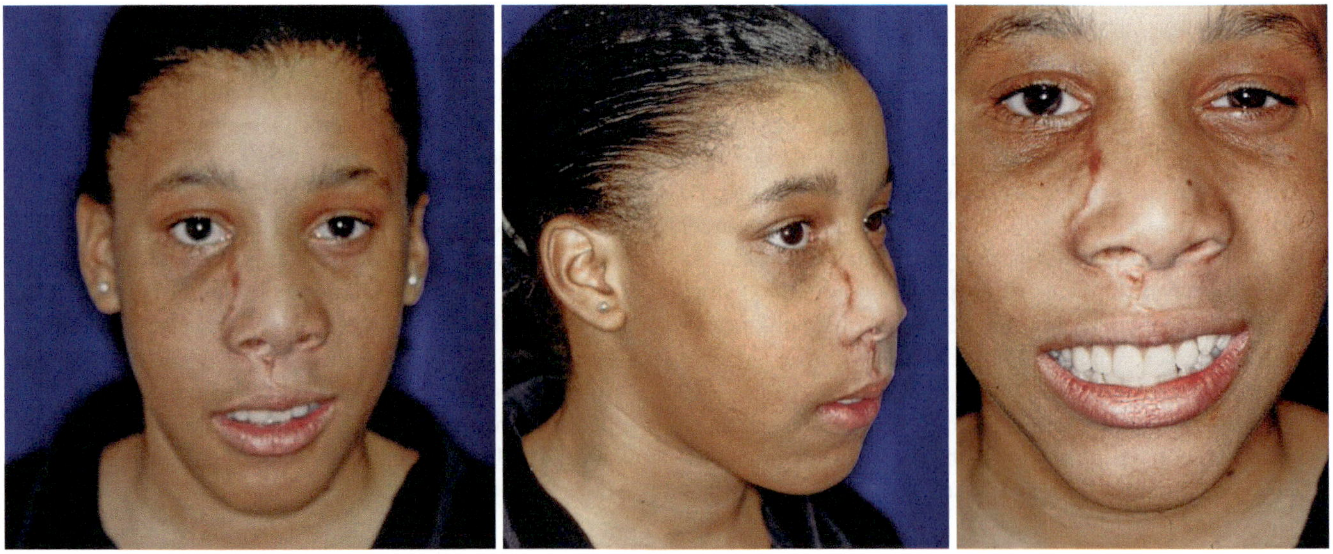

Some residual fullness of the right cheek remains. Dental rehabilitation has been accomplished with implants with a good aesthetic result. The Weber-Ferguson incision scar is visible. Postoperative CT imaging is not provided. No residual visual compromise is evident in the right eye.

Critique

A follow-up ophthalmic assessment and CT scan is mandatory to detect residual tumor, if any, and to determine the degree of incorporation of bone grafts. The ophthalmic assessment is to ensure no ongoing compromise of visual function is present.

A considerable amount of nonvascularized bone grafts have been harvested. An alternate approach could be vascularized fibula with osteotomies to reconstruct both the alveolar deficit and a separate bone island of fibula for the inferior maxilla. The orbital floor and rim could be reconstructed, as was performed in this case, with non vascularized bone and titanium mesh.

Case 3: Craniofacial Deformity

Case-Based Conference

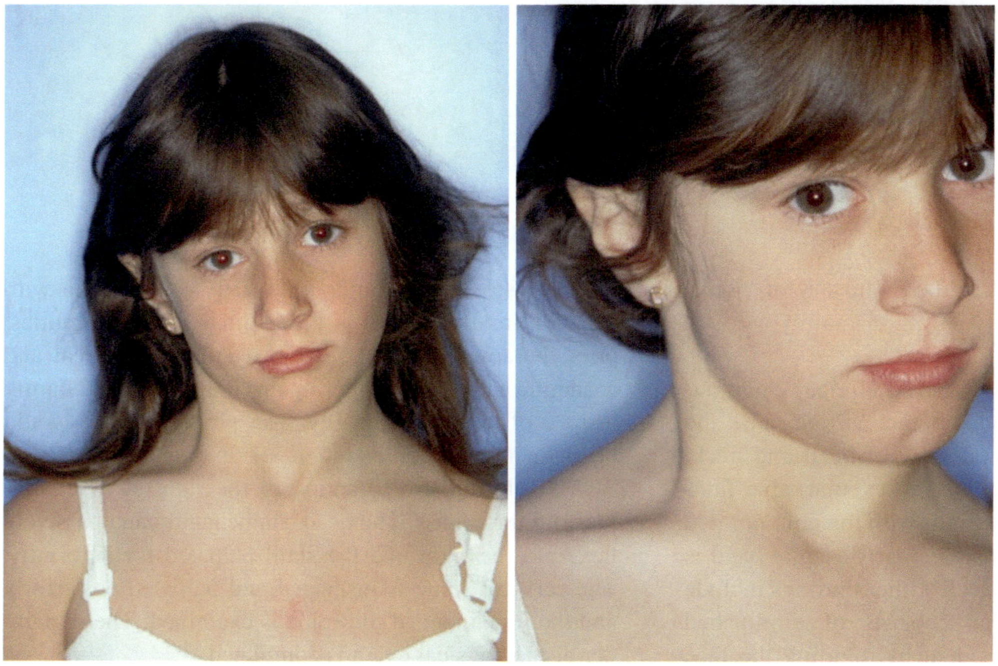

A 14-year-old whose parents described a history of "looks funny."

1. Describe the slide(s). Add a focused clinical examination.
   (a) Are any tests indicated? Justify.
2. What is the pathogenesis and pathologic anatomy of the patient's findings? Give a differential diagnosis.
3. Outline a treatment plan and give a prognosis or probability of success. What would have been your management if seen as an infant?

Case-Based Conference: Discussion

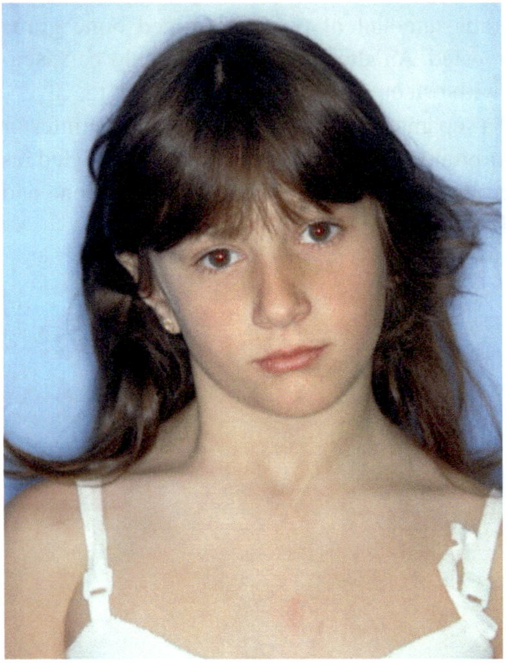

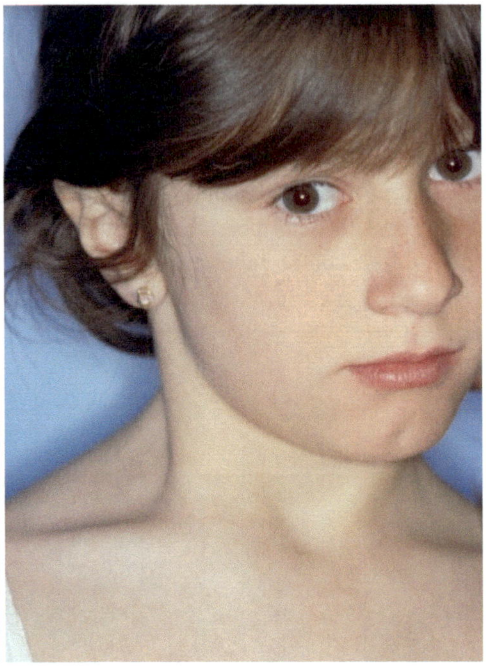

A 14-year-old whose parents described a history of "looks funny."

1. Describe the slide(s). Add a focused clinical examination. (The two photos provided depict a young girl, the first of which is a full frontal view of head and neck, shoulders, and upper chest. The most remarkable finding is the head is tilted to the right with the chin pointed to the opposite or left side and a clearly visible band is present in the right anterior neck. Other findings include some facial asymmetry that consists of diminished facial width on the right, evident by dividing the face into vertical fifths. The other elements of facial asymmetry include a greater vertical height of the left lateral face compared to the right and a slight decrease in the width of the right palpebral aperture. No other deformities or findings are evident. The contour of the posterior shoulder created by the trapezius appears normal. The eyes are symmetrical and in central gaze. The patient has a full head of hair and the contour of the skull cannot be ascertained. The second view consisting of a partial right oblique but with the patient looking toward the camera, adds little. The right eye is in full lateral gaze, accompanied symmetrically by the left. The right anterior cervical band is evident and apparently extends from the mastoid to the clavicle. No skin changes are evident. An additional finding is a deep and pronounced concha of the right ear.

   The history is essential. Questions would begin with age and first perception of the findings, birth difficulties, prior therapy, treatment for hip dysplasia, physical and academic activity, vision problems diagnosed, and family history of similar deformity. The physical exam would begin with a demonstration of extraocular motions, EOMs followed by palpation of the right sternocleidomastoid for a mass. The head can be gently and passively flexed to the right and the skull palpated for deformity. The cervical spine is inspected and palpated posteriorly and the remainder of the spine is examined. The remainder of the physical exam is completed.)

   (a) Are any tests indicated? Justify. (A CT scan can depict any associated skull abnormalities as well as determine the skeletal components of the facial findings. Plain films of the pelvis should detect any hip dysplasia. Cervical spine films are indicated to determine a primary or secondary alteration in the cervical vertebrae. An ophthalmic exam is mandatory to detect any ocular findings as well as estimate any dysfunction with correction of head posture. The full frontal photo should be utilized to calculate the cant angle of the head. The angle is calculated by a vertical plumb line of the photo, not the face, and a transverse line drawn between both pupils when used in conjunction with torticollis secondary to cervicothoracic scoliosis, is termed the Cobb angle. The angle may be of some prognostic value of surgical release.)

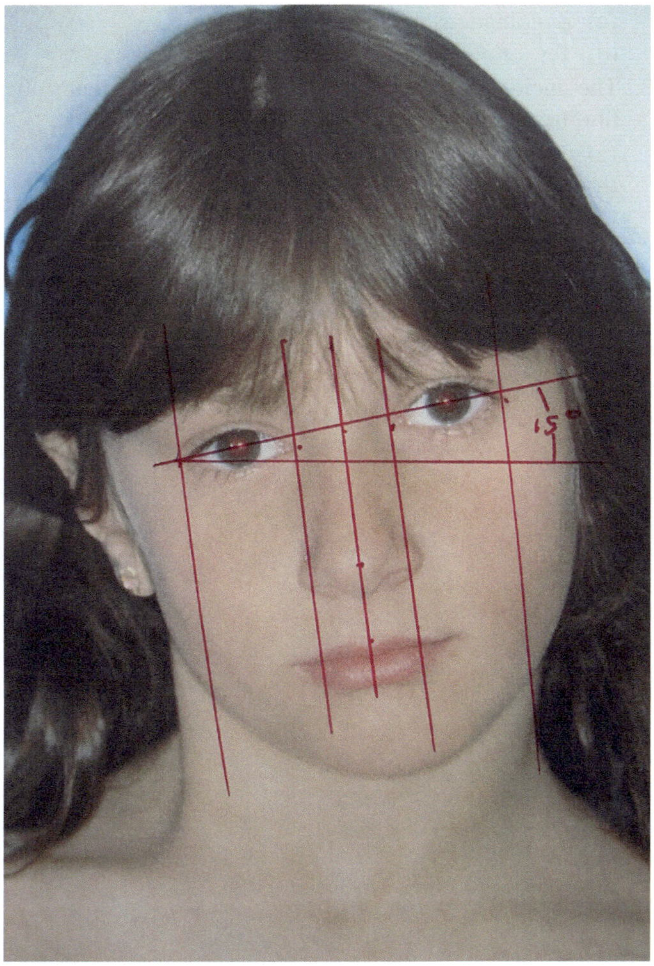

2. What is the pathogenesis and pathologic anatomy of the patient's findings? Give a differential diagnosis. (The pathogenesis of torticollis, assuming onset at birth and not recently, is not well-defined. A disproportionate number of patients report a history of difficult delivery so birth trauma has been implicated as well as uterine malposition and oligohydramnios. Cervical spine abnormalities, particularly of C1 and C2 such as hemiatlas may be causative. Although rare, ocular torticollis is the primary etiology and head posture and ipsilateral cervical contracture secondary. Ocular torticollis is marked by the absence of the lateral rectus and superior oblique on the affected side.

   The pathologic anatomy is fibrosis of the sternocleidomastoid. Additional pathology, inflicted by the long-term effect of shortening of the ipsilateral neck and hip posture, may consist of ipsilateral plagiocephaly, shortening or contracture of the scalene and trapezius muscles, recession of the ipsilateral zygoma as well as reduction of the height of the mandibular ramus. The angle of inclination in this patient is approx. 15°. Because the development of the cerebral visual cortex under the influence of the head posture since infancy has determined the "normal" plane of binocular visual axis to be in this instance 15°, reversion to the true horizontal may create significant vision disturbances.

   The differential diagnosis of congenital muscular torticollis, the presumptive diagnosis in this case, includes Klippel-Feil syndrome or other cervical spine abnormalities and, as mentioned above, a primary ocular causation.)
3. Outline a treatment plan and give a prognosis or probability of success. What would have been your management if seen as an infant? (Treatment should begin with physical therapy and passive head positioning in an effort to address and stretch the sternocleidomastoid. Unfortunately, the outcomes of conservative treatment of physical therapy and passive head positioning beyond infancy or early childhood is not rewarding. Injections of Botulinum toxin may have some efficacy but evidence is scant and fragmentary. Operative intervention should be given careful consideration of both pro and con. If accomplished, although an endoscopic approach has been described, consists of either a uni- or bipolar release of the sternocleidomastoid, the difference determined by a single or double release of the two heads of the muscle, sternal and clavicular. If a single release is elected, a low transverse incision 1–2 cm superior to the clavicle will provide both access and a satisfactory scar. Bipolar release adds an additional transverse superior cervical incision. To preserve integrity of the principal motor innervation, cranial nerve XI, attention should be directed toward the course of the spinal accessory nerve. The branch to the sternocleidomastoid enters the deep surface about 4 cm inferior to the mastoid. Although injury to the sternocleidomastoid branch is probably not of major consequence in a patient with a dysfunctional muscle, injury to the main trunk of the nerve would produce a major complication, paralysis of the trapezius, the result of a significant shoulder disability.

   Postoperatively, the patient should be splinted in the corrected head and neck posture. The duration of the necessity for sprinting is unknown. As suggested earlier, correction of head posture may induce vision difficulties including diplopia and loss of biocular vision that may require prismatic correction with glasses.)

In-Service Examination

1. Findings in Treacher-Collins syndrome include the following **EXCEPT:**
   (a) Tessier cleft IV
   (b) Class III occlusal relationship
   (c) Hypoplastic TMJ
   (d) Acute gonial angle
2. Derivation of the second branchial arch include:
   (a) Incus
   (b) Stylohyoid muscle
   (c) Zygomaticus major
   (d) Tensor veli palatini
3. The incidence of malignant conversion in monostotic fibrous dysplasia is:
   (a) 0.5–1%
   (b) 5–10%
   (c) 25%
   (d) 5%

Congenital Anomalies of the Head and Neck: Craniosynostosis

20

Bibliography

Persing JA, "Management Considerations in the Treatment of Craniosynostosis", *Plast. Reconstr. Surg.*, (2008); 121(4):**1–10 (Overview).**

Xue AS, Buchanan EP, and Hollier LH "Update in Management of Craniosynostosis", *Plast. Reconstr. Surg.*, (2022);149:**1209e–1221e.**

Humphries L.S., Swanson J.W., Bartlett S.P., Taylor J.A., "Craniosynostosis: Posterior Cranial Vault Remodeling", *Clin. Plast. Surg.*, (2021); 48:**455–61 ONLY.**

Forrest CR and Hopper RA, "Craniofacial syndromes and surgery", *Plast. Reconstr. Surg.*, (2013); 131(1):**86e Videos 1, 2 ONLY.**

Buchanan EP, Xue AS, and Hollier LH, "Craniofacial syndromes", *Plast. Reconstr. Surg.*, (2014); 134(1):**128e Videos 1, 2 ONLY.**

Sawh-Martinez R, Steinbacher DM, "Syndromic Craniosynostosis", *Clin. Plast. Surg.*, (2019); 46:**141–151.**

Losee M.D., J. E. and Mason M.D., A. C., "Deformational plagiocephaly: diagnosis, prevention, and treatment", *Clin. Plast. Surg.*, (2005); 32(1):**53–59, Figure 9 ONLY.**

Fearon J.A., Griner D., Ch. 25 "Hypertelorism", Principles and Practice of Pediatric Plastic Surgery Second Edition, Quality Medical Publishing (2017), Bentz M.L., Bauer B.S., Zuker R.M., (2017), **pgs. 649–659.**

Mundinger GS, Rehim SA, Johnson III O, et al., "Distraction Osteogenesis for Surgical Treatment of Craniosynostosis: A Systematic Review" *Plast. Reconstr. Surg.*, (2016);138:**657, 664–67 ONLY.**

Faculty Discussion and Study Guide

Overview of Craniosynostosis

1. As an overview, what is the principal difference or differences between syndromic and nonsyndromic synostoses? (The term synostosis references the premature fusion of cranial sutures and the resultant inhibition of perpendicular bone formation. The syndromic patients have multiple suture involvement of the coronal ring that includes the cranial base and also have a genetic, autosomal dominant, component. Nonsyndromic patients usually have but an isolated suture involved and the occurrence genetically is sporadic.)
2. In the epidemiology of craniosynostosis, what is the ratio of occurrence of syndromic versus nonsyndromic synostosis? (Most, 80%, are nonsyndromic.)
3. Rank in terms of frequency of occurrence the following: sagittal, unilateral coronal, unilateral metopic, bilateral lambdoid. (Sagittal is about 50%, unilateral coronal is about 10%, and the remaining are about 5% each.)
   (a) Gender proportion? (Sagittal is substantially more common in males, 4:1.)
4. What are the genetics of the two most common syndromic craniosynostosis, Aperts and Crouzons? (Autosomal dominant related to fibroblast growth factor receptors, FGFR.)
   (a) Saethre-Chotzen? (TWIST gene.)
5. Briefly discuss the theories about the interplay between fetal-neonatal dura and calvarial suture lines. (Briefly, the dura must play a role in premature fusion of calvarial suture lines. Experimentally, transplantation of normal dura from a normal to a craniosynostosis rabbit model will maintain the patency of synostotic suture lines, once opened.)
6. Discuss generally the pathological anatomy in synostosis. (Premature fusion of the cranial suture lines and restriction in growth in the transverse axis to the direction of the particular suture line. Compensatory overgrowth in the long axis of the particular suture line occurs.)
   (a) Define the specific suture line or lines involved:
      - Scaphocephaly (Sagittal)
      - Trigonocephaly (Metopic)
      - Plagiocephaly (Anterior unilateral coronal)
      - Plagiocephaly (Posterior unilateral lambdoid)

E. Luce, *A Curriculum for Plastic Surgery*, https://doi.org/10.1007/978-3-031-62087-4_20

- Brachycephaly (Bilateral coronal)
- Brachycephaly, turricephaly (Bilateral coronal)
- Kleeblattschädel (Pan)

7. Contrast or not the incidence of developmental delay in nonsyndromic vs. syndromic synostosis. (Incidence of developmental delay is quite high in syndromic synostosis and substantially less so in nonsyndromic synostosis particularly in more mild forms.)
8. What are the functional problems, cause of same, and frequency in synostosis? (The incidence of blindness and/or significant neurodevelopmental/intellectual delay is about 50% in multiple suture line fusion, 14% in single suture line fusion. The underlying cause is increased intracranial pressure.)
   (a) The correct statement of the following describes the occurrence of increased cranial pressure, ICP, in single suture synostosis or nonsyndromic synostoses: rare, occasional, frequent, nearly universal. (Probably occasional, 10–15%.)
   (b) True or false: In the absence of increased intracranial pressure neurocognitive developmental delay does not occur. (If the yardstick is as gross as neurocognitive developmental delay, the answer could be true, however, more complex cerebral dysfunction can certainly occur in the absence of increased intracranial pressure.)
9. What findings might indicate ICP? (Papilledema, tense fontanelle, changes in skull X-ray.)
10. What are the salient points in the history of an infant with craniosynostosis? (Failure to thrive, failure to achieve developmental milestones, obtundation, family history.)
11. What are the potential ocular problems in craniofacial dysostosis syndromes? (Shallow orbits with exophthalmos, corneal exposure, and vision loss.)
12. In summary, what is the preoperative assessment? (Multidisciplinary. Ophthalmology and neurosurgery consults for examination, probable CT scan. Of course, pediatrics and genetics will be involved as well. The patients are optimally managed with a craniofacial team.)
13. What is the justification for surgery in infancy? (To prevent the development of associated facial deformities, increased intracranial pressure, and calvarial deformities. Optimally performed at less than a year of age when the cranial bone is more malleable, to advantage the more rapid brain growth in the first year, and the ability of the calvarium to fill defects with new bone in the first year of life. Ordinarily, surgery for correction of synostosis is performed between the ages of 3–6 months, particularly to prevent the development of facial deformity in the more severe forms. On the other side of the risk-benefit equation is a major operation and blood loss in an infant.)
    (a) Give some specific milestones. (By age 18 months, 75% of skull growth has occurred and the ability to ossify cranial defects is markedly diminished after the age of 18 months.)
14. In general terms, what is the frequency of hydrocephalus in craniosynostosis? (Uncommon in nonsyndromic.)

Syndromic Craniosynostosis (Table 20.1)

1. A 6-year-old is seen in the craniofacial clinic with exorbitism, hypertelorism, maxillary hypoplasia, a class III relationship, and a relative mandibular prognathism. The academic performance is above average. What is the probable diagnosis? (Crouzon's) Genetic pattern? (Autosomal dominant, with a high penetrance.) Skull findings? Suture involvement? (Bilateral coronal with a resultant brachycephaly or turribrachycephaly, although a variety of calvarial deformities may be present.)
   (a) Differentiate from Apert's. (Apert's is frequently delayed in mental development and with hand findings such as syndactyly as well as frequent cleft palate.)
   (b) Why does exorbitism occur in both of these conditions? (Shallow orbits secondary to premature fusion of cranial base and sphenoid suture lines. As a result, proptosis and exposure to keratitis are significant risks.)
2. What constitutes Pfeiffer syndrome? (Similar facial features and hand findings as Apert's except the craniofacial deformity is usually not as severe and Pfeiffer's patients have broad thumbs and large toes and usually have normal intellectual development. Cardiac anomalies are more likely in Pfeiffer's syndrome.)

Table 20.1 Surgical algorithm options for syndromic craniosynostosis

Under 3 months	Strip craniectomy if evidence of elevated ICP, multisuture synostosis
6–8 months	Posterior vault distraction as first stage
10–13 months	Definitive cranial vault correction/fronto-orbital advancement
5–9 years	Le Fort III, Le Fort I distraction osteogenesis (early mixed dentition, aimed at correcting exorbitism, midface hypoplasia)
9–12 years	Le Fort III/monobloc advancement 1 stage (late mixed dentition)
15–20 years	Orthognathic surgery to set occlusion, facial balance

Sawh-Martinez R, Steinbacher DM, "Syndromic Craniosynostosis", *Clin. Plastic Surg.*, (2019); 46:146. (Reprinted with permission)

3. Carpenter syndrome is also a craniofacial dysostosis. What are the specific features? (Coronal synostosis, hypertelorism, epicanthal folds, flat nose, brachysyndactyly.)
4. What are the complications of syndromic synostosis that may dictate the timing of operative intervention? (Essentially three: increased intracranial pressure, corneal exposure secondary to the exorbitism, and to a lesser degree associated respiratory problems of airway obstruction with significant sleep apnea. The specific point is, compared to nonsyndromic or involvement of an isolated suture, syndromic craniosynostosis is substantially more likely to have an increase in intracranial pressure.)
5. Discuss the procedures generally including timing, and extent performed in Crouzon's and Apert's. (Craniectomy in infancy, subcranial midface advancement at age four, although posterior vault distraction osteogenesis will probably replace these traditional procedures. The necessity for craniotomy does arise in early infancy in some patients. Airway problems may dictate tracheostomy and increased intracranial pressure may mandate early intervention with cranial vault operative procedures. In general, multiple suture involvement is much more likely to require earlier intervention than single suture. Early intervention for multiple suture involvement addresses the impact of increase in intracranial pressure and may minimize craniofacial dysmorphism.)
   (a) What is the increased urgency and necessity to advance the midface at an earlier age? (Persistent respiratory problems, such as obstructive sleep apnea, and severe exorbitism with ocular complications.)
6. What are the variations on types of midface advancement? (A subcranial LeFort III with orbital bipartition or monobloc advancement. Monobloc advancement refers to an osteotomy across the cranial base in combination with craniotomy. A LeFort I osteotomy may be necessary after completion of facial growth with or without a concomitant mandibular osteotomy, an operation usually performed in the late teens. The evolution of distraction osteogenesis may be the "standard" method of management of these patients.)
7. What is the role and timing of posterior vault distraction? (The procedure of posterior vault distraction, initiated at age 3–6 months, offers expansion of the cranial vault in an address of the intracranial pressure and modification of the cranial and/or facial dysmorphology.)
   (a) What are the advantages compared to frontal cranial procedures? (Shorter operative time and a favorable morbidity profile.)
8. Does the performance of posterior vault distraction osteogenesis in infancy obviate the necessity for additional craniofacial procedures? (No. A variety of operations including monobloc, fronto-orbital advancement, midface advancement, and others may and probably will be required at some point later in childhood. Particulars will vary from patient to patient.)
9. Distraction osteogenesis has some inherent disadvantages. List. (Distraction osteogenesis requires a second operation for removal of the apparatus and has a prolonged treatment period. Distraction of the cranial vault is in a single vector so craniofacial deformities can only be addressed in one direction. Very young patients have thin bone. In older patients, the bone is less pliable. Pin track infections and scarring can occur.)

Editor's Note: A comprehensive discussion of the surgical approach to the different varieties of craniosynostosis, isolated or syndromic, is beyond the scope of this guide. The role of suturectomy, even performed endoscopically, followed by postoperative helmet remodeling has been principally limited to isolated involvement of the sagittal suture. Posterior vault distraction can be initiated early, at 4–6 months, followed by a second stage definitive cranial vault remodeling from 12 to 15 months. The use of spring-mediated cranioplasty, similar in concept to distraction osteogenesis, has been successful in a number of centers. Notable exceptions to this sequence are infants with severe respiratory problems, obstructive sleep apnea, or exposure keratitis, all of which mandate early operative intervention aimed toward the frontal-orbital-facial area.

Isolated Craniosynostosis (Fig. 20.1)

1. Sagittal synostosis is the most common, 50%. Give the physical exam findings. (Increase in the AP index of the skull, bifrontal bossing and occipital protrusion.)
   (a) Treatment. Discuss strip craniectomy vs. more aggressive or definitive correction. (Strip craniectomy is an older procedure and often results in incomplete correction of the associated secondary calvarial deformities. As a result, craniofacial surgeons have become more aggressive in definitive address of the frontal bossing and occipital protrusion.)
2. What are physical findings in brachycephaly and the causation? (Bitemporal widening, decrease in the anterior-posterior distance, recession of the frontal-orbital bar. Exorbitism may exist. Definitive correction requires address of the deformities of the frontoparietal bones as well as advancement of the frontal-orbital bar. The etiology is bilateral synostosis of the coronal suture.)

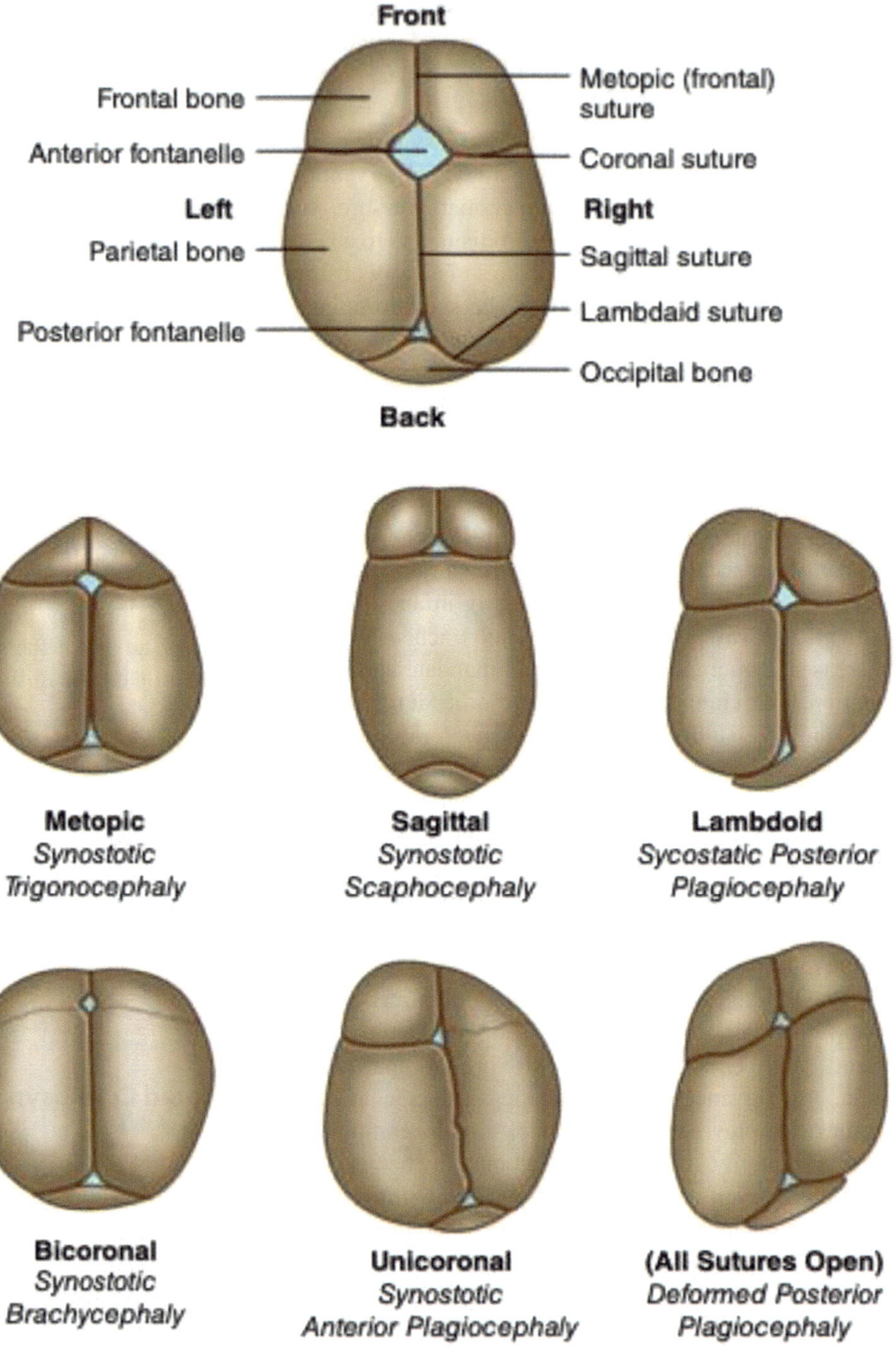

Fig. 20.1 Types of craniosynostosis

3. Describe the physical findings, including the orbit, in metopic synostosis. (Trigonocephaly is characterized by reduction in the transverse growth of the frontal bones, which results in narrowing of the anterior cranial fossa and a decrease in the interorbital distance. The distance between the lacrimal crests is diminished as well as the inter canthal distance, yet, the interpupillary distance remains the same so true hypotelorism does not exist.)
   (a) Discuss the necessity for surgical intervention. (The mildest forms may not require any cosmetic correction and in some mild deformities can be treated with burring of the midline V-shaped frontal bone deformity. More significant involvement and deformity will require craniectomy and reorientation of the frontal bone as well as release at the lateral skull base.)
4. Give the physical and X-ray findings in unilateral coronal synostosis or frontal plagiocephaly. (A recessed forehead and fronto-orbital rim on the ipsilateral side and contralateral bossing of the forehead and fronto-orbital rim. The

ipsilateral or involved side, the eyebrow is raised and perhaps the palpebral fissure is increased with vertical dystopia. The X-ray or CT findings are dubbed the "harlequin" sign. On physical examination both the nose and chin will be deviated to the contralateral side.)

(a) What explains the increased vertical height of the ipsilateral orbit? (Restricted growth of the greater wing of the sphenoid.)

(b) Briefly, describe the goals of operative correction. (The supraorbital bar on the involved side will need to be advanced. The flattening of the involved side and bossing of the contralateral side will need address, and the height of the ipsilateral orbit may need to be reduced by excision of bone at the frontozygomatic and nasomaxillary suture lines.)

5. Give the physical and X-ray findings in occipital plagiocephaly. (Fusion of the lambdoid suture line will result in flattening of the involved occipital skull with contralateral bossing as the result of deviation of the posterior cranial base to the involved side. The ear and external auditory canal are pulled posterior toward the involved suture line. The principal differential diagnosis is deformational plagiocephaly; see below.)

Deformational Plagiocephaly

1. Give a classification of plagiocephaly. (Synostotic or nonsynostotic, namely deformational and synostotic, anterior versus posterior or coronal vs. lambdoid.)
   (a) The frequency of posterior synostotic or lambdoid plagiocephaly is rare, occasional, or frequent. (Quite rare).
2. What is the underlying cause and demographics of deformational plagiocephaly? (Interestingly, the frequency of deformational posterior plagiocephaly increased substantially with the public campaign of pediatricians to keep infants in a supine rather than prone position. The cause, presumably, is prolonged pressure on one side of the skull as the baby lies with the head turned in a "comfort" position.)
3. Differentiate "true" lambdoid synostosis and deformational plagiocephaly in the following:
   (a) Timing and frequency. (True plagiocephaly is more likely to be seen at birth and deformational later in infancy.)
   (b) Orientation of the skull base. (The posterior skull base is transverse in deformational synostosis and slanted upward to the side of the synostosis in true posterior or lambdoid synostosis.)
   (c) Shape of skull. (Parallelogram in deformation plagiocephaly, more square in craniosynostosis.)
   (d) Location of compensatory overgrowth. (True: ipsilateral mastoid, and the opposite occipital and parietal. Deformational: no mastoid increase but the opposite occipital and ipsilateral frontal are increased.)
   (e) Facial changes. (True—none. Deformational—prominence of the ipsilateral orbit/cheek. In deformational plagiocephaly the ear mastoid region is displaced anteriorly as opposed to true lambdoid synostosis in which the ear and mastoid are displaced *posteriorly*.

   In summary, in deformative plagiocephaly in addition to unilateral occipital flattening has the ear and mastoid displaced anteriorly without an increase in bulging of the mastoid. Viewed from posteriorly, the skull resembles a parallelogram. The ipsilateral orbit, cheek, and forehead may be displaced anteriorly.)
4. Outline an algorithm for treatment based on age and severity. (Of course, synostotic or true plagiocephaly will require surgery. Deformational plagiocephaly of less than 3 months of age is unlikely to require any intervention; three to 6 months of age and if only moderate, simply repositioning the baby to look for improvement; moderate to severe or failure of positioning may require orthotic cranioplasty with a helmet. Those babies who present 6–18 months and have moderate or severe deformational plagiocephaly would require an orthotic cranioplasty. Finally, those babies who present greater than 24 months with severe deformity will require surgery, although this late presentation is distinctly uncommon.)

Orbital Deformities

1. Comprehension of orbital deformities includes the ability to differentiate a variety of conditions. Define the following:
   (a) Dystopia? (Malposition of the globe within the bony orbit)
   (b) Telecanthus? (Lateral displacement of the medial canthus)
   (c) Hypertelorism? (Lateral displacement of the bony orbit)
   (d) Epiphora? (An overflow of tears from the eyelid)
2. Differentiate the intercanthal distance (ICD) from the interorbital distance (IOD). How is that distance pertinent in traumatic, for example, nasoethmoid orbital fractures and deformities? (The IOD is actually a radiologic measurement from the medial wall of one orbit to the medial wall of another. The ICD is an external measurement from medial canthus to medial canthus. The latter, ICD, is increased in traumatic deformities but IOD is normal. In congenital deformities such as hypertelorism, both the IOD and ICD are increased. The normal ICD is 30–32 mm,

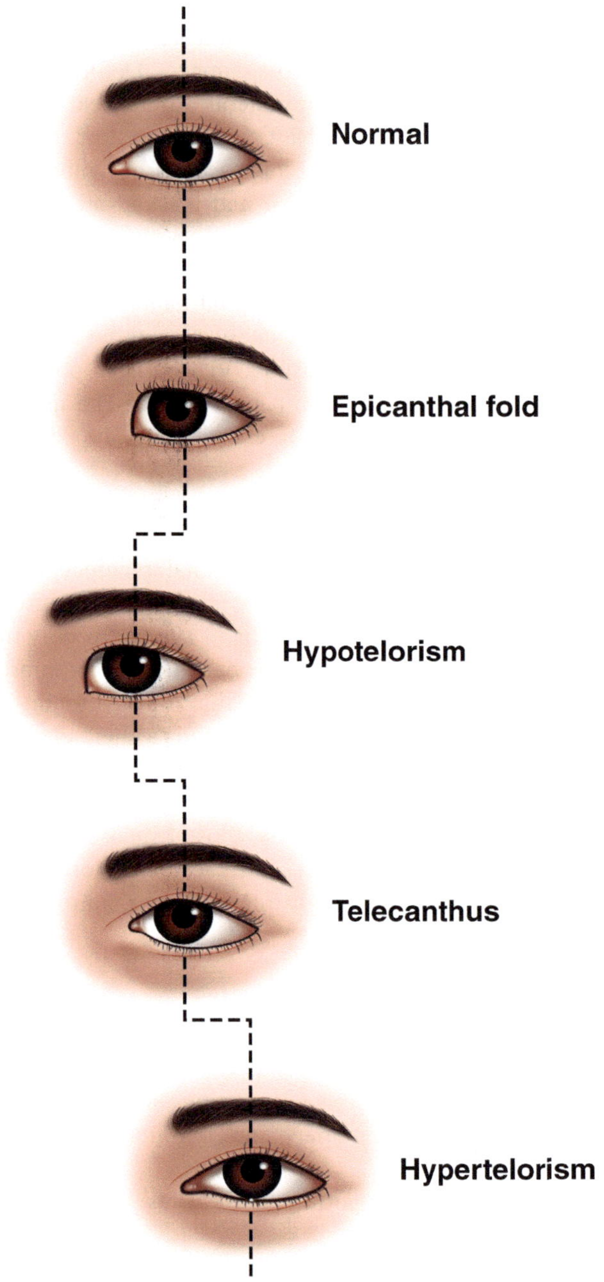

Fig. 20.2 Depiction of Deformation of Orbital Soft Tissue or Bone

although some gender and racial differences exist.) (Fig. 20.2)

3. Given that the descriptive term hypertelorism may be associated with a number of conditions and varies in severity, what are the general operative approaches? (In general, either some combination of orbital wall osteotomies or facial bipartition.)
4. What is the relationship of the nose and midface to the perception of hypertelorism? (A flattened nasal dorsum and midface hypoplasia accentuate the appearance of hypertelorism. Correction improves the overall perception and is an essential component of the treatment of hypertelorism.)
5. Differentiate four wall osteotomy from facial bipartition. (Four wall osteotomy, as the name implies, is medial movement of the orbits by a roof, lateral, and medial wall osteotomies as well as a transverse osteotomy across the superior maxilla bilaterally. Facial bipartition substitutes a pterygomaxillary disjunction for the transverse maxillary osteotomy.)

In-Service Examination

1. The genetic factor responsible for Aperts and Cruzon's syndrome is:
   (a) TWIST
   (b) TGIF-alpha
   (c) TGIF-beta
   (d) FGFR
2. The skull deformity in bilateral coronal synostosis is termed:
   (a) Brachycephaly
   (b) Plagiocephaly
   (c) Scaphocephaly
   (d) Trigonocephaly
3. The occurrence of increased intracranial pressure in non-syndromic craniosynostosis is:
   (a) Rare 1–2%
   (b) Occasional 10–15%
   (c) Frequent 40–50%
   (d) Nearly universal
4. An infant of 2 years old has hypertelorism, maxillary hypoplasia, Class III occlusal relationship, and broad large toes and thumbs. The most likely syndromic diagnosis is:
   (a) Crouzon
   (b) Apert
   (c) Pfeiffer
   (d) Saetr-Chotzen

21 Cysts, Sinuses

Bibliography

Li W, Reinisch JF, "Cysts, Pits, and Tumors", *Plast. Reconstr. Surg.*, (2009); 124(1S):**106e–111e.**

Moses MA, Green BC, Cugno BC, et al., "The Management of Midline Frontonasal Dermoids: A Review of 55 Cases at a Tertiary Referral Center and a Protocol for Treatment", *Plast. Reconstr. Surg.*, (2015); 135(1):**187–196 ONLY.**

Rohrich RJ, Lowe JB, Schwartz MR, "The role of Open Rhinoplasty in the Management of Nasal Dermoid Cysts", *Plast. Reconstr. Surg.*, (1999); 104(7): **2163–70.**

Rada E.M., Dorafshar A.H., Chapter 37 "Pediatric Head and Neck Masses" in Principles and Practice of Pediatric Pediatric Plastic Surgery Second Edition, Bentz M.L., Bauer B.S., Zucker R.M., (2017), CRC Press, **pgs. 1121–1129 ONLY.**

Prosser JD, Myer CM, "Branchial Cleft Anomalies and Thymic Cysts", *Otolaryngol. Clin. N. Am.*, (2015); 48:**1–9 ONLY.**

Faculty Discussion and Study Guide

Frontonasal Cyst

1. What is the pertinent anatomy relevant to the management of frontonasal cysts and masses? (Essentially, the three-dimensional anatomy of the skin-soft tissue of the glabella, the paired nasal bones, the articulation of the anterior portion of the ethmoid plate with the deep or posterior surface of the nasal bones, and more cranial and posterior is the anterior crista galli, foramen cecum, a bony aperture at the most anterior portion of the crista galli, and dura.)
2. What is the differential diagnosis of cysts and/or masses of the nasal area in an infant or young child? (Epidermal inclusion cysts, dermoids, gliomas, meningocele, meningoencephalocoele; teratoma in a neonate.)
   (a) Differentiate pathologically between epidermal inclusion cysts and dermoids. (Epidermal inclusion cysts as the name implies consist of epidermis and do not contain the adnexal structures. Dermoids originate in the dermis and contain hair follicles and sebaceous glands. In the absence of prior trauma, the occurrence of epidermal inclusion cysts in a young child would be distinctly uncommon, although dermoids of the glabella are uncommon as well. The presence of a punctum with discharge of "cheesy" material can occur with both. The presence of hairs would indicate a dermoid.)
3. What is a glioma? (Glioma as the name implies are ectopic nests of glial tissue. See below.)
4. What is the embryologic explanation for the occurrence of dermoids, gliomas, meningocele, and meningoencephalocele in this area? (In the embryo during nasal development, the dura extends as a diverticulum, transiently, into and superficial to the cartilaginous mass that will become nasal bones and septum. The space is the prenasal space and becomes obliterated with the retraction of the dura. The residual structure is the foramen cecum in the midline just anterior to the anterior limit of the crista galli. A dermoid may result from retention of ectodermal remnants in the obliterative process. Similarly, gliomas, meningoceles, and meningoencephaloceles result from a failure of the obliteration of the diverticulum and space. See Fig. 21.1.)
5. How might clinical examination differentiate a dermoid from a meningo- or meningoencephalocele? (The history or presentation of a draining sinus tract suggests dermoid. Since the latter two entities presumably have an intracranial connection, the mass should become more tense with Valsalva such as crying. The performance of the Furstenberg maneuver, namely observation during bilateral occlusion of the jugular veins, is not recommended. Given the possibility of a small but therapeutically important communication, a false negative

E. Luce, *A Curriculum for Plastic Surgery*, https://doi.org/10.1007/978-3-031-62087-4_21

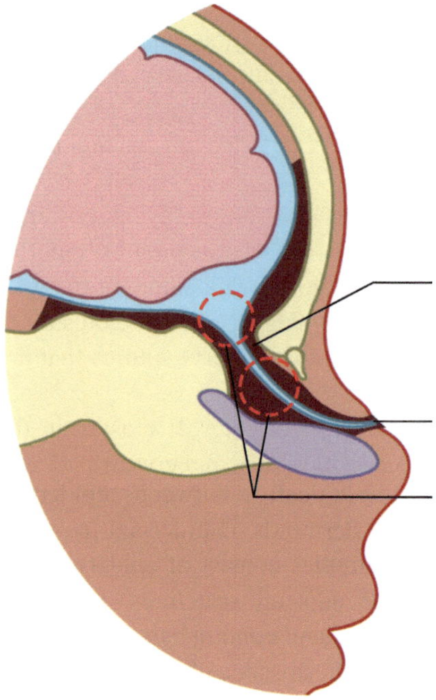

Fig. 21.1 Dermoid cyst

finding is misleading and the pressure placed on the anterior cervical region could also occlude the carotid.)

6. Outline the appropriate workup beyond clinical examination of a frontonasal cyst and/or mass. (The key question is the necessity for imaging, and in particular the fact that CT scan alone may not demonstrate the soft tissue relationships and a subsequent MRI may be necessary. Regardless, in a young child, general anesthesia may be required, not an inconsequential decision. If the mass is apparently with a high degree of certitude to be subcutaneous in location, imaging may not be obtained. Yet, in the vast majority of cases, particularly in the young child, imaging should be performed.)
7. Describe the operative management of a nasal dermoid. (Assuming the imaging does not suggest an intracranial extension, excision can be accomplished with a vertical midline glabellar incision, incorporating any sinuses. Smaller lesions, particularly located more inferior on the nasal dorsum, could be excised with an open rhinoplasty approach, particularly in young patients, <5 years of age, who by nature have a short nose. Endoscopic removal via a scalp approach has been described.)
8. Describe the operative management of meningocele and meningoencephocele. (Gliomas are usually a diagnosis established on the pathological examination of the specimen. Intraoperatively, careful dissection of the mass posterior and superior should ascertain the presence or not of a stalk that continues intracranially. The diagnosis of a meningo- or meningoencephalocele will most universally require a frontal craniotomy and possibly, depending on the magnitude of the defect, reconstruction.)
9. Although the emphasis is on the management of frontonasal cysts and masses, what is the *most common* location of a dermoid in the head and neck? (Lateral brow—over 50%.)
   (a) How to manage? (Direct excision. An endoscopic approach through a scalp incision is an alternative.)
10. One entity, rare, is a frontonasal teratoma. What are the important characteristics? (A teratoma of the frontonasal may be well—or poorly—differentiated, and the latter has elevated serum beta-human chorionic gonadotrophins. Teratomas have a high potential for malignant conversion, particularly those that are poorly differentiated or immature, and nearly always diagnosed in a neonate. Prompt resection is recommended.)

Cervical Cysts and Sinuses

1. Outline briefly the embryology of a thyroglossal duct cyst. (A ventral diverticulum forms from the pharyngeal pouch at the base of the tongue and migrates inferiorly to form the hyoid and the pyramidal lobe of the thyroid. Obliteration or failure of the same permits the encompassed cells to continue to secrete. The normal obliterative process leaves a proximal remnant, the foramen cecum.)
2. The clinical presentation of a thyroglossal duct cyst and or sinus? (A midline anterior cervical cyst, possibly mobile with swallowing or with protrusion of the tongue, smooth and nontender. Since the cyst communicates and possibly is contaminated by oral flora, such can result in infection in a third of the cases and even rupture with drainage. Physical examination should ascertain the presence of a thyroid gland discrete from the cysts.)
3. Besides clinical examination, is further workup indicated? (Barring worrisome findings on exam, the most relevant determination is the presence of a normal thyroid. Doubt would dictate the performance of a nuclear thyroid scan and TSH levels. An ultrasound can confirm the presence of a cystic rather than a solid structure. Management of ectopic thyroid and/or thyroid carcinoma is beyond the discussion of this submodule.)
4. Briefly describe the management of a thyroglossal duct cyst. (If actively infected, prior to excision, control with antibiotics is indicated. Excision is performed through a transverse cervical incision, circumferential mobilization of the cyst, and dissection superiorly, perhaps aided by cannulation of the tract with a nasolacrimal duct probe. Since the tract may be anterior within the body or posterior to the hyoid, a small segment of central hyoid bone is excised with the tract and specimen, termed the Sistrunk procedure. Further dissection superior may be necessary to the origin at the foramen cecum at the base of the tongue.)

5. Give a brief description of the embryology of second branchial cleft cyst and sinus. (The second branchial cleft, located in the embryo between the second and third branchial arches, contributes to the palatine tonsil and fossa. A cyst or sinus results from retention of the cleft or pouch in migration inferiorly.)
6. What is the clinical presentation of the same? (Either a cystic mass or draining sinus at the anterior border of the lower 1/3 of the sternocleidomastoid. The initial clinical presentation may be one of infection.)
7. Describe the relevant anatomy of a second branchial cleft cyst/sinus. (The relevant anatomy is the path of the underlying tract superiorly. The cyst and sinus courses superiorly between the internal and external carotid and lateral to the hypoglossal nerve but variations are not uncommon. More superiorly, if present, the tract is medial or deep to the stylohyoid and posterior belly of the digastric, terminating through the medial portion of the superior pharyngeal constrictor and into the tonsillar fossa.)
8. Describe the key operative steps. (A transverse cervical incision at the anterior border of the lower one-third of the sternocleidomastoid, release of the fascia and circumferential resection of the cyst and/or sinus, cannulation of the tract with a nasolacrimal duct probe and dissection, if necessary, into the carotid sheath. Further dissection will be dictated by the course of the tract as outlined by the question in anatomy. "Stair-step" incisions placed transversally and superiorly will facilitate exposure and dissection. See Figs. 21.2 and 21.3.)
9. How does the pertinent embryology of a first branchial cleft cyst or sinus differ from the above? (Although 95% of the branchial cleft-related cysts and sinuses are from the second branchial arch, origin from the first can occur as well. As the name states, the particular structures derived from the first branchial arch cleft are the external auditory canal, middle ear cavity, eustachian tube, and a portion of the external ear, as well as the tympanic membrane, incus, and malleus of the middle ear.)
10. Describe the relevant anatomy of the first branchial cleft cyst/sinus. (The relevant anatomy is the relationship of the sinus, if present in addition to a cyst, in relationship to the facial nerve. The tract may course lateral or superficial to the nerve or medial and deep. The other pertinent anatomical aspect is whether the tract originated in the external auditory canal. See below.)
11. What is the clinical presentation of a first branchial cleft cyst and/or sinus? (A pre- or intra-auricular sinus tract or cyst, perhaps complicated by infection.)
12. Surgical management of the same? (As described above, the relationship to the facial nerve is critical to the surgical approach. If dissection reveals a completely superficial course, exposure of the nerve will not be necessary. If not, dissection and exposure of the main extratemporal trunk, similar to the maneuver performed in the course of a parotidectomy, will facilitate further identification and dissection of the tract. Also, as mentioned above, excision of a small button of the cartilaginous external auditory canal may be necessary.)

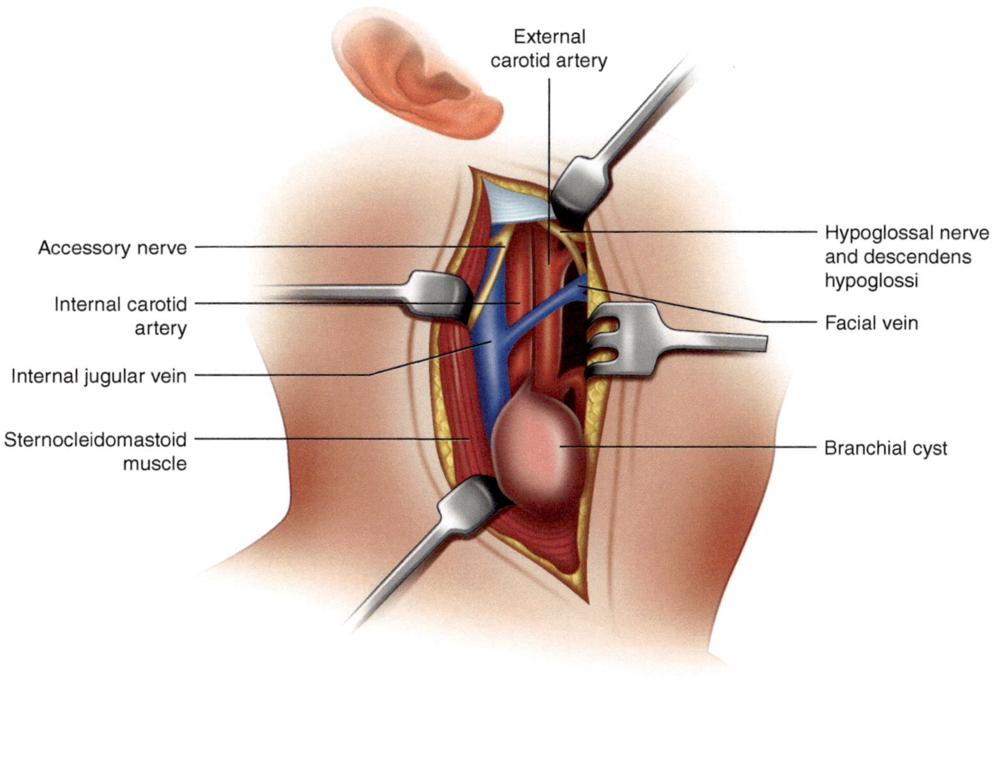

Fig. 21.2 Vertical cervical incision

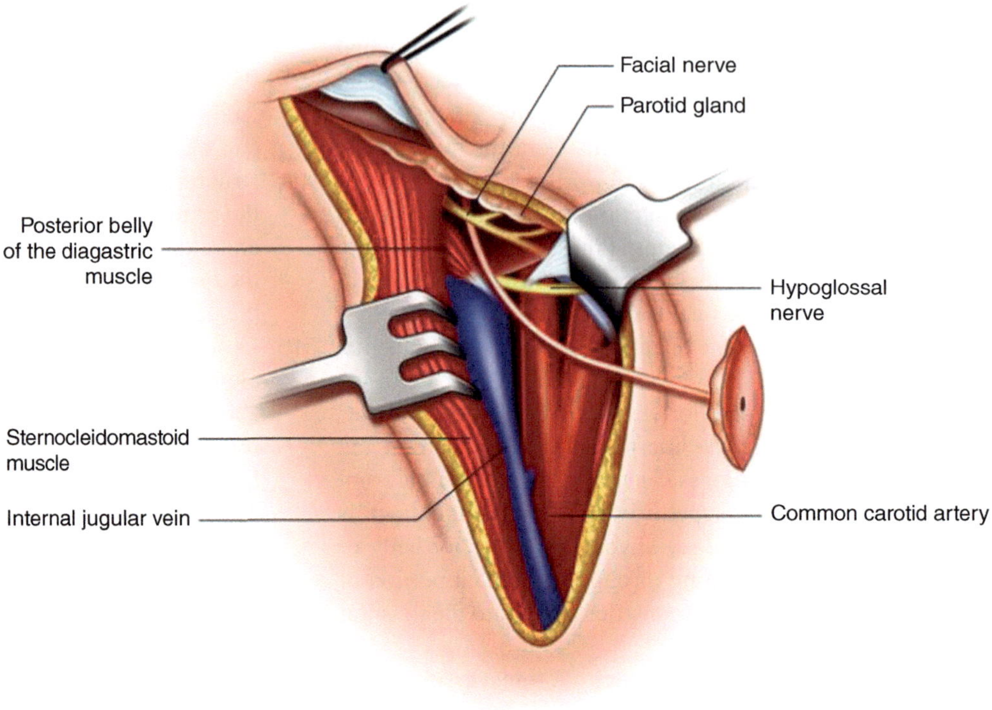

Fig. 21.3 Superior and vertical cervical incision

Case 1: Glabellar Mass

Case-Based Conference

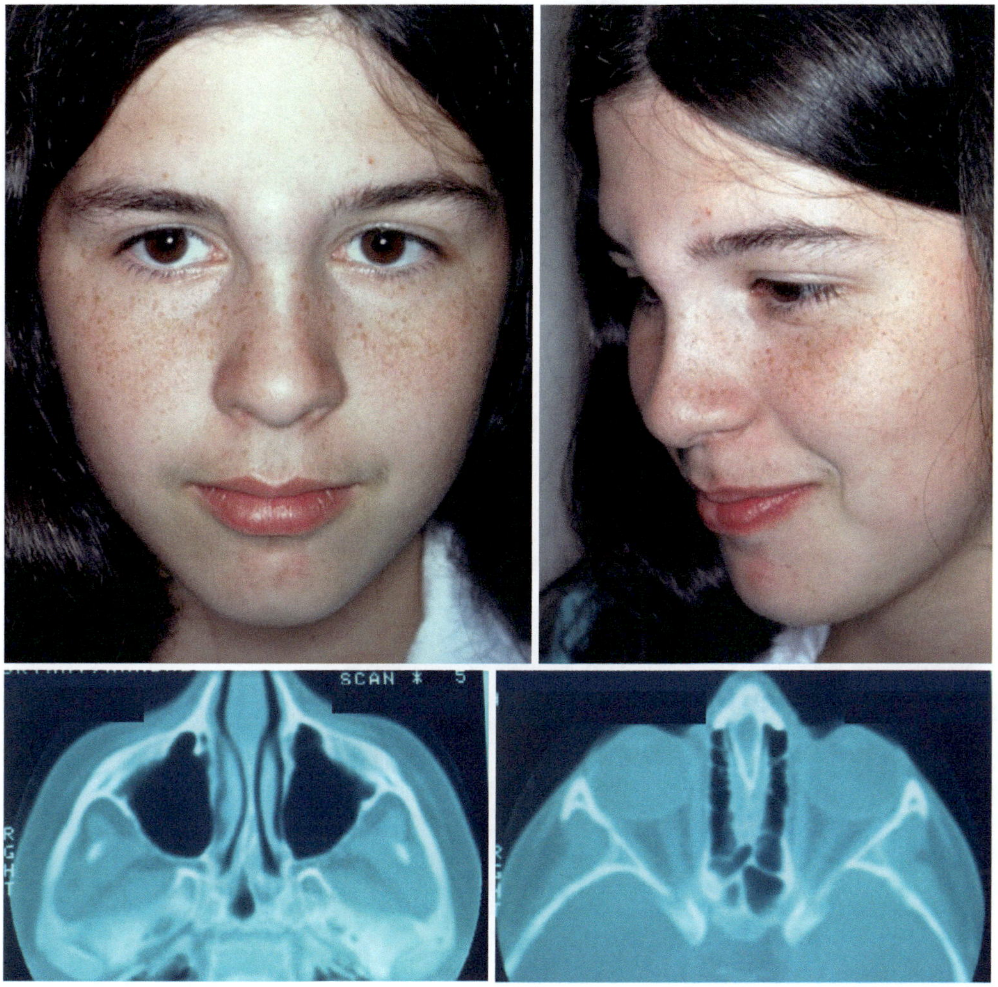

A 15-year-old with a “bump” present since infancy.

1. Describe the clinical slides and add a focused clinical examination. Describe the findings on the two slices of the axial CT scan. What additional slices do you desire?
   (a) Any tests indicated? Justify.
2. Based on photos and examination give a differential diagnosis. Add how the tests ordered will assist in diagnosis.
3. Describe the pathologic anatomy of each of the possible differential diagnoses and include pathogenesis if appropriate.
4. Outline a treatment plan for each.

Case-Based Conference: Discussion

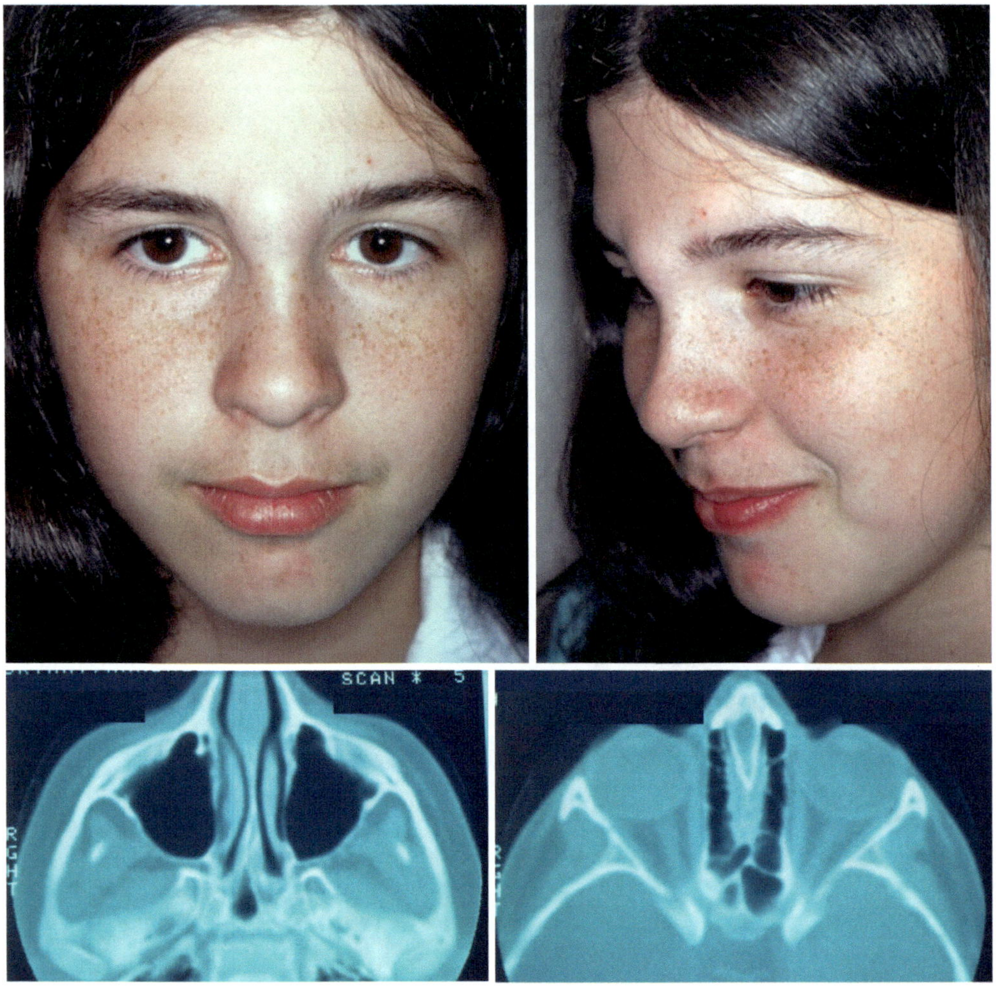

A 15-year-old with a "bump" present since infancy.

1. Describe the clinical slides and add a focused clinical examination. Describe the findings on the two slices of the axial CT scan. What additional slices do you desire? (Two views are provided, the first a full frontal of the face of a girl or young woman. The vertical facial proportions are normal, the central equal to the intercanthal distance with no evidence of telecanthus or intermedial canthal widening. The transverse facial proportions are also normal. No masses or deformities are evident in this view, a limitation perhaps of a two-dimensional photo. The second view is oblique with the patient's head tilted slightly downward. In contrast to the anterior-posterior, this view clearly depicts a glabellar mass, smooth, without skin involvement, rounded borders, and approximately 1.5–2.0 cm in size. Again, no other masses or deformities are visualized and the facial proportions appear normal.

   The history portion of a clinical examination is of some importance. Although the preamble relates the mass present since infancy, questions about the recent or remote increase as well as fluctuation in size should be posed and if positive, further details elicited. A history of nasal drainage and/or obstruction would be of value in assist of establishment of a diagnosis. Additional questions about drainage or inflammation of the mass would be of value. A focused physical exam would include palpation of the mass for firmness and compressibility. The mass should be observed for any change in characteristics with Valsalva. The skin should be closely inspected for the presence of a central punctum. The head and neck should be closely examined as well for the presence of other masses and the remainder of the physical exam completed. The two axial slices of the CT scan are at the level of the mid-maxillary sinus and mid-orbit, respectively. The former demonstrates a uniform widening of the anterior septum, the latter a worrisome splaying of the septum beneath intact nasal bones. Between the two splayed, ethmoid bone plates is a space filled with tissue of the same radial density as soft tissue. The medial walls of both orbits are composed of ethmoid air cells.)

(a) Are any tests indicated? Justify. (The most essential test is imaging, most particularly of the skull and maxillofacial. The imaging modalities include CT scan, contrast-enhanced, and MRI. The practice in many centers is an initial CT scan because of better resolution of bony anatomy, reserving MRI for more exact definition of soft tissue relationships. A provision of a detailed explanation of possible imaging findings is beyond the scope of this discussion. The essential determination is the presence or not of intracranial involvement as well as possible extension into either the ethmoidal or cartilaginous component of the septum. Findings indicative or suspect for dural involvement include a bifid crista galli or ethmoid plate, enlarged foramen cecum, and widened nasal bones or cartilaginous septum. The incidence of false positives is not insignificant in younger children.)

2. Based on photos and examination give a differential diagnosis. Add how the tests ordered will assist in diagnosis. (The differential diagnosis of a midline glabellar mass is epithelial inclusion cyst, nasal dermoid cyst, nasal glioma, and meningoencephalocele. An epidermal inclusion cyst would presumably have an onset or origin considerably later than infancy, perhaps as a result of adolescent acne. A vascular formation or infantile hemangioma is a remote possibility in the absence of any skin color alterations. The distinction among the remaining three possible diagnoses pivots to a large degree on the results of imaging. The absence of any of the bony abnormalities listed above signals little likelihood of intraosseous or intracranial extension. See below. As mentioned, false positives must be considered in young children. Tension evident on Valsalva provokes concerns of an extracranial extension of a meningo- or meningoencephalocele.)
3. Describe the pathologic anatomy of each of the possible differential diagnoses and include pathogenesis if appropriate. (The pathologic anatomy is better understood and explained with a discussion of the pathogenesis of the entities of nasal dermoid, glioma, and encephalocele and begins with embryology of the frontonasal region. In the fetal state, the aperture between the paired frontal bones permits dural extension inferiorly to nasal skin and in the prenasal space. The aperture is termed the foramen cecum. Regardless, with fetal maturation the dural diverticulum retracts, the prenasal space is obliterated, and the aperture fuses as the nasal frontal suture. Failure of this process of retraction and obliteration explains nasal dermoid or retention of the ectodermal element including the adnexal structures of skin; nasal glioma, retention of the glial elements; and meningocele or meningoencephalocele, a complete bony diastasis and migration of the frontal intracranial contents extracranially.)
4. Outline a treatment plan for each. (The operative approach will hinge entirely on the provisional diagnosis, facilitated substantially by the CT/MRI findings. Imaging results highly suggestive of extension intracranially mandates a combined intracranial-extracranial approach via bifrontal craniotomy with preservation of a supraorbital bar. That exposure can be enhanced perhaps by osteotomies performed at the nasal frontal portion of the supraorbital bar centrally. Any herniation of intracranial contents is reduced, dural repair accomplished if necessary, and the intranasal component dissected—perhaps between the leaves of the ethmoid and cartilaginous septum—and excised en toto. Nasal gliomas imply a somewhat greater risk of extension of the sinus tract and dermoid cysts and yet both in the absence of suspicious imaging findings can be approached extracranially. Several routes have been described and are available. Minimally invasive endoscopic excision through a remote hairline approach yields an optimal cosmetic result but may be problematic for excision of an intraseptal component. An open rhinoplasty can provide adequate access, particularly in younger patients with a shorter nose and distance to the nasal dorsum but may be inadequate for a glabellar lesion, particularly if sizable and the necessity for exposure of any proximal sinus tract. Direct excision by a vertical glabellar excision ultimately will yield a cosmetically satisfactory scar if somewhat limited exposure. If a punctum is present, such must also be excised, regardless of the approach. The concern in this case is the findings on the CT slices provided. The CT scan of a further cranial ward may assist in the implications for treatments, but given the findings evident at mid-orbit, the likelihood is that additional information will be indeterminate. One option in the circumstances of ambiguous imaging is the bicoronal flap that enables the performance of a frontal craniotomy if necessitated by intraoperative findings.

   The complete excision of cyst and sinus tract is of paramount importance. Residual epithelial remnants are the nidus for recurrence, inflammation and possible osteomyelitis and intracranial infectious sequelae.)

In-Service Examination

1. An infant presents with a preauricular cyst and sinus into the external auditory canal. These structures are derived from what embryological structure?
   (a) First branchial cleft
   (b) Second branchial cleft
   (c) Third branchial cleft
   (d) Second branchial cleft and associated hillock

2. A 10-year-old presents with a midline dorsal nasal mobile, noncompressible mass. What is the most likely diagnosis?
   (a) Meningocele
   (b) Dermoid
   (c) Teratoma
   (d) Epidermal inclusion cyst

Vascular Tumors

22

Bibliography

Gampper TJ and Morgan RF "Vascular Anomalies: Hemangiomas", *Plast. Reconstr. Surg.*, (2002); 110:**572–578 ONLY.**

Mulliken JB and Young AE, Chapter 3: "Diagnosis and Natural History of Hemangiomas", Vascular Birthmarks: Hemangiomas and Malformations, W.B. Saunders Co., (1988) **pp 41–62.**

Greene AK, Phillips JH, Ch. 11 "Vascular Anomalies", *Pediatric Plastic Surgery Second Edition,* CRC Press, Bentz M.L., Bauer B.S., Zuker R.M., (2017); **pgs. 199–211 ONLY.**

Szychta P, Stewart K, Anderson W, "Treatment of Infantile Hemangiomas with Propranolol: Clinical Guidelines", *Plast. Reconstr. Surg.*, (2014); 133(4):**852–862.**

Faculty Discussion and Study Guide

Editor's Note: A useful classification of vascular anomalies is a division into two broad groups: tumors and malformations. This module is constructed as Chap. 22 (present chapter) and Chap. 23.

Diagnosis, Pathology, and Natural History of Hemangiomas

1. Give the classification of congenital vascular anomalies. (Essentially, the division is: one, tumors which consist entirely of hemangiomas, and two, malformations. With respect to hemangiomas, the three types are infantile, "congenital", and kaposiform. The vast majority of infantile hemangiomas are involute. The congenital variety is fully developed at birth, may involute partially or not at all, and is considered noninvoluting. One variant is termed rapidly involuting and generally completely regresses by age two. The malformations side of the division, discussed in Chap. 23, consists of tissue types of capillary, venous, lymphatic, or a mixture of all. The vascular malformations are further divided into low flow and high flow but from a practical standpoint, virtually all high flow vascular malformations are arterial venous. Slow flow is either capillary or venous in nature.)
   (a) Describe a molecular biology differentiation between infantile and congenital hemangiomas. (Infantile hemangiomas express the protein GLUT1 and congenital hemangiomas do not.)
2. What is the epidemiology of infantile hemangiomas in neonates: frequency, gender ratio, single versus multiple (4–10% by age 1 year, 3:1 female to male ratio, 80% are single. Congenital have no gender predisposition.)
   (a) Significance of multiple cutaneous hemangiomas (Some patients may also have visceral hemangiomas. Visceral hemangiomas almost always have multiple cutaneous lesions but not necessarily the opposite.)
3. Describe the "herald spot" or macular stain? (Infantile hemangiomas may first appear on examination of the neonate as an erythematous or blanched flattened area or telangiectasia of the skin without any initial tumor formation or distortion, although 70–90% are evident by age 2–4 weeks.)
4. Explain the phrase "not all hemangiomas look like strawberries" and "not all strawberries are hemangiomas". (The two phrases explain the differentiation of hemangiomas and vascular malformations: a hemangioma may lie deeply within the subcutaneous tissue and hence the skin has a bluish color, yet a hemangioma if located more superficially in the dermis would indeed appear more as a "strawberry". The other phrase describes that what appears to be a strawberry hemangioma may actually be a superficial vascular malformation which as described below will behave differently.)
5. What are some of the differentiating characteristics of hemangiomas versus vascular malformations? (Most hemangiomas have little external evidence at birth other

E. Luce, *A Curriculum for Plastic Surgery*, https://doi.org/10.1007/978-3-031-62087-4_22

than a herald patch or macular stain, then rapid growth in the first year of life is termed the proliferative phase, versus malformations which are present at birth but exhibit little change other than growth with growth of the child. With time a change in color in hemangiomas occurs but not so with vascular malformations. Also, hemangiomas are firm and rubbery versus malformations which are easily compressible and may become tense with Valsalva.)

6. We've already discussed some of the clinical findings in differentiating hemangiomas from malformations. A malformation and a rapidly proliferating hemangioma in two different 6-month olds are biopsied. How would the essential histology differ in these two? (Under the influence of vascular endothelial growth factor, VEGF, a true hemangioma will have immature, rapidly proliferating endothelial cells. A vascular malformation will be populated by mature normal-appearing endothelial cells.)
   (a) What cell may be present in abundance in an involuting hemangioma? (Mast cell; 30–40 times expected.)
7. Discuss involution of hemangiomas including clinical hallmarks, appearance, and timing. (Of those hemangiomas that involute, one-half do so by age 5 and three-fourths by age 7, and then perhaps some additional involution by age 10 or 12. Indications that the process of involution is underway are indicated by lightning and/or violaceous color, decrease in tenseness with Valsalva, overall diminution in the tenseness of the lesion, and the appearance of wrinkled skin. Hemangiomas have rapid growth in the early months of life, plateau at about age 1 year, then begin the process of involution.)
8. Discuss imaging in hemangiomas and vascular anomalies. (The diagnosis of hemangiomas can be established clinically. If some other pressing indication for imaging such as an indeterminate diagnosis, imaging may be indicated. The vascular anomalies are best defined with MRI but will require sedation or general anesthesia, so a balanced consideration in an infant or young child must be made. If the clinical exam is equivocal, ultrasound is the first tier of imaging. If embolization is considered in an arteriovenous malformation, a formal angiogram will be necessary.)

Clinical Picture

1. You receive a call from the resident who relates he has seen a 1-year-old in the clinic with a "cavernous" hemangioma who, on further questioning from you, relates that this is a bluish mass of the parotid region without discrete skin changes. In all likelihood, what is the lesion and how do you correct the resident's terminology? (The readings describe the so-called "cavernous hemangiomas" are simply hemangiomas in a subcutaneous location with intact skin. The intact skin renders a bluish hue to the mass, so in all likelihood, this represents a venous malformation.)
   (a) If so, then what accounts for the color difference between, for example, a blue and a bright red hemangioma? (Location and level of skin involvement. Bright red hemangiomas tend to lie in papillary dermis or superficial layers of the dermis. Blue hemangiomas are either in deep reticular dermis or perhaps even the subcutaneous tissue.)
2. Parents bring in their firstborn child, a 6-month-old girl, with a mass of the cheek. Outline your clinical approach (Pertinent history of the lesion change over time?; present at birth?, increase in size?, any bleeding? Then physical exam; appearance including the skin, compressible, firm versus hard).
   (a) The skin is bluish but intact, compressible, 4x4 cm. in size; present since birth, with the possible increase in size perhaps with growth of the child. (This lesion is probably a vascular malformation).
   (b) Further workup indicated? (Probably not. MRI or CT scan would require sedation or general anesthesia; and angiography is rarely indicated, observation with return visits.)
3. You are consulted on an infant with a sternal cleft and cardiac anomalies because of a facial hemangioma. The presence of what other anomalies should be suspected? (Eye and intracranial as the PHACES syndrome: posterior fossa abnormalities, hemangioma, arterial intracranial anomalies, cardiac, eye, sternal cleft.)
4. What is the typical clinical presentation including the age of the Kasabach-Merritt syndrome? (The age of onset is 5–6 weeks with either multiple hemangiomas or a single hemangioma >5 cm., typically outside of the head and neck. In contrast to routine hemangiomas, the gender ratio is equal in Kasabach-Merritt syndrome. The onset is sudden and a rapid increase in size with tenseness of the overlying skin possibly with petechiae; concomitant evidence of systemic coagulopathy with bleeding, for example, purpura, GI bleeding, etc. The presence of purpura is evidence of profound thrombocytopenia. The diagnosis can be confirmed with MRI which has a distinctly different appearance than garden variety hemangioma.)
   (a) Presumed pathology and name? (The current thought is that this lesion represents a unique hemangioma from the garden variety type hemangioma. Kaposiform hemangioendothelioma is identifiable as a discrete lesion and about one-half are complicated by a coagulopathy due to platelet trapping within the lesion.)
   (b) What is the treatment of choice? (Vincristine is the agent of choice but the presence of Kasabach-Merritt syndrome may require more rapid therapeutic effect

and systemic steroids can be employed. Heparin is contraindicated. Heparin and the administration of platelets only exacerbate the coagulopathy.)

5. You are consulted on a 6-week-old who has been admitted with congestive heart failure of unknown etiology because he has multiple cutaneous hemangiomas. How can you help with diagnosis and management? (Palpate hepatomegaly. If present, particularly if the infant is also anemic, consider hepatic hemangiomas. If the primary response by the consulting service to your finding is that the hepatomegaly is due to congestive heart failure, suggest a CT scan and/or ultrasound of the abdomen. The CHF may be due to shunting and high-output failure.)
6. Parents bring a 2-year-old child to the office with a history of a rapidly growing mass of the thigh. On exam is a firm, rubbery mass with overlying red-blue skin in the mid-thigh. Plain X-rays provided by the parents demonstrate distortion and scalloping of the adjacent femur. Most likely diagnosis? (Sarcoma or other soft tissue tumor; bony distortion in the presence of hemangioma is extremely uncommon.)
7. Describe the clinical picture of pyogenic granuloma. (In a child, most commonly located on the head and neck or extremities, and usually does not have an antecedent history of trauma. Repeated bleeding episodes occur and no lesion existed prior to the appearance. On excision, a characteristic pathological picture would indicate extensive fibrosis and inflammation, not the appearance of a hemangioma. Recurrence is not uncommon. Treatment is by excision and cautery of the base with silver nitrate. Repeated application of silver nitrate may be necessary.)

Treatment

1. Discuss the treatment of hemangiomas with the following:
   (a) Steroids (Propanol is evolving into the first line treatment below, but may be contraindicated in some patients and steroids may be employed. Usually reserved for specific indications such as visual or airway obstruction, recurrent severe bleeding which is uncommon, Kasabach-Merritt syndrome, and severe distortion of the facial features. Mulliken has recommended deferral, if possible, of initiation of steroid therapy until after the age of 3 months to minimize complications. The initial dosage is 2–3 mg/kg/day of prednisone. At least a week to 10 days may be required to observe a response and expected response rate is dramatic in one-third, partial in one-third, and none in one-third. The dosages are quite high and require at least 10 days to 2 weeks for a response. One protocol consists of administration of steroids for 6 weeks then a pause and/or tapering, yet the average duration of steroid administration in Mulliken's series was 6 months. The complications were cushingoid facies in 3/4 of the children and growth retardation in 1/3, although growth was resumed after cessation of steroid therapy.)
   (b) Interferon (Actually, is of mostly historical interest because of the high incidence of severe side effects such as spastic diplegia. The principal disadvantage besides the severe side effects is the prolonged period of treatment needed, 12–18 months).
   (c) What is the conceptual and therapeutic problem with treatment of hemangiomas with lasers? (Depth of the laser is only 1.5 mm and frequent ulceration occurs.)
2. What patient is a candidate for systemic propranolol therapy? (The same indications as for systemic *steroid* therapy: visual obstruction, upper respiratory obstruction, or rarely, persistent bleeding.)
   (a) What is necessary pre-treatment? (Cardiac clearance in the form of EKG and a cardiology consultation; blood glucose.)
   (b) What are some contraindications? (The PHACES syndrome, congenital heart disease, asthma, and possibly blood glucose abnormalities.)
3. Give a dose/time regimen. (The therapeutic dose is 2 mg/kg divided into three daily dosages with continuance on the average of 6 months with a subsequent 2-month weaning period. An advisable regimen is to gradually increase the daily dosage with a target of 2 mg/kg/day.)
4. Give three complications. (The cardiac complications of bradycardia and hypotension, hypoglycemia, and bronchospasm.)
5. What is the management of periorbital hemangiomas, for example, a 6-month-old who presents with a growing hemangioma of the upper eyelid. The sclera and cornea are still visible on the affected side. (Mulliken recommends retinoscopy to determine if a refraction error is present. Presumably, one could also perform an evoked brainstem response. Regardless, any obstruction of vision for any length of time over 2 weeks can result in permanent damage and repeated ophthalmologic exams may be necessary.)
   (a) Why does permanent damage occur and what is the treatment? (Cortical blindness, amblyopia, and/or deformation of the cornea. The treatment used is currently propanol.)
   (b) What are the hazards of intralesional injections? (Blindness).
6. Manage the following problems:
   (a) A 6-month-old with increasing stridor of 2 weeks duration with an MRI that demonstrates a subglottic hemangioma. (Use systemic steroids first, then tracheostomy if necessary, and/or possibly propanol.)

(b) A hemangioma of the nasal tip of 2 cm in size. (Recent enthusiasm has emerged over the excision of facial hemangiomas of limited size. A number of authors have described excision +/– local reconstruction of smaller hemangiomas.)

Editor's Note: Quite recent publications (two) have indicated efficacy for the use of sirolimus, an immunosuppressive agent, in the treatment of the proliferative stage of infantile hemangiomas. The work requires confirmation from other teams to achieve mainstream status.

Case-Based Conference

Case 1A: A Vascular Anomaly in an Infant

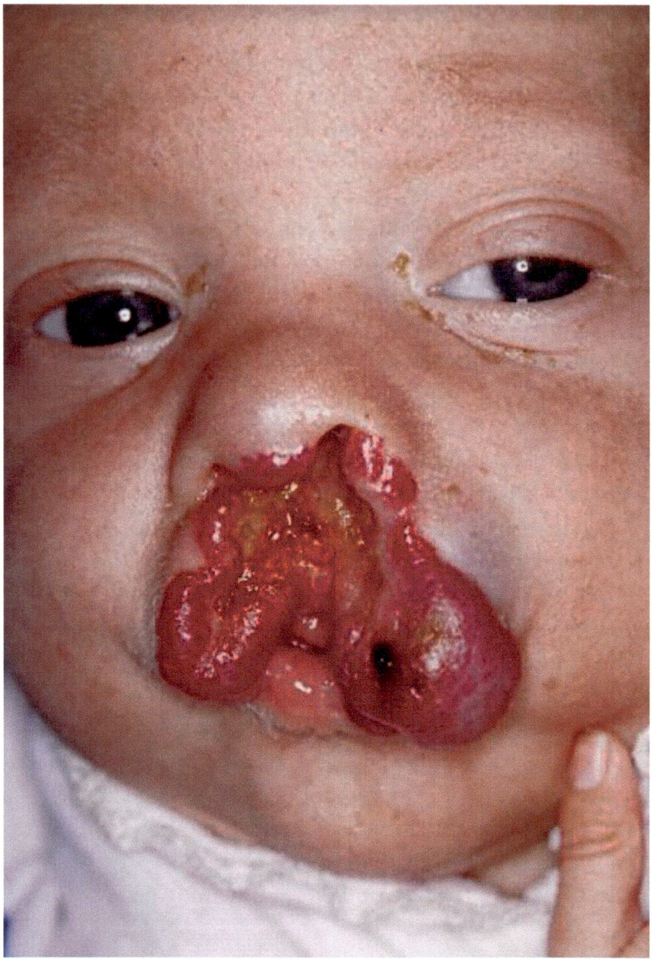

A 3-month-old with a rapidly growing, ulcerated mass.

1. Describe the slides. Add a clinical examination.
   (a) Are any tests indicated? Justify.
2. Give a classification system, a differential diagnosis, and your preferred diagnosis.
3. Explain the pathophysiology and pathologic anatomy.
4. Outline a treatment plan including your counseling of the parents.

Case 1B: The Infant Is Now One Year of Age After Your Treatment Plan

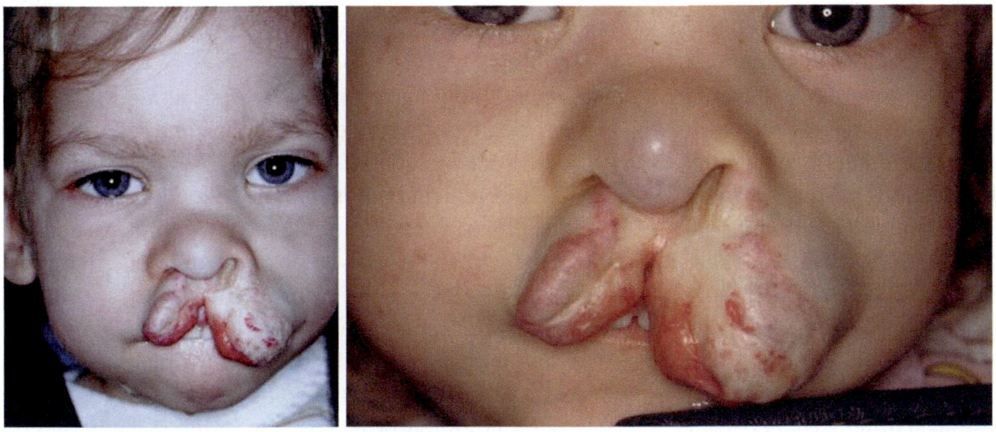

1. Describe the slides and add an exam.
2. Interpret the results and outline the continuation of your treatment plan.

Case-Based Conference: Discussion

Case 1A: A Vascular Anomaly in an Infant

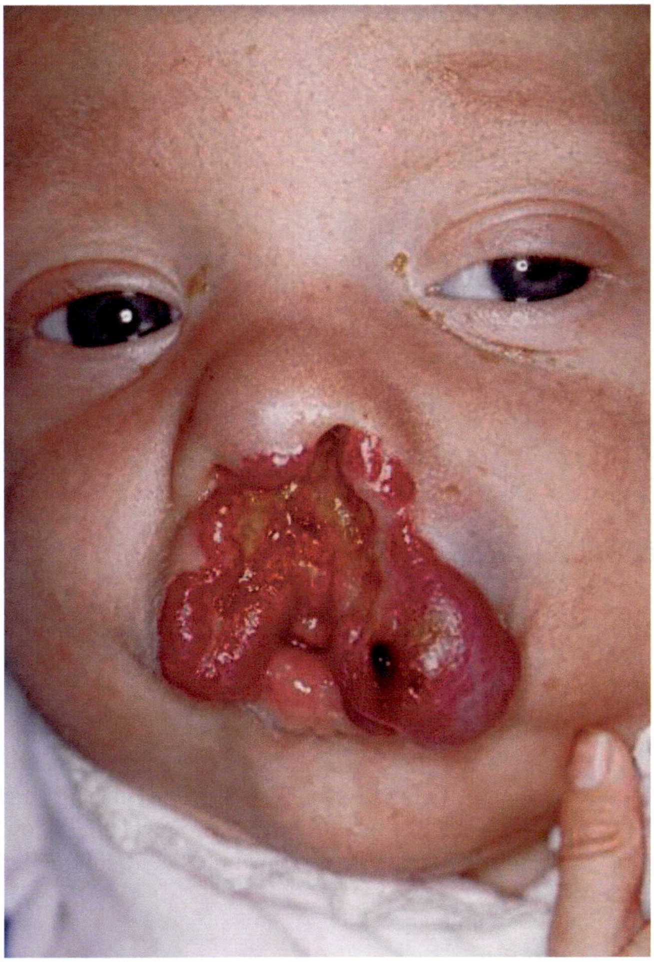

A 3-month-old with a rapidly growing, ulcerated mass.

1. Describe the slides. Add a clinical examination. (The single slide provided is a frontal view of a Caucasian infant that includes the central face from lateral canthus to lateral canthus and mid-forehead to just beneath the chin. The principal and dramatic finding is a large mass, deep red in color and exuberant in appearance that appears to have replaced the upper lip. The mass consists of two lobules that have a central cleft and are sufficiently sessile that only the central portion of the lower lip is visible. The mass process extends into the skin of the columella, the left ala, and in all likelihood, into the floor of the nose on the left. Because of the angle of the photo, the right nostril is mostly obscured by the mass. No active or recent bleeding is evident. No other lesions are apparent. The eyes are open and appear normal. The facial proportions are normal and no deformities are seen.

   The clinical examination would begin with questions about the appearance of the patient as a neonate and in particular, if a lesion was present, and if not, if the lip was intact. The preamble states that the lesion has rapidly grown, so additional questions center on bleeding episodes, if any, the ability of the baby to feed, and weight gain. A history of other congenital diagnoses, central nervous system or cardiac, might point toward syndromes such as PHACES: posterior fossa abnormalities, hemangioma, arterial intracranial anomalies, cardiac and eye anomalies, and sternal cleft. The history of frequency, severity, and management of bleeding episodes should be elicited. The physical exam must determine as much as possible the extent including the intramucosal involvement, palpate for thrills, and a complete inspection of the trunk and extremities for other hemangiomas.)
   (a) Are any tests indicated? Justify. (Although imaging is of value in some instances of vascular anomalies, imaging of this patient is not appropriate. The single test of possible utility is genetic testing. An infantile

hemangioma, see below, will express the protein GLUT1 and congenital hemangiomas will not, but the history should easily discern the difference.)

2. Give a classification system, a differential diagnosis, and your preferred diagnosis. (Classification of congenital vascular lesions has some element of overlap and can be confusing. The two broad types of vascular anomalies are tumors and malformations and this anomaly is within the tumor type, hemangioma. Based on the history of rapid growth, the patient's lesion is an infantile hemangioma rather than congenital. Congenital hemangiomas are much less common, fully formed at birth, and enlarge with growth of the infant. Further, an assumption in this case is that no other hemangiomas are present. The presence of multiple hemangiomas would raise a concern about concomitant visceral lesions, particularly hepatic.)
3. Explain the pathophysiology and pathologic anatomy. (The essential biologic pathophysiology of infantile hemangioma is unknown. Angiogenic cytokines such as vascular endothelial growth factors are elevated and diminish with involution. In many instances, only a macular stain is present at birth, a "herald" spot that within the first month of life rapidly proliferates. At age 1 year, infantile hemangiomas begin to involute and the involution progresses over the subsequent 3–4 years. Complete involution is frequent but not invariable. Regardless, further resolution beyond the age of 5–6 years is not likely. Intralesional mast cell cytosis is present in the involutional phase.

   The pathologic anatomy is the destruction of the normal upper lip with involvement of the columella and possibly the floor of the nose.)
4. Outline a treatment plan including your counseling of the parents. (The contemporary management of hemangioma attended by visual or airway obstruction or other complications as this instance of a destructive lesion, consists of the administration of a beta-blockade such as propranolol. Contraindications include congenital cardiac disease, asthma, and intracranial pathology. The dosage is variable but a common protocol is an initial 0.1 mg/kg TID for 3 days, increased to 0.3 mg/kg and 0.6 mg/kg TID for 3 days each, and continuance of a 2 mg/kg daily until the therapeutic effect has been obtained.

   Counseling the parents of the patient should center on two aspects: one, avoid surgical intervention until maximal degree of involution has occurred, and second, a significant deformity of the upper lip will be the residual of the involution process.)

Case 1B: The Infant Is Now One Year of Age After Your Treatment Plan

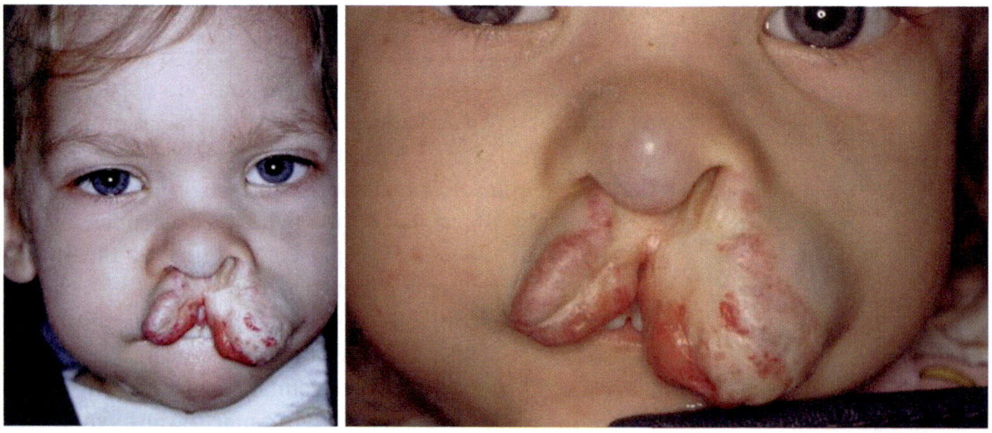

1. Describe the slides and add an exam. (Two similar slides are provided, each of a frontal central facial view. Substantial involution of the lesion has occurred both in size and appearance. The exuberant and florid redness of the surface has been mostly replaced by pale white and flattened tissue. Some of the upper cutaneous lip is visible and the floor of the right nostril has normal-appearing skin. The remaining mass is considerably larger on the left. A further close-up confirms these findings as well as a mostly normal floor of the left nostril. An asymmetrical fullness of the lip on the left beneath the intact skin is more readily apparent on this view as well as a superior and lateral displacement of the left alar base. The nasal lobule has a faintly violaceous hue that may represent a photographic artifact or possibly underlying hemangioma. The tip is not deformed. Two maxillary incisors are seen beneath the two lobules of the lesion which are now clearly separate with skin visible at the labial-columellar junction.)

2. Interpret the results and outline the continuation of your treatment plan. (The photos depict a partial but considerable involution of the hemangioma, either pharmacologically induced or spontaneous. Since the infant is only 1 year of age, the natural history of spontaneous involution at this early age would seem improbable but possible. Although pharmacological treatment could be continued in all likelihood, if improvement and appearance have plateaued, surgical intervention is appropriate.

   The procedure would have several reconstructive goals: one, debulk tumor or the fibrofatty tissue as a residual of the involution process, preserve the intact cutaneous lip, and address the cleft between the two lip segments. To do so would require excision of tissue at the base of the columella. If possible, the left elevated and laterally displaced alar base should be advanced medially and inferiorly with excision of redundant nasal floor, similar to the nasal repair of an incomplete cleft lip. The parents should be counseled about the probable necessity of future revisions.)

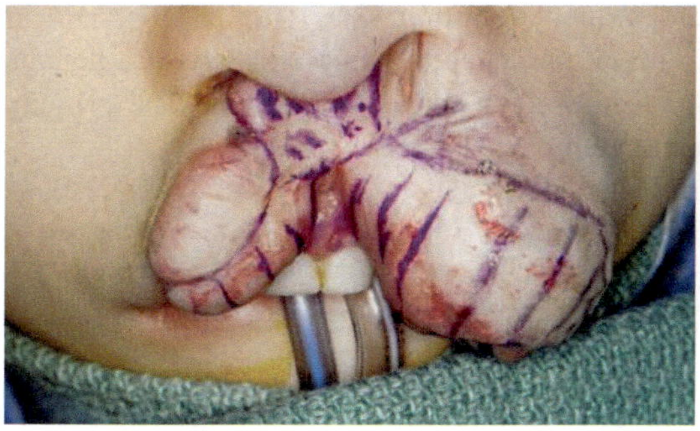

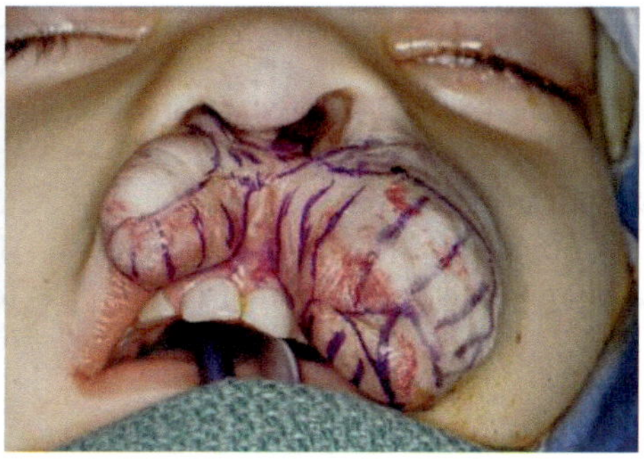

Two intraoperative photos are provided. These include a partial submental vertex and an anterior-posterior closeup. Multiple pen marks would indicate incisions, presumably, tissue for excision. The close-up focus demonstrates a plan for transverse incisions for the entire length of the two segments of the lip, placed at the junction of the intact cutaneous and the more inferiorly positioned remnant of the hemangiomatous process. Medially, the incisions curve vertically into the nasal sill and upward into the floor. The medial and inferior nasal floor is stippled to suggest a planned incision. On the left alar base, a short transverse incision is also marked. The superior extent of the intramucosal excision and the character and amount of mucosa retained in the labial sulcus is not evident.

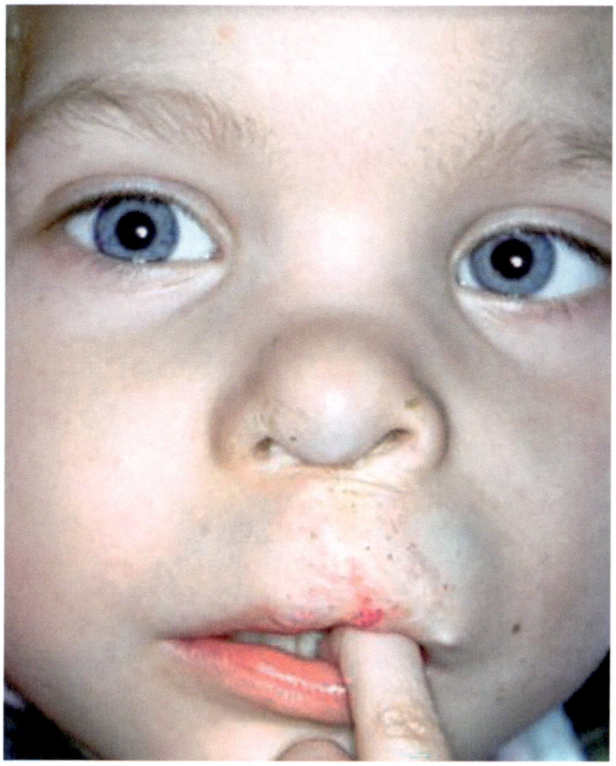

Postoperative

The upper lip is intact. The left side is nearly normal in appearance, if perhaps somewhat long. The mucosal component is present and of normal configuration with a suggestion of a cupid's bow. No philtrum is present but rather some flattened scarred skin that occupies the central one-third of the lip. The mucosa of the left side of the lip is attenuated with a small dogear laterally and inferior. The overall vertical height of the lip is probably increased. The left alar base-nasal sill is moderately widened and defaced as well as still positioned above the transverse level of the right side. The tip is bulbous and the columella is shortened.

Critique

How the right lip was lengthened is not readily apparent from the intraoperative drawings. If not performed, the left alar base advancement would have benefited from an alar cinch suture to the septum. Some lengthening of the columella could have been accomplished by utilization of the excised, stippled, skin.

In-Service Examination

1. A distinguishing genetic feature of infantile or involuting hemangiomas is the presence of:
   (a) TGIF-alpha
   (b) TGIF-beta
   (c) TWIST
   (d) GLUT 1
2. A significant complication of the treatment of hemangioma with propranolol is:
   (a) Increased intracranial pressure
   (b) Hypoglycemia
   (c) Tachycardia
   (d) Frequent vomiting
3. An infant has a rapid increase in size of a hemangioma, GI bleeding, and thrombocytopenia. The primary treatment agent is:
   (a) Heparin
   (b) Vancomycin
   (c) Recombinant VEGF
   (d) Vincristine

Vascular Malformations

23

Bibliography

Thehinia A.H., Upton J., Chapter 37: "Dysplasias-Tumorous Conditions of the Upper Extremity", Neligan PC, Plastic Surgery, Elsevier 5th Edition, (2023), Volume 6: **pg. 868.**

Arneja JS and Gosain AK, "Vascular Malformations", *Plast. Reconstr. Surg.*, (2008); 121(4):**195e–204e.**

Greene AK, Perlyn CA, and Alomari AI, "Management of lymphatic malformation", *Clin. Plast. Surg.*, (2011); 38:**75–82.**

Greene AK, Alomari AI, "Management of Venous Malformations", *Clin. Plast. Surg.*, (2011); 38: **pgs. 83–91 ONLY.**

Greene AK and Orbach DB, "Management of arteriovenous malformation", *Clin. Plast. Surg.*, (2011); 38(1):**95–101 ONLY.**

Faculty Discussion and Study Guide

Editor's Note: A useful classification of vascular anomalies is a division into two broad groups: tumors and malformations. This module is constructed as Chap. 22 – Vascular Tumors and Chap. 23 – Vascular Malformations.

Vascular Malformation of the Head and Neck

1. Give a brief classification of vascular anomalies. (Hemangioma or vascular malformation—see Chap. 22: **Hemangiomas** are divided into involutional and non-involutional. Vascular malformations are divided into high and low flow; high consists of arteriovenous malformations. Low flow is further subdivided into capillary, lymphatic, venous, categories and mixed.)
2. From a biological perspective why is a capillary malformation present at birth and doesn't grow but a vascular tumor proliferates in the postnatal period and infancy? (The difference is a stable endothelium in a malformation and a proliferative endothelium in vascular tumors. Of course, cytokines are active in the latter.)
3. What are the findings in capillary malformation? (A pinkish to deep red hue to the skin in infants and young children.)
   (a) What changes can be anticipated in capillary vascular malformations over the years? (A progressive cobblestone appearance with deepening of the color from deep red to progressively more purple, particularly in the third and fourth decades.)
4. Define the following capillary malformation syndromes:
   (a) Sturge-Weber syndrome (Facial capillary malformation in the distribution of the ophthalmic division of cranial nerve V, leptomeningeal vascular malformations with possible associated seizures, and possible retinal involvement.) What workup is indicated? (MRI and pediatric ophthalmologic and neurologic consults.)
   (b) Klippel-Trenaunay syndrome (Capillary or lymphatico-venous malformation of the trunk and/or extremities and hemi-hypertrophy with increase in length of the involved bony skeleton).
   (c) "Stork's bite" (Extremely common macular stains in neonates of the nape of the neck, upper eyelid, and glabella that fade slowly)
   (d) Rendu-Osler-Weber (Autosomal dominant of telangiectasias of mucous membranes of the upper aerodigestive and gastrointestinal tract.)
   (e) Maffucci (Multiple hemangiomas and enchondromas with a 20% incidence of chondrosarcoma.)
5. An infant presents with what appears to be a capillary malformation of the lower cheek and chin on the right side of the face. Is a CT scan or MRI scan of the brain indicated? (Theoretically no, since leptomeningeal involvement with vascular malformations is only seen if the skin distribution of the port-wine stain involves the

E. Luce, *A Curriculum for Plastic Surgery*, https://doi.org/10.1007/978-3-031-62087-4_23

ophthalmic division of cranial nerve V. Of course, practically, the answer may be different.)

   (a) The significance of a "port wine" stain of the midline lower back? (May signal presence of spina bifida occulta or a tethered spinal cord.)

6. Which imaging modality is preferred for congenital vascular lesions? (MRI with T_1 and T_2 weighted images, although CT provides a CTA if necessary.)
7. Treatment of choice for capillary malformations? (The pulsed-dye laser at 585 mm with multiple treatments. The chromophore at this wavelength is hemoglobin. Lightening of the lesion can be accomplished but not eradicated. Some evidence exists that intense pulsed light may also be efficacious.)
8. At what period in embryonic development do malformations of the lymphatic system probably occur? (Between 6 and 9 weeks, the time of the development of the cervicofacial lymphatic system.)
9. Give a classification for lymphangiomas. (A classification that has therapeutic application is a division into macrocystic and microcystic variety. The somewhat arbitrary division is 5 mm. Macrocystic is, as the name implies, large fluid-filled cysts. The large cysts enable treatment with aspiration and sclerotherapy. Microcystic again, as the name implies, consists of much smaller cysts and compact tissue that may require resection rather than non-operative treatment. Combined or mixed are quite common.)
10. Lymphatic malformations are most commonly seen in the newborn nursery. Where does a "cystic hygroma" occur anatomically, and what step(s) are necessary in the diagnostic workup? (The cervico-facial region. Ultrasound in addition to chest X-ray to document mediastinal involvement.)
    (a) If not present at birth, what are the milestones for presentation? (50% at birth, 80% by age 1 year, 90% by 2 years of age.)
    (b) Do lymphangiomas regress? (Essentially, no.)
11. Do lymphangiomas that increase in size after birth do so by the same mechanism as hemangioma? If not, how? (They do not. Hemangiomas increase by proliferations of the vascular channels, lymphangiomas increase in size by fluid accumulation, and cellulitis, with secondary obstruction by fibrosis of the anomalous lymphatic channels.)
    (a) A 4-year-old with a diagnosis of a lymphangioma of the head and neck since age one presents with upper respiratory obstruction and a history of rapid increase in size. Explain the pathophysiology. (A rapid increase in size of a lymphangioma may be due to lymphangitis, obliteration of the few remaining lymphatic channels, and rapid accumulation of fluid and increase in size. In a 4-year-old that event may have been precipitated by an upper respiratory tract infection. For treatment, see questions below.)
12. Skeletal changes in hemangioma are extremely rare. Is this true for lymphangioma? A-V malformations? (The presence of skeletal hypertrophy is common in the presence of a soft tissue lymphangioma, for example, hypertrophy of the maxilla or mandible may occur in conjunction with a lymphatic anomaly of the face. Skeletal *destruction* of the mandible or maxilla is not common but can certainly occur as an intraosseous lesion in facial A-V malformations, a different entity (see below). Skeletal and soft tissue overgrowth is not uncommon in lymphangiomas of the extremities, particularly in Klippel-Trenaunay syndrome.)
13. What is one most serious complications in lymphangioma, besides airway obstruction? (Infection in the lesion.) Why? (Acute infections are usually those of cellulitis and the usual problems of acute infections. But, more importantly, each infection leads to fibrosis, obstruction of whatever lymphatic pathways exist, and enlargement of the lesion. Prompt management with antibiotics of any lymphangitis is quite important and family counseling needs to be accomplished.)
    (a) What is another common complication? (Intralesional bleeding in about one-third of the cases.)
14. Discuss excision of lymphatic malformations or lymphangiomas in terms of timing, indications, size or type most amenable, and success rates. (Discussion of timing is a little vague in the readings, but generally, most advocate a plan of watchful waiting unless some specific indications arise. Indications would include the obvious ones of vision or airway and small well-localized lesions are clearly more amenable than large diffuse lesions of the head and neck or extremities. Essentially, indications are either functional or aesthetic. The technique is one of tedious dissection but complete resection, if possible, is necessary. Recurrence is quite common, probably due to undetected anomalous lymphatic channels outside the field of dissection. The first line of therapy in lymphatic malformations is sclerotherapy by aspiration of cyst and injection of a sclerosing agent such as bleomycin, doxycycline, or sodium morrhuate. Sclerotherapy is more likely to be successful in those lesions that are macrocystic than microcystic for the obvious reason that the larger the cyst the more likely the sclerosing agent can be efficacious. Nevertheless, the recurrence rate is significant, 20–40%. One treatment for the microcystic variant, if anatomically possible, is compression.)
    (a) What is lymphangioma circumscriptum? (A lesion of the skin with multiple warty cutaneous lesions and clear drainage that is required to prevent recurrence en-bloc excision to the level of fascia and either flap or split-thickness skin graft coverage.)

15. What are the recommendations for treatment of the following problems:
    (a) A large neck cystic hygroma with respiratory obstruction (Needle decompression for fluid drainage, initiation of antibiotics, and observation unless the situation is immediately life-threatening. Consider the administration of a sclerosing agent if imaging determines the cystic hygroma is macrocystic. The sclerosing agent may produce a transient edema for the first 24–48 h so careful monitoring of the airway is important. Recurrent episodes may lie in the future and some consideration should be given to prophylactic tracheostomy. A significant percentage will ultimately require tracheostomy in infancy or early childhood.)
    (b) Macroglossia (Wedge excision or possibly radiofrequency ablation).
    (c) A fronto-orbital lesion with vision obstruction (Excision).
16. What is the clinical picture of a venous malformation, also known as a cavernous hemangioma? Some typical locations? (A typical appearance is a soft and compressible lesion but expands with Valsalva. The skin usually has a bluish hue and is not directly involved although it may occur. Pain and tenderness may exist. Phlebolith or thrombosis in large lesions can result in firm, painful masses. The recommended prophylaxis is aspirin 80 mg. If the lesion expands rapidly in size following puberty, pregnancy, or trauma and an arteriovenous component is evident, reclassification may be indicated. A typical locations include intramuscular and intraosseous, although venous malformation may occur virtually anywhere in the body including mucosa, muscle, and within the viscera. Most are low flow. Mixed lesions of both lymphatic and venous malformations can also occur.)
17. What is the treatment for a low flow or venous anomaly of the head and neck? (The definitive treatment is total excision for cervicofacial venous anomalies. Workup including delineation of the extent is a necessity preoperatively. Observation as an initial treatment may be indicated. Sclerotherapy is a valid option as well as compression for extremity lesions.)
    (a) What is the radiologic appearance and management of an intraosseous venous malformation of the mandible? (Typically, a honeycomb appearance on X-ray with expansion of the cortices but not osseous destruction as more typically seen in an A-V malformation. The treatment of choice is mandibular resection and reconstruction.)
18. In a short sentence, discuss the essence of the pathophysiology of A-V malformation. (Multiple low-resistance arteriovenous shunts divert regional blood flow from the capillary bed and promote collateral formations and dilatation with involvement of the adjacent vascular tree. The venous component, because of the lower vascular resistance, becomes the preferential route for arterial flow and can become "arterialized".)
    (a) List five clinical characteristics of A-V malformations. (Pain, warmth, palpable thrill, bruit, skin necrosis, and destruction of adjacent bone. Congestive heart failure is late.)
19. Discuss imaging of A-V malformations. (Imaging can be accomplished with color duplex Doppler. More sophistication and detail particularly with extensive soft tissue involvement is obtained with MRI and contemporary CT angiography with 3-D reconstruction. Formal angiography is implemented as a preoperative modality in conjunction with embolization. See below. Until recently, formal angiography has been a "gold standard" to achieve anatomic detail in A-V malformations.)
20. Give a clinical classification (Most common is the Schobinger staging system:

    I Quiescent—pink-blue, arterio-venous shunt detected on Doppler.

    II Expansion—add enlargement, pulsations, thrill/bruit, engorged veins to I.

    III Destruction—add to II ulceration/bleeding, soft tissue necrosis.

    IV Decompensation—stage III plus congestive heart failure.

    Arteriovenous malformations may not be evident until childhood, although are present at birth. Progression through the stages will occur over time, perhaps accentuated in adolescence.)
21. How would you counsel a patient or parents of a patient who is under consideration for resection of a high flow A-V malformation? (Besides the obligatory discussion of intra-and postoperative complications, counseling should also include the high recurrence rate at 5 years—perhaps as high as 80%. Optimal results are obtained with Stage I and II lesions.)
22. Comment on the following treatment for high flow A-V malformation: proximal ligation of the external carotid, embolization of feeding vessels, resection. Characterize resection in terms of magnitude and scope and cure rate. (A proximal ligation of the external carotid is never indicated as a primary treatment modality and simply encourages collateral circulation, perhaps even from the internal carotid system that will make subsequent resection with the recurrence more difficult. Embolization as a preoperative maneuver that will facilitate resection 48 h later is quite useful but is also not indicated as a primary treatment. Resection needs to be considered as an en bloc or extirpative oncologic-type operation with the appropriate reconstruction.)

Vascular Malformations of the Extremities

1. The readings outlined the differential diagnosis and treatment of primary lymphedema. What are the diagnostic and treatment considerations? (Primary lymphedema will have a delayed onset after birth and even into early childhood. MRI imaging may help distinguish it from other anomalies such as a venous or mixed venous-lymphangioma. Primary lymphedema is optimally managed with nonsurgical methods such as compression stockings. Operative intervention is accomplished by liposuction with or without actual soft tissue excisions since the lymphedema process is extrafascial in location. Associated hypertrophy of the bone similar to lymphangiomas elsewhere, may produce lower extremity overgrowth.)
2. Name two syndromes that may appear similar in clinical picture to primary lymphedema. (Klippel-Trenaunay and Parkes Weber. Klippel-Trenaunay syndrome is a mixed lymphatic venous lesion and may have associated varicosities as a diagnostic clue. Parkes-Weber is relatively rare and has arteriovenous anomalies, progressing to fistula and a high flow lesion, associated with enlargement of the extremity.)
3. Summarize the problematic nature of venous malformations of the extremities. (Even if initially asymptomatic, venous malformations are inherently progressive and enlarge with time. The secondary problems of musculoskeletal changes including hypertrophy eventually will require treatment. Other issues include possible nerve compression, functional impairment, and even ulceration for which conservative treatment will be inadequate. The available treatment modalities include sclero therapy, pharmacologic management with sirolimus has demonstrable efficacy. Surgical excision directed toward specific symptomatic lesions can afford relief and in some instances, functional improvement. A significant proportion of patients will sustain localized intravascular coagulopathy and develop phleboliths.)

Case 1: Large Mass of Cheek

Case-Based Conference

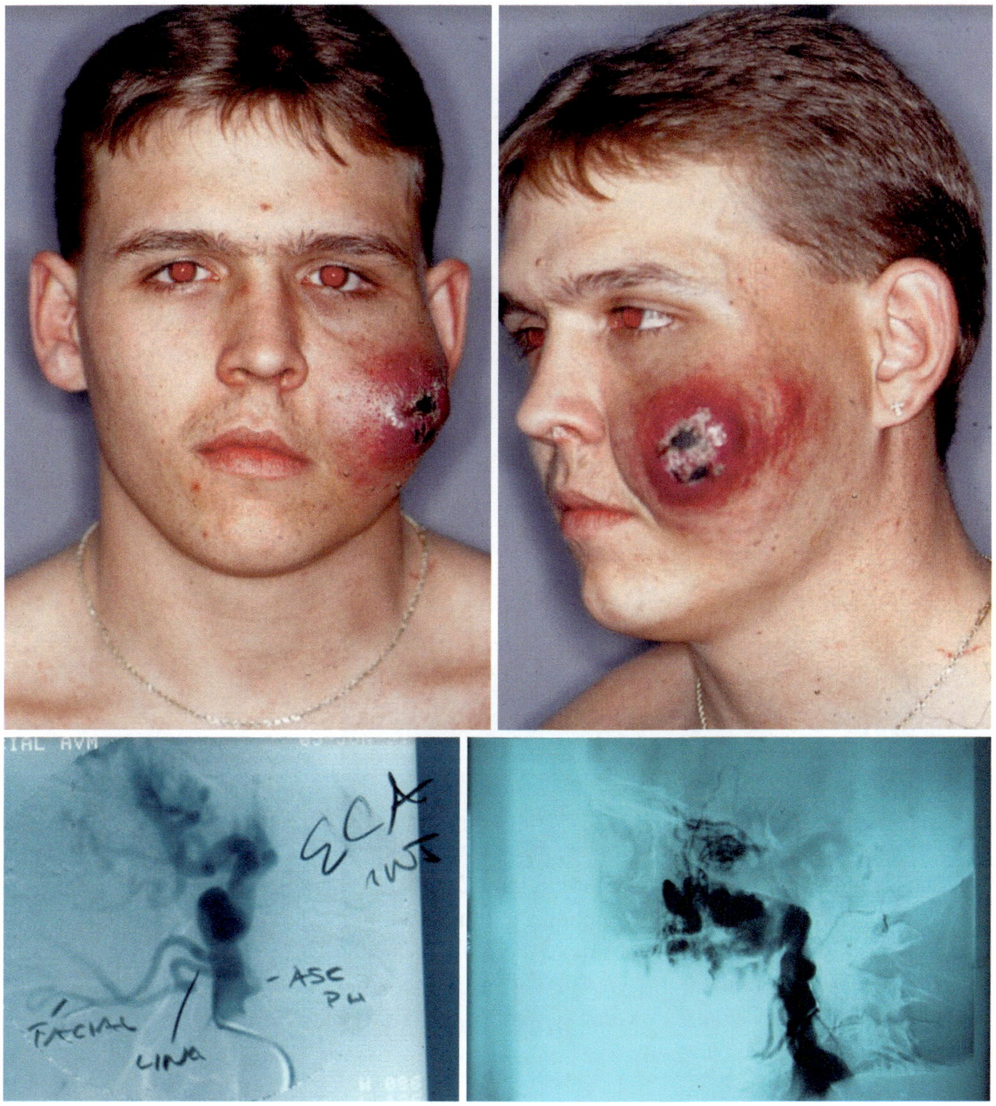

An 18-year-old who presents with a mass of the left cheek, present since birth. Over the past several years the mass has increased in size and over the past year has become ulcerated and bled on several occasions requiring transfusions. Provided are several views. In the last view (picture with head extended), the patient is performing a Valsalva maneuver. CT Scan demonstrates no bony abnormalities.

1. Describe what you see on the slides. Obtain a *pertinent* history and physical examination.
   (a) To the best of your ability, interpret the angiogram. What additional views of the angiogram would you have considered *essential* for the diagnosis/treatment (the venous phase was interpreted as extremely rapid)? Any additional diagnostic tests?
2. What is your diagnosis? What is the pathophysiology of your diagnosis?
   (a) What is the natural history of this lesion?
3. Outline a treatment goal. Outline your treatment plan, operative or non-operative.

Case-Based Conference: Discussion

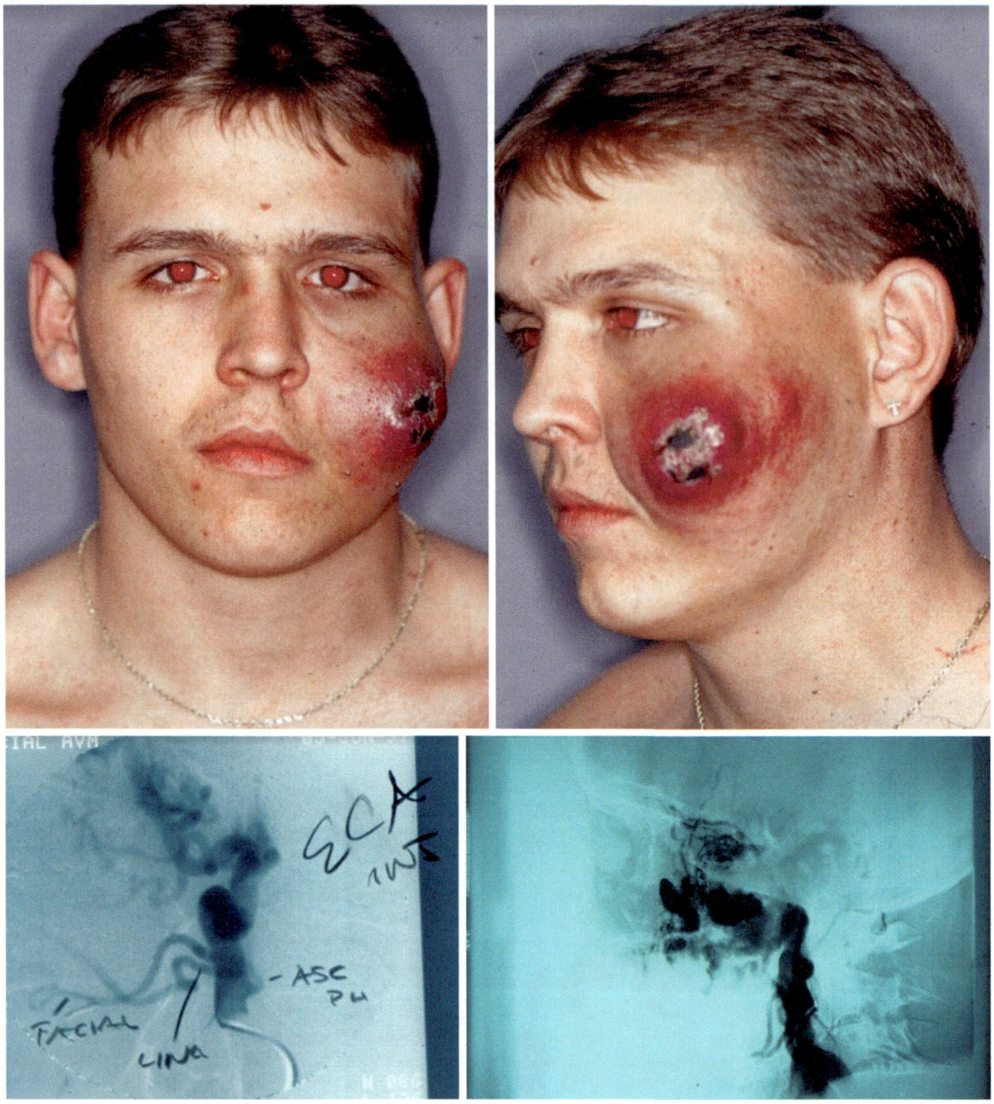

An 18-year-old who presents with a mass of the left cheek, present since birth. Over the past several years the mass has increased in size and over the past year has become ulcerated and bled on several occasions requiring transfusions. Provided are several views. In the last view (picture with head extended) the patient is performing a Valsalva maneuver. CT Scan demonstrates no bony abnormalities.

1. Describe the slide(s). (Young man with an obvious mass of the left cheek, ulcerated and erythematous, occupying the entire cheek with a rim of spared apparently normal skin in the preauricular area. The eye, nose, and adjacent lips are spared. The neck view with the patient's head turned to the opposite side demonstrates a prominent, large vein consistent with the external jugular.) Add a focused clinical examination. (The history would focus on the evolution re: present in early childhood, bleeding episodes, transfusions, specifics of past treatment including embolization and/or vessel ligation in the neck; assessment of the functional level by history with respect to exercise tolerance and/or any history suggestive of congestive heart failure; any history of intraoral bleeding with tooth extraction. The physical exam would focus on facial nerve functioning, palpation of the mass firmness, and a palpable thrill; palpate and auscultate the neck for a bruit. Intraoral exam for evidence of extension including involvement of the mandible.)
2. What is the pathologic anatomy/pathophysiology? (The mass probably represents a vascular anomaly, in particular an arteriovenous fistula, high flow. As Dr. Mulliken has described, a congenital nidus exists that contains A-V communications that usually lie dormant in early child-

hood. This stage is known as Schobinger I. Under perhaps hormonal or other influences, growth occurs in late childhood with perhaps multiple bleeding episodes, Schobinger II. Apparently, the channels or a-v communications enlarge and perhaps proliferate. Since the flow is from an arterial to a low-resistance venous system without passage through a capillary bed, a bed of higher resistance, the regional flow is increasingly preferential through the A-V malformation or fistula. As the fistula flow becomes dominant, a secondary cardiovascular effect occurs, consisting of increased cardiac output of increased heart rate and stroke volume which can culminate in congestive heart failure, Schobinger IV. The secondary cardiovascular effect can be demonstrated with a positive Nicolandi-Branham sign, bradycardia, and elevated diastolic followed by an increase in systolic blood pressure with digital compression placed on the a-v fistula, more commonly seen with a-v fistulas of a traumatic origin.

The pathologic anatomy of a head and neck A-V fistula consists of structures involved by the process such as the maxilla and/or mandible and the soft tissues of the parotid, masseter, and adjacent soft tissue.)

3. Outline a treatment plan. (Imaging should delineate the vascular anatomy as well as involvement or not of the skeletal structures. With respect to vascular imaging, the feeder vessels are outlined as well as the venous drainage. In this case, as depicted on the case images, the arterial feeders are derived from both the external carotid, lingual and facial, as well as the *internal* carotid through the ophthalmic artery, ethmoids, and in the case of a scalp A-V malformation, abnormal transosseous branches via the middle meningeal. The choice of modalities is the conventional arterial angiogram but more recently the use of both MRI and CT angiograms have been described. The latter, CTA, allows 3-D computer reconstruction, which, perhaps, allows more precise preoperative planning.

As described, the images demonstrate large arterial feeders from both the external and internal carotid with nearly instantaneous filling of the venous system including the external and internal jugulars. The maxilla and mandible are not involved. Since a portion of the arterial flow is from feeders from the internal carotid, preoperative (24–48 h) embolization, otherwise an optimal therapeutic modality, would not be useful in this situation. Similarly, percutaneous suture ligation of feeder vessels at the periphery of the lesion prior to resection would be of limited value, although has been described and would have little downside. The margin of the resection is the uninvolved skin-soft tissue but a preliminary cervical incision and identification of the carotid system would be advisable, should vascular clamping be a necessity for a life-saving maneuver in face of torrential hemorrhage. Resection should be accomplished en bloc with soft tissue margins placed in grossly uninvolved skin. Reconstruction in this instance is accomplished with free tissue transfer of a fascio-cutaneous flap such as the radial forearm.

Postoperative (4 Months)

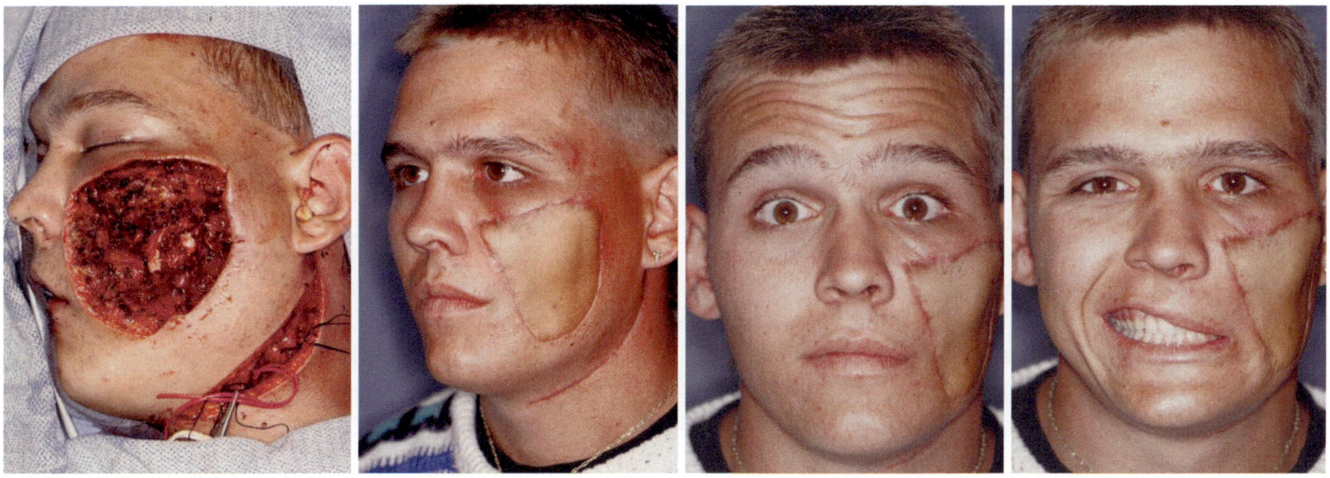

The single intraoperative photo demonstrates the operative approach which consisted of an initial cervical incision, identification, and isolation of the carotid vessels, and dissection of the recipient artery, the facial. The resection of the lesion was considered as an en-bloc excision, analogous to an oncologic operation. The postoperative photos include an oblique view of a well-healed flap and neck incision. The two additional frontal views depict intact facial nerve function with the notable exception of the buccal branch.

Critique

The principal criticism is the poor color match of the radial forearm flap. An option would have been a pre-expanded supraclavicular artery flap, harvested either as a pedicled or free flap for "blush" area skin.

In-Service Examination

1. A 10-year-old presents with venous malformation and multiple enchondromas. The syndromic diagnosis is:
   (a) Sturge-Weber
   (b) Parkes-Weber
   (c) Rendu-Osler-Weber
   (d) Maffucci
2. An infant has a large macrocystic lymphangioma of the upper arm. Treatment with what agent may be efficacious?
   (a) Doxycycline
   (b) Propranolol
   (c) Steroids
   (d) Recombinant VEGF
3. What is the appropriate treatment for an enlarging A-V malformation of the cheek?
   (a) Sclerosing agent and compression
   (b) Ligation of the ipsilateral carotid artery
   (c) Angiographic embolization
   (d) Angiographic embolization and surgical resection

Ear Deformities: Anatomy, Embryology, Otoplasty

24

Bibliography

Porter, C. J. W. and Tan, S. T., "Congenital Auricular Anomalies: Topographic Anatomy, Embryology, Classification, and Treatment Strategies", *Plast. Reconstr. Surg.*, (2005); 115(6):**1701–1706 ONLY**.

Larrabee, W.F. and Makielski, K.H., Chapter 15: "Ears" Surgical Anatomy of the Face, Raven Press, (1993); **pp 177–85.**

Beahm EK and Walton RL, "Auricular reconstruction for microtia: Part I. Anatomy, embryology, and clinical evaluation", *Plast. Reconstr. Surg.*, (2002); 109(7):**2473–2475 ONLY**.

Janis, J., Rohrich, R.J., Gutowski, K.A. "Otoplasty", *Plast. Reconstr. Surg.*, (2005); 115:**60e–72e.**

Hoehn, J.G. and Ashruf, S. "Otoplasty: Sequencing the Operation for Improved Results", *Plast. Reconstr. Surg.*, (2005); 115:**5e–16e.**

Thorne CH and Wilkes G, "Ear Deformities, Otoplasty, and Ear Reconstruction", *Plast. Reconstr. Surg.*, (2012); 129(4):**701e–703e and Video 1.**

Savetsky IL, Cohen JM, Avashia YJ, Byrd HS, "Revisiting Primary Otoplasty: Surgical Approach to the Prominent Ear", *Plast. Reconstr. Surg.*, (2021); 148(1): **Videos 2, 3, 4 ONLY.**

Comments: Read Porter section on embryology first. Then read Larrabee for an overview and the first five pages of Furnas. The Hoehn reference is for details on otoplasty as is the video from the Thorne reference.

Faculty Discussion and Study Guide

Anatomy, Embryology

1. Discuss the embryology of the ear. (Six hillocks, three on each side of the first branchial cleft. The external ear is derived from the first or mandibular arch and the second or hyoid branchial arch. The first arch contributes to the tragus, the root, and the anterior superior helix. The second arch contributes to the antihelix as well as the remaining helix and lobule. Second arch derivatives develop into the lobule, concha, and the antihelix including the inferior crus. The free ear fold develops into the superior crus, scapha, and the remainder of the helical rim. See Fig. 24.1.)
   (a) What are the implications for lymphatic drainage? (The derivatives of the first or mandibular arch drain toward the parotid and anterior cervical nodes; the derivatives of the hyoid or second arch drain posteriorly into mastoid and posterior cervical nodes.)
2. Discuss the normal dimensions and measurements of the external ear as well as the normal location on the skull. In particular, what are the key elements for the correct positioning of the ear on the skull? (The height of the male ear in the adult is about 6.2 cm with a width of about 55% or 3.5 cm. The normal distance from the helical rim to the skull or mastoid is 12, 16, and 20 mm respectively at the superior, middle, and conchal helical rim locations. The ear is located approximately one ear length from the lateral canthus and sits 15° off vertical in a posterior direction. Finally, a line drawn from the lateral canthus intersects the superior and middle one-third of the ear.)
   (a) The ear has achieved 85% of adult size by what age? (3 years). The vertical height of the ear is attained at the level of 90% of the adult by what age? (approximately at age 5, 55/62 mm)
3. Label the particular topographical landmarks on the following drawing of the external ear. See Figs. 24.2 and 24.3.
4. Anatomy: Innervation
   (a) If you pick your ear with a toothpick you might cough. Why? (Innervated by Arnold's nerve, a branch of cranial nerve X.)
   (b) A postoperative parotidectomy patient complains of numbness of the tragus and anterior ear. Why? (Auriculo-temporal branch of cranial nerve V is resected with the parotidectomy)

E. Luce, *A Curriculum for Plastic Surgery*, https://doi.org/10.1007/978-3-031-62087-4_24

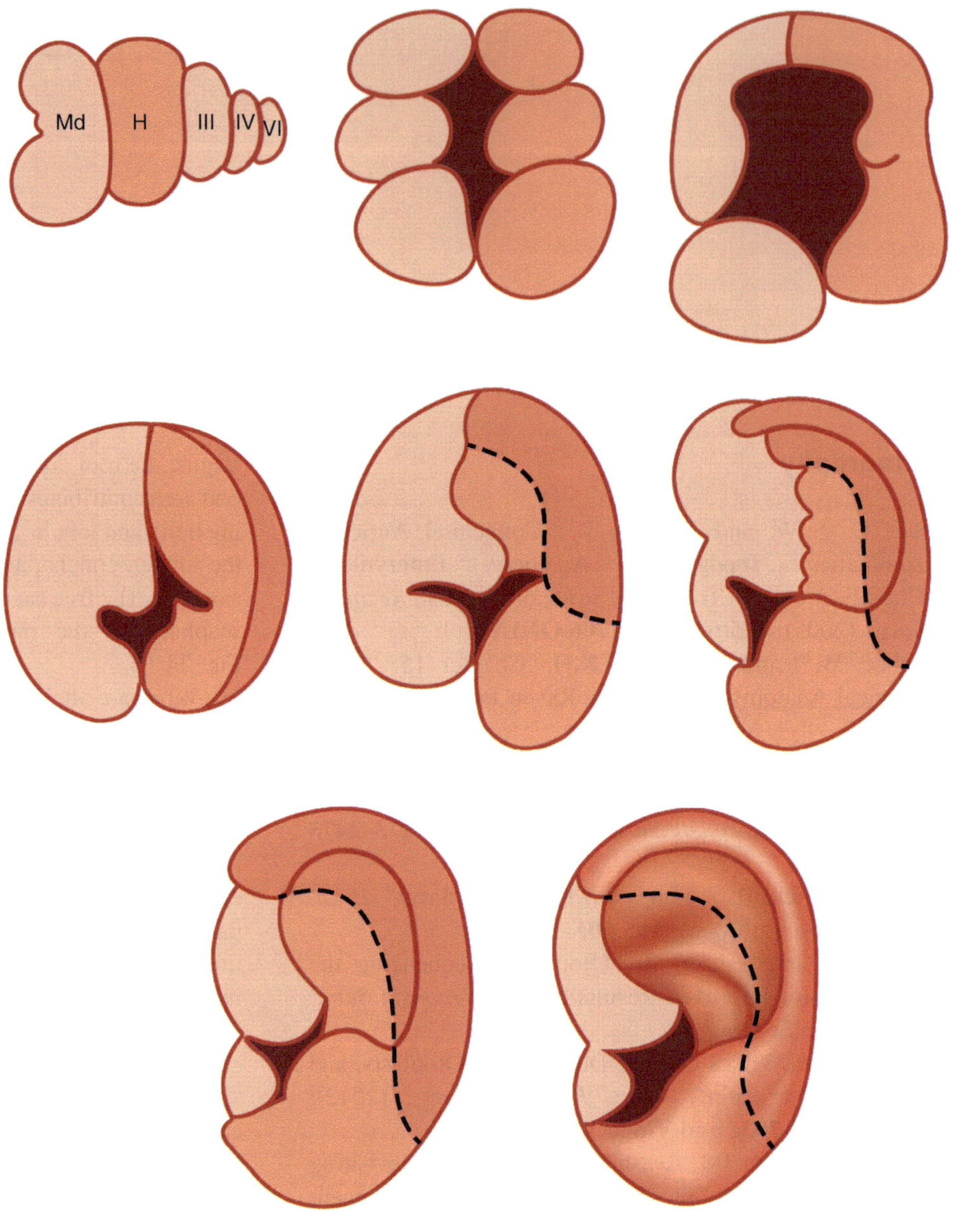

Fig. 24.1 Embryology of the ear

(c) The postoperative face/neck lift complains of numbness of the lobule. Why? (The greater auricular nerve branch of the cervical plexus has been damaged)

5. A patient has a clean transection of the external ear. In the OR you identify two named arteries for reimplantation. What are they? (Superficial temporal and the posterior auricular arteries.)

Otoplasty

1. Describe the anatomical basis of the prominent ear. (Several factors play a role in the prominent ear: (1) conchal excess or deep conchal bowl; (2) inadequate antihelical fold particularly the superior and perhaps inferior crus with absence of a triangular fossa; (3) a conchal scaphal angle of >90°. Of course, all of these factors can coexist in the same patient.)
2. What are the anatomical goals of otoplasty? (1) A smooth, rounded, and well-defined antihelical fold including both superior and inferior crus; (2) a helical/scaphal angle of 90° or slightly less; (3) reduction of the conchal-mastoid angle or height of the lateral lip of the concha. Other anatomical considerations include lateral projection of the helical rim beyond the visible antihelix and correct posterior orientation of the lobule.

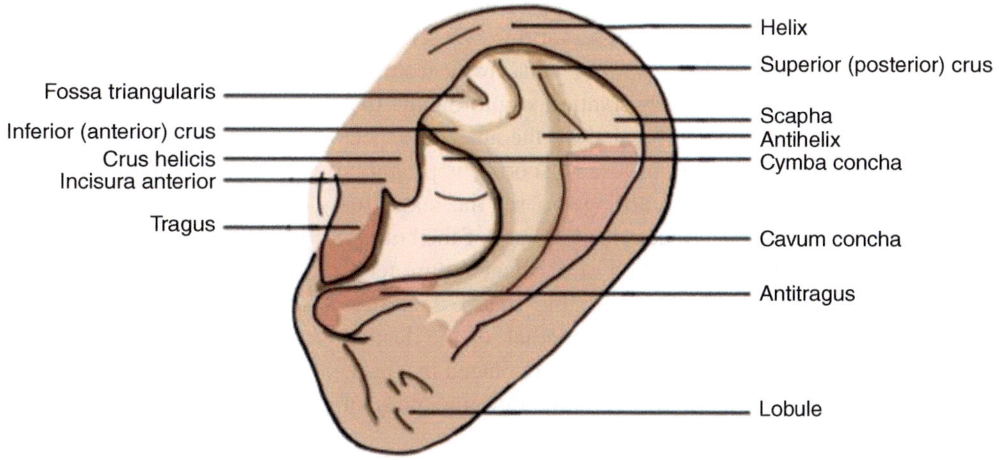

Fig. 24.2 Topographical landmarks

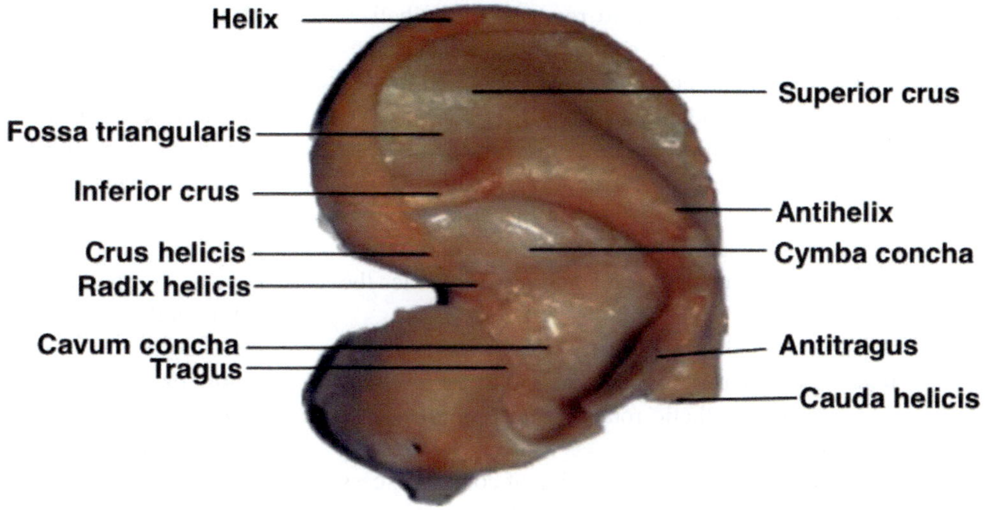

Fig. 24.3 Topographical landmarks of the cartilage

3. Discuss nonsurgical correction of prominent ears including timing. (Taping or molding may accomplish correction but only if begun within a few days postnatal.)
   (a) What is the explanation for the urgency of initiation of taping? (Probably the presence of circulating maternal estrogens in the immediate postnatal period.)
   (b) Outline the protocol described in the readings. (The newborn with an ear deformity is observed for about 1 week for spontaneous resolution which can occur in up to one-third of the cases. The ear conformer is built as described in the article and remains in place for approximately 2 weeks with three cycles performed over a total of 6 weeks. Some skin irritation and, uncommonly, ulceration can occur.)
4. Briefly, describe the contributions to otoplasty of the following: Luckett, Stenstrom, Mustardé, Furnas. (Luckett over 100 years ago described the basic pathology of protruding ears; Stenstrom described scoring of the cartilage on the anterior surface, following the concept of Davis and Gibson who hypothesized the cartilage will warp in the opposite direction of scoring or trauma; Mustardé described the use of cartilaginous sutures to produce the missing antihelical fold and superior crus. Furnas contributed to the use of concha–mastoid sutures for the prominent conchal bowl.)
5. What is the appropriate timing for an otoplasty in a child? (Probably 5–7 years, although certainly could be performed at age 4. A series has been published of otoplasties performed at age 2 with an unacceptably high recurrence rate.)
6. Describe access. (Most commonly, a postauricular sulcus incision or excision with undermining to the edge of the helical rim.)
7. Describe the main technical features of creation of the antihelical fold. (Scoring of the cartilage and suture fixation. Other techniques rely upon full thickness incision of the cartilage using parallel incisions to recreate the fold and may create undesirable sharp edges.)

(a) Scoring of the cartilage as a component of otoplasty rests on what scientific observation? (Observation that cartilage tends to warp or bend away from the injured surface. This observation would dictate that scoring should be performed on the anterior aspect of the cartilage. The purpose of scoring is probably more to weaken the cartilage to set the stage for suture techniques. Access is at the tail of the helix.)

8. Describe the Mustardé method of cartilage suture technique. (Placement of nonabsorbable mattress sutures placed on either side, lateral and medial, of the desired curve of the cartilage. These sutures are placed in a horizontal mattress fashion through the full thickness of cartilage.)
9. How would you determine if conchal excess or a "deep" concha exists? (One method is to simply fold the ear back into a normal position to recreate an antihelical fold and then examine the concha. Absolute measurements do exist as outlined in the anatomical portion of this discussion and study guide.)
10. Describe a method of reduction of the conchal excess. (A description by Furnas consists of nonabsorbable, full thickness mattress sutures placed in the posterior conchal cartilage and suturing into the mastoid fascia thus rotating the concha medially and anteriorly to reduce the height.)
    (a) What is the potential hazard? (Reduction and perhaps obstruction of the external auditory canal as well as an unaesthetic rotation and prominence of the tragus.)
11. Describe another technique. (Excision of conchal excess can be performed as well. These procedures are usually carefully measured as to the magnitude of the excision and the incision placed through a posterior approach to the conchal bowl. The excision site is then repaired and usually, the anterior skin is allowed to contract without concomitant excision. Anterior incisional scars are visible.)
12. You have performed cartilage scoring, Mustardé sutures, and a conchal excess resection and viewed the results. What is apparent is that the lobule is rotated anteriorly and projecting. What is the problem and the correction? (Not an uncommon scenario particularly in the presence of correction of conchal access. The solution is relatively simple and consists of an initial rotation of the tail of the helix posteriorly and sutured to the conchal bowl. Excision of excess lobule skin from a posterior approach usually through a fishtail excision design can be added if necessary.)
13. Instead of the scenario described in the previous question, you detect a "telephone" deformity. What is the problem and how can be corrected? (Telephone deformity refers to the prominence of both the lobule inferiorly and the superior helical rim. The correction of the lobule is as described in the prior question. Correction of the helical rim requires additional cartilage scoring as well as replacement of the Mustardé sutures to ensure that the helical rim is more medially or posteriorly placed. The middle one-third of the ear should be carefully inspected to determine if overcorrection with sutures has occurred with the helical rim not visible over the antihelix. Most commonly the technical error of superior rim prominence is failure to undermine sufficiently superior to enable placement of the first Mustarde suture superior or cephalad to satisfactorily recreate the superior crus.)
14. Give a postoperative management regimen (Hematoma can be a disastrous occurrence and the operative dressing is designed to minimize the potential for hematoma. Saline or glycerin cotton balls are molded into the ear contours and a large bulky head dressing is then applied. The dressing remains in place for 5 days, followed by the use of a sweat headband that is worn 24/7 for the next month to 6 weeks.)
15. What would you quote the parents of a child on whom you will do an otoplasty about complications with respect to recurrence and or reoperation? (Figures vary widely. The recurrence rate with Mustardé sutures alone without cartilage scoring is about 15% and is higher than combined scoring and sutures. The overall recurrence rate on average of several series is about 7%. Reoperation for scar revision, recurrence, and suture sinus is approximately 8–10%. Uncommonly, the posterior auricular sulcus incision hypertrophies.)

Case 1: Protruding Ears

Case-Based Conference

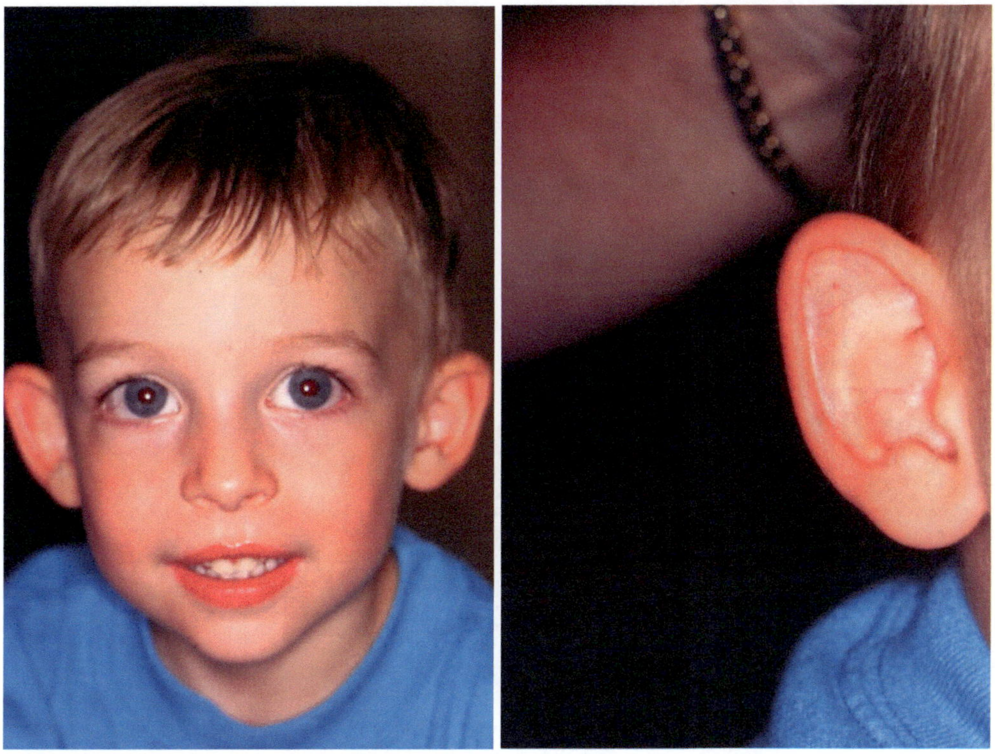

A 4-year-old referred by the pediatrician.

1. Describe the slides, and add a clinical exam.
   (a) What views are missing that would be helpful in the determination of the treatment plan?
   (b) Are any tests indicated? The child has normal hearing.
2. Assume you see the child at the age of 1 month. What would be the treatment plan?
3. What is the pathologic anatomy?
4. Give a menu of treatment options. Select one and justify, then describe.

Case-Based Conference: Discussion

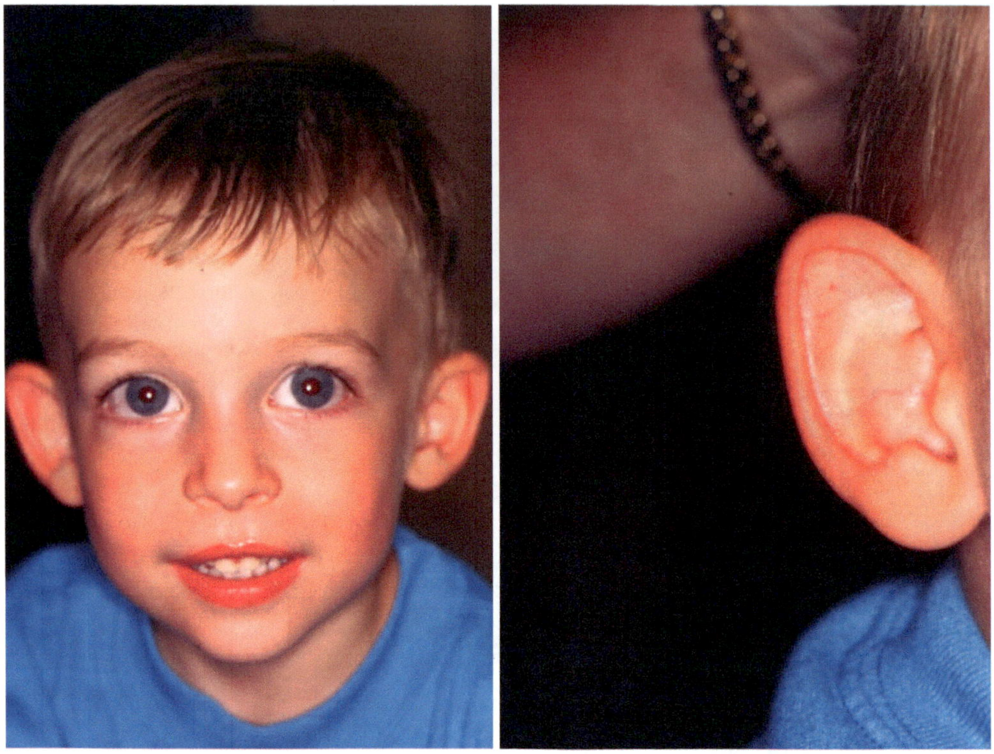

A 4-year-old referred by the pediatrician.

1. Describe the slides and add a clinical exam. (Two photos are provided, a frontal view of the head and neck and an anterior close-up of the right ear. The full face, with the exception of the ears, is of a normal-appearing young boy of his stated age. No facial skeletal deformity, specifically hypoplasia of the zygomas nor mandible, is evident. The periorbital structures appear normal without evidence of epibulbar dermoids. The ears are slightly blurry in the photo but clearly are protruding bilaterally and symmetrical. The close-up of the right ear illustrates several features of the protruding ear. The helical rim, lobule, tragus, and antitragus are normal and a suggestion of the inferior crus is present. No superior crus is evident and the scaphoid, although flat, is broader than in a normal ear. The conchal scaphal angle is >90°. A crus of the helix dividing the concha into a cymba and cavum is absent and as a result, the concha is featureless and also deep. The lobule is rotated somewhat anteriorly.

   The clinical examination would initially pursue any diagnosed congenital comorbidities including cardiac and renal. A short review of the child's developmental milestones would be appropriate as well. The preamble states the child has normal hearing. The physical exam focused on the ear will assist in the evolution of an operative plan. Observation followed by some key measurements including the vertical height and three points of the distance from the helical rom to the skull and mastoid. The three points are superior, the junction of superior and middle one-third, and at the level of the mid concha. The normal dimensions are 12, 16, and 20 mm, respectively. The ear should be gently folded posteriorly to recreate, if possible, the superior crus, assess the contribution of the conchal excess to the protuberance, and the element of the anterior rotation of the lobule.
   (a) What views are missing that would be helpful in the determination of the treatment plan? (The essential photographic documentation is the full frontal face, anterior and lateral views of each ear, and a view from the posterior.)
   (b) Are any tests indicated? The child has normal hearing. (In the absence of comorbidities, no.)
2. Assume you see the child at the age of 1 month. What would be the treatment plan? (The timing of nonsurgical management of ear deformities is as a neonate. The cartilage is malleable because of the influence of circulating maternal estrogens which diminish rapidly in the postnatal period. A number of systems are available to implement ear molding. At 1 month a partial correction may be obtained but parents should be counseled that surgical correction will ultimately be necessary, deferred until childhood.)
3. What is the pathologic anatomy? (As embodied in autologous microtia reconstruction, the cartilage framework

consists of three tiers in different planes: the helix and lobule; antihelix, tragus, and antitragus; and the concha. The Y-shaped configuration of the antihelix is crucial to the topography of the external ear. The stem of the Y parallels the helical rim inferiorly and then courses superior and anterior into a superior and inferior crus with an intervening triangular fossa. The scaphoid fossa or scapha is located between the superior crus and the superior helical rim. The bases of the protruding ear have in part lost a portion of the antihelix, most notably the superior crus. The other important component is a prominent concha science even in the presence of well-defined antihelical superior crus, a prominent concha can be solely responsible.)

4. Give a menu of treatment options. Select one and justify, then describe. (To list the procedures described for the correction of prominent ear recapitulates the history of the development of otoplasty. Luckett described the pathology but attempted correction with skin excision only. The principal contribution of Stenstron was to utilize the observations of Gibson and Davis that cartilage abraded perichondrium on one surface will tend to warp in the direction of opposite or intact perichondrium. Mustarde managed otoplasty by utilization of posterior sutures to recreate the missing superior crus and antihelical fold. The use of Mustarde sutures alone has been attended by a significant incidence of recurrence. The optimal treatment plan in this patient must address the components of the deformity, listed in the response to question 3. Accordingly, the operative sequence would be a postauricular incision with perhaps a conservative skin excision, an approach to the anterior surface of the cartilage via the tail of the antihelix, an abrasion of the anterior cartilage consistent with the principle of Stenstron. Once abraded, the cartilage is folded posteriorly and secured with horizontal mattress sutures of permanent material, the Mustarde sutures. The suture location is determined by a transcutaneous needle with the ear folded into the desired position and then ink marks are created in the cartilage by methylene blue placed within the lumen of the needle. Three locations, superior, middle, and inferior corresponding to the measurement sites described above will permit a sequential approach. A single knot in each enables the determination of adequate correction.

   The final two components are the address of the concha and lobule, in that order. Prior to the final secure of the Mustarde sutures, a decision is reached if the anterior rotation of an intact concha by the use of conchal-mastoid sutures will be sufficient. The principal limiting factor is the progressive encroachment of the external auditory canal by aggressive conchal-mastoid sutures. If so, conchal resection is necessary to accomplish by a posterior approach. A 4–5 transverse segment of the mid portion of the bowl is excised and repaired with 2–3 sutures. Anterior skin excess will plicate but resolve with time rather than a direct excision and the result is an invisible scar. Anterior lobule rotation can be repaired with a posterior skin excision by a variety of designs.

   Prior to placement of the compressive headdressing, the result should be judged from several perspectives. The optimal result, judged anteriorly, is an outcome marked by a helical rim just visible above the antihelix and readily a discernible superior crus. The unacceptable "telephone" deformity is represented by an abnormal anterior rotation of the superior helical rim and anterior rotation of the lobule. Both must be corrected. The latter is discussed above, and the former, protrusion of the helical rim is usually secondary to the need for a more superior and anterior undermining and placement of an additional Mustarde suture.

   A dressing carefully molded into the topographic configuration of the reconstructed ear and design for comfort is applied and remains in place for 5 days.)

Postoperative

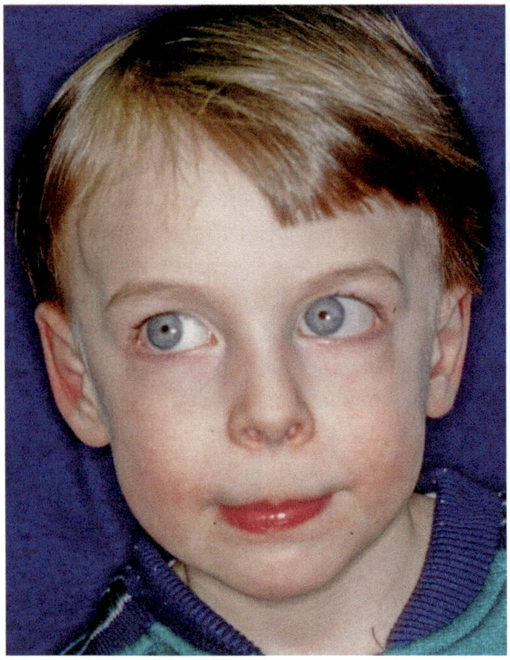
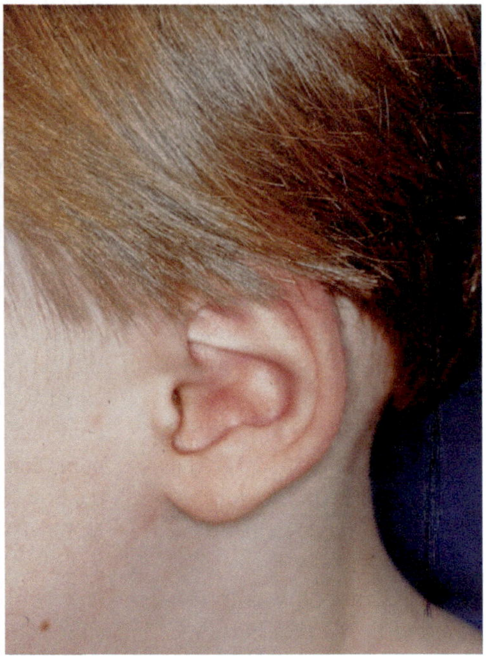

Two postoperative photos are those of a frontal head and neck that fills the frame of the photo and a close-up lateral view of the left ear. The most superior aspect of the helical rim is partially obscured by some hair. The former depicts an excellent aesthetic with the aesthetic criteria of correction of the protruding ears, preservation of the helical rim visible just lateral to the antihelical rim, correction of the conchal access, rotation of the lobule into a vertical position, and symmetry. The lateral close-up represents a recreation of the superior crus and a resemblance to a helical crus.

In-Service Examination

1. A postoperative patient complains of numbness of the tragal area. What nerve is involved?
   (a) Nerve of Arnold
   (b) Auriculotemporal
   (c) Facial
   (d) Anterior branch of the greater auricular
2. Furnas contribution to otoplasty is:
   (a) Description of the basic pathology
   (b) The anterior abrasion of ear cartilage
   (c) The use of conchal-mastoid sutures
   (d) The use of helical-antihelical cartilage mattress sutures
3. Cryptotia describes which of the following ear anomalies?
   (a) Absence of external auditory meatus
   (b) Upper pole helical rim buried beneath mastoid skin
   (c) Notching of the superior helical rim
   (d) Contralateral scapha with lidding of the helical rim

25 Ear Deformities: Congenital Deformities

Bibliography

Beahm, E.K. and Walton, R.L., "Auricular Reconstruction for Microtia: Part I. Anatomy, Embryology, and Clinical Evaluation", *Plast. Reconstr. Surg.*, (2002); 109(7):**2475–82 only**.

Wilkes, G.H. M. D., et al., "Microtia Reconstruction", *Plast. Reconstr. Surg.*, (2014); 134: **464e–476e. Including Videos 1–4.**

Thorne C.H., Wilkes G., "Ear Deformities, Otoplasty, and Ear Reconstruction", *Plast. Reconstr. Surg.*, (2012);129(4):**701e, 705e–714e ONLY, and Videos 2–5.**

Yamada, A., Chwa, E.S.; Boctor, M.J., "Update on Total Auricular Construction", *Plast. Reconstr. Surg.*, (2024);153(5):**1011e, Figure 1 ONLY.**

Reinisch J, Tahiri Y, "Polyethylene Ear Reconstruction: A State-of-the-Art Surgical Journey", *Plast. Reconstr. Surg.*, (2018); 141(2): **Videos 2–4, 461–470.**

Daniali, L. N. M.D., et al., "Classification of Newborn Ear malformations and their treatment with EarWell Infant Ear Correction System", *Plast. Reconstr. Surg.*, (2017); 139:681 **Videos ONLY.**

Paredes, Jr., A.A., et al., "The Constricted Ear", Elsahy, N. I., Clinics in Plastic Surgery, Elsevier Saunders, (2002); 29:**289–299.**

Bauer BS, Ch. 32 "Nonmicrotia", *Pediatric Plastic Surgery, Second Edition, Volume II,* (2017); **956–68 ONLY.**

Thorne MD, C. H., Brecht, L. E., Bradley MD, J. P., et al., "Auricular Reconstruction: Indications for Autogenous and Prosthetic Techniques", *Plast. Reconstr. Surg.*, (2001); 107(5):**1241–1251.**

Joukhadar N, McKee D, Caouette-Laberge L, "Management of Congenital Auricular Anomalies", *Plast. Reconstr. Surg.*, (2020); 146(2):**206e–207e, 212e–214e.**

Supplemental

Walton, R.L. and Beahm, E.K., "Auricular Reconstruction for Microtia: Part II. Surgical Techniques", *Plast. Reconstr. Surg.*, (2002); 110(1):**234–244 Only**.

Faculty Discussion and Study Guide

Clinical Exam and Workup Microtia

1. What are the types of microtia? (Lobular—absence of the ear with exception of the lobule; concha-type—presence of concha, lobule, acoustic meatus, tragus, and incisura; small concha—lobule and conchal indentation only. Anotia is complete absence.)
2. Give Tanzer's clinical classifications of auricular defects.
   (a) Anotia
   (b) Complete hypoplasia (microtia)
      - With atresia of the external auditory canal
      - Without atresia of the external auditory canal
   (c) Hypoplasia of middle third of auricle
   (d) Hypoplasia of superior third of auricle
      - Constricted (cup and lop) ear
      - Cryptotia
      - Hypoplasia of entire superior third
   (e) Prominent ear
3. Microtia can be considered as a part of the spectrum of what other craniofacial anomaly? (Hemifacial microsomia. Even though clinically no associated mandibular or temporal bone anomalies are evident in a patient with microtia, radiologic or imaging may detect underlying deformation.)

E. Luce, *A Curriculum for Plastic Surgery*, https://doi.org/10.1007/978-3-031-62087-4_25

4. What is the VECTER syndrome? (The syndromic picture has the following anomalies: vertebral, ear as microtia, cardiac, tracheo-esophageal, and renal.)
5. What ethnic groups have a high, relative, incidence of microtia? (Native American, Japanese.)
6. What, besides the ear, should the clinical exam include? (Associated anomalies of the mandible, facial nerve, occlusion, and the maxilla. Attempt to determine the presence of cardiac or renal defects.)
7. Besides a clinical exam, what diagnostic tests are indicated? (CT scan of the temporal bone and the status of the middle ear; MRI if indicated based on CT findings for the course of the facial nerve; audiologic including brain-stem evoked response. To determine the degree of conduction or sensorineural hearing loss.)
8. What is the nature of the hearing loss in microtia patients? (80–90% is conductive in nature, but 10–20% is sensorineural. So, in addition to the imaging studies discussed above audiologic including a brain-stem evoked response is indicated. In addition, the status of an atretic external auditory canal should be accomplished, particularly to rule out a cholesteatoma.)
9. A patient with bilateral microtia is seen by you at 3 months of age. What is the priority in the management? (To be fitted for hearing aids and evaluated for possible middle ear surgery. If the more contemporary implantable bone-anchored aids are selected that procedure needs to be coordinated with respect to stages, incisions, etc. Since the otologist would prefer the placement of the bone-anchor device in the post-auricular skin, a conflict may exist. A cutaneous bone conduction hearing aid may be used as a bridge in individual cases.)
10. As traditionally viewed, is middle ear surgery indicated in unilateral atresia with contra lateral normal hearing? (Not necessarily. More contemporary thought is given that children with only unilateral hearing loss appear to be at risk for delayed language development, etc. Some consideration should be given to middle ear surgery despite normal hearing in the opposite ear.)
    (a) True or false: A strong correlation exists between the external deformity and the degree of hearing loss. (In general, no.)
    (b) What are the approximate success rates of middle ear surgery in unilateral microtia? Bilateral? (70% and 50% respectively.)

Reconstruction of Microtia

1. One reading generally classifies ear anomalies into deformational when all components are present but deformed and malformational when some components are missing. What are the treatment implications of that classification? (Conceptually, deformational ear anomalies should be successfully treated as a neonate or in early infancy with nonsurgical means such as taping and molding, as discussed later. Clearly, if components of the external ear are absent surgery will be required.)
2. What is the appropriate timing for reconstruction of microtia and what are the factors? (Age 7 seems to be the consensus, but some more contemporary thought particularly in Asia is perhaps as late as 10 years old, see below. The three factors are the achieved height of the normal ear at a particular age, the potential for peer group abuse in school, and chest-wall deformity produced by harvest of the costal cartilage)
    (a) Do reconstructive ears grow? (Yes, the evidence from Brent's study is that over half of the ears grow "substantially," 40% "some" and 10% not at all.)
3. Contrast autologous versus alloplastic reconstruction of the ear (Donor site versus retention/safety. Autologous reconstruction requires harvest of cartilage with the potential for growth deformity as well as complications such as pneumothorax. Alloplastic reconstruction obviously does not require a donor site but may have a significant extrusion rate and long-term retention problems with the inevitable trauma of childhood. The final score is still out.)
4. What are the complications related to the rib donor site? (Deformity, pneumothorax)
    (a) How minimized (Retain the posterior perichondrium)
5. What are the central components of the four stages of Brent's reconstruction (Carving autologous cartilage from lateral costal 6–8 ribs, implantation, rotating the lobule remnant, elevation of the framework from the mastoid, and construction of the tragus and concha.)
    (a) What are the common criticisms of Brent's technique? (The number of reconstructive stages involved, lack of definition of the concha into cymba and cavum, loss of projection over time.)
6. Which ribs are used for what parts of the framework? (The "floating" rib 8 is used for the helical rim, the synchondrosis of ribs 6 and 7 for the concha, and the antihelix or base of the ear.)
7. How does the Brent method address the following situations?
    (a) A low hairline (Brent simply implants the ear cartilage in the desired and correct position on the skull and deals with the hair overlying the superior portion of the ear construction with electrolysis or in more severe cases with resurfacing with a skin graft and/or ablation of the hair. Minor degrees can be addressed with creation of a slightly smaller ear.)
    (b) Secondary reconstruction (Excision of the auricular scar, placement of sculpted autogenous rim cartilage

graft, and coverage with a temporoparietal fascial flap and skin graft.)
 (c) Exposure of the framework (Acutely, exposure of the underlying cartilage in the framework before vascularization is complete can be problematic. Exposure considerably later in the postoperative course, weeks or months, of a relatively small area can be managed simply with dressings to allow granulation tissue and secondary contracture and/or small graft. Exposure of alloplastic reconstruction is almost certainly doomed to failure.)

8. Outline the relative merits of Brent's technique vs. Nagata. (Each technique has their proponents. In Brent's hands, the results are excellent. Criticism is some loss of projection of the ear in some cases with the second stage or elevation of the cartilage framework from the skull. Nagata addresses this potential shortcoming with an accentuated height of the initial cartilage framework. Nagata's technique requires harvest of considerably more cartilage than Brent and to avoid chest wall deformity he defers reconstruction until the age of 10.)
9. What is specifically different about Nagata's technique of ear reconstruction? (Incorporation of the tragus into the initial framework rather than as a second stage, higher cartilage relief, use of more costal cartilage, use of temporoparietal flap in every case, two rather than three stages.)
 (a) How does Nagata achieve increased ear projection? (Incorporation of three levels or "floors" of cartilage framework; base or concha, crus and scapha, and triangular fossa as the second, and the antihelix and helical rim and tragus as the third; thus duplicating more closely the normal ear cartilage framework.)
10. What is accomplished with the second stage of the Nagata approach? (Increased projection of the ear by a posterior incision, placement of a wedge of banked ear cartilage, application of a temporoparietal fascial flap and full-thickness skin graft. This corresponds to Brent's elevation of the ear cartilage and placement of the full-thickness skin graft.)
 (a) What are the criticisms of Nagata's technique? (The magnitude of costal cartilage harvested and possible chest wall deformity, perhaps an increased incidence of skin necrosis because of the stress placed on the skin envelope by the accentuated height of the cartilage framework, use of the temporoparietal flap at the second stage ordinarily reserved for salvage procedures by other surgeons.)
11. What is the role of tissue expansion in ear reconstruction? (Currently, controversial. The criticism of the use of expanded skin is that the capsule obscures the fine details of a cartilage framework and even with excision of the capsule a similar criticism applies. Certainly, the attempt to expand scarred skin is inadvisable.)
12. Prosthetic ear reconstruction is discussed in Chap. 31. What are some appropriate indications in the microtia patient? (The failed reconstruction with a heavily scarred skin envelope. Severe skeletal and soft tissue hypoplasia. A familial decision after counseling may occur in select circumstances.)
 (a) The principal advantage is the absence of a donor site and attendant deformity as well as the ability to provide an ear at an early age. The disadvantages include the necessity for daily care and periodic prosthetic replacement.)
13. Alloplastic ear reconstruction is an alternate option to autogenous. Describe the key elements. (A large temporoparietal fascia flap, 10 × 13 cm, is utilized to cover a prefabricated porous polyethylene framework. The posterior or medial surface is covered with a full-thickness skin graft harvested from the groin, and the lateral or anterior surface with anterior ear skin remnant and mastoid skin. The entire construct is covered with a compression dressing.)
 (a) Advantages and disadvantages? (The principal advantage are construction of an ear at a relatively early age which has substantial psychosocial benefits. A chest wall donor site is avoided. Disadvantages relate to the propensity of alloplastic materials to become exposed and once exposed are usually condemned to loss. A thin skin envelope predisposes to such minor trauma. Alopecia can occur in the scalp donor site.)
14. Comment on the four videos from the Thorne paper.

 Videos 2 and 3—A comparison of the two methods of autogenous ear reconstruction: A more detailed carving by Wilkes included incorporation of a tragus and an increased height which appeared to enhance the final result similar to Nagata.

 Video 4—Alloplastic reconstruction with a Medpor framework was a single-stage procedure with simultaneous reconstruction of the ear canal. Use of multiple full-thickness skin grafts to ensure soft tissue coverage. Good result but the follow-up was 9 months only.

 Video 5—A prosthetic ear reconstruction that consisted of a comprehensive detailed step-by-step construction of the actual prosthesis, with less detail about the preparation of the recipient site. Prosthetic ear reconstruction will be covered more fully in the skin cancer module.

Other Ear Deformities, Cup or Constricted Ear

Editor's Note: Partial ear defects secondary to trauma or cancer resection are discussed in the skin and soft tissue tumor (Chap. 31).

1. What is a common thread? (Helical lidding with flattening of the helical arch, collapse of the scapha and triangular fossa, particularly the superior crus, upper pole compression, as well as reduction in the vertical height of the ear. The spectrum is one of a mild degree to one of severe deficiency of both skin and cartilage, absence of the triangular fossa and scapha and significant shortening of the vertical height of the ear. Failure to recognize these components is probably what leads to inadequate or failed correction.)
   (a) Extra Credit: Not specifically mentioned by the reading but what other component of the deformity becomes increasingly evident with worsening of the severity of the deformity? (Positioning of the ear on the skull more inferior)
2. What are the principal features of the cup ear? (As above. Deep concha, deficient superior helical rim and superior crus of the antihelix, and downward rolling of the helical rim and scapha to cover the superior pole of the ear. Or expressed differently, helical rim overhang with flattening and shortening of the circular arch formed by the rim, vertical compression of the scapha and triangular fossa, loss of the antihelix, and protrusion of the ear from the mastoid.)
   (a) What factor is responsible for a decrease in the vertical height of the ear; helical rim length or scapha-fossa compression or both? (Both)
3. Tanzer-Cosman classification of cup ear deformity provides a guide for surgical correction. Describe. (I—lidding of the helical rim only; IIa—more severe lidding of the helical rim and scapha, IIb—as in IIa but the necessity for adding additional skin and soft tissue, III—severe with significant reduction in the vertical height to the ear. The emphasis is on restoration, as much as possible the normal vertical height of the ear.)
   (a) What is another method or dimension to the classification? (Lidding, but <1 cm of vertical height discrepancy, 1–1.5 cm discrepancy, >1.5 cm discrepancy)
   (b) Treatment implications? (If <1 cm, can simply do excision and posterior suture technique; if 1–1.5 cm. cartilage rearrangement but no skin addition would be necessary; if >1.5 cm, the same plus skin flaps are necessary.)
4. How can one demonstrate conceptually what must be accomplished to correct a cupped ear? (Manually raising the helical rim overhang or lidding superiorly demonstrates that the scapha is compressed vertically and deficient and probably the helical circumference is inadequate. Once those two components are corrected then something still must be done to restore the antihelical crus and fossa.)
5. In the analysis of what is required for reconstruction, in addition to correction of cartilage deformity or deficiency, what other primary decision must be made? (Skin rearrangement and/or addition since a skin deficiency may exist as well. Excess skin is present posteriorly but deficient anteriorly.
6. Define cryptotia. (Cryptotia is the congenital deformity of the superior helical rim that consists of concealment beneath the adjacent temporal scalp.)
   (a) A repair? (A skin deficiency exists that can be addressed by the release of the retracted helical cartilage and placement of the full-thickness skin graft. On occasion the cartilage may be sufficiently deformed and require an address.)
7. Discuss the nonsurgical management of congenital ear deformities. (The only opportunity for nonoperative management is as a neonate with a limit of 4–6 weeks of age. The use of conformers that can be adjusted as the deformity is corrected can be optimally applied to prominent ears but have been utilized to treat other deformities as well.)
   (a) What is the explanation of the time limitation? (Circulating maternal estrogens).
8. What is Stahl's ear and how is it corrected? (Stahl's is an abnormal third crus that projects transversely from the antihelix toward the helical rim, usually at the junction of the superior and middle third. The result is some malformation of the scapha and helical rim. Operative correction consists of excision of the third crus from the rim, repair of the helix and scapha, and plus or minus augmentation of the superior crus with the cartilage.)

Case 1: Ear Deformity

Case-Based Conference

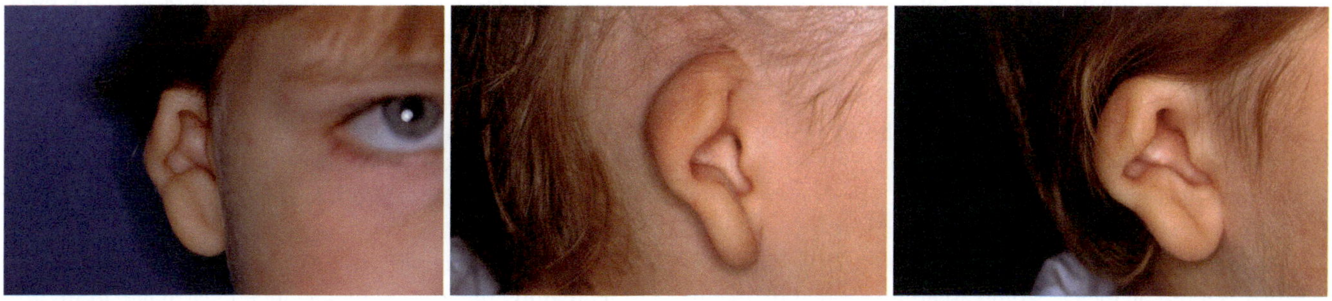

A 5-year-old with an ear deformity since birth. The vertical height of the ear is 3.1 cm. The other ear is normal in appearance.

1. Describe what you see in the slides. Do the slides eliminate other associated facial deformities? If so, what and what not?
   (a) Add a pertinent physical exam.
   (b) Are any imaging and/or lab studies indicated?
2. Describe the pathologic anatomy and relate same to the normal anatomy.
3. Outline a treatment plan including operation(s). Begin by citing the overall goal(s).

Case-Based Conference: Discussion

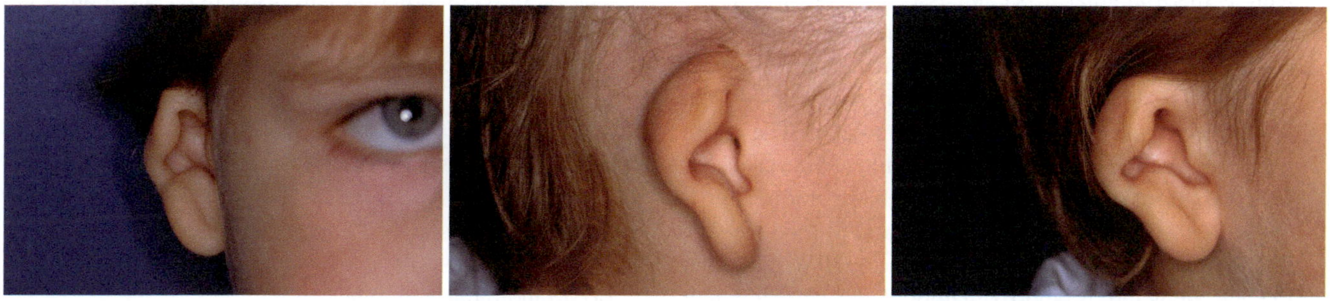

A 5-year-old with an ear deformity since birth. The vertical height of the ear is 3.1 cm. The other ear is normal in appearance.

1. Describe what you see in the slides. Do the slides eliminate other associated facial deformities? (Three views of an ear are provided. The frontal view includes the ear and just the lateral portion of the eye and adjacent temporal region. Several components of the deformity contribute to the configuration of the ear. The entire ear appears small vertically and anteriorly rotated. If a horizontal line is drawn from the lateral canthus, the position of the ear on the skull is approximately normal. The lobule is present and normal or perhaps large in size and anteriorly rotated. The concha is present but without a division into a cavum or a cymba. No discernible superior portion of the ear exists including the scapha, superior and inferior crus, and triangular fossa. A short portion of the medial superior helical rim is evident and the remainder consists of approximately 1–1.5 cm of what appears to be skin and soft tissue alone. The remaining two views are lateral and anterior oblique, both of which confirm impressions from the frontal view. The lateral view detects an external auditory meatus that may be stenotic and demonstrates the magnitude of the anterior rotation, particularly the lobule. The superior one-half of the ear, in contrast to the impression from the frontal view, appears to have a rim of cartilaginous support. The lower one-half of the ear is entirely lobule. A tragus and antitragus is present. No preauricular pits or sinuses are seen in any slide.) If so, what and what not? (No, although in the small portion of the visible lateral face, the area of the lateral zygoma and zygomatic arch appears normal. The diagnosis of Treacher Collins, craniofacial microsomia, and Goldenhar syndromes all

associated with congenital ear anomalies, are all possible. Missing is a posterior view of which would be of benefit to design the reconstruction.)

(a) Add a pertinent physical exam. (The past medical history would center on the detection of any cardiac, pulmonary, or renal congenital anomalies. The thrust of the initial consultation would be the determination, if possible, of the impact of the deformity on the child as well as the presence of a hearing deficit in the involved ear. The head and neck component of the physical exam would assess facial bones, mandible in particular, but also midface and zygoma. Attention centered on the ear would ascertain the height, manually lift the upper 1–1.5 superiorly and posteriorly, and examine the external auditory meatus. Otoscopic exam would complete the clinical evaluation.)

(b) Are any imaging and/or lab studies indicated? (In the absence of any associated facial anomalies, no imaging is indicated. Routine chemistries would be advisable including BUN and creatinine as well as CBC.)

2. Describe the pathologic anatomy and relate it to the normal anatomy. (The clinical scenario depicted in the slides is a moderately severe cup or lopear. The principal pathologic anatomy is compression and loss of the scapha as well as the triangular fossa and associated crura or complete superior pole collapse. The severely shortened helical rim has significant lidding, overhang, and anterior rotation. The lobule is enlarged out of proportion to the remainder of the ear and is anteriorly rotated. The entire ear protrudes from the skull and is quite short vertically. If two assumptions are established; one, the normal vertical height of the adult ear is 6.2 cm and second, by age five the growth of the ear is 90% of the adult height, then the ear depicted is approximately 2–2.5 cm deficient vertically.

   The Tanzer classification of the deformity is IIb or sufficiently severe to require the addition of both cartilage and skin envelope. Another classification, Cosman, determines the *measured* magnitude of the vertical deficiency. If <1 cm, managed with suture techniques alone, 1–1.5, cartilage and skin rearrangement, >1.5 cm the necessity for addition of skin and cartilage.)

3. Outline a treatment plan including operation(s). Begin by citing the overall goal(s). (The goals of the reconstruction are to increase the height of the upper pole or overall height of the ear, restore the scapha and fossa, rotate the reconstruction into a more normal auricular-cephalic angle, and rotate the lobule posteriorly. To do so, since the vertical deficiency is 2–2.5 cm, the design and approach will need to provide for the addition of cartilage and skin envelope. Since an excess of skin exists posteriorly, an approach performs incisions on the posterior aspect of the ear to create an inferior-based flap of 2 cm in width that incorporates some adjacent mastoid skin. The tip of the flap is located at the most medial aspect of the helical rim and scalp, the base at the point of an additional incision at the level of the external auditory meatus, transversely through both skin and cartilage, if present, to the lip or edge of the concha. The posterior flap is raised inferiorly and the anterior skin is superiorly to expose the underlying deformed and deficient cartilage. The cartilage is carved and released with a "barrel-stave" or "wagon wheel" configuration adding cartilage to increase the vertical height, linking and recreating the rim with an added cartilage graft also harvested from the opposite ear. The now-assembled cartilage is rotated and sutured to the skull-mastoid fascia. The resultant skin envelope deficit is addressed by rotation of the previously raised inferior-based post-auricular flap horizontally and anteriorly into the transverse incision. The inferior and posterior edge of the anterior skin flap is rotated into the flap defect. This design resembles a Z-plasty.

   A second stage addresses the dogear of the flap at the mid-helical rim and adds a full-thickness skin graft if necessary for release of the post-auricular sulcus. This method of reconstruction will result in an ear about 1 cm shorter than the opposite, presumably normal ear, a difference not perceptible to the observer.

In-Service Examination

1. Microtia has associated congenital defects of the following **EXCEPT**:
   (a) Mandibular hypoplasia
   (b) Preauricular pits
   (c) Inner ear
   (d) Cervical spine
2. Successful neonatal ear folding is possible because of what hormone?
   (a) Prolactin
   (b) Estrogen
   (c) Progesterone
   (d) Growth hormone
3. An 8-year-old male, status-post 2 months first stage autologous rib cartilage reconstruction presents with a 1 cm area of cartilage exposure. What is the appropriate treatment?
   (a) Dressing changes
   (b) VAC
   (c) OR for irrigation, debridement, and secondary closure
   (d) Graft removal

Part III

Skin, Soft Tissue Tumors

26 Skin, Soft Tissue Tumors: Pathogenesis, Work-Up, Syndromes

Bibliography

Mancebo SE, Hu JY, Wang SQ, "Sunscreens: A review of health benefits, regulations, and controversies", *Clin. Plast. Surg.*, (2014); 32:**721–31 ONLY.**

Netscher DT, Spira M, "Basal Cell Carcinoma: An Overview of Tumor Biology and Treatment", *Plast. Reconstr. Surg.*, (2004); 113(5):**74e–82e.**

Mendez BM, Thornton JF, "Current Basal and Squamous Cell Skin Cancer Management", *Plast. Reconstr. Surg.*, (2018); 142(3):**373–81.**

Netscher, DT, Leong M, Orengo I, et al., "Cutaneous Malignancies: Melanoma and Nonmelanoma Types", *Plast. Reconstr. Surg.*, (2011); 127(3):**37e–48e ONLY (including video 2 up to "Melanoma")**

Burton K, Ashack KA, and Khachemoune A, "Cutaneous Squamous Cell Carcinoma: A Review of High-Risk and Metastatic Disease", *Am. J. Clin. Dermatol.*, (2016); 17:**491–501 ONLY.**

Cumberland L, Dana A, Liegeois N, "Mohs Micrographic Surgery for the Management of Nonmelanoma Skin Cancers", *Facial. Plast. Surg. Clin. N. Am.*, (2009); 17:**325–335.**

Connolly KL, Nehal KS, Disa JJ, "Evidence-Based Medicine: Cutaneous Facial Malignancies Nonmelanoma Skin Cancer", *Plast. Reconstr. Surg.*, (2017); 139:**181e (Video 1 ONLY)**.

Knackstedt TJ, Knackstedt RW, Djohan M, et al., "New Developments in the Management of Cutaneous Squamous Cell Carcinoma", *Plast. Reconstr. Surg.*, (2021); 147(3):**499e–500e (To Advanced Disease) ONLY.**

Ahmad FI, MD, Su SY, Gross ND, "The Role of Sentinel Lymph Node Biopsy in the Management of Cutaneous Malignancies", *Facial. Plast. Surg. Clin. N. Am.*, (2019);27:**119–126 ONLY.**

Faculty Discussion and Study Guide

Sunscreens, Epidemiology

1. Outline the three components of UV light; what portion of the UV spectrum do they each respectively occupy and the significance of each. (C: 1–290 mm and absorbed completely by the stratosphere; B: 290–320 for the part blocked by the stratosphere but highly erythemic and responsible for most skin cancer; A: 320–400 and is 95% of UV light that strikes the earth's surface but is not thought in the past to be a significant agent in skin cancer. Currently, the thought is that UVA can play a symbiotic role with UVB in skin cancer by impairment of the immune rejection of UVB-induced malignant mutations. UVA may be the principal agent in solar-induced skin aging.)
2. Environmental factors that increase the UVR exposure? (Latitude, altitude, time of day, season.)
3. How do we measure the effectiveness of sunscreen? (SPF, sun protective factor).
   (a) What is it? (Ratio of a fixed dose to produce minimal erythema in protected versus unprotected skin exposed to UVR or the MED.)
4. For the most part, commercial sunscreens with SPF values have been developed to block what UV rays? (UVB.)
   (a) What wavelength? (290–320 mm). What is the wavelength of UVA? (320–400 mm.)
5. The lifeguard at the pool has a thick white sunscreen cream on his nose, what is it? (Zinc or titanium oxide.) What is the advantage if any? (A physical agent that blocks all UV rays and has little incidence of allergic or contact sensitivity.)
6. Your postoperative facelift patient relates an allergy to sunblocks. In all likelihood, what is the agent responsible? (PABA, or para aminobenzoic acid or a derivative.

E. Luce, *A Curriculum for Plastic Surgery*, https://doi.org/10.1007/978-3-031-62087-4_26

Since 2012, most, if not all, sunscreens do not contain PABA.)

7. Give the Fitz Patrick classification of skin types. (A classification from 1 to 6 of a spectrum that consists of the most pale skin that burns readily and never tans through six which consists of deeply pigmented skin that never burns.)
   (a) White, always burns, never tans
   (b) White, usually burns, difficulty tanning
   (c) White, sometimes mild burns, moderate tans
   (d) Moderate brown, rarely burns, easily tans
   (e) Dark brown, rarely burns, easily tans
   (f) Black, no burns
8. What is the current theory about the role of UV light in the production of skin cancer? (Ultraviolet light may create breaks in the DNA and allow these to be perpetuated by DNA replication. Alteration in the p53 suppressor gene may also occur. These breaks are mutagenic and represent a cancer phenotype.)
   (a) Besides the induction of DNA replication errors, how else does UV play a role in skin cancer? (Possibly immunosuppression by loss of Langerhans cells and increase in suppressor T cells.)
9. How does the geographic and anatomic distribution of squamous cell carcinoma, SCCa, versus basal cell carcinoma, BCCa, support the hypothesis that solar exposure plays a larger role in etiology of the former compared to the latter? (Those areas of the globe that have greater direct sunlight exposure, such as the equator, have a higher incidence as well as those areas of the body that have a higher amount of solar exposure.)
   (a) What is one possible histological explanation? (BCCa arises from the basal or deeper layers of the skin while SCCa arises from the Malpighian or more superficial layer.)
10. Actinic keratoses are the epidermal precursors of squamous cell cancer (SCCA) and basal cell cancer (BCCa) True or False? (False—SCCa only.)
11. Discuss arsenical keratosis in terms of body distribution, appearance, and precursors to what specific pathologic entity. (Usually acral or palmar/plantar, punctate lesions that lead to Bowen's disease but can also occur elsewhere in a non-solar exposure distribution.)
   (a) How might a patient be exposed to arsenic? (In the past most commonly medicinal solutions; otherwise industrial contact.)
12. Name two conditions present at birth that will set the stage for development of basal cell carcinoma, BCCa. Explain each. (Xeroderma pigmentosum: autosomal recessive that is a congenital inability to repair UV-induced DNA damage; basal cell nevus syndrome-skin is prone to basal cell development in young adults.)
   (a) EXTRA CREDIT: Name a third. (Sebaceous nevus of Jadassohn.)
13. In addition to the two congenital conditions mentioned earlier what are the other systemic and local predisposing causes for nonmelanotic skin cancer (Immunosuppression, chronic arsenic exposure; local radiotherapy, chronic wound, sebaceous nevus, porokeratosis, PUVA therapy.)
   (a) Which carcinoma predominates in immunosuppressed or scar cancer patients? (Squamous cell carcinoma.)
   (b) What are the findings in basal cell nevus syndrome? (Bifid ribs, keratocysts of the mandible, multiple basal cells, and red-brown nevi particularly an occurrence in young patients with a diagnosis of BCCa especially in non-sun exposed areas. The basal cell nevus syndrome is autosomal dominant.)
   (c) Describe the appearance of sebaceous nevus in early childhood. (Early in childhood the appearance of a plaque-like yellow slightly pebbled lesion that in later childhood and adolescence becomes more pigmented and more verrucous appearance.)
   (d) What is the treatment? (Excision because of a conversion rate of 20% to BCCa.)
   (e) Describe the defect and clinical picture in xeroderma pigmentosa. (Clinical picture is that of a young child deeply freckled with photophobia and perhaps already the development of either basal cell or squamous cell cancer. The defect is a congenital one of failure to repair ultraviolet light DNA damage. Xeroderma pigmentosa is autosomal recessive with a diminished life expectancy secondary to the development of melanoma and SCCa.)
14. What is Bowen's disease? (A superficial erythematous plaque of various sizes frequently distributed in a non-solar distribution that on histological examination is a squamous cell carcinoma in-situ but 3–11% can become invasive. An association with visceral cancers is controversial but may occur if the etiological agent in Bowen's disease is arsenical exposure.)
   (a) What is erythroplasia of Queyrat? (Genital Bowen's variant but perhaps a higher percentage of invasive conversions than Bowen's disease elsewhere on the body.)
   (b) EXTRA CREDIT: Link this discussion to London chimney sweeps and Percival Potts.
15. True or False: The increased incidence of skin cancer in renal transplant patients is primarily basal cell. (False, renal transplant patients have a markedly increased incidence of squamous cell carcinoma.)
   (a) What skin lesions coexist in these patients? (Multiple keratoses and keratoacanthomas.)

Basal Cell

1. What is the evidence from proportionate head and neck distribution of primary and recurrent BCCa that illustrates the point that either excision is compromised in certain areas *or* such areas are intrinsically predisposed to recurrence? (Lower eyelid, nasal tip and nostril, nasolabial, pre- and postauricular, medial canthus have a disproportionate number of recurrent lesions.)
2. What are some explanations for the ability of some aggressive basal cell carcinomas to spread sub-clinically, i.e., well beyond the clinically evident border? ("Path of least resistance" so periosteum, perichondrium, fascia, tarsal plate are resistant, and bone and cartilage are invaded late; embryonic fusion lines of philtrum, nasolabial fold, medial canthus, post and pre-auricular.)
3. In summary, what is a recommended approach to the classification of BCCa? (Classify grossly first, for example, nodular-ulcerative, superficial scaling, morpheaform, pigmented; then classify histologically as circumscribed or diffuse.)
4. Describe the gross appearance of the following: superficial scaling, morpheaform, nodular. (Nodular is as the name implies a well circumscribed nodule, at times ulcerated, lesion; superficial scaling is again as the name implies a scaling lesion with indistinct border, horizontal rather than vertical growth; morpheaform has a flat, ill-defined border often of considerable size.)
5. Discuss methods of biopsy including pros and cons. (An excisional biopsy with adequate, 2–4 mm margins can be done for well-defined nodular basal cell carcinoma and accomplish both diagnosis and treatment in the same procedure. This method can be applied if no functional or cosmetic deficit is thus created. The most common incisional biopsy technique is a punch biopsy which gives a pathological diagnosis without lesion excision in toto. Shave biopsy is commonly done by dermatologists.)
6. List the factors you would consider in the determination of margins. (Size, location, primary versus recurrent, gross appearance or type, histological appearance.)
7. Discuss two or three treatment modalities including the pros and cons of each:

   (Curettage and desiccation: no pathology report and scars are often hypopigmented. The only pro is the simplicity which explains why the vast majority of dermatologists use this modality. Cryotherapy: only good for patients with so many lesions that excision is not possible. 5-FU, Retin-A, and imiquimod all share the same cons, namely, marked inflammatory response and are not curative for skin cancer. The pro is that these agents eradicate other actinic changes and may define skin cancers more fully. Radiation therapy: the principal pro is that no operation is required. Many cons include the absence of pathology report, concealment of persistence-recurrence, and long-term radiation damage. Excision: pro is excision eradicates the cancer in 95–98% of the cases. The principal con is the necessity in some instances for reconstruction and the resultant scarring. Moh's: Actually, shares the same pros and cons as excisional therapy *except* presumably may achieve more complete extirpation.)
8. Describe the recommended margins in the following: 1 cm nodular BCC of cheek (3–4 mm), 1 cm morpheaform of the cheek (6 mm), 2 cm nodular BCC of the forehead (6 mm), 1 cm recurrent BCCa of the postauricular sulcus (10 mm).
   (a) What margin is recommended in a nodular basal cell 2.0 cm in diameter? (6–10 mm, depending on the site.)
   (b) With that margin what will be the percent of adequately excised lesions? (96–98%.)
9. One of your cosmetic patients seeks your opinion about a small basal cell of the cheek that the dermatologist has recommended curettage and desiccation. (Curettage has a tendency for hypopigmentation and hypertrophic scarring, apparently a high recurrence rate in the head and neck, may miss aggressive basal cell carcinomas. Not recommended for lesions >5 mm and/or poorly-defined borders. Appears to be popular with dermatologists.)
10. Outline the role of radiotherapy in the management of BCCa. (The overall cure rate appears to be somewhat lower than either excision or Mohs technique. The results are poor in recurrent lesions and not indicated in aggressive BCCa. Radiotherapy appears best for a frail patient with a small lesion in an essential area such as eyelid, but other surgeons would favor excision with the appropriate anesthesia. The underlying problem is concealment of persistent-recurrent disease as well as the deterioration in appearance over long periods of time.)
    (a) A patient who had a recurrent BCCa of the temple was excised with flap reconstruction. The final pathology revealed a close or positive margin. Tumor board has recommended radiotherapy. What is your decision? (Radiation therapy is not appropriate management of a positive margin in basal cell carcinoma. If approximately 1/3 of peripheral positive margins in BCCa excision will eventually recur, one treatment option is observation. Another option, of course, is re-excision. Re-excision is probably mandated in a positive deep margin.)
    (b) If not radiotherapy, what is the appropriate management? (The factors in decision to re-excise are histologic appearance, i.e., aggressive morpheaform and infiltrating strands of tumor versus pushing borders, horizontal, diffuse growth pattern without periph-

eral palisading, magnitude of margin involvement, deep rather than peripheral margin, and finally, patient compliance.)

11. Estimate the risk of new lesions in basal cell carcinoma and squamous cell carcinoma patients. (5-year incidence of 18% in squamous cell carcinoma and 45% in basal cell carcinoma.)

Squamous Cell

1. Express some figures that illustrate the aggressive behavior of recurrent SCCa. (30% metastasis rate, overall mortality in recurrent lesions is 25% which is a sum of the mortality rate in metastatic disease, 20%, plus 5% mortality in nonmetastatic).
2. Give the T classification in SCCa of the skin.
   T1 is a lesion <2 cm in diameter.
   T2 is 2–4 cm in diameter.
   T3 is more than 4 cm in diameter.
   T4 invasion into muscle or bone.
   (a) What is the approximate metastasis rate of a T2 SCCA of the skin? (30%.)
3. What are the histological variables that indicate the propensity, or lack of, for recurrence and metastasis in SCCa? (Degree of differentiation, depth of invasion, perineural invasion.)
   (a) Define objectively the risk of regional metastasis versus depth. (If >4 mm, risk of regional metastasis increases dramatically.)
4. What are other risk factors for recurrence and metastasis? (Particular location on the face such as the ear and mask or midface; size >2 cm; rapid growth; immunosuppressed patient, recurrent lesions, and occurrence in a chronic scar or ulcer.)
5. What is the propensity for and significance of lymph node metastases? (The incidence is 4–6%, higher in SCCa of the ear, immunosuppressed patients, scar carcinoma, and perineural invasion. Lymph node metastases have a significant adverse impact on survival, 30% at 5 years.)
6. Explain the role, if any, of sentinel lymph node biopsy of squamous cell carcinoma, SCCa, of the skin. (High-risk cutaneous SCCa have a rate of nodal metastases as high as 10–20%, depending on the characteristics of the cohort. Sentinel lymph node (SLN) biopsy, and detection of possible occult lymphadenopathy have a potential role but the available data is limited. Consideration should be given, if the experience is available, to SLN biopsy in SCCa with features of thickness >4 mm, size >2 cm, poorly-differentiated, and recurrent lesions.)
7. You have a patient with a 3 cm SCCa of the temple with palpable parotid nodes. What is your management? (Fine needle aspirate of the parotid nodes; resection with a superficial parotidectomy plus modified radical neck dissection plus postoperative radiotherapy; 30% probability of positive cervical nodes if the parotid has positive nodes; palpable nodes almost always signifies extracapsular extension which is an indication for irradiation.)
   (a) If a metastasis does develop with squamous cell carcinoma of the head and neck, when will most of those occur? (90%, 3 years from the initial diagnosis.)
8. The readings outline margins for excision of SCCa: (Size-dependent, <2 cm in size, well differentiated on histology without fat invasion, and <4 mm depth of invasion, would recommend 4 mm margins which should yield a 95% cure rate. Consider risk factors as less histologic differentiation, >2 cm in size, invasion >6 mm into the fat—all of which may dictate 6 mm or perhaps more margins, particularly if larger than 2 cm.)
9. You excise a 2 cm SCCa of the cheek and reconstruct it with a sliding cheek flap. The final pathology examination reveals a positive margin at one edge. The residents suggest radiation therapy. (Radiation therapy probably is not an appropriate option because of the overall relatively poor control for recurrence and the concealment of possible recurrence by the fibrosis of radiation changes. In contrast to BCCa, positive margins in SCCa should never be managed by observation. Overall mortality, as noted above, in recurrent lesions is 25%. Re-excision and reconstruction should be accomplished.)
10. You are requested to see a patient with giant condyloma of the vulva. After excision and split thickness skin graft the pathology returns as carcinoma in-situ, the GYN consultant advises p.o. RT to prevent recurrence. Good idea? (No). Why? (Convert to aggressive SCCa.)
    (a) Name of entity? (Buschke-Lowenstein.)
11. What is the typical history and physical findings in keratoacanthoma? (The history is that of very rapid appearance and growth, literally in weeks, with possibly some spontaneous regression. The appearance is that of an exophytic well-defined lesion with a keratin plug and microscopic findings of in situ SCCa.)
12. You are referred to a patient with a biopsy proven squamous cell carcinoma in an old burn scar of the thigh. The lesion is about 3 cm in size. What are the considerations in management? (The principal consideration is the aggressive nature of burn scar carcinoma in terms of recurrence and regional metastasis. A wide excision as well as therapy directed toward the inguinal nodes, at least a sentinel lymph node biopsy, is indicated. These lesions are referred to as Marjolin's ulcers and can occur

in not only old burn scars but chronic osteomyelitis and even chronic leg and perineal wounds. The lag time is substantial, 25–30 years, but becomes shorter with advancing age of the patient with the original injury.)
   (a) What are the indications for biopsy? (Rolled and elevated edges, surrounding induration, recent change, a diagnosis of pseudoepitheliomatous hyperplasia.)
13. What is the entity of pseudoepitheliomatous hyperplasia? (A pathological diagnosis seen in Marjolin's ulcers and scar cancer and may be a precursor of SCCa.)
   (a) Spindle cell cancer? (Highly undifferentiated and may be difficult to distinguish from sarcoma; poor prognosis.)
14. The readings briefly describe a regimen of oral agents that may be effective in a highly selective population of patients with advanced SCCa. What are they? (Retinoids and interferon.)

Mohs Micrographic Surgery

Describe the advantages and technique of Mohs micrographic surgery contrast with other conventional methods of tissue sectioning from microscopic examination. (Mohs micrographic surgery is a method of immediate frozen tissue examination of the specimen. The specimen is ordinarily sectioned horizontally, instead of the vertical sections performed with conventional histologic examination. Sampling of the lesion site is done until all three-dimensional aspects are cleared of tumor. The principal advantages of micrographic surgery are immediate examination of all potential interfaces of the tumor with normal tissue, an office setting, use of local anesthesia, and finally examination of the tissue by the surgeon instead of a second party. Vertical sectioning or sampling techniques of the specimen may miss peripheral margin involvement between vertical sections. This method is purported to yield lower recurrence rates. Other methods include total marginal control which consist of excision of the tumor, a relatively narrow margin followed by additional 2–3 mm excision and deep margin which is then examined pathologically by frozen section.)

Case 1: Analysis of Extensive Basal Cell Including Medial Canthus

Case-Based Conference

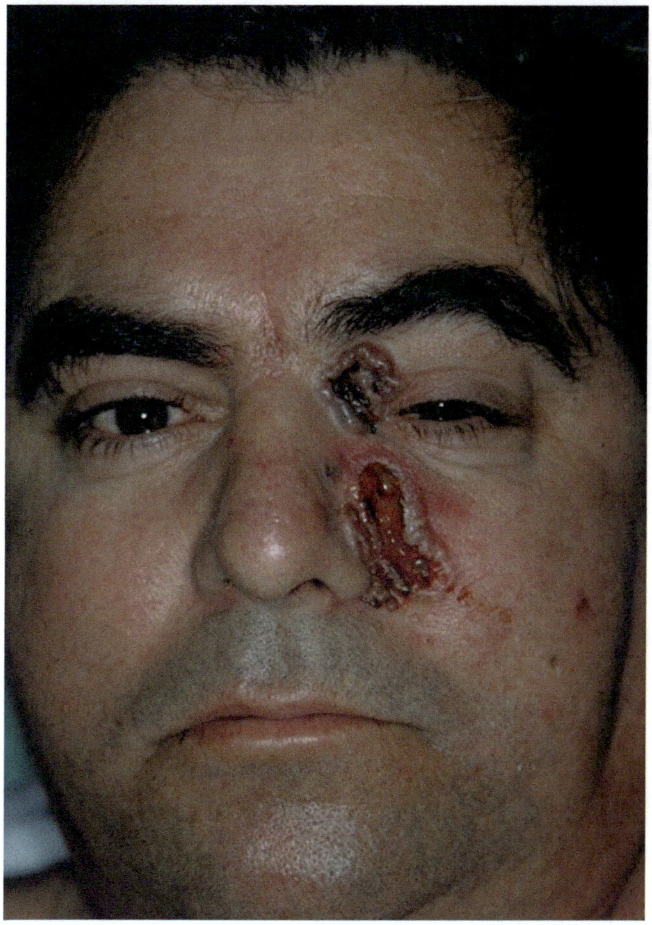

A 45-year-old with a history of ulcerated lesions of the face of unknown duration. No health problems.

1. Describe the slides and add a focused clinical examination.
2. Any tests indicated? Justify.
3. Outline the excision. Draw the proposed margins.

Case-Based Conference: Discussion

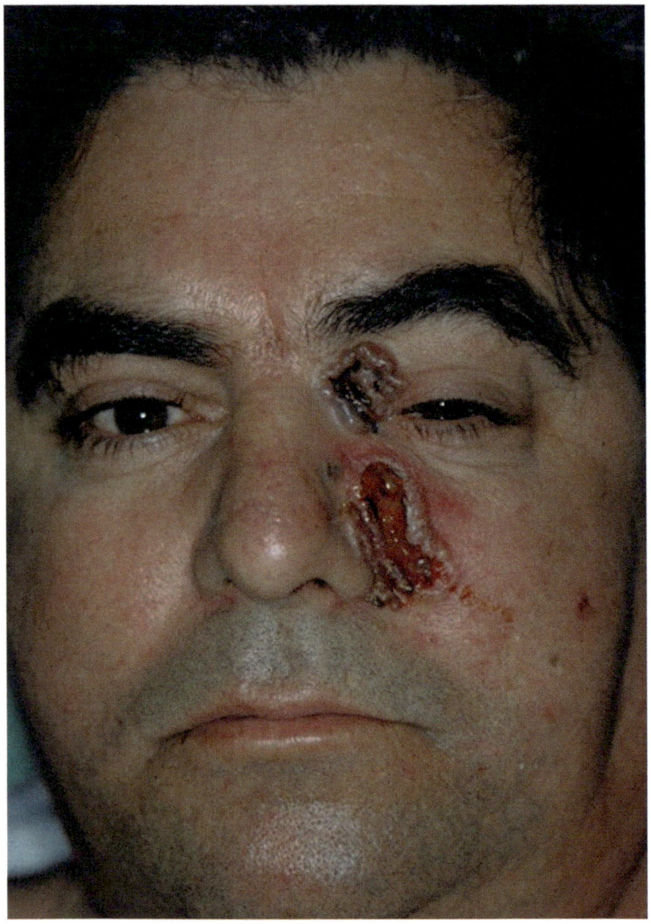

A 45-year-old with a history of ulcerated lesions of the face of unknown duration. No health problems.

A 47-year-old patient otherwise in good health. Biopsy reveals basal cell carcinoma.

1. Describe the slides and add a focused clinical examination. (A single slide is provided of a white male, a frontal view that includes the face only. The view is slightly tilted to the left and downward. The most noteworthy finding is two ulcerated lesions with heaped up or raised edges occupying the left face. One is located on the medial cheek encroaching upon the lateral aspect of the nose. The lesion appears to be 2–2.5 cm in cranial-caudal length and approximately 1.5 cm wide. The ulcerated portion is not superficial. The lesion extends from the alar-upper lip fold to medial lower lid skin but not to the lash or lid margin. An additional lesion of similar characteristics but smaller, 1–1.5 cm is located in the medial canthal and medial brow region. The lateral aspect borders on the medial eyelid commissure, the inferior medial brow, and the superior nasal sidewall. No other lesions are evident. In toto, the two ulcerated lesions occupy the medial cheek, medial canthal, lateral nasal, and medial upper lid aesthetic subunits. The palpebral aperture of the left eye is narrowed significantly with the lash margin at mid-pupil. The brow appears to be possibly elevated.

   The pertinent historical questions begin with the presence of pain, nature of pain if present, past treatments, if any, the duration and constancy of the left lid ptosis, comorbidities and current medications. Possible causes of immunosuppression should be pursued. A social history completes the historical portion of the clinical assessment. Physical examination would include a touch test for sensation over the distribution of the infraorbital and superior trochlear nerves and palpation of both lesions for mobility versus fixation to the underlying structures. Eversion of the upper lid, perhaps with corneal anesthesia, will determine the possible involvement of the conjunctiva. Voluntary elevation of the upper lid is tested.)
2. Are any tests indicated? Justify. (The most essential test, unless a history of comorbidities mandates further investigation, is a CT scan. If any suggestion of infraorbital or supratrochlear nerve involvement arises during the clinical exam, a more detailed imaging of the bony course of those nerves should be included. Of course, if a biopsy had not been previously obtained, a 4 mm punch biopsy at the edge of one of the lesions is performed.)
3. Outline the excision. Draw the proposed margins. (In all likelihood the pathological diagnosis will be basal cell carcinoma of the nodular-ulcerative morphological subtype. The site is within one of the embryologic fusion lines, notorious for subclinical extension. As such given the size, the margins should be generous, 8–10 mm. The deep plane of excision in all likelihood will be upon bone with the latter structure exposed without periosteum.)

Intraoperative

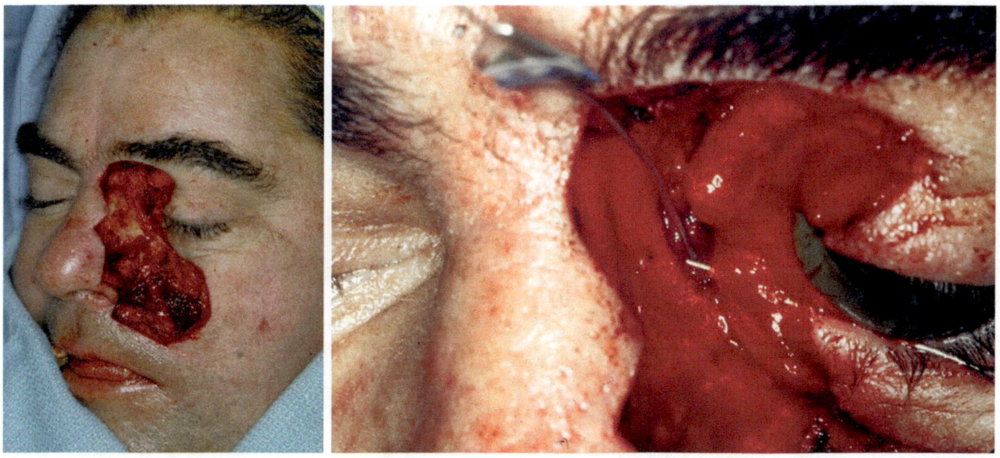

The operative defect is consistent with an excision with a 1 cm margin. The defect will require reconstruction of aesthetic subunits of the medial cheek, lateral nasal, medial canthal, and medial upper and lower eyelid. The photo on the right demonstrates lacrimal duct probes in both canaliculi that have been transected.

Case 2: Multiple Basal Cell Cancers

Case-Based Conference

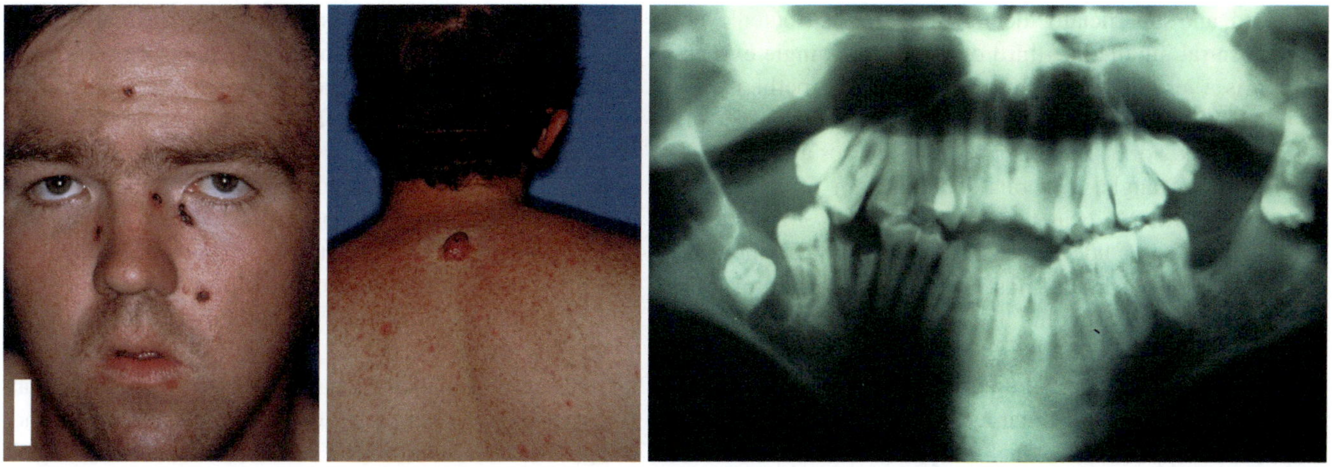

A 33-year-old with a 1-year history of multiple facial and truncal lesions.

1. Describe the slides and add a clinical exam.
   (a) Interpret the Panorex. Any other tests indicated?
2. Give a provisional diagnosis. What is the pathologic anatomy/pathogenesis of your diagnosis?
3. Outline a comprehensive treatment plan.

Case-Based Conference: Discussion

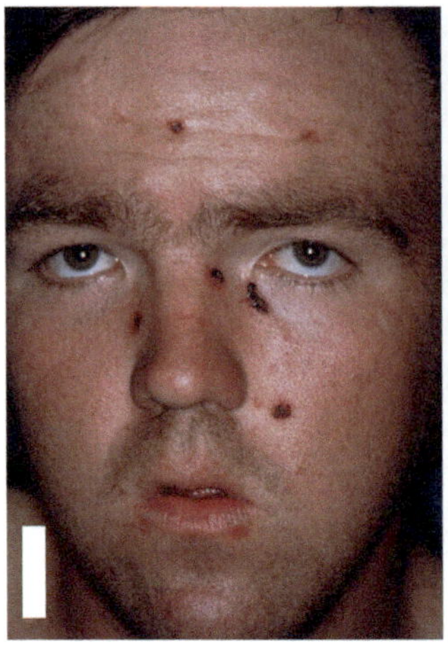
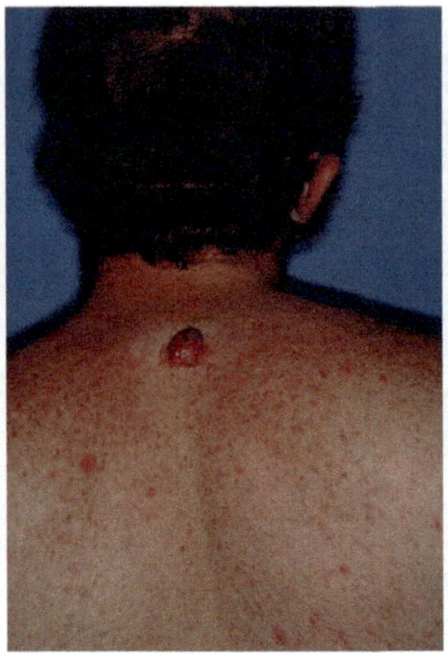
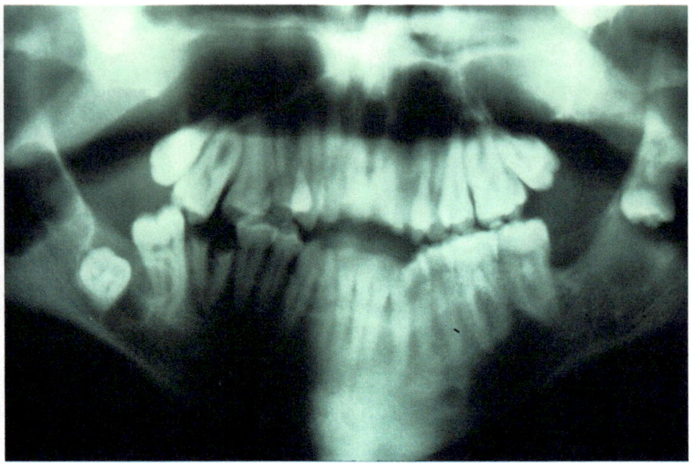

A 33-year-old with a 1-year history of multiple facial and truncal lesions.

1. Describe the slides and add a clinical exam. (Two clinical slides are provided. The first is of the head and neck but limited to a frontal facial view with a small portion of the right lateral to the lateral canthus not included. The patient is Caucasian and appears of stated age. The most remarkable finding is that of multiple small, 5–6 mm, raised, and superficially ulcerated lesions distributed over the central middle one-third of the face. A single exception is a lesion on the central forehead and perhaps the left forehead. The overall complexion appears to be of Fitzpatrick 2 or 3. The other finding, perhaps a product of the camera angle, is a bilateral 2–3 mm of lower lid scleral show. No evidence exists of either conjunctiva inflammation or lid scarring. The other clinical photo is of the upper back and most of the posterior scalp. The most remarkable finding is a flesh-colored exophytic, broad based lesion of 1.5–2.0 cm in the midline of the lower cervical-upper thoracic region. Several other 3–4 mm superficial papular lesions are scattered over the posterior upper trunk. A halo of pale skin surrounds the midline lesion and the post shoulders appear sun tanned as well as the posterior cervical area.

   The clinical examination would be initiated with questions about past lesions treated and then information elicited regarding past medical history and current medications. The dental history and current complaints also should be questioned. The family history is pertinent, specifically, a history of skin cancer in first-degree relatives. Social history including tobacco use completes the history. The physical exam will require a total body skin assessment for the detection of other lesions. An intraoral examination evaluates dentition and the presence of intraoral lesions. Given the provisional diagnosis, see below, the clinical evaluation should include questions about neurologic-based symptoms as well as a basic neurologic exam.)

   (a) Interpret the Panorex. Are any other tests indicated? (The accompanying Panorex is of overall poor quality because of over-exposure and blurring. The film demonstrates an impacted right lower third molar with a well-defined cyst on the distal aspect extending beneath the adjacent molar. The opposite mandibular third molar is absent but a smaller, also localized cyst is present. The status of the cysts and evaluation of the mandible and maxilla should be imaged with a CT scan and should include the head to determine the presence or not of intracranial lesions. If a prior biopsy has not been performed, one of the facial lesions should be excised. The necessity and implications of a genetic diagnosis are discussed in the treatment questions. Multiple consultations including cardiology and medical genetics are indicated.)

2. Give a provisional diagnosis. What is the pathologic anatomy/pathogenesis of your diagnosis? (The clinical findings are consistent with a basal cell nevus or Gorlin's syndrome. Basal cell nevus syndrome is a relatively uncommon autosomal dominant disorder. The characteristics include those seen in this patient of diagnosis at a younger age, multiple lesions at the time of presentation, a distribution of non-solar exposure as well as sun-damaged skin. Other findings include odontogenic keratocysts of the mandible, evident in this patient, bifid ribs, palmar and plantar pits, and calcification of the falx cerebri. Some association with other tumors particularly ovarian fibromas in a majority of female patients and medulloblastoma in a small percentage of children with the diagnosis. The genetic lesion is a mutation of the 9q22, PTCH, that affects a tumor suppressor gene. The

pathology of the consequent basal cell carcinomas is identical to that of the garden or sporadic variety.)

3. Outline a comprehensive treatment plan. (The treatment considerations for the individual lesions does not differ substantially from treatment of basal cell carcinoma in general. Radiotherapy should not be utilized given the high carcinogenic propensity in basal cell nevus syndrome patients. Standard surgical margins apply to the patient's presumed facial basal cell carcinomas as well as the lesion on the back.

   Prophylaxis is indicated in patients with a diagnosis of basal cell nevus syndrome. Agents described include isotretinoin, imiquimod, and, most recently, the immunomodulating agent vismodegib. All have a significant side effect and complication profiles. Other prophylactic measures include comprehensive and vigorous UV protection including clothing, eyewear, and sunscreen agents. Genetic testing is crucial for several reasons. Conformation of the diagnosis will enable the implementation of the above prophylactic measures but also initiate testing of primary relatives, particularly children. Approx. 20% of children with basal cell nevus syndrome will develop medulloblastoma prior to age 5 so screening is essential.

   The care of the basal cell nevus syndrome patient is multidisciplinary and will require the services of a medical oncologist and medical geneticist.)

In-Service Examination

1. The carcinogenic effect of the components of ultraviolet light is:
   (a) 1–290 nm
   (b) 290–320 nm
   (c) 320–400 nm
   (d) 400–480 nm
2. The findings in basal cell nevus syndrome include the following **EXCEPT:**
   (a) Mandibular cyst
   (b) Sternal cleft
   (c) Bifid ribs
   (d) Occurrence of basal cell carcinoma in early adulthood
   (e) Autosomal recessive inheritance
3. The risk for skin cancer in renal transplant patients is:
   (a) Increase of basal cell and squamous cell carcinomas
   (b) No increase in risk of either basal cell or squamous cell carcinoma compared to the normal population
   (c) Increase for squamous cell carcinoma but not basal cell carcinoma
   (d) Increase for basal cell carcinoma but not squamous cell carcinoma
4. Of the following what is the indication for routine rather than Mohs excision of a skin cancer of the face?
   (a) Recurrent tumor
   (b) Squamous cell carcinoma of 2.0 cm in diameter
   (c) 1.0 cm basal cell carcinoma of the cheek
   (d) Morpheaform basal cell carcinoma

27 Eyelid

Bibliography

McCord Jr. CD and Codner MA, Chapter 1: "Classical Surgical Eyelid Anatomy", Eyelid and Periorbital Surgery. Quality Medical Publishing, (2008), **pp. 3–46. (pp 1–13, 28–38 inclusive)**.

Zide BM and Jelks GW, Chapter 3: "The Eyelids", Surgical Anatomy of the Orbit. Raven Press (1985): **pp 21–32.**

Stein JD, and Antonyshyn OM, "Aesthetic Eyelid Reconstruction", *Clin. Plast. Surg.*, (2009); 36(3):**379–396. (Skip 379–382)**.

Alghoul M, Pacella SJ, McClellan WT, and Codner MA, "Eyelid Reconstruction", *Plast. Reconstr. Surg.*, (2013); 132(2):**288e–302e.**

Codner MA, McCord CD, Mejia JD, Lalonde D, "Upper and Lower Eyelid Reconstruction", *Plast. Reconstr. Surg.*, (2010); 126(5):**234e–238e ONLY and Videos.**

5 Videos from Codner MA, McCord CD, Mejia JD, Lalonde D, "Upper and Lower Eyelid Reconstruction", *Plast. Reconstr. Surg.*, (2010); 126(5):**231e (Videos ONLY).**

1. Tenzel-Stewart Flap
2. Hewes Flap
3. Hard Palate grafts
4. Hughes and bipedicled Trippier flaps
5. Mustarde' and Trippier flaps

Chang EI, Esmaeli B, Butler CE, "Eyelid Reconstruction", *Plast. Reconstr. Surg.*, (2017); 140(5):**724e–735e. (Video only; Actually a slide presentation of Hughes and Cutler-Beard flaps)**.

Faculty Discussion and Study Guide

Editor's Note: Eyelid anatomy is also included in Chap. 43 and Chap. 97.

Anatomy

1. Describe the composition of the lamella of the upper and lower lids. (The lower lid is composed of the anterior lamella of skin and orbicularis muscle, the middle lamella is the septum, and the posterior lamella is capsulopalpebral fascia and conjunctiva. The tarsus is considered part of the posterior lamella. In the upper lid, the anterior lamella consists of skin, orbicularis muscle, and the orbital septum; the levator aponeurosis is considered the posterior lamella as well as Muller's muscle and conjunctiva. The tarsus is considered part of the posterior lamella.)
2. Height of the palpebral fissure? Width? (10 mm and 32 mm).
3. Compare and contrast the upper and lower lid in attachment of the septum to the tarsus. (The upper lid septum actually fuses with the levator aponeurosis superior to the tarsus with a difference in the superior attachment between Caucasian and Asian eyelids. See blepharoplasty module. In the lower lid the septum directly attaches to the inferior border of the tarsus after a fusion first to capsulopalpebral fascia, the lower lid analog of

E. Luce, *A Curriculum for Plastic Surgery*, https://doi.org/10.1007/978-3-031-62087-4_27

the levator aponeurosis, and then both as a conjoined structure to the inferior border of the tarsal plate.)

(a) Describe the relationship of the lash margin of the lower lid to the iris and upper lid? Relationship of the lateral to the medial canthus in a transverse plane? (The lash margin of the lower lid is just at or 1 mm above the inferior limbus of the iris while the upper lid margin is 1–1.5 mm below the superior limbus. The lateral canthus sits about 2 mm higher than the medial canthus and at a level of the inferior limbus of the pupil with a considerable variation with ethnicity.)

(b) Describe the configuration of the scleral "white" areas medial and lateral to the iris. (These areas are referred to as the medial and lateral scleral triangles. The medial is slightly smaller than the lateral and relatively fixed from person to person, the lateral is more variable. The overall aesthetic appearance of the eyelid is adversely affected by a change in the configuration of the lateral scleral triangle.)

4. Discuss the anatomic relationship between the levator aponeurosis, tarsal plate, the preseptal orbicularis, and the dermis of the upper eyelid. Describe differences between the Caucasian and Asian anatomy. (The levator aponeurosis inserts onto the superior edge and the anterior aspect of the tarsal plate, as well as fascial fibers inserting into the deep aspect of the preseptal orbicularis muscle and dermis, which is responsible for the formation of the palpebral fold, usually 10 mm above the lash margin. The low-lying fusion of the orbital septum with the levator aponeurosis and even more inferiorly on the anterior surface of the tarsus and the absence of dermal and orbicularis attachments to the tarsus at a more superior point creates either an absent or low palpebral fold in the Asian upper eyelid, since the orbital septum may insert quite inferiorly on the levator aponeurosis. Preaponeurotic fat can be located quite inferiorly on the lid as well in the Asian upper eyelid.)

(a) What is the height of the superior tarsus? Inferior tarsus? (9–10 mm for the superior, 4–5 mm for the inferior.)

(b) What is responsible for the palpebral or supratarsal fold? (See above. The attachments of levator aponeurosis fibers insert into pretarsal orbicularis and even dermis. The fold is produced by the folding of superior unattached skin about 10 mm above the lash margin. The attachment of the septum may play a passive role in the formation of the palpebral fold.)

5. Describe the medial configuration of the pretarsal orbicularis. (The pretarsal orbicularis divides into a deep and superficial head or posterior and anterior head with respect to the relationship to the lacrimal sac. The anterior or superficial head becomes a portion of the anterior limb of the medial canthal tendon while the posterior head, also known as Horner's muscle, inserts into the posterior limb of the medial canthal tendon. Both of these heads may play an active role in the lacrimal pump system as does an additional extension of the preseptal orbicularis, or Jones muscle, that inserts on or posterior to the lacrimal sac proper.)

(a) What is the clinical demonstration that virtually all of the blinking mechanism of the eyelid is due to medial canthal orbicularis? (Myomectomy when performed for blepharospasm, now of historical interest, demonstrates that even if all the muscle except for the most medial portion is excised the blinking mechanism as well as lid posture is retained.)

(b) What is the role of a secure medial canthus in eyelid closure? (Provides the anchoring point for the transverse curvilinear fibers of the orbicularis to act upon and thus raise the lid as a process of muscle contracture. In the absence of a secure canthus the eyelid simply "fish mouths".)

(c) What are the inferior and superior retinaculum? (The individual fibrous condensations of the lower and upper lids respectively fuse to become the medial and lateral canthi.)

6. What is the bony-soft tissue relationship at the medial canthus provided by the medial canthal tendon? (The anterior limb of the medial canthal ligament inserts on the anterior lacrimal crest and the posterior limb, probably the more important of the two in terms of lid adherence, inserts on the posterior lacrimal crest. Between those two crests is the lacrimal fossa containing the lacrimal gland.)

7. In summary, what are the structures that compose the medial canthus? (Medial canthal ligament, medial horn of levator aponeurosis, medial condensation of both Whitnall's and Lockwood's ligaments, check ligament of the medial rectus.)

(a) Lateral canthus? (Replace "medial" with "lateral".)

8. What is Whitnall's ligament? Tubercule? (Whitnall's ligament is a transverse condensation of fascial fibrous tissue that courses horizontally about 8–10 mm superior to the levator aponeurosis and is the principal supporting ligament of the upper lid. The medial origin is from the trochlear fascia and laterally extends to the fascia about the orbital lobe of the lacrimal gland. The Whitnall's tubercle is the bony prominence just posterior to the lateral orbital rim, important for the insertion of the lateral canthal tendon.)

(a) Lockwood's ligament? (Analogous structure to Whitnall's ligament in the lower lid, medial origin is indistinct, laterally into the lateral retinaculum.)

9. Where are Eisler's fat pad and recess? (At the lateral canthus deep to the orbicularis, superficial to the lateral canthal tendon.)
10. Discuss anatomically in terms of the aging process the difference between pretarsal and the palpebral or septal portion of the orbicularis. (The principal difference is that the pretarsal is tightly adherent to the underlying tarsus and so seems to undergo less redundancy with the aging process than the palpebral portion. Advanced changes in the latter can produce festoons.)
11. Explain the functional relationship between orbicularis and levator and outline how you can prove it. (The levator opens the eye, the orbicularis closes it; paralysis of cranial nerve III will produce ptosis, and paralysis of cranial nerve VII results in passive, by relaxation of the levator, closure of the upper lid only and laxity of the lower lid.)
12. Protection of the cornea is primarily provided by: (A static lower lid of adequate height and an upper lid with sufficient inferior extent. Dynamically, by a functioning orbicularis.)
13. What is the analog of the levator aponeurosis and Muller's muscle in the lower lid? (The capsulopalpebral fascia investment of the inferior rectus and oblique muscles is the analog of the levator aponeurosis and actively lowers the lid at the moment that the globe is rotated downward. The levator originates from the fascia of the *superior* rectus. The non-striated inferior palpebral muscle in the lower lid is the analog of Muller's muscle.)
    (a) What is Muller's muscle? (A non-striated muscle originating from the posterior aspect of the levator and courses posterior to the levator aponeurosis into the superior border of the tarsus; the muscle is innervated by the sympathetic nervous system and is quite intimate to the conjunctiva throughout its course.)
14. Describe the points of anastomosis between the internal and external carotid systems. (Supratrochlear, supraorbital, and medial palpebral are terminal branches of the ophthalmic artery, part of the internal carotid system. Those branches anastomose with terminal branches of the angular artery, a portion of the external carotid system.)
15. How can a supraorbital or glabellar injection produce blindness? (A rare occurrence but if a substance is injected with pressure inadvertently into the supraorbital or supratrochlear artery the bolus can travel retrograde into the ophthalmic artery and then subsequently antegrade into the central retinal artery.)
16. The marginal arterial arcade can serve as the vascular supply to an upper or lower eyelid flap. What is the source of the marginal artery of the upper and lower eyelid? (Medial and lateral palpebral arteries.)
    (a) Source of the medial and lateral palpebral arteries? (Ophthalmic and lacrimal arteries, respectively, both branches of the internal carotid.)
    (b) Location of the transverse arcades on the upper and lower eyelids, respectively, is where? (The marginal upper lid arcade is located about 2 mm above the lash margin and just deep or posterior to the tarsus. An additional more superior transverse arcade termed the peripheral arcade, lies on the upper eyelid 1–2 mm superior to the superior border of the tarsus and between the levator aponeurosis muscle and Muller's muscle posteriorly. The lower lid has only one well-defined transverse arcade which is at the inferior border of the tarsus about 4 mm from the lash margin.)
17. In the process of excising fat from the medial compartment in an upper lid blepharoplasty, you encounter substantial bleeding from deep within the compartment. What is the probable source? (Superior medial palpebral artery. See Fig. 27.1.)
18. A squamous cell ca of the lateral lower lid will drain to what lymph nodes? (Parotid.)
19. Besides the areas of sensory innervation, what is the principal difference between the supratrochlear and zygomaticofacial nerves? (The supratrochlear is a branch of the first or ophthalmic division of the trigeminal, cranial nerve V, and the zygomaticofacial a branch of the second division, the maxillary.)

Reconstruction Upper Eyelid

1. Approximately, what proportion of the upper eyelid lost with a full-thickness defect can be closed directly? (Approximately 20% in young patients, up to 30% in older patients, but the risk is excessive tension and ptosis of the lid margin.)
    (a) Describe the technique. (Closure in layers, posterior lamella with buried fast absorbable sutures, anterior lamella repaired with a key 6° silk suture at the gray line. Particular attention is directed toward closure of the tarsus with interrupted 6° Vicryl sutures that are buried away from the conjunctiva.)
    (b) What maneuver may facilitate direct closure in the upper limits of those guidelines and concerns if performed? (Release of the superior retinaculum of the lateral canthal tendon. To do so may create rounding of the lateral palpebral fissure and an unaesthetic lateral scleral triangle.)
2. Describe the appropriate resection of an upper lid lesion to facilitate primary closure. (Resection should be designed as a pentangle rather than a wedge or V-shaped defect. The latter will predispose to a lid margin notching defect because of greater tension on the tarsus.)

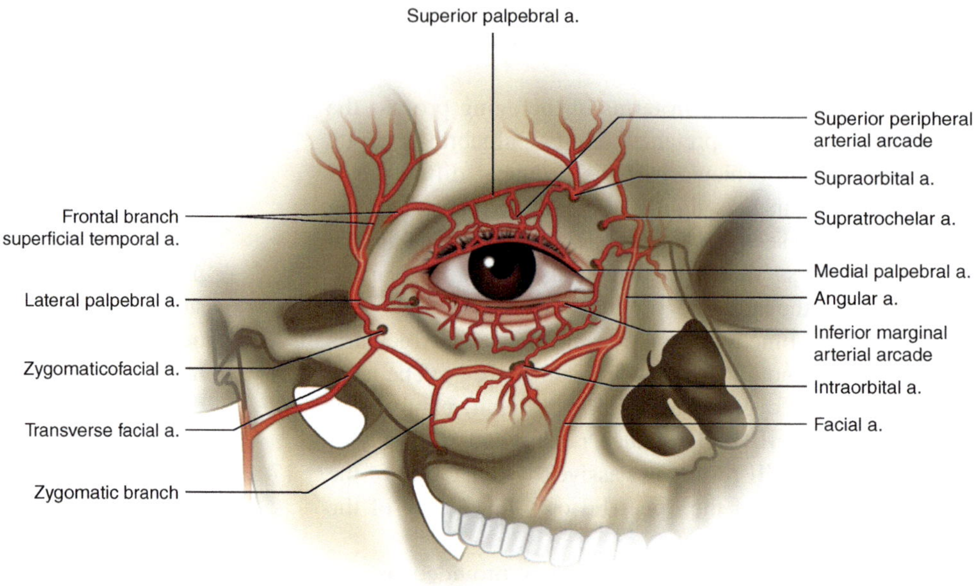

Fig. 27.1 Superior medial palpebral artery

(a) If the defect is sufficiently large, what are the functional considerations in reconstruction? (If primary closure is not possible and local skin flap reconstruction is necessary, consideration must be given to tarsus replacement, preferably by ear conchal cartilage or palatal mucoperiosteum depending on the status of available conjunctiva.)

3. What are the options in reconstruction of a 50% central full-thickness defect of the upper lid? (Either a Tenzel-Stewart flap, a superiorly-based lateral musculocutaneous flap incorporating the remaining lateral lid including tarsus and conjunctiva and utilizing a lateral canthotomy of the superior retinaculum only *or* a full-thickness Cutler-Beard flap from the lower eyelid, preserving the lash margin and 4 mm of anterior lamella of the lower lid intact. Ear cartilage graft is added for tarsal support between conjunctiva and skin and suturing the cartilage graft superior edge to levator aponeurosis and horizontally to the tarsal remnants. Conjunctiva can be reconstituted with buccal or septal mucosa. The flap will require division and inset at 3–6 weeks. Another option is a lower lid-sharing flap. See Figs. 27.2, 27.3, and 27.4. The Tenzel flap is essentially an upper lid-sharing flap and results in absence of lashes laterally.)
   (a) A 50% defect of the lateral one-half of the upper eyelid? (Not a Tenzel-Stewart, perhaps Cutler-Beard or a Mustarde lower lid-sharing flap. The lower lid-sharing procedure is essentially the eyelid analog of an Abbé flap, a pedicled lower lid flap based medially and rotated into the defect. If the flap is limited to 10 mm or less, primary closure of the lower lid donor site is possible. Otherwise, closure can be accomplished by advancement of the lateral lower lid with a lateral cantholysis. A secondary division will be necessary in 3 weeks.)
4. What are the available non-flap options of reconstruction of the posterior lamella? (Mucoperiosteal graft from the hard palate; chondro-mucosal graft from the nasal septum, conchal cartilage graft and buccal mucosa if placed within a flap reconstruction of the anterior lamella.)
   (a) Flap options? (Sliding or advancement tarsal-conjunctival flap.)
5. A method to reconstruct a total full-thickness upper eyelid loss? (Inferiorly—based paramedian forehead flap combined with a septal mucoperichondrial graft or a Fricke flap. A Fricke flap is a cutaneous flap, laterally-based of suprabrow area that will require posterior lamella reconstruction. Both are quite thick for lid reconstruction and will require secondary revision.)
6. The most common complications in upper eyelid reconstruction? (Lagophthalmos, lid ptosis.)

Lower Eyelid

1. How would you estimate if direct closure of a lower lid defect can be accomplished? If the defect is too large what result would be duplicated by this maneuver? (A temporary suture is placed into each of the transected edges of the tarsus medially and laterally and advanced to simulate primary closure. If the defect size is prohibitive, a notching defect will be evident.)
2. Describe the key elements of the Hughes flap. (Use of a posterior lamella, tarsal-conjunctival, flap based superiorly from the upper eyelid leaving 4 mm of the inferior portion of the upper lid intact to preserve the marginal

Fig. 27.2 Lateral rotational flap (Tenzel flap) for upper lid closure

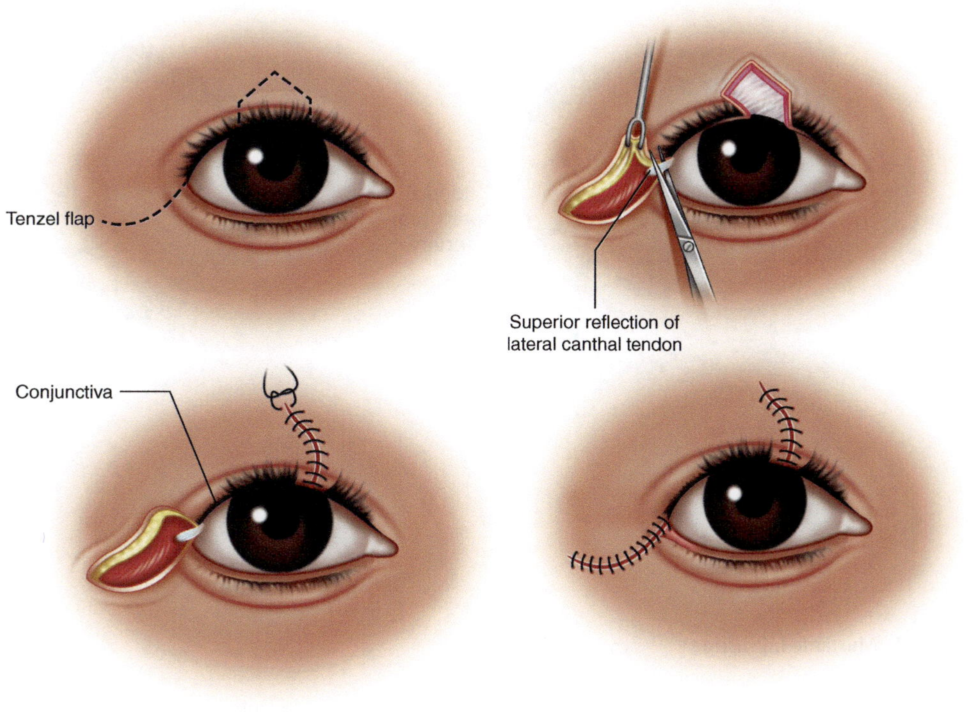

Fig. 27.3 Cutler-Beard lower lid sharing

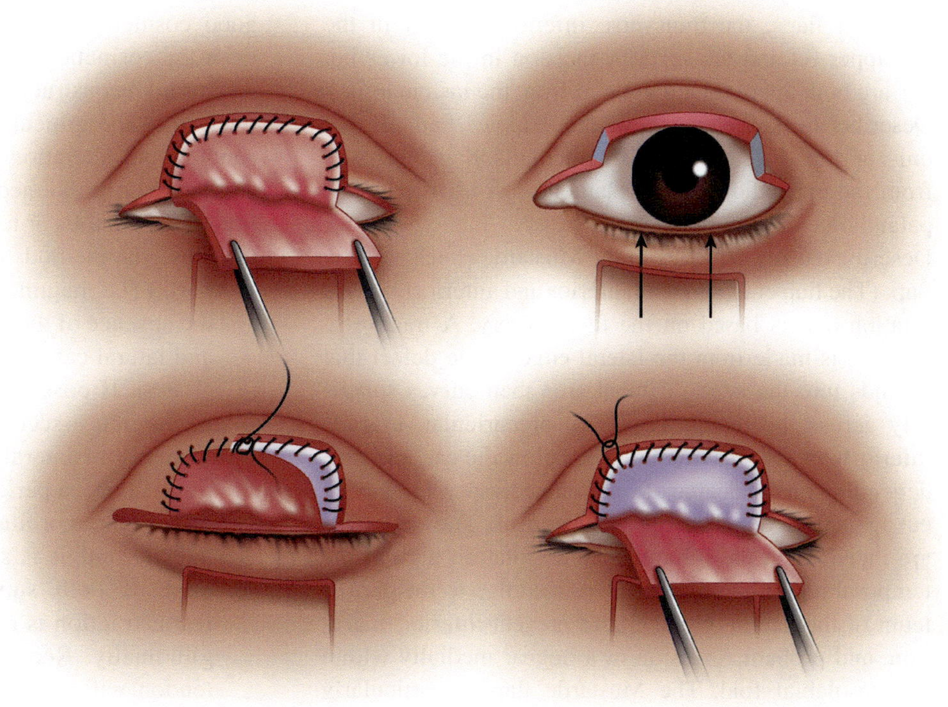

arcade and an element of tarsus, transferring the flap beneath the upper lid margin into the defect; anterior lamella reconstruction with a full-thickness skin graft division and inset at 3 weeks.)

(a) What is the vascular explanation for the difference in design of flaps from the upper and lower lid? (The presence of a single transverse vascular arcade in the lower lid at the inferior margin of the tarsus, 4 mm,

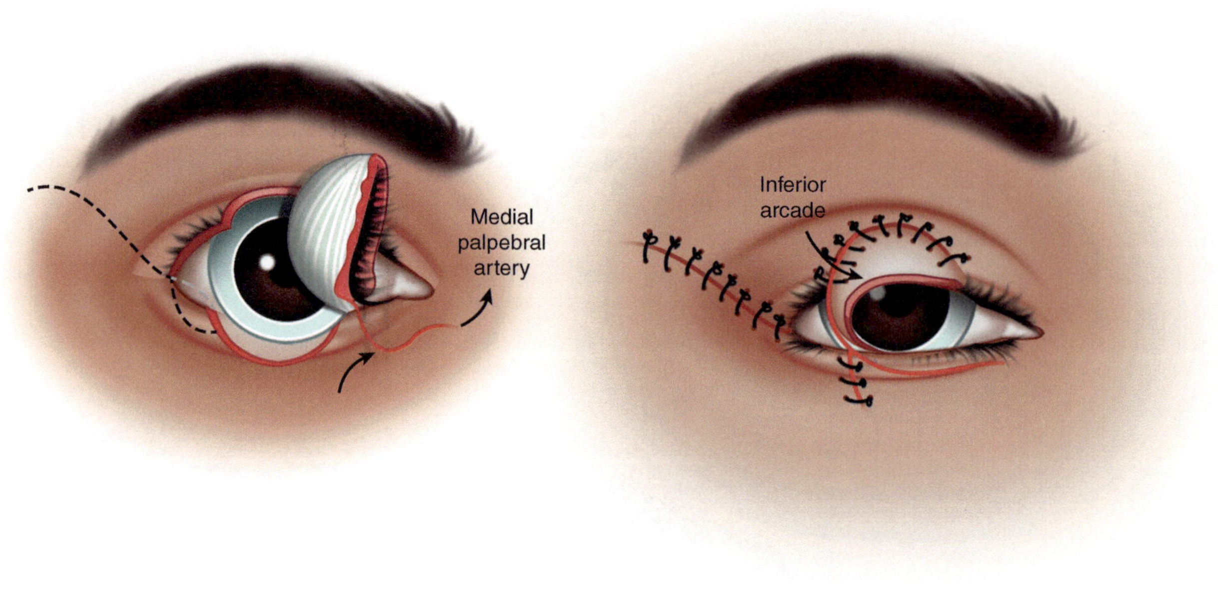

Fig. 27.4 Mustarde lid sharing

vs. the double transverse vascular arcades in the upper lid the more superior, the superior palpebral artery, located 10–11 mm superior to the lash margin. Practically, at least in the design of cross-lid advancement flaps, the transverse inferior incision in the upper lid and the superior incision in the lower lid, are both approximately 2 mm from the lash margin.)

3. Describe the key elements of the Trippier flap. (Either uni- or bipedicled skin and orbicularis flap harvested from the upper lid, posterior lamella reconstructed with palatal mucoperiosteal graft.)
4. Describe the key elements of the Mustarde cheek rotation flap. (The flap consists of an inferior and anteriorly-based rotation and is based on the facial artery. A transverse incision is made from the lateral edge of the defect that extends into the lateral canthal area then curves superiorly across the temple region to preauricular, extends inferiorly in the preauricular fold, below the ear, and then depending on the degree of rotation necessary, has a back cut again transversely in the superior neck. The key points are incisions in the sub-ciliary line, rotation high in the temporal region, anchoring the rotated flap to the periosteum of the lateral orbital rim to prevent inferior migration, and probable excision of a dogear medially within the nasolabial fold. The Mustarde flap is particularly suited for more vertical defects. The flap is elevated superficial to the SMAS or if vascularity is of concern then dissection is deep to the SMAS but to do so places branches of the facial nerve at risk. Posterior lamella reconstruction is achieved with septal mucoperichondrium. See Table 27.1.)
5. Although not discussed above, proper reconstruction of the lateral and medial canthus is necessary to achieve a good cosmetic result. What occurrences might detract from the cosmetic result? (If the tarso-ligament component of lid reconstruction is ignored, the persistent medial traction of the orbicularis will produce rounding of the canthus and alteration of the lateral scleral triangle. A similar error in the medial canthus will create lateralization of the canthus or telecanthus.)
   (a) Describe methods to restore tarso-ligamentous support. (The magnitude of the defect of the tarsus and the absence of the retinacular elements of the medial and lateral canthal tendons will dictate the methods chosen. If possible, advancement of the remaining tarsus into a secure anchor in bone, lacrimal bone medially or lateral orbital rim, is the most expeditious. If not, a periosteal-temporal fascia flap, based on the lateral orbital rim and wall with respect to the lateral canthus is sutured to the medial tarsal remnant. If both superior and inferior retinaculum reconstruction is required, the flap can be split longitudinally. Reconstruction of the medial canthal tendon will require a free fascial graft such as the temporalis deep fascia. A separate consideration in reconstruction of the medial canthus region is the possible necessity for reconstruction of the nasolacrimal system as well.)

Table 27.1 Indications, Advantages, and Disadvantages of Different Flaps Used for Eyelid Reconstruction

	Indications	Advantages	Disadvantages
Flaps for upper eyelid reconstruction			
• Direct closure	Defects of 20–30% of upper lid	Lash continuity	Tight closure can cause ptosis
• Sliding tarsoconjunctival	Medial or lateral posterior lamella defects	One-step procedure; composite flap (tarsus and conjunctiva)	No lash restoration; requires anterior lamella coverage
• Bridge (cutler-beard)	Full-thickness defects of the entire upper lid	Reconstruction of total upper lid defects	Two-stage procedure; no lash restoration; risk of lower lid ectropion; need for tarsal replacement
• Lower lid-sharing (Mustardé)	Broad, shallow, full-thickness marginal defects of 30–60% of the upper lid	Lash continuity	Two-stage procedure; Tenzel flap may be needed to close donor site
• Semicircular rotational (Tenzel)	Anterior lamella defects of up to 60% of the eyelid	Reconstruction of large anterior lamella defects	No lash restoration; requires posterior lamella coverage
• Temporal (Fricke)	Anterior lamella defects of the entire upper lid	Reconstruction of large anterior lamella defects	Two-stage procedure; donor skin very thick; risk of frontal branch lesion
Flaps for lower eyelid reconstruction			
• Direct closure	Defects of 20% of the lower lid	Lash continuity	Tight closure can cause ectropion
• Advancement tarsoconjunctival (modified Hughes)	Posterior lamella defects of the entire lower lid	Reconstruction of large posterior lamella defects; composite flap (tarsus and conjunctiva)	Two-stage procedure; requires anterior lamella coverage
• Tarsoconjunctival (Hewes)	Large, shallow, posterior lamella defects of the lid	Reconstruction of large posterior lamella defects; composite flap (tarsus and conjunctiva)	Two-stage procedure; requires anterior lamella coverage
• Semicircular rotational (Tenzel)	Anterior lamella defects of up to 60% of the eyelid	Reconstruction of large anterior lamella defects	No lash restoration; requires posterior lamella coverage
• Vertical myocutaneous cheek lift	Broad shallow defects of the anterior lamella	One-stage procedure; natural result	Requires anterior lamella coverage; risk of lower lid malposition; no lash restoration
• Tripier	Anterior lamella defects of the entire lower lid	Reconstruction of large anterior lamella defects of the lower lid; thin donor skin	Two-stage procedure; requires posterior lamella coverage; distal part of the unipedicled flap may be unreliable
• Rotation cheek (Mustardé)	Deep vertical defects of the entire lower lid	Reconstruction of large anterior lamella defects of the lower eyelid	Thick donor skin; risk of lower lid malposition; requires posterior lamella coverage
• Temporal (Fricke)	Anterior lamella defects of the entire lower lid	Reconstruction of large anterior lamella defects	Two-stage procedure; donor skin very thick; risk of frontal branch lesion; requires posterior lamella coverage

Condner MA, McCord CD, Mejia JD, Lalonde D, "Upper and Lower Eyelid Reconstruction", *Plast Reconstr Surg.*, (2010); 126(5):232e. (Reprinted with Permission)

Videos

Codner *PRS,* (2010); 126:231e.

Video 1

A Tenzel reconstruction of a lateral one-third defect of the upper lid. No apparent reconstruction of the posterior lamella. Essentially, a small reversed Mustarde but limited to temporal skin only. Plan is to allow conjunctiva to re-epithelialized. Excised dog ear transversely in the lid fold. Donor site closed. Suture periosteum to the deep aspect of the Tenzel flap, considered a canthopexy, to stabilize the lateral canthus and prevent rounding. Otherwise, no tarsal reconstruction was performed. Flap donor site closed by advancement.

Video 2

Hewes flap plus a vertical skin flap for a defect of the lateral one-half of the lower lid *but* 2–3 mm of lateral canthus preserved. Constructed a flap of tarsus-conjunctiva that includes the superior palpebral artery laterally, but preserving the lower 4 mm of posterior lamella. Flap is *lateral*-based and uses a piece of 6-0 silk into the tarsus. Closed the anterior lamellar defect by advancement with medial and lateral subciliary sutures.

Video 3

Hard palate grafts.

Large defect of two-thirds of the upper and lower lid of both posterior and anterior lamellae. Harvested a single large palatal graft. Added a buccal mucosa graft but the location of the donor site was not clear. Also, closed the anterior lamella with apparently a Mustarde for lower lid but upper lid closed with "excess skin". Second case was a graft plus a lateral Tripier flap, myocutaneous. Requires a second stage if medially based. Advocated an obturator. Claimed by the narrator that healing occurs in a "week or two". Considerable discussion about bleeding from the palatal donor site. Entropion release of posterior lamella and closure of resultant defect with palatal graft.

Video 4

Hughes plus a bipedicled Tripier flap.

Central one-half defect of both lamella of the lower lid. Reserved 4–5 mm of inferior upper lid to retain some tarsus in the marginal arcade. Advanced a flap of tarsus and conjunctiva, namely the Hughes flap, into the defect and provided skin coverage with the bipedicle Tripier flap. Returned 3 weeks later for division and inset of the Hughes and apparently, some inset-revision of the Tripier flap.

Video 5

Large defect of four-fifths of the lower lid, full thickness, but also a portion of the adjacent cheek. Residual fragment of a few millimeters of medial canthus in lid. Reconstruction with ear cartilage from the concha, cheek defect with the Mustarde flap and anterior lamella with a lateral-based Tripier. Apparently, conjunctival defect closed by advancement from the sulcus. Also, Tripier will require a second-stage revision. Critique-Mustarde design perhaps was not sufficiently superior to provide lateral support.

Case 1: Ca of the Lower Eyelid

Case-Based Conference

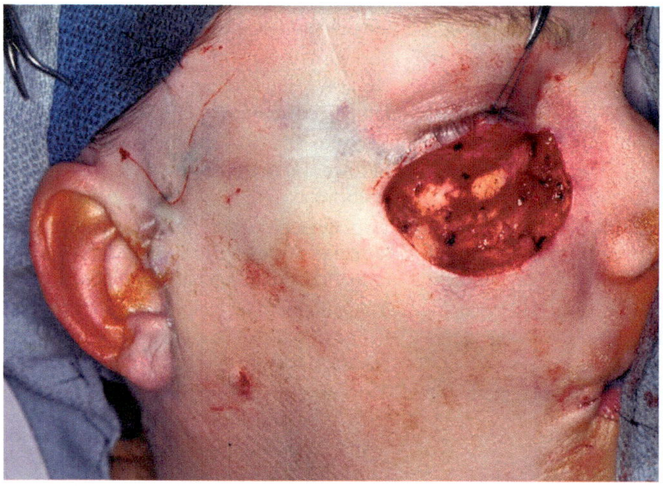

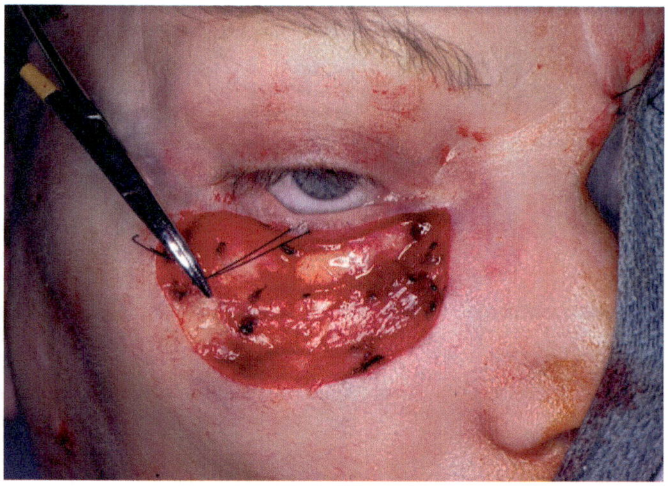

A 55-year-old who is immediate post-op resection of a recurrent bcca. Margins are widely clear on final pathology.

1. Describe the slides. Perform a clinical exam. Do you plan adjuvant therapy?
   (a) Any tests indicated? Justify.
2. Describe the defect in terms of aesthetic units and pathologic anatomy.
3. Outline and draw a reconstructive plan.

Case-Based Conference: Discussion

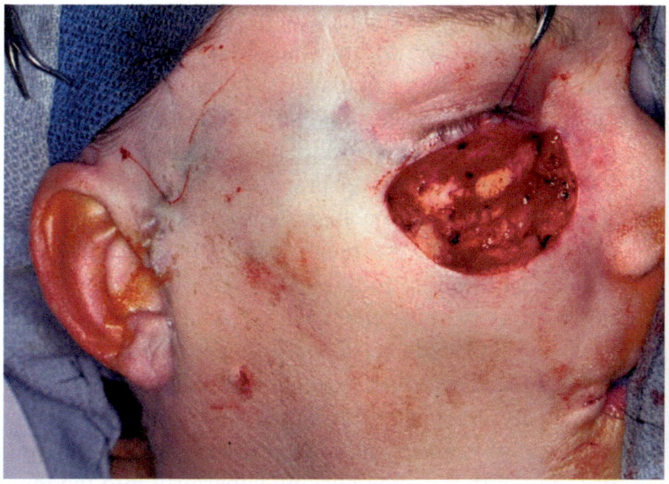

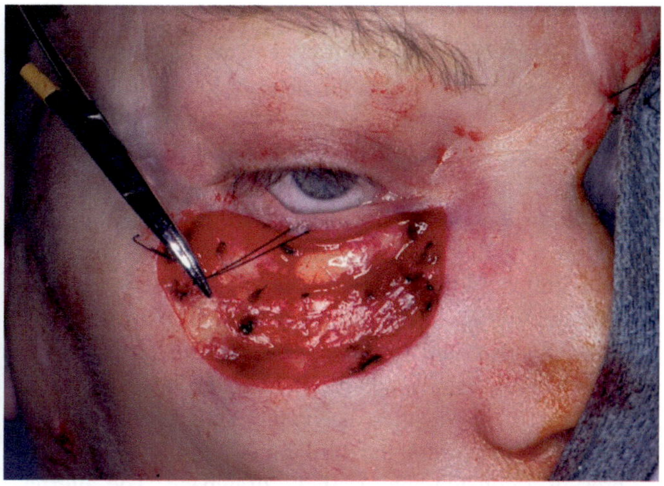

A 55 year-old who is immediate post-op resection of a recurrent bcca. Margins are widely clear on final pathology.

1. Describe the slides. Perform a clinical exam. Do you plan adjuvant therapy? (Two slides are provided and in both the patient appears to be under general anesthesia, probably in the Operating Room. The first a frontal-oblique view, limited to the right side from brow to just superior to the mouth. The most remarkable finding is a substantial-sized apparently fresh defect of the lower lid, infraorbital area, and immediately adjacent cheek. The defect, which spares the lash margin, extends from the medial canthus to a centimeter or so beyond the lateral canthus transversely and inferiorly for approximately 4 cm. The medial extent is the nasolabial groove and the lateral limit is 6–7 cm. Several small dark spots are present consistent with coagulation. The infraorbital rim is not visible; however, infraorbital fat, retained by the orbital septum can be visualized superiorly. Overall, the wound is shallow and the inferior half consists of soft tissue, orbicularis muscle. No other findings are evident. A long suture, tagged with a hemostat has been placed through the lash margin at the midway point. The suture appears to be under traction, yet the tarsus-lash unit appears for the most part, adhered to the globe. The second view is lateral with the same proportion of the face exposed, including the ear. No other information is garnered from the nature or the extent of the defect. A scratch mark is present in the right temple indicative of the temporal hairline.

   Given the preamble, a reasonable scenario is that the patient was seen preoperatively with freshly-performed Mohs defect. If so, the consultation would center on establishment of overall health status, assessment of the defect, and discussion with the patient of a treatment plan. The history would consist of questions about comorbidities, if any, hints of the presence of a coagulation disorder such as easy bruisability, history of transfusions, or multiple miscarriages. The past medical history is reviewed as well as current medications including over the counter. A social history is recorded including tobacco, alcohol, and drug use. The physical exam would determine the dimensions and characteristics of the defect as outlined above and an inspection for any additional lesions. If a complete physical is included in the realm of the practitioner, the heart, lungs, and abdomen are examined.

   The diagnosis is basal cell carcinoma and an indication for additional treatment is either a positive or very close, 1 mm, margin. If so, to render postoperative radiotherapy is an error in judgment. Those pathologic findings are indications for additional resection.)

   (a) Any tests indicated? Justify. (Imaging is not indicated nor testing unless the clinical examination or the past medical history determines the presence of comorbidities.)
2. Describe the defect in terms of aesthetic units; pathologic anatomy. (The defect consists of the aesthetic units of the lower eyelid, which extends to the infraorbital rim and a portion of the cheek subunit which consists of the anterior cheek from the nasolabial fold to the preauricular region which is an additional subunit, and inferiorly to the third subunit, the area of the cheek inferior to the oral commissure, anterior to the preauricular and superior to the mandible. The pathologic anatomy is absence of the anterior lamella of the entire lower lid, loss of the adjacent cheek skin-soft tissue but an intact lash margin. As such, the conjunctiva is intact and at least a proportion of the tarsus. Since lower lid tarsus is approximately 5–7 mm centrally and 7 mm laterally, presumably several mm of tarsus remains intact. Bone is not exposed in the depths of

the wound. In summary, the pathologic anatomy is an anterior lamella defect of the entire lower lid as well as an adjacent cheek defect.)

3. Outline and draw a reconstructive plan. (Although formidable in size, a critical component of lower lid composition and a challenge for reconstruction, the posterior lamella, is intact. So, the reconstructive plan must meet the needs of the pathologic anatomy. Two options present, flap or skin graft coverage. To address the graft option, probably not a satisfactory choice, a full-thickness skin graft would be necessary to avoid secondary contracture and a consequent ectropion. Although a reasonable color match could be accomplished with harvest from somewhere, usually cervical within the head and neck blush area, the vagaries of complete take and the failure to address the contor, the third dimension or depth, would present a considerable aesthetic drawback. The alternative option, flap reconstruction, obviates these disadvantages. The local flap available, the Mustarde cheek rotation, mandates observation of several important principles that include design, dissection plane, and recognition of contraindication variables.

   The Mustarde cheek flap has become the workhorse of subtotal and total lower lid reconstruction. The vascular basis of the Mustarde is the facial artery and as such the pedicle is designed inferiorly and anteriorly. A transverse incision is made from the lateral edge of the defect that extends into the lateral canthal area then curves superiorly across the temple region to preauricular, extends inferiorly in the preauricular fold, below the ear and then, depending on the degree of rotation necessary, has a back cut again transversely in the superior neck. The key points are: incisions in the sub-ciliary line, rotation high in the temporal region, anchoring the rotated flap to the periosteum of the lateral orbital rim to prevent inferior migration, and probable excision of a dogear medially within the nasolabial fold. The Mustarde flap is particularly suited for more vertical defects. The flap is elevated superficial to the SMAS or if vascularity is of concern then dissection is deep to the SMAS but to do so places branches of the facial nerve at risk. As in all rotation flaps, a dog ear inferior to the defect will result, the magnitude dictated by the total degrees of rotation. In this instance, combined with the inherent laxity of the cheek lateral to the nasolabial fold, a substantial-sized excision of a dog ear medially can be anticipated. The dog ear excision should be designed to permit closure in the nasolabial fold. Other important technical points include, as mentioned above, the design of a flap with the apex curving superiorly into the temporal skin-soft tissue, extension vertically and inferiorly into the preauricular fold, and then a rotation incision placed into the natural relaxed skin tension line in the neck. As the incision is extended anteriorly to facilitate rotation consideration should be given to the presence of the facial vessels as pedicled at the mid-mandibular point. An additional technical point is stabilization of the flap to prevent inferior migration by placement of a suture from the deep aspect of the flap to the periosteum, just lateral to the lateral canthus. With respect to contraindications, the occurrence or incidence of flap necrosis in those patients who smoke has been significant. As mentioned above consideration could be given to a subSMAS dissection but only performed by those with the intimate knowledge of the location and distribution of the facial nerve.)

Postoperative: Intra- and Six Months Postoperative

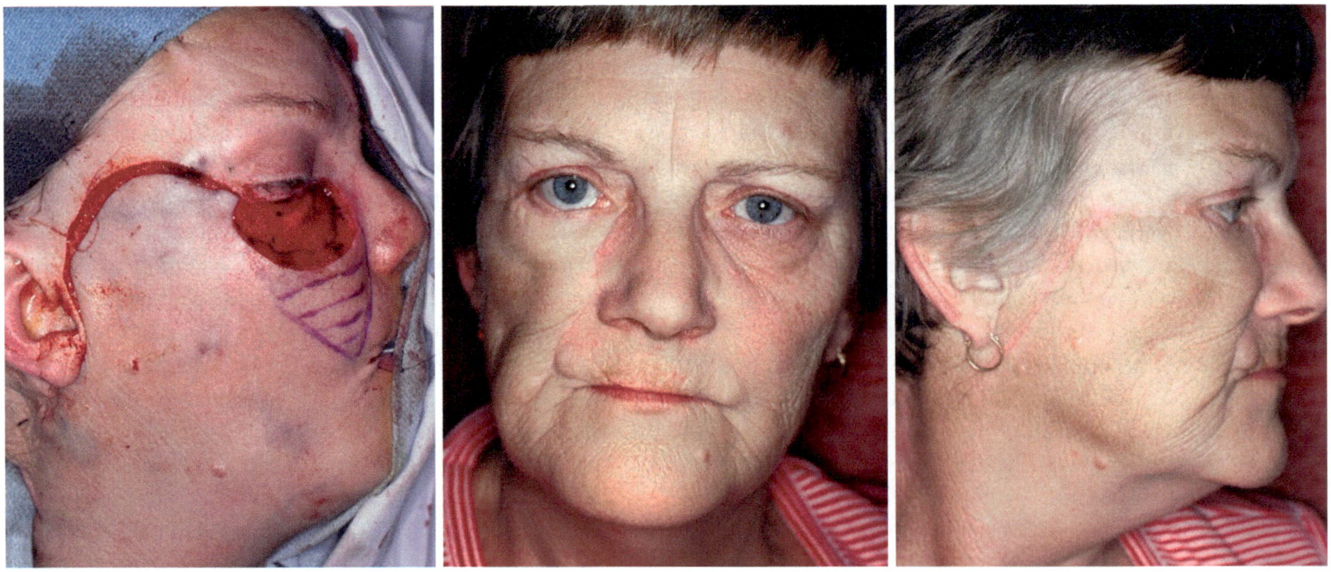

The single intraoperative slide depicts the initial component of the operative plan, rotation of an inferior-anterior cheek flap, the Mustarde flap. Also, the surgical markings indicate the plan for a substantial-sized dog ear excision. The two postoperative views demonstrate a satisfactory reconstruction with a 1–2 mm scleral show but no evidence of exposure conjunctivitis. Some asymmetry because of some element of concavity of the inferior and lateral cheek is also evident. The lateral view depicts a 1–2 cm wide well-healed skin graft in the immediate preauricular area. The color match is excellent and was probably harvested from the opposite neck. Interestingly, no extension of the flap incisions anteriorly into the neck was necessary to achieve sufficient rotation.

Critique

The patient has a 2 mm scleral show but no evidence of any exposure keratoconjunctivitis. A full-thickness skin graft is present in the preauricular area that appears to be a good skin match. Preservation of the lash margin and a portion of the adjacent tarsus facilitated reconstruction. Perhaps the final result would have benefited from a lateral canthal procedure.

Case 2: Ca of the Lower Eyelid

Case-Based Conference

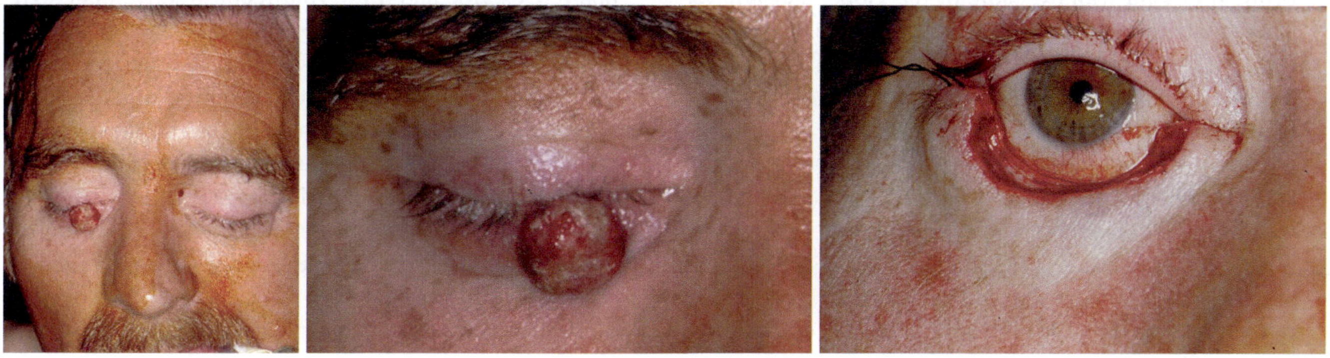

A 56-year-old in good health with a 2 year history of a growing lesion of the eyelid. Biopsy is diagnostic for basal cell carcinoma.

1. Describe the slide(s), add a focused history and physical examination.
   (a) Any tests indicated? Justify.
2. In anatomical terms, describe the pathology.
3. Based on your description in question two, outline a treatment plan. Including the sequence in any operative procedure, incisions, and draw your proposed resection on the board. Describe and draw your reconstructive plan.

Case-Based Conference: Discussion

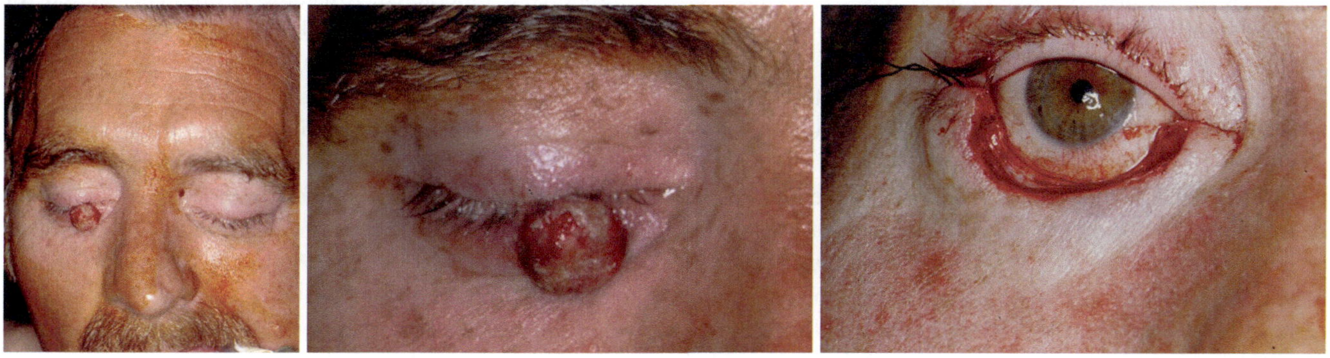

A 56-year-old in good health with a 2 year history of a growing lesion of the eyelid. Biopsy is diagnostic for basal cell carcinoma.

1. Describe the slide(s), add a focused history and physical examination. (Two photos are provided—the first is a frontal three-fourths of the face from the hairline to the mouth. The eyes are closed. The most remarkable finding is an exophytic mass, non-ulcerated and well-defined, approximately 1 to 1¼ cm of the mid-portion of the right lower lid, oriented slightly more medial. No other lesions are visible and the patient's complexion appears to be a Fitzpatrick 2. The second slide is a closeup view of the right periorbital area and immediate adjacent inferior cheek. The remarkable finding is a full-thickness defect of the lower lid with exposure of the globe, and inferior sclera that is about 1.5 cm in depth. Although not particularly well-visualized, approximately 1 cm of intact lid is present laterally with a loop of silk suture placed superior to the lash margin. Medially, a segment of intact lid is present that would appear to be about 5 mm or less in size. The wound margins of the defect are fresh and not bleeding. The inferior bulbar conjunctiva is injected. Again, no other lesions are evident.

   The pertinent history would establish the presence of eye complaints if any, as well as any past eye diagnosis or surgery. Questions about comorbidities (preamble states patient is in good health), past operations, current medications and social history completes the history component of the clinical examination. The physical is focused on the right eye and in particular the lesion. With loupe magnification the adjacent lid is assessed for induration or erythema including the conjunctiva. Function of both upper and lower lid including levator of the upper lid and orbicularis is evaluated. Vision is tested on both eyes either with a Snellen card or by confrontation.)
   (a) Any tests indicated? Justify (Imaging is not indicated nor testing unless the clinical examination or the past medical history determines the presence of comorbidities.)
2. In anatomical terms, describe the pathology. (The pathologic anatomy consists of the magnitude of the defect in relation to the percentage of the normal transverse dimension of the lower lid, approximately 32 mm, the involvement of the structures in a cross-section of the lid, and the inferior extent of the defect. Although an exact measurement of the transverse length is not possible, the defect appears to incorporate about ½ or 15–16 mm. The defect is full-thickness namely both anterior lamella that consists of skin and orbicularis; middle lamella of the orbital septum and; posterior lamella of tarsus and conjunctiva. An additional question is the involvement of the inferior punctum and canaliculus of the lacrimal collecting system, not distinguished on the close-up photo. The depth of inferior extent of the defect would appear as judged by comparison to the transverse dimensions, to be 15 mm. A thorough understanding of the blood supply to both lids is essential in devising methods of reconstruction. The lower lid has a single transverse arterial arcade at the level of the inferior border of the tarsus, termed the inferior marginal arcade. The upper lid, in contrast, has two interrelated transverse arcades, a marginal also distributed just superior to the lash margin and more peripheral located between Mueller's muscle and levator above the superior edge of the tarsus.)
3. Based on your description in question two, outline a treatment plan. Including the sequence in any operative procedure, incisions, and draw your proposed resection on the board. Describe and draw your reconstructive plan. (The treatment plan begins with the assurance of clear margins and then implements reconstruction. Reconstruction in this scenario would require reconstitution of all lamellae after determination of the status of the inferior punctum and canaliculus, optimally performed in the OR by lacrimal duct probes. This scenario assumes an intact system. Options available include tarso-conjunctival flaps, harvested from the upper lid, pedicled superiorly, and covered with full-thickness skin, termed a Hughes flap; a flap of similar composition but pedicled laterally, termed a Hewes flap; a semicircular rotational flap of skin of the lateral canthus and crow's foot area that includes the lateral lid remnant, termed a Tenzel flap; a transversely oriented skin-muscle flap of the upper eyelid either bipedicled or pedicled laterally, termed a Trippier flap; and a sliding cheek flap, termed a Mustarde flap. Each of these options pose advantages and disadvantages. Both the Hughes and Hewes flaps require two stages and anterior lamella coverage and the latter can be difficult to orient into the defect. The Tenzel and Trippier flaps require posterior lamella reconstruction in addition and the latter may be unreliable if unipedicled and of somewhat limited mobility if bipedicled. Mustarde is optimally suited for subtotal defects of the lower lid and also will require posterior lamella reconstruction.

   The defect is central and probably lends well to a cross-lid flap of the upper lid incorporating tarsus and conjunctiva or perhaps full-thickness of both posterior and anterior lamella. The conventional Hughes flap is tarsal-conjunctiva with an immediate full-thickness skin graft, harvested from the upper lid or postauricular. The procedure, performed under local or general anesthesia, begins with a horizontal upper lid conjunctival incision, the length dictated by the transverse size of the defect, and placed about 3–4 mm superior to the gray line of the lid to preserve some element of the tarsus. The dissection is trans-tarsus and between

Mueller's muscle and the levator, both of which will be dissected free of the incorporated tarsus. Two parallel vertical incisions create the flap to be advanced inferiorly into the defect. The tarsus is secured into the most inferior aspect of the lower lid defect and the full-thickness skin graft is applied. The second stage, accomplished 2–3 weeks later, severs the flap and repairs the conjunctiva of the donor site. An alternate method is the construction of a full-thickness flap, anterior and posterior lamella, advanced and secured into the defect. The flap can be divided and inset at 2 weeks with a concomitant repair of the donor site of the upper lid. The concern with harvest of a full-thickness flap is the possible complication of ptosis because neither the levator nor Mueller's are repaired. Yet, the medial or lateral horn of the levator aponeurosis remains intact, and, in all probability, both adhere to the remaining upper tarsus.)

Postoperative (Intra- and Three Months Postoperative)

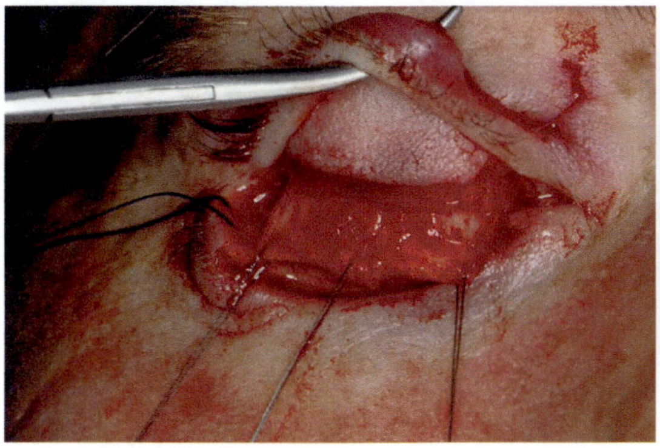

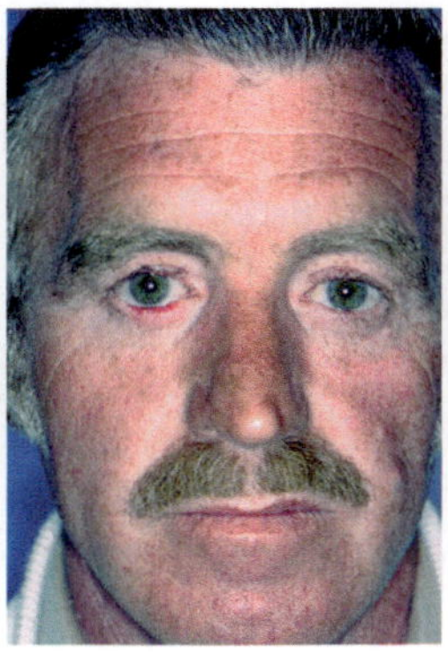

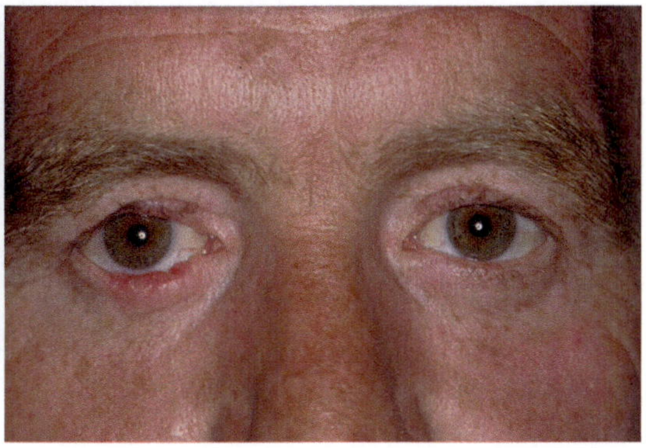

The intraoperative photos depict an operative plan of advancement of a Hughes flap from the upper lid, in this instance composed of both anterior and posterior lamellae. Harvest of both hinges on the conviction on the part of the surgeon that sufficient skin exists in the upper lid so that lagophthalmos will not be complicated in the final outcome. The two postoperative slides of a full face frontal and close-up demonstrate a satisfactory reconstruction with little scleral show and no evidence of exposure conjunctivitis. The reconsted portion of the lid lacks a lash margin.

Critique

Given the harvest of both lamellae with the donor flap, from an aesthetic and functional perspective the outcome appears excellent. An additional view with lid closure would have demonstrated the absence of lagophthalmos.

Case 3: Upper Eyelid Lesion

Case-Based Conference

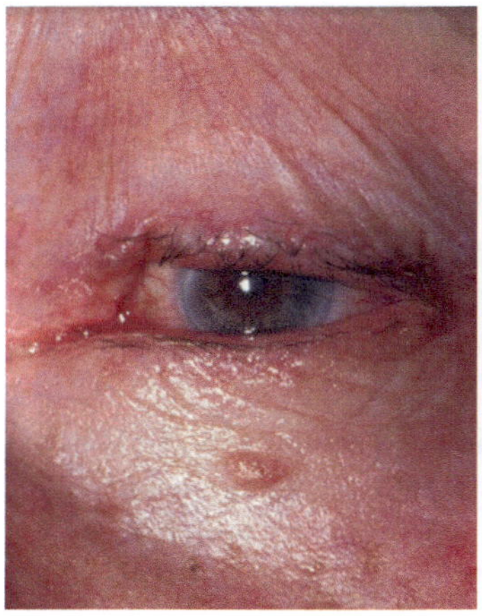

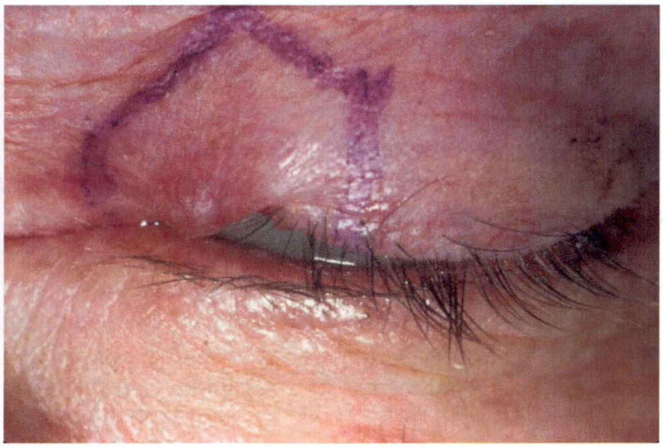

A 65 year-old with a 3-month history of a lesion of the medial upper eyelid that has grown in size. Biopsy is diagnostic for basal cell carcinoma. Your treatment plan will include resection and reconstruction.

1. Describe the slide(s). Add a focused clinical exam.
   (a) Any tests indicated? Justify.
2. What are the considerations in the resection? What is your anticipated defect? Would the pictured excisional design be yours? Why or why not?
3. Summarize the pathologic anatomy.
4. List a menu of options, select yours, and describe and/or draw.

Case-Based Conference: Discussion

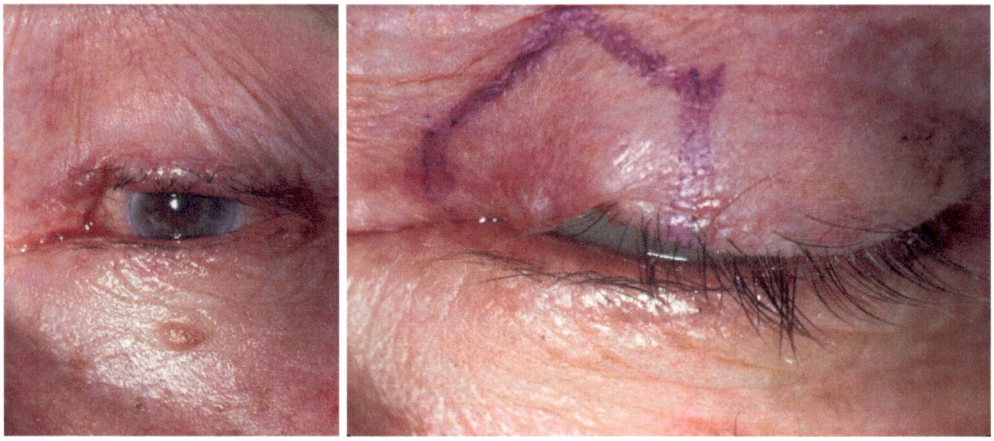

A 65 year-old with a 3-month history of a lesion of the medial upper eyelid that has grown in size. Biopsy is diagnostic for basal cell carcinoma. Your treatment plan will include resection and reconstruction.

1. Describe the slide(s). Add a focused clinical exam. (Two photos are provided—the first is limited to the left, presumably, periorbital area, and is sufficiently close up that neither the medial canthal nor the brow region is included. The most remarkable finding is a contracture and V-shaped or notching deformity of the medial one-fourth of the upper lid. On the skin edge of the contracted lid is a poorly-defined nodular pink lesion that appears to be approximately 3–4 mm. The adjacent bulbar conjunctiva is injected, the adjacent skin is non-erythematous. The overall skin color of the patient, though, is pink. On the lower lid in the mid-pupillary line a cm from the lash margin is a well-circumscribed 5 mm papular, non-ulcerated lesion. Some scattered lentiginous skin changes are evident at the lateral canthus. The second photo depicts yet a more limited view, restricted essentially to the upper and lower eyelids. In this photo, the lids are closed except for the medial notched deformity. The skin nodule at the lash margin is again seen but in this view is accompanied by some immediately adjacent erythema. The lentiginous changes of the lateral one-fourth of the upper lid are visualized. The additional finding in this view is the presence of ink marks in the form of a pentangle, the base at the lash margin with the nodule incorporated, and several mm medial and lateral to the lesion of uninvolved lid is also included.

   The clinical examination begins with questions designed to determine the initial appearance and additional questions about vision changes or epiphora as well as past diagnoses of eye diseases. The past medical history is ascertained, current medications and any questions regarding symptoms indicative of the presence of comorbidities are posed to the patient. A social history including tobacco and alcohol use is documented. The physical exam determines the extent to the degree possible of the lesion, including conjunctival involvement. Although the histological diagnosis in this instance is basal cell carcinoma, the regional lymph node drainage, the parotid, should also be examined. The remainder of the head and neck is examined for the presence of other skin lesions. A standard heart, lungs, and abdomen examination complete the physical.)
   (a) Any tests indicated? Justify. (Imaging is not indicated nor testing unless the clinical examination or the past medical history determines the presence of comorbidities.)
2. What are the considerations in the resection? What is your anticipated defect? Would the pictured excisional design be yours? Why or why not? (Given the diagnosis of basal cell, a reasonable margin is 3 mm, although a marginal control by sequential frozen section diagnosis

would be essential if that option is selected. The indistinct nature and appearance of the lesion may dictate a two-stage approach, resection and delayed reconstruction following permanent histologic examination of margins. Although the diagnosis in this instance is basal cell, one must be aware of other neoplastic entities that occur in the upper lid, including sebaceous adenoma and carcinoma arising from the Meibomian glands and the glands of Zeis. The pattern of lymphatic drainage from adnexal carcinomas of the upper lid is into the intra parotid lymph nodes. The design of lesion excision should encompass vertical parallel excisions through skin and lash margin and the vertical height of the underlying tarsus included. Triangular or wedge-shaped incisions set the stage for a notching defect. The design pictured, pentangular, is the recommended option even if primary closure is not anticipated.)

3. Summarize the pathologic anatomy. (The pathologic anatomy of the case is the magnitude of the defect and the lid structures involved. The dimensions of the ultimate defect are not immediately apparent. Excision of the lesion with adequate margins will in all likelihood create a defect of the transverse upper lid of 10–12 mm. That magnitude of defect is not amenable to primary closure without the creation of notching of the upper lid. Regardless, if involvement of the conjunctiva is clinically evident, a full-thickness resection will be necessary that will encompass the anterior lamella, skin, orbicularis, and orbital septum as well as the posterior lamella of tarsus and conjunctiva. An additional element of the resection defect is the superior punctum and canaliculus located in the medial lid and within the confines of the planned resection. In summary, the reconstruction needs are anterior and posterior lamella constituting approximately one-third of the medial upper eyelid and loss of the upper canaliculus lacrimal drainage system.)
4. List a menu of options, select yours, and describe and/or draw. (Since primary closure is not feasible for defects greater than one-fourth of the transverse dimension of the upper lid, 30–32 mm, tissue transfer will be necessary for reconstruction. A number of options are available for reconstruction of this defect and include: a sliding tarso-conjuctival flap from the adjacent lid; a bridge or advancement flap from the lower lid, a Cutler-Beard flap; a rotation flap from the canthus, a Tenzel flap; a pedicled rotational flap from the lower lid, and a composite graft harvested from the opposite lower lid. Each has advantages and drawbacks. The bridge Cutler-Beard and rotational flaps both require a second-stage for division and inset, the sliding tarso-conjunctival flap does not reconstruct the anterior lamella and utilizes tissue from an already compromised lid; a composite graft requires a lower lid donor site and implies successful vascularization of the graft. The position of the defect, substantially medial, would obviate a Cutler-Beard flap and the dimensions tilt away from a sliding tarso-conjunctiva flap. Construction of a pedicled rotational flap, harvested from the lower lid is feasible. The design should be >5 mm in vertical height to ensure inclusion of the principal feeding vessel, the inferior marginal arcade. The dimensions should be slightly smaller than the defect and limited to 30% of the lower lid or 9 mm. Second-stage division and inset is performed in 3 weeks. The dimensions of the composite grafts are similar only the donor site is the opposite lower lid. Marked skin changes can be anticipated during the process of vascularization of composite grafts. Whatever method of reconstruction is selected, due consideration must be given to reconstitution of tarsal integrity to prevent bowstringing of the lid laterally.

   The last item is the management of the lacrimal collecting system. Although the issue is somewhat controversial, perhaps the preponderance of lacrimal drainage is more into the inferior punctum, which will of course remain intact in this instance, than the superior punctum. As such intubation and reconstitution of the superior canaliculus may not be indicated.)

Intraoperative

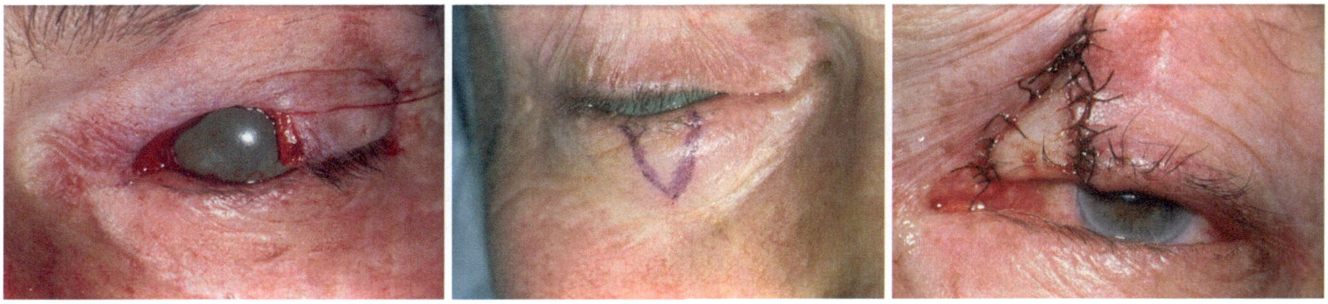

The intraoperative defect is similar in dimensions to the preoperative drawing and appears 12–15 mm. A composite graft of a "V" or wedge shape has been outlined in the central portion of the opposite lower lid that is approximately 9–10 mm. A subsequent photo, also intraoperative, the graft has been sewn into the defeat.

Postoperative (Six Months)

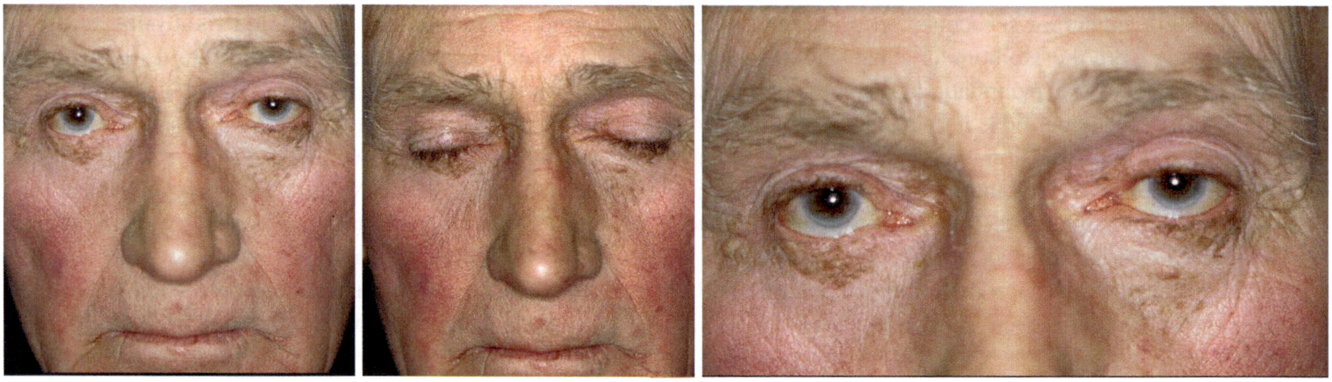

In the three postoperative photos, a full face with lids open and closed and a close-up of the orbits only, the graft is imperceptible and the upper lid closes completely without notching. Lash growth in the grafted lid is evident. Two millimeters of scleral show is present bilaterally without associated keratoconjunctivitis.

In-Service Examination

1. The anatomical analog of the levator aponeurosis in the lower lid is:
   (a) Orbital septum
   (b) Jones's
   (c) Capsulopalpebral fascia
   (d) Lockwood's ligament
2. Arterial bleeding is encountered in excision of the medial lower lid fat pad. What is the artery?
   (a) Lacrimal
   (b) Medial palpebral
   (c) Supratrochlear
   (d) Inferior transverse
3. A 50% defect of the lower lid is optimally reconstructed with:
   (a) Primary closure with lateral canthal release
   (b) Hughes flap
   (c) Fricke flap
   (d) Cutler-Beard
   (e) Tenzel

28 Cheek

Bibliography

Menick MD, F. J., "Reconstruction of the Cheek", *Plast. Reconstr. Surg.*, (2001); 108(2): **496–504**.

Rapstine, E. D., Knaus, W. J. II, Thornton, J. F., "Simplifying Cheek Reconstruction: A Review of Over 400 Cases", *Plast. Reconstr. Surg.*, (2012); 129: **1291–1299**.

Mureau MAM, Hofer SOP, "Maximizing Results in Reconstruction of Cheek Defects", *Clin Plastic Surg*, (2009); 36:**461–75.**

Cohen, J.M., Zide, B., "Facial Expansion: A Blueprint for Coverage",*PlastReconstrSurg.*,(2023);151(6):**1286–1292 ONLY.**

Boutros, S., Zide, B. "Cheek and Eyelid Reconstruction: The Resurrection of the Angle Rotation Flap", *Plast Reconstr Surg.*, (2005); 116(5):**1425–29 ONLY.**

Sami P. Moubayed, Akram Rahal, Tareck Ayad, "The Submental Island Flap for Soft-Tissue Head and Neck Reconstruction: Step-by-Step Video Description and Long-Term Results", *Plast. Reconstr. Surg.,* (2014); 133(3): **684–686 (Including Videos).**

Vinh VQ, Anh TV, Ogawa R, Hyakusoku H, "Anatomical and Clinical Studies of the Supraclavicular Flap: Analysis of 103 Flaps Used to Reconstruct Neck Scar Contractures", *Plast. Reconstr. Surg.*, (2009); 123(5):**1471–80.**

Cordova A, Pirrello R, D'Arpa S, et al., "Vascular anatomy of the supraclavicular area revisited: Feasibility of the free supraclavicular perforator flap", *Plast. Reconstr. Surg.*, (2008); 122(5):**1399, (Figure 12 only).**

Pallua N, Kim BS, "Pre-expanded Supraclavicular Artery Perforator Flap", *Clin Plastic Surg*, (2017); 44: **49–54.**

Faculty Discussion and Study Guide

Cheek Reconstruction: Local Flaps

1. Describe the borders of the cheek as an aesthetic facial unit. (The peripheral posterior superior border begins at the anterior edge of the sideburn and then courses inferiorly along the preauricular fold to the angle of the jaw. At that point the inferior border courses transversely along the body of the mandible. The superior transverse border is at the junction of the cheek and lower lid skin. The medial border is the junction of the nasal sidewall with the cheek then coursing inferiorly along the nasal labial fold to the marionette line, the juncture of the upper and lower lips, and finally, transversely across the anterior mandible to join the inferior transverse border.)
2. Describe the zones of the cheek, the landmarks, and the significance of each. (The readings describe three zones, Zone 1 is the infraorbital region bordered by the nasolabial fold medially and extends over the malar eminence laterally. The lid cheek junction is the superior border. Inappropriate tension at this point can lead to ectropion; incisions medially can be camouflaged to the nasolabial fold. Zone 2 is the preauricular and adjacent posterior cheek region, an area of less mobility of skin and soft tissue. Zone 3 is the inferior anterior cheek and adjacent chin. Excessive tension can distort the commissure and lateral upper lip. See Fig. 28.1.)
3. What are corollaries or general principles in reconstruction of the cheek including the priority of color, texture, and the necessity to respect the aesthetic unit? (Reconstruct the entire unit if involved as a unit; avoid if possible skin grafts and distant flaps because of the color mismatch; use if possible local and regional flaps. The important principle is the necessity for uniformity of skin color and texture, so local and adjacent regional flaps are preferable and skin grafts are not. Distant microvascular flaps may be necessary but result in a poor color match. In contrast to the nose, uninvolved skin is not excised to reconstruct an aesthetic unit.)
   (a) What are the guidelines about the direction of incisions? (Vertical incisions medial to the lateral canthus attract the viewers and are unaesthetic. Transverse incisions should be below the horizontal

E. Luce, *A Curriculum for Plastic Surgery*, https://doi.org/10.1007/978-3-031-62087-4_28

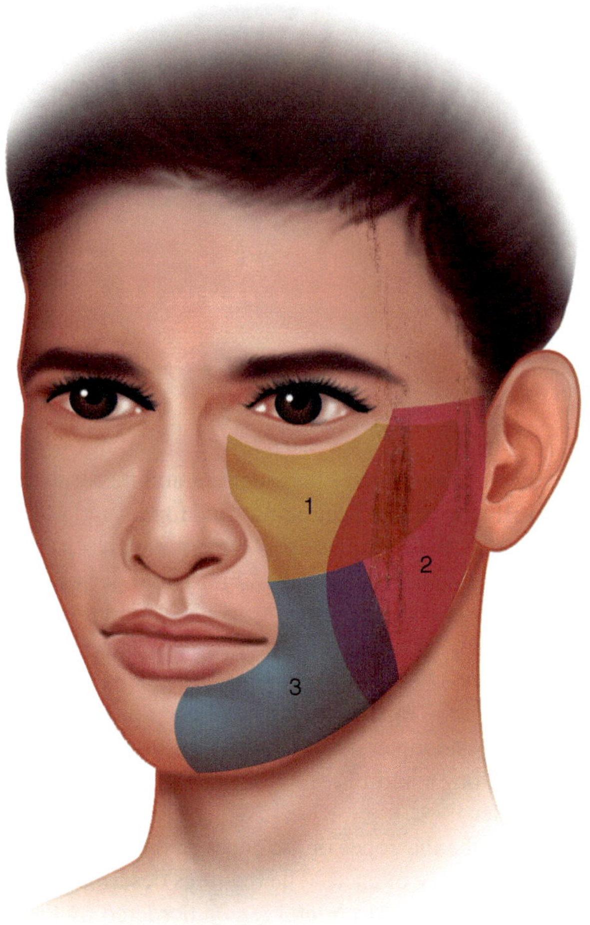

Fig. 28.1 Zones of the cheek

mandibular body and above the zygomatic arch-temple region.)

4. In addition to the general principles outlined in the above question, how does the particular site of the defect influence the design of the skin flap for closure/reconstruction? (Smaller anterior defects can be repaired with posteriorly-based rotation advancement flaps. Large anterior defects or posterior defects are optimally resurfaced with anteriorly-based rotation advancement flaps also described as the Mustarde' cheek flap. The division is somewhat arbitrary since posterior-based flaps are more superior and anteriorly-based flaps are inferior in direction.)
5. Describe the design of an anterior or posterior-based cervicopectoral flap. (See Fig. 28.2.)

   (Although the design of both anterior and posterior based or viewed differently as anterior and inferior vs posterior and superior, flaps, as represented in the drawings, depict extension of the incision well into the pectoral area to harvest cervical and pectoral skin, the posterior cervical limb is subject to hypertrophy, and the chest extension may not be necessary. An alternative and perhaps more attractive option is extension into the neck and transversely in the inferior cervical skin either posterior for a posterior-superior-based flap or anterior for an anterior-inferior flap. If the facial artery is left intact, sufficient well-vascularized soft tissue and skin should be available.)
6. Outline two methods of elevation of an inferiorly/anteriorly-based cervicofacial flap. (One is a Mustarde' flap which is a skin-only flap and the other is a sub-SMAS or deep plane flap that presumably permits enhanced blood supply. The benefit of the increase in vascularization with a dissection in the deep plane carries the risk of injury to the branches of the facial nerve. Both are designed similarly with respect to skin incisions.)
7. What are the key elements in the construction design and use of the Mustarde' flap? (If the incision crosses into the infraorbital area at least 1+cm of lateral skin at the lateral canthus should be left intact for proper lymphatic drainage of the residual eyelid skin; the incision across the temple should curve in a convex direction superiorly, arching superior to the lateral canthus. The flap should follow the preauricular fold and then curve posteriorly beneath the lobule of the ear. Anchoring the flap to the periosteum of the lateral orbital rim is important to prevent inferior flap traction and ectropion. The superior transverse incision is optimally placed in the subtarsal crease rather than subciliary.)
8. What modification may permit closure of a posterior donor site defect as a result of rotation of a Mustarde flap into a large anterior defect? (Use of postauricular and cervical skin as a separate "bilobed" flap rotated from the postauricular area into the preauricular donor site defect or full-thickness skin graft harvested from the supraclavicular area.)
9. For a large Mustarde flap, closure of the preauricular donor site, if not possible primarily, may be accomplished with a full-thickness skin graft harvested from the opposite neck. What is another option? (Another option is the use of postauricular skin, designed as an additional inferiorly-based flap, referred to in the readings as an "angle" or Schrude flap.)
10. Critique by pros and cons of the use of transposition or bilobed flaps for closure of small cheek defects. (Although local skin is used, some of the incisions by definition will cross the relaxed normal skin tension lines of the cheek and the methods violate the cheek as an aesthetic unit. Nevertheless, in elderly patients these techniques may suffice because of the minimal scarring and lax facial skin in this age group.)
11. Tissue expansion can be utilized to address cheek-soft tissue defects. What are some of the principles with

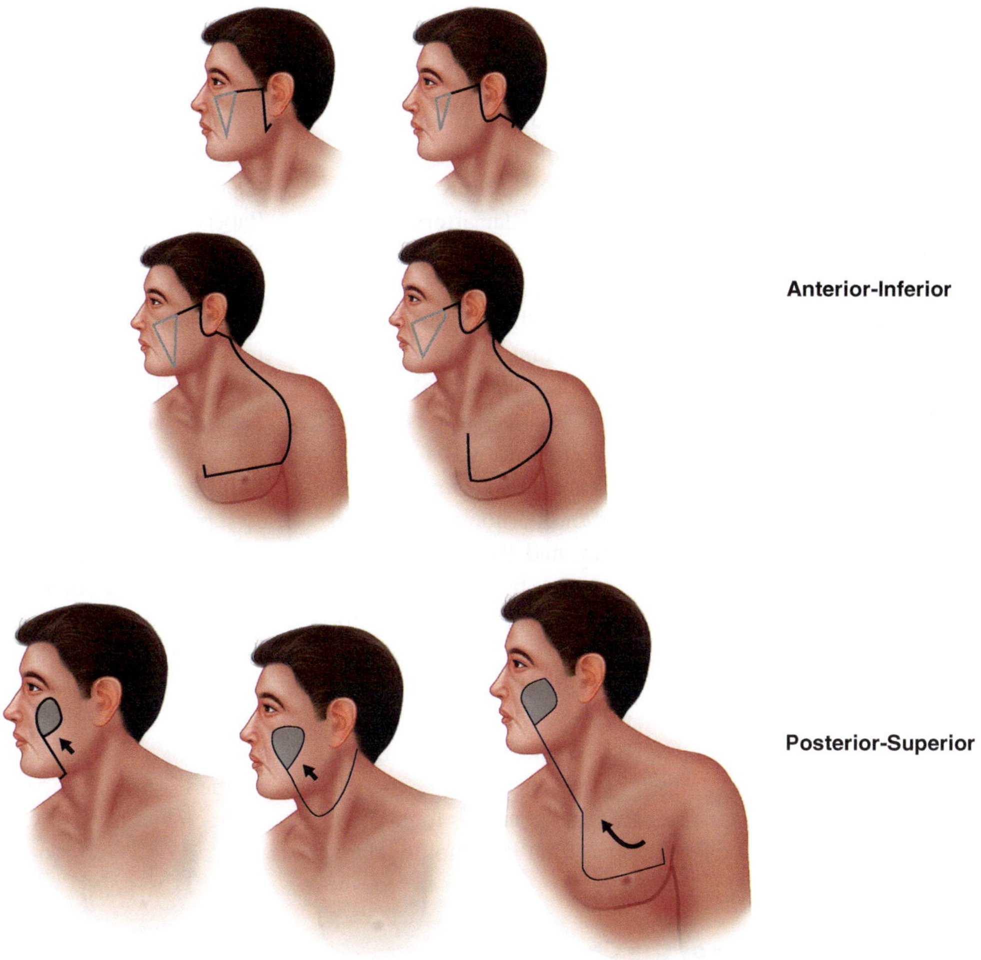

Fig. 28.2 Cervicopectoral flap

respect to expander type, size, and flap design? (The recommendations include the selection of rectangular rather than round or crescentic expanders, the base dimensions as large as the defect or modestly larger, and an expanded flap design of rotation rather than advancement.)

(a) Where should the tissue expander be placed? (Even though the uninvolved cheek skin may be available, the expander should be placed in the upper neck skin. In general, tissue expanders located within the cheek itself have a prohibitively high complication rate.)

Regional Flaps

1. The submental artery flap is, as the name implies, based on the submental artery. Describe the source vessels and subsequent course of the artery. (The submental arises from the facial artery shortly after the latter exits from the submandibular gland and before the facial traverses vertically over the mandible. The submental artery arises deep and proximal to that point and subsequently courses over the mylohyoid and provides branches to that muscle.)
   (a) What nerve is at risk in the harvest of a submental artery, SMA, flap? (The mandibular branch of VII. Not described in the readings but since the mandibular gland is either mobilized and/or excised, the lingual nerve is also in the surgical field.)
2. Describe the steps in the harvest of the SMA flap. (The initial incision is the inferior limb of the proposed transverse submental skin island and is used to access the ipsilateral submandibular gland and identification of the facial artery and vein. The branches to the submandibular gland are ligated and the gland is excised. The inferior limb of the proposed flap is extended to the opposite side and the flap is dissected subplatysmal retrograde and superficial to the contralateral anterior belly of the digastric muscle. The ipsilateral digastric will be incorporated into the flap. As the flap is elevated, the superior course of the facial vessels will be ligated and transected, which enables the flap to be pedicled essentially on the origin of the facial vessels from the external carotid artery.)
3. Readings are provided about the supraclavicular flap and variants of the same. Describe the vascular anatomy of

the "standard" supraclavicular flap. (The principal arterial supply is from the transverse cervical artery, a branch of the thyrocervical trunk that originates from the subclavian artery. The transverse cervical artery in turn is the origin of the supraclavicular arising, in 90% of the instances, at the mid-third of the clavicle. In the remaining 10%, the origin of the supraclavicular artery was at the lateral one-third of the clavicle.)

4. What is the angiosome of the supraclavicular flap? (Reliable to the tip of the shoulder. Further extension over the deltoid encroaches on the vascular territory of the posterior humeral circumflex and entails a preliminary delay.)
5. What are some anatomical landmarks to assist in location? (A general location in the posterior cervical triangle is formed by the lateral border of the sternocleidomastoid muscle, the external jugular vein, and the clavicle. The origin of the transverse cervical artery from the thyrocervical trunk is approximately 4 cm from the sternoclavicular joint and the origin of the supraclavicular artery from the transverse cervical artery is another 4 cm.)
6. Where is the supraclavicular artery with respect to the deep, deltoid, and fascia? (The vessel, after piercing the deltoid fascia approximately 4 cm distal to the takeoff from the transverse cervical artery, can be found just superficial to the fascia. Harvest of the flap should incorporate the deltoid fascia and the pedicle can be lengthened by dissecting to the origin of the transverse cervical artery from the thyrocervical trunk and ligating the vessel, the transverse cervical artery to increase pedicle length, distal to the origin of the supraclavicular artery. Of course, this procedure enables the harvest as a free flap.)
7. One variant is termed the supraclavicular artery perforator flap. What is the blood supply? (The term is somewhat confusing. The perforator is actually a branch of the transverse cervical artery, proximal to the origin of the supraclavicular and a more correct term would be a transverse cervical artery perforator flap. The pedicle by definition is shorter than the supraclavicular fasciocutaneous flap.)
8. A separate reading described a variant that also incorporated pre-expansion to harvest a larger flap. What was the design and vascular supply? (The flap was a rectangle with the long axis more oriented over the upper medial arm than the supraclavicular fossa. The blood supply is an anterior branch of the transverse cervical artery, exiting between the sternal and clavicular head of the sternocleidomastoid. Of course, pre-expansion can also be performed on the supraclavicular skin pedicled on the supraclavicular artery.)

Case 1: Skin Cancer of the Cheek

Case-Based Conference

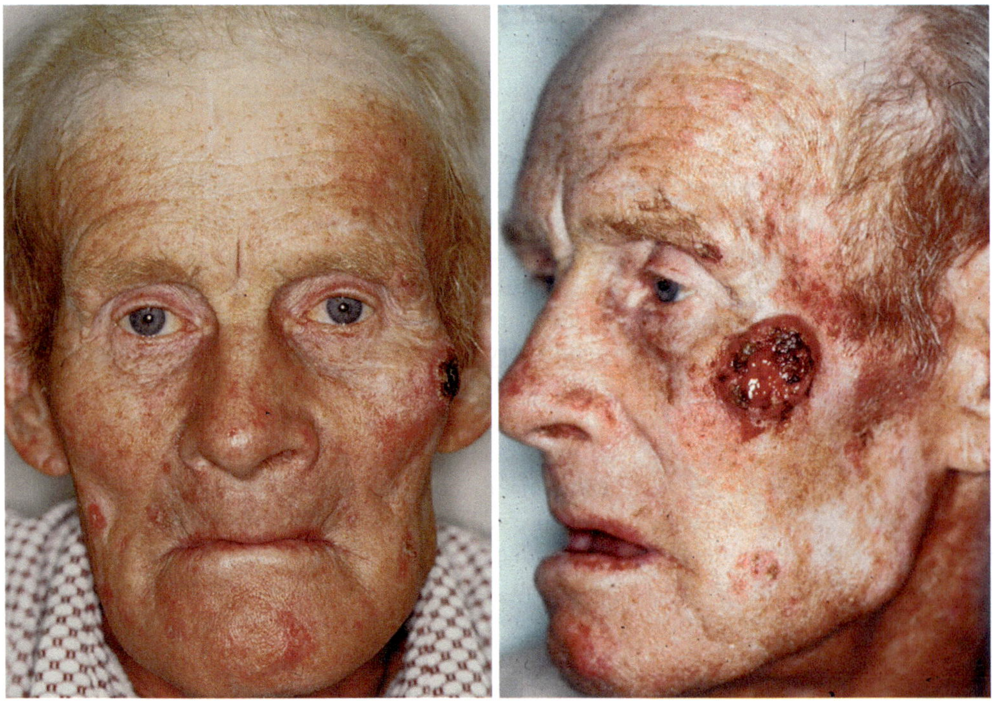

A 66-year-old man with an ulcerated lesion of 1-year duration that has increased in size. A preliminary biopsy by the dermatologist reveals squamous cell carcinoma. The patient is in good health.

1. Describe the slides and add a focused clinical examination.
   (a) Are any tests indicated? Justify.
2. Outline the pathologic anatomy and describe your operative excision. Draw your margins on the board.
3. Outline a reconstructive plan.

Case-Based Conference: Discussion

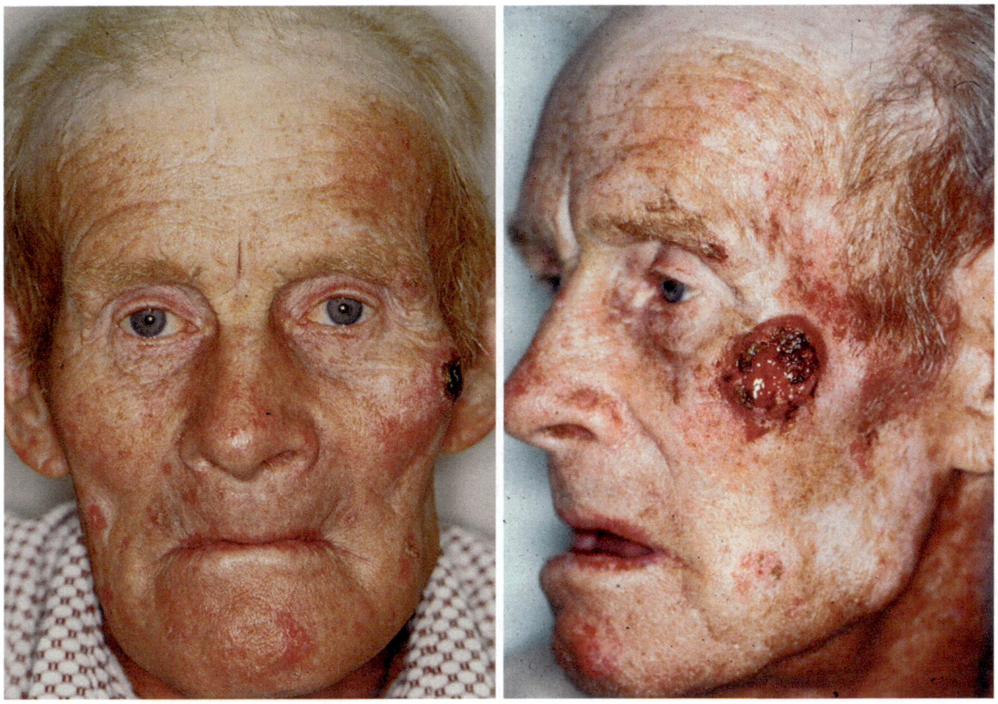

A 66 year-old man with an ulcerated lesion of 1-year duration that has increased in size. A preliminary biopsy by the dermatologist reveals squamous cell carcinoma. The patient is in good health.

1. Describe the slides and add a focused clinical examination. (The two photos provided are a frontal and left lateral view of a male who appears his stated age. The predominant finding in both views is a large ulcerated lesion on the left cheek. In the frontal view, the lesion is only visualized in profile and contains an overlying eschar. The underlying malar eminence appears somewhat more prominent than the opposite. A number of other small superficial scaling lesions are present on the inferior right cheek, upper lip, and chin. The left lateral view depicts the cheek lesion, located midway between preauricular and the nasolabial line, approximately 3 cm in width and 4 cm in length, larger than anticipated on the frontal view, and clearly ulcerated. The superior tip encroaches on the left temple. Another superficial small scaling lesion is present on the inferior cheek. The eye has no evidence of conjunctivitis or evidence of eyelid dysfunction.

   The clinical examination begins with questions to reaffirm the duration and the recent behavior with respect to the increase in size. Additional questions would focus on associated pain, if any, the pattern of distribution of such pain, and any symptoms of left eye inflammation. Systemic symptoms of weight loss and malaise are explored. The preamble states the patient is in good health but a past medical history of operations, medications, and procedures should be obtained as well including a social history of smoking and current occupation. The physical exam begins with an assessment of the seventh cranial nerve function particularly the zygomatic and temporal branch as well as palpation of the preauricular and anterior cervical areas for the presence of lymphadenopathy. The lesion is gently manipulated to determine mobility including inserting an examining finger into the labial sulcus. A careful head and neck skin exam will complete the physical.)

(a) Are any tests indicated? Justify. (Some consideration should be given to imaging the bone, the zygoma, underlying the lesion. Findings in the clinical examination of radiating facial pain would favor further assessment of the possibility of tumor involvement of the maxillary division of V. Review of the pathology report will yield information about the histology beyond diagnosis, particularly the degree of differentiation.)

2. Outline the pathologic anatomy and describe your operative excision. Draw your margins on the board. (The pathologic anatomy is a large ulcerated infiltrative squamous cell carcinoma of the left cheek, situated in Zone 2 in an elderly male in good health. The lesion lies directly over the course of the zygomatic branch of the facial nerve as well as the zygomatic-facial of the maxillary division of the trigeminal nerve. The peripheral skin margins for a squamous cell carcinoma of this dimension, 4 by 3 cm, should be a minimum of a centimeter. After infiltration of local anesthesia, the excision would begin posteriorly to identify the parotidomasseteric fascia to determine the deep plane of dissection and, if possible, preservation of the branches of the facial nerve. The exception might be if clinical and/or imaging examination would indicate fixation and involvement or at least proximity to the underlying bone. The other option is a superior incision, deepening to the level of the deep temporal fascia. Regardless, in both instances, the dissection would proceed directly over the bone. Using the posterior incision the deep dissection would progress until incision of the additional peripheral margins becomes necessary. The lesion is tagged for pathological examination.

   An additional consideration is the inclusion of a sentinel lymph node biopsy. The size of the primary and the degree of differentiation will assist in that judgment process and perhaps favor a formal assessment of the status of the regional lymph nodes. To do so would require a decision preoperatively for the injection of radionuclide for lymphoscintigraphy. The sentinel node will be preauricular or a high jugulodigastric.)

3. Outline a reconstructive plan. (The execution of the reconstructive plan will hinge on the elements of oncologic management. If a single-stage reconstruction is adopted, assurance of tumor-free margins will be obtained from the results of frozen sections. A more conservative approach is meticulous scrutiny of the adequacy of the resection, particularly the deep margin, with two-stage management by application of a dressing, permanent section examination, and reconstruction in 24–72 h.

   Successful reconstruction demands adherence to the general principles of avoidance of skin grafts or distant flaps and, if possible, vertical incisions in Zone 1. In the selection of local flaps for closure, the two possibilities are inferior or superior-based flaps. Inferior flaps, vascularized by the facial artery, are somewhat more anterior than superiorly oriented posterior flaps, vascularized by the transverse facial and directly and indirectly by the superficial temporal artery. In this instance, given the location and size of the defect, a more posterior or lateral flap design would facilitate closure. The anterior vertical limb would descend into the nasolabial fold, over the chin and mandible, and into the neck. The location of the facial artery bisecting the mandible should be ascertained with a handheld Doppler if a performance of a back cut in the submandibular region is necessary to obtain sufficient length at the superior most inset. See critique. Regional options include the submental and supraclavicular artery perforator flaps but the defect appears too large for the former and too anteriorly located for the latter.

   The other consideration is the procedure of tarsorrhaphy. Given the overlap between the buccal and zygomatic branches of the facial nerve, if the deep dissection was directly on the zygomatic periosteum, the decision about the necessity of a tarsorrhaphy could be deferred until postoperative assessment of lid closure. If lid closure was inadequate, a temporary tarsorrhaphy could be accomplished at the same setting as the flap reconstruction.)

Intraoperative

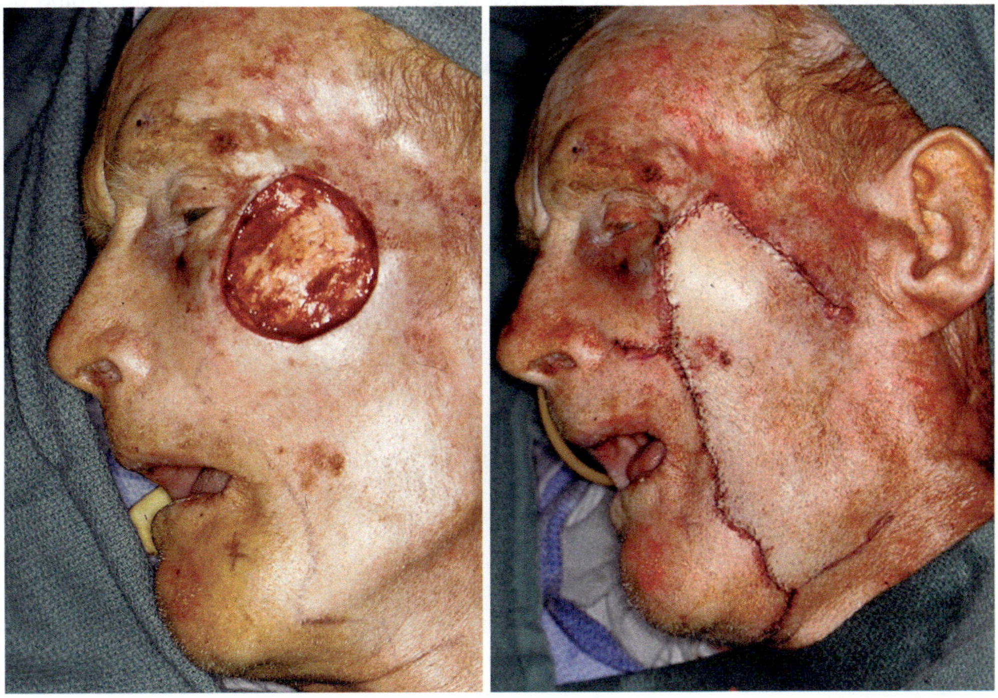

The intraoperative photo depicts the post excisional defect. Although the malar eminence of the zygoma is exposed, a thin layer of overlying soft tissue is present. The following photo demonstrates the inset of a large facial-cervical flap, based posterior and inferior. The defect has been closed but the flap is distinctly pale over the distal one-fourth.

Postoperative (Six Months)

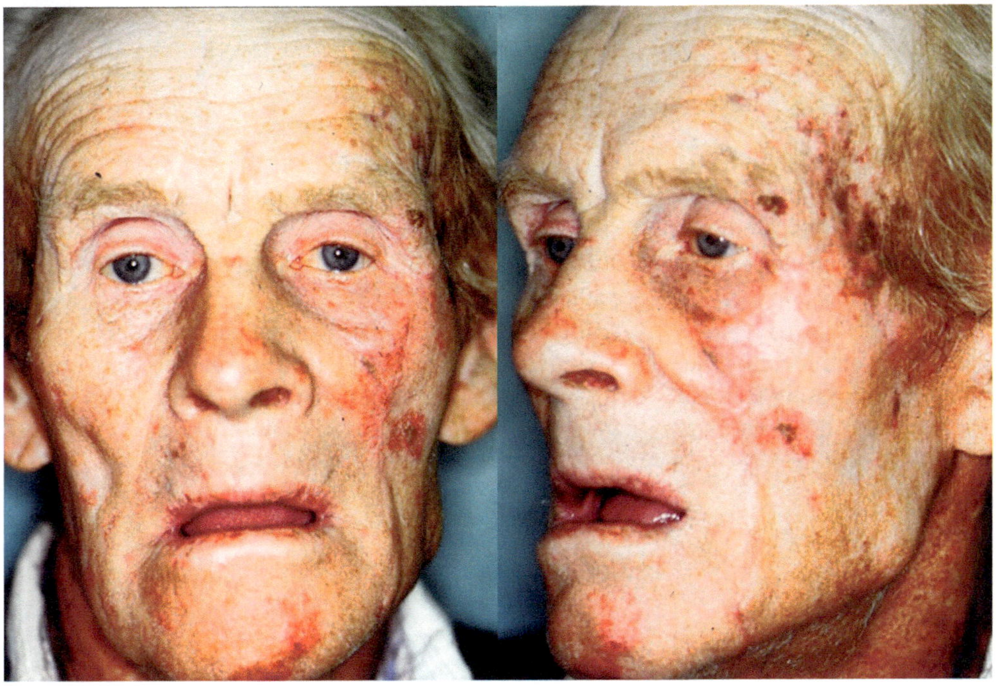

In the frontal and left oblique view, the reconstruction has been successful and the incisions are nearly imperceptible. No ectropion of the lower lid is evident. The most pronounced finding, particularly on the oblique view, is that of scattered areas of melanosis in the temple.

Critique

The result is satisfactory. The lower lid function is intact. If tension of the distal inset was perceived, extension of the anterior incision further inferiorly into the neck, if needed, and a posterior back cut would be of value. Care would be taken with the back cut not to encroach upon the course of the facial artery. Intraoperative application of nitroglycerine paste would be efficacious to address the paleness of the flap.

The patient, judged by the appearance at 6 months, would have benefited from a program of skin care, incorporating a short course or courses of 5-FU cream or imiquimod.

Case 2: Ca of the Face

Case-Based Conference

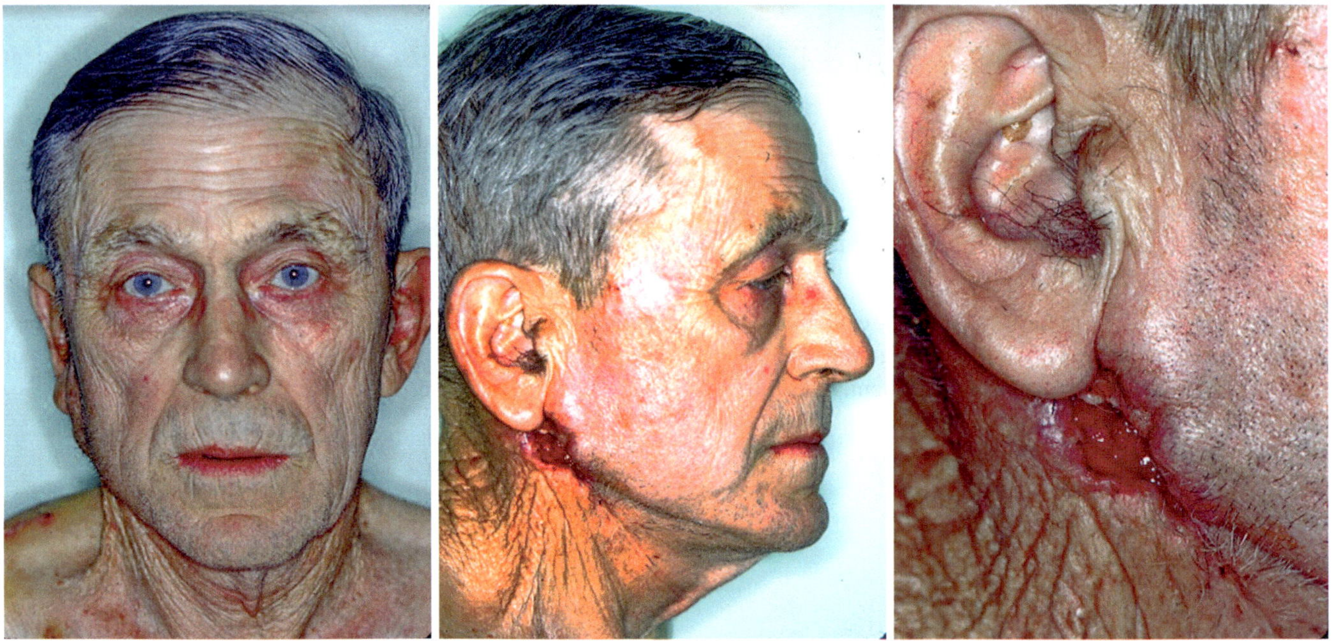

A 64-year-old man who had a "skin cancer" excised from the same area 18 months ago and received postoperative radiotherapy because a tumor was present at the margins. A biopsy has revealed poorly differentiated squamous cell cancer. CT scan demonstrates no mandibular involvement.

1. Describe the slides. Add a clinical exam and focus on the following historical items: possible predisposing factors. Add a physical examination.
   (a) Any additional imaging? Justify.
   (b) Discuss the appropriateness of radiotherapy as employed above.
2. Based on the information that you have describe the pathologic anatomy.
3. Outline a treatment plan that includes the oncologic or resective aspects as well as reconstruction. Give options for reconstruction, select yours, and justify.

Case-Based Conference: Discussion

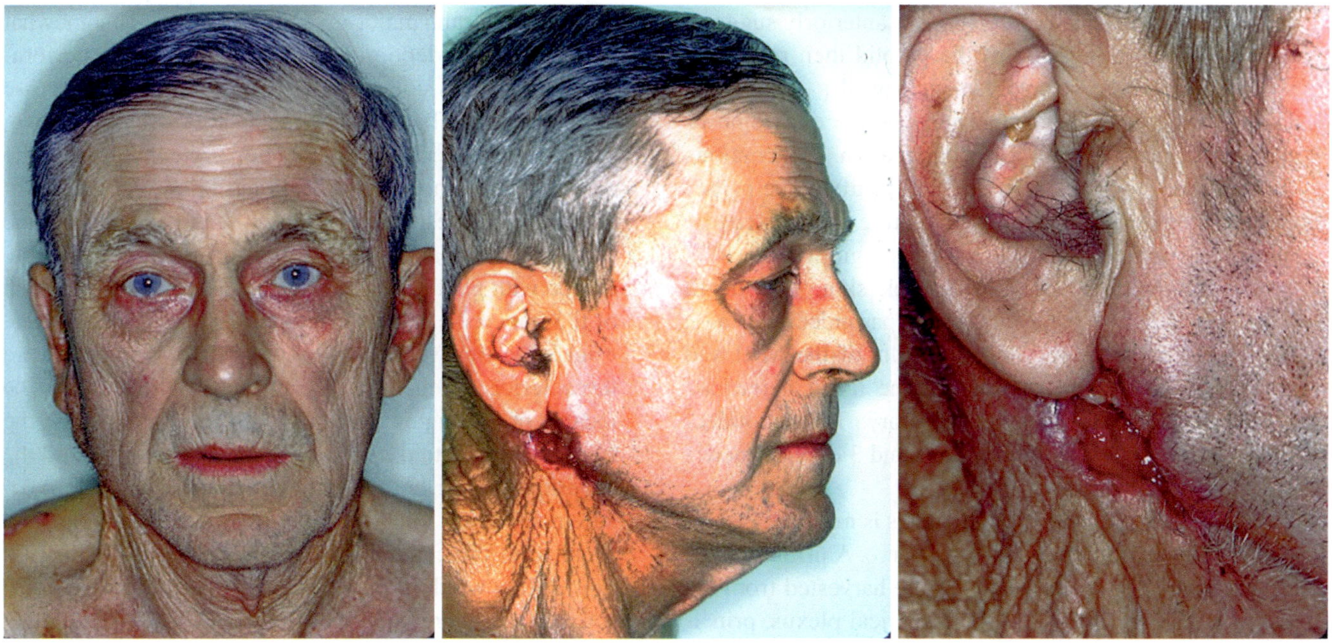

A 64-year-old man who had a "skin cancer" excised from the same area 18 months ago and received postoperative radiotherapy because tumor was present at the margins. A biopsy has revealed poorly differentiated squamous cell cancer. CT scan demonstrates no mandibular involvement.

1. Describe the slides. Add a clinical exam and focus on the following historical items: possible predisposing factors. Add a physical examination. (Male who appears stated age. The frontal view is largely unremarkable except for a slight bulge or prominence suggested in the right posterior cheek. The lateral view including close up demonstrates a deeply ulcerated lesion beneath and inferior to the lobule of the ear that appears to be approximately 2 cm in size with an area of skin thickening for an additional cm anterior to the body of the ulcer. The adjacent superior lateral neck skin appears mildly contracted. No other skin lesions are visible. In the frontal view, forehead furrows are present, the right lower eyelid is in normal position as well as the oral commissure, all indicative of a functioning or intact facial nerve.) Add a focused history and physical examination. (Further detail from the history should be elicited of the size, location, and method of excision of prior cancer, the number of weeks of radiotherapy, and the appearance of the ulceration and presumably subsequent growth. The patient should be questioned about current symptoms of pain or trismus. The past medical history is completed with a review of possible comorbidities. The physical exam focuses on facial expression or movement, a demonstration of mobility or lack of same of the lesion, mandibular excursion, and facial sensation. Palpation is accomplished of the preauricular, submandibular, and anterior cervical region for adenopathy.)
   (a) Any additional imaging? Justify. (MRI is a more sensitive imaging modality for determination of soft tissue extent of the carcinoma. Particular attention should be directed toward detection and degree of involvement of the parotid. CT scan, as the preamble has stated, can more accurately detect bony involvement, in this instance the angle of the mandible.)
   (b) Discuss the appropriateness of radiotherapy as employed above. (Re-excision is the preferred and recommended option for a positive margin after removal of squamous cell carcinoma of the skin. Given the high probability of recurrence with the attendant morbidity and mortality observation alone is contraindicated. The use of adjuvant or postoperative radiotherapy in extensive squamous cell cancer may provide better local control than resection alone but that conclusion assumes negative pathological margins. Should tumor recur after excision and postoperative radiotherapy then the treatment scenario, as in the case under discussion, becomes substantially more complex.)
2. Based on the information that you have describe the pathologic anatomy. (The lesion represents an aggressive,

poorly differentiated, recurrent squamous cell, post excision, and radiotherapy. The deep ulceration inevitably involves the parotid while the fullness anteriorly suggests tumor extension. Invasion of the parotid then raises the specter of facial nerve involvement as well.)

3. Outline a treatment plan that includes the oncologic or resective aspects as well as reconstruction. Give options for reconstruction, select yours, and justify. (The pathologic anatomy dictates the radical nature of the excision. Wide local excision entails a 2–3 cm margin which would encompass adjacent cheek and neck skin. The depth would include at least a superficial parotidectomy and, hinging to some degree on the results of the MRI and operative exploration, sacrifice of the facial nerve and total parotidectomy may be necessary. The parotidectomy will provide access to level 2 and 3 cervical nodes for excision as well.

   The reconstruction of two elements is necessary: skin-soft tissue and, if sacrificed, facial nerve. A primary graft to reconstitute the facial nerve can be harvested from the donor site of the branches of the cervical plexus, principally the greater auricular nerve, easily accessed through the neck incision. A lateral tarsorrhaphy is advisable in this age group for corneal protection since several months are required for nerve regeneration and facial muscle recovery. Even if full facial nerve function is not attained, partial return may be of benefit.

   A variety of flaps are available for the skin-soft tissue defect either free or pedicle. The two donor site options for pedicle flaps are the chest and shoulder. The pectoralis major, delto-pectoral, or internal mammary perforator are all pedicle flap options. The internal mammary perforator may not have sufficient length, the delto-pectoral would require delay and has some element of unpredictability, and the pectoralis major myocutaneous flap is somewhat bulky. The shoulder options are a supraclavicular perforator flap or cervicohumeral as an extended transverse trapezius flap. The supraclavicular artery flap, pedicled, perforator, or free with or without pre-expansion is the contemporary choice for cheek and lateral facial reconstruction. Harvested as a fasciocutaneous option, the supraclavicular artery, SCA, flap offers a thin, pliable choice with good skin color match. The SCA is a branch of the transverse cervical, derived from the thyrocervical trunk. The transverse cervical artery courses anterior to the anterior scalene muscle and the SCA branch can be located in a triangle formed by the posterior border of the sternocleidomastoid anterior, the clavicle inferior and the superior anterior border of the trapezius. Absolute measurements are 8 cm from the sternoclavicular joint and 3 cm from the clavicle. The Doppler can assist in location. A flap width of up to 7 cm will permit primary closure of the donor site in most patients. Reaching a defect higher on the cheek may require an extension beyond the deltoid insertion that encroaches on the posterior humeral circumflex angiosome. A 1-week delay of the distal one-third can minimize the possibility of ischemic necrosis. The flap should be harvested in the subfascial plane. Transfer and inset can be accomplished by tunneling or incision and release of cervical skin. Of course, a number of free fasciocutaneous flaps are available including the radial forearm. The supraclavicular artery perforator flap offers the optimal combination of thinness, pliability, and color match.)

Intraoperative

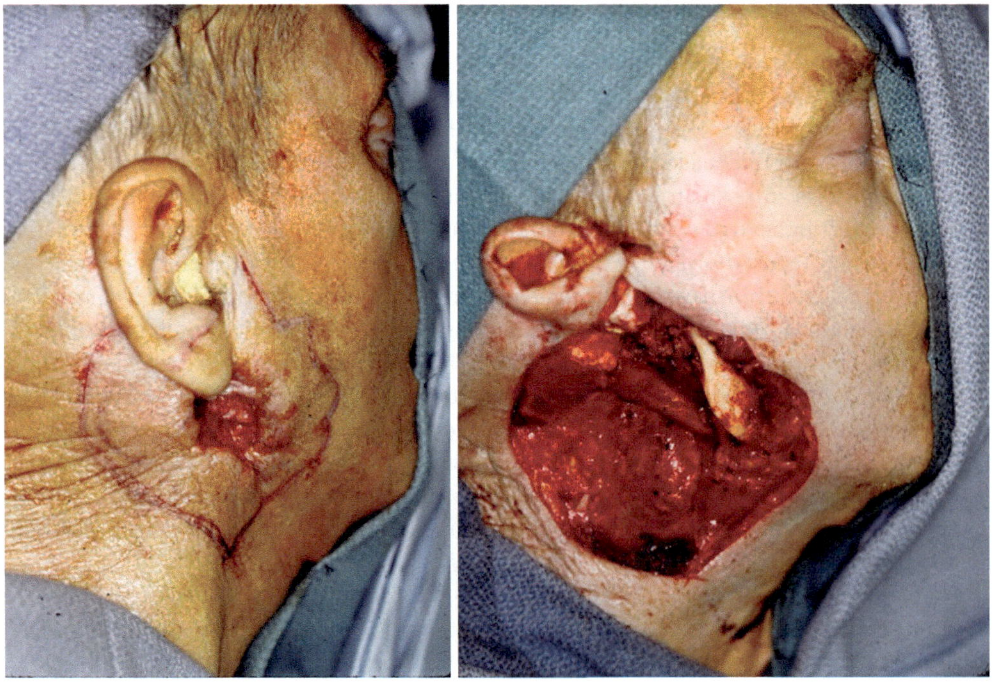

The first slide depicts the operative resection plan that consists of a diamond-shaped excision directed vertically. The dimensions appear to be 10 × 10 cm. The second intraoperative photo demonstrates the defect with a skeletonized mandibular angle and the posterior belly of the digastric muscle. No facial nerve is visible.

Postoperative (Early and Late)

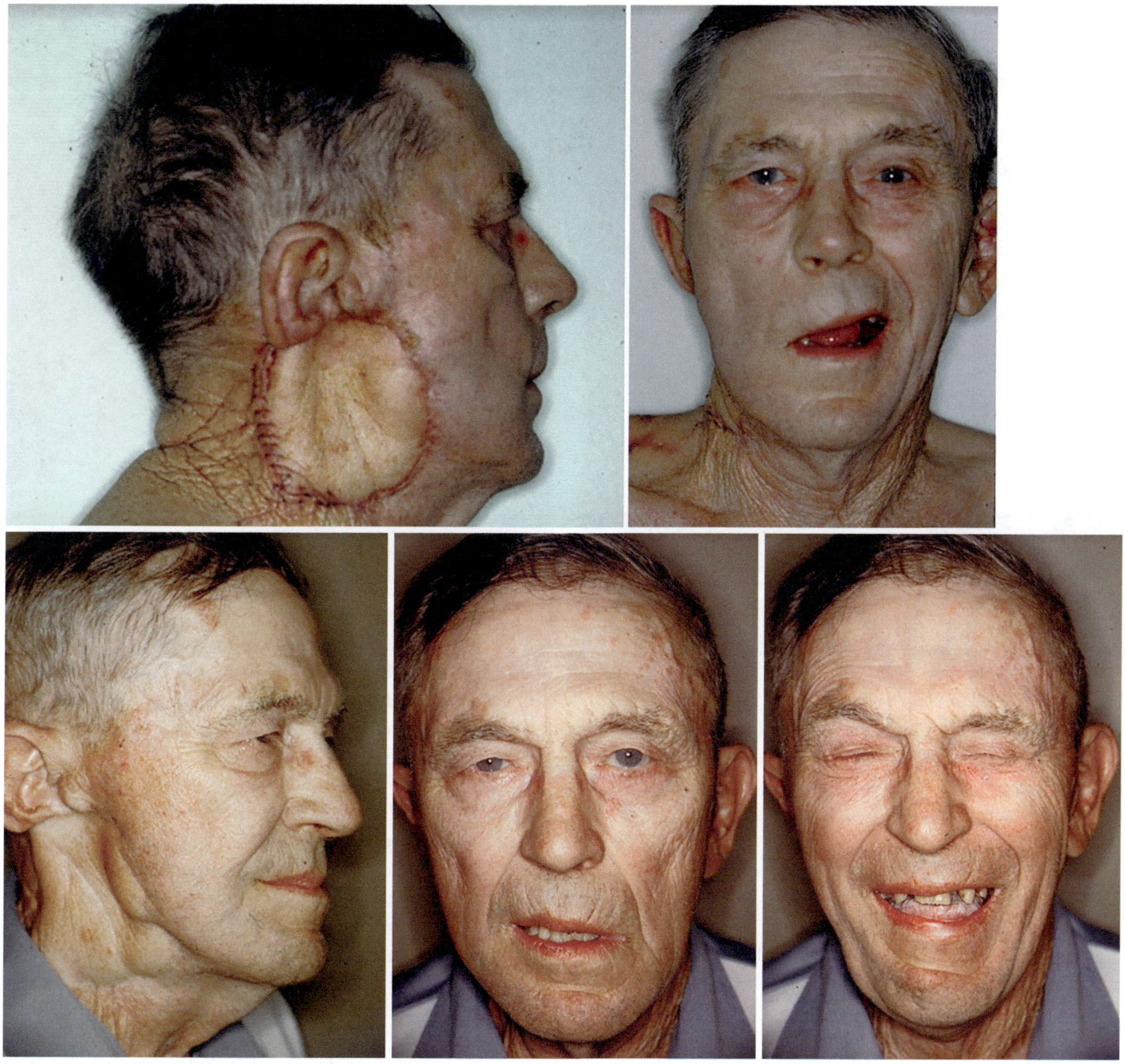

The first two photos are a lateral view of inset of a large, well-vascularized flap with sutures in place, followed by a frontal view that illustrates the absence of function in the temporal and buccal branches of the facial nerve, indeterminate of the zygomatic and mandibular branches. The late follow-up photos are those of a well-healed flap and intact cranial nerve function and all facial branches.

Case 3: Large Lip-Cheek Defect

Case-Based Conference

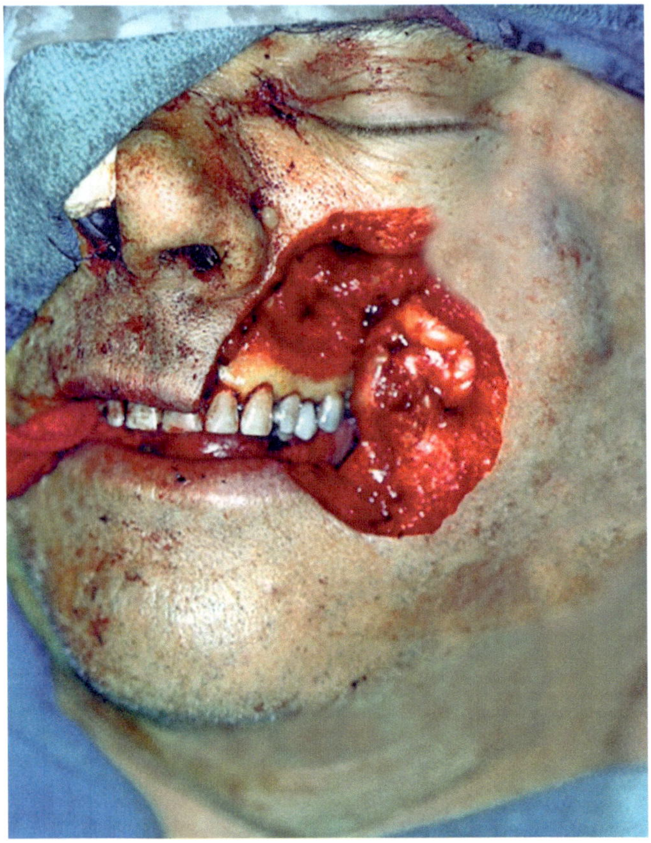

A 60 year-old with multiple medical problems including significant PVD, peripheral vascular disease, and immediate-post resection of recurrent squamous cell ca of the lip-commissure performed by the surgical oncologist.

1. Describe the slide. Add any pertinent clinical information not already provided above.
2. Describe the defect.
3. List the reconstructive needs and outline a reconstructive plan.

Case-Based Conference: Discussion

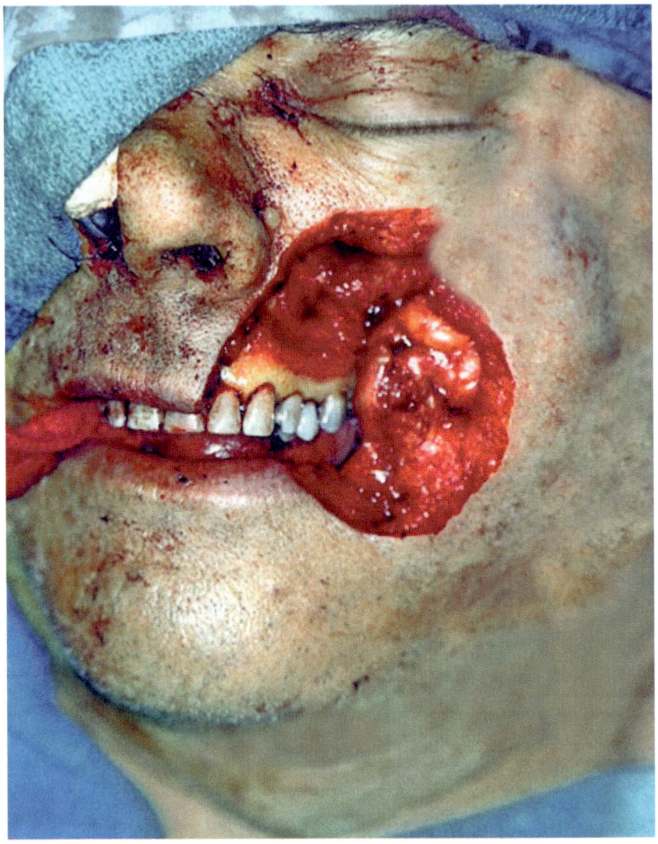

A 60-year-old with multiple medical problems including significant PVD, peripheral vascular disease, immediate-post resection of recurrent squamous cell ca of the lip-commissure, performed by the surgical oncologist.

1. Describe the slide. Add any pertinent clinical information not already provided above. (No photo of the preoperative appearance of the lesion is available, rather a photo of the intraoperative defect. Presumably, the reconstructive surgeon had the opportunity to examine the patient. If so, the initial history should establish prior treatment of the original lesion including the extent of excision and any adjuvant treatment, particularly radiotherapy. The initial history would ascertain if the patient experienced pain and if so, the character and distribution. Significant pain and the distribution of the divisions of the trigeminal nerve should raise concerns about neurovascular extension. The severity of the associated comorbidities should be explored including diagnosis and medications. A social history would include tobacco, alcohol, or substance abuse. The thrust of the physical exam is to determine as much as feasible the anticipated defect including an intraoral exam for the degree of mucosal involvement. Facial nerve function is ascertained and documented. The

parotid and cervical node-bearing areas are palpated. The presence of the facial and superficial temporal arteries are palpated or examined with a handheld Doppler, particularly if the decision has been established that the reconstruction will be performed with local and not free flaps.

The assumption is that the surgical oncologist will pursue imaging as well as any additional testing to clarify, if necessary, the severity of the comorbidities. Presumably, the surgical oncologist will also decide on the efficacy of a sentinel lymph node biopsy.)

2. Describe the defect. (The single intraoperative photo, an oblique view, demonstrates a substantial-sized defect that encompasses the entire lateral subunit of the left upper lip, perhaps the lateral one-fourth or approximately 2 cm of the lower lip, the commissure, and the adjacent medial cheek. The superior extent is to a point halfway between alar base, which is intact, and the infraorbital rim. The buccal and maxillary alveolar ridge mucosa is absent with exposure of the detention from medial to the medial incisor to distal of the first molar. The orifice or papilla of Stensen's duct may have been resected.)
3. List the reconstructive needs and outline a reconstructive plan. (The deficit includes full thickness of the lateral subunit of the upper lip, the lateral lower lip, commissure, and inferior one-half of Zone 2 and superior portion of Zone 3 of the cheek. The buccal sulcus has been sacrificed and possibly the orifice of Stensen's duct. The reconstructive plan must include a reconstitution of a portion of the lip deficit. Although an inevitable degree of microstomia will result, the lower lip could serve as a donor site. If the transverse width of the upper lip is approximately 8 cm and the philtrum 2 cm, each lateral unit is 3 cm. The lateral unit is divided into a medial fixed portion relatively less mobile because of attachment to the nasal sill and alar crease, a distance of about 1.5 cm. The remainder of the lateral unit is the mobile subunit. The upper lip deficit appears to be about 2.5–3.0 cm, a critical-sized defect. Of the 7 ½ cm of a normal lower lip transverse width, approximately 6.5 cm appears to remain, providing about 1–1.5 for an Abbë flap. A 1.0 to 1½ cm Abbë flap can reconstruct the medial element of the lateral unit of the upper lip, the mobile subunit reconstituted with the flap option that is utilized for reconstruction of the cheek defect. The latter, the cheek, would probably be optimally addressed, at least in this patient, with a Mustarde flap. Some of the details about the design and harvest of the Mustarde flap are included in Case 1-Chap. 27. Briefly, the flap is placed on the facial muscles elevated superficial to the SMAS or sub-SMAS if perfusion is a concern as for example in a smoker, but should transition superficial once the zygomaticus major is encountered. An inferior and medial dogear with the result. The rotation will require a combination of the preauricular incision into the neck transversely and directed anteriorly into a relaxed skin tension. The flap is stabilized with a suture from the deep aspect to the periosteum of the zygoma or into the deep temporal fascia. If the posterior donor site deficit is considerable, closure with a full-thickness skin graft harvested from the ipsilateral or contralateral neck will be necessary. The Mustarde flap seems to be susceptible to necrosis and smokers so a concerted effort should be directed toward tobacco cessation. The buccal sulcus was realigned with a posteriorly-based mucosal flap. The saliva secretion through Stensen's duct is passively allowed to seek passage into the intraoral cavity.)

Intraoperative

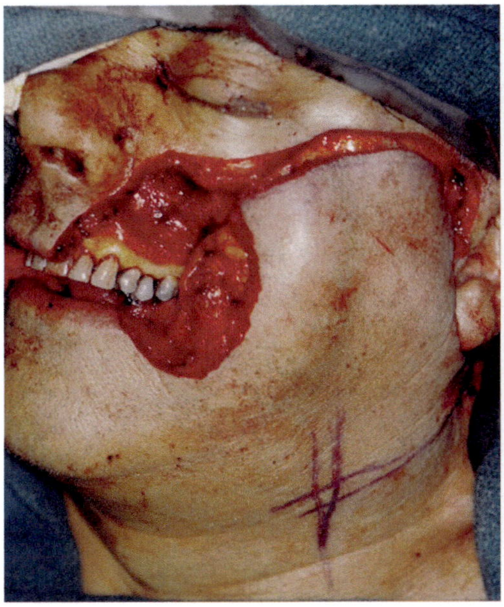

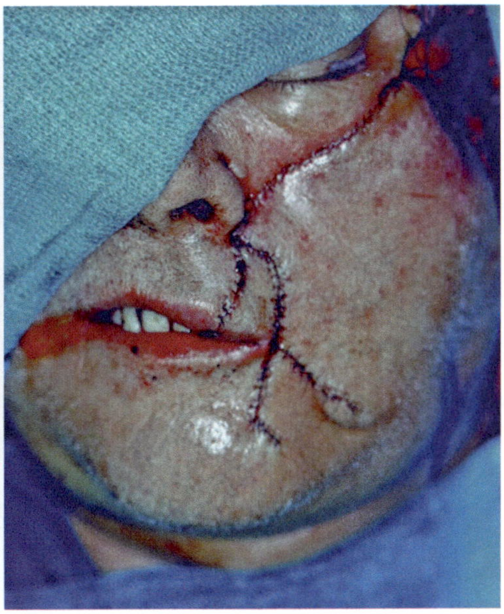

The two intraoperative photos illustrate the superior incision portion of the cheek flap that, judging by the thickness, is certainly sub-SMAS in configuration. The superior limb arches obliquely and superiorly into the inferior temporal area and then courses preauricular. Surgical ink markings over the mandibular body appear to designate the course of the facial vessels. In the following photo, the defect has been closed with an Abbë flap to the upper lip, and the remainder of the defect with a cheek flap. The dogear has been excised medially and inferior.

Postoperative (Six Months)

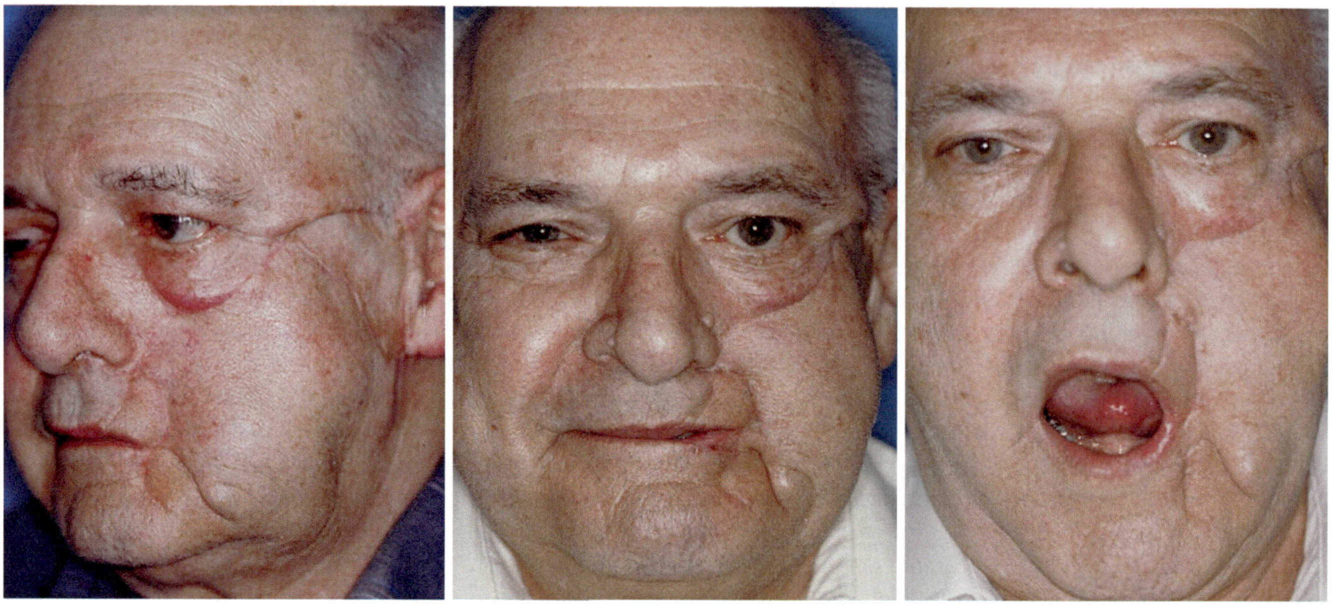

A total of three photos provide the postoperative follow-up. An oblique view depicts a fully-healed wound without deficit except for some residual edema of the infraorbital region superior to the inset of the cheek flap. A frontal view confirms the findings including the absence of ectropion or scleral show of the left lower lid. The final slide with the patient opening his mouth depicts minimal microstomia.

Critique

Since a full native dentition is present, difficulty with denture insertion is not a problem and a small dogear exists that could be excised with local anesthesia if the patient so desires.

29 Nose

Bibliography

Editor's Note: Some overlap exists in the Menick references.

Parrett, B. M., Pribaz J. J., "An Algorithm for Treatment of Nasal Defects", *Clin. Plastic Surg*, (2009); 36:**407–420.**

Taghinia A. H., Pribaz J. J., "Complex Nasal Reconstruction", *Plast. Reconstr. Surg.*, (2008); 121(2):**15e–20e.**

Menick F. J., "Nasal Reconstruction with a Forehead Flap", *Clin. Plastic Surg*, (2009); 36:**443–459.**

Menick F. J., "The Evolution of Lining in Nasal Reconstruction", *Clin. Plastic Surg*, (2009); 36:**421–438.**

Menick F. J., "Practical Details of Nasal Reconstruction", *Plast. Reconstr. Surg.*, (2013); 131(4):**613e–630e. (Including videos)**

Thornton J. F., Griffin J. R., Constantine F. C., "Nasal Reconstruction: An Overview and Nuances", *Semin Plast Surg*, (2008); 22(4):**257–265. (Good technical points)**

Faculty Discussion and Study Guide

1. Draw the aesthetic subunits of the nose (Fig. 29.1).
   (a) What is another method to anatomically separate the areas of the nose? (Division by thirds; into an upper one-third, the glabella and medial canthi; a middle one-third, the dorsum, and nasal side walls; and the lower one-third, the tip and alar side walls.)
   (b) Structurally, besides location, what are the reconstructive considerations in complex nasal defects? (Which, if not all, of the three layers—skin, skeletal support, and lining—are involved.)
   (c) How does the division of the nose into a superior two-thirds and inferior one-third impact reconstruction? (In two ways—the skin of the dorsum and side walls is thin and mobile and the tip and alae are thicker, more sebaceous, and more tightly adhered to the underlying skeletal framework. In addition, the envelope, skin and soft tissue, are supported by cartilage, lower lateral, and the upper two-thirds by more rigid bone and septum.)
2. What is the reconstructive principle incorporated into the aesthetic subunit concept? (Optimally, any reconstruction should encompass an entire aesthetic subunit because the margins of the reconstruction will be camouflaged to some degree by the borders of the aesthetic subunit.)
   (a) When is the application of that principle not appropriate? (The application of the necessity to reconstruct an entire aesthetic subunit is less rigorous in the superior one-half to two-thirds of the nose, namely the aesthetic subunits of the medial canthi, nasal side walls, and dorsum. The application of the principle is more rigorous in those areas where the borders are much better defined by the underlying contour, namely, the tip and alar rim region.)
3. Essentially, what is the functional role of skeletal support and the necessity for replacement of the same? (Central skeleton, nasal bones, and septum maintain the rigidity of the nasal cavity for passage of airflow. The alar rims and domes prevent collapse on inspiration.)
4. Conceptually, divide the reconstruction of the nasal support elements into two components and discuss. (Skeletal-median support and alar-columellar support. Skeletal support is central and replaces missing septum or, uncommonly, bony defects. Alar and dome support is accomplished with conchal cartilage. The cartilage grafts are employed as batten, columellar strut, and tip or shield grafts.)
   (a) What are the options for the former? (Bone, cranial or rib, costal or septal cartilage)
   (b) The latter? (Conchal or septal cartilage)
5. List the four most commonly employed flaps used for skin coverage in nasal reconstruction? Briefly describe each. (The frontonasal flap, bilobe, nasolabial, forehead,

E. Luce, *A Curriculum for Plastic Surgery*, https://doi.org/10.1007/978-3-031-62087-4_29

Fig. 29.1 Aesthetic subunits

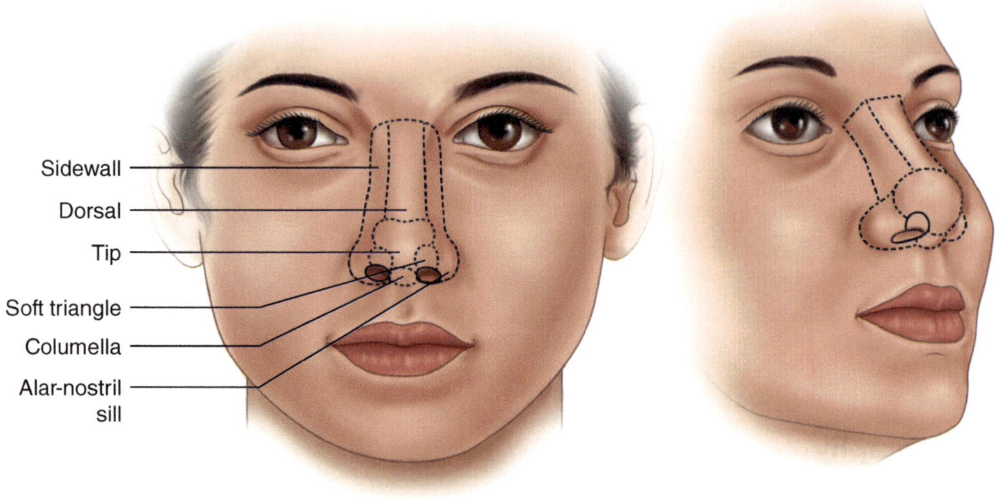

and glabellar flap. Glabellar flaps are short, triangular shaped in design and intended to replace nasal dorsum and medial canthal defects. Fronto-nasal flaps are based on branches of one angular artery and consist of rotating the remaining dorsal nasal skin and glabellar skin into the defect. Nasolabial flaps are based superiorly and utilized for lateral alar rim defects. Inferiorly-based nasolabial flaps when utilized for nasal reconstruction almost uniformly require a second-stage revision or revisions and are best avoided. Bilobed flaps on the nose are similar to those designed elsewhere and are primarily indicated for small, 1.5 cm or less, defects of the dome. Larger defects of the nasal tip reconstructed with bilobed flaps tend to pin cushion.)

(a) Any role for V-Y advancement flaps? (Relatively small defects of the lateral middle third can be closed with an island-type V-Y advancement flap with incorporation of the lateral nasal branch of the angular artery. Shortcomings are the tendency, if insufficient advancement is performed, of lateral tension and distortion. See Fig. 29.2.)

6. Outline options for the following defects.
   (a) Nasal sidewalls. (Small defects can be closed with a full-thickness skin graft with an acceptable result. Larger defects, particularly more superior may require a rotational glabellar flap.)
   (b) Central nasal upper one-third. (More superior and smaller defects can be closed with a glabellar flap, larger defects probably will require a forehead flap. Full-thickness skin grafts are feasible in elderly patients.)
   (c) Middle third central or lateral. (Frontonasal rotational flap.)
   (d) Alar. (If lateral, a rotational superiorly-based nasolabial flap unless the defect is <1.5 cm, than a composite graft.)
   (e) Dome or central tip. (Frontonasal or bilobed flap. Larger defects will require a staged forehead flap.)
7. A composite graft is optimally used for what defect and size? (Alar rim defects that require both lining, support, and coverage of a maximal size of 1.5 cm, probably less. The helical rim is the most common donor site for such grafts. The readings also describe a free flap harvested from the most anterior portion of the helical rim and based on the superficial temporal vessels, probably the superior auricular artery, not advisable except in extreme circumstances.)
8. Describe, in all three dimensions, the blood supply of the forehead flap. (The blood supply is based on the supratrochlear artery and vein which exits through the supratrochlear foramen or notch 1.5–1.7 cm lateral to the midline. The artery after exit from the foramen becomes supraperiosteal about 2 cm superior to the superior orbital rim, enters the frontalis muscle, and ultimately becomes subdermal in location at the most distal portion of the flap.)
   (a) What ramifications does that description have for raising the flap? (The pedicle can be as narrow as 1.5 cm, although described as 1–1.2 cm in one of the readings, and the course of the artery allows aggressive thinning of frontalis muscle and subcutaneous fat in the distal portion of the flap if a two-staged approach is planned. As the flap is raised the most proximal or inferior portion of the dissection should be directly on the periosteum or even subperiosteal in depth.)
   (b) Describe the orientation of a forehead flap for a right heminasal defect. (An ipsilateral orientation of the flap on the supratrochlear artery, rotated medially, will provide greater length than a contralateral.)
9. Describe the two- and three-stage forehead flap for nasal reconstruction. (Two stage is placement of the flap and then division of the pedicle. To do so does not permit an intermediate stage, described below, and is useful per-

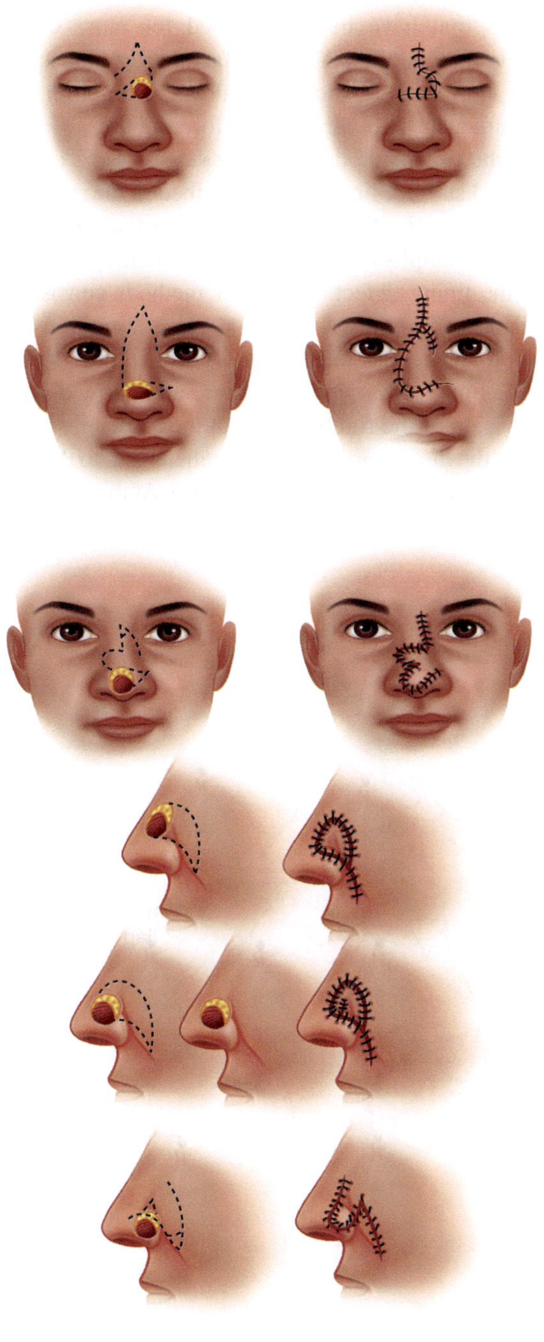

Fig. 29.2 V-Y advancement flaps

haps for small defects and requires thinning of the distal portion at the first stage. Although additional thinning is possible at the second stage, division of the pedicle must be limited to the more proximal inset to avoid devascularization. In addition, cartilage grafting must be buried within the flap unless a well-vascularized lining is present. Three-stage forehead flap as described by Menick consists of rotation of the full-thickness of the flap including frontalis muscle, a 4-week interval, detachment of the flap from the recipient site with radical defatting of both the flap and the residual tissue on the recipient site, and then an additional 4-week interval. The final stage is the division of the pedicle and inset of the flap.)

10. In the reconstruction of tip-alar defects with a three-stage forehead flap, at what stage are cartilage grafts placed and why? (Cartilage grafts are placed in the second or intermediate stage, primarily because the thinning of the flap is performed at this stage. If well-vascularized lining is present at the onset, cartilage grafts can be placed and covered with a first-stage forehead flap.)
11. What are the most critical errors in reconstruction of the nose? (Inadequate lining).
    (a) Why? (Wound contracture of inadequate lining or raw areas of nasal lining will inevitably distort the overlying skin cover unless those areas lie extremely high in the nasal vault, not an area that is ordinarily reconstructed.)
12. The readings discuss options for nasal lining, one of which is a septal mucoperichondrial flap. Describe including blood supply. Critique. (The hinged or pivot septal mucoperichondrial flap is hinged inferiorly and anteriorly and consists of septal mucosa and the underlying perichondrium. The flap is then pivoted and rotated into the lining deficit, usually the lower one-third of the nose. The flap can be used to line a middle vault donor defect when a bipedicled bucket handle flap is rotated inferiorly into the defect. The flap will obstruct the nostril and denude cartilage which with time will remucosalize. Larger bilateral pedicled flaps that include septal cartilage will create a permanent fistula and are probably not recommended.)
    (a) What is the blood supply of the septal mucoperichondrial flap? (The septal branch of the superior labial artery.)
13. What is the management of the raw area of the septum, consequent of the harvest of a pivot or hinged flap? (Usually is left raw and will reepithelize if the cartilage is intact. Bipedicled mucosa flaps in contrast usually require placement of a full-thickness skin graft or a septal flap.)
    (a) Critique (The use of intranasal flaps can distort the intranasal anatomy and produce nasal obstruction or nostril stenosis. In addition, the dissection in the limited area of the nasal cavity is difficult and tedious.)
14. Give some options for small or moderate-size lining defects with the benefits and liabilities. (If well-vascularized native skin coverage is present, quite uncommon, a simple full-thickness skin graft can be performed. More likely is the necessity to provide lining such as a bipedicled mucosal or bucket handle flap. The flap is based both laterally on the alar mucosa and medially on the septal tissue and rotated inferiorly with possibly a skin graft to close the donor site defect. An additional option is placement of a skin graft on the raw aspect of the tip of a forehead flap at the first-stage inset.

A third option is placement of a skin graft on the forehead flap in situ and allowing a week to 10 days for a "take" before rotation. A final additional option are turnover of flaps of skin based on the edges of the defect.

The disadvantages of the bipedicled flap are limited operative exposure, limited size defect, and the possibility of nostril stenosis. Skin grafts placed on the raw surface of the forehead flap often become thickened and inflexible as the readings detail. Turnover flaps of residual skin based on the edge of the defect are of tenuous blood supply and inadequate for larger defects. In fact, all of the options listed are probably best suited toward a 1.0–1.5 cm defect. See Figs. 29.3 and 29.4.)

15. Outline additional options for more extensive defects. (As Menick describes, his workhorse has become the fold-over distal extension of a forehead flap with thinning and debulking at a second stage. See below. Other options that have been described for more extensive defects include the FAMM or facial artery musculomucosal flap and for total nasal reconstruction, lining accompanied with a free radial forearm flap.)
16. Describe two methods including stages of the use of the forehead skin for lining. (As described in the readings, an extension of the forehead flap even beyond the hairline can be accomplished with the extension designed for inset into the lining defect. The other methods consist of the excision of frontalis muscle and galea at the most distal portion and replacement with a full-thickness skin graft for the lining. Both options require an intermediate stage of division of the forehead flap at the alar rim with defatting of the distal portion of the forehead flap to the level of the subdermis and sculpting of the tip. At the intermediate

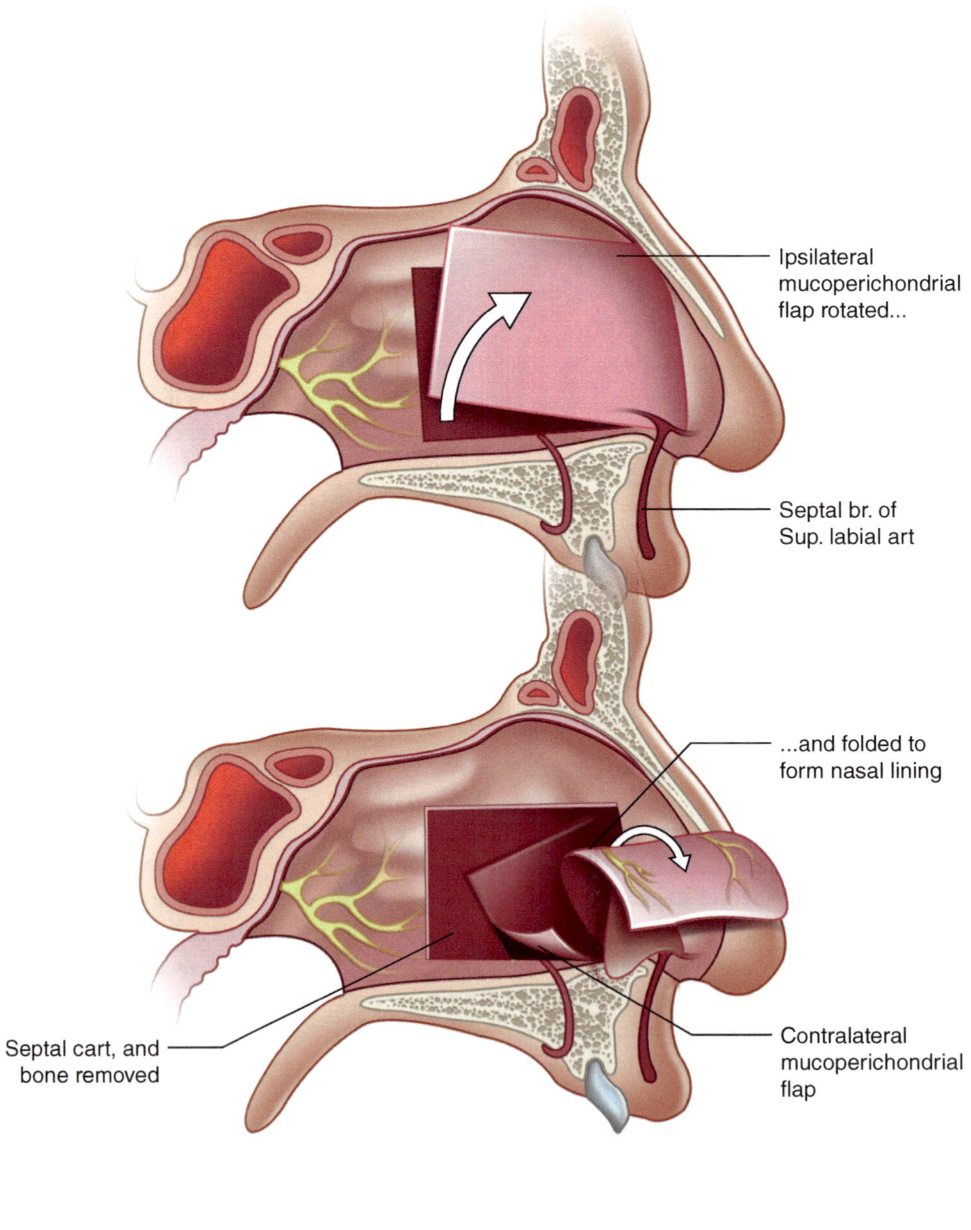

Fig. 29.3 Bipedicled mucosal flap (Redrawn from Burget G.C. and Menick F. J. "Nasal Support and Lining: Marriage of Beauty and Blood supply", *Plast Reconstr Surg.*, (1989);84:189. (Reprinted with Permission))

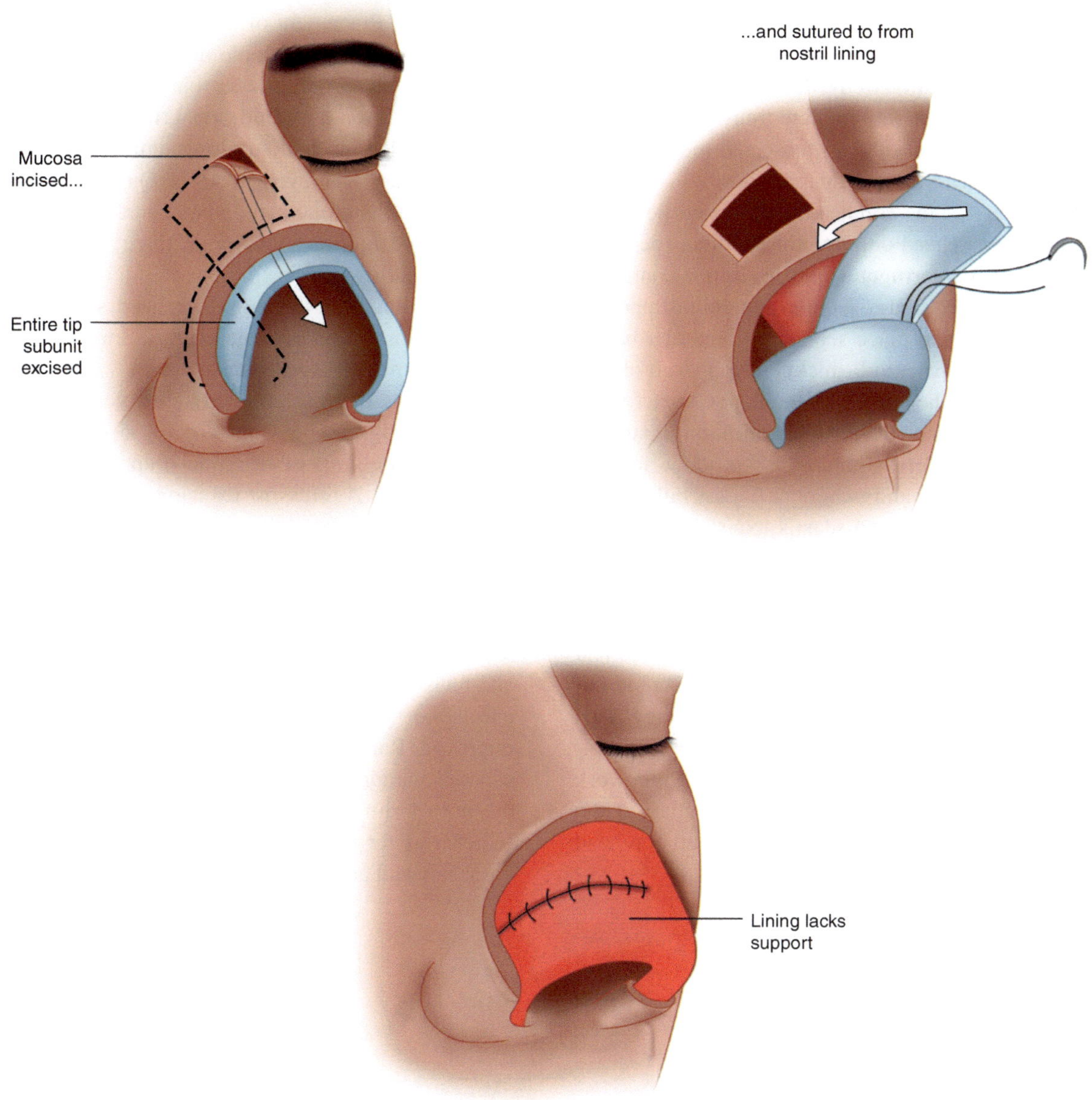

Fig. 29.4 Bucket handle flap. (Redrawn from Burget G.C. and Menick F. J. "Nasal Support and Lining: Marriage of Beauty and Blood supply", *Plast Reconstr Surg.*, (1989);84:189. (Reprinted with Permission))

stage, the forehead flap is reset into the tip. The third stage consists of division and inset of the pedicle.)

(a) What defect or indications are appropriate for the full-thickness skin graft method? (Only moderate-size defects, perhaps an upper limit of 1.5 cm. Also, elderly or debilitated patients may not be able to tolerate the nasal obstruction that's inevitable with a staged extended forehead flap.)

17. Although certainly uncommon in the average plastic surgeon's practice, what are the general dictates of reconstruction of massive nasal defects that involve all three components? (Free flap reconstruction with the radial forearm flap is performed for lining the nasal vault, cantilever bone graft for dorsal support and cartilage grafts for tip, and forehead flap for external coverage. Free flap for coverage instead of forehead flap should be avoided because of color mismatch. Although not discussed by the readings, frequent skeletal support is also necessary for the adjacent maxilla.)

Videos from Menick

Menick MD, F. J., "Nasal Reconstruction with a Forehead Flap", *Plast Reconstr Surg.*, (2013) 131:63e. Videos 1–7.

Video 1—Lateral alar defect from full-thickness tissue necrosis consisting of the entire alar subunit from dome laterally with extension into the tip subunit. Marked out all landmarks. Created template of both subunits. No Doppler of the superficial temporal artery-? included

Plan/forehead flap. Recreation of the defect. Excised remaining tip defect. Contralateral template transferred to forehead flap. Lateral border of flap transected medial brow. Developed the flap 1.5 cm inferior to brow.

Video 2—Stage one of the forehead flap; lining defect as extension of the forehead flap into the hairline. Elevation with division of the corrugator *but* dissection continued superficial to the periosteum. No cartilaginous support at this juncture except did place septal cartilage alar batten graft. Flap was quite pale. Full-thickness skin graft placed on the raw aspect of the pedicle of the flap. Gauze for the superior aspect of donor defect with primary closure of the inferior portion. *Point*—short flaps produce tension that leads to contracture and ischemia. Excess bulk on the lining including frontalis and scar is excised, limited to the lining extension only.

Video 3—One month later. Stage two; Intermediate elevation, debulking of flap, and right alar rim support. The flap is elevated but retains the lining in place. Elevation of just 3 mm of thickness of the distal tip of the flap. Excision of fat and frontalis from the defect; "intranasal lining flaps rarely utilized." "Intermediate thinning is safer than thinning at the first stage." Placed alar batten graft framework harvested from the concha and divided the flap at the juncture of the lining appendage. The thinned forehead flap is replaced onto defect.

Video 4—Must always provide cartilage support. Stage two (continued); Placement of alar batten but also included a portion of the residual dome in the graft. Placement of a tip shield graft for increased projection. The template dictated the excision of an additional rim margin off the forehead flap. Flap inset and quilting sutures placed into reset forehead flap. Removed at 48 h. Quilting sutures were placed across the planned division site.

Video 5—One month later. Stage three; Pedicle division. Nostril a little stenotic. Reopened inferior midline forehead closure. Excised entire forehead scar. Inset was a *short*, almost imperceptible scar. Tailored the base that contained medial brow to inset.

Video 6—Stage three (continued); Recipient inset. The flap is elevated aggressively to within 1.5 cm of the nostril margin. Debulking of proximal flap inset over tip and nasal dorsum. *Aggressive* excision of scar from the flap and the bed of the dorsum. More quilting sutures and additional skin excision from the intact dorsum. Define alar-cheek junction by buried deep stitches. The flap is purple at the end.

Video 7—Four months later; Late revision—"Most will require late revision mostly quilting sutures to further define alar-nasolabial definition and nostril narrowing." Some improved. Raise the flap inset on two margins: one, at the superior margin or alar crease and thinned same; second, at the nostril rim to improve nostril stenosis by debulking. Indications for late revision are slightly bulky, junction of nasal sidewall and ala indistinct, nostrils slightly stenotsic.

Case 1: Nasal Lesion

Case-Based Conference

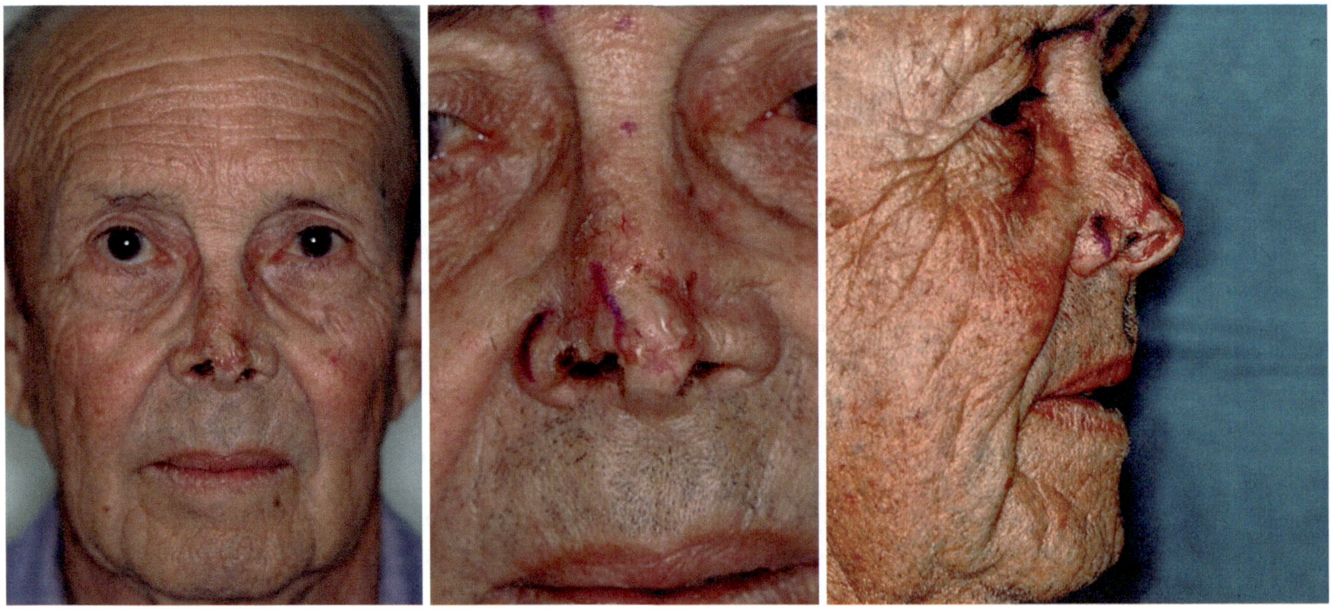

A 69-year-old with a history of a nasal lesion, biopsied with pathology of "basal cell with marked inflammation." Past history of "skin cancers" removed. The patient is otherwise in good health and a non-smoker.

1. Describe the slide(s) and add a focused clinical exam.
   (a) What tests do you want?
2. For your most likely diagnosis, outline the anticipated defect in aesthetic terms. Draw the defect.
3. Outline a treatment plan including sequence and incisions. Begin with a menu of possibilities and then choose your entree(s). Justify.

Case-Based Conference: Discussion

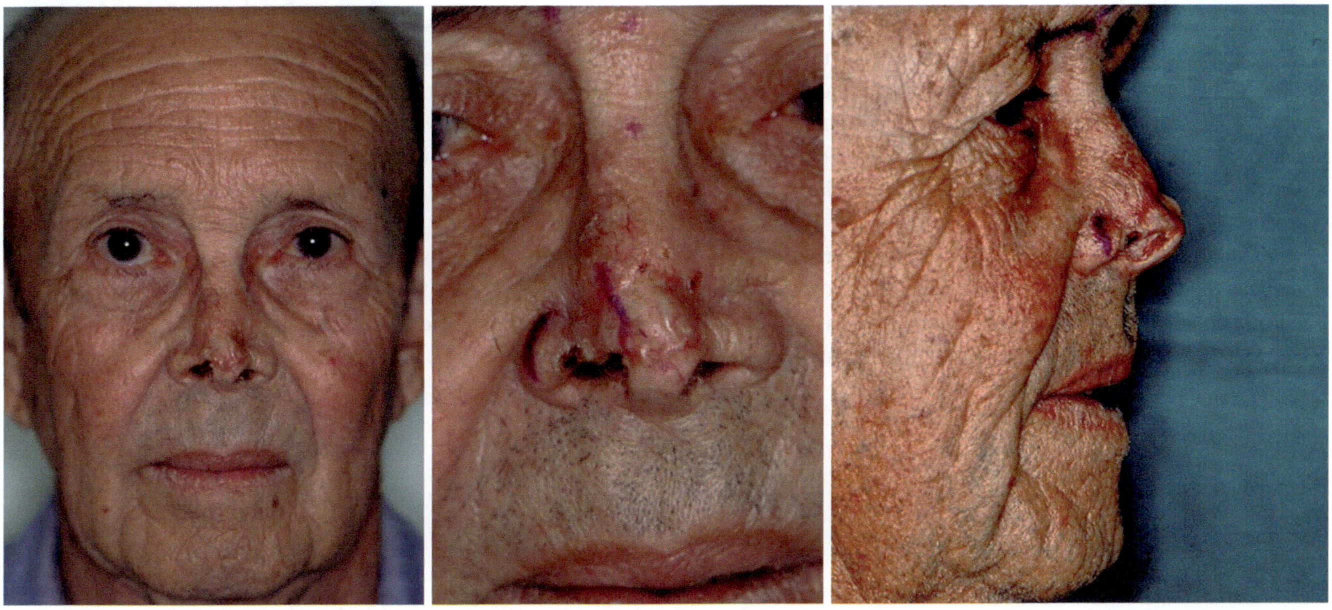

A 69-year-old with a history of a nasal lesion, biopsied with pathology of "basal cell with marked inflammation." Past history of "skin cancers" removed. The patient is otherwise in good health and a non-smoker.

1. Describe the slide(s) and add a focused clinical exam. (Two views, frontal and lateral, are available. The frontal view demonstrates a distal nasal lesion that has replaced the lobule with pearly nodularity-type changes and occasional telangiectasia. A small area of superficial ulceration is evident superior and lateral. A crusting lesion is evident on the mid-third of the dorsum. The right alar rim and medial alar unit have skin changes that blend onto the lobular lesion. The remainder of the face has no discernible lesions. The lateral view demonstrates advanced deformity of the distal third of the nose including destruction of the soft tissue configuration and skeletonization of the tip. The alar rim is retracted with the marked columellar show.

   The history would focus on the past treatment including extent of prior excision and, most importantly, if radiation therapy had been administered. Performance status, smoking history, and medications would complete the history. The physical exam of the nose would include a careful assessment of the involvement or not of the underlying alar cartilages and also a nasal speculum exam.)
   (a) What tests do you want? (If a tissue diagnosis had not been offered in the preamble, an incisional biopsy of the pearly white area of the lobule would be advisable.)
2. For your most likely diagnosis, outline the anticipated defect in aesthetic terms. Draw the defect. (The treatment scenario posed by the patient is somewhat diagnostic although mostly therapeutic. If not previously performed, an incisional biopsy will confirm the clinical diagnosis of skin cancer, basal or squamous cell. The recurrent nature of the lesion and the location, the nose, would probably dictate management by Mohs surgery, yet for purposes of discussion the presumption is that the plastic surgeon will provide resection as well as reconstruction. The treatment scenario is one of provision of coverage and possibly support and lining as well for a defect of the distal one-third of the nose. The anticipated defect, though, is not only the entire tip but also the middle one-third as well as the lower lateral cartilage and lining on the right. In essence, the patient's aesthetic desires would dictate some of the

treatment plan. Excision of the involved areas consists of lobule and alar subunits and will extend from one nasolabial fold to the other namely, the skin coverage of the tip, alar subunits, and distal nasal dorsum. If possible, the alar cartilage and nasal lining should be preserved but sacrificed if so indicated. Reconstruction would await pathological clearance, probably at 48 h or "slow Mohs".)

3. Outline a treatment plan including sequence and incisions. Begin with a menu of possibilities and then choose your entree(s). Justify. (A paramedian forehead flap will provide coverage, bilateral ear conchal grafts, and septal mucosal flaps can reestablish support and lining, respectively. If cartilage grafting is warranted, placement of the conchal grafts at the first or second stage can be accomplished. If the lining defect on the right does not extend beyond the limits of the lower lateral cartilage, an additional option is extension of the forehead flap into the hairline and use of the tip extension for recreation of lining. A median extension will be necessary for reconstruction of the columella. This extension, as well as the forehead flap proper, will require aggressive thinning at the intermediate stage. Two different approaches or designs of the forehead flap afford the opportunity for a sculpted or contoured reconstruction that simulates or duplicates the fine details of the nasal tip. The first is an excision of the frontalis and subcutaneous fat from the distal 2–3 mm of the flap at the time of flap creation and inset with two stages, the second-stage transection and inset. The second option is the addition of an intermediate stage following flap reconstruction and rotation into the defect. The intermediate stage, performed 2–3 weeks after inset, consists of detachment of the flap, an extensive excision of fat, frontalis or thinning of the distal flap, and then reinset. Both methods divide the flap and inset 3–4 weeks later. If an extension of the forehead flap is employed for lining, the 2–3 weeks hiatus is necessary to ensure vascularization of the extension prior to the second stage, when the flap will be raised but the lining extension remains behind.

   The forehead flap offers an elegant reconstruction of this patient's anticipated defect.)

Intraoperative

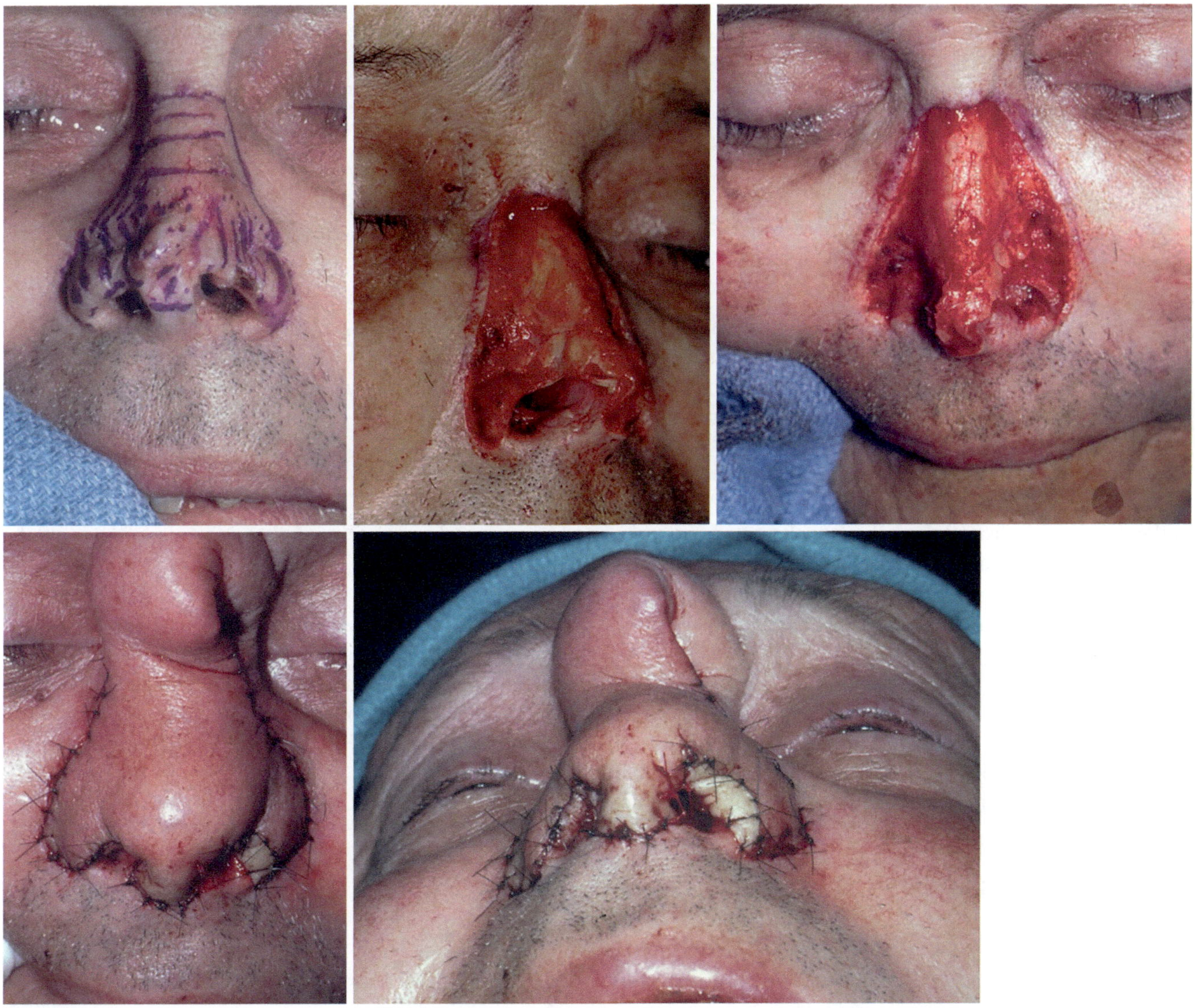

The five intraoperative slides illustrate in turn the proposed excision, the excised defect from a full frontal view and right oblique, and last, a forehead flap inset into the defect. The excision consists of the entire skin envelope from sub glabella area superiorly, nasolabial fold laterally, both alar rims to the alar base laterally, and to mid or the total columella. The nasal aesthetic units of the dorsum, side walls, tip, alar-nostril sill, and most of the columella, all are planned for excision. The extirpative photos demonstrate what remains—the osseocartilaginous framework only. In the final intraoperative slide the forehead flap has been inset and freshly sutured with complete reconstruction of the columella, nostrils, and remainder of the nose with the pedicle intact. Cartilage grafts have been placed and a small full-thickness skin graft added to the alar lining on the left.

Postoperative (Four Months)

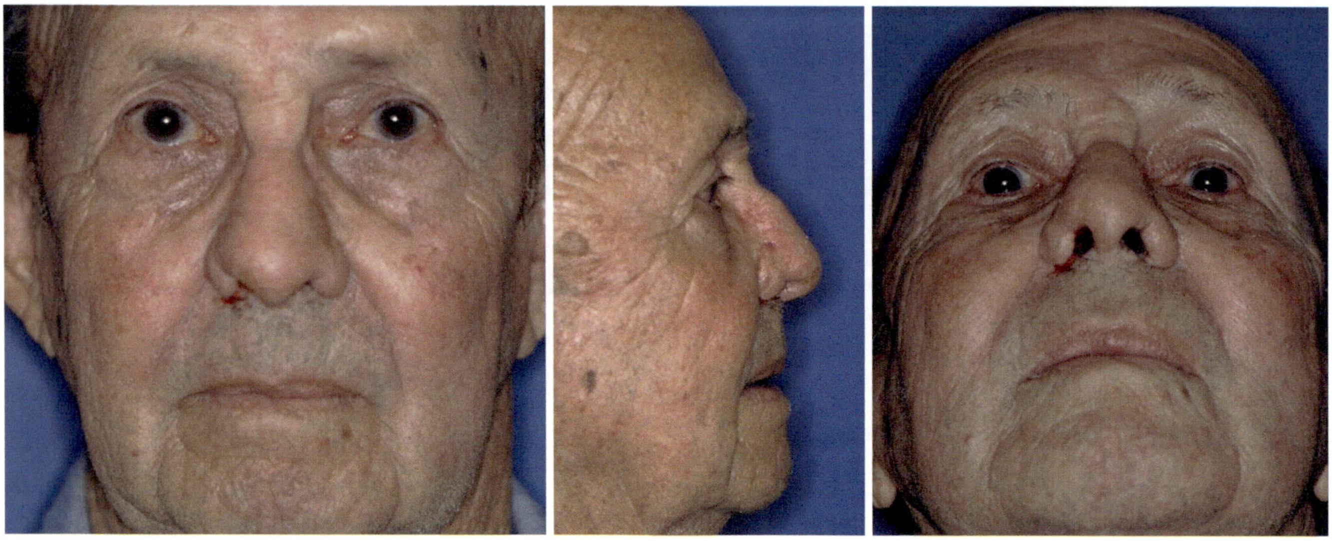

In the three views, frontal, lateral, and submental vertex the shape symmetry and aesthetics of the reconstructed nose are good. Conchal cartilage provided bilateral batten grafts to reinforce alar support and prevent external nasal valve collapse.

Crique

Reconstruction was accomplished in two stages at the request of the patient. A three-stage approach would have permitted defatting of the flap and ultimately better definition of the tip.

A minor notching defect of the right alar rim could be addressed with revision.

Preamble If the forehead flap is classified as a regional option the following series of cases illustrate the use of local flaps for nasal reconstruction. The description of the cases and clinical examination have been truncated but the principles outlined earlier of assessment of the defect and the patient still pertain.

Case 2: Nasal Lesion

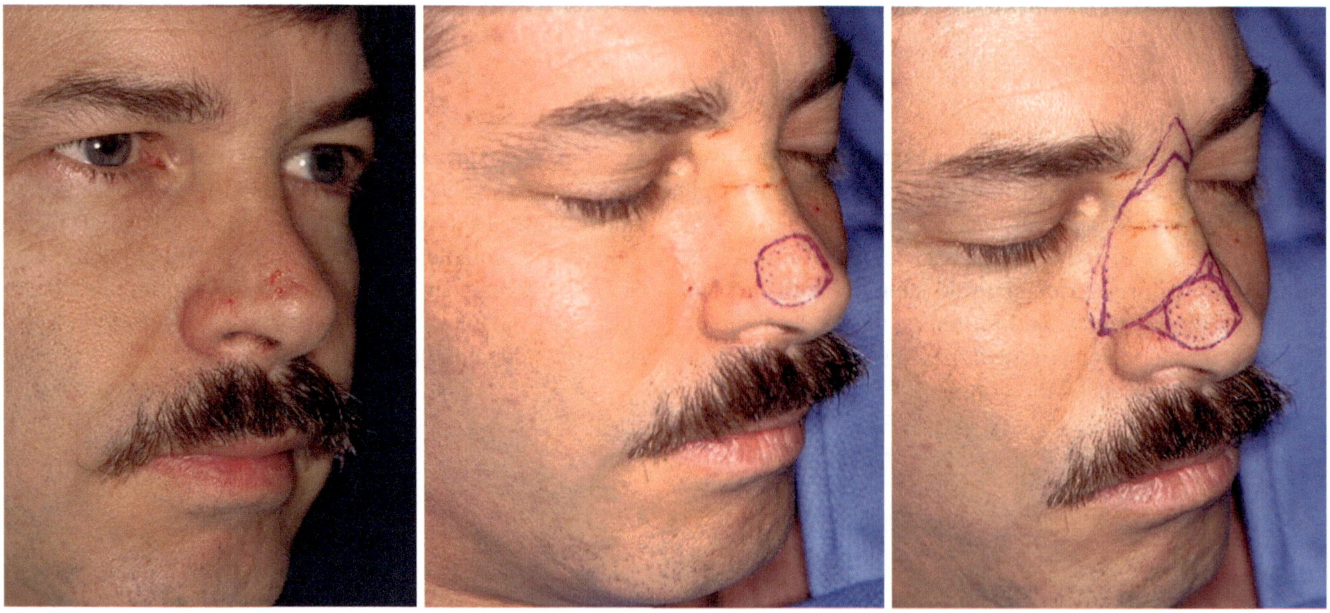

A 41-year-old man with a basal cell carcinoma of the right nasal tip aesthetic unit and also encroaches on the dorsum.

The anticipated defect will be substantial and some consideration should be given to a delayed reconstruction after final pathology has assured the excisional margins are not involved. The options for reconstruction are, remotely, a forehead or a frontonasal.

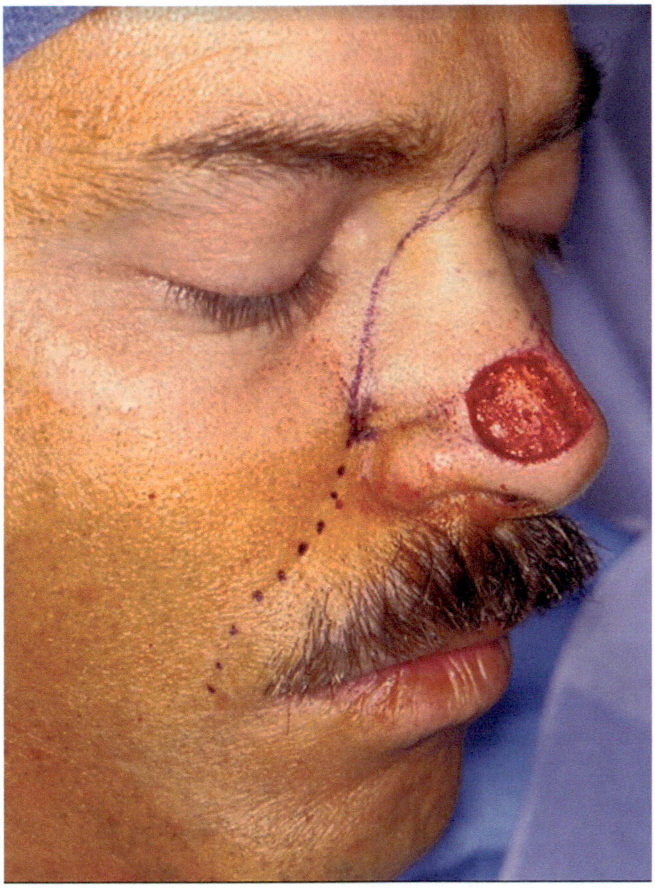

The markings indicate a surgical plan for a frontonasal flap. The frontonasal flap is based on branches of the angular artery, particularly the lateral nasal, and a vessel of the internal carotid system, the dorsal nasal artery. Originally described as a V-Y type advancement flap with utilization of a glabellar component, the frontonasal flap functions optimally as a rotation, with little or no 'V' in the glabella.

Intraoperative

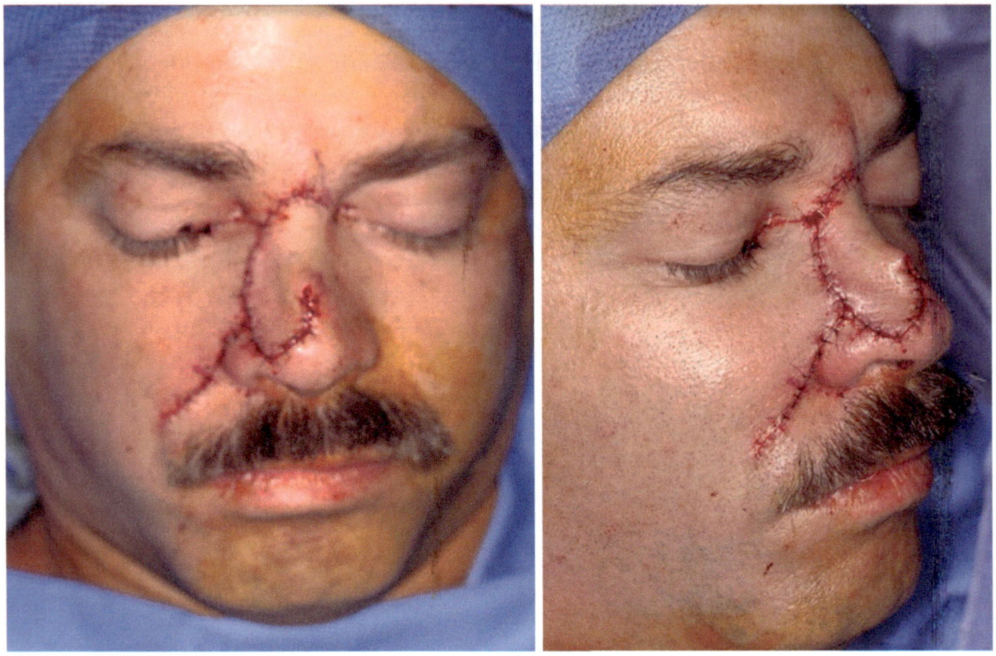

The flap is elevated in the immediate supraperiosteal or perichondrial plane, with the dissection continued over the opposite lateral side wall. Once rotated into the defect, a dogear is inevitable that will flatten and rarely, if ever, require excision. Little or no glabellar skin has been harvested.

Postoperative (Four Months)

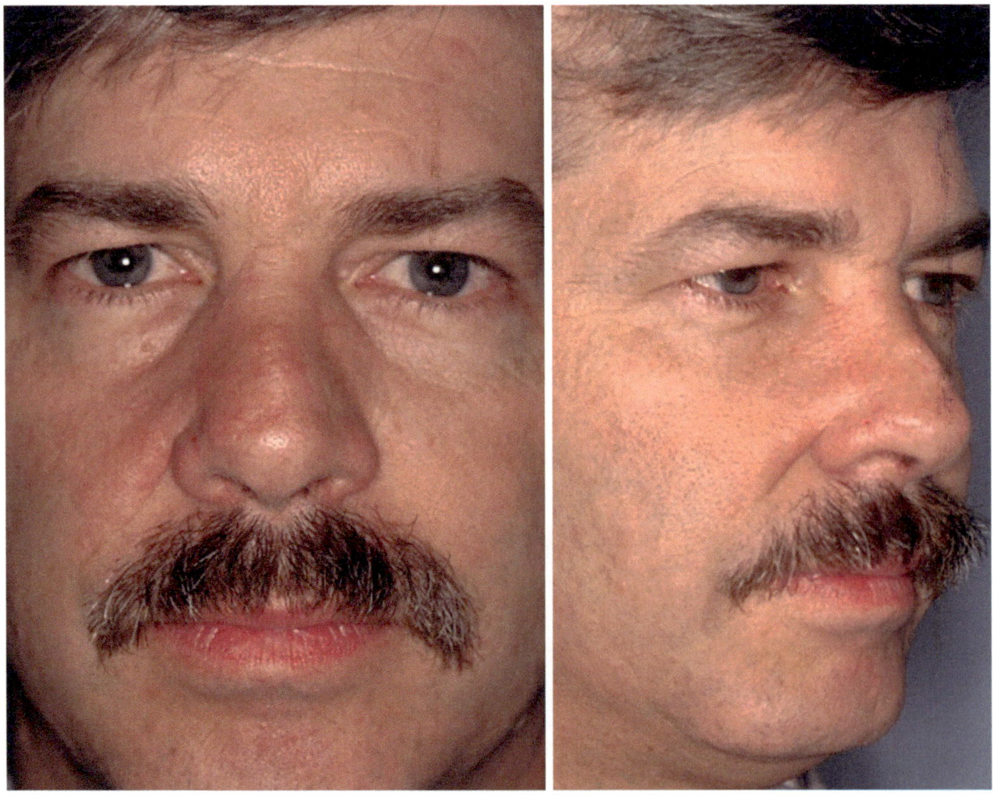

The flap is blended imperceptibly into the adjacent nasal skin, the tip highlights have persevered, and the dogear has resolved.

Case 3: Nasal Lesion

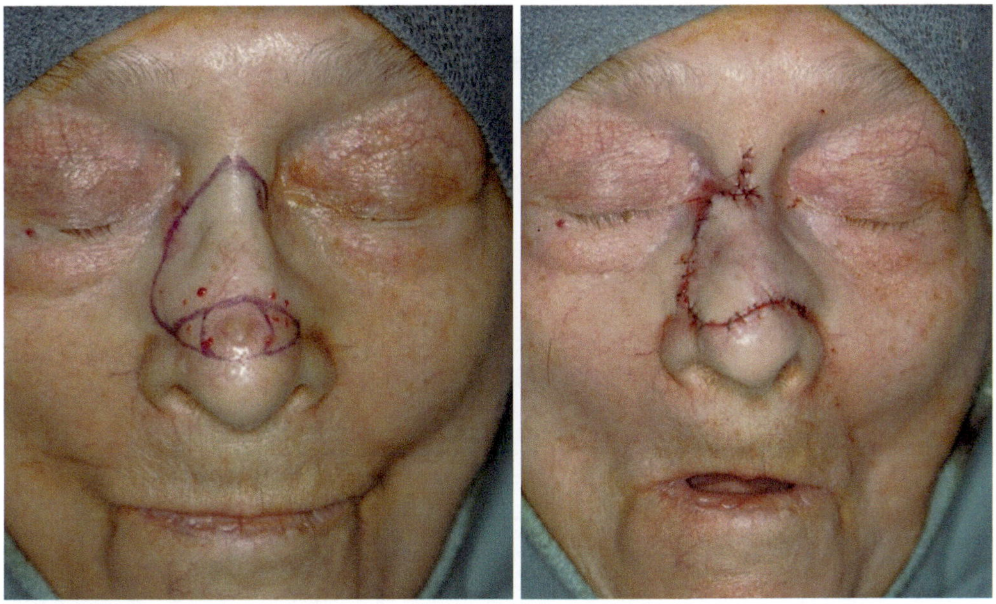

A 68-year-old woman with a basal cell carcinoma of the supra tip aesthetic unit. The markings indicate a surgical plan for a transverse elliptical excision to facilitate closure with a frontonasal flap. The flap incisions follow the aesthetic lines, junction of the cheek and nasal side, traversing the glabella in a relaxed skin tension line of the transverse furrow and into the opposite cheek-dorsum junction. The rotation arch can be enhanced by extension of the incision inferiorly, not necessary in this case.

Postoperative (Six Months)

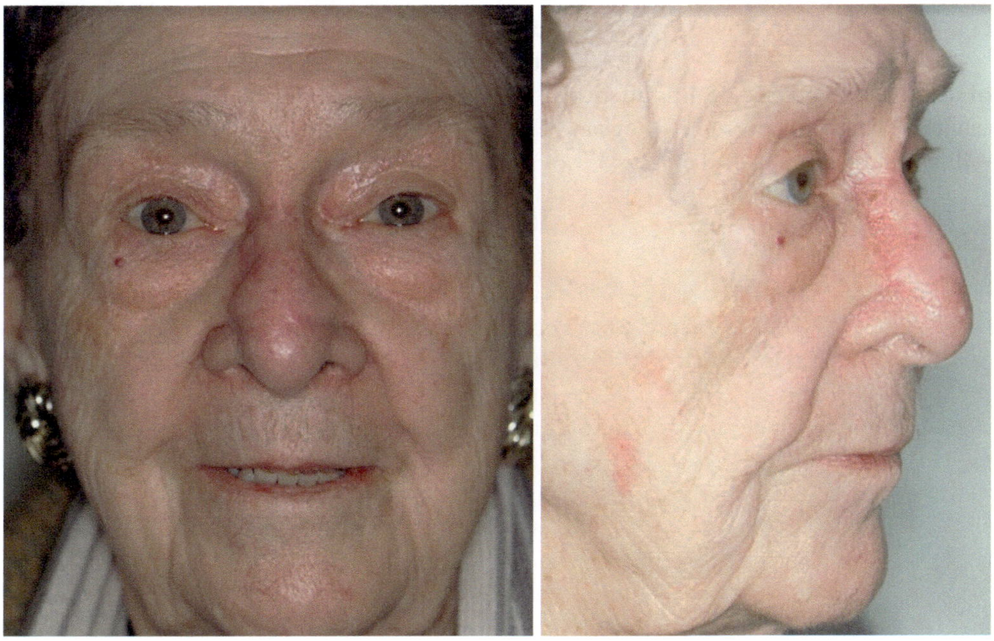

In the frontal view, the aesthetics of the nose have been preserved and on lateral the nasal tip has not been retracted cephalad.

Case 4: Nasal Lesion

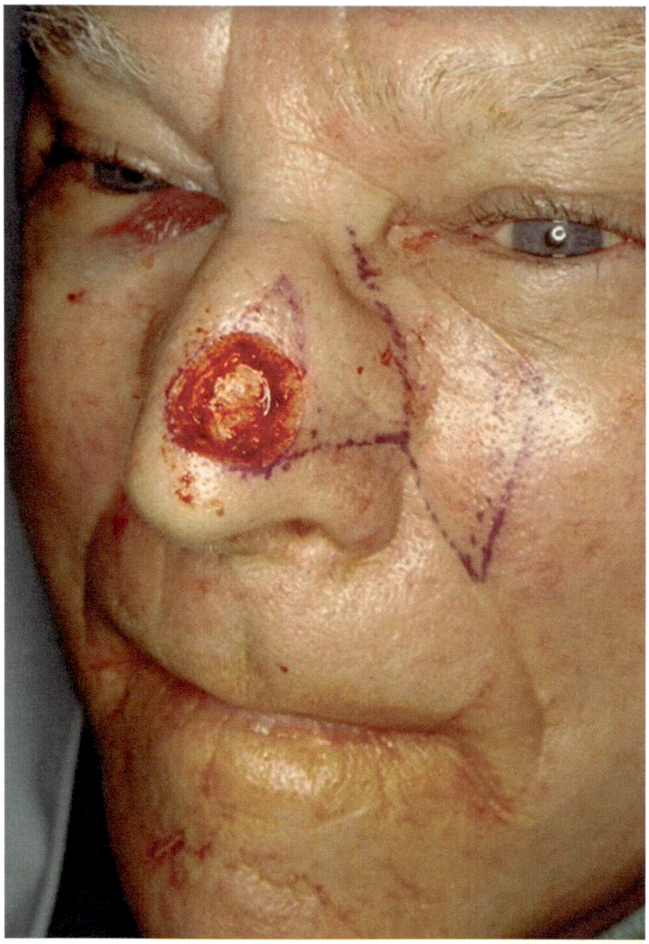

A 64-year-old with an excisional defect accomplished 48 h prior. The defect involves the subunits of the left tip, dorsum, and a portion of the nasal sidewall, beyond the limits of the frontonasal flap. An option is excision of the remaining left nasal tip and a forehead flap for reconstruction. In this instance, a superiorly-based nasal sidewall flap has been designed to reconstruct the defect and a nasolabial flap to close the donor site. If possible, cheek advancement will obviate the necessity of the second flap.

Intraoperative

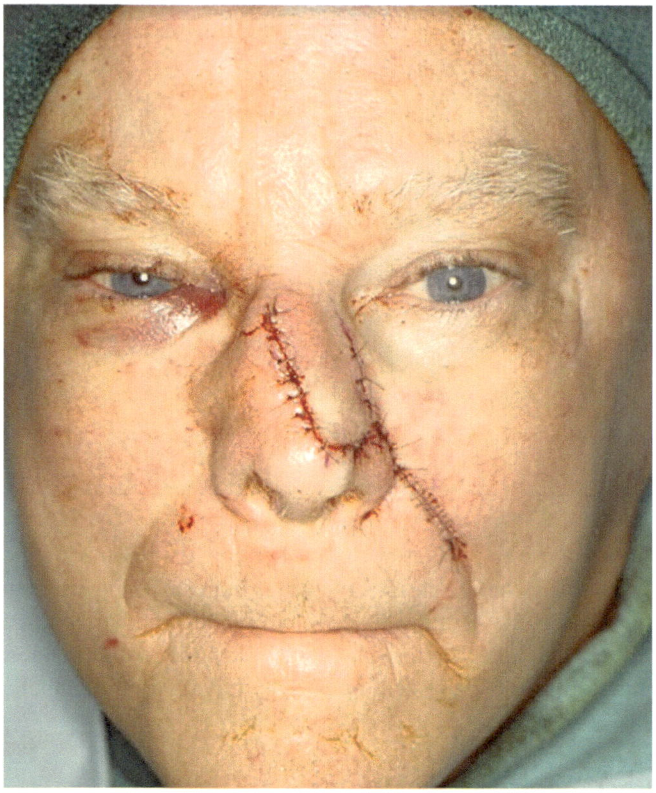

The nasal flap has been rotated into the defect and the cheek advanced to close the donor site. Extension of the incision inferiorly is necessary to permit advancement and avoid dogear.

Postoperative (Three Months)

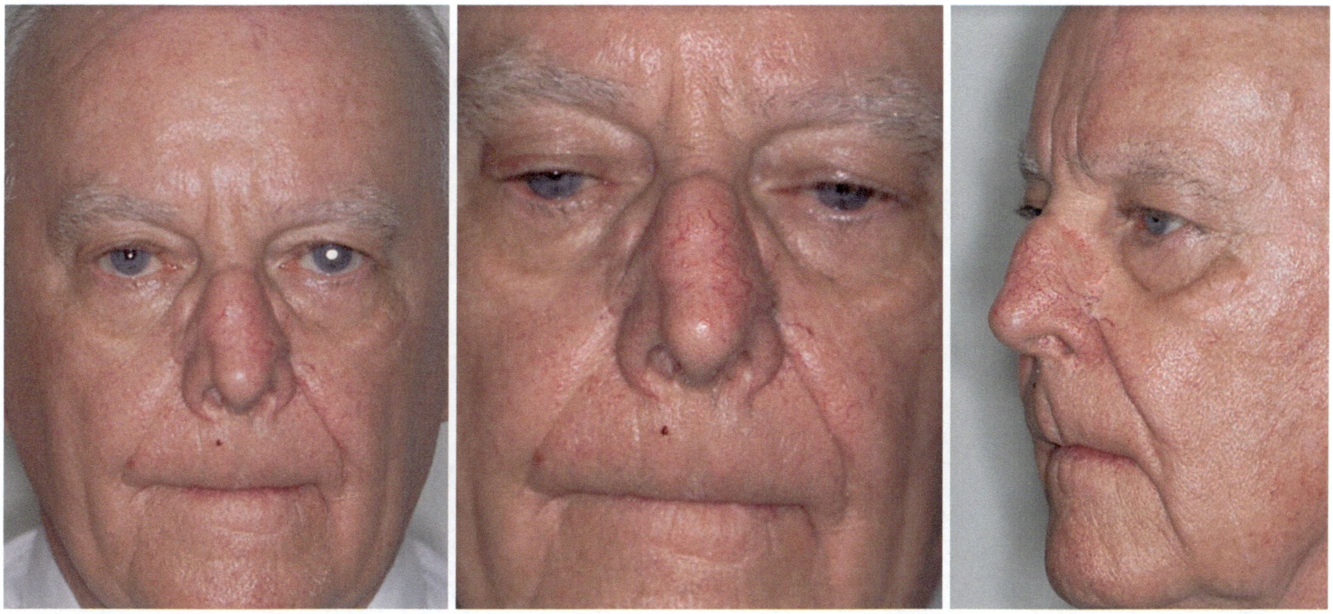

The outcome is good without aesthetic deficit.

Case 5: Nasal Lesion

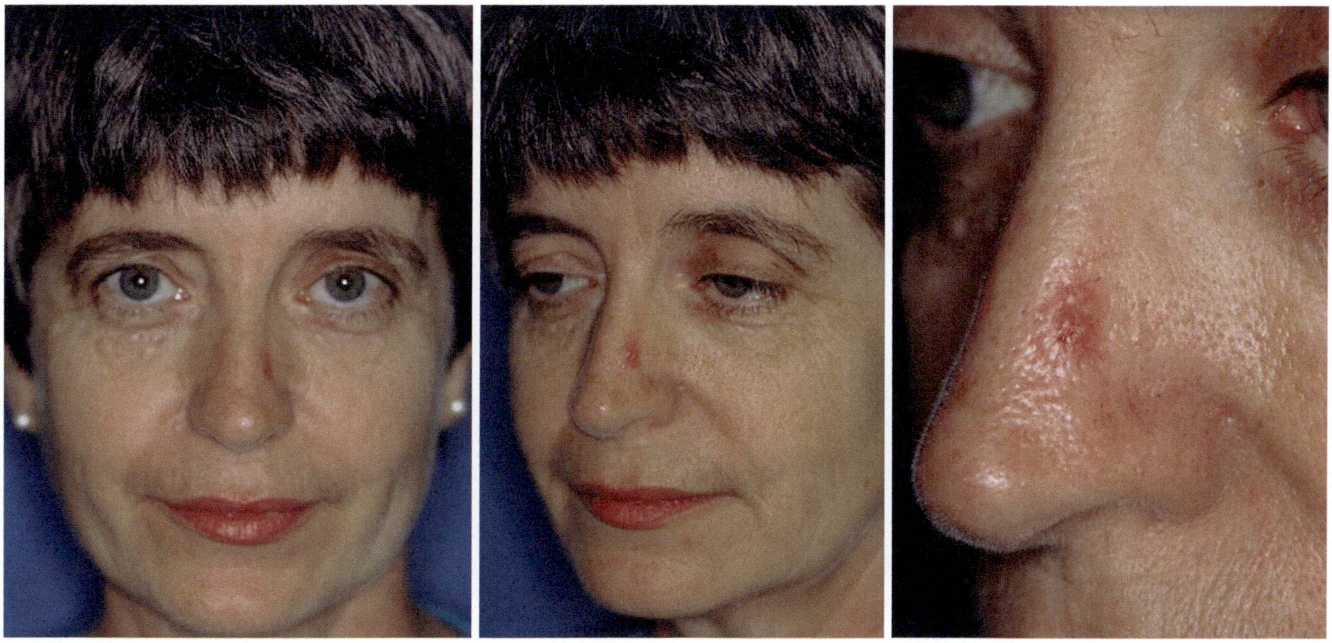

A 44-year-old with a basal cell carcinoma of the middle third of the nose.

Intraoperative

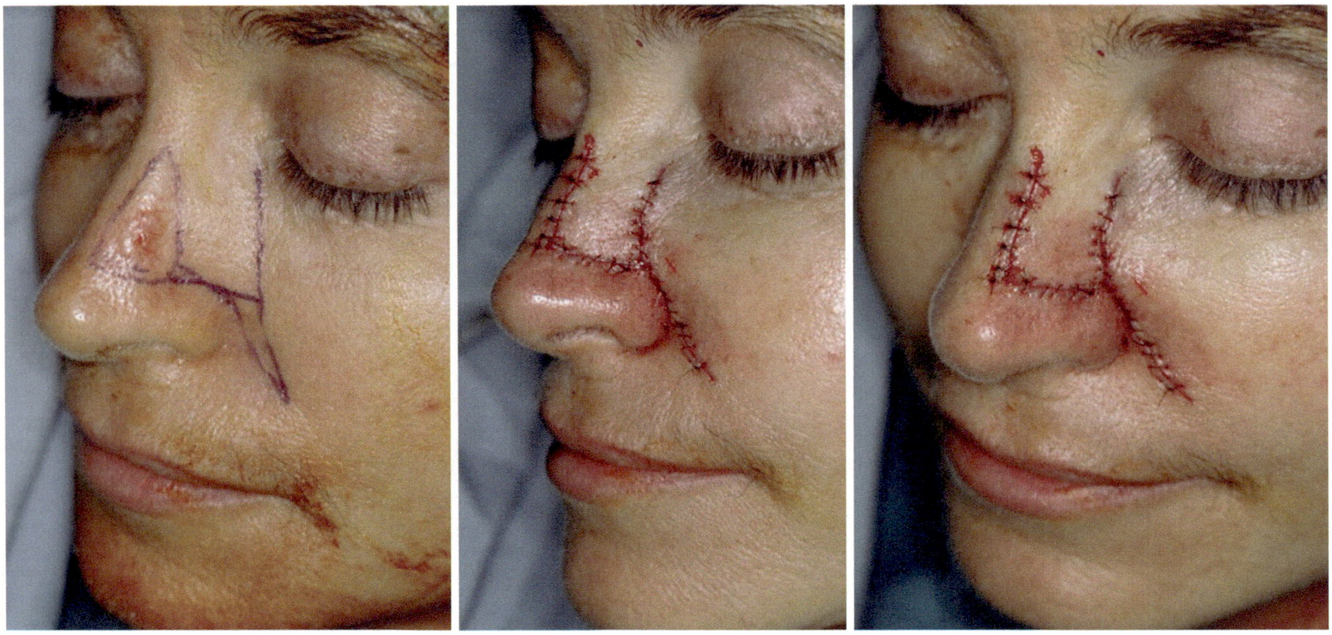

Although a frontonasal flap is certainly an option for the anticipated defect, a superiorly-based flap combined with cheek advancement has been designed. Extension of the incision inferiorly into the nasolabial fold will permit tension-free closure of the cheek advancement with the lateral incision proposed to ultimately lie in the nose-cheek junction.

Postoperative (Three Months)

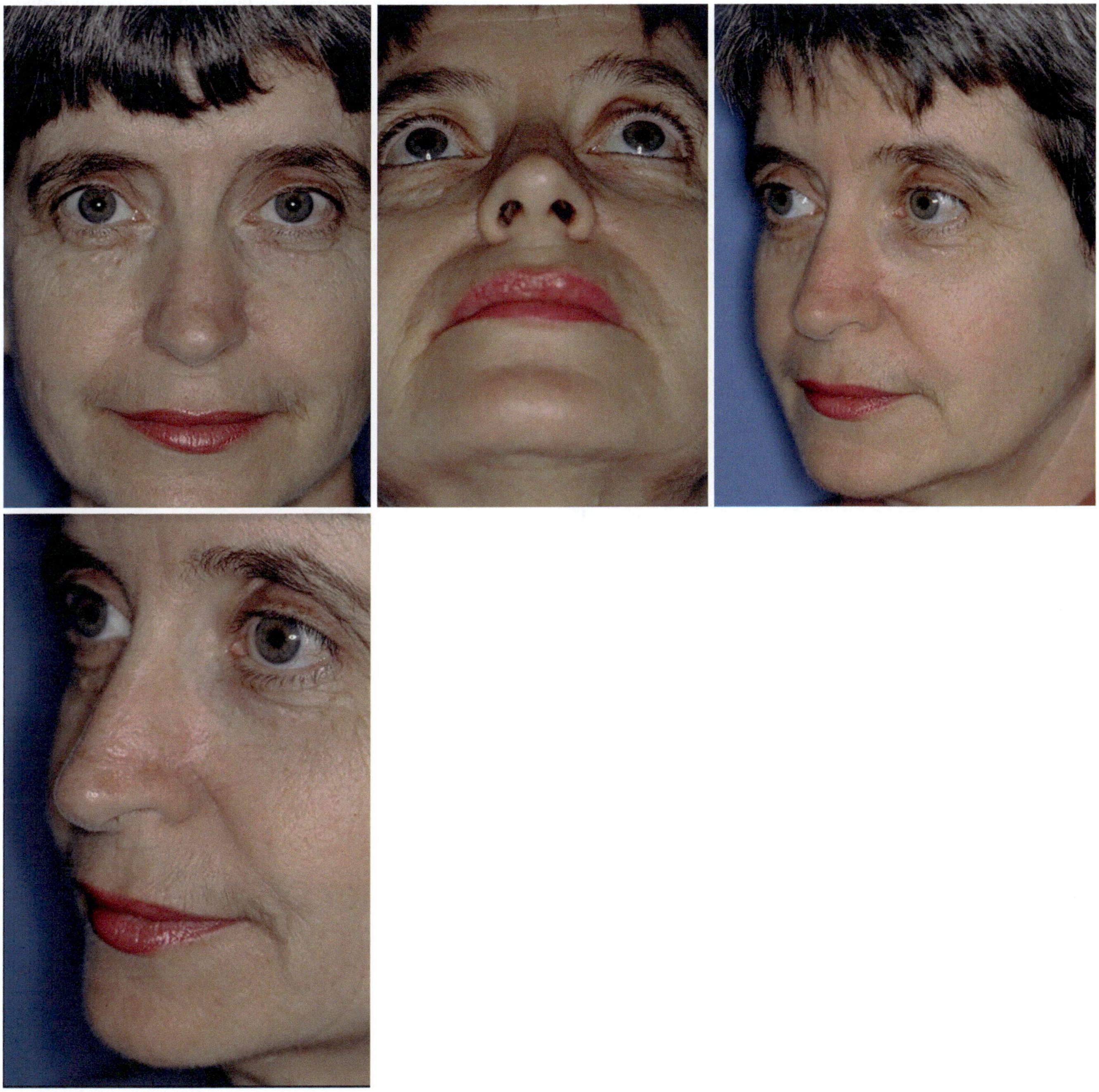

The borders of the flap inferiorly and laterally are within the aesthetic unit junction, the dorsal inset is not perceptible, and nostril configuration has not been altered.

Case 6: Nasal Lesion

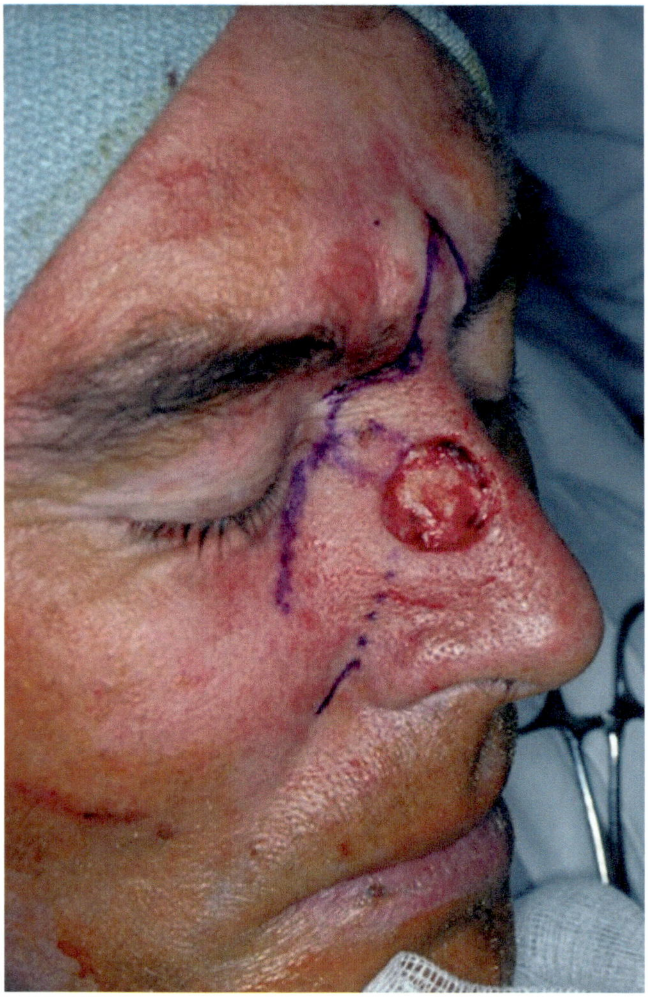

A defect of the junction of the superior and middle one-third on the lateral nasal sidewall but also with the involvement of an adjacent dorsum. A full-thickness skin graft may have yielded a satisfactory result but judged by the depth of the defect some concavity and depression of the final result could be anticipated. In this case, a bilobed flap design of medial canthal and glabellar skin has been outlined. The principles of bilobed flaps, outlined in I.E.2., until a careful consideration of the axis of both flaps. The medial canthal flap, utilizing the thin skin will reconstruct the nasal defect, not unlike a full-thickness skin graft, and the glabellar flap will close the donor site.

Postoperative (Three Months)

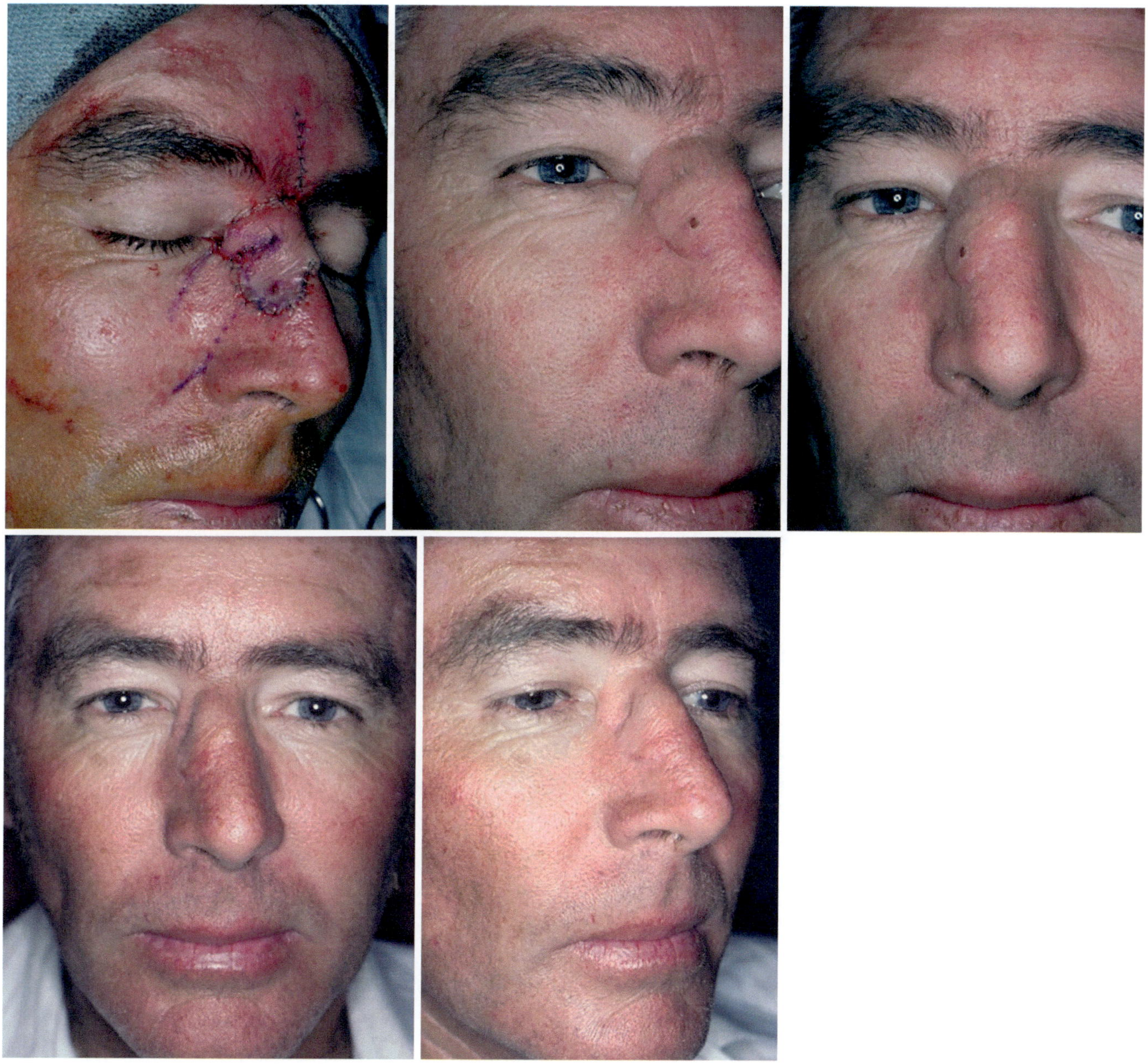

Some pin cushion effect is evident, not an uncommon finding in bilobed flaps that usually resolves with time.

Summary

Although a variety of algorithms have been offered, perhaps a more utilitarian approach is the acquisition of experience and facility with a handful of flaps including forehead, frontonasal, nasolabial, and in quite limited circumstances, bilobe. The incisions necessary for the rotation of the two flaps in a bilobed design can create a cluster of scars on the tip that are not acceptable and application is usually limited to the superior one-third. The superiorly-based nasolabial flap is optimally applied to the lateral alar defects with a minimal arc of rotation necessary. Attempts to increase the arc of rotation to address more anterior defects will inevitably result in a second-stage revision.

In-Service Examination

1. The principal arterial blood supply to the frontonasal flap is:
   (a) Supratrochlear
   (b) Dorsal nasal
   (c) Branch of the sphenopalatine
   (d) Angular
2. Tip defects of 2 cm with resection of both medial crura are optimally reconstructed with:
   (a) Frontonasal flap and cartilage graft
   (b) Parmedian forehead flap only
   (c) Parmedian forehead flap and cartilage graft
   (d) Inferior-based nasolabial flap and cartilage graft
3. A 1 cm full-thickness defect of the alar rim is optimally reconstructed with:
   (a) Bilobed flap with conchal graft
   (b) Primary closure
   (c) An auricular composite graft
   (d) Inferior-based nasolabial flap

30 Scalp and Forehead

Bibliography

Mericli A.F., Selber J.C., Chapter 2 "Scalp and forehead reconstruction", Neligan PC, Plastic Surgery, Elsevier 5th Edition, (2023), Volume 3: **pg. 39–51.**

Luce EA, Chapter 8: "Reconstruction of the Scalp and Forehead", *Non-Melanoma Skin Cancer and Cutaneous Melanoma*, Othon Papadopoulos, Springer, (2020):**265–293.**

Iblher N, Ziegler MC, Penna V, et al., "An algorithm for oncologic scalp reconstruction", *Plast. Reconstr. Surg.*, (2010); 126(2):**450–458.**

Corradino B and Lorenzo SD, "An algorithm for oncologic scalp reconstruction", *Plast. Reconstr. Surg.*, (2011); 127(6):**2506–2507 ONLY**.

Seitz IA and Gottlieb LJ, "Reconstruction of scalp and forehead defects", *Clinics in Plastic Surgery*, (2009); 36:**355–373.**

Van Driel AA, Mureau MA, Goldstein DP, et al., "Aesthetic and oncologic outcome after microsurgical reconstruction of complex scalp and forehead defects after malignant tumor resection: An algorithm for treatment", *Plast. Reconstr. Surg.*, (2010); 126(2):460–470. **(Read Discussion ONLY – pgs. 464–469).**

Silberstein E, Pagkalos VA, Landau D, et al., "Aplasia cutis congenita: Clinical management and a new classification system", *Plast. Reconstr. Surg.*, (2014); 134(5):**766e–771e.**

Sadigh PL, Chang LR, Hsieh CH, etal., "The Trapezius Perforator Flap: An Underused but Versatile Option in the Reconstruction of Local and Distant Soft-Tissue Defects", *Plast. Reconstr. Surg.*, (2014); 134(3): **449e–456e.**

Uğurlu, K., Özçelik, D., Hüthüt, İ., Yildiz, K., Kilinç, L., Baş, L., "Extended Vertical Trapezius Myocutaneous Flap in Head and Neck Reconstruction as a Salvage Procedure.", *Plast Reconstr Surg.*, (2004);114(2):**339–349 (Skip Case Reports and Results pgs 342–346).**

Faculty Discussion and Study Guide

Anatomy

Editor's Note: The detailed anatomy of the brow region is addressed in the module on Chap. 99.

1. Describe the vascular supply to the scalp including the origin of the principal vessels. (The paired vessels consist of the supraorbital and supratrochlear vessels originating from the ophthalmic artery and internal carotid, the superficial temporal and post auricular vessels originating from the external carotid and posteriorly the occipital vessels, originating also from the external carotid.)
   (a) In what layer of the scalp is the principal vascular supply?
2. Describe the principal sensory innervation of the scalp. (The deep branch of the supraorbital nerve innervates the anterior or frontal and parietal scalp; the auriculotemporal and zygomatico-temporal, both branches of the maxillary division (just superficial to the galea) of the trigeminal nerve, provide sensation to the temple. The occipital region is supplied by the greater and lesser occipital nerves, branches of C_2.)
3. Describe the principal sensory innervation of the forehead. (Innervation is provided by the supraorbital and supratrochlear nerves exiting from their respective foramina.)
   (a) Outline the course of the supraorbital nerves. (Approximately 1.5 cm superior to the superior orbital rim the supraorbital nerve divides into a deep and superficial branch. The deep branch runs along the deep aspect of the frontalis and the more superficial branch is on the anterior surface of the frontalis.

E. Luce, *A Curriculum for Plastic Surgery*, https://doi.org/10.1007/978-3-031-62087-4_30

The superficial branch provides sensory innervation of the forehead and the deep branch to the scalp as described above.)

4. The galea is contiguous with what other structures? Describe for 180° beginning anteriorly at the midline of the forehead. (The galea interfaces with the superior edge of the frontalis muscle in the frontal region, the superior portion of the temporoparietal fascia laterally and the occipitalis, the fascia overlying the superficial portion of the trapezius, posteriorly.)
   (a) How does the galea interface with the frontalis? (The galea splits at the superior border of the frontalis into a deep and superficial layer on either aspect of the frontalis and then fuses approximately 2 cm above the supraorbital rim where the galea blends with the periosteum. The last anatomical fact, the fusion point at 2 cm above the superior orbital rim, necessitates in the process of raising a bicoronal flap, a switch in transition from a supra-periosteal dissection to subperiosteal dissection.)
5. What anatomical fact explains the resistance of the scalp to primary closure of defects? (The tight adherence of the dermis of the skin to the underlying subcutaneous tissue and, importantly, to the galea.)
6. What is and what creates the superior temporal fusion line? (The superior temporal fusion line is the bony ridge created by the interface of the convex frontal bone with the more concave anterior aspect of the temporal bone. The temporal hollow is filled by the temporalis muscle.)
7. What is the anatomical relationship of the frontal or temporal branch of cranial nerve VII both topographically and in cross-section in the temporal region? (The course of the frontal branch of the facial nerve into the frontalis muscle is approximately 1.5 cm superior to the superior orbital rim at the level of the lateral canthus. In cross-section, the nerve after crossing the zygomatic arch lies deep to the temporoparietal fascia.)
8. What are the implications of the development of a bicoronal flap? (The nerve must be protected as the dissection progresses inferiorly and temporally. That protection is accomplished by utilizing the split of the deep temporal fascia into a superficial and deep portion approximately 3 cm or so superior to the zygomatic arch. By incision of the superficial portion, one accesses the superficial temporal fat pad and continues the dissection further inferiorly. The nerve is now superficial to the plane of dissection.)
9. What is the single most important consideration in free flap reconstruction of the forehead? (The necessity to reconstruct the entire aesthetic unit of the forehead. Otherwise, the placement of the flap with retention of a portion of the native forehead skin presents a patchwork appearance.)

Non-oncologic Defects

1. What is the single-most important factor that dictates treatment in aplasia cutis congenita? (An associated skull defect that occurs in approximately 25% of patients with exposure to the underlying dura. Since the defect commonly involves the midline, the sagittal sinus will be exposed in aplasia cutis congenita. The probability of skull defects rises in direct proportion to the size of the overall soft tissue defect.)
2. Describe the options and appropriate application of the same. (Conservative treatment, and dressing changes, may be appropriate for small defects without exposed dura or dural veins. For larger defects the potential for desiccation and bleeding is substantial. Split-thickness skin grafting, particularly if performed early, does provide closure and given the osteogenic capability of the neonate dura, no further procedures may be necessary. For larger defects with incomplete osseous regeneration, the difficulty of the dissection of the skin graft for a cranioplasty can be formidable. Full-thickness skin grafts do provide an additional dermal layer as a buffer. More recently, Integra® has been utilized for aplasia cutis congenita and may be the optimal approach for larger defects.)
3. Describe in dimensions how size dictates the management in aplasia cutis congenita. (If the defect is <15 cm^2 without an associated skull defect and no involvement or exposure of dural veins then conservative treatment with wet dressing changes until epithelialization occurs is perfectly appropriate. Skin-soft tissue defects of >15 cm^2 with an associated cranial defect and exposed dura as well can also be managed conservatively if no dural veins are involved. Some difference of opinion exists with a more aggressive approach with urgent, <24 h, coverage provided. Any defect with exposed dura and sagittal sinus with exposed veins should have emergency coverage with either skin substitute or autologous skin graft. See Table 30.1.)
4. Describe options and appropriate application of same in a full-thickness, soft tissue and bone, burn injury of the scalp. (If intervention occurs prior to an established infection of the bone, provision of soft tissue coverage alone will enable the bone to function as a perfect in situ bone graft. That soft tissue coverage can be accomplished by regional or distant microvascular flaps.)
   (a) Discuss the role of decortication in the management of selected non-oncologic bone defects. (In younger patients with trauma-related full thick thickness and periosteum soft tissue defects, one option is decortication of the outer cortex, exposure of the diploic cavity, and delayed skin grafts. Yet another variant of this option is placement of Integra® with delayed thin

Table 30.1 Proposed classification for aplasia cutis congenita of the Scalp

Type	Size of defect	Layers involved	Involvement of veins	Immediate treatment	Late treatment
0	Any	Intact epidermis without skin appendages (scarred, hairless area on the scalp)	No	None	Hair transplantation, serial excision, or tissue expansion and flap reconstruction according to final defect size
I	<15 cm^2	Skin defect, no skull bone defect	No	Conservative treatment until complete epithelialization	
II	>15 cm^2	Skull bone defect, exposed dura	No	Conservative treatment until complete epithelialization; emergency coverage may be considered	
III	Any, usually large	Skin and skull defect with exposed dura and sagittal sinus	Enlarged exposed veins	Emergency coverage with allograft, skin substitute, or autologous skin graft	
IV	Any, usually large	Skin, skull, and dura defect with brain exposure	Any, usually with enlarged exposed veins	Flap reconstruction	

Modified from Silberstein E, Pagkalos VA, Landau D, et al., "Aplasia Cutis Congenita: Clinical Management and a New Classification System", *Plast Reconstr Surg.*, (2014) Nov;134(5):766e–774e. (Reprinted with Permission)

skin grafts after a 2–3 week hiatus. This last variant addresses the friability of skin grafts placed directly onto cranial bone.)

Oncologic

1. The readings provide algorithms to direct the decision process. What are the factors to consider in the selection of a treatment option? (Location—temporal versus frontal, occipital versus vertex. Size—critical limits for primary closure, local scalp flap, or free flap. Defect character—pericranium intact, partial or full thickness bone loss, hardware present, nature of wound as infected and/or irradiated.)
2. In general, what is the upper limit of defect size of the scalp that can be closed primarily? (2.5 cm. In one of the readings larger defects, 3–4 cm, were listed as potential for primary closure, yet the largest defect in the series closed primarily was 24 mm.)
   (a) What maneuver can be incorporated into undermining? Give the pros and cons and limits. (The use of galeal scoring or cross-hatching in order to provide additional extensibility is a possible option. The blood supply to the scalp lies just superficial to the galea and can be damaged with galeal scoring.)
3. Describe the Orticochea method of scalp closure. (The entire remaining scalp is mobilized in either three or four flaps all based inferiorly and on a main blood supply. Laterally-based flaps are perfused by the superficial temporal arteries and posterior by the occipital arteries. Similar to peeling a banana the flaps are then interposed in advance to close defects listed as large as 6 cm. Defects of the vertex lend themselves to this method if adopted. The principal difficulty with application of the Orticochea method is that once the flaps are completely developed and closure is still not possible a bridge has been burned. See Fig. 30.1.)
4. In the choice of a split-thickness skin graft for an anticipated oncologic defect of the scalp, what factors should be considered? (The presence or absence of prior radiation or the necessity of postoperative radiation; the absence or presence of the periosteum.)
5. What is the principal disadvantage of skin grafting a decorticated skull either primary or secondary? (Lack of long-term durability. Skin grafts directly over decorticated bone have little resistance to the wear and tear of everyday life and ulcerate easily with poor healing. As described earlier, the use of Integra® in an intermediate stage may address this particular disadvantage or drawback.)
6. What are some general caveats in the use of tissue expansion for scalp defects? (Probably the maximum defect is 50% of the scalp. Placement of the incision for access differs among surgeons but if an incision is utilized at the interface of the defect and the proposed scalp expansion a layer closure should be accomplished as well as a mandatory 2-week hiatus before expansion. Also, the expander is placed with minimal initial volume, 30 cc or less. The patient should be advised, that particularly with multiple expansions, the density of hair follicles will be reduced as a result of thinning of the hair.)
7. What defect dimensions, the upper limit of which raises a consideration of use of free tissue transfer for closure? (6–8 cm centrally, 4–5 cm laterally or at the hairline.)
   (a) What are other indications for free tissue transfer? (Prior irradiation, full-thickness resection with exposed dura, multiple scars from prior excisions.)

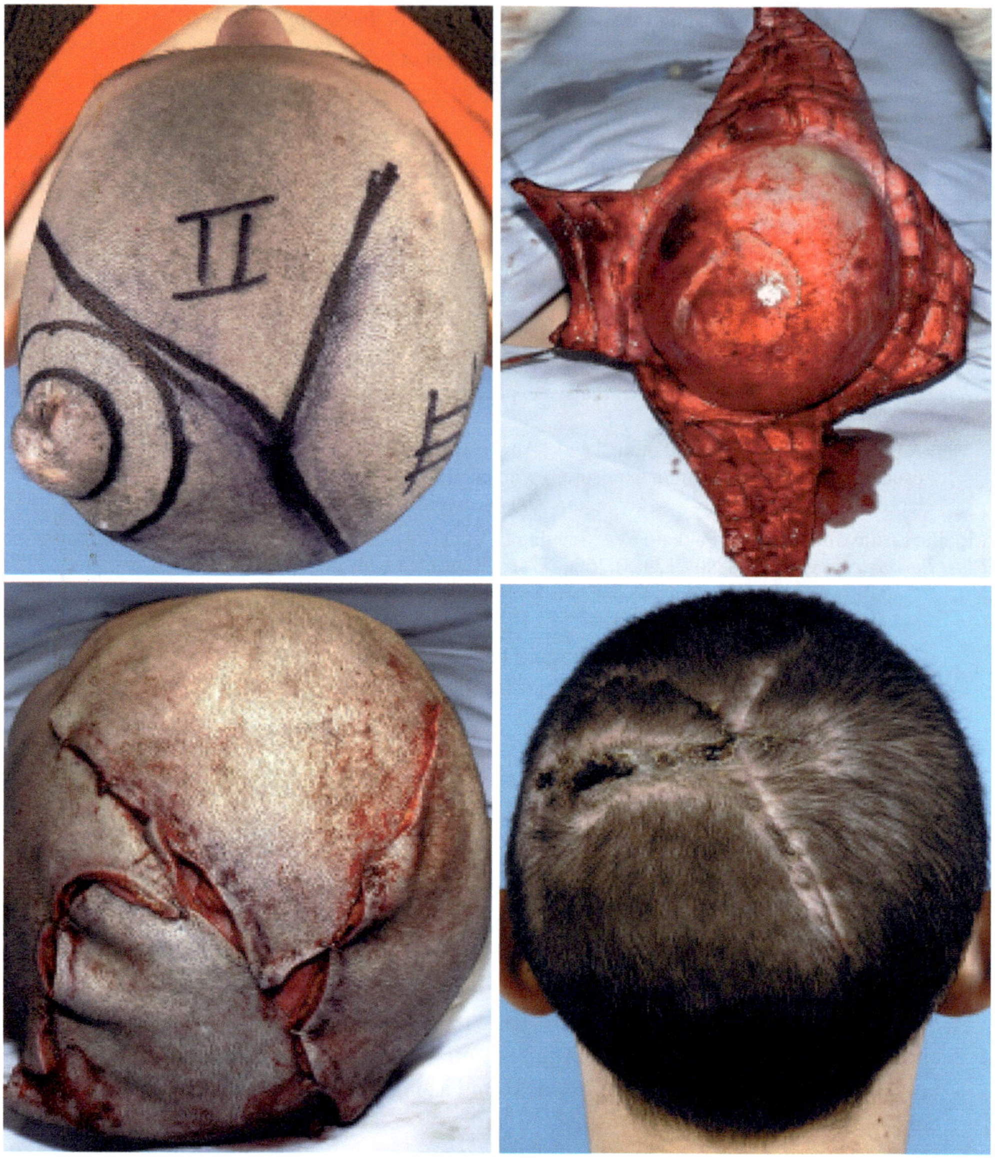

Fig. 30.1 Case 2, type C reconstruction with Orticochea flap in a 23-year-old woman with a fibrohistiocytic sarcoma. (*Above, left*) Preoperative planning. (*Above, right*) Flap mobilization and scoring of galea. (*Below, left*) Wound closure. (*Below, right*) Early postoperative result at 4 weeks postoperatively. Iblher N, Ziegler MC, Penna V, et al., "An algorithm for oncologic scalp reconstruction", *Plast Reconstr Surg.*, (2010); 126(2). (Reprinted with Permission)

8. What is the one anatomical exception to the general rule that regional pedicled flaps are not suitable for larger scalp defects? (The occipital region.)
   (a) Describe the two possible options for the use of pedicle flaps harvested from the posterior thoracic region for coverage of occipital defects. (The two options are posterior trapezius and dorsal scapular flaps. The former is vascularized by the descending branch of the superficial cervical artery, a tributary of the transverse cervical. The latter, the dorsal scapular is perfused by perforators from the dorsal scapular artery, a deep branch of the transverse cervical artery. The course of the descending branch of the superficial cervical artery is, as the name implies, superficial to the rhomboids and levator scapulae. The dorsal scapular artery courses deep into the levator scapulae in the rhomboids. Ordinarily, the posterior trapezius is harvested as a myocutaneous flap and the dorsal scapular, as described in the readings, as a perforator flap. With proximal dissection to the origin of the superficial cervical artery, the arc of rotation of the trapezius can permit reconstruction of occipital skull defects. Dissection of the dorsal scapular artery flap can be tedious, as in all perforator-based flaps, and the arc of rotation will be limited to a point between the rhomboid major and minor.)
9. What are the main considerations in the choice of microvascular flap reconstruction of the scalp? (Muscle alone plus skin graft vs. musculocutaneous favors muscle plus skin graft because of bulk issues. The length of the pedicle needs to be considered because of the necessity to access the superficial temporal artery and vein in the preauricular region. In summary, latissimus dorsi alone

with skin graft is favored over the use of the anterolateral thigh or DIEP flap unless one is committed to debulking. Another flap choice for smaller or medium-sized defects is the radial forearm flap.)

10. Describe the use of an Integra® dermal template for reconstruction of scalp defects. Outline the pros and cons. (Integra® or dermal template can be utilized to close a scalp defect as a two-stage procedure. The first stage consists of placement of Integra® on a vascularized bed with two options. One, retention of pericranium, and two, granulation tissue after removal of the outer cortex. The second stage is performed 3 weeks later with removal of the silicone outer layer and placement of thin autografts. Vascularization of the Integra® is facilitated by the use of negative wound pressure therapy. The advantages of this approach obviously are less complexity compared to free tissue transfer or split-thickness skin graft directly over pericranium or vascularized bone. Split-thickness skin grafts alone lack the thickness of dermis provided by a dermal template. Disadvantages are cosmesis except in the bald individual and two-stage approach. See Figs. 30.2 and 30.3.)

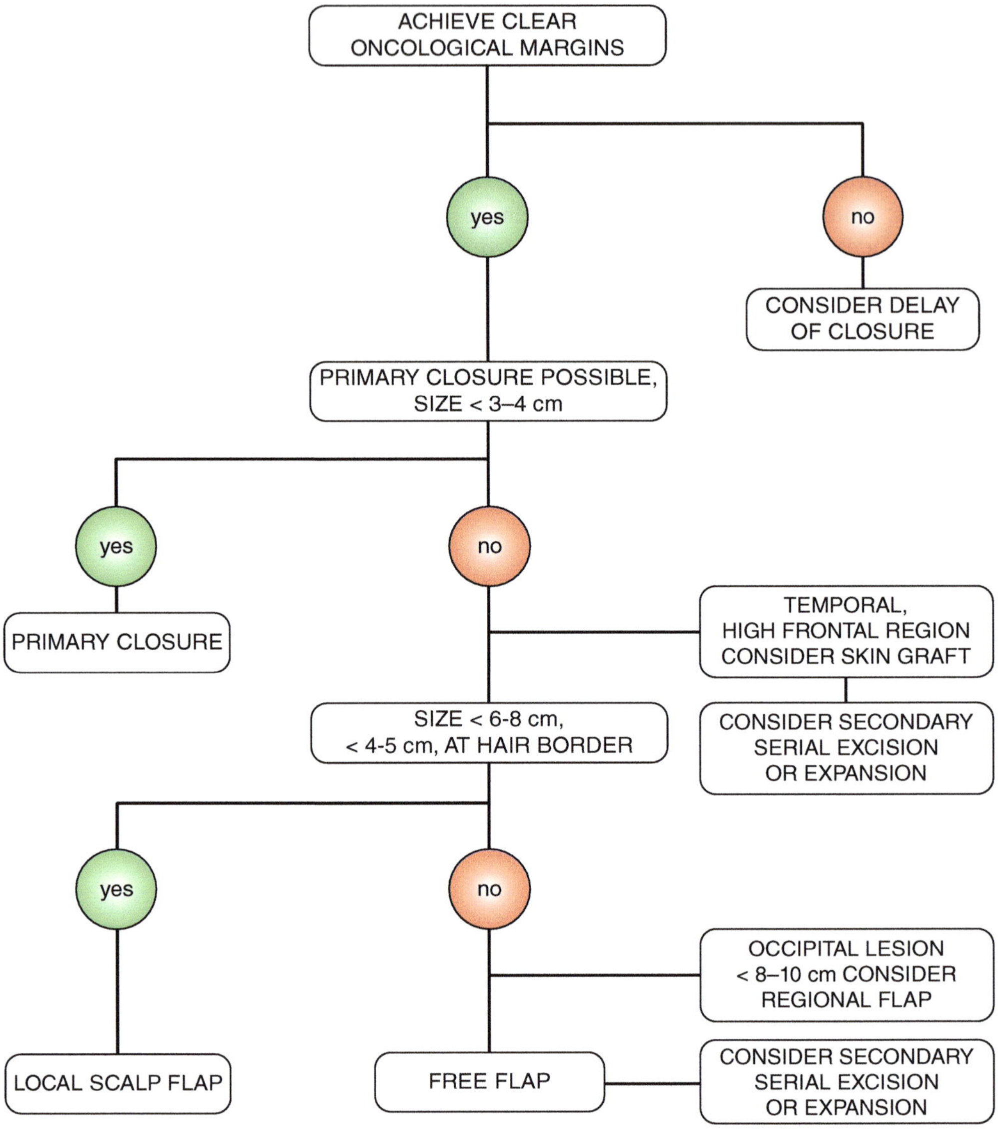

Fig. 30.2 Algorithm for oncologic scalp reconstruction in schematic form. (Iblher N, Ziegler MC, Penna V, et al., "An algorithm for oncologic scalp reconstruction", *Plast Reconstr Surg.*, (2010); 126(2):450–459. (Reprinted with Permission))

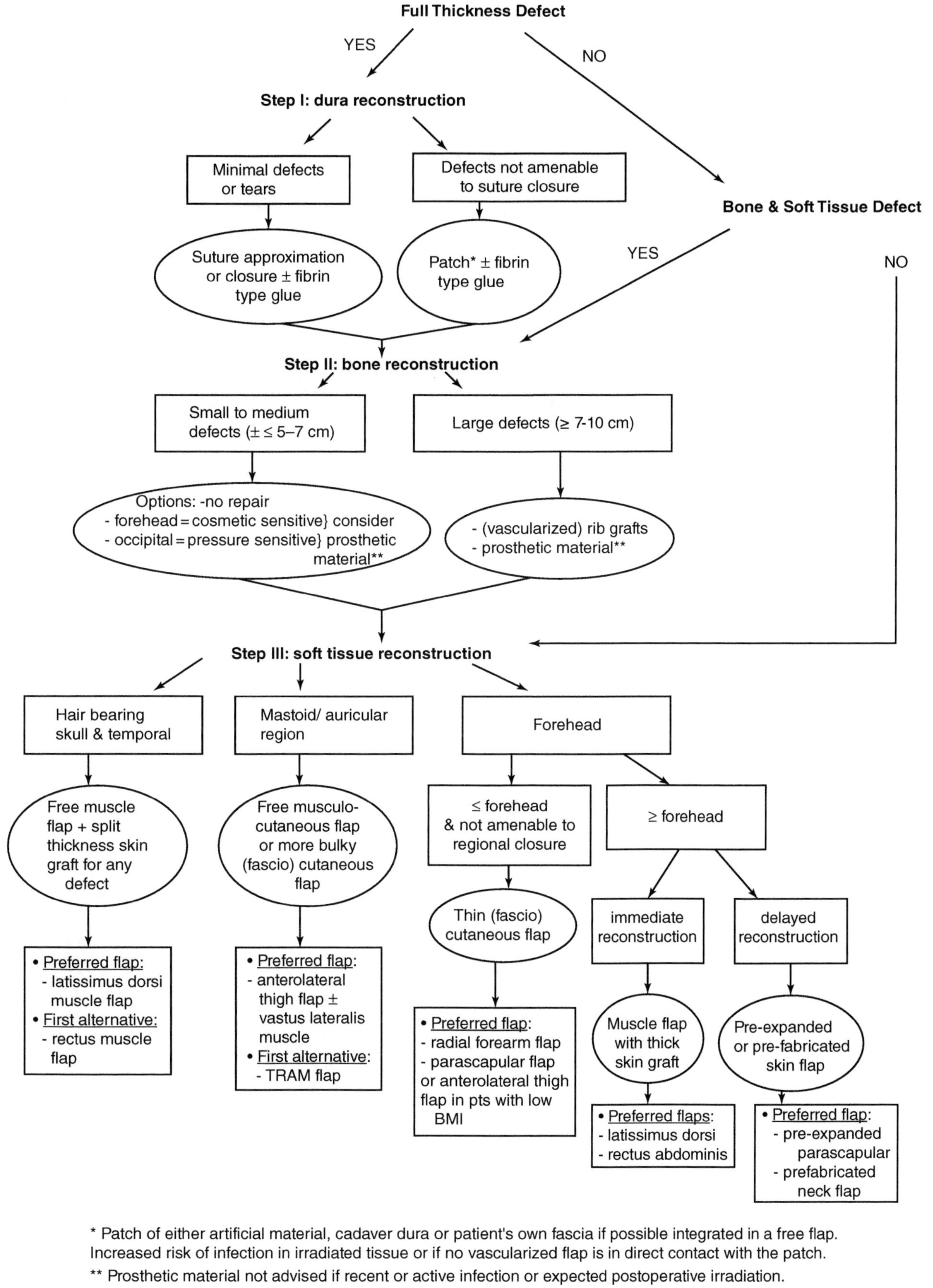

Fig. 30.3 Algorithm for oncologic scalp reconstruction in flow form. (Van Driel AA, Mureau MA, Goldstein DP, et al., "Aesthetic and oncologic outcome after microsurgical reconstruction of complex scalp and forehead defects after malignant tumor resection: An algorithm for treatment", *Plast Reconstr Surg.*, (2010); 126(2):460–470. (Reprinted with Permission))

Case 1: Recurrent Ca of the Scalp

Case-Based Conference

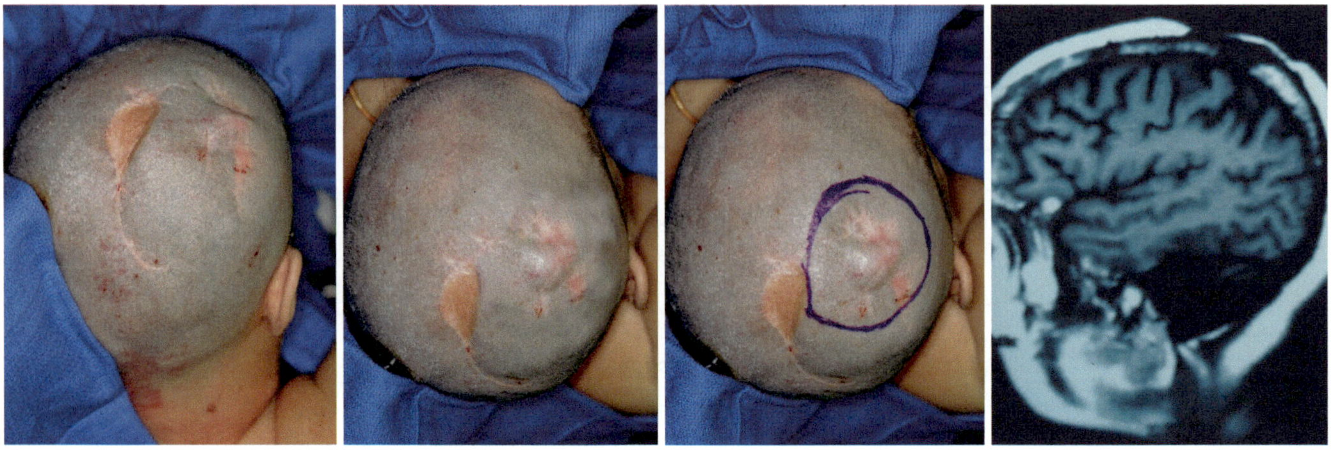

A 48-year-old woman with recurrent fibrosarcoma of the scalp who has just completed prolonged chemoradiotherapy. Her original resection was 2 years ago.

1. Describe the slide(s). Add a focused clinical exam.
   (a) Tests indicated? The MRI demonstrates no dural involvement.
2. What is the pathologic anatomy? Explain in detail how your analysis affects the treatment plan.
3. Outline your treatment plan.
   (a) Manage the patient both oncologically as well as the reconstruction.

Case-Based Conference: Discussion

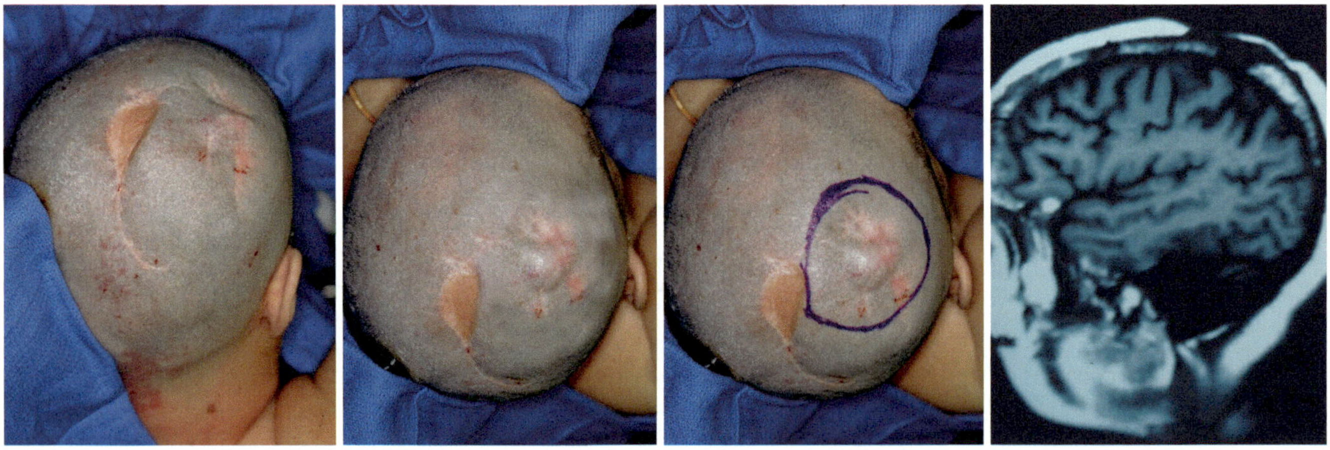

A 48-year-old woman with recurrent fibrosarcoma of the scalp who has just completed prolonged chemoradiotherapy. Her original resection was 2 years ago.

1. Describe the slide(s). (Patient probably located in the OR in a prone or lateral decubitus position with shaved scalp and old postoperative changes indicative of an inferiorly-based occipital flap and skin graft. A probable mass is located on the lateral and distal, anterior limb of the flap without evident skin ulceration. The second view is mostly superior and demonstrates the aforementioned mass that appears to be about 2 cm in size and not well-defined. No alopecia is evident.)
   (a) Clinical exam? (The history would focus on the past treatment records including histological information including cell type, differentiation, and size of the original primary. The same focus on the histology of the present recurrence would be gleaned from the

path report. The patient questions would consist of the methods of diagnosis of recurrence, the particulars of chemoradiation as number of cycles and weeks of treatment as well as adverse responses. The date of completion of radiation therapy should be elicited. Other history includes comorbidities and smoking. An important component of the history is to establish the functional status by questions about the activities of daily living as well as weight loss, if any. The physical exam of the mass would ascertain if fixed or mobile. The posterior cervical nodal basin is examined.)

(b) Test indicated? (An MRI has been performed. Imaging should include a CT scan to better define the bony defect evident on MRI. A PET scan was performed, presumably, prior to the initiation of neoadjuvant therapy.)

(c) Interpretation of the MRI? (Bony defect directly underlying the tumor mass. No apparent dural involvement.)

2. What is the pathologic anatomy? (The two elements of the pathologic anatomy is the nature of the tumor and the current anticipated defect. The cell type and grade will be a rough yardstick of the magnitude of resection although the tumor is recurrent and will require an aggressive excision.

   The other element or component is the eventual defect. The soft tissue excision will encompass a 2–3 cm margin given the diagnosis of fibrosarcoma. The MRI indicates a full-thickness bony defect, size indeterminant and although the MRI is read as "no dural involvement", the possibility of dural involvement by tumor must be included in the reconstructive plan. The pathologic anatomy includes the presence of irradiated tissue. The etiology of the bone defect could be osteoradionecrosis or direct tumor involvement and dissolution of bone. In summary, the oncologic plan should be wide soft tissue resection, a margin of bone resection, and consideration of the necessity of dural excision and replacement.)

3. Outline your treatment plan. (The soft tissue margins outlined on the slide appear inadequate since the soft tissue reconstruction will probably require a free flap, the size of the defect to some degree becomes irrelevant, and generous margins should be planned. Whether the etiology of the bony loss in the skull is osteoradionecrosis, ORN, or tumor is also immaterial. The bone margins should be resected for an additional 2 cm. The specimen should be excised as an en bloc resection, and the dura inspected as the specimen is lifted free.

   Reconstruction begins with the dura, if necessary, and reconstitution with a dural substitute of which bovine pericardium is one frequent choice. Although the dural replacement will be within a previously irradiated field, the coverage will be a well-vascularized flap. The options for reconstitution of the skull defect are non-vascularized autogenous bone as harvested as split cranioplasty bone, vascularized bone within a free flap, and alloplastic reconstruction. Of the last, alloplastic, the options are methyl methacrylate, polyethylene such as PEEK and titanium mesh. Given the milieu, the use of titanium mesh is probably the method of choice if alloplastic reconstruction is the option selected. If vascularized bone is selected then the free flap options by definition would be a composite flap. Possibilities include fibula, scapular, and deep iliac. The fibula including a skin island would be a bulky flap replacement for the scalp soft tissue and may create some technical challenges in orientation of the skin island and bone into the defect. The scapula might require repositioning of the patient, the deep iliac is a difficult dissection, and the skin island may be less reliable than other options. On balance, the use of nonvascularized bone, obtained by use of a full-thickness cranial bone flap, split with one-half for closure of the defect and the other for the donor site is probably the preferable option.

   Certainly, the soft tissue defect can be addressed with a myocutaneous or fasciocutaneous free flap, utilized also as coverage over the skull reconstruction. If so, the next decision in the algorithm in flap selection is muscle alone plus skin graft or a musculocutaneous flap. Choices include latissimus or serratus anterior as muscle alone or as a musculocutaneous flap in the instance of the latissimus. Serratus anterior, lower slips, plus skin graft would be an acceptable option. The addition of the skin island to the latissimus muscle might be bulky as would the use of the anterolateral thigh flap as an option. Rectus abdominis, muscle alone is another option but would probably require a change in position. Length of vascular pedicle is a consideration. The superficial temporal vessels are in close proximity to the defect but may not be suitable because of friability, particularly the vein. If so, the pedicle must be of sufficient length to reach the neck.)

Intraoperative

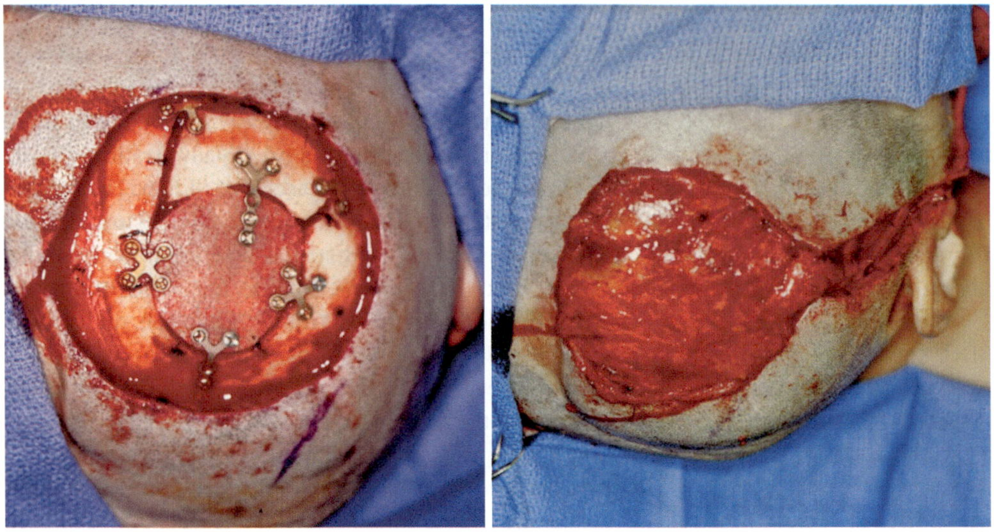

The two intraoperative views illustrate the excised defect that included skin-soft tissue and full-thickness skull. A split calvarial graft has been secured. In the following slides, a muscle flap covers the bone and adjacent cranium. The pattern of resection would indicate a wider skin and soft tissue margin than that employed for the bone. A preauricular incisional wound enabled access to the superficial temporal vessels.

Postoperative (Two Months)

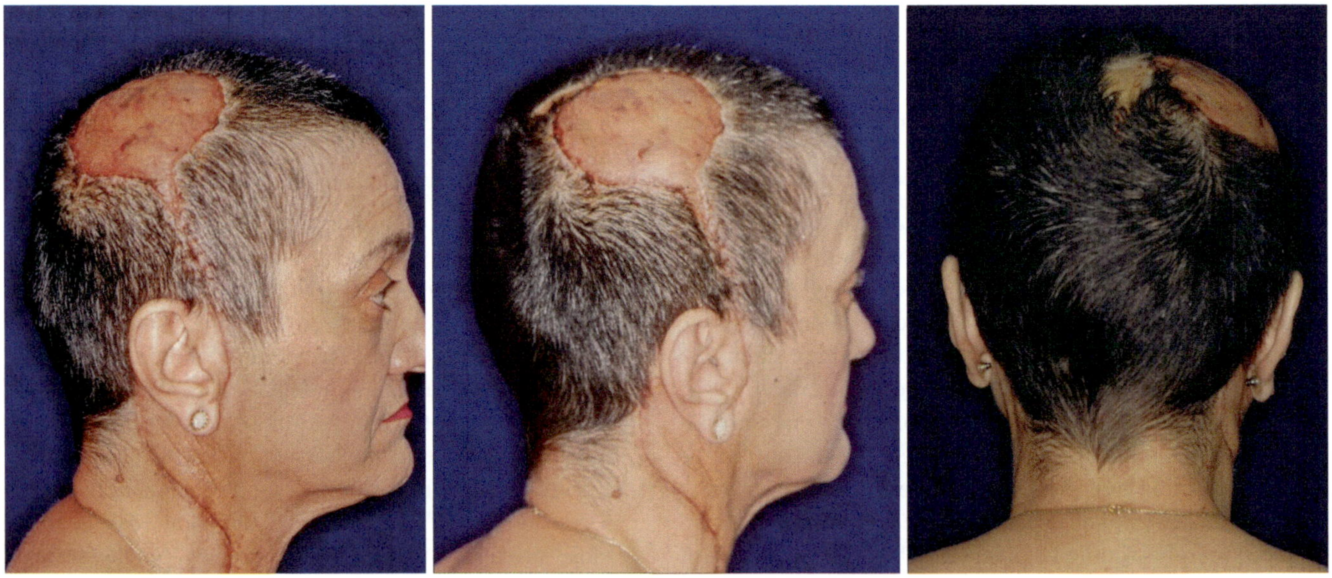

Several photos provide anterior, posterior, and oblique views of the result. The wounds are well-healed and clearly as judged by appearance and posture the patient is functioning. The cervical incision would indicate the recipient vessels were not the superficial temporal, not an anticipated occurrence. Not unanticipated since on occasion both the artery and vein are thin-walled and friable. Planning should routinely include a long donor vascular pedicle, if possible. In this instance, although the latissimus was the donor muscle, vein grafts were still necessary, a necessity that increased the complication rate.

Case 2: Scalp Reconstruction

Case-Based Conference

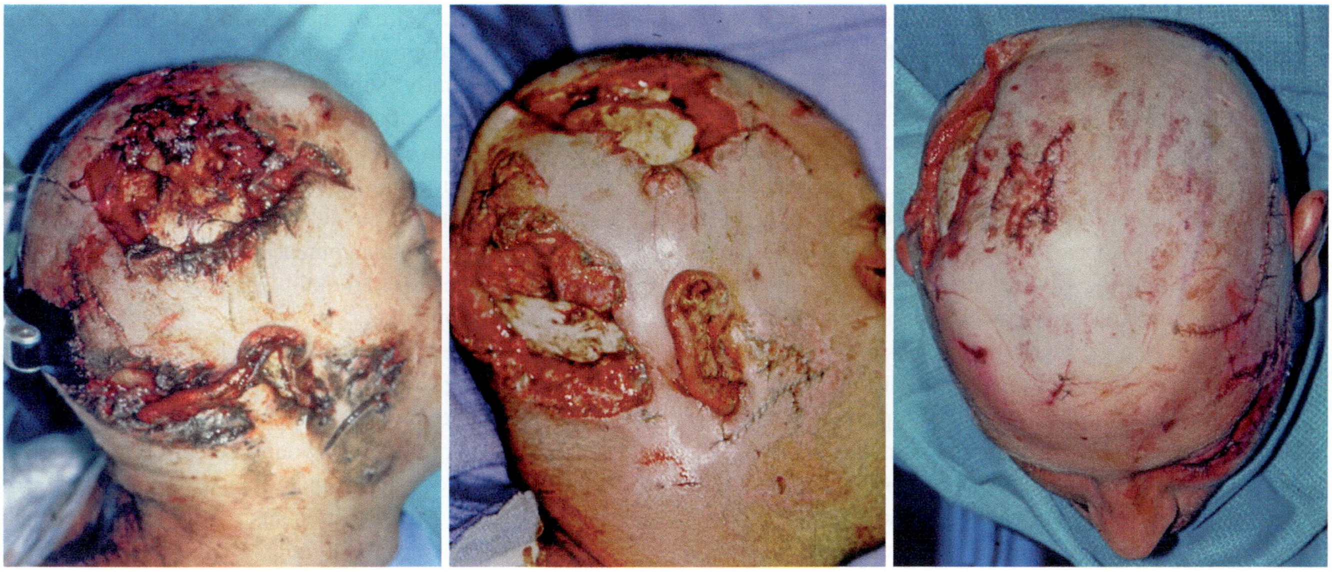

A 25-year-old male involved in an MVA currently in OR for treated liver laceration. Stable and no other injuries.

1. Describe the slide(s). Add a focused clinical exam.
   (a) Are any tests indicated? The third slide demonstrates appearance after closure of facial lacerations.
2. What is the pathologic anatomy? Explain in detail how your analysis affects the treatment plan.
3. Outline your treatment plan.

Case-Based Conference: Discussion

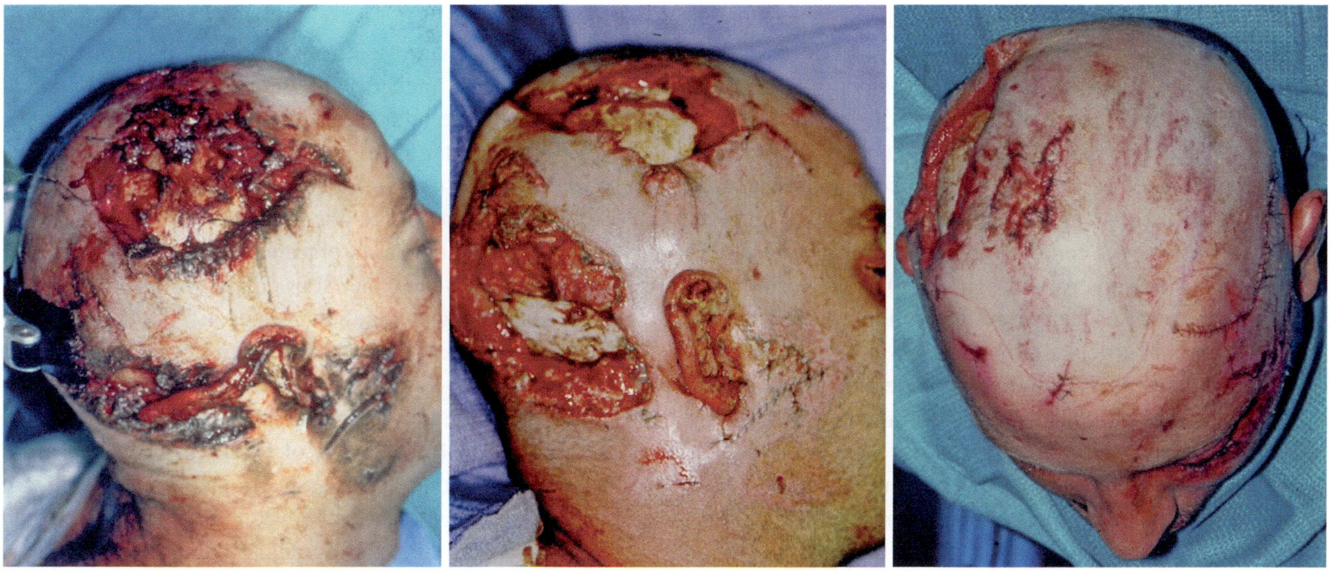

A 25-year-old male involved in an MVA currently in OR for treated liver laceration. Stable and no other injuries.

1. Describe the slide(s). Add a focused clinical exam. (Three photos are available. The first is a right lateral with the head suspended by a Mayfield head tong. The dominant findings are several. A large full-thickness soft tissue defect is evident on the right parietal scalp, encroaching on the adjacent temporal and occipital scalp, measuring perhaps 8 × 10 cm. The exposed skull is clearly present in about one-half of the defect, but the bone coverage of the remaining skull appears traumatized and of dubious value. Embedded into the wound edges as well as the wound itself is foreign material, gravel, or road dirt. Further inferiorly, overlying the region of the mastoid and right inferior occiput is another area of soft tissue loss with perhaps bone exposure. Again the wound is impregnated with dark foreign material. The right ear is traumatized but the view does not permit further characterization. In the preauricular area several lacerations, were also heavily contaminated. In the second and third slides, wound toilet and debridement have been accomplished. The second photo is essentially the same perspective as the first. The exposed skull view encompasses the majority of the parietal wound. The remaining soft tissue appears healthy. The mastoid and occipital wounds have a substantial-sized area of bone exposure, probably 4 × 6 cm in the center of a larger wound at least twice that size. The ear is intact and the facial lacerations have been closed. The third photo pictures a view from above the patient, illustrating the remaining frontal, left temporal, and parietal scalp. The occipital scalp is not visible. No additional tissue loss is evident, although a laceration has been closed that courses from the left lateral superior forehead posteriorly into the temporal scalp just superior to the ear.

   The history should be obtained from the medical records and the trauma team to establish approximate time and mode of injury, loss of consciousness upon arrival and results of facial and head CT scans if obtained as well as known comorbidities and current meds. The preamble states the patient is in the OR so determination of the presence of facial fractures will hinge on physical exam, and in particular palpation.)
   (a) Tests indicated? The third slide demonstrates appearance after closure of facial lacerations. (Certainly, if CT scans of the head and face were not obtained because of the urgency of the clinical situation, such should be performed promptly in the postoperative period.)
2. What is the pathologic anatomy? Explain in detail how your analysis affects the treatment plan. (The pathologic anatomy is an avulsive wound consistent with extensive abrasion from a motor vehicular accident. The wound characteristics are those of heavy contamination by impregnated road material and devitalized tissue. The initial objective at this juncture, the intraoperative consultation, will be debridement of the wounds, copious irrigation, and closure of the lacerations. If dirt has been penetrated into the bone, removal by burring will be necessary. Importantly, substantial areas of the skull have been denuded of soft tissue coverage. The wounds have been incurred in a patient setting of a serious life-threatening injury and the recovery would dominate the nature and timing of the subsequent treatment plan. The objective of the management will be to accomplish coverage of the exposed skull and wound closure in an expeditious manner.)
3. Outline your treatment plan. (If stable, the patient returns to the operating room at 48–72 h, saline wet dressings or negative wound pressure therapy administered during that hiatus. A longitudinal wound closure-reconstructive plan should be developed including stages. A number of options exist for the components of the treatment plan. From simple closure to complex are the following: first, closure of the wounds with scalp flaps with split-thickness skin grafting of the donor sites. Lacking a view of the left side and central posterior scalp, the ability to design said flaps from the photos is handicapped somewhat. Regardless, the parietal defect could be optimally closed with a large rotation flap, harvested from the remaining frontal, temporal, and parietal scalp based anteriorly. Of the two pedicle options, anterior or posterior, anterior would be selected for two reasons—first, placement of the grafted donor sites posterior rather than more conspicuously anterior, and; second, the necessity to close the right occipital defect with a second scalp flap, pedicled inferiorly harvested from the remaining intact occipital scalp. The incision for the tip of this flap would interface and be adjacent to the tip of the first flap. The second stage after a sufficient hiatus, would consist of the insertion of tissue expanders, an expansion process, and eventual excision of the donor site skin grafts.

   The second option is placement of burr holes and/or decortication to the cancellous cavity, followed by a program of dressing changes and/or negative wound pressure therapy and after sufficient time when granulation tissue is present, split-thickness skin graft closure. Perhaps followed by, if the patient and surgeon mutually select, tissue expansion for excision of the skin graft. The third option incorporates free tissue transfer. The bridge of viable skin and soft tissue between the two defects could be divided and the two fragments rotated clockwise and counterclockwise respectively into the parietal defect. Or the reverse direction to accomplish closure of the occipital defect, at least coverage of the bone. The parietal defect, now either enlarged by the latter option or smaller with the former, could be managed with a free muscle flap, preferably the latissimus and split-thickness skin graft. Again, the option exists for eventual use of an expanded scalp to excise skin graft and, probably, muscle. The last consideration is the use of a posterior trapezius myocutaneous or dorsal scapular artery perforator flap. The posterior trapezius is based on the descending branch of the transverse cervical artery and requires the harvest of the muscle and skin as a composite flap. Preoperative planning dictates an assurance that the flap will reach the defect. Although the trapezius muscle extends to the level of the T_{10-12}, the most inferior portion of the muscle will not sustain a skin island. The dorsal scapular artery perforator flap, in contrast, is composed of skin and soft tissue based on as the name implies the dorsal scapular artery. The artery courses deep and exits between the rhomboids. The lengthening of the pedicle would require division of the rhomboideus minor. The same prerequisite of planning applies to this flap as well.

In selection of the appropriate treatment option, the benefits and liabilities need to be carefully weighed. The option of rotational flaps, followed possibly by tissue expansion for aesthetic reasons is the least complex. The principal drawback is the likelihood of a complication of the expansion process, not rare in the head and neck. Decortication, granulation tissue emergence, and skin graft options are also relatively simple. The liability is the possibility of infection, colonization of the exposed bone, and development of osteomyelitis. Cranial osteomyelitis can result in sequestration of bone and/or epidural abscess. The use of free tissue transfer plus/minus a posterior thoracic pedicled flap is clearly the most complex and is subject to the vagaries of ischemia and flap failure.

The pros and cons of each of the above need to be weighed carefully and discussed in depth with this patient.

Postoperative (One Year)

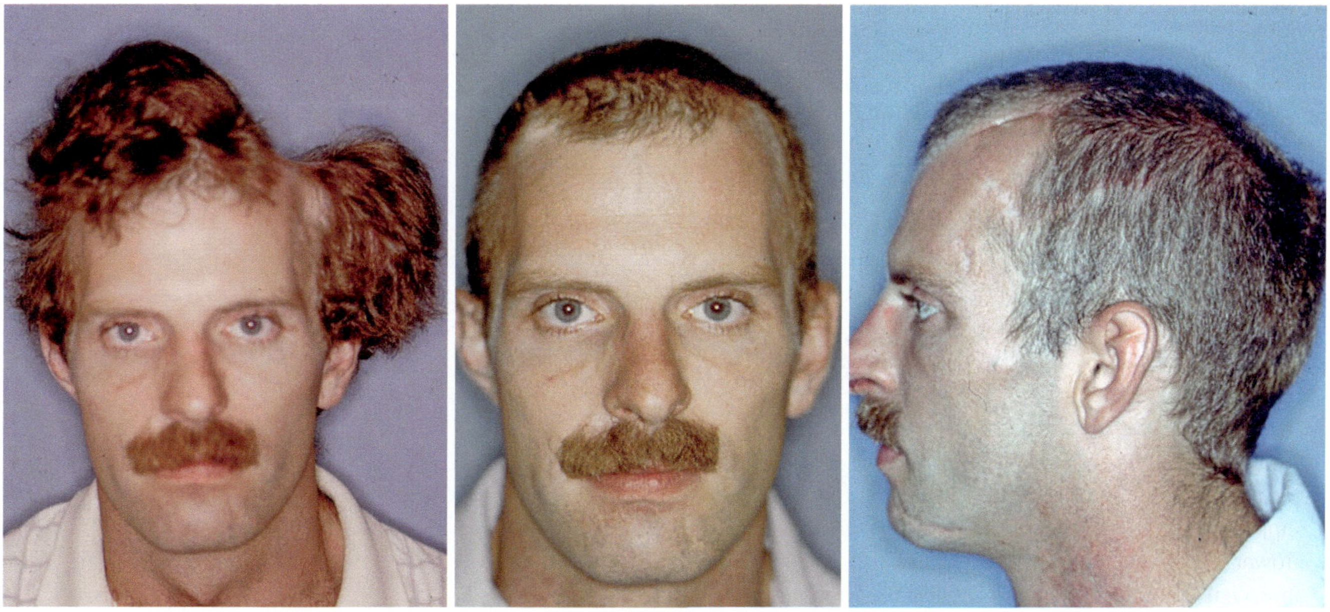

The first photo is a frontal view of the patient. Two apparently fully expanded tissue expanders are in place, one in the left temporal scalp, and the other in the right parietal area. The overlying hair-bearing scalp depicts hair growth of substantial length and thickness, consistent with a duration of 1 year. The final two photos reflect the accomplished postoperative result, with the restoration of a normal hairline.

In-Service Examination

1. The location or the depth of the frontal or temporal branch of the facial nerve superior to the zygomatic arch is:
   (a) Subcutaneous
   (b) Superficial to the temporoparietal fascia
   (c) Deep to the temporoparietal fascia
   (d) Deep to the superficial layer of the deep temporal fascia

2. A neonate in the NICU has a full-thickness and skull defect of 3 cm. Appropriate management is:
   (a) NWPT
   (b) Local wound care
   (c) Free muscle only flap within 3–5 days
   (d) Scalp flaps and delayed tissue expansion reconstruction

3. The vascular supply of a large full-thickness defect of the occipital scalp is:
   (a) Thoracodorsal
   (b) Thoracoacromial
   (c) Dorsal scapular
   (d) Occipital

31 Ear

Bibliography

Shonka D.C., Park S.S., "Ear Defects", *Facial Plast Surg Clin N Am,* (2009);17:**429–439.**

Sanniec, K., Harirah, M., Thornton, J.F., "Ear Reconstruction after Mohs Cancer Excision: Lessons Learned from 327 Consecutive Cases", *Plast Reconstr. Surg.*, (2019);144(3):**722–728, Figures 1 and 2 ONLY.**

Jackson, I. T., Ch. 6 "Ear Reconstruction", Local Flaps in Head and Neck Reconstruction, Quality Medical Publishing, (2007); pp. **317–337**.

Thorne C. H., Brecht, L. E., Bradley J. P., et al., "Auricular Reconstruction: Indications for Autogenous and Prosthetic Techniques", *Plast. Reconstr. Surg.*, (2001); 107(5): **1241–1251**.

Giot J. P., Labbe D., Soubeyrand E., et al., "Prosthetic Reconstruction of the Auricle: Indications, Techniques, and Results", *Seminars in Plastic Surgery*, (2011); 25(4): **265–272**.

Faculty Discussion and Study Guide

Anatomy, Embryology

Editor's Note: Ear anatomy is also discussed in Chaps. 24 and 25.

1. If you pick your ear with a toothpick you might cough—Why? (Innervated by Arnold's nerve, a branch of cranial nerve X which provides sensation to the external auditory canal and concha.)
   (a) A postoperative parotidectomy patient complains of numbness of the tragus and anterior ear—Why? (The auriculo-temporal branch of cranial nerve V, resected with the parotidectomy, provides sensation to the anterior helical rim and triangular fossa as well as the superior one-half of the helical rim.)
   (b) The postoperative face/neck lift complains of numbness of lobule—Why? (The greater auricular nerve branch of the cervical plexus has been damaged. The lesser occipital nerve may provide some overlap.)
2. Anatomy: Lymphatic drainage, describe the classical concept (Concha and meatus into the parotid nodes and into the anterior cervical nodes; auricle and canal into the mastoid and superior posterior cervical nodes, consistent with the embryologic origin of each.)
3. Discuss the embryology of the ear. (Six hillocks, three on each side of the first branchial cleft. The external ear is derived from the first or mandibular arch and the second or hyoid branchial arch. The first arch contributes to the tragus, the root, and the anterior superior helix. The second arch contributes to the antihelix as well as the remaining helix and lobule. Second arch derivatives can be further divided into the free ear fold which develops into the lobule, concha, and the antihelix including the triangular fossa and the remaining portion of the second arch to the scapha and helical rim.)
4. Orient the ear topographically on the skull. Do so in terms of position on the skull, axis, and the distance from the orbit. (The external ear is about 15° posteriorly inclined from the vertical, 6 cm in height in the adult, located one ear length posterior to the lateral canthus; a transverse line drawn through the lateral canthus intersects at the junction of the superior one-third and inferior two-thirds of the ear; the top of the ear is at the brow, the lobule at the base of the columella.)
5. The principal blood supply to the external ear is derived from what two vessels? (Superficial temporal and posterior auricular arteries).
6. A significant proportion of skin cancer of the ear is squamous cell carcinoma. What are some treatment corollaries? (First, 4 mm margins in well-differentiated, smaller lesions; 6 mm margins in less differentiated lesions; in

E. Luce, *A Curriculum for Plastic Surgery*, https://doi.org/10.1007/978-3-031-62087-4_31

larger lesions, >2 cm, perhaps 1 cm margin. Second, management of the lymphatics. In the absence of palpable lymph nodes, some consideration has been given recently to the performance of SNL biopsy in high-risk lesions, defined as >2 cm, poorly-differentiated, depth of invasion >4 mm, and recurrent. The efficacy is debatable.)

Ear Reconstruction

1. What particular part of the ear, after excision of skin cancer, favors a skin graft and what site does not? (*If* perichondrium is intact the concha and the post-auricular areas lend well to a skin graft, perhaps the scapha as well.)
   (a) Why? (Both areas are relatively featureless as opposed to the antihelix or superior or inferior crus all of which have surface landmarks.)
   (b) What type of skin graft? (Full-thickness harvested from the "blush" area above the clavicles is preferable to avoid secondary contracture from a split-thickness skin graft. Consider the opposite ear as a donor site.)
   (c) If perichondrium is not intact, is skin graft an option? (Yes, if the defect is <1.5 cm in size, since the graft will survive and be taken as a composite graft. Excisions that result in defects larger than 1.5 cm usually result in sacrifice of the underlying cartilage.)
2. Describe three methods of single-stage helical rim repair after skin cancer excision including limitations. (Primary wedge closure, star excision, and helical rim advancement flap. Wedge closure is simply a triangular resection and reapposition of the cartilage and skin and is limited to defects of 1 cm or less. Larger defects of 1 to 1.5 cm can also be closed primarily but require a star or vertical excision of antihelical cartilage both superiorly and inferiorly-see accompanied diagram. Perhaps the points of the star should consist of excision of cartilage only with resolution of the excess skin with time. A third method, perhaps up to a 1.5 cm defect, is an Antia rim advancement-see diagram. Rim advancement consists of a full-thickness incision through anterior skin and cartilage as well as posterior perichondrium but maintenance of the post-auricular skin intact. Rim advancement procedures work optimally for superior helical rim defects. These three techniques wedge, star, and rim advancement should be considered as points on a continuum. See Figs. 31.1 and 31.2.

   A small, 1 cm, composite graft can be harvested from the opposite ear for modest defects.)
   (a) Limitations? (All three methods will shorten the vertical height of the ear somewhat but a smaller ear is not particularly aesthetically noticeable. Attempts to extend the indications to a defect >25% are at risk for severe anterior cupping of the ear and an unacceptable appearance.)
3. Describe a method for a full-thickness, skin and cartilage, defect of the concha. (Two options exist. One, a full-thickness skin graft onto the raw area created by the

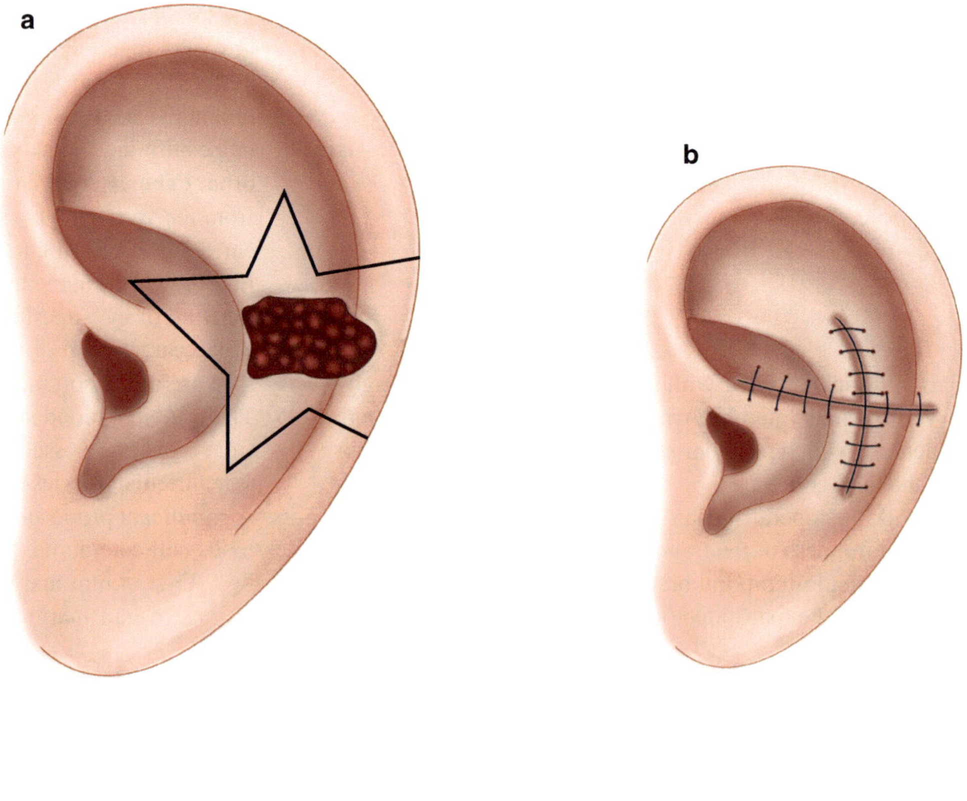

Fig. 31.1 Primary wedge closure (**a**) Star-shaped design of excision, (**b**) Closure

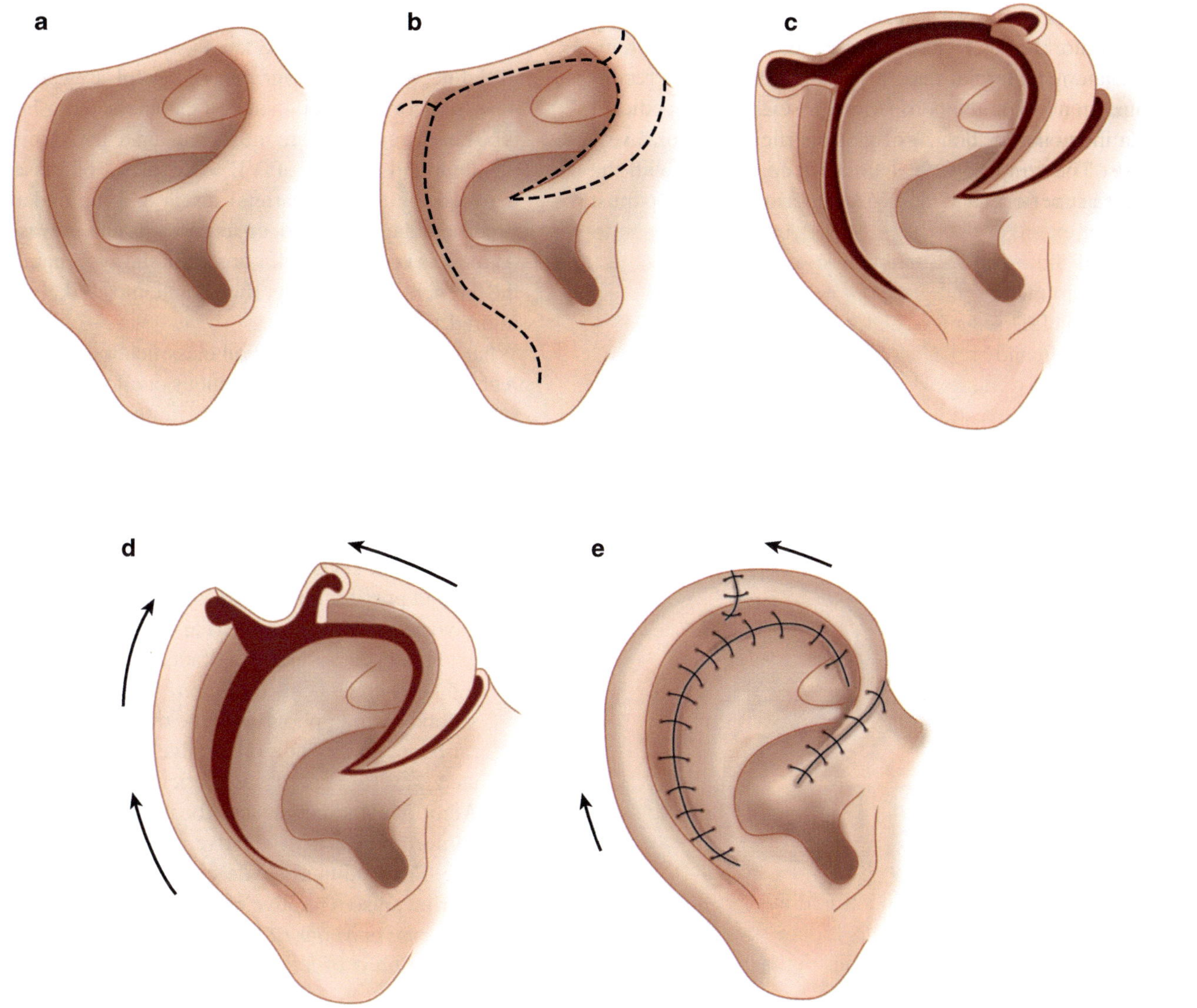

Fig. 31.2 (**a**) Crumpled helical rim, (**b**) Outline of Antia-Buch rim advancement flap, (**c**) Incisions, (**d**) Advancement of flap, (**e**) Closure

removal of the conchal cartilage, and two, a revolving-door flap of post-auricular and adjacent scalp mastoid skin, designed as an island flap. The anterior edge of the island is sutured to the medial portion of the conchal defect at the external auditory meatus and the posterior edge of the island is sutured to the lateral edge of the ear defect at the antihelical rim. Perhaps a preferable method is a full-thickness skin graft but the repair with the graft at the external auditory meatus must be meticulous to avoid stenosis. If that graft is <1.5 cm, the grafts can be placed onto conchal cartilage bare of perichondrium.)

4. How does a defect of the different be repaired? (For the superior defect, hairless skin is often not available so some consideration has to be given for the provision of hairless skin such as a temporoparietal fascial flap +/− cartilage graft dependent on defect size plus full-thickness skin graft. For defects in the inferior two-thirds the post-auricular skin is available as a flap.)
5. Describe a method for a full-thickness middle one-third defect. Outline two types of designs. (One method consists of a tube vertically oriented of post-auricular skin that is raised and transferred in three stages. The second and third stages consist of attachment to the superior and inferior edge of the defect, respectively. The other option is a post-auricular flap based posteriorly, raised and sutured to the superior and inferior as well as the anterior edges of the defect, and is divided and inset at a second stage. See Figs. 31.3 and 31.4.)
   (a) Of the two, which appeals to you intuitively? Why? (The post-auricular flap for ease of transfer, two-

stage instead of three, easier to incorporate an autogenous or alloplastic strut for support.)

6. What are the key technical aspects of the use of the temporoparietal fascial flap in partial and total ear reconstruction? (The temporoparietal fascial flap is pedicled on the posterior branch of the superficial temporal vessels. The temporoparietal fascia is contiguous with the galea superiorly and the SMAS inferiorly. The flap must be raised just deep to the hair follicles and alopecia is a complication. Once the fascia is secured over the underlying cartilage framework, key tacking or bolster sutures to define surface contour can be useful as well as the necessity for subfascial suction catheters and a bolster-type head dressing. Care must be taken to avoid injury to the temporal branch of VII. The plane of dissection between the temporoparietal fascia and the underlying superficial layer of the deep temporal fascia is avascular. At the level of the superior border of the zygomatic arch, the branch is more superficial and most likely to be injured.)
7. What are two or three general classifications of total ear reconstruction? (Either autogenous or alloplastic and the second can be further subdivided into a prosthetic and alloplastic framework such as Med-Por plus autogenous coverage.)
8. What are the indications for prosthetic ear reconstruction? (The readings provide four: failed autogenous reconstruction, severe soft tissue and/or skeletal hypoplasia, and post-traumatic or post-ablative.)
   (a) Give an example of each. (Failed autogenous is self-explanatory; severe hemifacial microsomia with tight deficient skin and severe concave hollowing secondary to hypoplasia of the mandible and temporal bone; a traumatic or ablative defect that has created severe soft tissue deficiency and scarring. Additional indications may be the presence of severe comorbidities, post-ablative irradiation, both relative. The readings also describe a low or unfavorable hairline, also a relative contraindication.)
9. Give the pros and cons of prosthetic reconstruction. (The reconstruction is of a finite nature and requires replace-

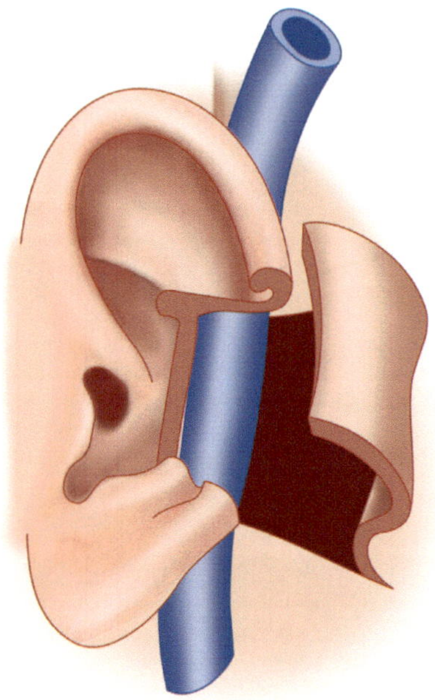

Fig. 31.3 Post-auricular flap (Superior)

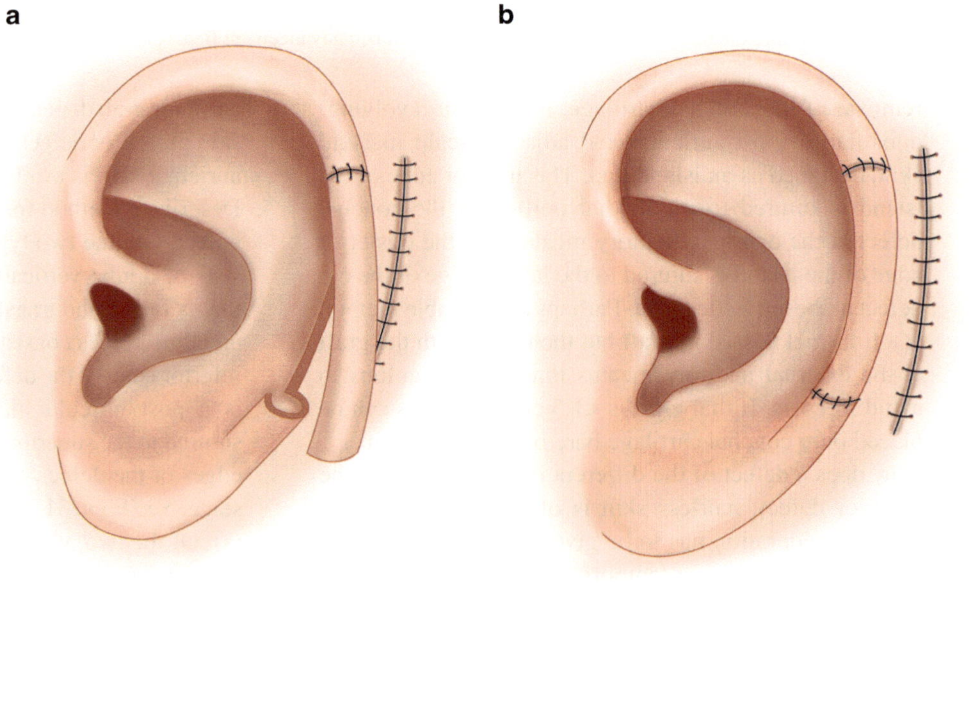

Fig. 31.4 (**a**) Flap attached initially superior, (**b**) Inset

ment every 3–5 years with the attendant cost. The psychological overtones of the necessity for patients to remove or replace the ear on a daily basis, the possibility of trauma to the fixation posts with sporting activities etc., and a bridge can be burned if soft tissue is excised to create a thin bed for the prosthetic bone posts. Regardless of the degree of perfection in aesthetic quality, the texture and color can not match normal skin.)

10. Briefly, list the steps in placement of an osseointegrated prosthetic ear reconstruction. (Essentially three stages. After a CT scan is performed, the first stage is placement of the titanium bone implants. The second stage is the placement of the fixtures onto the screw implants done 6–8 months after the first stage to allow bone integration into the screws, capped to prevent soft tissue ingrowth, and finally, construction and application of the prosthesis, after an additional 2 months before the second stage fixtures can be loaded.)
    (a) What are some desirable characteristics of the soft tissue for prosthetic reconstruction? (Thin perhaps even a skin graft, bone thick enough, >3 mm, to allow for retention of the titanium screws, and of course absence of any ulceration or infection.)
    (b) What if the patient has had prior radiotherapy to the temporal bone? (Osseointegrated prosthetic ear reconstruction is still feasible. The use of hyperbaric oxygen may be necessary.)

Case 1: Ca of the Ear

Cased-Based Conference

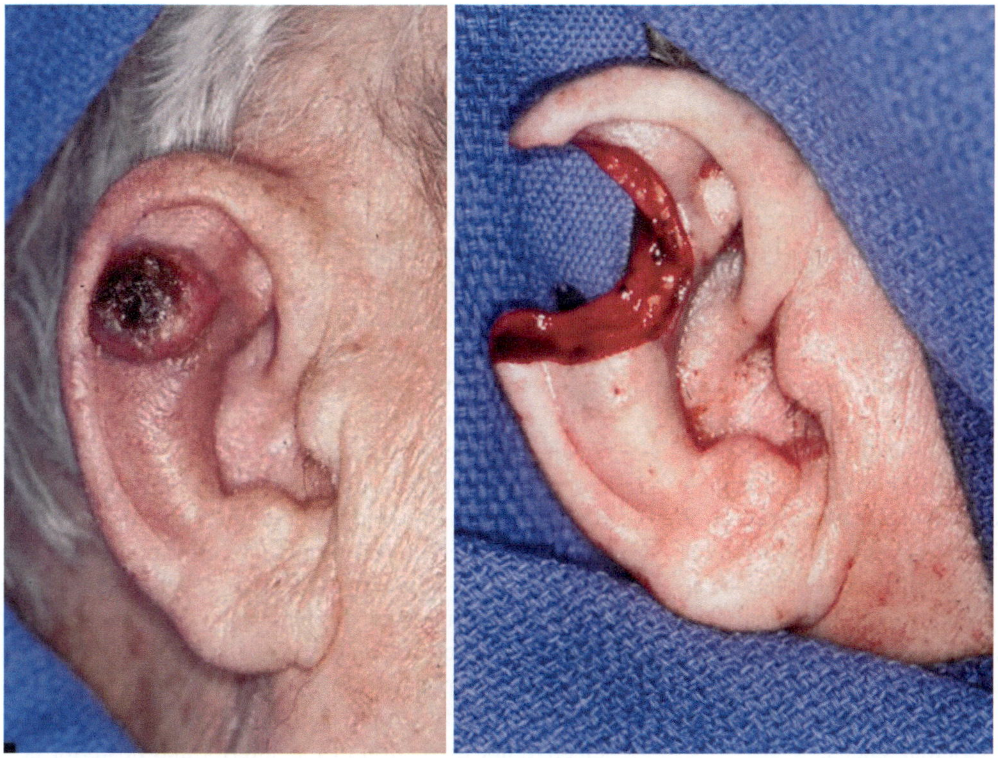

A 68-year-old with a biopsy-proven poorly-differentiated squamous cell carcinoma of the ear. The patient is in good medical health.

1. Describe the findings on the slides and add a focused clinical examination.
    (a) Are any tests indicated? Justify.
2. Describe the pathologic anatomy. Does the poorly-differentiated nature dictate additional treatment? What?
3. Outline a treatment plan based on your response to Questions 2 and 3.

Cased-Based Conference: Discussion

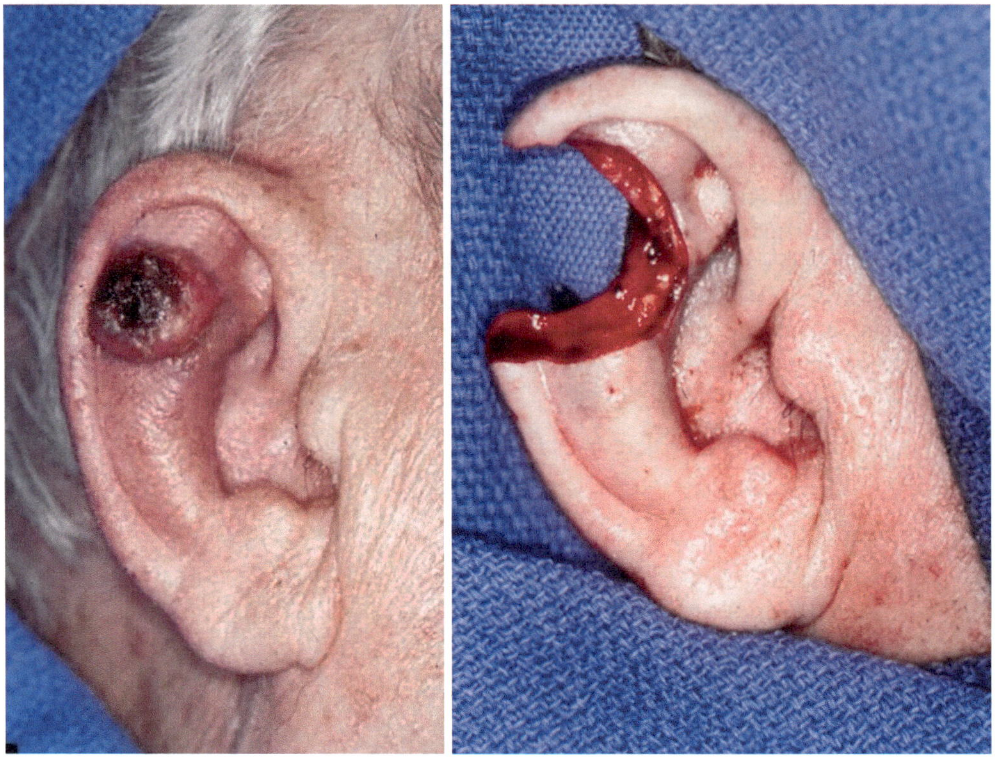

A 68-year-old with a biopsy-proven poorly-differentiated squamous cell carcinoma of the ear. The patient is in good medical health.

1. Describe the findings on the slides and add a focused clinical examination. (On anterior or lateral view is an exophytic lesion that appears about 2 cm in size, located in the superior one-third of the ear. Specifically, occupying the scapha, triangular fossa, and abutting the helical rim. A segment of the superior helical rim and scapha and root of the helix do not appear involved. The remainder of the ear does not appear abnormal, although the antihelix seems edematous with a blunted appearance of the normal contour. Also, the usual division of the concha into cybum and cavum is not present. On the posterior or medial view, which is blurred, the lesion involves the rim and extends toward but not into the post-auricular sulcus.

   The intraoperative view of the defect is discussed in question 4.

   The clinical exam would include a history of duration, facial pain, and tobacco use. The patient is in good medical health. The physical exam would begin with palpation of the lymph node-bearing areas pertinent to this lesion, namely, the post-auricular or mastoid, posterior cervical, and anterior cervical as well as the parotid nodes. Attention directed toward the ear would attempt to determine the nature of the edema, if actually present.)

   (a) Are any tests indicated? Justify (Probably not. A case could be established for CT scan of the neck for detection of adenopathy. If the lesion had not been previously biopsied, an incisional biopsy at the periphery, perhaps posteriorly could be performed. An argument can be also made that given the appearance a definitive excision with margins as diagnosis and treatment is an option.)
2. Describe the pathologic anatomy. Does the poorly-differentiated nature dictate additional treatment? What? (A poorly-differentiated squamous cell carcinoma of the external ear of approximately 2 cm in dimensions with full-thickness involvement of skin and cartilage. The size of the lesion and histology point toward possible occult metastatic lymphadenopathy. The probability is not sufficient to justify prophylactic neck dissection, neither selective nor dissection of the anterior and posterior cervical triangles. Widespread adoption of the experience with the use of sentinel lymph node (SLN) in melanoma of the head and neck in non-melanoma skin cancer of the face has not occurred and only small case reports are in the recent literature. If performed, a SLN would dictate a prior lymphoscintigraphy and use of radioactive colloid as well as a hand-held gamma probe for intraoperative detection. The therapeutic conundrum is that both lymph node basins, anterior and posterior, are possible sites of the SLN.)

3. Outline a treatment plan based on your response to questions #2 and 3. (A wedge resection with 5-6 mm margins would result in a defect of about one-third or more of the ear (See slide 3). A hierarchy of reconstructive procedures are available. Closure with or without the use of a "star" pattern of additional cartilage excision probably will not be sufficient. The reduction in ear height plus the production of an anterior cupping deformity of the remaining ear will be unacceptable. Some reduction and vertical height is tolerable, cupping deformity is not. For any given defect, that determination can be made with a simple suture to oppose the edges of the defect and examination for anterior cupping. The next rung of the reconstructive ladder would be the Antia-Buch procedure, advancing the inferior and superior rim segments, a procedure that essentially recruits tissue from the lobule and the root of the helix. Although an Antia-Buch approach would reconstruct the rim satisfactorily, the scaphal and antihelical defect would not be addressed.

   If local flaps are warranted, a flap of post-auricular skin, based posteriorly, could be sutured to the anterior edge of the defect. Structural support could be provided by a strut of cartilage or Medpor tunneled beneath the base of the flap. The second stage would raise the superior and inferior limbs of the flap including the respective tips of the buried strut. The edges of the strut are sutured to the superior and inferior cartilage remnants respectfully, and the flap skin is closed to the adjacent auricular skin. The third stage is division of the posterior base of the flap of sufficient length to fold into the post-auricular sulcus and sutured to the anterior edge of the defect posteriorly. The resultant flap donor site defect is closed with a thick split-thickness graft harvested from the neck.)

Case 2: Ca of the Ear

Cased-Based Conference

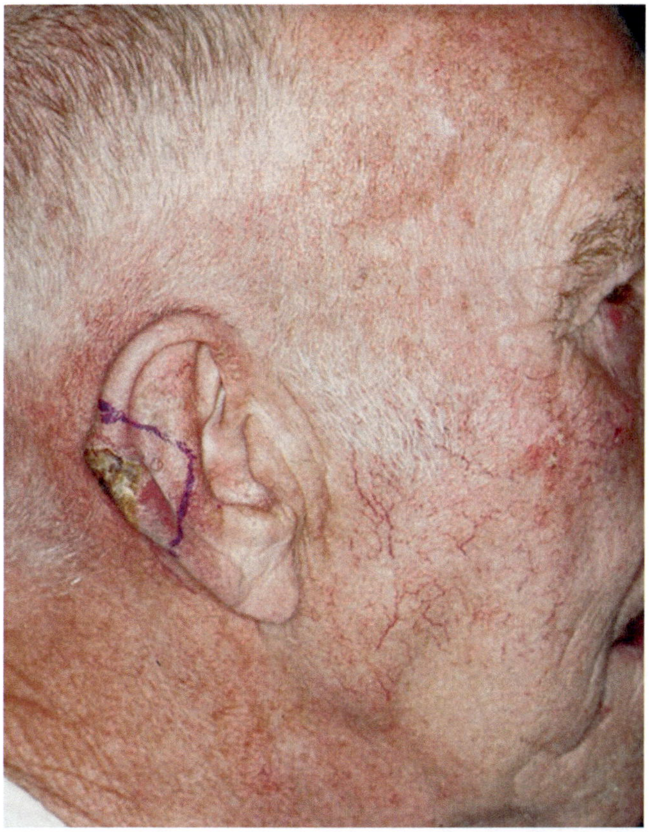

A 68-year-old with a biopsy-proven poorly-differentiated squamous cell carcinoma of the ear. The patient is in good medical health.

1. Describe the findings on the slides and add a focused clinical examination.
   (a) Are any tests indicated? Justify.
2. Describe the pathologic anatomy.
3. Does the poorly-differentiated nature dictate additional treatment? What?
4. Outline a treatment plan based on your response to questions #2 and 3.

Cased-Based Conference: Discussion

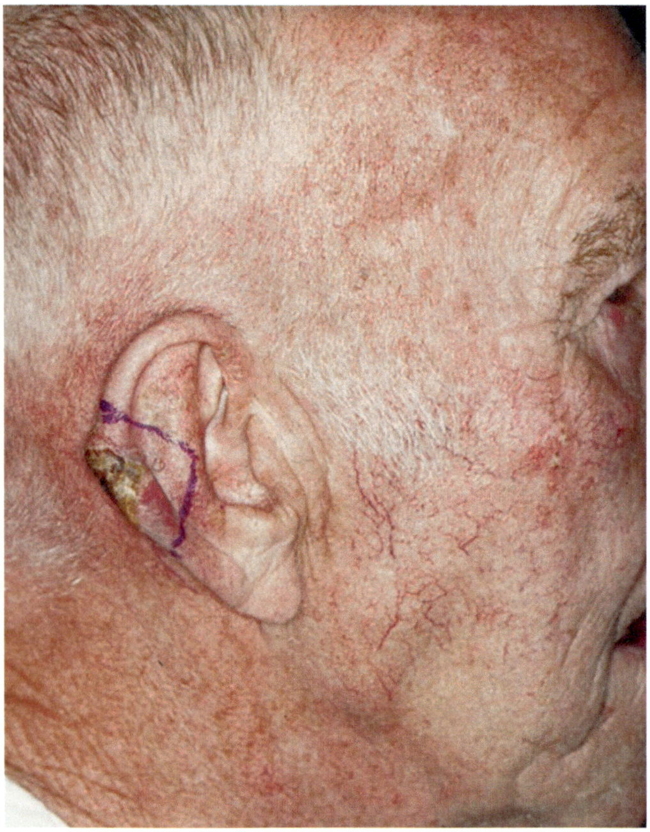

A 68-year-old with a biopsy-proven poorly-differentiated squamous cell carcinoma of the ear. The patient is in good medical health.

1. Describe the findings on the slides and add a focused clinical examination. (On anterior or lateral view is an exophytic lesion that appears about 2 cm in size, located in the superior one-third of the ear. Specifically, occupying the scapha, triangular fossa, and abutting the helical rim. A segment of superior helical rim and scapha and root of the helix does not appear involved. The remainder of the ear does not appear abnormal, although the antihelix seems edematous with a blunted appearance of the normal contour. Also, the usual division of the concha into cybum and cavum is not present. On the posterior or medial view, which is blurred, the lesion involves the rim and extends toward but not into the post-auricular sulcus.

   The intraoperative view of the defect is discussed in question 4.

   The clinical exam would include a history of duration, facial pain, and tobacco use. The patient is in good medical health. The physical exam would begin with palpation of the lymph node-bearing areas pertinent to this lesion, namely, the post-auricular or mastoid, posterior cervical, and anterior cervical as well as the parotid nodes. Attention directed toward the ear would attempt to determine the nature of the edema, if actually present.)
   (a) Any tests indicated? Justify (Probably not. A case could be established for CT scan of the neck for detection of adenopathy. If the lesion had not been previously biopsied, an incisional biopsy at the periphery, perhaps posteriorly could be performed. An argument can be also made that given the appearance a definitive excision with margins is an option.)
2. Describe the pathologic anatomy. (A poorly-differentiated squamous cell carcinoma of the external ear of approximately 2 cm in dimensions with full-thickness involvement of skin and cartilage.)
3. Does the poorly-differentiated nature dictate additional treatment? What? (The size of the lesion and histology point toward possible occult metastatic lymphadenopathy. The probability is not sufficient to justify prophylactic neck dissection, neither selective nor dissection of the anterior and posterior cervical triangles. Adoption of the experience with the use of biopsy of the sentinel lymph node (SLN) in melanoma of the head and neck in non-melanoma skin cancer of the face has not occurred and only small case reports are in the recent literature. If performed, an SLN would dictate a prior lymphoscintigraphy and use of radioactive colloid as well as a hand-held gamma probe for intraoperative detection. The therapeutic conundrum is that both lymph node basins, anterior and posterior, are possible sites of the SLN.)
4. Outline a treatment plan based on your response to questions #2 and 3. (A wedge resection with 5–6 mm margins would result in a defect of about one-third or more of the ear (See slide 3). A hierarchy of reconstructive procedures from simple closure to the use of local flaps will be necessary. Closure with or without the use of a "star" pattern of additional cartilage excision probably will not be sufficient. The reduction in ear height plus the production of an anterior cupping deformity of the remaining ear will be unacceptable. Some reduction and vertical height is tolerable, cupping deformity is not. For any given defect, that determination can be made with a simple suture to oppose the edges of the defect and examination for anterior cupping. The next rung of the reconstructive ladder

would be the Antia-Buch procedure, advancing the inferior and superior rim segments, a procedure that essentially recruits tissue from the lobule and the root of the helix. Although an Antia-Buch approach would reconstruct the rim satisfactorily, the scaphal and antihelical defect would not be addressed.

If local flaps are warranted, a flap of post-auricular skin, based posteriorly, could be sutured to the anterior edge of the defect. Structural support could be provided by a strut of cartilage or Medpor tunneled beneath the base of the flap. The second stage would raise the superior and inferior limbs of the flap including the respective tips of the buried strut. The edges of the strut are sutured to the superior and inferior cartilage remnants respectfully, and the flap skin closed to the adjacent auricular skin. The third stage is division of the posterior base of the flap of sufficient length to fold into the post-auricular sulcus and sutured to the anterior edge of the defect posteriorly. The resultant flap donor site defect is closed with a thick split-thickness graft harvested from the neck.)

Case 3: Ca of the Ear

Cased-Based Conference

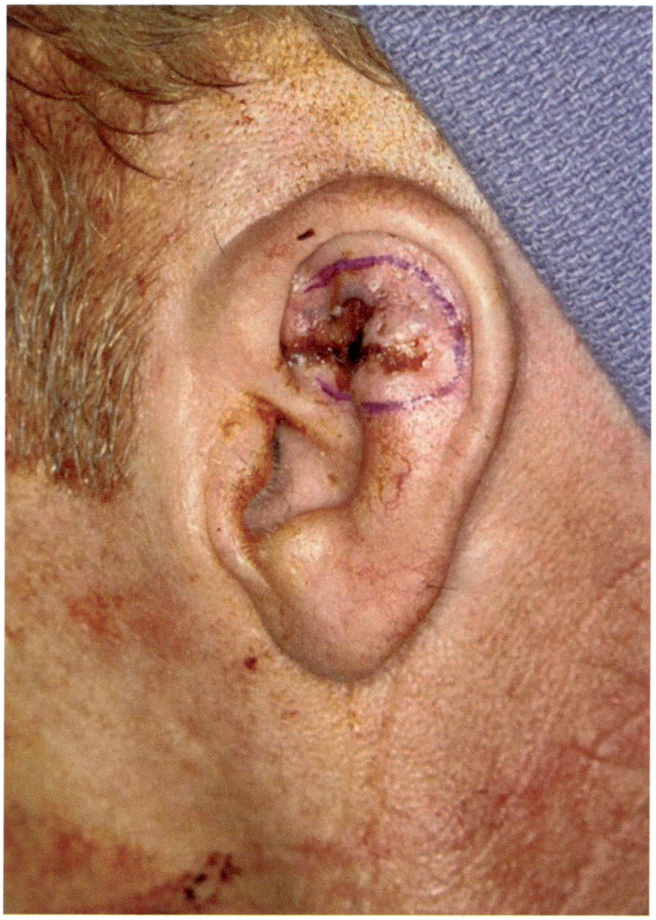

A 68-year-old with a biopsy-proven well-differentiated squamous cell carcinoma of the ear. The patient is in good medical health.

1. Describe the findings on the slides and add a focused clinical examination.
   (a) Are any tests indicated? Justify.
2. Describe the pathologic anatomy.
3. Outline a treatment plan based on your response to questions #2 and 3.

Cased-Based Conference: Discussion

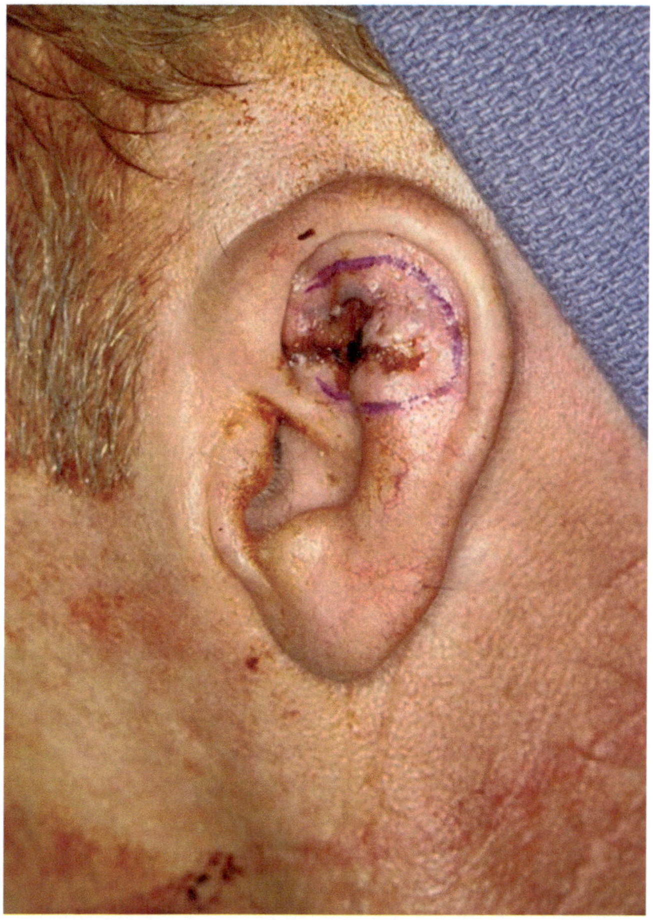

A 68-year-old with a biopsy-proven well-differentiated squamous cell carcinoma of the ear. The patient is in good medical health.

1. Describe the findings on the slides and add a focused clinical examination. (A single photo illustrates an ulcerated lesion of the ear. The view is lateral and restricted mostly to the ear. A surgical marking outlines the extent of the lesion. The lesion occupies the scapha, the superior half of the antihelix, and has obliterated the superior and inferior crus and triangular fossa. The normal configura-

tion of the antihelix is absent. Although in general nodular in appearance, the anterior central portion in the region of the superior crus, the carcinoma is ulcerative and penetrates the underlying tissues. A thin rim of scapha and the adjacent helix are not involved. A limited view of the adjacent scalp and neck skin does not contain additional lesions.

The clinical exam should begin with a history of duration, associated pain, if any, and character and distribution if pain is present, followed by any history of treatment of other skin cancers. The preamble states the patient is in good health but otherwise, a routine past medical history would pursue the presence of comorbidities and both prescription and over-the-counter medications. A social history of tobacco, alcohol, and substance abuse completes the history. The physical exam attempts to ascertain the depth of the penetration although the photo suggests the upper portion of the ear is probably fixed to the underlying tissue and not mobile. The face and neck are examined for the presence of other lesions and the anterior and posterior lymph node basins are palpated for lymphadenopathy. The area of the ear, inferior to the lesion, absent of a normal antihelix is palpated for edema. The opposite ear is examined for comparison.)

(a) Are any tests indicated? Justify. (The probability of occult lymph node metastasis is quite low and does not justify the performance of a CT scan. The pathology report should be reviewed for determination of depth of invasion.)

2. Describe the pathologic anatomy. (The pathologic anatomy is that of a squamous cell carcinoma of the lateral or anterior ear with involvement of skin and cartilage of the scapha and superior antihelix. In addition, a portion of the carcinoma has penetrated a soft tissue medial to the ear, perhaps into the underlying deep temporal fascia. A small rim of intact scapha and adjacent helix may provide sufficient framework support if the skin deficit is addressed. Excision of the lesion will create a through-and-through defect.

The other pathological consideration is the propensity for lymphatic metastasis. Given the size of the primary and the well-differentiated characteristics, the probability is quite low. If the histologic pathology was poorly-differentiated, some consideration should be given to a sentinel lymph node biopsy. Other concerns that may arise from the pathology include presence of lymphovascular invasion and depth, >4 mm, of invasion. The clinical situation is rendered somewhat more complex, given the variability of the normal lymphatic drainage of the ear. The embryologic origin of the area of the ear involved in the second branchial arch and a pattern of retromastoid and posterior cervical lymph node involvement would not be unusual. Drainage into the intraparotid lymph nodes is plausible as well. If a sentinel lymph node biopsy is selected as a therapeutic option, highly debatable, preliminary lymphoscintigraphy would be of value.)

3. Outline a treatment plan based on your response to questions #2 and 3. (The gross margins of the lesions have been marked and an additional 4 mm margin is mandatory. The use of a frozen section will be compromised by the presence of cartilage in the specimen so excision, application of a dressing, and a wait for the final pathology examination would be prudent. The excision would encompass anterior skin, the underlying cartilage, the medial or posterior skin of the inferior portion of the defect, and the underlying retroauricular soft tissue in the more superior aspect of the defect. Certainly, an argument could be established of amputation of the entire superior 40% of the ear and a decision might tilt in that direction if the histology was one of poor differentiation as discussed above or if the path reveals a positive margin or margins.

The reconstructive need is reconstitution of the skin envelope if the helical rim has been retained. For the lower one-half of the defect, the area of through-and-through tissue loss, an option is to suture the edges of the defect to the retroauricular mastoid, prepared by de epithelialization of a rim of mastoid skin to permit placement of sutures. The superior half of the defect, consisting of a bed of soft tissue, could be closed with a full-thickness skin graft harvested from the opposite ear. A second stage would release the ear and a small graft placed on the mastoid donor site.)

Intraoperative

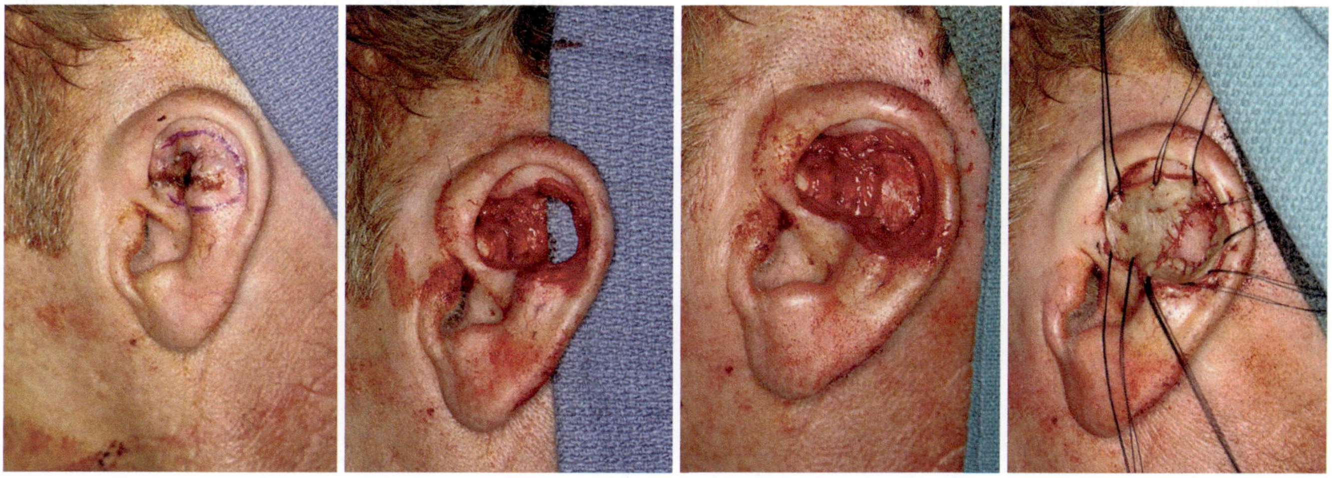

The first photo demonstrates a full-thickness or through-and-through defect of the scapha as well as the adjacent medial component of the defect created by excision of skin and cartilage. The subsequent photo depicts the full-thickness defect sewn into retroauricular skin, and finally, a full-thickness skin graft closes the remainder of the anterior ear skin defect.

Postoperative

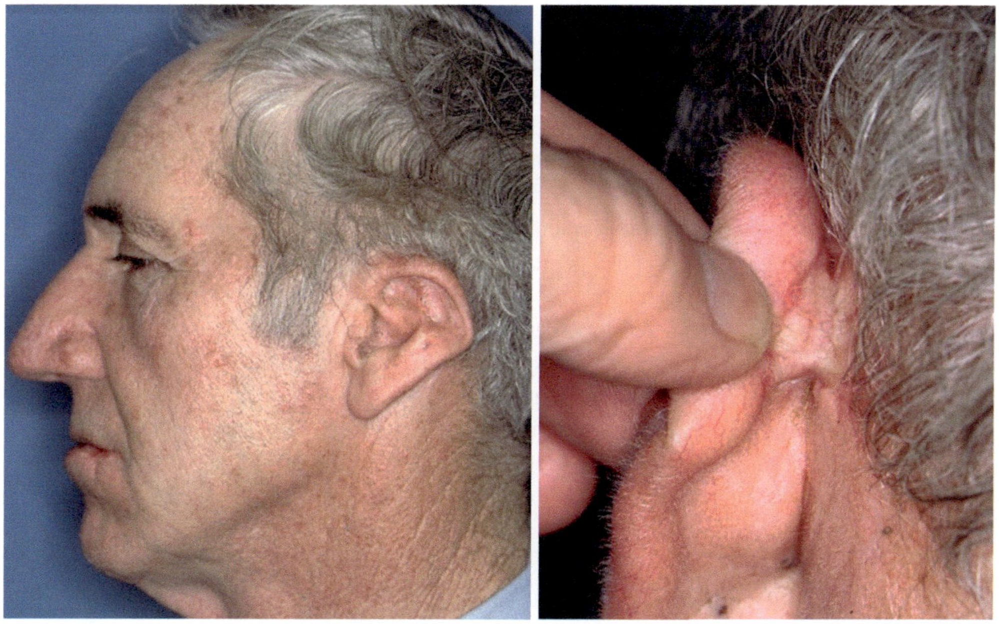

In two photos, a full lateral and a post-auricular perspective, some distortion of the inferior helical rim is evident, perhaps from some anterior cupping. In the post-auricular closeup, the ear is still adhered to the mastoid, so apparently the second stage is yet to be performed.

In-Service Examination

1. During otoscopic removal of ear cerumen the patient begins to cough. What nerve has been stimulated?
   (a) Posterior branch of the greater auricular
   (b) Nerve of Arnold
   (c) Auriculotemporal
   (d) Stapedial

2. A 2.5 cm defect of the middle one-third of the ear is optimally reconstructed with:
   (a) Temporoparietal flap plus autologous rib graft
   (b) Temporoparietal flap and alloplastic porous polyethylene
   (c) Wedge closure
   (d) Antia-buch
   (e) Post-auricular flap and conchal graft
3. A 2 cm defect of the superior helical rim is optimally reconstructed with:
   (a) Wedge closure
   (b) Antia-Buch flap
   (c) Temporoparietal fascia plus full-thickness skin graft
   (d) Composite graft from the opposite ear

32 Melanoma

Bibliography

Dźwierzyński WW, "Managing Malignant Melanoma", *Plast. Reconstr. Surg.*, (2013); 132(3):**446e–460e (Skip 450e–455e but include Table 3, Skip staging tables-outdated)**.

Knackstedt T, Knackstedt RW, Couto R, Gastman Brian, "Malignant Melanoma: Diagnostic and Management Update", *Plast. Reconstr. Surg.*, (2018);(142):**202e–212e and Video 1**.

Cochran AM, Buchanan PJ, Bueno Jr. RA, Neumeister, MW, "Subungual Melanoma: A review of Current Treatment", *Plast. Reconstr. Surg.*, (2014); 134: **259–262 (to literature review), 271–272**.

Upadhyaya S.N., Knackstedt R.W., Ko J.S., Gastman B.R., The Use and Technique of Sentinel Node Biopsy for Skin Cancer, *Plast Reconstr Surg.*, (2022);149(5):**995e–1005e ONLY**.

Pavri SN, Clune J, Ariyan S, Narayan D, "Malignant Melanoma: Beyond the Basics", *Plast. Reconstr. Surg.*, (2016); 138(2):**330e–338e ONLY**.

Supplemental

Ariyan S and Berger A, Ch. 31: "Melanoma", Neligan PC, Plastic Surgery 3rd Edition (2013); 1:**748–771, 776–784 ONLY**.

Faculty Discussion and Study Guide

Pathology, Epidemiology, Staging

1. What are the documented risk factors for the development of melanoma? (Family history, dysplastic nevus syndrome, history of frequent severe childhood sunburn, Fitzpatrick 1 or 2 complexion.)
2. Classify melanoma morphologically? (Nodular, superficial spreading, lentigo, and acral lentiginous.)
   - (a) Differentiate histologically and survival. (Superficial spreading as the name applies is a relatively thin lesion until a vertical growth phase occurs. Nodular is a thick lesion with a significant and early vertical growth phase. Lentigo is by definition a carcinoma-in-situ until basement membrane invasion occurs and then the lesion is designated as lentigo maligna melanoma. Finally, acral lentiginous is a lesion confined to fingers or toes or palms and soles of the hand as well as subungual areas. Survival is best for lentigo followed by superficial spreading, nodular, and worst for acral lentiginous.)
   - (b) What is characteristic of a lentigo maligna melanoma? (Occurs within a lentigo lesion in sun-exposed areas, most commonly on the head and neck known as Hutchinson's freckle in an elderly patient. Essentially, lentigo maligna is an in-situ lesion with intact basement membrane. Lentigo maligna melanoma is an invasive or vertical growth pattern into the dermis.)
   - (c) Give some specific epidemiological features of each. (Superficial spreading has a gender predilection for women and a younger age group than the other types, lentigo maligna is seen in the elderly patient, and acral lentiginous is seen disproportionally in African Americans.)
3. In the conversion of radial growth into a vertical pattern of melanoma, when viewed in a cross-section of skin what has occurred? (Invasion of the basement membrane of the epidermis by malignant melanocytes. So histologically, the melanocytes have actively invaded the dermis or a vertical growth pattern.)
4. What are the prognostic factors in melanoma? (Tumor thickness, presence of ulceration, lymph node metastases, and mitotic index. Gender and trunk vs. extremities may be independent prognostic variables. The mitotic index as a prognostic variable has only been established for thin, <1 mm, melanomas and is no longer considered in staging.)

E. Luce, *A Curriculum for Plastic Surgery*, https://doi.org/10.1007/978-3-031-62087-4_32

5. What is desmoplastic melanoma and what other entity can be confused with desmoplastic melanoma clinically? (Desmoplastic melanoma is a neurotropic lesion, lacks pigmentation, and clinically can appear to be a dermatofibroma. Histologically, the lesion is dominated by the presence of fibrosis and spindle cell orientation of the cellular component.)
   (a) Desmoplastic melanoma should be differentiated from a similar-appearing lesion. (Amelanotic melanoma)
   (b) Clinical behavior of desmoplastic melanoma? (Although histologically appears to be less of a differentiated lesson, the risk of metastasis to the regional lymph nodes is low but the risk of systemic metastasis is much higher than garden variety melanoma and viewed from this perspective, desmoplastic melanoma behaves more as a sarcoma than an epithelial skin cancer.)
6. Discuss the features of acral lentiginous melanoma. (As mentioned, a disproportionate distribution in African Americans, on the plantar and palmar aspect and the occurrence in the neomatrix as subungual. Mucosal melanomas, distinctly rare in comparison, are considered as variant. Characteristically, acral melanomas present in a more advanced stage.)
   (a) What is Hutchinson's sign? (The presence of pigment in the adjacent skin is highly suggestive of a subungual melanoma.)
   (b) What is the prognosis in general: worse, better, or the same as other types of malignant melanoma? Explain. (Worse. Delay in diagnosis, perhaps because of location and a significant proportion are amelanotic.)
7. What is the typical presentation, management, and outcomes of subungual melanoma? (The digit most commonly involved is either the thumb or the large toe but any finger or toe can be involved. The presentation is of a pigmented lesion that streaks throughout the nail and is often mismanaged as an infection or fungus until quite advanced. A biopsy is necessary which can be performed by a window in the nail. Subsequent management traditionally has been amputation but a thin 1 mm or less lesion can be addressed with excision and full thickness skin graft. More thick lesions should probably be amputated at the next joint. Of course the same indications for SLN exist.)

Assessment, Excision

1. What is the A, B, C, D, E criteria for suspicion of a malignant melanoma? (Asymmetry, border irregularity, color, diameter, elevation of lesion.)
   (a) What is the significance of depigmentation within a nevus suspected of melanoma? (This should heighten suspicion since those areas may well represent spontaneous regression and signal a host or immunologic response.)
   (b) What is the significance of depigmentation within a halo lesion? (Halo nevus is not malignant and the surrounding pale or halo area is characterized histologically by lymphocytic infiltration but no pigment.)
2. What is the value of excisional biopsy vs. incisional? (Areas of deeper invasion may exist in the lesion not incorporated in an incisional biopsy. Thus, accurate staging requires excision of the entire lesion, if possible.)
   (a) However, if the excisional biopsy is preferred, what are the indications for an incisional biopsy? (In some areas particularly with a larger lesion, cosmetic and/or functional reasons may dictate an incisional biopsy.)
   (b) If incisional biopsy is selected, how performed? (One can do a punch biopsy with emphasis on any papules or more deeply pigmented lesions, preferential for an incisional biopsy.)
   (c) Shave biopsy techniques are frequently used in non-melanoma skin cancer. Is such appropriate for malignant melanoma? (Absolutely not. Will give no information about the depth of the lesion.)
3. Differentiate the Clark and Breslow systems of the depth of invasion. (Clark is I–V and is determined on histology as I—intraepithelial, II—into the papillary dermis, III—into the interface between the papillary and reticular dermis, IV—invasion to the reticular dermis, V—into the subcutaneous fat. Breslow's classification is an absolute measurement of the depth of thickness as expressed in millimeters or tenths of a millimeter. Breslow's system has largely supplanted the older Clark system.)
4. Define the 2018 TNM staging system for melanoma.

T classification	Thickness	Ulceration status	Stage
Tis	NA	NA	Stage 0
T1	≤1 mm	(a) Without ulceration (b) With ulceration	IA IB
	<0.8 mm	(a) Without ulceration (b) With ulceration	IA IB
	0.8–1.0 mm	(a) Without ulceration (b) With ulceration	IB IB
T2	1.0–2.0 mm	(a) Without ulceration (b) With ulceration	IB IIA
T3	2.0–4.0 mm	(a) Without ulceration (b) With ulceration	IIA IIB
T4	>4.0 mm	(a) Without ulceration (b) With ulceration	IIB IIC
T1A–T4A, N1			IIIB/C
T4B			IIID

N classification	No. of metastatic nodes	Nodal metastatic mass
N1a	1 node	(a) Micrometastases are detected by SLN biopsy only
N1b	1 node	(b) Clinically evident
N2a	2–3 nodes	(a) Micrometastases are detected by SLN biopsy only
N2b	2–3 nodes	(b) Micrometastases clinically evident
N3a	4 or more metastatic nodes	(a) Micrometastases is detected by SLN biopsy only
N3b	4 or more metastatic nodes	(b) Clinically evident

5. What is the recommendation for a workup of primary melanoma with a clinically negative physical examination of the lymph node basin? (None. Certainly, a case can be established for CBC, LDH, and chest X-ray.)
6. A patient presents with an incisional biopsy of 1.5 mm thickness of melanoma of the calf and palpable inguinal lymphadenopathy. What are the diagnostic procedures to be performed? (The presence of nodal metastases may signal occult systemic disease. Chest X-ray, liver function tests and/or LDH, CT scan of the abdomen and chest or a PET scan, needle biopsy of the inguinal lymphadenopathy.)
7. What is the role of PET/CT scan? (The initial development of PET scans was to demonstrate metastases in patients with advanced disease. Subsequently, the performance of PET/CT scans evolved as a baseline to measure response to chemotherapy in similar patients. Currently, the utility value may be in initial surveillance in Stage II C and higher, namely, the presence of nodal metastases and more clearly in Stage III. Practitioners may encounter difficulty in pursuit of insurance coverage for PET scans in early-stage melanoma.)
8. Give a wide local excision margin for the following thickness in malignant melanoma: 1.0 mm, 1.0–2.0 mm, and 4.0 mm. (1 cm, 1–2 cm, and 2 cm, respectively.)
9. What is the role of Moh's in malignant melanoma? (At this juncture, none until evidence indicates Moh's is comparable to wide local excision. May have a yet-to-be-defined role in lentigo maligna.)
   (a) Management of a positive margin in pathology? (Perhaps a role for Moh's but re-excision carries an increased possibility of a repeat positive margin.)
10. What is the potential management of melanoma-in-situ at the surgical margin after re-excision of a prior positive margin? (Consideration should be given to the administration topically of imiquimod, an immunomodulator that provokes an inflammatory response directed toward the atypical melanocytes.)
11. Give the approximate 10-year survival for the following: T1b, T4a, N0, N1a (T1b approximately 90%, slightly lower than T1a; T4a 50%, N0 80%, N1a 60%)
12. Give the hierarchy or primacy of lesion characteristics vs. lymph node status. (If the lymph nodes are positive that prognostic factor overwhelms any characteristic of the lesion such as thickness.)

Regional Lymphnodes

1. A patient presents with a 2 cm axillary lymph node which on a needle biopsy is positive for malignant melanoma. No lesion is apparent on the upper extremity or trunk. What are two likely explanations? (One is spontaneous regression, the other much less likely is a conversion of a lymph nodal nevus to melanoma.)
2. What are Sappey's lines? (The pattern of lymphatic drainage in the trunk. A transverse or horizontal band of approximately 5 cm centered on the umbilicus can drain either superiorly or inferiorly. Superior to that zone, the lymphatic drainage is to the axillary nodes and inferiorly to the inguinal nodes. Though considerable variation occurs clinically.)
3. Briefly discuss the definition of and controversy of elective dissection of regional lymph nodes in melanoma. (Elective regional lymph node dissection, ELND, means the removal of the lymph nodes in the setting of a clinically negative exam for adenopathy. The controversy centers on whether survival was enhanced by the removal of the non palpable yet pathologically present metastases in the lymph nodes. Survival was enhanced in those ELND patients who had clinically negative but pathologically positive nodes on examination in comparison to patients who were observed and subsequently developed adenopathy in follow-up, yet some morbidity attends the performance of lymph node dissection including chronic lymphedema. The controversy has been addressed by the development of the concept of a sentinel lymph node biopsy. In addition, studies that match the two groups in terms of prognostic variables such as tumor thickness, etc. the incidence of subsequent development of lymph node metastasis in the observed group was *lower* than anticipated from the percentage of pathologically-positive lymph nodes in the ELND group. The assumption is that spontaneous regression of a certain percentage of the clinically negative but pathologically positive lymph nodes in the observed group occurred. Interesting observation but the debate has been successfully addressed by the development of SLN biopsy.)
   (a) What are the probabilities of a negative or non palpable lymph node actually positive on microscopic

exam and, conversely, nodes that are palpable, but negative on final pathology? (Approximately 20% in each group but the essential point is the incidence of pathologically positive, clinically negative lymph nodes to a substantial degree hinges on the thickness of the lesion. Also, palpable hyperplastic nodes are more frequent in the groin than the axilla.)
   (b) What is the most likely explanation of the 4% of patients who have a negative SLN but later develop clinically evident positive lymph nodes on follow-up? (Occult metastasis missed on pathological examination of the SLN.)
4. What is the value of lymphoscintigraphy? (Identifies the nodal basin, particularly in truncal or midline lesions; identifies the location of the sentinel lymph node; and, in truncal lesions, may also identify an in-transit node.)
   (a) The common practice is the scheduling of lymphoscintigraphy on the morning of surgery. Why? (Half-life is quite short, 6 h, and identification of the sentinel lymph node or nodes may be quite difficult after 18–24 h.)
5. What are the indications for performance of a SLN biopsy? (In general, a lesion of 1 mm thickness or thicker. A thinner lesion may warrant SLN biopsy if ulceration is present, the mitotic rate is high, or a vertical growth phase exists.)
6. Give a hierarchy probability for a positive SLN in the following lesions. (a) Less than 1.0 mm (5%). (b) 1–2 mm (15%). (c) 2–4 mm (30%). (d) >4 mm (50% or greater)
7. What is the underlying concept, philosophy, and premises as the foundation for the performance of a sentinel lymph node, SLN, biopsy? (The physiologic fact that enables the performance of a sentinel lymph node biopsy is that an ascending hierarchy of lymphatic nodal drainage exists and that the lymph node closest to the primary tumor is the first echelon or level of lymph node metastases. If that lymph node can be identified and biopsied then the pathological diagnosis can be established. A negative SLN implies no other nodal metastases exist and that an SLN pathologically negative is truly negative.)
   (a) What is the essential argument(s) for the use of SLN in the management of patients with malignant melanoma? (Possible enhanced intrinsic survival if the sentinel lymph node is positive which then would lead to a regional lymph node dissection; perhaps use of adjuvant therapy and prognostic information for patient counseling. Currently, investigation and discussion are underway regarding the necessity or lack of same for completion of a regional lymph node dissection in patients with a positive SLN biopsy. See below.)
8. Outline the basic steps in performance of sentinel lymph node biopsy? (A preoperative mapping of the lymphatic drainage and lymph nodes by means of lymphoscintigraphy with the injection of a radioactive colloid. In the operating room, an injection of lymphazurin blue or isosulfan blue into the dermis of the primary is accomplished, the primary tumor is excised and a sentinel lymph node is identified by means of a handheld collimator or gamma probe for identification of the area of high radioactivity versus the background level as well as confirmation by visualization of a blue lymph node.)
   (a) Is the lymph node submitted for a frozen section? (No) Why not? (Pathologists have difficulty in identifying metastatic melanoma in a lymph node, a valuable amount of pathological material is lost with the frozen section, and no capability exists to test for biological markers such as S-100.)
9. You perform an SLN on a melanoma 2.1 mm thickness and the node is positive. What is the probability of additional lymph nodes positive? (Virtually none. In fact, only 15–20% of which most are derived from thicker lesions, will have additional positive lymph nodes on completion node dissection. These numbers are the argument for an SLN biopsy only for intermediate-risk lesions.)
   (a) Do multiple positive nodes imply an impact on prognosis? (Yes. A single positive node on SLN vs. multiple positive nodes on ELND carries a lower 5-year survival.)
10. You operate on a cheek melanoma of 1.5 mm thickness. A preoperative lymphoscintigraphy indicates the SLN is in the preauricular area as does the intraoperative gamma probe. What is the next step? (Not a lock-step superficial parotidectomy. Rather an adequate preauricular incision should be made, a skin flap developed, a probe used to localize the point of radioactivity, and a lymph node directly excised.)
11. Comment on the timing of wide local excision and the performance of sentinel lymph nodes. (The wide local excision should be done at the same time as sentinel lymph node. Prior wide excisions can lead to scarring and failure of identification of the lymphatic drainage basin.)
   (a) How would you manage a patient who is referred to you with a 2.0 mm lesion that was previously widely excised and skin-grafted? (If possible try to use lymphoscintigraphy to identify a drainage basin and subsequently perform a SLN biopsy. If a SLN cannot be identified, choose between the performance of an elective nodal dissection of the nodal basin most likely involved but the preferential course is one of observation.)
12. What role will molecular biology play in SLN management of the melanoma patient? (Yet to be determined,

but perhaps we will define a subset of patients who are negative on routine histological examination and yet positive on PCR and are at more risk than patients who are negative both on routine and molecular examination of the lymph nodes.)

Advanced Disease

1. Define an in-transit metastasis, comment on prognosis, and treat the same in the lower extremity. (An in-transit metastasis is a nodule present at least 2 cm or more from the primary and in the direction of lymph node drainage. The prognosis is quite poor, N3 disease, with an 80% 5-year mortality. The only treatment besides systemic chemotherapy is regional extremity perfusion with melphalan or other cytotoxic agents. The morbidity of regional extremity perfusion can be quite substantial. The philosophy is not to improve survival but rather to avoid severe limb disability, dysfunction, and pain.)
2. Briefly, describe the use of nonsurgical modalities in the treatment of melanoma. (Interleukin-L is a chemotherapeutic agent used for metastatic disease by activation of the host immune system. The efficacy of other chemotherapeutic agents, other than immunomodulators and targeted molecular therapy, see below, in malignant melanoma is either little or none.)
3. What is a contemporary approach to metastatic melanoma? (The advent recently of molecular targeted therapy and immunomodulation have provided an option rather than radiation. One-half of melanomas have the BRAF genetic mutation and are potentially susceptible to molecular targeted therapy. A more broad address of metastasis is immunomodulation. Both of these modalities have a significant incidence of systemic side effects and the secondary development of nonmelanoma skin cancers in the instance of BRAF-inhibitory agents.)
4. What is the role of radiation therapy in melanoma? (Limited. The indications for address of the regional lymph node basins postoperatively are patients with bulky nodes, extracapsular extension of the nodal metastasis, and four or more lymph nodes as well as the characteristics of the primary neurotropism and, possibly, desmoplastic melanoma. When radiation is added to therapeutic lymph node dissection, the incidence of lymphedema, particularly in the lower extremity, is quite high. Melanoma is relatively radioresistant and radiotherapy may be of limited efficacy.)

Editor's Note: The landscape of the management of the advanced disease of melanoma is in flux. These patients are optimally presented to a tumor or skin neoplasm board.

Video Notes

Dźwierzyński WW, "Managing Malignant Melanoma", *Plast. Reconstr. Surg.*, (2013); 132(3):446e, Videos 1–4.

- Four short videos of the dye injection, use of the gamma probe on intact skin, SLN excision, and gamma probe counts. Fair quality, adequate narrative.

Case-Based Conference

Case 1: Melanoma

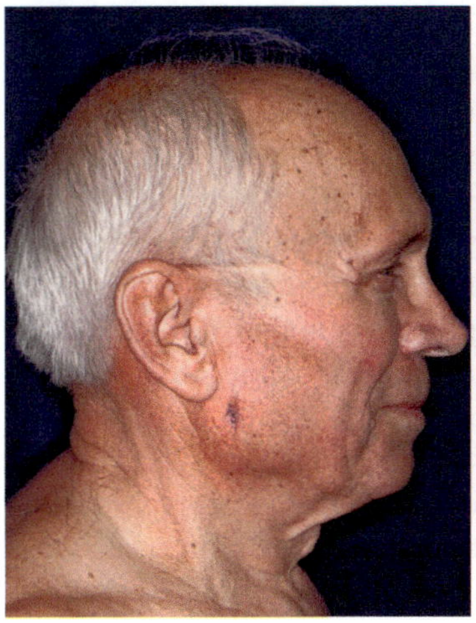

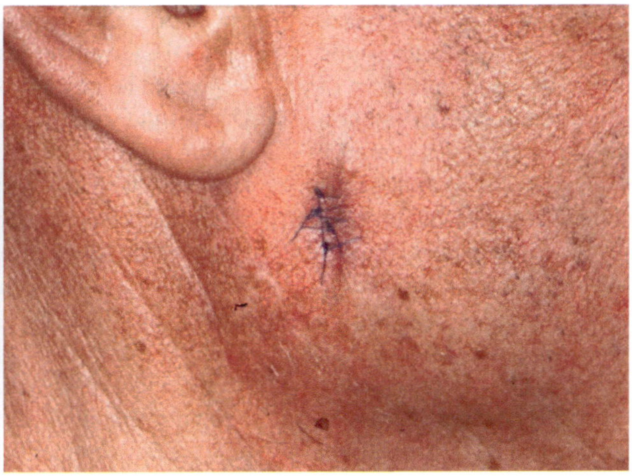

A 61-year-old male with excisional biopsy-proven melanoma of 1.1 mm thickness who is in otherwise excellent health.

1. Describe the findings on the slide(s) and add a *pertinent* clinical examination.
   (a) Are any tests indicated other than routine labs? Justify.
2. Discuss the value of the excisional biopsy in this case vs. a punch or incisional biopsy.
3. You are responsible for the oncologic and reconstructive management of this patient.
   (a) Outline your operative treatment plan including steps and sequence.
   (b) Draw on the board your anticipated defect and reconstruction.

Case-Based Conference: Discussion

Case 1: Melanoma

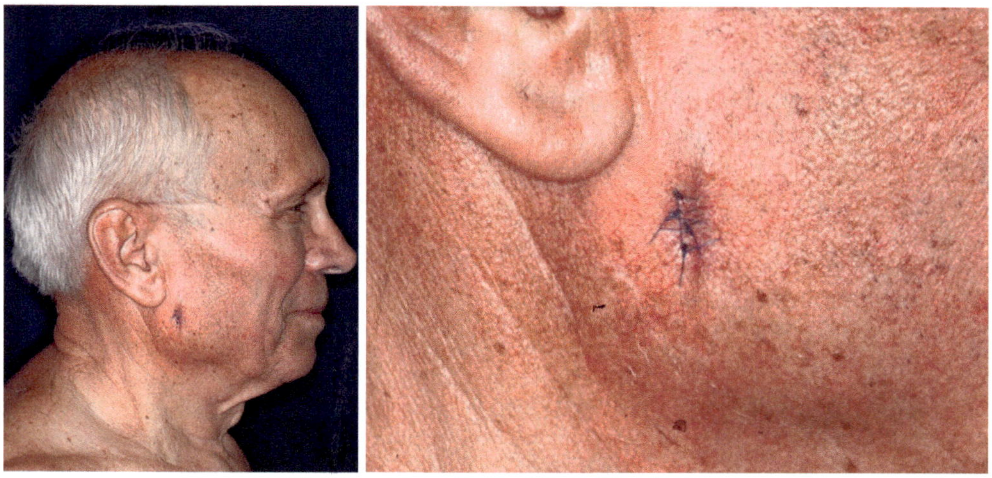

A 71-year-old male with excisional biopsy-proven melanoma of 1.1 mm thickness who is in excellent health.

1. Describe the findings on the slide(s) and add a *pertinent* clinical examination. (Lateral view of an elderly male with a 1 cm sutured vertically-oriented incision located in the posterior-inferior cheek approximately 1–2 cm below and 1–2 cm anterior the level of the lobule. A few scattered small, less than 1 cm light brown nevi are present over the forehead and temple. The clinical exam would elicit more historical information of value indicative of metastatic disease as systemic symptoms such as abdominal pain, bone pain, and CNS symptoms. The appearance de novo or changes in a preexisting nevus as well as the rate of growth should be elicited. Inquiry about prior ulceration will assist in management and prognosis. Additional family history would focus on the occurrence of melanoma although that will not significantly affect the patient's management. Physical examination would be concentrated in the head and neck, in particular to determine if palpable parotid or neck nodal disease is present. The most likely site of neck nodal disease would be in the level 2 or level 3 nodes in the anterior cervical triangle. If not completed by the dermatologist, the trunk and the extremities are subject to a clinical skin scan. As in all preoperative patients a history of possible coagulopathy e.g. Leiden factor, protein c deficiency as perhaps characterized in general by multiple miscarriages, bleeding gums, or easy bruisability.)
   (a) Are any tests indicated other than routine labs? Justify. (Assuming that the patient would have a chest X-ray and CBC perhaps liver function test as LDH. Given the early stage of the disease, a PET scan would be ordered on protocol only.)
2. Discuss the value of the excisional biopsy in this case vs. a punch or incisional biopsy. (For a relatively small lesion, excisional biopsy is advisable if the procedure will not inflict a cosmetic deficit simply from biopsy alone. Punch or incisional biopsies may not provide a complete pathological picture, particularly if variegation of thickness exists within the lesion.)
3. You are responsible for the oncologic and reconstructive management of this patient. (Schedule for lymphoscintigraphy for mapping of the lymph node basin. The patient will need a sentinel lymph node biopsy and a radioisotope injection on the morning of surgery will be required.

Lymphoscintigraphy and the radioisotope injection can be accomplished simultaneously.)

(a) Outline your operative treatment plan including steps and sequence. (The patient should be consented to wide local excision and sentinel lymph node biopsy. The operative draping should consist of the face, neck, and upper chest. An injection of 1 cc of isosulfan or lymphazurin blue should be accomplished prior to prepping and draping. The excisional margin of this lesion would be 1–1.5 cm with the appropriate plans for reconstruction/closure. The handheld gamma probe is used to localize the site of the probable sentinel node. One should be prepared in this instance for both an intraparotid and anterior cervical neck node excision since either site can be the location of the sentinel node. The incision is made over the location of the highest count obtained with the gamma probe and the blue staining of the node is used as confirmation of the sentinel node. The next therapeutic step is the performance of a superficial parotidectomy if one is unable to clearly identify the sentinel node. At this juncture the resident should provide the basic procedural steps in a superficial parotidectomy.)

An area of controversy is the frozen section which is only performed in a few centers since most pathologists are not comfortable with frozen section diagnosis of a positive sentinel lymph node in melanoma. Permanent or delayed pathologic examination implies if a positive node exists histologically a completion or staged regional node dissection will be necessary. In scenarios where a non-palpable sentinel node is a microscopically positive, clinically, negative, pathologically positive nodal disease, in 80% of the instances the remaining nodes are negative. As a result, the necessity for completion of nodal dissection is currently under review and the preponderance of opinion is that the additional procedure is not warranted.)

(b) Draw on the board your anticipated defect and reconstruction. (Given a margin of 1–1.5 cm the total defect will be approximately 2.5–3 cm in transverse diameter. The posterior limb of a vertically-oriented excision would be incorporated in the preauricular incision for parotidectomy. The parotidectomy incision would extend inferiorly and anteriorly into the neck. The result would be a cervico-facial flap that would allow the remaining anterior cheek and adjacent neck skin into the defect with closure.)

Intraoperative

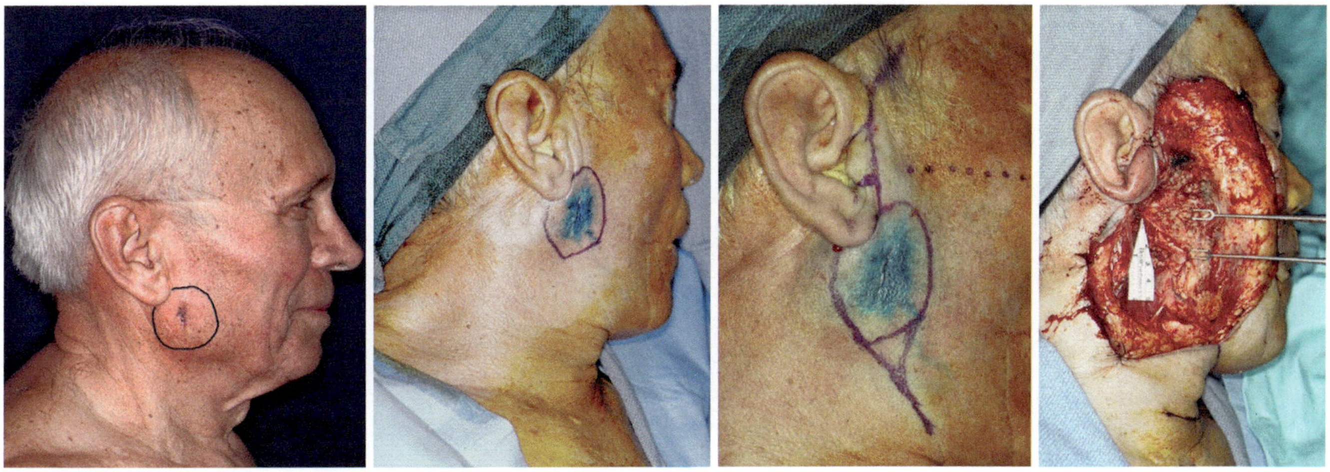

A series of photos depict the preoperative proposed margins and intraoperative view of a more vertical reorientation of the proposed excision to ensure adequate margins at the superior and inferior limits of the biopsy scar and permit elliptical closure. The stain of a vital dye in preparation for a sentinel lymph node, SLN, biopsy is evident. The subsequent photo outlines the incision for a parotidectomy, if necessary. In the final intraoperative photo, a superficial parotidectomy has been accomplished. The pointer indicates the proximal trunk of the facial nerve.

Postoperative

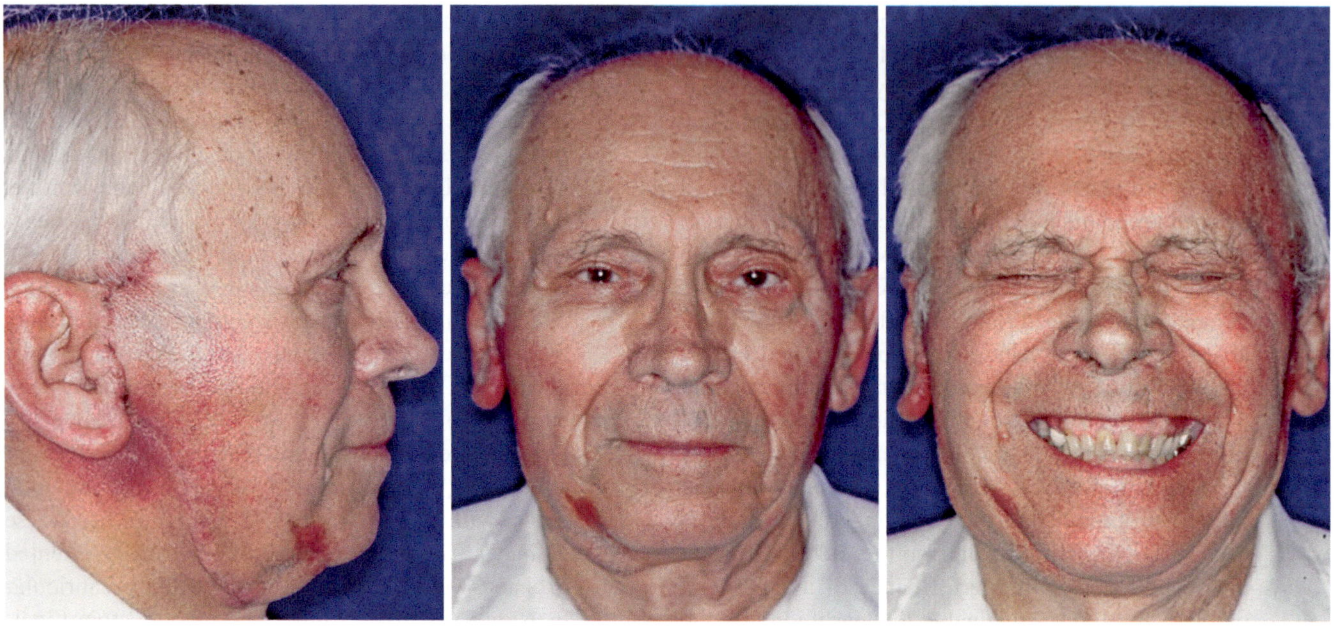

A recent postoperative series of three views demonstrate a healing, primary closure of the wide local excision and parotidectomy. The repose and facial animation indicates intact facial nerve function. In most instances in skilled hands, intraparotid sentinel lymph node biopsy can be accomplished without a formal parotidectomy. If not, injury to the facial nerve is minimized by the identification of the proximal trunk and elevation of the superficial lobe of the parotid.

Case-Based Conference

Case 2: Melanoma

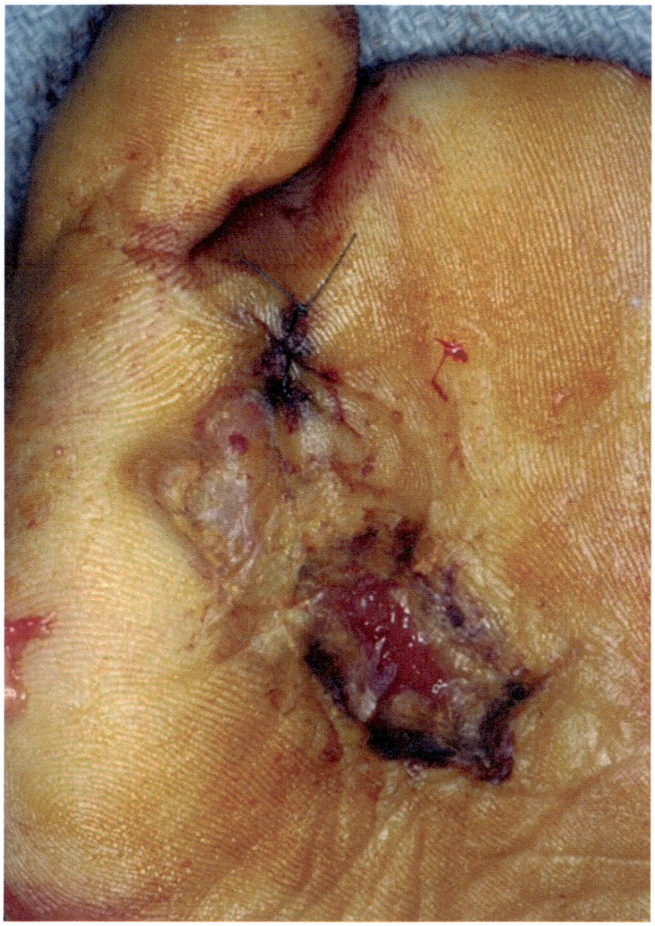

A 62-year-old male with a pigmented lesion of 2 years duration and a 4–5 month history of ulceration. With the exception of some hypertension and elevated cholesterol, in good health. A recent biopsy (suture) revealed malignant melanoma of indeterminate depth.

1. Describe the slide and add a clinical examination.
   (a) Are any tests indicated? Justify.
2. What is the pathologic anatomy?
3. Outline an oncologic and reconstructive plan. Describe in detail including the reconstructive challenges.

Case-Based Conference: Discussion

Case 2: Melanoma

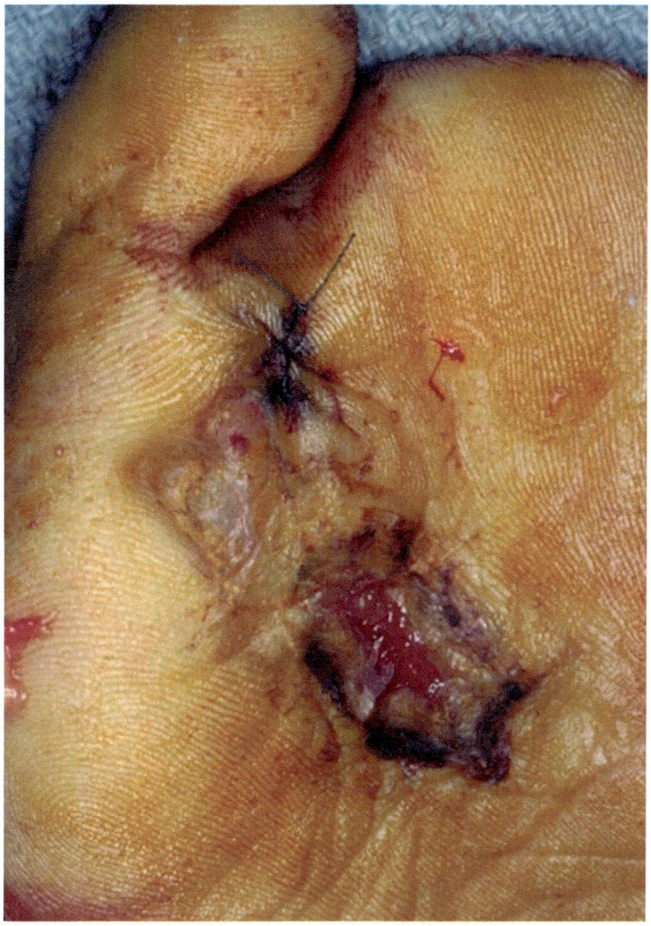

A 62-year-old male with a pigmented lesion of 2 years duration and a 4–5 month history of ulceration. With the exception of some hypertension and elevated cholesterol, in good health. A recent biopsy (suture) revealed malignant melanoma of indeterminate depth.

1. Describe the slide and add a clinical examination. (A single photo is a close-up view of the plantar aspect of the right foot, restricted to the fifth toe and adjacent sole to perhaps the midline medially and distal instep proximally. The remaining toes have been draped and are not

visible. The most notable features are a deeply pigmented area at the base of the fifth toe and a single suture in place. Further proximal is an ulcerated area of 1 × 1 cm, surrounded by a zone of an additional centimeter of dark pigmentation. Just medial is an area of several millimeters of hypopigmentation with a pinkish hue that is clearly different than the surrounding plantar skin. No other lesions are evident.

In addition to the history given in the preamble, other information to be solicited from the patient would include symptoms elsewhere including bone pain, particularly back or ribs, headache, swelling in the groin and systemic symptoms of recent weight loss or malaise—all in quest of possible metastatic disease. Other past medical history include skin lesions treated or other medical problems or operations. The family medical history would include melanoma. Social history includes alcohol, tobacco, or substance abuse. The physical exam includes palpation of the groin for lymphadenopathy, the abdomen for an enlarged liver or masses, and the skin for other pigmented lesions.)

(a) Any tests indicated? Justify. (The primary thrust in this case of the necessity of laboratory tests and imaging is the detection of occult metastatic disease. Although some controversy exists about the efficacy as a screening modality, the use of PET-CT scan, positive emission tomography in more advanced local disease has garnered some support. Elevated serum lactic dehydrogenase is also an independent prognostic variable. Since the biopsy yielded only indeterminate results of the depth, the other question is if repeat biopsy would be efficacious. The likelihood of a thin melanoma in this clinical scenario is quite small. Assuming a thickness of greater than 1 mm and in the presence of ulceration, the magnitude of the wide local excision of the primary and the indications for sentinel lymph node biopsy are the same, regardless of thickness.)

2. What is the pathologic anatomy? (The pathologic anatomy of melanoma is the staging, a system that has therapeutic and prognostic implications. The two local tumor factors are lesion thickness, namely the Breslow level, and presence of ulceration or not. Assuming a thickness of greater than 1 mm in the presence of ulceration, the staging of the primary is T2 or 3b and stage IIA or B. The other element, clinically, is the presence of palpable lymphadenopathy. Of the variants of types of melanoma, the case in this instance is an example of acral melanoma. Acral lentiginous melanomas can also occur in subungual locations. In general, acral melanomas present in a more advanced stage, such as this case, and have a correspondingly poorer prognosis.)

3. Outline an oncologic and reconstructive plan. Describe in detail including the reconstructive challenges. (The principal oncologic management is wide local excision of the primary and sentinel lymph node biopsy. Of concern in addition to peripheral margins is the involvement by the ulceration of tissue planes beneath skin and a peripheral margin of 2 cm will probably place the fifth toe in jeopardy and a consideration should be lent to incorporation of amputation within the specimen. If so, the amputation level could be a metatarsophalangeal disarticulation but excision at the level at the distal metatarsal will provide a smoother contour of the lateral aspect of the foot. The deep margin incorporates the plantar fascia as the first tumor barrier. The digital nerves and vessels will be exposed as well. The performance of a sentinel lymph node biopsy is clearly indicated because of the significant incidence of occult lymphatic metastasis in the stage, T2 or 3b, of this lesion. Preliminary lymphoscintigraphy will be of assistance. In the operating room an injection of lymphazurin blue or isosulfan blue into the dermis of the primary is accomplished, the primary tumor is excised and a sentinel lymph node identified by means of a handheld collimator or gamma probe for identification of the area of high radioactivity versus the background level as well as confirmation by visualization of a blue lymph node.

Reconstruction of the plantar aspect of the foot is always a challenge. The weight-bearing plantar aspect in ambulation stresses any type of tissue transfer or grafts. In gait analysis, the weight-bearing surfaces in the forefoot are principally the first and fifth metatarsal heads and with some secondary on the second. With loss of the fifth, the fourth metatarsal will become the site of lateral forefoot weight-bearing in the push off phase of gait. Reconstructive options include skin graft and free tissue transfer with a thin fasciocutaneous flap as the radial forearm. Each is insensate, although perhaps a skin graft will gain some protective sensation, and depending on the plantar padding that remains, are nearly equal in durability.)

Intraoperative

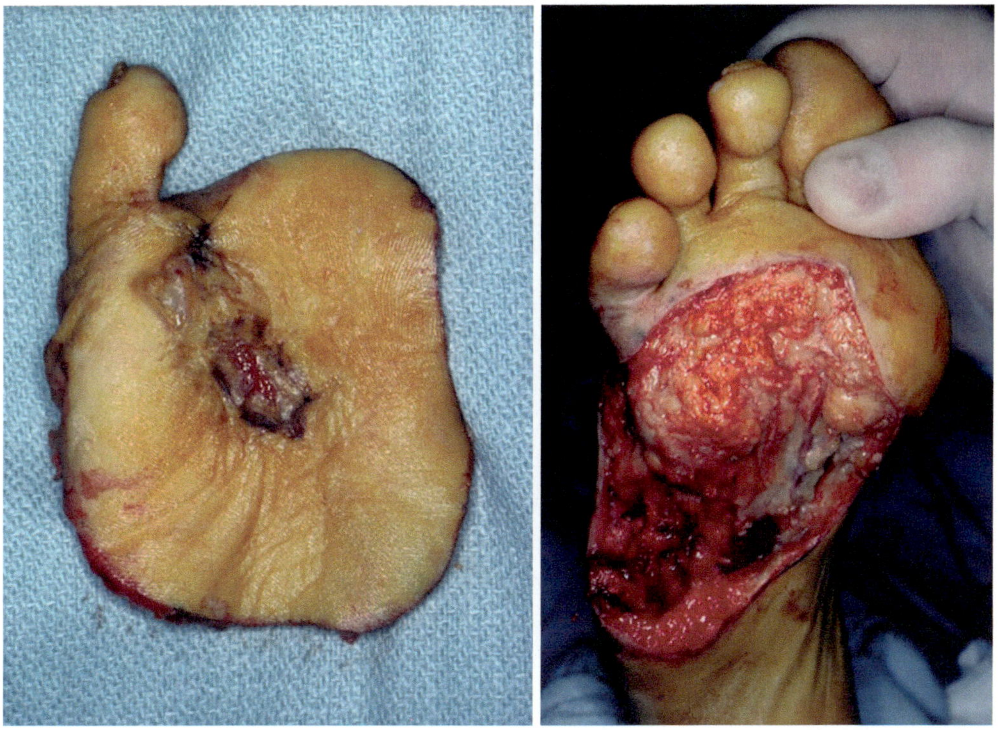

The two intraoperative photos depict the specimen of the lesion and generous margins as well as a fifth toe amputation en bloc. The defect illustrates excision of plantar fascia and distal aponeurosis. The heads of the second metatarsal are well covered with soft tissue.

Postoperative (6 Weeks and 6 Months)

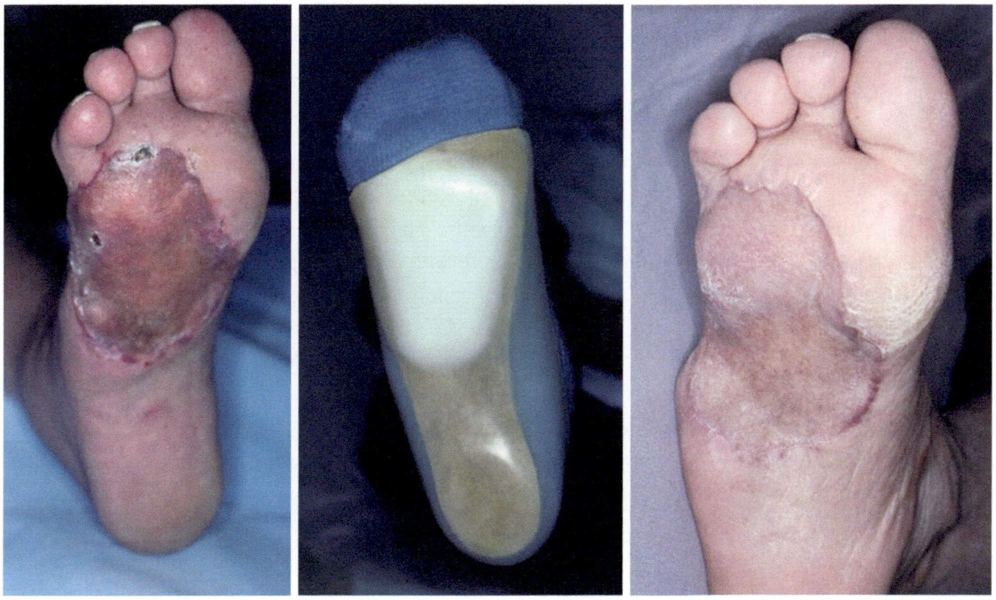

The defect has been closed with a skin graft, healed with a couple of small crusts. The following photo is of a foot orthotic within an inset, the dimensions of which duplicate the defect. Rehabilitation by use of orthotics can offload weight-bearing to areas less susceptible to chronic injury. The last photo is of a mature skin graft without evidence of ulceration.

In-Service Examination

1. A hierarchy of survival from best to worst among the morphological types of melanoma is:
   (a) Acral, superficial spreading, nodular, lentigo
   (b) Superficial spreading, nodular, lentigo, acral
   (c) Lentigo, superficial spreading, nodular, acral
   (d) Lentigo, acral, superficial spreading, nodular
   (e) Superficial spreading, lentigo, nodular, acral
2. Appropriate margins of melanoma of 1.6 mm in thickness are:
   (a) 5 mm
   (b) 1.0 cm
   (c) 2.0 cm
   (d) 3.0 cm
3. Sentinel lymph node biopsy is indicated in which of the following situations?
   (a) Lentigo maligna of the cheek
   (b) A 1.2 mm thick melanoma of the forearm
   (c) A subungual melanoma in situ
   (d) All of the above

33 Pigmented Lesions

Bibliography

Salopek, T. G. and Friedman, R. J., "Ch. 16: Dysplastic Nevi", Cancer of the Skin, Rigel, D.S., et al., Elsevier Saunders, (2005); **pgs. 203–215**.

Arneja, J. S. and Gosain, A. K., "Giant Congenital Melanocytic Nevi", *Plast. Reconstr. Surg.*, (2009); 124(1S):**1e–11e**.

Moustafa D., Blundell A.R., Hawryluk E.B., "Congenital Melanocytic Nevi", *Current Opinion in Pediatrics*, (2020);32(4): **491–497**.

Arad E, Zuker RM, "The Shifting Paradigm in the Management of Giant Congenital Melanocytic Nevi: Review and Clinical Applications", *Plast. Reconstr. Surg.*, (2014); 133(2):**367–376**.

Bauer B.S., Few J.W., Chavez C.D., Galiano R.D., "The role of tissue expansion in the management of large congenital pigmented nevi of the forehead in the pediatric patient", *Plast Reconstr Surg.*, (2001);107(3):**668–75**.

Chang, C.J., Kou, Ching-Song, "Comparing the effectiveness of Q-switched Ruby laser treatment with that of Q-switched Nd:YAG laser for oculodermal melanosis (Nevus of Ota)", *J. Plas. Recon. & Aesth. Surg.*, (2011); 64: **339–340, 342–344**.

McGuire, L. K., Disa, J. J., Lee, E. H., Klaus, J. B., et al., "Melanoma of the Lentigo Maligna Subtype: Diagnostic Challenges and Current Treatment Paradigms", *Plast. Reconstr. Surg.*, (2012); **288e–297e**.

Lyon VB, "The Spitz Nevus: Review and Update", *Clin Plastic Surg*, (2010); 37: **21–24, 29–30 ONLY**.

Supplemental

Marghoob Ashfaq A., M.D. Chapter 17: "Congenital Melanocytic Nevi." *Cancer of the Skin*. Rigel, D.S., et al., Elsevier Saunders, (2005) 120(5):**221–241**.

Faculty Discussion and Study Guide

General

1. Differentiate pathologically the following benign nevi: junctional, intradermal, compound, blue. (Junctional nevus has active melanocytes at the epidermal/dermal junction; an intradermal nevus is entirely within the dermis; a compound nevus is an intradermal nevus that has migrated into the epidermis and is probably the most common; the blue nevus is simply a nevus that has a blue color usually in a intradermal location.)

Dysplastic Nevi

1. What is the clinical definition of a dysplastic nevus, namely specific features? (A size usually greater than 5 mm, variegated pigmentation, irregular and indistinct borders, multiple nevi of various sizes, all features similar to that of melanoma)
   (a) What is the risk with the presence of dysplastic nevi and a positive family history of melanoma? (Although the incidence varies, the risk is high, perhaps even as high as 100%, since the patient may qualify for the diagnosis of dysplastic nevi syndrome—see below.)
   (b) Histology? (Large nuclei, marked junctional proliferation at epidermal-dermis interface, irregular nests of cells, lymphocytic infiltration.)
   (c) What is the approximate risk over 5–10 years? (Approximately 10% in the absence of a family history.)
2. What is the clinical definition of familial dysplastic nevi or B-K mole syndrome? (A family history in primary or secondary relatives of malignant melanoma, large number of nevi usually more than 50 with a gross appearance as defined above with a disproportionate number on the

E. Luce, *A Curriculum for Plastic Surgery*, https://doi.org/10.1007/978-3-031-62087-4_33

trunk as opposed to the extremities and head and neck, and some distinct histological features.)

3. You excise a single dysplastic nevus from a patient without other suspicious nevi and a negative family history. Is the risk for malignant melanoma increased in this patient? (Yes, probably twofold since the dysplastic nevus is a tumor marker.)
   (a) Comparable to dysplastic nevus syndrome, namely a positive family history? (No. a markedly higher risk in dysplastic nevus syndrome since the positive family history suggests a genetic predisposition.)
   (b) Does a histologic hierarchy exist in dysplastic nevi from less to more of a concern? (Yes. The degree of dysplasia from mild to severe.)
4. On clinical grounds, you establish a diagnosis of dysplastic nevus syndrome. What is the recommended management? (A periodic follow-up should begin in late adolescence or early 20s since the conversion of dysplastic nevi to melanoma at a younger age is extremely rare. That follow-up, dependent on risk factors such as family history and number of nevi, should be at least every 6 months. The traditional technique, in addition to physical examination, for follow-up is total body photography. Total body photography is then used for comparison purposes on return visits, initially 3–6 months, perhaps ultimately a year. The more recent innovation has been the ability to digitize photographs and software is available for that purpose. Other techniques include the use of dermoscopy or enhanced magnification of the direct examination of nevi.)
   (a) Recommend genetic testing? (No.)
   (b) Perform excision for pathologic confirmation? (No, not necessary if a clinical diagnosis has been established, but is confirmatory and of value for patient counseling.)
   (c) Perform multiple excisions to reduce overall risk? (No, dysplastic nevus is a *marker* for malignant melanoma risk which most frequently arises de novo and would require excision of 140–220 dysplastic nevi to excise a single undetected malignant melanoma.)
   (d) Other measures initiated in follow-up? (The patients need to be scrupulous in the use of sunblocks and avoidance of excessive sun exposure.)
5. You are referred to a patient by a dermatologist with an incompletely excised dysplastic nevus for further excision. Management? (Probably should re excise simply to differentiate between a dysplastic nevus and malignant melanoma which is not possible without complete excision. The decision can hinge on the degree of dysplasia as discussed above.)
6. Is laser a recommended treatment for dysplastic nevi? (No, does not eliminate melanocytes deep within the dermis.)

Congenital Melanocytic Nevi

1. Define and characterize a congenital melanocytic nevus pathologically. (Present at birth, benign proliferation, histology of involvement of the superficial and deep dermis and even the subcutaneous fat as well as an extension of nevus cells around adnexal structures within the deep dermis.)
   (a) Define a giant congenital melanocytic nevus. (Various criteria were offered by the readings but offer 20 cm or more in greater diameter achieved in adulthood, corresponding to approximately 6 cm on the infant's body and 9 cm on the infant's head. A criterion of 1% or 2% of the total body surface area was also offered.)
   (b) Classify by size small, medium, and large. (Small <1.5 cm, medium 1.5–19 cm, large >20 cm.)
2. What is known about the genetics of congenital melanocytic nevus, CMN? (Info about genetic mutation is limited to giant CMN in whom NRAS or BRAF mutations, principally NRAS, occurred in the majority of the patients so examined.)
3. How do you explain the occurrence embryologically of leptomeningeal melanoma in the same patient with a congenital melanocytic nevus, CMN? (Neural crest origin of melanocytic stem cell; although it also explains neurotropism in melanomas)
   (a) Give another anatomical location of the same phenomenon. (Retinal melanoma)
4. What is the natural history of congenital melanocytic nevus? (The development of dark, coarse hair at age 1–2 years followed by elevation of the lesion with verrucous and hyperkeratotic changes about the age of 10 years.)
5. Comment and define the risk of transformation of malignant melanoma in congenital melanocytic nevus. (Again, the incidence appears to be controversial and lacking a consensus. Nevertheless, the most common percentage cited from the readings was 4–8%, 0–5% for small-medium, 4–10% for large lesions. Some recent evidence indicates no increase in risk for small and medium-sized congenital nevi in the absence of satellite lesions. The principal risk is in giant-sized nevi.)
   (a) What risk factors besides size? (Multiple lesions, papular or nodular changes within the nevus, heterogeneous pigmentation, axial location.)
6. How does the epidemiology of malignant melanoma in congenital melanocytic nevus in smaller lesions differ from that of large lesions? (In smaller lesions, a lower incidence of melanoma conversion and a majority of melanomas occur at puberty or later in contrast to large congenital melanocytic nevi in whom the majority of melanomas occur before the age of 10 and one-half by

age 3. The behavior of the latter can be aggressive with significant mortality.)

   (a) How do small vs. large lesions differ in ease of the diagnosis of malignant melanoma if such should occur? (Development of malignant melanoma in smaller lesions tends to be more superficial, namely in the superficial dermis and more readily diagnosed clinically. Melanoma in large and giant congenital melanocytic nevi frequently occur in deep dermis or even the subcutaneous fat and may not be detectable in the early stages which may be a partial explanation for the observed aggressive behavior.)

7. What is the importance of the findings of multiple satellite nevi in a patient with a large congenital melanocytic nevus? (May yield a higher disposition to conversion to malignant melanoma within the large congenital melanocytic nevus, although malignant melanoma does not occur in satellite nevi but can occur in non-involved skin.)
8. In the office, a new patient, a 3-month-old infant, presents with multiple truncal nevi and two nevi located over the sagittal suture line of the skull. The parents relay the infant has been treated symptomatically by the pediatrician for two seizure episodes. What is one likely explanation? (Leptomeningeal involvement and possibly, although remotely at age 3 months, a melanoma.)
   (a) What is the next step? (MRI imaging of the meninges and brain; ophthalmologic examination for possible retinal melanoma, accomplished by age 6 months. As discussed in the readings, infants with giant congenital nevi even though asymptomatic should probably be imaged before 6 months of age. The two reasons are general anesthesia is not required, and after the age of 6 months, the progressive myelination of the CNS may obscure detection of melanocytosis.)
9. You see a 4-year-old in the office with a nevus of the entire dorsum of the forearm. The parents desire removal because of cancer concerns and have been told that the laser is the preferred modality. Your counseling? (Unfortunately, a nevus of that size will have melanocytes that penetrate through dermis even into the subcutaneous fat. A laser will only remove epidermis and superficial dermis and leave residual melanocytes.)
   (a) Regarding the advisability of excision? (If excision is the option, the only definitive procedure is done at the level of the fascia. The other option is observation since by definition this nevus is large and has a risk, perhaps 10%, and the parents should be so advised)
10. Discuss the essence of the argument for and against excision of congenital melanocytic nevus in infancy or early childhood. (As discussed above, the risk is dependent on size and the other risk factors outlined above. Conversion to malignant melanoma is 4–8%. The problem with observation is twofold: One, the parents even once informed of that risk level are commonly intolerant of observation; two, with age, usually in early adulthood, verrucous changes occur within the nevus that become increasingly less acceptable from a cosmetic aspect. In childhood even with shaving of the dark hair the appearance of the nevus may provoke peer group abuse. Clearly, the excision, which should include the subcutaneous fat, is a significant undertaking and the provision of coverage is a challenge to provide a cosmetically acceptable result, particularly on the extremities since excision is at the level of the fascia. The use of tissue expansion, Integra, etc. in the reconstruction is covered in other modules.)
11. The readings outline the use of tissue expansion in addressing large pigmented nevi of the forehead in children. The readings outlined an approach that favored transposition over advancement flaps. Why? (The advancement of expanded skin appeared to create more aesthetic landmark distortion such as the brow and hairline than transposition flaps.)
12. Comment on the following in the management of pediatric giant pigmented nevi:
   (a) Incision placement
   (b) Amount of fill on the O.R. table
   (c) Use of drains
   (d) Timing of postoperative fill initiation
   (e) Overexpansion

   (By photographs, the surgeons appeared to place the incisions at the border of the lesions and added a “comfortable intraoperative fill” to smooth the expander and fill the dead space on the O.R. table. Expansion was begun 7–10 days postoperatively and used butterfly drains and appeared to over expand and use multiple expanders rather than a single expander. Fill did not begin until 2 weeks post-placement and overfill was common.)
13. What were the general principles with respect to the management of congenital nevi of the forehead and scalp? (Respect aesthetic landmarks such as the eyebrows and hairline; use transposition flaps rather than advancement; create brow ptosis rather than elevation since the former is much more readily corrected.)
14. What other measures, besides excision and grafting, can be utilized in the treatment of large congenital nevi of the face? (A variety of lasers, predominately the Q-switched ruby and Nd:YAG and, more recently, the picosecond alexandrite. The demonstration of superiority and efficacy awaits larger clinical trials.)

Editor’s Note: This topic is also discussed in Chap. 9.

Spitz Nevus

1. In general, what characterizes Spitz nevus? (A melanocytic lesion that most frequently occurs in children and has melanoma-like features microscopically but in most instances has a benign clinical behavior.)
2. Typical clinical appearance of a Spitz nevus? (A pink round papule, usually as small as 5–6 mm. on the face of a child, characteristically pink because of a lack of melanin, although pigmented Spitz nevus can occur.)
   (a) Common differential? (In a child, pyogenic granuloma or dermatofibroma.)
3. Discuss non-invasive methods of evaluation. (The modality available is dermoscopy or the examination of tissues by enhanced means such as magnification and oil immersion as well as the use of polarizing light. Another modality is the use of polarizing light or confocal microscopy.)
4. What are the essential pathologic features? (The hallmark feature is the presence of large spindle-shaped melanocytes with an admixture of epithelioid cells. The neoplastic findings of concern such as disorderly pattern, frequent mitosis, or loss of lateral demarcation are absent.)
5. What is the essence of the controversy with Spitz nevus? (The problem is the ambiguity generated by the presence of atypical microscopic findings and the difficulty in discernment of melanoma from a benign nevus. Atypical features in a lesion excised from a child are likely to be regarded as benign, the same findings in an adult more likely to be diagnosed as melanoma.)
6. What is the definitive diagnostic test? (Of course, excisional biopsy.)
   (a) Role of molecular studies or biologic markers? (Unclear at this time. A pattern of results with a number of assessments may be helpful but not diagnostic. No bright line exists between benign and malignant lesions with the use of such studies.)

Lentigo Maligna

1. Define lentigo maligna including pathology, characteristics, and epidemiology. (Characteristically, the lesion is a tan to deep brown perhaps black lesion of the head and neck in older, even elderly, seventh or eighth decade, patients. The historical name is that of Hutchinson's freckle. Pathologically, the lesion is a melanoma-in-situ, namely, cytologically malignant but lacking basement membrane invasion.)
   (a) Differentiate between lentigo maligna and lentigo maligna melanoma. (The principal differentiation is invasion by the malignant melanocytes into adjacent normal tissue, the dermis.)
   (b) What is the most likely differential diagnosis? (Seborrheic keratosis, although the appearance in the elderly of seborrheic keratosis is considerably more raised and verrucous than melanoma.)
2. What is the significance of a raised, more deeply pigmented papule within a macular lentigo maligna? (May well signify a conversion to melanoma with a vertical growth phase.)
   (a) Approximately what percentage of lentigo maligna harbor areas of lentigo maligna melanoma? (15–18%)
3. Since most lentigo maligna lesions of the face are frequently quite large, what are the guidelines for performance of a biopsy? (The biopsy should be directed toward the darkest or certainly the most palpable area of the overall lesion. Multiple biopsies may be necessary.)
4. Describe the typical histopathology in lentigo maligna. (An increased number of melanocytes along the junction of the dermis and epidermis with perhaps extension into the adnexal structures, large nuclei, irregular nest of melanocytes. Molecular biology immunostains markers such as S-100 can be performed as well.)
5. Discuss the appropriate margin in lentigo maligna and lentigo maligna melanoma of the head and neck. (Although 20 years ago a consensus conference recommended a 5 mm margin, subsequent investigations have determined that a 5 mm margin will fail to clear disease in a significant percentage of cases of lentigo maligna. Although the numbers vary, a 10 mm margin would be necessary to obtain clear margins in 95+% of the cases. The issue is particularly pressing if a single-stage excision followed by immediate reconstruction is adopted since a positive margin on final pathology will require re-excision and possible compromise of the reconstruction. The margin in lentigo maligna is dictated by the thickness of the lesion similar to other types of melanoma.)
6. Because of the controversy outlined in the above question, Mohs micrographic surgery has been recommended in the management of lentigo maligna and lentigo maligna melanoma. Discuss. (The pros clearly are that the magnitude of the excision potentially can be limited by a Mohs approach. The problem is twofold: one, frozen section even in the hands of the experienced pathologist is difficult and inconsistent in lentigo maligna; two, by definition the margins are extremely close since Mohs attempts to obtain a single section free of disease which may be as narrow as 1 mm or less.)
7. What methods have been adopted to address the paradox outlined in the above questions? (Two approaches, "slow Mohs" and a staged approach to address the paradox. Slow Moh's consists of rapid preparation of the sections with results available in 24 h. A staged approach simply allows the return of the final pathology results using a

conventional time frame with reconstruction deferred until margins are negative. Nevertheless, the pathologic examination should be conceptually the same as dermatographic surgery and not by the conventional "bread-loaf" technique. The timeblock should be a consecutive 2 perhaps 3 days to allow for re-excision of positive margins. A relatively novel approach is to do a circumferential excision of margin only, perhaps 10 mm, with the central lesion intact. Once margins are clear the bulk of the central lesion can then be excised. This approach minimizes the issue of dressings for the patient.)

8. Outline non-surgical methods of treating lentigo maligna including the drawbacks. (A variety of techniques including the use of the laser, immunomodulation with imiquimod, chemical peels, and cryotherapy all attempt to destroy the lesion yet retain sufficient dermis to allow spontaneous healing. The problem is that deeply-seated residual malignant cells in the dermis are responsible for persistent/recurrent melanoma. Healing may be incomplete and produce a considerable degree of scaring. All of these modalities should be considered inappropriate in the treatment of lentigo maligna and/or melanoma. Radiotherapy has apparently been utilized but restricted to infirm patients who can not tolerate surgery. Melanoma in general is considered relatively radioresistant. Aldara® or imiquimod is particularly controversial. Use can eradicate the pigment, yet the architecture may remain unchanged and the readings cite that the risk is not diminished. Further investigation is necessary.)

Case-Based Conference

Case 1: Pigmented Lesion

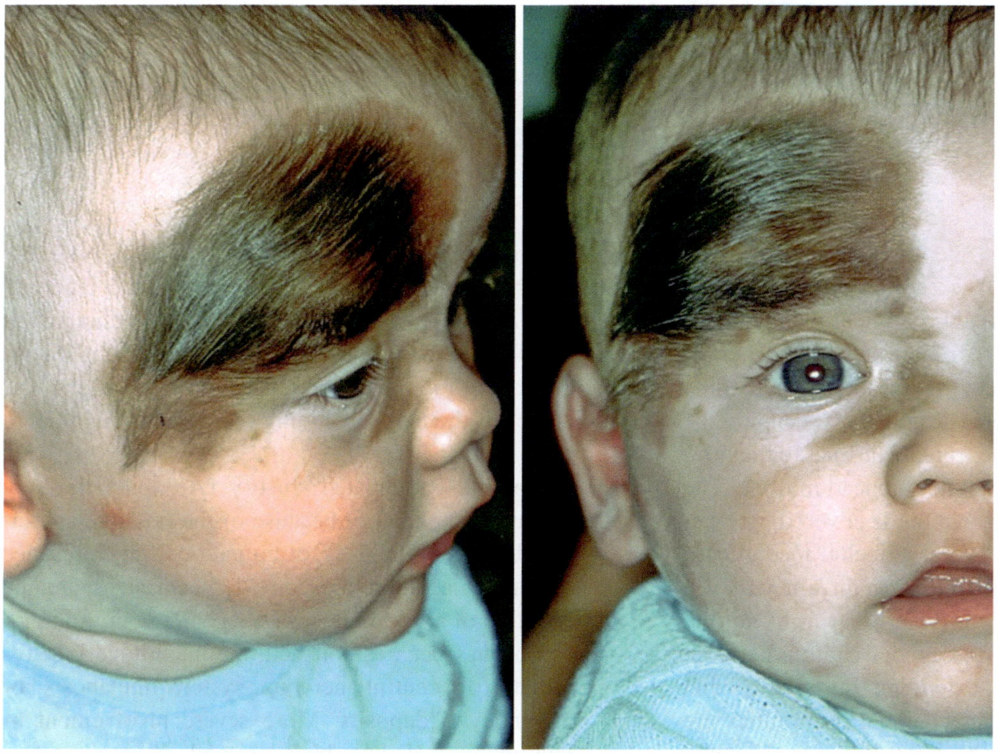

A 1-year-old with a facial nevus.

1. Describe the two slides and add a clinical examination.
   (a) Are any tests indicated? Justify.
2. What is the pathologic anatomy?
3. Treatment indicated, apart from aesthetic concerns? Discuss.
4. Outline a treatment plan. If surgical procedure(s) are a component, describe.

Case-Based Conference: Discussion

Case 1: Pigmented Lesion

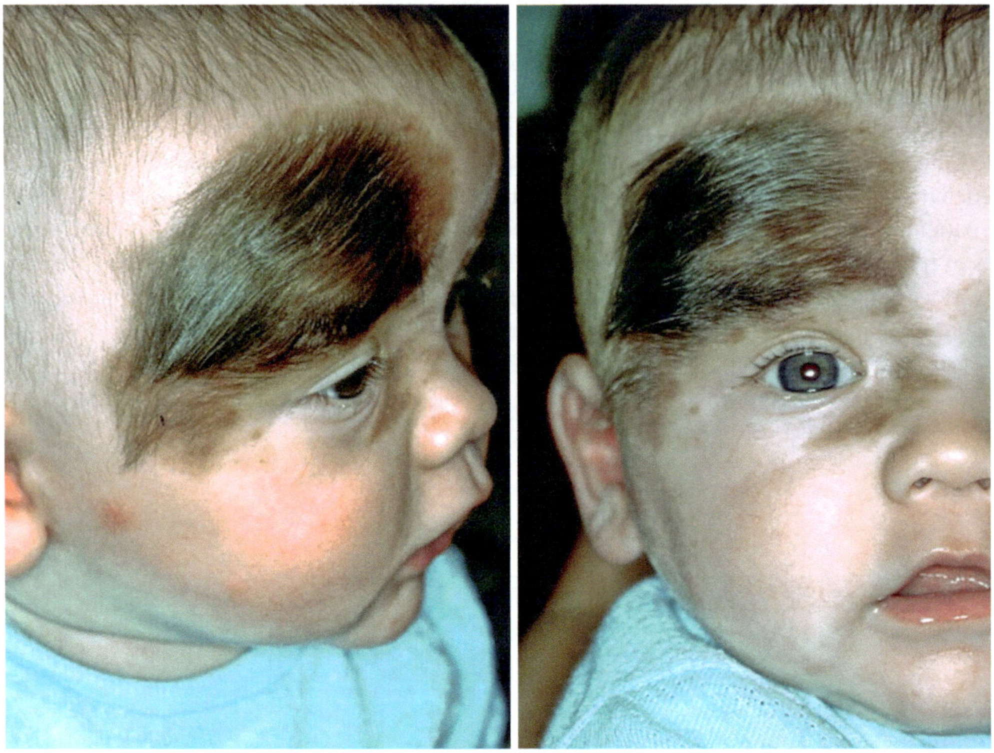

A 1-year-old with a facial nevus.

1. Describe the two slides and add a clinical examination. (Two photos are provided. A frontal and oblique facial view. The frontal view does not include the left side of the face. Depicted is a pigmented lesion that occupies the entire right forehead from the frontal hairline, to the inferior margin of the brow, and to the forehead midline. The nevus appears to be tan or brown but is covered by long, nearly black hair. The right lateral glabella, medial canthal, and medial infraorbital areas contain a nevus of a similar tan hue but absent hair. A narrow rim of normal skin free of nevus is present in the medial canthus between nevus and epicanthal fold, extending into the medial lower eyelid. No other lesions or facial deformities are evident. The visible sclera, the right, is a normal white without evidence of lesions. The oblique view lends little additional information. The extension of the forehead nevus into the right temple is illustrated. Again no other lesions are evident.

   The clinical exam is primarily directed toward an assessment of coexisting diagnosis and would begin with a history from parents or guardians of developmental milestones, any history of seizures, and, if physician referred, any past diagnostic tests or lab work performed. Questions posed should establish if the lesion was present at birth as implied by the preamble or has emerged recently. A history of similar lesions and/or melanoma in the family is important. The physical exam should include an intraoral inspection of the palate and the remainder of the body including the back for pigmented lesions.)

   (a) Are any tests indicated? Justify. (An ophthalmology consult is mandatory because of the possible associated lesions of the uvea, examination for the presence of glaucoma, and retinoscopy. The central test and the question of appropriateness is an MRI scan. An association has been established, the magnitude indeterminate of central nervous system melanosis or melanocytic deposits. More severe involvement as leptomeningeal has been termed neurocutaneous melanosis and may, rarely, result in CNS symptoms and/or melanoma. In the presence of giant congenital melanocytic nevus, satellite lesions, and post-axial distribution, an indication may exist for the performance of an MRI in infancy. That indication is not universally agreed or consensually derived in the asymptomatic patient. A specific association of nevus of Ota and CNS melanocytosis has not been established.)

2. What is the pathologic anatomy? (The pathologic anatomy can be described grossly and microscopically. The occurrence of a congenital pigmented lesion in the distribution of the trigeminal nerve, in this instance the ophthalmic division, is termed a nevus of Ota—contrasted with a nevus of Ito limited to the area of the lateral antebrachial cutaneous nerve and posterior shoulder. Most commonly, conjunctiva and sclera are involved, hence the term also of ocular dermal melanosis. Involvement of these structures is not apparent in the photos and the patient may represent a variant. Microscopically, the distribution of the melanocytes is distinctly abnormal, including presence in the dermis, eccrine glands, hair follicles, and in large lesions, the subcutaneous fat. As discussed above CNS involvement may be present as well. Finally, the biogenetic profile is BRAF or NRAF mutations.)

   Treatment indicated, apart from aesthetic concerns? Discuss. (The question centers on the possible risk or predisposition toward the occurrence of malignant melanoma. Studies with conflicting results have been published but the risk appears to increase with increasing size of the congenital nevus. The general classification is small, less than 1.5 cm, intermediate less than 20 cm^2, and giant. The patient's risk of a medium-sized lesion is 1–3%. The low incidence will not reassure the family and the necessity of treatment will be dictated by aesthetic concerns.)
3. Outline a treatment plan. If surgical procedure(s) are a component, describe. (Of the two modalities available, surgical and non-surgical, both have benefits and liabilities. The only non-surgical treatment with demonstrable efficacy is the laser. Several lasers have been utilized and described to treat melanocytic nevi including the Q-switched Nd:YG and Q-switched alexandrite. More recently, the pico-second laser has been employed with reportable effectiveness. Numerous permutations are possible including wavelength, fluency, and fractional combinations. Although considerable enthusiasm accompanies the reports of the use of the various lasers, an assessment is elusive. Because of the depth of some melanocytes, the reticular dermis, residual pigmentation may remain particularly in dense lesions as in the case discussed. Regardless, multiple sessions will be required. Laser treatment will require general anesthesia in a young child but is probably the first choice of treatment if no other indications are present.)

   Excision in the application of skin graft is the most definitive and is a single stage but may be less aesthetic than tissue expansion of native skin. Tissue expansion avoids a donor site but requires multiple procedures and incisional scars as well as the summative development of complications. Achieving the optimal result with excision and closure with skin grafts will mandate minimization of a color difference with native facial skin and avoidance of hypertrophic scarring of the donor site. A preliminary expansion of supraclavicular skin may be of benefit.

   An additional factor in the non-surgical-surgical equation is that laser therapy does not reduce the possibility of the development of melanoma.

   If surgical excision is elected, the timing is a consideration. Neurodevelopmental delay in children who have been subjected to general anesthesia, particularly lengthy procedures on multiple instances, has raised concerns about the advisability of elective procedures at a young, perhaps less than 3 years of age. In this case, treatment can be deferred until age 3–4 years and still accomplish completion of reconstruction by preschool. Similar conclusions apply to laser therapy.

Postoperative (Age 5)

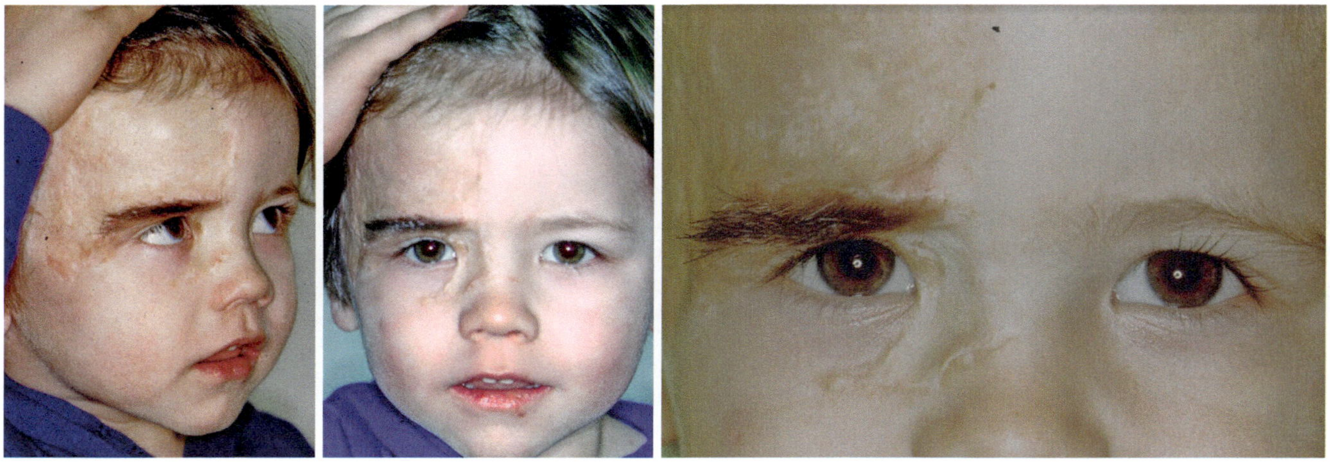

Three photos are provided: a full face frontal, oblique, and a view encompassing both and limited to both periorbital regions. Excision and reconstruction with a skin graft have been performed with a good to excellent color match with native forehead skin. The oblique view confirms this. The eyebrow is distinctly darker than the opposite. The glabellar-medial canthal lesion has been replaced by an apparent full-thickness skin graft with also an excellent color match but some thickening of the graft borders. The epicanthal fold is present but also somewhat more prominent than the contralateral side.

In-Service Examination

1. Nevus of Ota refers to:
   (a) A congenital scalp lesion with a significant predilection for conversion to basal cell carcinoma
   (b) A congenital nevus of the sacral region
   (c) A congenital nevus of the face over the distribution of the trigeminal nerve
   (d) A large melanoma on the face in the elderly
2. A newborn with a Mongolian spot or a 5 × 5 cm pigmented lesion of the lumbosacral area should be evaluated for what?
   (a) Cardiac anomalies
   (b) Renal and collecting system anomalies
   (c) Visceral vascular malformations
   (d) Occult spina bifida
3. Multiple cafe au lait spots in a child may be suggestive of:
   (a) Multiple neurofibromatosis
   (b) Parks-Weber syndrome
   (c) Klippel-Traunnay syndrome
   (d) Weber-Feguson syndrome

34 Adnexal Tumors, Sarcomas, Miscellaneous

Bibliography

Misra A, Mistry N, Grimer R, Peter F, "The management of soft tissue sarcoma", *J. Plast. Recon. & Aesthetic Surg.*, (2009); 62:**161, Table 2 ONLY**.

Maldonado A.A., German G.K., Sauerbier N., Ch. 4: "Lower Extremity Sarcoma Reconstruction", Neligan PC, Plastic Surgery, Elsevier 5th Edition, (2023), Volume 4: **pg. 128 and Figures**.

Bogucki, B, Neuhaus I, and Hurst EA. "Dermatofibrosarcoma Protuberans: A Review of the Literature", *Dermatologic Surg.*, (2012); 38(4):**537–547 (Ignore Tables 1–3)**.

Hollmig ST, Sachdev R, Cockerell CJ et al. "Spindle Cell Neoplasms Encountered in Dermatologic Surgery: A Review", Dermatol Surg 2012;38:**825–27, 833–37 ONLY. (Skim the Discussions on molecular biology.)**

Senchenkov A and Moran SL, "Merkel cell carcinoma: Diagnosis, management, and outcomes", *Plast. Reconstr. Surg.*, (2013); 131:**771e–778e**.

Faculty Discussion and Study Guide

Soft Tissue, Bone Sarcomas

1. Describe the epidemiology of soft tissue sarcomas in terms of most common type, age group, and relative frequency. (Soft tissue sarcomas are most commonly seen in young and middle-aged adults peaking at age 50 except for rhabdomyosarcoma which is most commonly seen in the pediatric group and is the most common soft tissue sarcoma in the pediatric group as well. Overall, soft tissue sarcomas are uncommon. The most common of all soft tissue sarcomas is malignant fibrous histiocytoma. Liposarcoma is next followed equally by fibrosarcoma and synovial sarcoma.)
   (a) Bone sarcomas? (In contrast, bone sarcomas are seen more commonly in teens and young adults and the most common bone sarcoma is osteogenic sarcoma followed by Ewing's sarcoma. The most common location is the metaphyseal area about the knee.)

Editor's Note: Bone sarcomas are exclusively in the province of orthopedic surgeons with a specialty interest in musculoskeletal oncology.

2. What are the three proven etiologies of soft tissue sarcomas? (Although a variety of noxious agents have been discussed such as chlorophenols, herbicides, and others, only prior external radiation, long standing lymphedema, and hereditary etiologies have been established.)
   (a) Discuss each of the three. (Criteria for establishing radiation-induced sarcomas are sarcoma within the radiation ports, a latency of greater than 5–10 years, and a histological diagnosis that's different from original cancer treated. The usual histology is fibrosarcoma.
   Lymphangiosarcoma occurs in long-standing lymphedema, acquired after regional nodal dissection, usually post-mastectomy axillary dissection and radiation therapy. A hereditary etiology is von Recklinghausen's disease or neurofibromatosis Type I with a development of neurofibrosarcomas both centrally and peripherally. Maffucci's syndrome, a clinical picture of multiple enchondromas and hemangiomas, can develop sarcomas.)
   (b) Most common location? (Extremities, mainly the thigh.)
3. What are the clinical features suggested in the presence of a soft tissue sarcoma? (Size greater than 5 cm, a location deep to the fascia, a history of an increase in size and pain, although pain is present in only about one-third of the cases. Also, tumor swelling that has persisted for longer than 4 weeks, a popliteal or groin location.)

E. Luce, *A Curriculum for Plastic Surgery*, https://doi.org/10.1007/978-3-031-62087-4_34

4. Describe the work-up, excluding biopsy, of a soft tissue sarcoma including imaging. Assess fixation to adjacent structures. (Physical exam would focus on the lymph node bearing areas in an extremity tumor, although the prevalent metastases are hematogenous usually pulmonary. An extremity soft tissue sarcoma deserves careful clinical assessment of nerve involvement, fixation to adjacent structures, and size.)
   (a) Discuss imaging of a sarcoma. (Plain films should be performed and MRI scans are important to evaluate the bony and soft tissue extent of the sarcoma. The CT provides superior imaging of bone involvement. A CT scan of the chest and abdomen for metastatic disease is important, particularly since CT is optimal for imaging lung metastasis, the predominant site of hematogenous dissemination. The advent of 3D CTA assists in the definition of vessel displacement, invasion, or occlusion.)
   (b) Blood work? (Alkaline phosphatase and lactic dehydrogenase are of some limited value as independent predictive factors.)
5. How should one approach the biopsy of soft tissue sarcomas? (Four methods of biopsy are available: FNA—good only for work-up of recurrence and requires an experienced cytopathologist. Varying degrees of differentiation are common and may be missed by this technique, information which is important for treatment planning, particularly in large tumors. Core needle biopsy if also an experienced pathologist is available and if multiple cores are submitted, can be satisfactory. CT-guided core needle biopsy may provide sufficient tissue for a histologic diagnosis including degree of differentiation but many sarcomas have areas of varying differentiation. Excisional biopsy is not advisable unless superficial in location, well defined, and is less than 3 cm in size. Incisional biopsy is the biopsy of choice since it yields an adequate amount of tissue to allow planning of the resection without compromising adequate treatment.)
   (a) What is the perspective on excisional biopsy? (As noted above, not advisable because the pseudocapsule is a false plane created by the compression of tumor cells and contamination of tissue planes can occur.)
6. What is the role of PET/CT scan? (The initial development was to demonstrate distant metastases in patients with advanced disease. Subsequently, the performance of PET/CT evolved as a baseline to measure response to chemotherapy in similar patients. Currently, the utility value may be in initial surveillance and workup in Stage IIB and higher. The efficacy has not been demonstrated to enable a routine recommendation.)
7. What is the advice about the placement of incisional biopsy sites? (Orient scar along the long axis of the extremity to allow resection with an ellipse of skin in the same direction. In the trunk, plan the orientation of the incision parallel to areas of skin laxity.)
8. Interpret the grading system as prognostic variables with respect to tumor recurrence? (The larger the tumor the greater the local recurrence rate and subsequent lower disease-free and overall survival outcome. More undifferentiated tumors have a high propensity for local recurrence as well. Good examples include the embryonal cell sarcoma, angiosarcoma, and malignant peripheral nerve tumors.)
9. In general, how are soft tissue sarcomas graded and staged? (Tumor size, location whether superficial or deep, histologic grade, namely degree of differentiation, evidence of regional, and distant metastases. Sarcoma grading systems do not include the histologic cell type. Histologic grading or differentiation uses the classic pathological criteria as the number of cell mitosis for high power field, pleomorphism, etc. See Table 34.1. Essentially, the staging factors are size, less than or greater than 5 cm, location as superficial or deep, and histologic grade.)
10. How are bone sarcomas graded and staged? (See Table 34.1. The classification system is essentially low-grade vs. high-grade and intra- vs. extra compartment.)
    (a) The clinical significance of grade and size? (Increasing grade, low to high, and size directly correlate with increased probability of metastasis, increased probability of recurrence, and diminished survival.)
11. What is the classification of surgical margins and the relevance of the same? (The classification is based on whether the resection was within the tumor, through or tangential to the pseudocapsule, through normal tissue but within the anatomical compartment, and lastly resected outside the anatomical compartment. The relevance is the respective anticipated recurrence rates of 100, 40–60, 10, and 0.5% for each. Small, 3 cm or less, and low-grade tumors can be excised with a 1 cm margin. Larger and high-grade tumors have a propensity for recurrence, attended by a higher rate of metastasis, and diminished survival that dictates wider margins.)
12. What pathologic feature(s) explain this finding or outcome based on the magnitude of resection? (Tumor compression of adjacent tissue creates a pseudocapsule that is surrounded by a reactive zone, a zone populated with nests of viable tumor cells. Hence, the necessity for wide surgical margins.)
13. What are the role and possible disadvantages of neoadjuvant therapy? (Neoadjuvant therapy or treatment given preoperatively is either chemo or radiotherapy or a com-

Table 34.1 Staging system for soft tissue [Sarcomas 8th Edition (2019)[a]]

Classification and staging	Characteristic
Primary tumor (T)	
T1	Tumor 5 cm or less in greatest dimension
T2	Tumor greater than 5 cm but less than 10 cm in greatest dimension
T3	Tumor greater than 10 cm but less than 15
T4	Tumor greater than 15 cm
Regional lymph nodes (N)	
N0	No evidence of nodal metastasis
N1	Nodal metastasis present
Distant metastasis (M)	
M0	No distant metastasis
M1	Distant metastasis present
Grade (G)	
G1	Total differentiation, mitotic count, and necrosis score of 2 or 3
G2	Total differentiation, mitotic count, and necrosis score of 4 or 5
G3	Total differentiation, mitotic count, and necrosis score of 6, 7, or 8
Musculoskeletal Tumor Society staging system	
Stage	*Characteristic*
IA	Low-grade, intracompartmental
IB	Low-grade, extracompartmental
IIA	High-grade, intracompartmental
IIB	High-grade, extracompartmental
IIIA	Low- or high-grade, intracompartmental with metatases
IIIB	Low- or high-grade, extracompartmental with metatases

[a] Modified from, *AJCC Cancer Staging Handbook*, 8th edition. Edge SB, Byrd DR, Compton CC, et al., Springer, New York, NY, (2019). (Reprinted with permission)

bination of both. The principal disadvantage is deferment of the definitive surgical resection and, in the case of radiotherapy, the presence of irradiated and compromised tissues that may affect wound healing. Currently, chemotherapy is given only on enrollment of a patient in a research protocol.)

14. Give the general surgical principles to be applied in the resection of soft tissue sarcomas. (Wide, usually 4–5 cm laterally and 2 cm on the deep aspect margins; on occasion a compartmental approach, namely resection of the entire fibromuscular compartment from origin to insertion, if possible, is necessary. Nerves and vessels should be preserved unless enclosed by the tumor.)
    (a) What are bone sarcomas? (A segmental resection approach is most commonly used for bone sarcomas with limb salvage and reconstruction as discussed below. Amputation is rarely, 5% or less, performed for either soft tissue or bone sarcomas.)
    (b) Discuss management of large vessel or nerve involvement. (Preservation of major nerves and vessels is preferable by stripping adventitia or perineurium. If resection is mandated by extensive tumor involvement then reconstitution by vein grafts or prosthesis for arteries and nerve grafts for nerve.)
15. What are some general principles of wound closure? (Most patients will require postoperative radiotherapy so closure under tension over large soft tissue open spaces is to be avoided by necessary tissue transfer. A wound VAC can be employed as a temporary or bridging modality.)
16. What is the role of postoperative radiotherapy? (Unless the tumor is quite small 3 cm or less and of low grade histologically, postoperative radiation therapy is recommended. The essence of this recommendation is that the vast majority of sarcomas will require adjuvant radiotherapy.)

Reconstruction

1. What is the hypothesis behind "limb salvage" techniques? (Combinations of surgical resection, pre and postoperative radiation therapy, brachytherapy, and chemotherapy are used to achieve cure rates with limb salvage equal to those of amputation of extremities alone.)
2. Summarize the conceptual evolution in treatment of extremity sarcomas from the reconstructive standpoint. (Prior to the microvascular and myocutaneous era, amputation was the treatment of choice for extremity sarcomas. The development of allografts and local flaps has been attended by a significantly high occurrence of infection, nonunion, and late fractures particularly with the use of postoperative radiotherapy. Microvascular reconstruction including the use of vascularized fibula grafts enables the reconstruction of bony and soft tissue defects with healthy vascularized tissue.)
3. Contrast and compare reconstruction of the musculoskeletal system after resection in the upper extremity vs. the lower extremity. (Maintenance of mobility for positioning of the extremity and space as well as excellent sensation are the principles for reconstruction of the upper extremity. The lower extremity, in contrast, requires stability and strength for weight bearing.)
4. When would vascularized fibula grafts be more appropriate and what circumstances would favor allograft or non-vascularized autograft in reconstruction? (An irradiated, fibrotic bed does not lend well to the use of non-vascularized tissue such as allografts or non-vascularized autografts because of the necessity of bone healing by creeping substitution. In the upper extremity weight bearing is not a necessity and in the pediatric instance, both favor reconstruction with the use of vascularized fibula. A notable exception in the absence of an irradiated or

fibrotic bed, are bony defects less than 6 cm that would favor non-vascularized bone grafts. The femur and the proximal tibia must be able to bear a significant load with weight bearing and as such perhaps a combination of vascularized fibula encased in a solid bone allograft sheath would be the preferred choice.)

Merkel Cell Carcinomas

1. What is a Merkel cell? Where are they predominantly located? (A specialized nerve or neuroendocrine cell of the basal epithelium over terminal nerve endings in the superficial dermis. The cell is perhaps a touch receptor located everywhere but abundant in the fingertip and tip of the nose.)
   (a) The Merkel cell carcinoma is similar to which other malignant neuroendocrine tumors? (Carcinoid, small cell cancer of the respiratory tree, bronchogenic)
2. What is the typical patient profile? (White, elderly, male: female predominance of 2:1, a distribution of about one-half on the head and neck.)
   (a) Conditions/diagnoses that may be predisposed to Merkel cell carcinoma? (Immunocompromised patients such as AIDS or organ transplant; psoriasis patients treated with methoxsalen and ultraviolet A. Based on geographic incidence, sun exposure is considered a risk factor.)
   (b) What is the virus associated with but not necessarily causative in the majority of patients with Merkel cell carcinoma? (A polyomavirus)
3. Characterize the behavior of Merkel cell carcinoma. (An aggressive malignant skin cancer with a high propensity for local recurrence and regional and distant metastasis.)
4. What is the appearance? (Rapidly growing, painless, blue-red nodule with overlying intact skin, most commonly in sun-exposed areas.)
5. Describe the pathologic picture. (The more differentiated are trabecular with high cellularity and large nuclei; the less differentiated are monotonous sheets of diffuse cells with little stroma.)
   (a) What do they resemble pathologically and can be confused with? (Small cell carcinoma of the lung, lymphoma)
   (b) What is the molecular biological marker most frequently detected? (Cytokeratin-20)
6. Give a differential diagnosis. (If superficial, may resemble squamous cell carcinoma, basal cell, amelanotic melanoma, or cutaneous lymphoma. If large and deep, adnexal tumors, skin metastases from a visceral tumor.)
7. What is the role of imaging? (A significant incidence of metastatic disease at presentation would indicate a CT scan of the chest and abdomen as appropriate. PET scan, similar to melanoma, is currently under investigation but certainly has the capability of diagnosis of metastatic disease.)
8. Stage at presentation? (Only two-thirds are localized, regional metastases are present in 30% although the majority of lymph node involvement is pathologic positive but clinically negative and 7% have distant metastases.)
9. What are the criteria utilized for staging purposes? (Size, involvement of adjacent structures besides skin, micro- or macroscopic involvement of the regional lymph nodes.)
10. What are the treatment recommendations? (Wide local excision with a 1 cm margin particularly for tumors >2 cm, sentinel lymph node biopsy and if positive a completion regional node dissection. Mohs is an alternative but may not offer an advantage over wide local excision. An exception may be aesthetically sensitive areas of the head and neck.)
11. What is the role of radiotherapy? (Merkel cell carcinoma is radiosensitive. If the primary was large and/or the margins were close, postoperative adjuvant radiotherapy would be indicated. Also, if extracapsular disease was present on lymph node excision or multiple lymph nodes were positive, radiotherapy would be advantageous. The incidence of chronic lymphedema of an extremity rises substantially following both regional lymph node dissection and postoperative radiotherapy. One therapeutic option in the presence of a positive sentinel lymph node is, if not previously assessed, imaging for distant metastasis, and if positive, radiotherapy to the regional lymph nodes rather than a completion node dissection.)
12. A typical clinical course? (1/3 recur in a year despite complete excision, 2/3 develop regional lymph node metastasis with about a 50% salvage rate. Close and continued postoperative follow-up is mandatory.)

Dermatofibrosarcoma Protuberans (DFSP)

1. Characterize dermatofibrosarcoma protuberans, DFSP, as a general description. (A slow-growing insidious uncommon soft tissue tumor with a high rate of local recurrence and uncommon metastasis.)
2. What is the typical patient profile in a patient with DFSP? (Middle-aged patients are perhaps more commonly African-American than white although this is somewhat controversial with an equal distribution between males and females. One-half of the lesions occur on the trunk. The head and neck location is somewhat uncommon,

15%, and acral lesions or the hands and feet are distinctly uncommon.)

3. What is the clinical picture and history of a DFSP? (The tumor is slow-growing and rarely metastasizes. The clinical picture is that of a subcutaneous tumor with perhaps a red-purplish discoloration of the overlying skin.)
4. Describe the histological appearance. (A bland appearance of dermal spindle cells with an appearance not unlike collagen bundles except for the storiform or cartwheel appearance. Importantly, tumor extension and tentacles of the tumor occur well beyond the body of the tumor.)
   (a) What are the implications for management? (The two ramifications of the histological appearance are first, the difficulty in marginal assessment, particularly with frozen sections, and secondly, the explanation for the high rate of local recurrence.)
5. What is a differential diagnosis for both the clinician and pathologist? (Probably the most common soft tissue tumor that is similar in clinical appearance and overlaps histological appearance with dermatofibrosarcoma is dermatofibroma.)
6. Describe the principles of management. (Wide resection is the mainstay of treatment. Margins as large as 3–4 cm have been recommended. The role of Mohs micrographic surgery has played a more prominent role more recently in management, particularly since the tumor extensions are asymmetrical in distribution. Yet, the difficulty in frozen section distinction of margins may be best addressed by the use of "slow Mohs" since that technique will allow examination of margins with permanent sections. Perhaps a useful compromise is a resection with narrow margins and the use of Mohs to define the ultimate margin of clearance of the tumor. The disadvantage is the potential necessity of multiple excisions.)
7. What are the pros and cons of the role of radiotherapy? (The pros are perhaps some opportunity for local control with the application of radiotherapy. The cons are reports that radiotherapy simply induces more aggressive sarcomatous changes in the tumor.)
8. What is a possible therapy for unresectable metastatic disease? (Molecular targeted therapy with imatinib. Potential patients should be tested for the mutation or fusion gene first.)

Malignant Fibrous Histiocytoma

1. Characterize the clinical behavior of malignant fibrous histiocytoma. (Locally aggressive tumor with a significant incidence of local recurrence and metastasis.)
2. Classification? (Confined to the subcutaneous tissue or superficial and deep within the involvement of fascia or muscle.)
   (a) Pathologic appearance? (Sheets of pleomorphic spindle cells.)
3. Management? (Imaging of the primary, regional lymph nodes, and detection of distant metastasis. Wide local surgical excision is the treatment of choice.)

Case-Based Conference

Case 1: Recurrent Ca of the Scalp

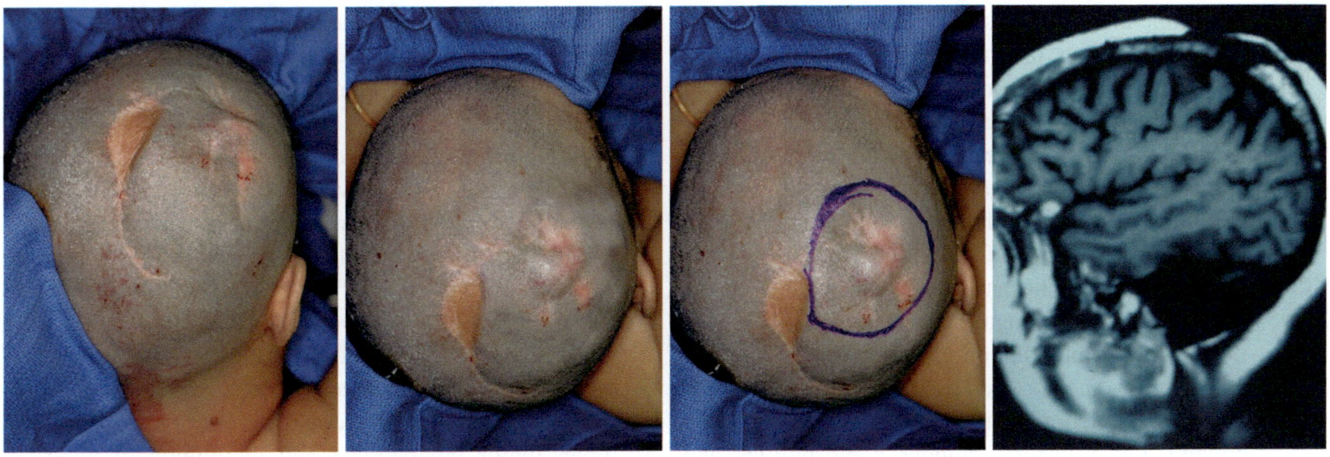

A 48-year-old woman with recurrent fibrosarcoma of the scalp who has just completed prolonged chemoradiotherapy. Her original resection was 2 years ago.

1. Describe the slide(s). Add a focused clinical exam.
   (a) Tests indicated? The MRI demonstrates no dural involvement.
2. What is the pathologic anatomy? Explain in detail how your analysis affects the treatment plan.
3. Outline your treatment plan.
   (a) Manage the patient both oncologically as well as the reconstruction.

Case-Based Conference: Discussion

Case 1: Recurrent Ca of the Scalp

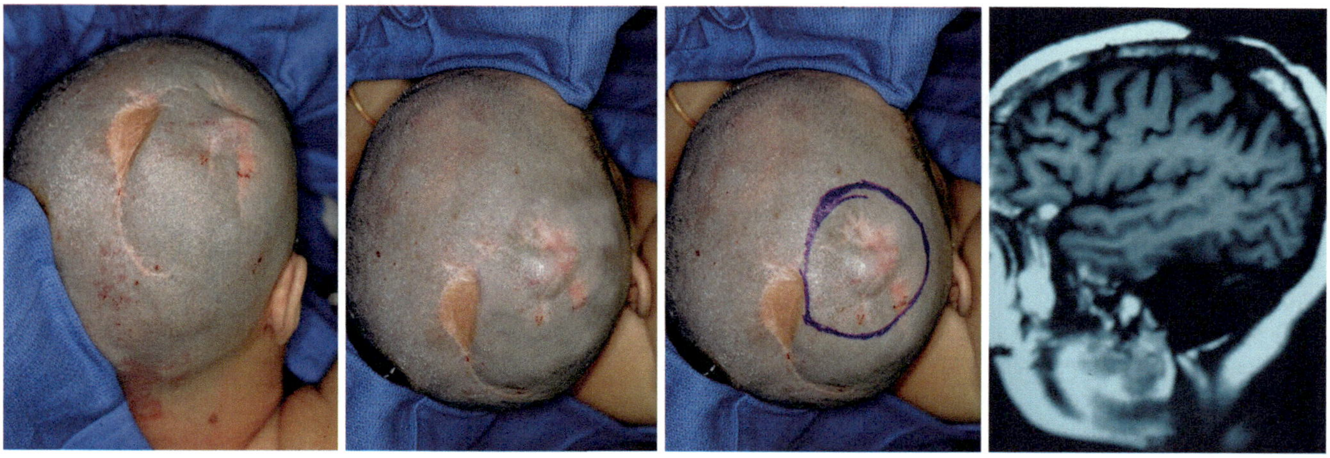

A 48-year-old woman with recurrent fibrosarcoma of the scalp who has just completed prolonged chemoradiotherapy. Her original resection was 2 years ago.

1. Describe the slide(s). (Patient probably located in the OR in a prone or lateral decubitus position with shaved scalp and old postoperative changes indicative of an inferiorly-based occipital flap and skin graft. A probable mass is located on the lateral and distal, anterior limb of the flap without evident skin ulceration. The second view is mostly superior and demonstrates the aforementioned mass that appears to be about 2 cm in size and not well-defined. No alopecia is evident.)
   (a) Clinical exam? (The history would focus on the past treatment records including histological information including cell type, differentiation, and size of the original primary. The patient questions would consist of the methods of diagnosis of recurrence, the particulars of chemoradiation as number of cycles and weeks of treatment as well as adverse responses. The date of completion of radiation therapy should be elicited. Other history includes comorbidities and smoking. The physical exam of the mass would ascertain fixed or mobile. The posterior cervical nodal basin is examined.)
   (b) Test indicated? (An MRI has been performed. Imaging should include a CT scan to better define the bony defect evident on MRI.)
   (c) Interpretation of the MRI? (Bony defect directly underlying the tumor mass. No apparent dural involvement.)
2. What is the pathologic anatomy? (The two elements of the pathologic anatomy are the nature of the tumor and the current anticipated defect. The cell type and grade will be a rough yardstick of the magnitude of resection although the tumor is recurrent and will require an aggressive excision.

   The other element or component is the eventual defect. The soft tissue excision will encompass a 2–3 cm margin given the diagnosis of fibrosarcoma. The MRI indicates a full-thickness bony defect, size indeterminant and although the MRI is read as "no dural involvement", the possibility of dural involvement by tumor must be included in the reconstructive plan. The pathologic anatomy includes the presence of irradiated tissue. The etiology of the bone defect could be osteoradionecrosis or direct tumor involvement and dissolution of bone. In summary, the oncologic plan should be wide soft tissue resection, a margin of bone resection, and consideration of the necessity of dural excision and replacement.)

3. Outline your treatment plan. (The soft tissue margins outlined on the slide appear inadequate since the soft tissue reconstruction will probably require a free flap, the size of the defect to some degree becomes irrelevant, and generous margins should be planned. Whether the etiology of the bony loss in the skull is osteoradionecrosis, ORN, or tumor is also immaterial. The bone margins should be resected for an additional 2 cm. The specimen should be excised as an en bloc resection, and the dura inspected as the specimen is lifted free.

   Reconstruction begins with the dura, if necessary, and reconstitution with a dural substitute of which bovine pericardium is one frequent choice. Although the dural replacement will be within a previously irradiated field, the coverage will be a well-vascularized flap. The options for reconstitution of the skull defect are non-vascularized autogenous bone as split autogenous cranial bone grafts, vascularized bone within a free flap, and alloplastic reconstruction. Of the last, alloplastic, the options are methyl methacrylate, polyethylene such as PEEK and titanium mesh. Given the milieu, the use of titanium mesh is probably the method of choice. If vascularized bone is selected then the free flap option by definition would be a composite flap. Possibilities include fibula, scapular, and deep iliac. The fibula including a skin island would be a bulky flap replacement for the scalp soft tissue and may create some technical challenges in the orientation of the skin island and bone into the defect. The scapula might require re-positioning of the patient and the deep iliac is a difficult dissection and the skin island is less reliable than other options.

   Certainly, the soft tissue defect can be addressed with a myocutaneous or fasciocutaneous free flap, utilized also as coverage over the skull reconstruction such as an alloplastic method. If so, the next decision in the algorithm in flap selection is muscle alone plus skin graft or a musculocutaneous flap. Choices include latissimus or serratus anterior, although the latissimus would appear to be quite bulky as is the anterolateral thigh flap as an option. Rectus abdominis, muscle alone, similar to the latissimus would be bulky. The length of vascular pedicle is a consideration. The superficial temporal vessels are in close proximity to the defect but may not be suitable because of friability, particularly the vein. If so, the pedicle must be of sufficient length to reach the neck. Serratus anterior, lower slips, plus skin graft would be an acceptable option.)

Intraoperative

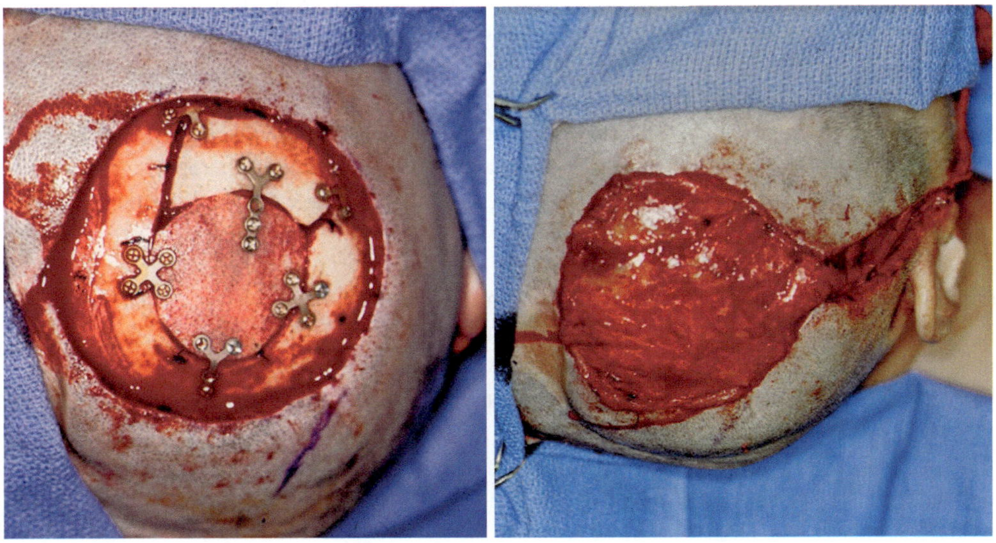

The two intraoperative views illustrate the excised defect that included skin-soft tissue and full-thickness skull. A split calvarial graft has been secured. In the following slides, a muscle flap covers the bone and adjacent cranium. The pattern of resection would indicate a wider skin and soft tissue margin than that employed for the bone. A preauricular incisional wound enabled access to the superficial temporal vessels.

Postoperative

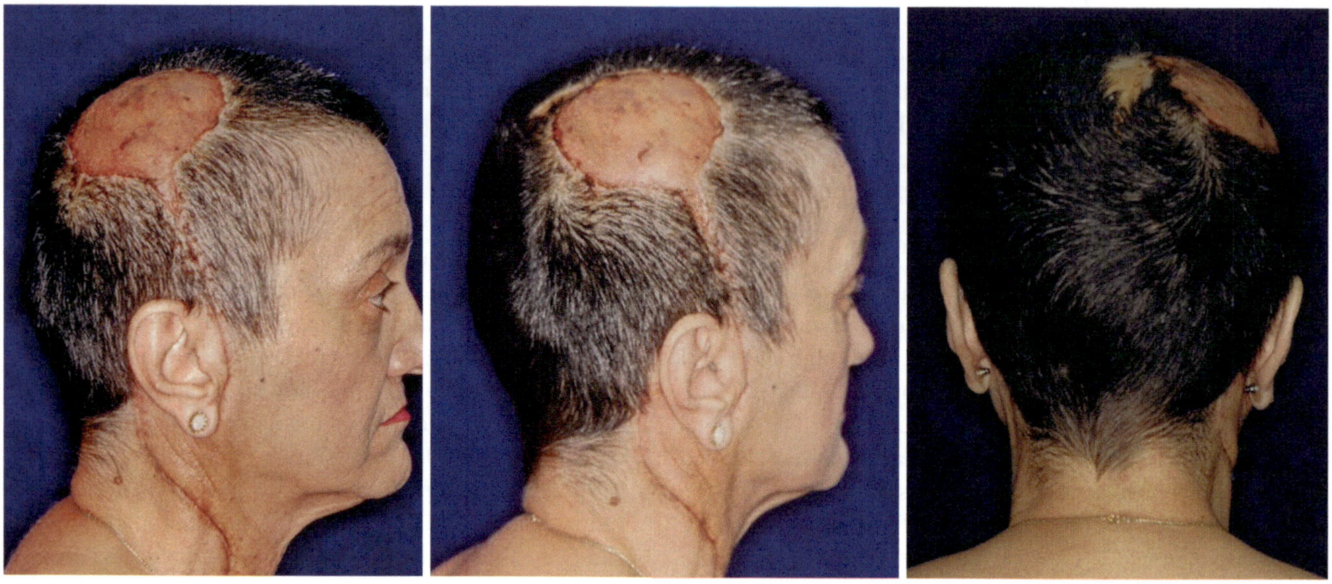

Several photos provide anterior, posterior, and oblique views of the result. The wounds are well-healed and clearly as judged by appearance and posture the patient is functioning. The cervical incision would indicate the recipient vessels were not the superficial temporal. Not unanticipated since on occasion both the artery and vein are thin-walled and friable. Planning should routinely include a long donor vascular pedicle, if possible. In this instance, although the latissimus was the donor muscle, vein grafts were still necessary, a necessity that increases the complication rate.

In-Service Examination

1. The tumor marker for Merkel cell carcinoma is:
   (a) Cytokeratin-20
   (b) S100
   (c) CD-30
   (d) Alpha Ketoglutarate
2. The appropriate management of a 2 cm Merkel cell of the dorsal forearm is:
   (a) Wide local excision with a 1 cm margin alone
   (b) Wide local excision with a 2 cm margin alone
   (c) Wide local excision with elective lymph node dissection
   (d) Wide local excision with a sentinel lymph node biopsy
   (e) Wide local excision with a sentinel lymph node biopsy and postoperative radiotherapy
3. Staging of sarcomas include the following variables **EXCEPT**:
   (a) Size
   (b) Anatomic location
   (c) Nodal metastases
   (d) Mitoses per high-powered field
   (e) Intra- or extracompartmental extension

Part IV

Head and Neck Tumors

Anatomy, Workup, Principles of Treatment, Including Radiation Therapy and Chemotherapy

35

Bibliography

Chow L.Q.M., "Head and Neck Cancer", *New England Journal of Medicine*, (2020); 382:**60–67 ONLY (to Metastatic)**.

Mathhew M, Goldenberg D, "AHNS Series: Do you know your guidelines? Principles of Surgery for Head and Neck Cancer: A Review of the National Comprehensive Cancer Network Guidelines", *Head and Neck*, (2016); 39:**1–5**.

Barnes, L. Edited by Myers, Eugene N. and Suen, J. Y. "Chapter 3: Pathology of the Head and Neck: General Considerations." *Cancer of the Head and Neck.* Third Edition. **pp 17–25**.

Ch'ng S., Morrison E., Rastogi P., Chen Y.R., Ch. 8: "Carcinoma of the Upper Aerodigestive Tract", Neligan PC, Plastic Surgery, Elsevier 5th Edition, (2023), Volume 3: **pg. 190–216 (Skip section on Lip and Salivary Gland Tumors)**.

Luce, E. A. MD. Chapter 31: "Modified and radical neck surgery." Operative Plastic Surgery. Evans, G. R. D., McGraw-Hill Medical Publishing Division. **pp 337–346**.

Savvides P, "The role of chemotherapy in the management of patients with head and neck cancer", *Seminars in Plastic Surgery*, (2010); 24(2):**137–39**.

Hussey, D. H., and Wen, B-Chen. Chapter 99: "Principles of Radiation Oncology." *Head & Neck Surgery-Otolaryngology*. Second Edition. **pp 1389–1400**.

Faculty Discussion and Study Guide

Anatomy

1. Define the anatomical limits of the following:
   (a) Oral cavity (The oral cavity begins at the vermilion border of the lips and extends to include the buccal cavity or mucosa, the anterior or mobile tongue, floor of mouth, hard palate, and the maxillary and mandibular alveolar ridges. The posterior border is the circumvallate papillae of tongue, demarcating the fixed and mobile portions of the tongue, and superiorly the posterior border of the hard palate and laterally the retromolar trigone.)
   (b) Pharynx—oropharynx (As implied previously, the fixed or posterior tongue which begins at the circumvallate papillae is the floor of the oropharynx which is limited posteriorly by the lingual aspect of the epiglottis. The soft palate is considered part of the oropharynx as well as the anterior and posterior tonsillar pillars, tonsillar fossae, and posterior and lateral pharyngeal walls.)
   (c) Nasopharynx (The skull base superiorly, the nasal cavity with the nasal aspect of the hard and soft palate, nasal side walls, adenoids, and associated portion of the superior posterior pharyngeal wall to the inferior limit of the adenoids or C1.)
   (d) Hypopharynx (The hypopharynx consists of the pyriform sinuses, the postcricoid area of the larynx, and the inferior lateral pharyngeal walls. The inferior limit of the hypopharynx, somewhat arbitrary, is the beginning or proximal end of the esophagus.)
2. Define five or six lymph node-bearing areas of the neck anatomically. (The mental and submandibular triangles, Zone 1; the superior anterior cervical or jugulodigastric, Zone 2; mid anterior cervical to the border of the inferior belly of the omohyoid nodes, Zone 3; inferior anterior cervical inferior to the inferior belly of the omohyoid nodes, Zone 4; posterior cervical nodes Zone 5; and the peri-tracheal nodes Zone 6. See Fig. 35.1.)
3. Although the overlap is substantial, what areas of the upper aerodigestive tract metastasize to the following lymph node basins: anterior level I, level IV, and level V? (Level I—lower lip, floor of mouth, uncommonly anterior tongue; levels II and III as an extension from level I, oral cavity; level IV—hypopharynx, larynx; level V—oropharynx, nasopharynx.)
4. Define the anatomical borders of the submandibular and posterior cervical triangles. (The submandibular triangle

E. Luce, *A Curriculum for Plastic Surgery*, https://doi.org/10.1007/978-3-031-62087-4_35

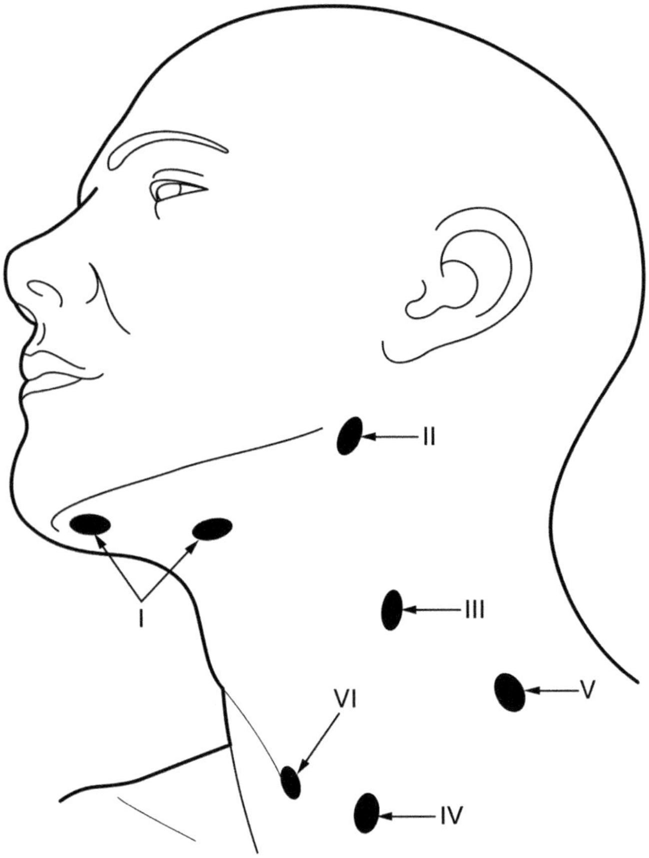

Fig. 35.1 Anatomy of the neck

is bounded anteriorly by the anterior belly of the digastric, inferiorly by the posterior belly of the digastric, and superiorly by the body of the mandible. The posterior cervical triangle is bounded anteriorly by the posterior border of the sternocleidomastoid, posteriorly by the anterior border of the trapezius, superiorly by skull base, and inferiorly by the clavicle.)

Evaluation, Classification, and Staging

1. What are the leading risk factors in the development of head and neck squamous cell cancer? (Tobacco, alcohol, Epstein-Barr virus, human papillomavirus.)
2. How can specific symptoms assist in the location of the tumor? (Hoarseness—larynx, dysphagia—hypopharynx and/or esophagus, unilateral hearing loss and/or pain—nasopharynx, mouth soreness—oral cavity. Of course, overlap of symptom complex is quite common.)
3. What are the specifics of the physical exam in the head and neck cancer patient? (Depending on the location, the essentials or basics of the physical exam are palpation of the lymph node basins, examination of cranial nerves V–VIII, intraoral exam including palpation, mirror indirect laryngoscopy or as is more common, and office endoscopic laryngoscopy.)
4. What is the workup, beyond the clinical examination, of the patient with a T_2 N_1 M_o carcinoma of the tongue? (FNA of the lymph node for confirmation of nodal metastasis can be utilized in skilled hands and with examination by a skilled cytopathologist, CT scan including chest, and rigid or flexible endoscopy with general anesthesia.)
   (a) Describe the technique of performance of FNA. (FNA, fine needle aspiration biopsy is performed with a small, usually a 22-gauge, needle attached to a 10 cc syringe used for aspiration. The cellular content of the tumor or mass is then done and placed on a microscopic slide or perhaps even a cell block for tissue processing. FNA has been primarily useful in salivary gland masses as well as thyroid nodules.)
5. What imaging modality would most effectively evaluate for tumor extent in the following?
   (a) A cancer of the floor of the mouth adjacent to the lingual aspect of the anterior mandible. (CT scan)
   (b) A carcinoma of the tongue with possible positive cervical nodes. (CT scan) Why? (To define the likelihood of metastatic involvement of the lymph nodes.)
   (c) A cancer of the ethmoid sinus with possible intracranial extension (CT scan and MRI)
6. A skin cancer of the lower eyelid with possible intraorbital extension (MRI.) Define the levels of T and N staging for the oral cavity (Fig. 35.2)

$T_1 < 2$ cm	N_1 lymph node <3 cm
T_2 2–4 cm	N_2a 3–6 cm single node or **a** node
$T_3 > 4$ cm	N_2b multiple modes <6 cm a **bunch** of nodes
T_4 invasion into adjacent structures	N_2c bilateral or contralateral nodes <6 cm
	$N_3 > 6$ cm

Editor's Note: Because of better survival in human papilloma virus (HPV)-positive oropharyngeal cancer, the most recent (2017) staging system relatively downgrades the stage of the disease. Nevertheless, less-intensive treatment on the basis of HPV-positivity is not currently recommended.

7. What is the stage of disease for the following?
   (a) T_2 tumor of the floor of mouth without palpable lymph nodes? (Stage II)
   (b) A T_4 of floor of mouth invading mandible without palpable lymph nodes? (Stage IV)

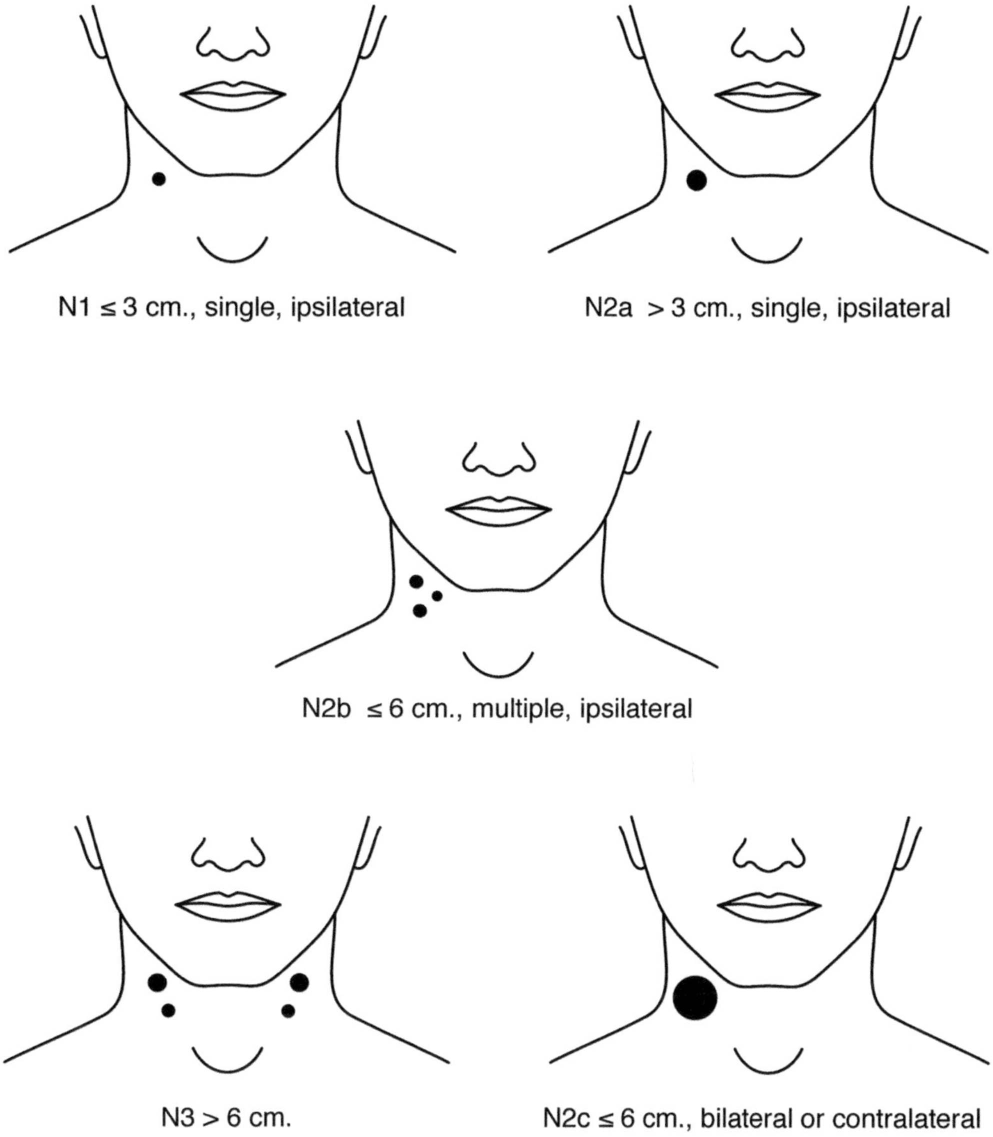

Fig. 35.2 Staging of oral cavity

(c) A T_2 tumor of the tongue with several palpable lymph nodes of the ipsilateral neck all measure less than 4 cm in diameter. (Stage IV)
(d) A T_2 tumor of the pharynx with a 6 cm ipsilateral lymph node. (Stage IV)

> **Editor's Note**: If N_0, the T size drives staging. If N_1, all are stage III, if N_2, all are stage IV.

8. What is a Karnofsky status or scale? (A performance scale that attempts to assess in a global or general sense the patient's ability to perform activities of daily living and is rated from 0 (dead) to 100 (normal)).

(a) A new consultation with head and neck cancer arrives in a wheelchair from a nursing home. What is the Karnofsky rating? (About 40)

Pathology of the Head and Neck

1. What is HPV-associated head and neck cancer including incidence and significance? (Human papilloma virus (HPV) is detected, when tested, in an increased percentage of diagnosed oropharyngeal cancers, perhaps a reflection of the increase in awareness. The significance, prognostically, is an enhanced response to chemo- and radiation therapy. The improved prognosis has resulted in a recent separate staging system for HPV-positive disease. Immunochemistry testing for p16 expression should be performed.)

2. List three pathologic features of the primary that may indicate an increased propensity for lymph node metastases and explain. (Thickness greater than 4 mm, perineural invasion as probably a reflection of intralymphatic tumor, blood vessel invasion, and to some degree, differentiation. By National Comprehensive Cancer Network (NCCN), guidelines, a minimum of 5 mm margin *pathologically* is considered adequate, less is defined close. The significance is reflected in recurrence and survival rates. Since specimen shrinkage occurs even without formalin preparation solutions, surgical margins should be, depending on the nature of the tumor, 1–2 cm.)
3. Discuss the problem with recurrence with a positive tissue margin. Explain why a negative margin may recur. (A positive microscopic margin may indicate two things: one, an inherent and intrinsic virulence of the tumor as well as perhaps simply an inadequate resection. Certainly, a negative margin may recur because of the incompleteness of any pathologic examination. Also, there is evidence from molecular biology that cells adjacent to the margin may be routinely histologically negative but positive by molecular biology. Regardless, a positive margin increases the recurrence rate by 2–3 times.)
   (a) What is the role of radiotherapy (RT) in management? (Little unless there is absolutely no other option. The preferable option is re-excision followed by radiotherapy.)
4. How would the recurrence rate compare if the frozen section is negative but the permanent section is positive? (Still a markedly increased recurrence rate.)
5. How does the presence and characteristics of the regional lymph node involvement affect the prognosis? (The presence of nodal metastases decreases the survival by about 50%; multiple and large lymph nodes diminish the survival substantially as does the level of neck involvement as well as contralateral neck involvement. Histological evidence of extracapsular extension has similar adverse consequences, although practically, involved lymph nodes greater than 2 cm almost universally have extracapsular extension.)
6. Comment on the importance of nodal metastasis with extracapsular extension in a lymph node. (Indicative of much more likely locoregional recurrence and radiotherapy is indicated.)
   (a) If you can palpate a clinically positive cervical lymph node, what is the probability of extracapsular extension? (If the assumption is that a node must be 1–1.5 cm in size to be palpable by a skilled examiner, the probability of extracapsular extension in a 1.5 cm node is approximately 75%.)
7. The expected survival duration, mortality of 90%, in a previously treated patient who developed pulmonary metastasis is what? (2 years)
   (a) What is the hiatus between resection of the cancer and recurrence or metastasis if that should occur? (90% are apparent in less than 2 years.)
8. In breast cancer, locoregional recurrence heralds the presence or subsequent occurrence of distant metastases in 90% of the patients, but conversely, the vast majority of breast cancer patients who develop metastasis do so without local or regional recurrence. Is that relationship true for head and neck cancer? (No. Distant metastases occur in only 10–20% of patients *without* concomitant locoregional recurrence.)
9. One of the diagnosis and treatment difficulties in the smoking head and neck cancer patient is the possibility of a coexistent cancer of the lung. What percent of head and neck cancer patients will have a coexistent neoplasm? What is the proper term? (Synchronous cancer. Figures vary but with the use of a CT scan of the lung and endoscopy, probably 10–15%)
   (a) What is a metachronous primary? (The *subsequent* development of a separate primary.) What is the usual interval? (26 months)
10. What tumor or tissue type is cytokeratin immunochemistry stain specific for? (Epidermoid neoplasm)
   (a) S-100? (Melanoma)

Clinical Application of Therapeutic Radiation

Editor's Note: The principles of therapeutic radiation are also discussed in Chap. 2.

1. The depth of tissue penetration for the radiation effect on the cancer is determined by what? (The energy of the beam such as 125 kV used in electron beam therapy for skin dosage, increased in CO_{60} delivered by cobalt beam to finally that of the linear accelerator from 4 to 24 MV which can focus the radiation intensity at 10–12 cm deep in the case of the latter.)
   (a) What is the importance? (Expression of skin-sparing effect or that only a small percentage of radiation is delivered to the skin with higher voltage sources from, for example, the linear accelerator.)
2. How does ionizing radiotherapy achieve the cancerocidal effect? (Depending on the particle energized, for example, photons, the energized particle is capable of breaking an electron free of orbit which can in turn inflict cellular damage, a direct effect. The particles can also react with oxygen to create free radicals that can also damage the DNA of the cell, rendering it incapable of replication, an indirect effect.)

3. What are the tumor and treatment variables in the use of radiotherapy? (Tumor "load," intrinsic nature of the virulence of the tumor such as cell doubling time, host environment as the degree of hypoxia, nature of the radiotherapy modality such as external beam versus brachytherapy, fraction dose as well as total dose.)
4. What is (are) the explanation for the diminished efficacy of radiotherapy with an increase in tumor size? (Two reasons: One, the number of cells killed is on a log scale, so, the same amount of radiation that reduced the number of cells from 1×10^{10} to 1×10^9 will be necessary to further reduce from 1×10^9 to 1×10^8, etc., until the reduction of 100 to 10 and then ultimately 10 to 1 cell. A greater volume of tumor implies a greater number of cells. Second, the central portion of large tumors is frequently hypoxic and the presence of oxygen is necessary to obtain a cell-kill effect.)
5. Define fractionation. (Simply, the total dose given over a period of time divided by the number of doses to be given. For example, 60 Gy may be given in doses over a 6-week period of time with 10 Gy per week, divided by 5 days or 2 Gy each day.)
6. Two different protocols are proposed for a head and neck tumor: (a) delivery 60 cGY over 3 weeks with a twice-a-day fractionation schedule, termed hyperfractionation and (b) a similar dose of over 6 weeks with once-a-day treatment. Which protocol will have the greater cancerocidal effect and why? (The first. The shorter, more intense schedule will minimize cell repopulation and reduce the possibility of sublethal injury.)
   (a) At what price? (A maximal overlap of therapeutic and morbidity curves with a higher probability of significant acute complications.)
7. How is the concept of sublethal injury translated into the selection of a fractionation treatment plan? (If the cell target is hit by insufficient ionization the sublethal injury can be repaired by the cell if no further hits occur. So, a greater total dose may be required to produce the biologic effect desired when given in multiple fractions rather than a single fraction. The greater the number of fractions, the greater the opportunity for cellular repair. Clearly, a single large dose of radiation is not feasible, except in intraoperative radiotherapy, IORT, but the fractionation schedule needs to be as short as tolerable.)
   (a) What is the concept of cell cycle in the selection of a treatment plan? (Cells in the S phase or the phase of DNA synthesis are much more radio-resistant than the other phases of the cell cycle. The clinical impact is a mathematical one, namely, the greater number of fractions and the greater probability of hitting cells in a radiosensitive phase during irradiation. One factor in that mathematical equation is the rapidity of cellular cycling and those cells that cycle rapidly such as skin and mucosa are more sensitive to radiation).

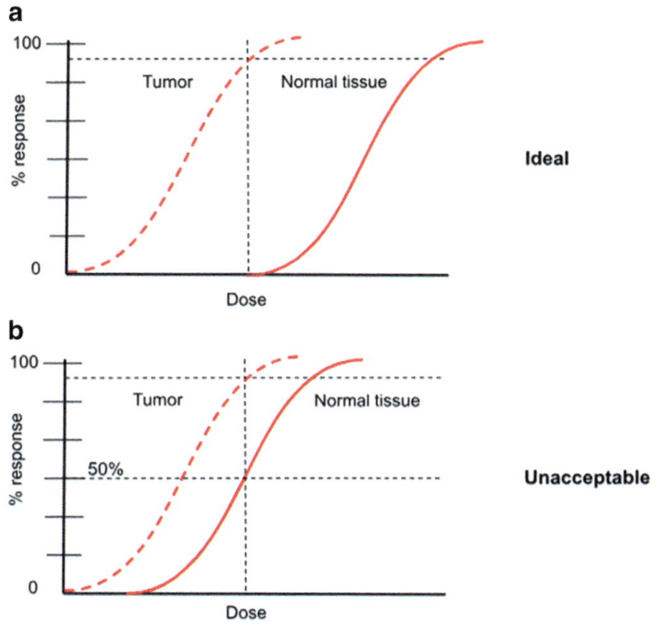

Fig. 35.3 Tumor control ratio

8. Discuss the "therapeutic ratio" in radiotherapy of the head and neck. (A relationship of the sigmoidal curve of therapeutic efficacy versus frequency or incidence of complications.)
   (a) Construct a curve that would yield a 10% complication rate for a 90% cure. Do the same for a 50% complication rate with a 90% prospect of cure (Fig. 35.3.).
   (b) The anticipated tumor control is of moderate probability but has a low incidence of complications.
   (c) A high probability of tumor control but a greater probability of complications.
9. A patient is treated with prostate cancer. Why will he more likely develop mucositis of the rectum before the necessary dose to control the cancer is achieved? (The rate of cell turnover determines the probability of cellular death by ionizing radiation. The epithelium mucosa has a much higher cell turnover rate than the cellular component of prostate cancer.)
10. What are the advantages of brachytherapy? (Confined to the implant volume, delivered continuously at a low rate).
    (a) Disadvantage? (Opposite, namely a limited amount or volume of tissue treated).
11. A T_4 cancer of the lip invades the mandible. How does this finding affect the efficacy of postoperative radiotherapy? (Markedly diminished because if tumor cells remain in bone after resection, control is not possible.)

   (a) Why? (Involvement and dissemination through the Haversian canal system as well as osteoclastic activity by the tumor cells. The therapeutic implication is that bone margins must be negative.)
12. You are consulting a patient with a 2 cm squamous cell cancer of the mobile tongue. He asks if primary therapy with radiotherapy is as efficacious as surgery, namely a hemiglossectomy. (Yes, for T_1 lesions in terms of *cure*, the two (surgery and radiotherapy) are equal.)
   (a) A 4.5 cm tumor of the tongue? (T3 lesion—No. Radiotherapy is not as efficacious as surgery for the reasons cited earlier, which include, principally, the tumor size.)
13. What are the pros and cons of preoperative radiotherapy? (The pros are the enhanced efficacy of radiotherapy in a well-oxygenated virginal environment and the control of peripheral microscopic extent is better with radiotherapy than in the more hypoxic, less well-vascularized central tumor that can be surgically resected. Yet, radiotherapy tissue damage sets the stage for much higher incidence of wound healing problems, necrosis, and complications with increased morbidity and mortality. Also, radiotherapy creates difficulty in the determination of positive margins. Finally, if margins prove to be positive, no recourse is available.)
   (a) Pros and cons of postoperative radiotherapy? (The opposite of the previous one. Namely, radiotherapy is less effective in the postoperative or hypoxic environment. Yet, the tumor has been resected which leaves the more peripheral microscopic extension for control with radiotherapy, and since the surgery was performed in a non-radiated field, a lower incidence of complications.)
   (b) Window of therapy? (Within 6 weeks of surgery for head and neck tumors.)
   (c) What are the dosage comparisons between pre- and postoperative radiotherapy? (For the reasons stated earlier, preoperative radiotherapy dosage is usually lower, 50 Gy, whereas postoperative radiotherapy is in the range of 55–60 Gy. Preoperative RT in head and neck cancer is rarely done.)
14. Outline the rationale for the combination of surgery and radiotherapy. (Surgery, of course, is effective for removing macroscopic tumors. Radiotherapy is effective for irradiation of microscopic disease at the tissue periphery. Unfortunately, this approach has been abused in the past by "debulking" tumors and application of radiotherapy. Postoperative radiotherapy is most efficacious when margins of resection are microscopically negative.)
15. What is the role of chemotherapy in the treatment of head and neck cancer? (The role is complex. Chemotherapy, usually high-dose cis platinum, may be employed in advanced disease with concomitant radiotherapy, offered to patients with no comorbidities and high functional status, reserving surgery for salvage. Because of the significant toxicity of high-dose cis platinum, the emphasis is on the selection of the appropriate patients. High risk is defined as more than one lymph node metastasis, extracapsular nodal extension, and/or microscopically positive mucosal margins in early-stage disease and locally advanced T_3 and T_4 tumors.
   Finally, induction chemotherapy refers to the use prior to definitive concurrent chemoradiation. Chemotherapy is also offered as a postoperative adjuvant therapy to high-risk patients. The term concurrent chemoradiation refers to a treatment that consists of a three-dose regimen of high-dose cis platinum administered intravenously once every 3 weeks concurrently with a 6-week course of radiotherapy for a total dose of 60 Gy. The regimen has been applied in both a neoadjuvant and adjuvant setting. Clearly, the complex interplay of the stage of disease, overall patient status, toxicity of the regime, and patient preferences mandate multidisciplinary assessment, conference discussion, and recommendations.)

Neck Dissection, Sentinel Lymph Node Biopsy

1. Differentiate the "classical" or "comprehensive" radical neck dissection from a selective neck dissection. (A classical, current term is comprehensive, radical neck dissection addresses and excises the lymph node-bearing areas in all five of the lymph node zones. That dissection will include the sacrifice of the sternocleidomastoid muscle, internal jugular vein, and spinal accessory nerve. Because of the morbidity and deformity resulting from the sacrifice of those structures, an effort has been developed for a more selective approach. The most common modification is preservation of the sternocleidomastoid muscle and spinal accessory nerve, or in some instances, the internal jugular vein as well. The Zone 5 or the posterior cervical triangle may not be dissected in instances of N_0 neck and an oral cavity primary. Another example of selective neck dissection is a supraomohyoid which essentially dissects Zones 1, 2, and 3, limiting the inferior extent at the level of the inferior belly of the omohyoid.)
2. What is the role of sentinel lymph node, SLN, and biopsy in SCCa of the head and neck? (Under investigation. The application of the SLN biopsy concept is in the clinical setting, breast, and melanoma, of N_0 status or no palpable lymphadenopathy. The inherent difficulty in the determination of a "sentinel" lymph node in the lymphatic drainage system of the upper aerodigestive tract, particularly the oral cavity and oropharynx is the multiple possible lymphatic drainage pathways.)

Case-Based Conference

Case 1: Malignant Neck Mass

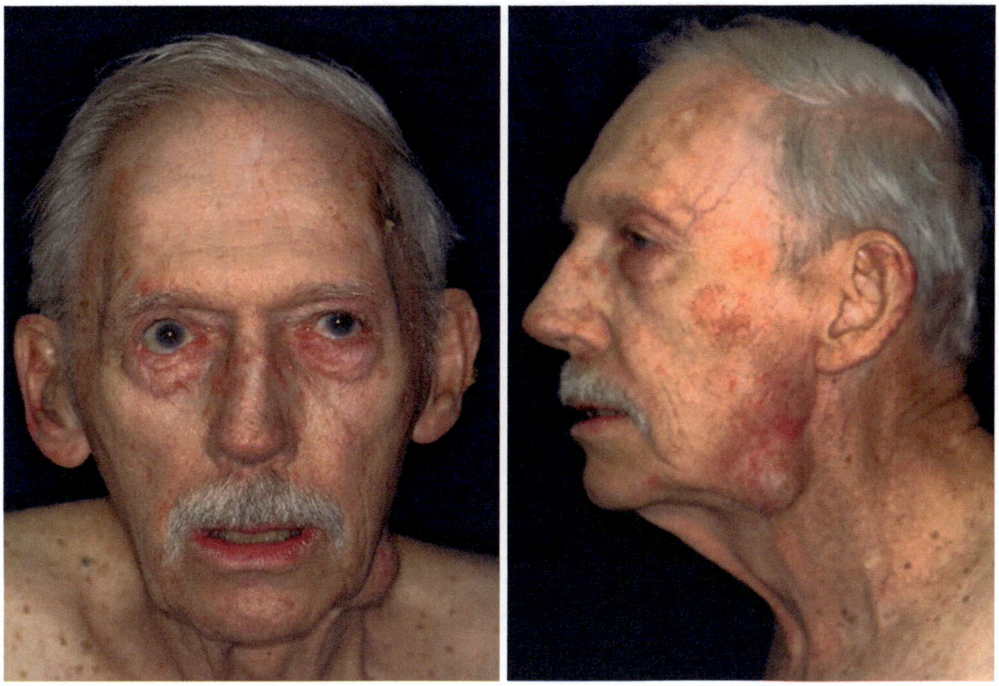

A 72-year-old man with a history of a mass of the left face/neck for 6 months with an increase in size. An FNA has revealed malignant cells. The patient is in surprisingly good health and has had a recent medicine and cardiology workup.

1. Describe the slides. Outline a brief, focused history. Perform a physical exam.
   (a) What additional tests and workups are necessary? Justify each.
   (b) Is any additional pathological information necessary beyond the FNA? If yes, why?
2. The workup to date is negative. What is the appropriate treatment at this juncture? Outline and detail. If surgical, describe.

Case-Based Conference: Discussion

Case 1: Malignant Neck Mass

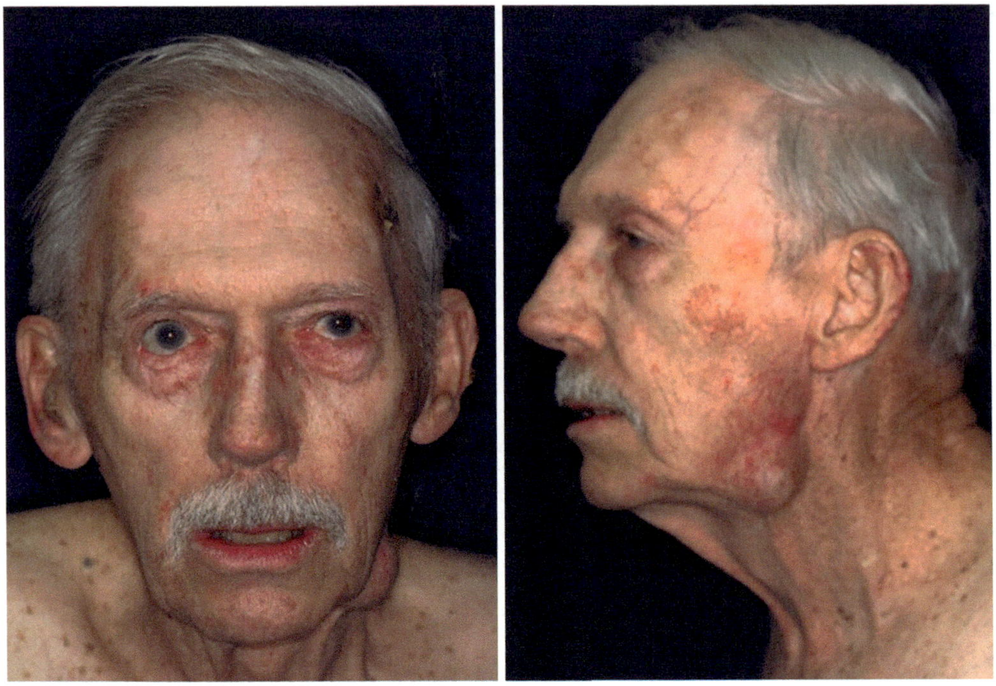

A 72-year-old man with a history of a mass of the left face/neck for 6 months with an increase in size. An FNA has revealed malignant cells. The patient is in surprisingly good health and has had a recent medicine and cardiology workup.

1. Describe the slides. Outline a brief, focused history. Perform a physical exam. (Elderly male in a frontal view with a visible mass lateral and inferior on his left neck. No skin lesions are apparent. The lateral view has an obvious mass of approximately 3 cm in size at and just below the angle of the mandible. The overlying skin is intact with some suggestion of erythema. No other masses are apparent.)

   Outline a brief, focused history. Perform a physical exam. (The history would focus on pathology of the upper aerodigestive tract: dysphagia and if positive can the symptoms be lateralized, hoarseness, otoalgia also lateralized, intraoral ulceration or mass, trismus as well as the constitutional symptoms of weight loss, and easy fatigability. Although the probability of a metastasis of a visceral, infraclavicular, primary is quite low, a history of cough, chest pain, or abdominal complaints would be important. However, the focus of this case is on the head and neck. Social history would include smoking. The physical exam would begin with palpation of the neck including the anterior and posterior triangles, supraclavicular fossa, the opposite neck, as well as the ipsilateral parotid. The neck exam would conclude with an evaluation of the neck mass for firmness and mobility. The next step in the assessment of the physical is an intraoral exam including inspection of the buccal cavity, anterior and lateral floor of mouth, tongue, the oral aspect of the hard and soft palate, and palpation of the mobile tongue. Indirect or laryngoscopy, if performed, will give a view, albeit somewhat limited, of the base of the tongue, lateral pharyngeal wall, vallecula, and false and true vocal cords.)

   (a) What additional tests and workups are necessary? Justify each. (If nothing is detected on a physical exam and since the probability of an oro- or hypopharyngeal primary is significant, the next step is imaging followed by direct visualization of these structures. Although that visualization can be accomplished endoscopically with local anesthesia, the likelihood of the concomitant biopsy dictates the necessity of general anesthesia in the operating room. In preparation for that procedure, the head and neck, chest, and abdomen should be imaged. A CT scan will assist in determining the presence of additional lymphadenopathy in the neck, detect a lesion in those regions not well visualized such as the nasopharynx, subglottic, and pyriform sinuses, and potentially ascertain the presence of a visceral primary.)

   (b) Is any additional pathological information necessary beyond the FNA? If yes, why? (If no other adenopathy is palpated elsewhere, axilla or inguinal, and no clues are apparent on the imaging studies. See the next section.)
2. The workup to date is negative. What is the appropriate treatment at this juncture? Outline and detail. If surgical, describe. (In the operating room, palpation of the base of the tongue, performance of nasopharyngoscopy, direct laryngoscopy, and, depending on the results of the CT scan, bronchoscopy and esophagoscopy may be necessary. Biopsies are obtained in the nasopharynx, base of tongue, and tonsillar fossa, at times a tonsillectomy rather than biopsy alone.

   After completion of the exam under anesthesia and if no primary is detected, an incisional biopsy is obtained. Planning the location of the incision is important since the incision performed must be subsequently incorporated and excised with a subsequent radical neck dissection. Core needle biopsies will not provide sufficient tissue for biological markers, particularly if the diagnosis is lymphoma. A portion of the specimen should be placed in saline rather than formalin to facilitate the testing of molecular markers, in particular, lymphoma.

   The most likely pathologic diagnosis is squamous cell cancer, but possibilities include the full list of soft tissue tumors such as adnexal carcinoma, sarcoma, or lymphoma. If the diagnosis of metastatic squamous cell, unknown primary, is sustained, the definitive therapy is a neck dissection, radical or modified. A modified neck dissection preserves most commonly the sternocleidomastoid treatment and the spinal accessory nerve. In some settings, the internal jugular vein may be preserved as well. A one-stage approach is possible with the collaboration of an experienced pathologist. If the surveillance biopsies are negative and an incisional biopsy is diagnostic of squamous cell carcinoma, a neck dissection can be performed, since in high likelihood, the unknown primary is within the head and neck. Lacking that assurance, a delay in acquiring a final tissue diagnosis, presumably of squamous cell carcinoma, will be necessary before a neck dissection is accomplished. Judged by the size of the nodal metastasis and stage III of the disease postoperative radiotherapy to the neck is indicated. Inclusion of the nasopharynx in the radiation ports has been described but variable treatment enthusiasm exists for this extension of adjuvant therapy.)

Editor's Note: The resident at this juncture should be able to describe the 10–12 essential steps in the performance of a radical neck dissection as well as management of the complications of skin flap necrosis, hematoma, and lymph fistula.

Case-Based Conference

Case 2: Posterior Neck Mass

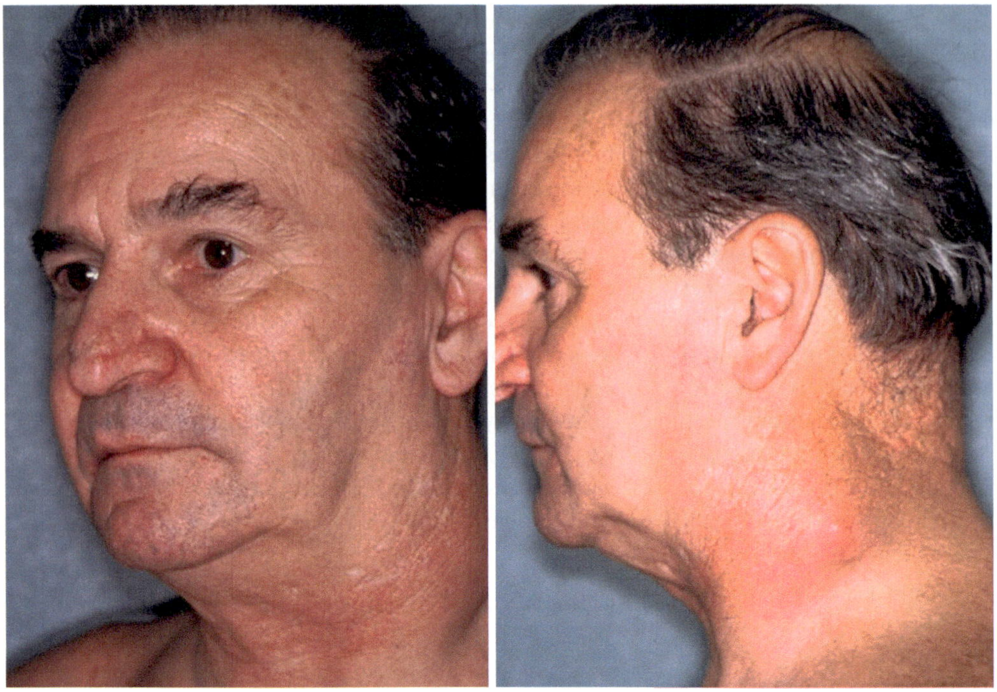

A 50-year-old with a complaint of an enlarging left neck mass of several months' duration. An FNA has revealed "malignant cells."

1. Describe the slides. Add a history and physical.
   (a) Testing? Imaging?
2. The workup is negative. Sum up the scenario at this junction and provide a differential diagnosis. What is the appropriate treatment plan at this juncture? Outline and detail. If an operative procedure is involved, describe it.

Case-Based Conference: Discussion

Case 2: Posterior Neck Mass

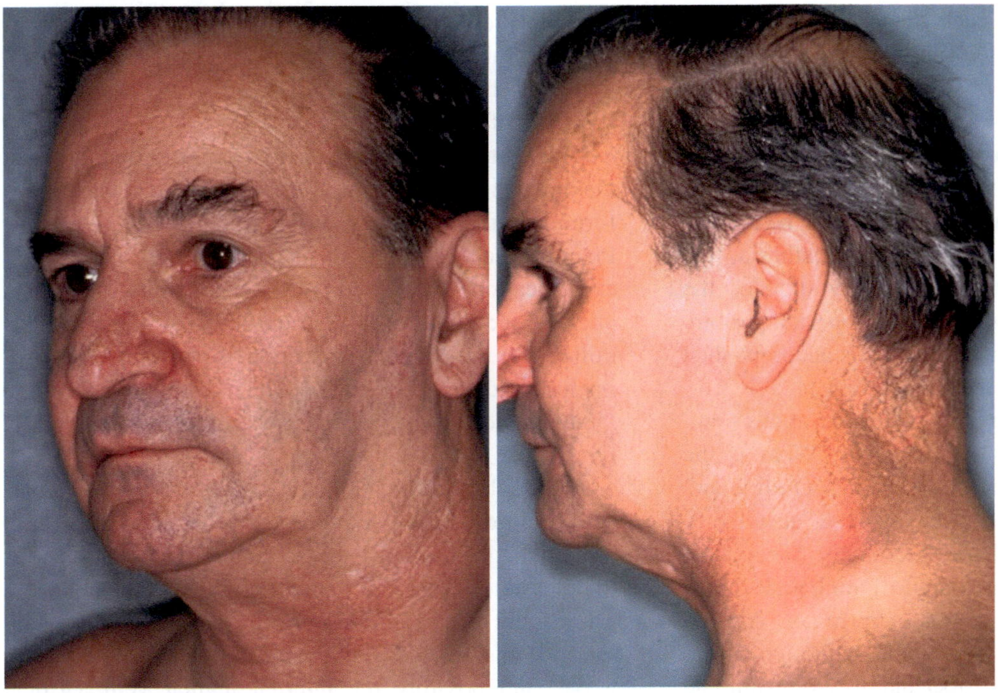

A 50-year-old with a complaint of an enlarging left neck mass of several months' duration. A FNA has revealed "malignant cells."

1. Describe the slides. Add a history and physical. (The photos depict a large mass of the left posterior neck. The lateral photo illustrates the extent of the mass more clearly than the oblique view. The limits are not discrete and well defined but appear to extend just superior to the supraclavicular fossa, posteriorly to the trapezius and the nuchal muscle mass, and superiorly to the level of the ear lobule. The anterior limits are perhaps better visualized on the oblique view. The overlying skin is essentially intact although a suggestion for slight erythema overlies a small area on the most inferior aspect on the lateral view. No other lesions or abnormalities are evident. The oblique photo lends some estimation of the overall dimensions, about 7 × 8 cm. In addition, the anterior extent of the mass appears to overlap at least a portion of the clavicular head of the sternocleidomastoid muscle. Although again no skin lesions are apparent, a suggestion of fullness in the submandibular region is present just anterior to the angle of the jaw.

   The history and physical would begin with questions related to possible pathology of the upper aerodigestive tract: pain and/or difficulty with swallowing, sores within the oral cavity, unilateral otoalgia and/or hearing loss, trismus as well as the constitutional symptoms of weight loss, malaise, easy fatigability, or night sweats.

   The physical exam would begin with palpation of the neck including the anterior and posterior triangles, supraclavicular fossa, the opposite neck as well as the ipsilateral parotid. The neck exam would conclude with an assessment of the neck mass for firmness, mobility, and tenderness. The intraoral exam includes inspection of the buccal cavity, anterior and lateral floor of mouth, tongue, the oral aspect of the hard and soft palate, and palpation of the mobile tongue. Indirect or laryngoscopy, if performed, will give a view, albeit somewhat limited, of the base of the tongue, lateral pharyngeal wall, vallecula, and false and true vocal cords. Consideration should be given to an alternate diagnosis than a tumor of upper aerodigestive tract, namely, intrathoracic or intraabdominal region. Another possibility is lymphoma or, more remotely, a non-neoplastic etiology. As such, a careful examination for adenopathy of the axillae and groin is mandatory. The abdomen is included in the examination for possible enlarged spleen, hepatomegaly, or masses. Finally, given the posterior cervical triangle as the drainage basin for the scalp, a careful examination of that region for the presence of a melanoma or adnexal tumor is also accomplished.)

   (a) Testing? Imaging? (If nothing is detected on a physical exam and since the probability of an oro-, naso-, or hypopharyngeal primary is significant, the next step is imaging. A CT scan with thin slices for the head and neck, thicker for chest and abdomen, will assist in determining the presence of additional lymphadenopathy in the neck, detect a lesion in those regions not well visualized such as the nasopharynx, subglottic, and pyriform sinuses, and potentially ascertain the presence of a visceral primary. Lacking detection of a primary at this juncture, a direct endoscopic examination of the upper aerodigestive tract is warranted. Although that visualization can be accomplished endoscopically with local anesthesia, the likelihood of the concomitant biopsy dictates the necessity of general anesthesia in the operating room. In some hands, an incisional biopsy is accomplished in the same setting. See the next section.)

2. The workup is negative. Sum up the scenario at this junction and provide a differential diagnosis. What is the appropriate treatment plan at this juncture? Outline and detail. If an operative procedure is involved, describe it. (The scenario is one of a large, presumably neoplastic mass, of the posterior cervical triangle, lymph node drainage basin level IV without an apparent primary. The differential diagnosis at this point is broad. Although in rare instances the supraclavicular fossa and, by extension, the posterior cervical triangle, can be occupied by a metastasis of a visceral primary, lung, or the lower gastrointestinal (GI) tract, lacking detection on imaging that possibility does not play a role in the subsequent treatment plan. The most likely diagnosis is squamous cell carcinoma of the upper aerodigestive tract. Although any of the locations within the oropharynx or hypopharynx may be the culprit, the more likely is a primary of the nasopharynx. Another substantially less likely possibility is a melanoma or adnexal tumor of the scalp as is a primary presentation of lymphoma.

The next step is acquisition of a definitive pathological diagnosis since the results of the FNA are not adequate to formulate therapy. An incisional biopsy is necessary. Planning the location of the incision is crucial since whatever location is selected, the incision must be subsequently incorporated and excised with the incisions utilized for radical neck dissection. A portion of the specimen should be preserved in saline rather than formalin to facilitate testing of molecular markers, particularly lymphoma.

Although, if the pathological diagnosis is squamous cell carcinoma, a one-stage approach based upon a frozen section diagnosis is possible, a more prudent approach is to defer a neck dissection until the final path is obtained. The patient will require a posterior neck dissection with sacrifice of the sternocleidomastoid, the spinal accessory nerve, and possibly the internal jugular vein. Critical structures to be identified and preserved include the upper portion of the brachial plexus.)

Intra- and Postoperative (10 Days)

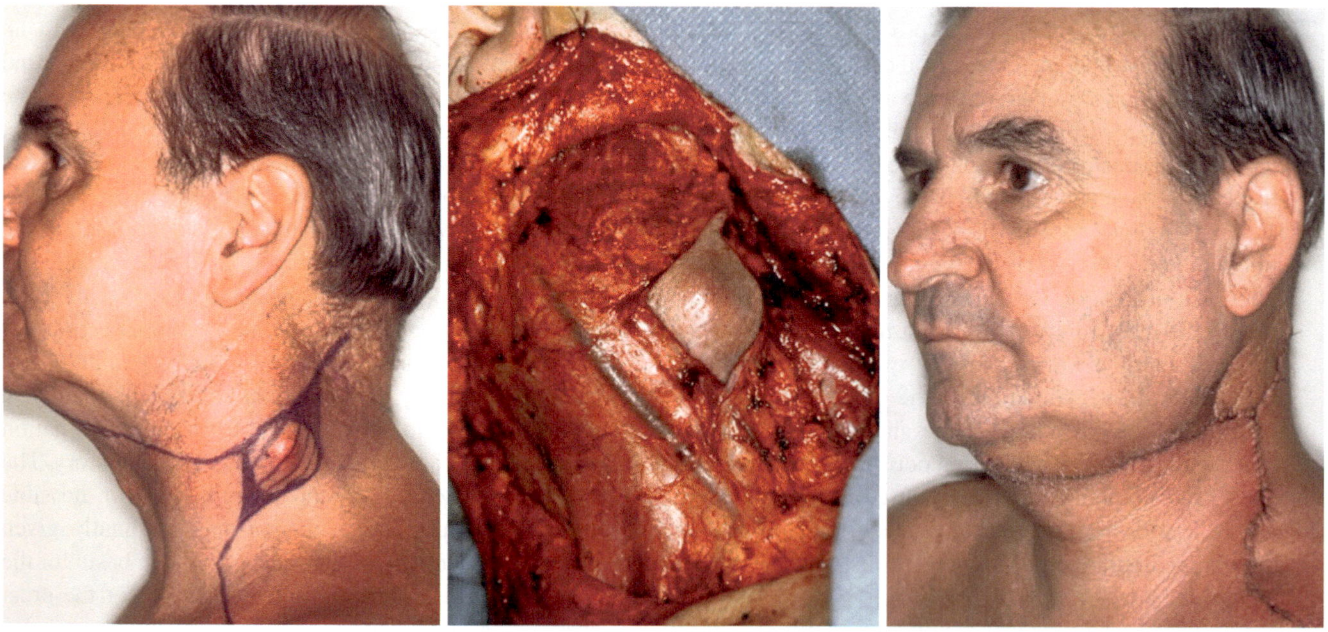

The first two photos demonstrate the planning for an excision of the area of redness and an outline of an anteriorly based cervico-pectoral flap for advancement into the skin defect. The second photo is after the elevation of skin flaps and prior to neck dissection. The third photo is 10 days postoperative.

In-Service Examination

1. The following structures are considered within the oropharynx **EXCEPT**:
   (a) Lingual aspect of the epiglottis
   (b) Anterior tonsillar pillar
   (c) Posterior tonsillar pillar
   (d) Uvula
2. The limits of the posterior cervical triangle include all of the following **EXCEPT**:
   (a) Skull base
   (b) Inferior belly omohyoid
   (c) Posterior border of the sternocleidomastoid
   (d) Anterior border of the trapezius
3. All the following are variables in the survival of squamous cell carcinoma of the upper aerodigestive tract **EXCEPT**:
   (a) Tumor thickness
   (b) HPV status
   (c) S-100 status
   (d) Presence or absence of lymph node metastases
   (e) Tumor size
4. A patient has a 2 cm squamous cell carcinoma of the floor of mouth with invasion of the lingual aspect of the mandible. The correct stage is:
   (a) I
   (b) II
   (c) III
   (d) IV

Lip

36

Bibliography

Anvar BA, et al., "Lip Reconstruction", *Plast Reconstr Surg.*, (2007) 120(4):**57e–64e**. **READ FIRST**.

McGregor IA and McGregor FM, Chapter 5: "The Lips." Cancer of the Face and Mouth. Churchill Livingstone Co. **pp 148–166**.

Luce EA, "Reconstruction of the Lower Lip", *Clinics in Plastic Surgery*, (1995); 22(1):**109–121**.

Sadove RC, Luce EA, McGrath PC, "Reconstruction of the Lower Lip and Chin with the Composite Radial Forearm-Palmaris Longus Free Flap", *Plast Reconstr Surg.*, (1991); 88(2):**210–214**.

Ninkovic M, Spilimbergo S, Ninkovic M, "Lower lip reconstruction: Introduction of a new procedure using a functioning gracilis muscle free flap", *Plast Reconstr Surg.*, (2007); 119(5):**1472–1480**.

Luce EA, "Upper lip reconstruction", *Plast Reconstr Surg.*, (2017); 140: **99–1007**.

Luce EA, Jing XL, Carlson T, "Abbe Flap Reconstruction of the Upper Lip", *Plast Reconstr Surg.*, (2020); 145(3):**606e–607e and Video**.

Supplemental

Salibian A., Zide B., "Elegance in Upper Lip Reconstruction", *Plast Reconstr Surg.*, (2019);143:**572–580**.

Faculty Discussion and Study Guide

Considerable amount of overlap existed among the articles. The following is a collation of questions for all of the articles.

Anatomy

1. The mouth is often described as a sphincter but also is an organ of facial expression. List the muscle(s) responsible for the former as well as the muscle(s) for the latter. (The orbicularis oris is mostly responsible for sphincter function and oral competency aided in a secondary way by the following muscles which are more responsible for facial expression: the depressors/elevators of each side of the lips as well as the depressors and levators of each angle of the mouth. Additional contributions come from the risorius and levator superioris alaeque nasalis. The zygomaticus major and minor contribute to the elevation of the upper lip.)
2. Distinguish between the two lips, upper and lower, in terms of form and function. (The lower lip is a key element of oral continence and has a dramatic amount of sphincter function but is otherwise featureless above the mental crease. The upper lip performs as a more static structure, perhaps as a curtain, and has a topographical landmark, the philtrum as well as some elements of fixation by the alar base(s) of the nose.)
   (a) Describe the aesthetic topography of the upper lip. (The upper lip is thought of as two aesthetic units: the philtrum as one unit and the remaining portion of the lip from philtral column to the nasolabial fold as a lateral aesthetic unit. From the reconstruction perspective, the lateral unit can be subdivided into medial and lateral subunits.)
   (b) Important in an estimation of the percentage of magnitude of a proposed defect, what are the transverse dimensions of the upper and lower lip? (Upper lip 8.0 cm, lower lip 7.5 cm although considerable variation exists. See Fig. 36.1.)

E. Luce, *A Curriculum for Plastic Surgery*, https://doi.org/10.1007/978-3-031-62087-4_36

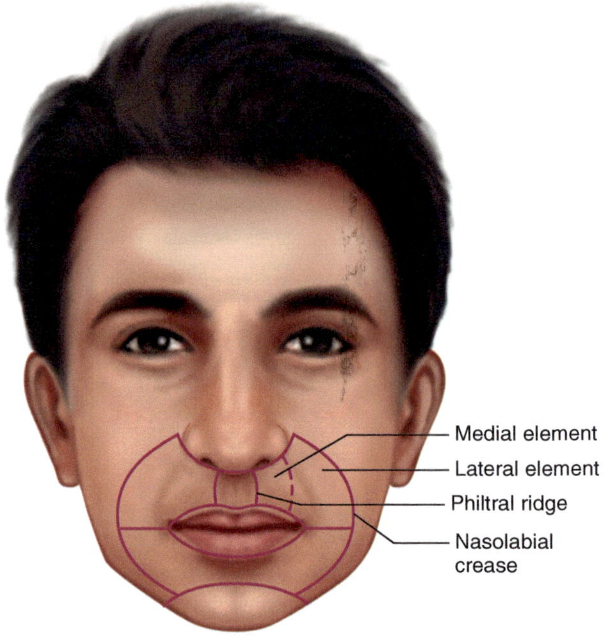

Fig. 36.1 Topography of the upper lip

3. Describe the sensory and motor innervation of the upper and lower lip. (Branches of the infraorbital nerve, a component of the maxillary division of the trigeminal nerve, provide sensory innervation of the upper lip; the mental nerve, the terminal branch of the inferior alveolar nerve, is a component of the mandibular division of the trigeminal and provides sensation to the lower lip. The motor innervation is via the facial nerve, the mandibular and buccal branches to the lower and upper lip, respectively.)
4. The principal blood supply to the lips is through the labial arteries as a branch of what artery? (Facial artery and vein.)
   (a) Where in the cross-section of the lower lip is the labial artery? (On the same transverse plane as the vermilion border *but* on the mucosal side, an important anatomical feature for construction of a cross-lip flap.)
5. What are the histological characteristics unique to the vermilion? (Serves as a junction between keratinized stratified squamous of the epidermis of the skin and the non-keratinized stratified squamous epithelium of the mucosa and is an important landmark that guides accurate alignment in coaptation.)
6. Describe and contrast the lymphatic drainage of the upper lip and lower lip. (The lower lip drains to both the submental and submandibular lymph nodes, yet the submental nodes drain only the very central portion of the lip. The cross-over to the opposite side can be significant even in medial lip lesions. Otherwise, the principal drainage of the lateral portion of the lower lip is to the submandibular nodes and then to the upper anterior cervical nodes or level II. The two halves of the upper lip are embryologically distinct with a central contribution of the fronto-median process and drain to the parotid and upper cervical or perhaps submandibular nodes without contralateral overlap. Contralateral metastasis from an upper lip squamous cell cancer does not occur. The lateral portion of the upper lip may drain in some instances only to the parotid.)
7. You want to launch a study of sentinel lymph node biopsy of carcinoma of the lower lip, using isosulfan blue dye only. What are your prospects for success? Why? (Quite low. Lymphatic drainage of the lower lip has considerable variability with respect to the primary echelon, the most likely location for the sentinel node including upper cervical vs. submandibular, *and* contralateral drainage in more medial lip lesions is not uncommon. In the absence of localization by a gamma probe, locating of the incision for the identification of the blue-stained node would be difficult. Little experience has been published using sentinel lymph node biopsy in carcinoma of the lower lip.)

Pathology

1. Discuss the distribution of squamous and basal cell cancers on the upper and lower lip. (A general figure to remember is that 90% of the basal cell carcinomas of the lips occur on the upper lip, while 90% of squamous cell carcinomas occur on the lower lip.)
2. What is the evidence for an actinic etiology in lower lip cancer? (Occupational, geographic both global and national, actinic changes seen in patients with lip cancer, and the spatial anatomy with respect to the angle of sun rays between upper and lower lip vermilion.)
3. Give a morphologic classification of squamous cell carcinoma of the lip. (Exophytic, ulcerative, verrucous)
   (a) What are some of the unique features of verrucous cancer? (Appearance, namely, exophytic well-defined lesion with usually a large keratin plug; histology is of a well-differentiated squamous cell cancer *without* basement membrane or lamina propria invasion. The behavior of verrucous cancer tends to be indolent and slow-growing with rare metastases.)
   (b) What is spindle cell cancer? (A highly undifferentiated lesion with stromal changes and a virulent clinical course and significantly higher mortality.)
   (c) What is the significance of the morphologic type? (The morphologic type is a general predictive variable of local recurrence and lymph node metastasis. Lymph node metastasis is nearly nonexistent in ver-

rucous cancer, uncommon in exophytic except in very large lesions, and more predominant in ulcerative lesions.)

4. What is Broder's classification of squamous cell cancer of the lip? (A four-level classification determined by the degree of differentiation with histological examination: 1—well, 2—moderate, 3—poor, 4—undifferentiated.)
   (a) Other histologic prognostic findings of importance? (Lymphovascular invasion, perineural invasion, infiltrating rather than pushing borders, thickness greater than 6 mm.)
5. Describe the T classification of lip tumor size. (T_1 less than 2 cm; T_2 2–4 cm; T_3 greater than 4 cm; T_4 invasion of adjacent structures such as the mandible.)
6. Besides the histological characteristics referenced above, what other factors may herald a poor prognosis? (Size greater than 3 cm, lymph node involvement either clinically or pathologically. See below.)
7. What are the predictive factors of the presence of lymph node metastases? (Size, differentiation, upper lip vs. lower lip, histopathology, thickness of tumor, perineural or lymphovascular invasion.)
   (a) Comment on the clinical utility for predicting lymph node metastasis of each. (Size is the most useful clinically. Although, differentiation is a consistent predictor if the lesion is undifferentiated as well as the presence of lymphovascular or perineural invasion. All three are quite, 2–3%, uncommon. As mentioned, thickness greater than 6 mm may herald the presence of lymph node metastasis. Recurrent lesions are also more likely to harbor lymph node metastases, although this factor has not been closely studied.)
8. Give the approximate percentage of lymph node metastases with the following primary size of carcinoma of the lip, assuming a well-differentiated and non-ulcerated primary: 1.5, 3, 4.5 cm. (T_1 1.5 cm—4%, T_2 3 cm—25%, T_3 4.5 cm—60%)
   (a) What are the treatment implications? (Certainly, an elective lymph node dissection cannot be justified in a T_1 or a small T_2 lesion. Serious consideration should be given to the performance of an elective neck dissection in lesions >3 cm. That lymph node dissection can be a suprahyoid or supraomohyoid performed bilaterally.)
9. Give a hierarchy from high to low survival rates in the following situation of lymph node metastases or absence, in a lower lip cancer: Clinically positive on presentation; clinically negative but pathologically positive on neck dissection at initial presentation; subsequently clinically positive on follow-up; remains clinically negative. (The best survival rate of 90–95% is seen in the patient who remains clinically negative. Development of metachronous metastases on follow-up is associated with a 50–60% survival. The patient who presents with clinically negative and pathologically positive nodes has approximately 40–50% 5-year survival. Finally, the most dismal prognosis is clinically positive lymph nodes on presentation which has about a 10% survival rate.)
10. What are the indications for postoperative radiotherapy? (Size, a T_3 lesion, undifferentiated and/or spindle cell with respect to primary tumor characteristics, extracapsular extension of and/or multiple nodal metastasis.)

Treatment: Lower Lip

1. What techniques are available for direct excision, design, and closure? Discuss each including the pros and cons. (Essentially, a V design versus a rectangle with "wings" or a W. V-shaped design is easiest to close but oncologically may be unsafe as the two limbs of the V narrow and diminish the size of the tumor-free margin. A rectangular design requires some type of inferior transverse Burrow's triangle to facilitate closure. The transverse inferior limb can parallel the mental crease and allow a more aesthetic closure than a vertical closure that extends beyond the mental crease.)
2. What is the evidence for a concomitant vermilionectomy or lip shave performed with the excision of a lip squamous cell primary? (The frequency of actinic and precancerous changes in the remaining vermilion—quite common).
   (a) Briefly describe technical maneuvers to avoid vertical notching or narrowing and thinning transversely with a vermilionectomy. (Lip shave is performed to remove severely dysplastic changes in the vermilion which by definition are limited to the mucosa. Excision of mucosa alone and not the immediately adjacent pars marginalis of the orbicularis is the appropriate procedure. Vertical notching can be avoided by the placement of deep sutures through the orbicularis as the primary advancement of the two segments and then the eversion of the skin closure similar to the lower eyelid. Narrowing or thinning transversely probably means a substantial amount of orbicularis and soft tissue have been inappropriately removed and may commit to an advancement tongue flap—not a desirable option.)
3. What is the appropriate margin for a well-defined exophytic lesion of the following size: 1.5, 3.0, 4.5 cm. (6 mm with a T_1 lesion, 8–10 mm with a mid-T_2 lesion, 10 mm or greater with a T_3 lesion of 4.0 cm. All of this assumes a well-defined nonulcerative, non-infiltrative primary.)

4. Draw and contrast a Gillies fan flap and a Karapandzic flap. (A Gillies fan flap attempts to redistribute the remaining lip segments as well as a portion of the upper lip-commissure region into the resultant defect. The donor site defect is closed by rotating the adjacent and lateral cheek tissue into the donor site defect. Karapandzic performs the same procedural maneuver but keeps the lateral and superior incisions more in the aesthetic lines of the face *and* preserves the neurovascular structures to the rotated lip segments. Similar mucosal incisions will provide lining.)
   (a) Limitations of the Karapandzic flap? (May reduce the oral stoma to the point of microstomia. This reviewer's critique is that the incisions extending superiorly and medially on the upper lip are not necessary. The classic Gillies fan flap rotates a denervated lip segment. See Fig. 36.2.)
5. Describe the Webster-Bernard cheek advancement closure of a lower lip defect. (Webster-Bernard consists entirely of bilateral cheek advancement flaps into the lower lip defect. The advancement is accomplished by the excision of Burrow's triangles in both nasolabial folds superiorly and a horizontal incision inferiorly that parallels the mentalis or mental crease. An additional set of Burrow's triangles is excised bilaterally at the lateral extent of the mental crease incision. Since the tension is maximal at the vertical closure of the two advancement flaps, the reconstructive outcome is often a lower lip drawn beneath the upper, rather than a pouting, everted posture.)
6. Describe an Abbé flap from the lower lip to the upper lip including design, blood supply, and inset. (The design can either be as a V, or more frequently, as a rectangle with W "wings," and is based on an intact labial artery and inset into the upper lip defect using the wings in perialar or nasal sill distribution. The flap should be designed to match the entire vertical height of the upper lip to avoid a patchwork appearance. So any individual

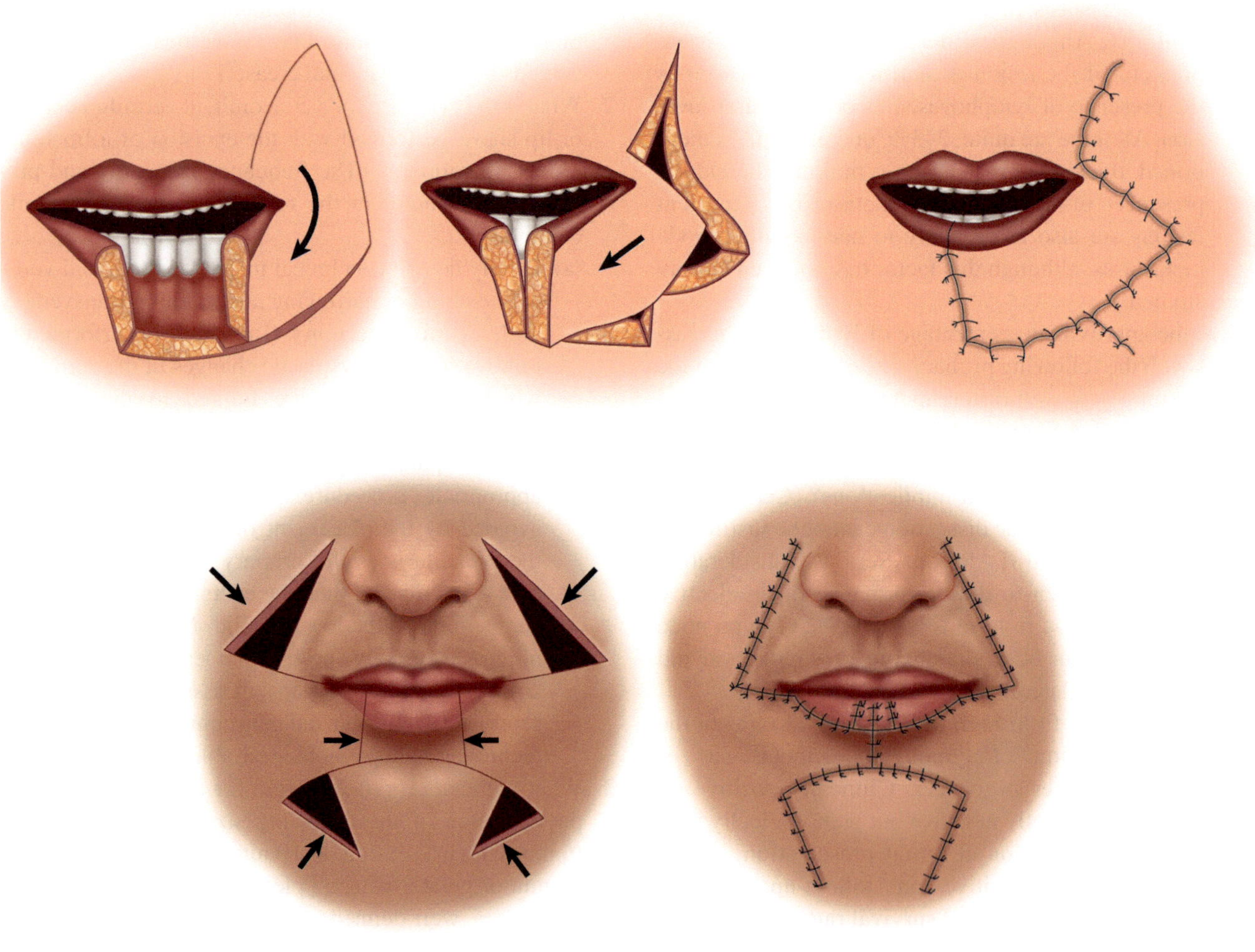

Fig. 36.2 Karapandzic flap

native lip at the alar sill should be excised to permit inset within the shadow of the same.)

(a) How does the design of an Abbé flap taken from the *upper* to the lower lip differ? (One must respect the donor site defect as more complex than the lower lip and usually requires a Burrow's triangle excision in the perialar area and advancement of the lateral upper lip segment into the donor site defect created by raising the Abbé flap. No more than one-fourth of the upper lip can be closed primarily without an undue degree of deformity. Because of the availability of other options, most notably Karapandzic, Abbé flaps are uncommonly harvested from the upper lip.)

7. Describe a reconstructive plan for primary of the following sizes: 1.5, 3.0, 4.5 cm. (For discussion: 1.5 cm—probably primary closure, 3.0 cm—either Abbé flap or if margins are larger, Karapandizic flap; 4.5 cm—assume a lower lip transverse width of 7.5 cm, nasolabial flaps, or free radial forearm flap.)
8. Discuss and describe the use of the radial forearm flap for total lip reconstruction. (Technical points are best relegated to a preoperative conference. In essence, the lower lip and soft tissue are removed as an aesthetic unit and reconstructed with the use of the plantaris tendon as a support sutured into each modiolus.)
9. You resect a carcinoma of the lower lip and close it. Two years later the patient has firm nodularity in the scar consistent with recurrence, but also complains of unremitting pain in the ipsilateral mandibular teeth and lower face with demonstrable diminished sensation over the same area. Diagnosis? (Perineural invasion through the mental nerve, extension along the inferior alveolar nerve, and perhaps extension proximal into the mandibular division of the trigeminal nerve. A CT scan will be necessary to diagnose and delineate.)
10. One of the readings describes the use of the gracilis muscle as a free flap for reconstruction of a total lower lip defect. What are the key points and potential advantages? (The obturator nerve of the gracilis is sutured to the proximal transected marginal mandibular nerve and the author describes as well implanting the stump of the mental nerve into the muscle. The groin flap coverage is provided by a skin graft harvested from the scalp or supra-clavicular area.)

Treatment: Upper Lip

1. Comment on the following for reconstruction of the upper lip: full-thickness skin grafts. (Full-thickness skin grafts in general are an unsatisfactory option for upper lip reconstruction. Even though the contraction of full-thickness skin grafts is minimal, reconstitution of a defect of an aesthetic unit that consists of skin and underlying orbicularis will have a contour deficit. Closure of small defects, less than 1 cm, within the shadow of the nasal sill is a notable exception or a superficial defect of the philtrum.

   Particular care should be undertaken in not excising lesions with an elliptical design. Because of the Rose-Thompson effect, a vertical lengthening will result in an upper lip that is too long and asymmetrical in comparison to the opposite side.)
2. What is the preferred method for closure of an 8 mm full-thickness defect of the philtrum? (Excise the remaining unit, 2–3 mm in females and 3–4 mm in males since the average width is 10 and 11 mm, respectively. The philtrum in toto is then reconstructed with an Abbé flap.)
3. Describe the reconstruction of a 10 mm defect of the medial portion of the lateral aesthetic unit. (Advancement closure can be accomplished with a perialar crescentic excision or Burrow's triangle. Particular attention should be directed toward the avoidance of inadvertent lengthening of the lip or narrowing of the ipsilateral nostril. See Fig. 36.3.)
4. What are the caveats for use, if any, of a nasolabial flap for upper lip reconstruction? (Use of the nasolabial flap should be reserved for subtotal or total defects of the aesthetic unit, should be inferiorly based, and combined with a buccal mucosal flap if lining needs dictate so.)
5. What are the indications for an Abbé flap? (As described above, for the reconstruction of the philtrum as well as defects of greater than 1.5 cm of the lateral unit, assuming a lip width of approximately 7.5 cm and a philtrum width in a male of 12 mm, a defect greater than 1.5 cm will be 50% or greater of that portion of the lip. See Table 36.1.)

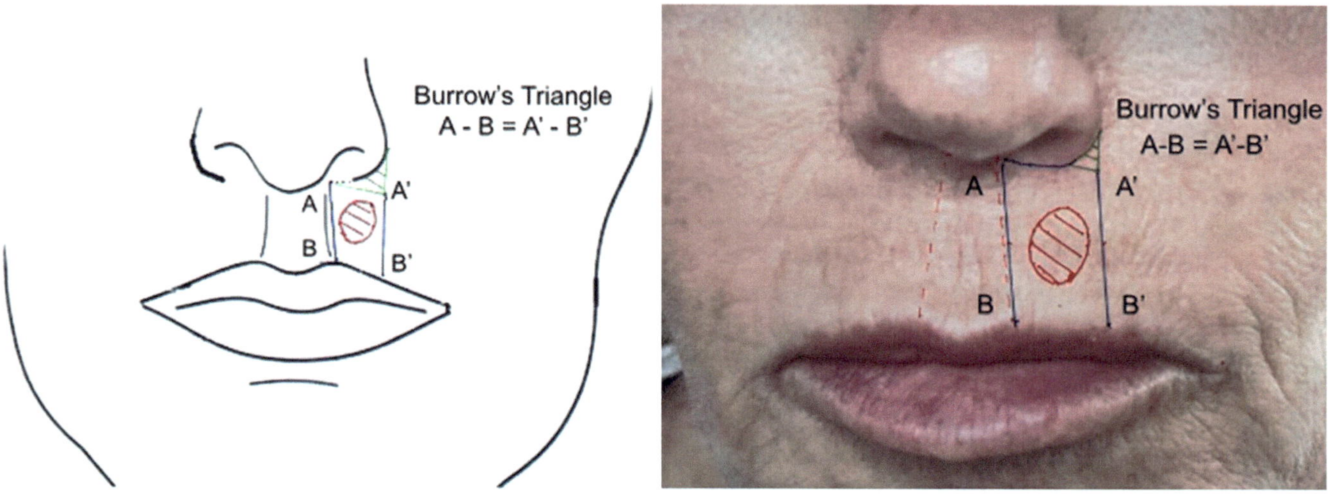

Fig. 36.3 Burrow's triangle

Table 36.1 Reconstructive options for various defects

Defect	Reconstructive options
Philtrum	Abbe flap
Lateral aesthetic unit	
Medial <1.5 cm	Advancement of remaining lip and Burrow Triangle
Medial >1.5 cm	Abbe flap
Lateral aesthetic unit	
Lateral <1.0–1.5 cm	Primary closure
Lateral >1.5 cm	Nasolabial flap

Luce E.A., "Upper Lip Reconstruction", *Plast Reconstr Surg.*, (2017);140(5):p 999–1007. (Reprinted with Permission)

Case-Based Conference

Case 1: Tumor of the Upper Lip

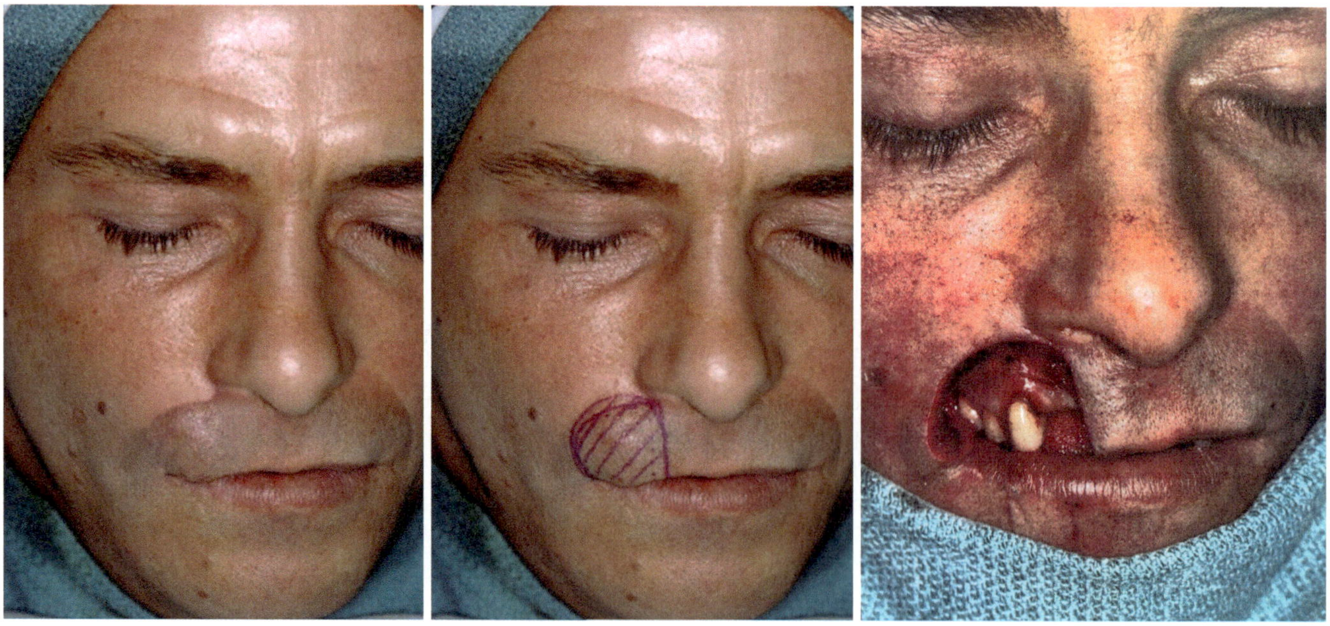

A 36-year-old with a biopsy-proven malignant "adnexal tumor" of the right upper lip.

1. Describe the slide(s), add a focused history (patient is in excellent health), and a focused physical examination.
   (a) Any tests indicated? Justify.
2. What are the oncologic considerations in this case? Consider the most frequent pathologic diagnosis and the anticipated defect in each.
3. Describe the post-resection slide and outline a reconstructive plan.

Case-Based Conference: Discussion

Case 1: Tumor of the Upper Lip

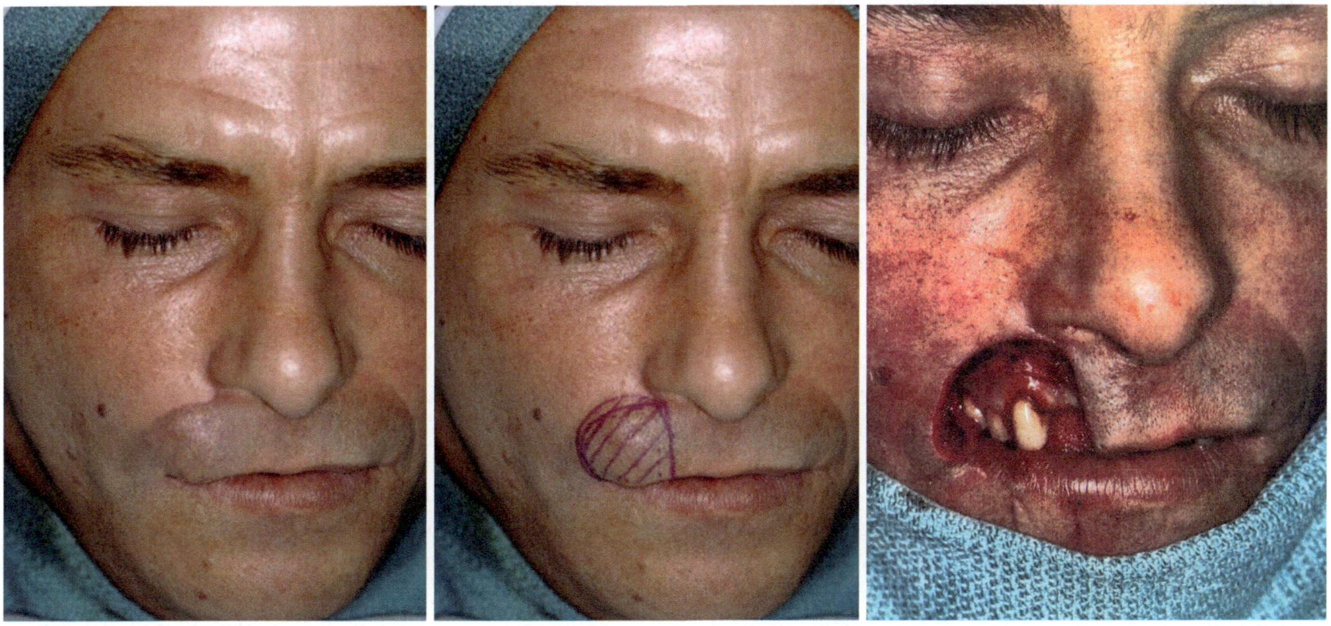

A 36-year-old with a biopsy-proven malignant "adnexal tumor" of the right upper lip.

1. Describe the slide(s), add a focused history (patient is in excellent health), and a focused physical examination. (The two photos demonstrate a full-facial view with a slightly oblique perspective to the patient's right—a white male who appears to be of the stated age. The eyes are closed. Given the preamble, attention is drawn to the right upper lip. The findings are subtle in a two-dimensional photo but a suggestion of fullness is present in the lateral aspect, particularly superior. The fullness would appear to be approximately 1.5 × 1.0 cm. No skin changes or ulcerations are evident except for a slightly violaceous transverse band of 1–2 mm crossing the length of the right upper lip. The color and appearance are sufficiently uniform that the presence may be an artifact. No other lesions or deformities are evident. The second slide adds lines drawn to outline the philtral columns. In addition, a dotted line has been drawn around the circumference of the palpable tumor that, again, appears to be 1.5 × 1.0 cm.

   The history of the present illness would include questions re duration as perceived by the patient, rate of enlargement if any, pain if present including distribution, and details about the biopsy including access. The past medical history questions are designed to detect comorbidities, medications, and a social history is obtained about tobacco/drug use and vocation. The physical exam would begin with observation of the lip during pursing and smiling and an examination of the labial mucosa by eversion of the lip. Bimanual palpation is accomplished with a finger intraoral and another externally to determine the firmness and mobility of the mass. Palpation of the lymph node basin includes parotid, submandibular, jugulo-digastric, and the remaining anterior cervical chain. A complete oral examination of the floor of the mouth, tongue, and hard and soft palate completes the head and neck assessment.)

(a) Any tests indicated? Justify. (The pathology should be reviewed and, if some ambiguity exists, a second opinion requested. An accurate pathologic diagnosis is crucial in the determination of the treatment plan. The justification of imaging would hinge to a substantial degree on the pathology. See below. If so indicated, an MRI, preferred to a CT scan, would delineate the extent of the tumor.)

2. What are the oncologic considerations in this case? Consider the most frequent pathologic diagnosis and the anticipated defect in each. (As mentioned above, the histopathologic diagnosis will substantially dictate the management plan. The term "adnexal tumor" is a catch-all phrase that could include a variety of pathologic entities of both skin adnexal structures and the minor salivary glands. Although neoplasms of the skin adnexal structures can be benign or malignant, the malignant tumors characteristically present with some elements of skin changes including nodular and/or ulcerative variants. A benign tumor conceivably could present as the clinical picture of this patient.

   Neoplasms of the minor salivary glands are substantially more likely to be malignant than benign. The most common benign tumor of salivary gland origin in the upper lip is pleomorphic adenoma or benign mixed tumor. The predominant malignant tumor is adenoid cystic carcinoma followed by mucoepidermoid. The aggressiveness of the latter, mucoepidermoid, hinges on the degree of differentiation on histologic examination or grade; high-grade lesions are substantially more likely to recur and metastasize. The former, adenoid cystic carcinoma, has a propensity for subclinical extension along the course of peripheral nerves with resultant repeated local recurrences. Because of the relentless nature of the disease, late survival of 10–15 years is dismal. A clinical clue in the scenario under consideration would be pain or dysesthesia over the distribution of the infraorbital nerve, perhaps further defined with an MRI.

   To anticipate the defect of these pathologic possibilities, the diagnosis of pleomorphic adenoma will require a full-thickness resection of the lip with a small margin of normal tissue since the apparent capsule is in reality a pseudo capsule created by compression of the tumor. The malignant diagnoses of adenoid cystic and mucoepidermoid require a minimum of 1 cm margin. Wider margins in adenoid cystic do not result in a lower recurrence rate. As such, the anticipated defect in pleomorphic adenoma is probably 2 cm, and given a malignant diagnosis, approximately 3 cm or the majority of the lateral subunit of the upper lip.

   The other oncologic consideration is the management of the regional lymph nodes with a diagnosis of a malignant primary. As discussed above, tumors of the minor salivary gland of the upper lip are predominantly malignant, most commonly adenoid cystic and mucoepidermoid. The former can metastasize to lymph nodes but does so late in the disease process and characteristically after repeated extensive local recurrences. The latter, mucoepidermoid, can frequently metastasize, particularly if poorly differentiated, and that potential must be considered in the development of the treatment plan. Given the distinct rarity of tumors of the minor salivary gland origin in the upper lip, little information is available to provide a treatment pathway. So, some generalities are necessary.

   If enlarged lymph nodes are clinically evident, neck dissection is indicated followed by postoperative radiotherapy. Palpable lymph nodes in the presence of a malignant primary almost universally represent a metastasis with extracapsular extension, setting the stage for recurrent regional disease and the necessity of administration of adjuvant therapy and therapeutic radiation. Management of a clinically negative neck, N_0, in the presence of a primary with a significant incidence of lymph node metastasis compels addressing the regional lymph nodes, in the instance of the upper lip, the parotid, and neck. Certainly, that objective can be accomplished with a selective neck dissection. Yet, the circumstances of a highly malignant tumor will dictate radiation of the primary after resection and reconstruction. If so, the therapeutic radiation ports can encompass the treatment of the regional lymph nodes as well as the primary. Adenoid cystic carcinoma is a notable exception. Adenoid cystic carcinoma is classified in descending order of differentiation as tubular or cribriform, mixed, and solid based on the histologic appearance. The indication for postoperative radiotherapy applied to the primary site can hinge on this histologic subtype. Regardless, postoperative radiotherapy to the lymph nodes is not indicated because of the infrequency of lymphatic metastasis until late in the course.

   More globally in head and neck oncology, some of the treatment quandaries in the management of the lymph node basin can be drawn from the management of squamous cell carcinoma. Determination of the presence of lymph node metastases in squamous cell carcinoma of the upper aerodigestive tract has been addressed with the utilization of sentinel lymph node biopsy. Although the practice has been adopted in some centers, principally European, the experience cannot be directly translated to this case.)

3. Describe the post-resection slide and outline a reconstructive plan. (The slide is the same view although perhaps slightly closer to the patient but with an obvious resection defect of the right upper lip. The defect is full-thickness with exposure of the underlying alveolar ridge

and dentition. The dimensions of the defect are considerable. The lateral extent is beyond and into a centimeter of the adjacent cheek and superiorly to the alar groove. The medial margin is slanted downward to a point on the vermilion several millimeters lateral to the cupid's bow on the right.

The aesthetic units of the upper lip consist of a central philtrum and a lateral unit, divided into a relatively fixed medial subunit and a more mobile lateral subunit. The magnitude of the defect can be quantified as a proportion of the right upper lip by an assumption that the lateral portion, lateral to the philtrum, is approximately 3 cm. The defect would appear to retain a remnant of approximately 0.5 cm inferiorly and 1.0 cm superiorly or 60–80% of the lateral lip plus a centimeter of cheek. Advancement repair or closure can inadvertently lengthen vertically the upper lip at the repair site. An elliptically oriented excision will, particularly if the excision includes skin only, lengthen the free border of the lip. A rectangular design with the superior transverse limb at the nasal sill is preferable. The inferior transverse limb of the rectangle is the free border of the lip. The height of the vertical lateral limb measured from the vermilion should equal the medial limb or the height of the philtral column as measured from the white roll to the base of the columella. The vertical excess lateral and superior is excised as a perialar crescentic or Burrow's triangle, also facilitating the advancement of the lateral lip remnant and adjacent cheek. The magnitude of the defect as pictured would appear to preclude an advancement repair.

If a two-stage lip switch or Abbé flap is deemed necessary, the size of the defect dictates the size of the flap. In this case, the anticipated defect of 2.5–3.0 cm implies a flap of 1.5 cm harvested from the central lower lip and pedicled on the ipsilateral labial artery. With the knowledge of the anatomical location of the vessel at the level of the vermilion but on the mucosal aspect, a near-definitive inset can be performed with a narrow pedicle, divided 2 weeks later.)

Intraoperative

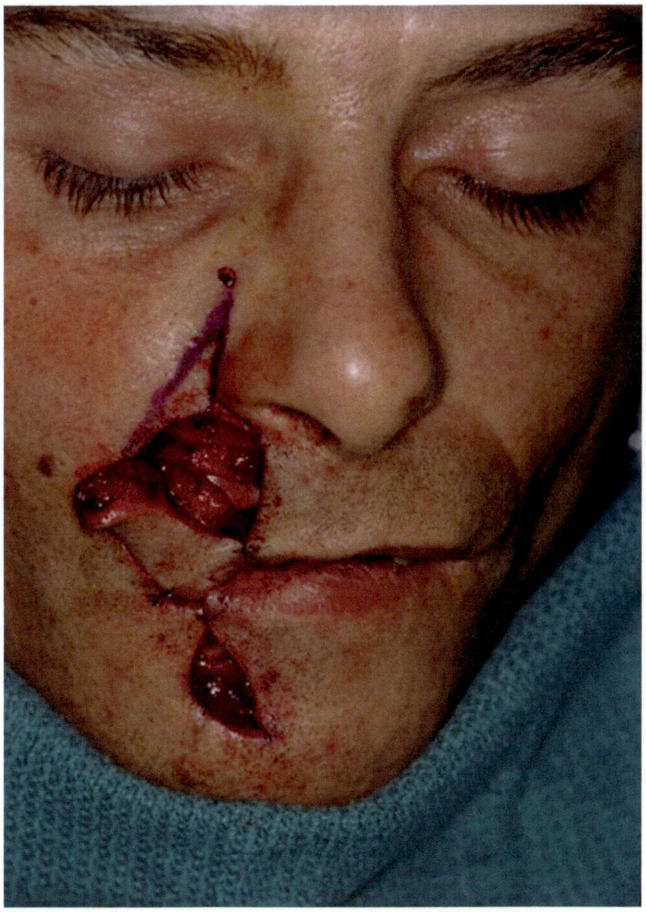

A single full-face frontal view illustrates the rotation of an Abbe flap harvested from the lateral lower lip, in preparation for inset into the defect. Also, the residual markings of the proposed Burow's triangle are evident, a testimony that cheek advancement was under consideration.

Postoperative (3 Months)

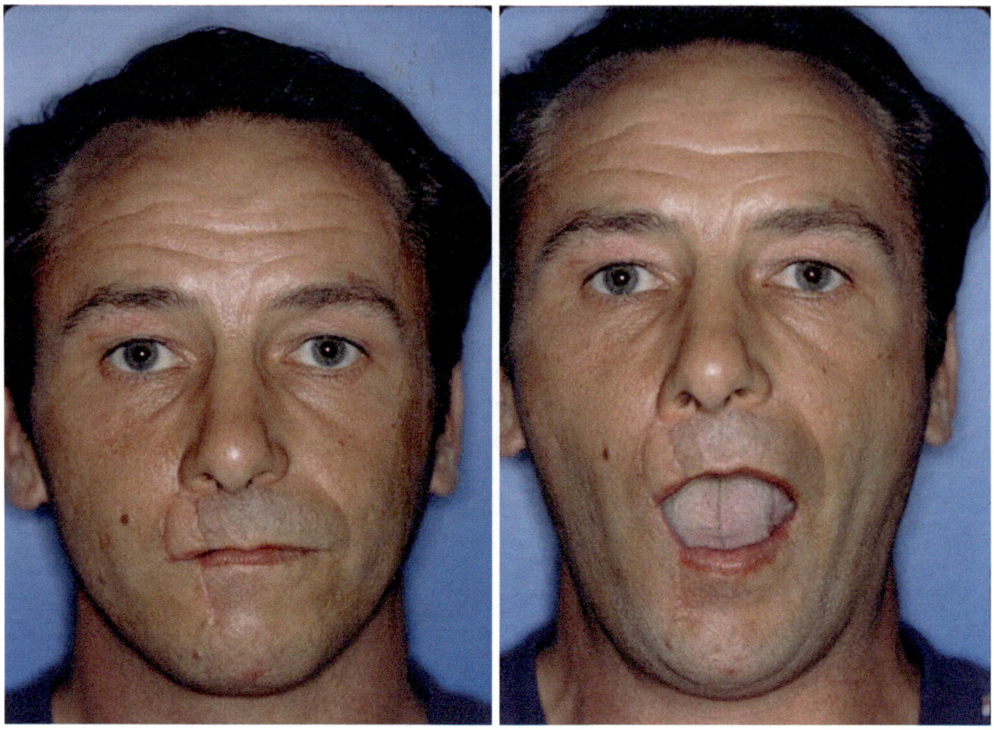

The two photos are with the lips closed and full mouth opening. In the first, the flap is well-healed with adequate restoration of transverse lip length, and there is no distortion of the anatomical landmarks, although the outline of the flap is perceptible. The donor site incisional scar is acceptable. The second photo demonstrates no limitation of opening or microstomia.

Case-Based Conference

Case 2: Ca of the Lower Lip

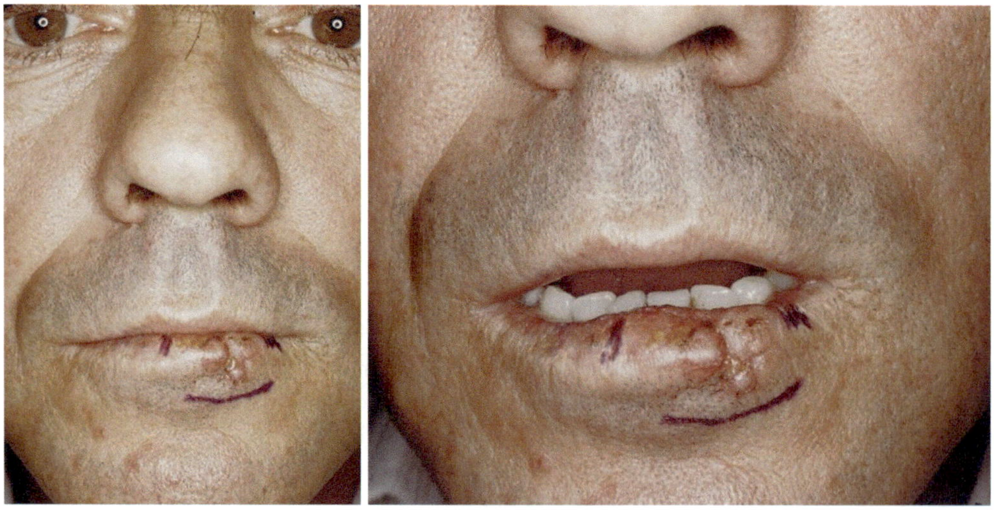

A48-year-old with a biopsy-proven recurrent squamous cell carcinoma of the lower lip. The ink marks delineate the extent of the induration.

1. Describe the slide(s), add a focused history (patient is in excellent health), and a focused physical examination.
   (a) Any tests indicated? Justify.
2. What are the oncologic considerations in this case?
3. Outline a reconstructive plan. Include a plan B if your inquisitor is not satisfied with plan A.

Case-Based Conference: Discussion

Case 2: Ca of the Lower Lip

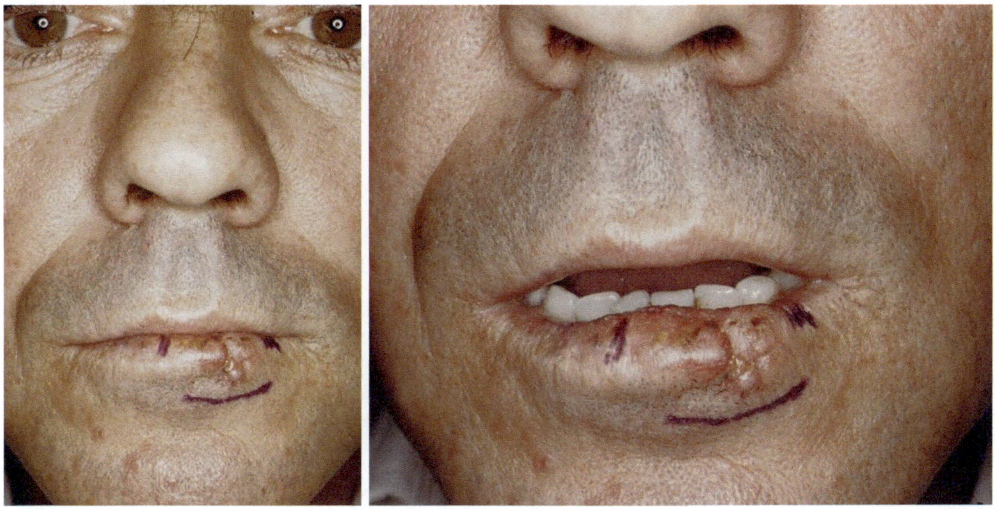

A 48-year-old with a biopsy-proven recurrent squamous cell carcinoma of the lower lip.

1. Describe the slide(s), add a focused history (patient is in excellent health), and a focused physical examination. (Middle-aged male without evident advanced actinic skin changes with a poorly defined lesion about 2 cm in size on the left lower lip that includes vermilion-mucosa with nodular extension into the adjacent skin. Has ink markings on the left lip about 5–7 mm short of the commissure, another horizontal ink mark above the mental crease, and an additional vertical ink mark about the mid-portion of the right lip. *No* scars are evident. Has several crusting changes on the remainder of the lip. Add a clinically focused exam. Patient is in good health. History re: last excision, any postoperative radiotherapy, presently any facial or dental pain, smoking; physical exam of palpation of the lesion, submental, submandibular, and cervical lymph node-bearing areas, the performance of a good intraoral exam including sensation over the distribution of the inferior alveolar nerve, possible indirect laryngoscopy.)
   (a) Any tests indicated? Justify. (In the absence of palpable adenopathy or a fixed status of the primary lesion, debatable. CT scan of the neck may detect occult lymphadenopathy. If a smoker, CT scan of the chest is justifiable.) Other tests? (Review of the histology on biopsy for differentiation, lymphovascular invasion, thickness greater than 6 mm.)
2. What are the oncologic considerations in this case? (The two considerations are the magnitude of the lesion resection and the status of the regional nodes. With respect to the latter, some predictive factors of regional lymph node metastasis have been described and include the degree of differentiation, thickness of the primary, namely, greater than 6 mm, the size of the primary as well as the gross characteristics; exophytic, less likely and ulcerative-infiltrative, more likely, and the presence of lymphovascular invasion. The grossly poorly defined nature of the lesion, apparent infiltration into the soft tissue of the skin, and the recurrent nature would all increase the likelihood of regional metastasis. The use of sentinel lymph node sampling in head and neck cancer in general and lip cancer specifically has not been widely adopted. Because of the cross-over of lymphatic drainage, lateralization of a prophylactic dissection is difficult, and bilateral neck dissection, even if selected, has some significant attendant morbidity. One compromise approach is bilateral suprahyoid neck dissection, namely, dissection of the level II

cervical nodes and contents of the submandibular and submental triangles.

The margins should be quite wide including inferiorly at the mental crease. A lip shave should be added excising the vermilion of the remaining lip, since vermilionectomy has appeared to lower the occurrence of new cancerous lesions. The photo would seem to indicate a resection of approximately 5 cm of the lower lip.)

3. Outline a reconstructive plan. Include a plan B if your inquisitor is not satisfied with plan A. (For a 7.5 cm lower lip, a 5 cm resection would be two-thirds or 67% of the lip. Available methods for reconstruction include an Abbe/or cross-lip flap and Karapandzic advancement. Both have benefits and liabilities. The maximal size Abbe from the upper lip and still allowing primary closure would be approximately 2 cm or one-fourth of the 8 cm transverse diameter upper lip. Supplementing the lower lip remnant of 2.5 cm, one-third, with an additional 2 cm creates a 4.5 cm lip, somewhat small particularly for a younger patient. The other liability is the two-stage nature of the reconstruction and the necessity of the two lips adhered for the requisite 2–3 weeks. A Karapandzic procedure offers a single-stage approach, preserves innervation in the advanced segments, but also may create microstomia. Free tissue transfer such as a radial forearm flap would be suitable for a larger defect, although perhaps a highly sophisticated treatment plan as an innervated prefabricated platysma flap would be an option in the future. Recent work centers on the use of the innervated gracilis flap with coverage with a supraclavicular pedicled flap.)

Intraoperative

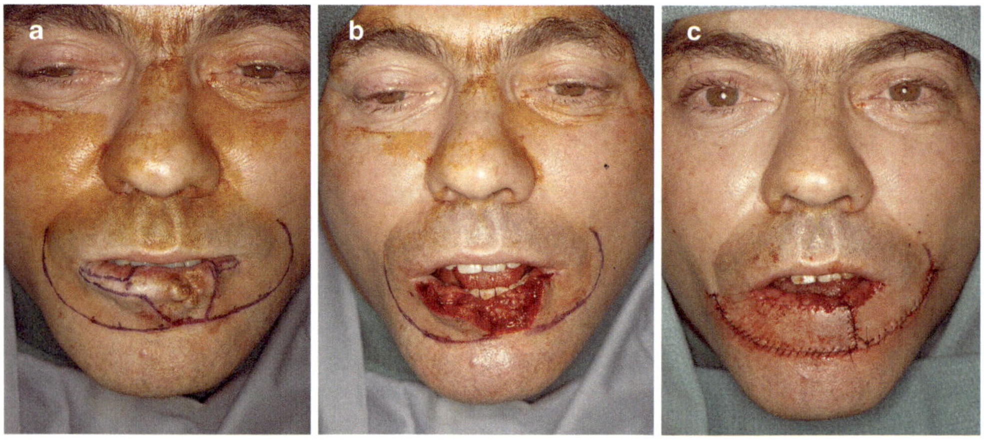

The three photos illustrate the proposed excision, defect, and reconstruction. The first outlines a wedge resection of the primary, en bloc with a total vermilionectomy. The resection appears to encompass about two-thirds of the lip. Also marked out is a Karapandzic rotation-advancement closure. The second photo is of the defect and the third closure. All three illustrate the performance of the procedure under local anesthesia.

Postoperative (6 Months)

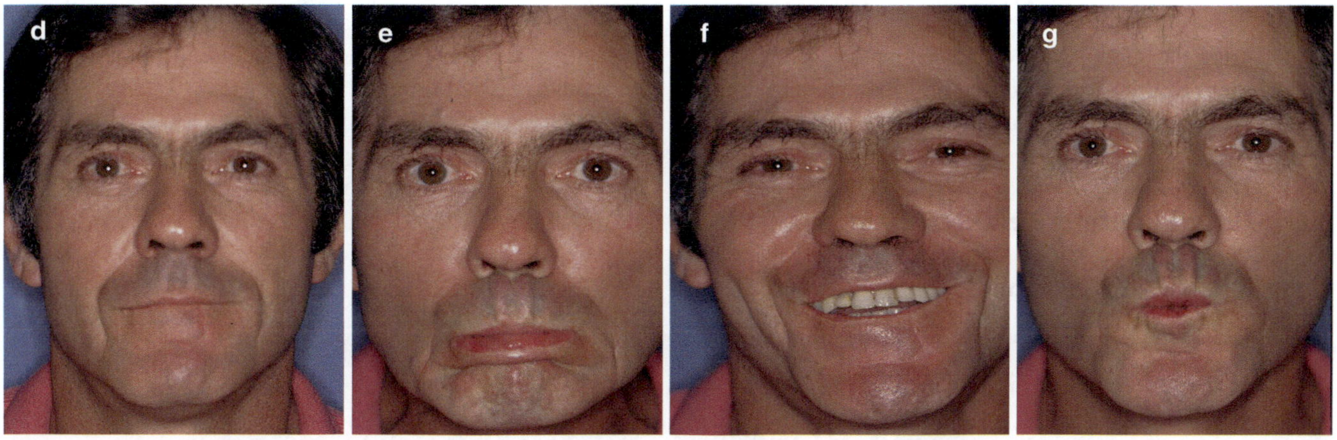

The two postoperative photos depict the result with a slight smile and lips closed, a broad smile, dynamic eversion of the lower lip, and puckering. The result is aesthetically and functionally excellent.

Case-Based Conference

Case 3: Basal Cell Ca Upper Lip

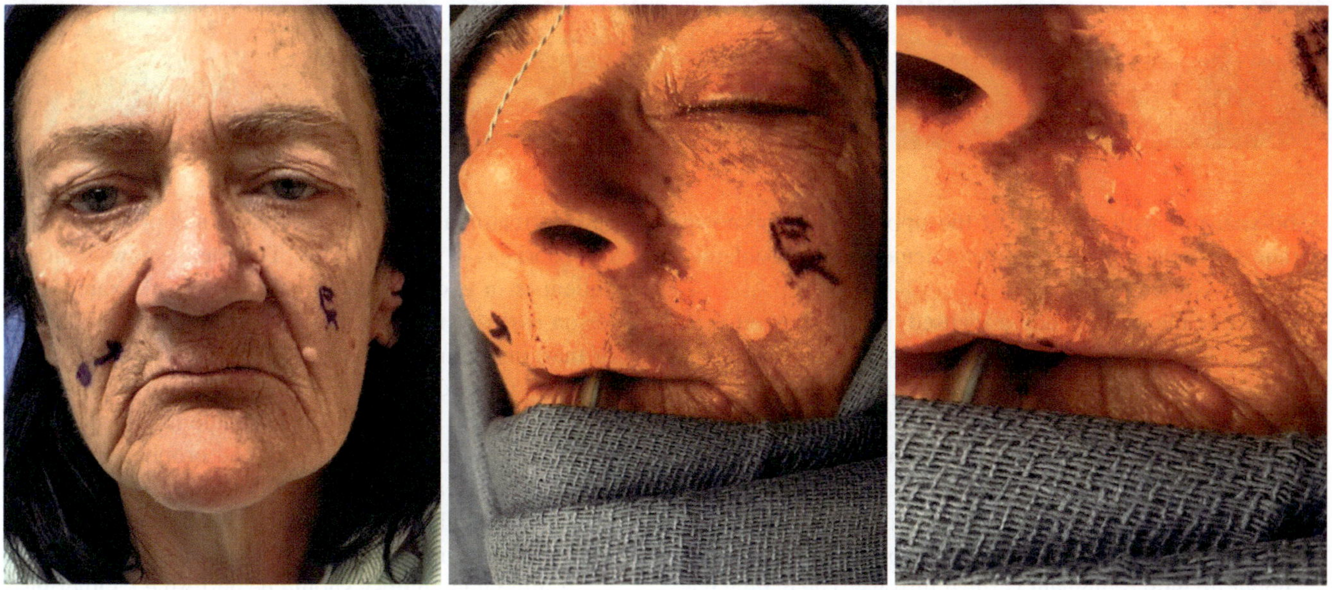

A 60-year-old with a lesion of the upper lip of unknown duration. Patient smokes ½ ppd and denies health problems.

1. Describe the slide(s), add a focused history (patient is in excellent health), and a focused physical examination.
   (a) Any tests indicated? Justify.
2. Describe the anticipated defect in aesthetic terms. What are the oncologic considerations in this case? The actual defect will be presented at the conference.
3. Outline a reconstructive plan. Include a plan B if your inquisitor is not satisfied with plan A.

Case-Based Conference: Discussion

Case 3: Basal Cell Ca Upper Lip

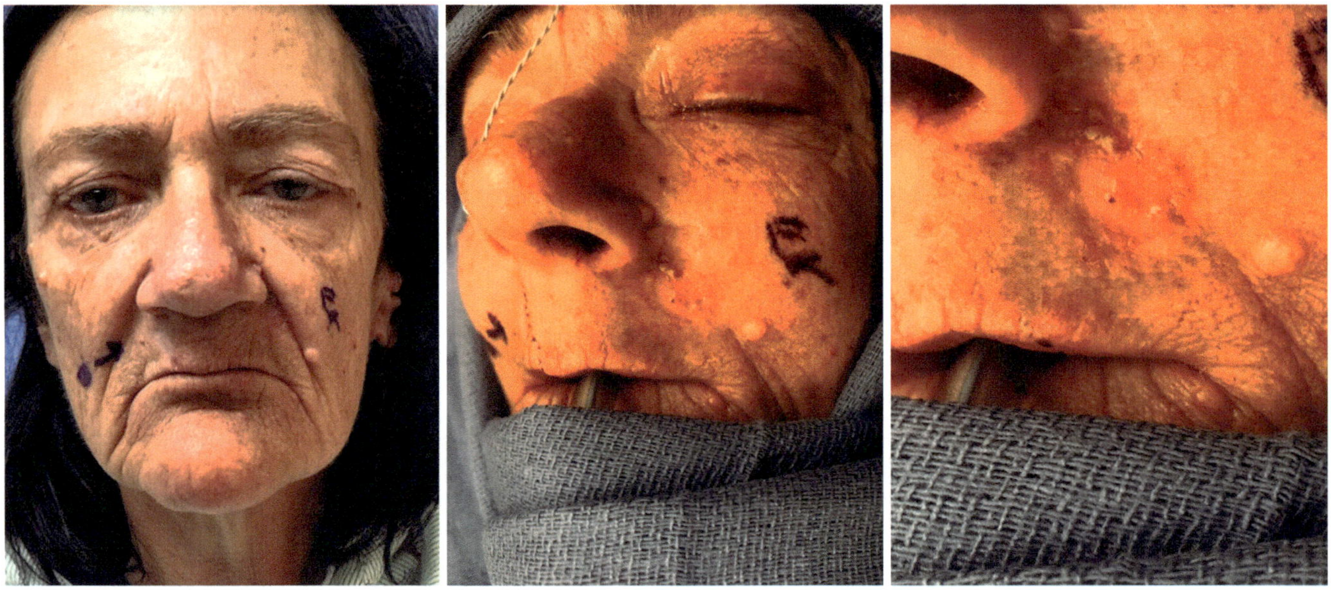

A 60-year-old with a lesion of the upper lip of unknown duration. Patient smokes ½ ppd and denies health problems.

1. Describe the slide(s), add a focused history (patient is in excellent health), and a focused physical examination. (The first slide demonstrates a woman who appears her stated age with a scaling lesion of the lateral upper lip and an adjacent deep nasolabial fold with some overhanging cheek skin. The other features are a small, 2–3 mm pink, shallow lesion of the medial right upper lip. Other notable features are signs of actinic and/or tobacco damage of the upper lip with prominent vertical furrows. The patient has lax upper eyelid skin and bilateral lid ptosis. The next two slides are intraoperative and the lesion in question is more apparent in a nearly full-face photo and a close-up of the left lip and immediately adjacent cheek. The lesion in question appears superficial and poorly demarcated. The dimensions are not distinct but appear to be approximately 1.5 cm. Two small, 1 mm, papillomatous changes are apparent at the superior border of the lesion.

   The history would mostly center on other skin cancers in the past and risk factors such as family history, prior cancer treatment with chemotherapy, and prior treatment for psoriasis with UV light. The stem shows that the patient is in excellent health. The physical exam of the lesion assesses for palpable thickness and ascertainment of margins with magnification. The facial skin is examined for the presence of synchronous lesions including the right upper lip. Given the probable long-term smoking history, a careful oral cavity and oropharynx examination as well as palpation of the lymph node-bearing areas of the neck is mandatory.)
   (a) Any tests indicated? Justify. (Lacking a diagnosis, a 2 mm punch biopsy should be performed. Otherwise, other than a screening chest X-ray, electrocardiogram (EKG), and routine labs, no additional tests are necessary.)
2. Describe the anticipated defect in aesthetic terms. What are the oncologic considerations in this case? The actual defect will be presented at the conference. (The lesion appears to be a non-melanotic skin cancer and given the location, most likely a basal cell carcinoma and more specifically, the morpheaform variant. A preliminary biopsy as mentioned above, will confirm that diagnosis. The

gross margins are outlined in the operating room with loupe magnification and 6 mm margins are added to the discernible edge of the lesion. The additional oncologic consideration is the depth which should include underlying muscle including the orbicularis and more laterally and superiorly the elevator of the upper lip. Mucosa and submucosa are retained. Given the morphologic subtype, morpheaform, the appropriate plan would be either a referral to a Mohs dermatologist or a delayed reconstruction after excision and placement of a dressing that permits a careful pathologic assessment of margins on permanent section. Reconstruction is performed 48–72 h later.)

3. Outline a reconstructive plan. Include a plan B if your inquisitor is not satisfied with plan A. (The aesthetic units of the upper lip consist of a central philtrum and a lateral unit, divided into a relatively fixed medial subunit and a more mobile lateral subunit. The anticipated defect in this instance is the entire medial subunit and a portion of the adjacent lateral subunit. The lesion appears to be approx. 1.5 cm and with the included margins the defect would be 2.5–2.7 cm, although the surgeon should be prepared for a very possible larger defect. Defects of this magnitude will probably require an Abbé flap harvested from the lower lip. The guidelines hinge from an assumption of an 8 cm transverse length of a normal upper lip that permits closure of a 25% defect or 2 cm primarily. Defects, other than the philtrum, of 1.5 cm or less can be addressed with advancement closure, 1.5–2 cm depending on the age of the patient, and laxity of remaining upper lip and cheek may also be closed with attention to detail as outlined below. Larger defects of >2 cm will probably require an Abbé flap.

   Advancement closure can inadvertently lengthen vertically the upper lip at the repair site. An elliptically oriented excision will, particularly if the excision includes skin only, lengthen the free border of the lip. A rectangular design with the superior transverse limb at the nasal sill is preferable. The inferior transverse limb of the rectangle is the free border of the lip. The height of the vertical lateral limb measured from the vermilion should equal the medial limb or the height of the philtral column as measured from the white roll to the base of the columella. The vertical excess lateral and superior is excised as a perialar crescentic or Burrow's triangle, also facilitating the advancement of the lateral lip remnant and adjacent cheek.

   If a two-stage lip switch or Abbé flap is necessary, the size of the defect dictates the size of the flap. In this case, the anticipated defect of 2.5 cm implies a flap of 1.5 cm harvested from the central lower lip and pedicled on the ipsilateral labial artery. With the knowledge of the anatomical location of the vessel at the level of the vermilion but on the mucosal aspect, a near-definitive inset can be performed with a narrow pedicle, divided 2 weeks later.)

Intraoperative

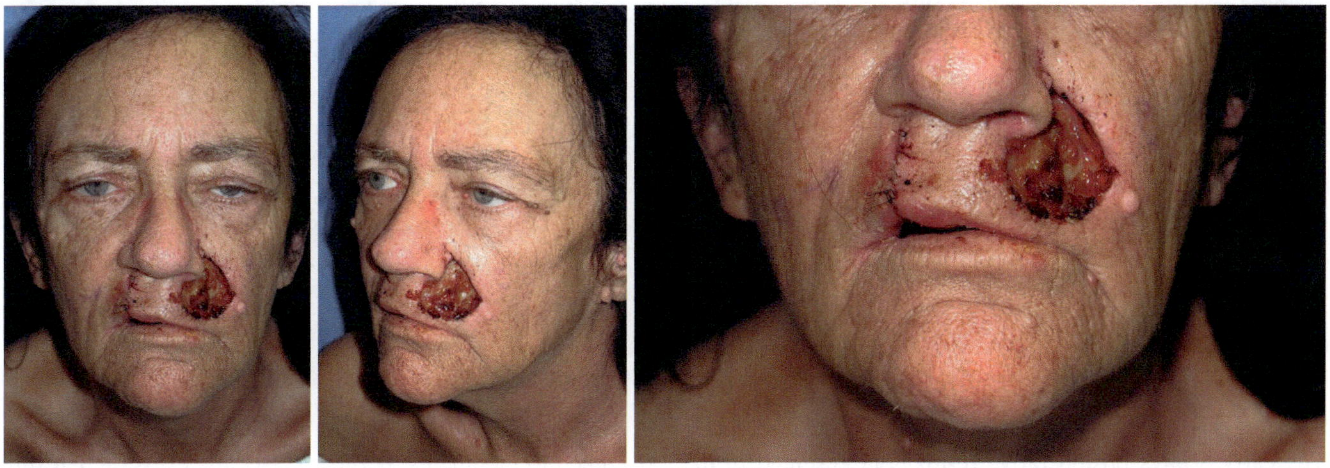

The three photos, full-face frontal, oblique, and close-up of nose, lips, and chin demonstrate the defect post-excision 48 h, with the final sections assuring the tumor was completely excised. A vertical primary closure has been completed on the right upper lip with some shortening. The defect of the left side extends from about 5 mm lateral to the philtrum to the nasal-cheek border with some extension, again 5 mm, into the medial cheek. The defect involves the entire vertical height of the lip with a vermilion and 3–4 mm of inferior cutaneous lip intact. Superiorly, the defect extends several millimeters above the alar base. The nasal sill and the mucosa are intact.

Since the philtrum on average is about 1.5 mm wide and the total upper transverse width is approximately 7.5–8.0 cm, the defect encompasses all of the lateral subunit and a majority of the medial subunit.

Postoperative (5 Days and 2 Months)

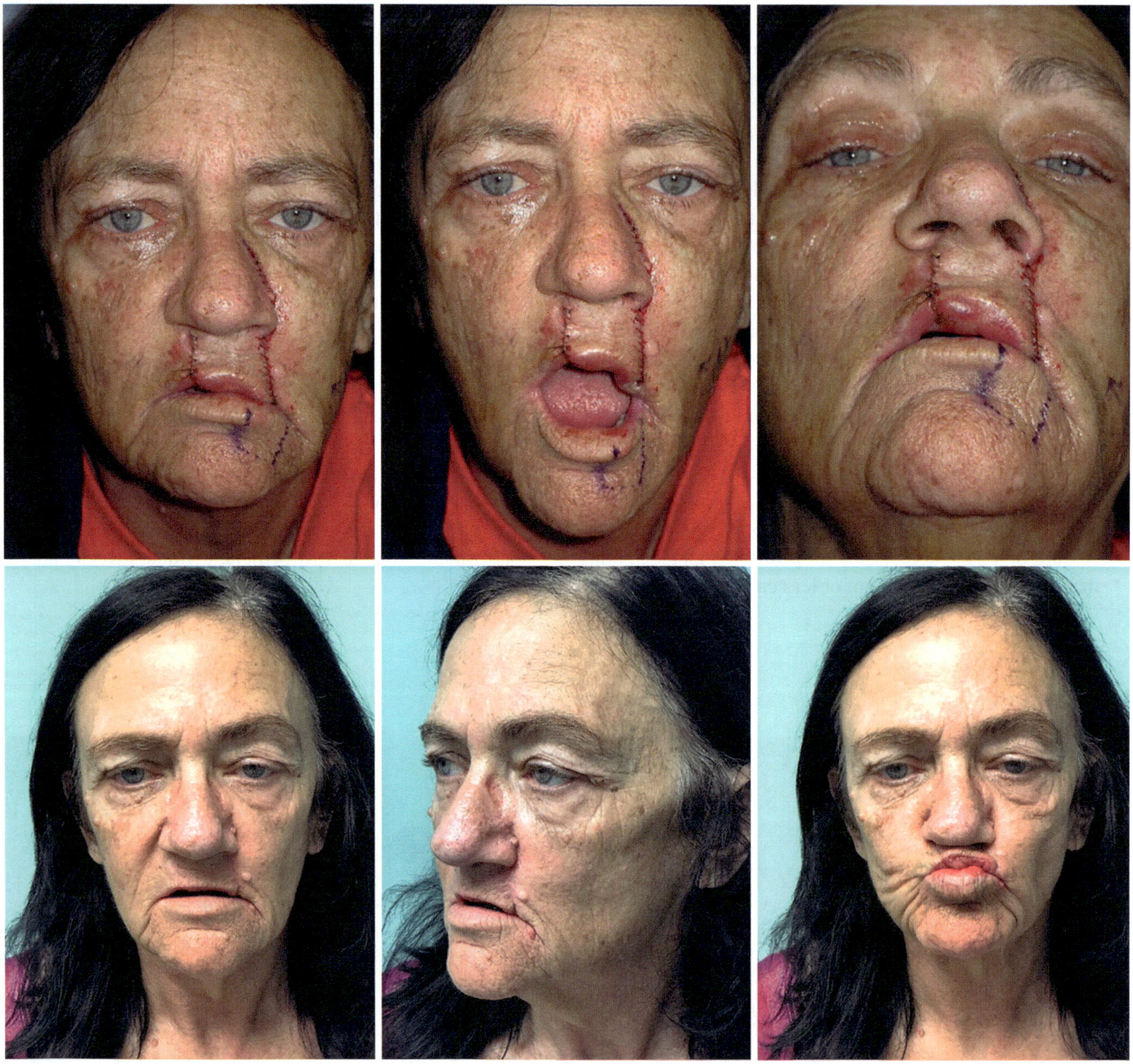

The early 5 days postoperative result is represented in the three photos, full face, oblique, and submental vertex. An Abbe flap has been marked on the left lower lip but closure has been performed with cheek advancement as indicated by the medial movement of the nevus located just lateral to the lateral edge of the defect and the intraoperative views. No Burrow's triangle was necessary since the defect was designed to include the perialar crescentic excision. Closure was continued superiorly in the nasal-jugal groove. In the submental vertex view some minor flaring of the alar base is present.

In the later postoperative, at 2 months, photos show that the shortening of the closure of the right lip has resolved. The reconstruction of the left lip with cheek advancement represents a highly satisfactory outcome with normal positioning of the commissure, symmetry of vermilion, mucosa, and white lip, no vertical or transverse deficiency, and a good functional result.

In-Service Examination

1. The lymphatic drainage to the regional lymph nodes of the upper and lower lip
   (a) Both drain to both the parotid and cervical nodes
   (b) The upper lip drains exclusively to parotid
   (c) The lower lip drains exclusively to the submental nodes
   (d) Upper lip drains to both the parotid and cervical nodes
2. What is the appropriate oncologic treatment for a T_3, 4.0 cm, squamous cell carcinoma lesion of the lower lip?
   (a) Radiotherapy
   (b) Wide local excision
   (c) Wide local excision, selective neck dissection
   (d) Wide local excision, selective neck dissection, and postoperative radiotherapy
3. An Abbe transposition flap to the upper lip:
   (a) Optimally designed to rotate clockwise into a left-side defect with counterclockwise to a right-side defect
   (b) Medial or lateral positioning of the pedicle is not a consequence
   (c) The blood supply is the angular artery
   (d) The pedicle can be located directly at the level of the vermilion

37 Mandibular Reconstruction

Bibliography

Potter JK, Chapter 60: "Mandibular Reconstruction", Bagheri SC, Bell RB, and Khan HA, Current Therapy in Oral and Maxillofacial Surgery, Elsevier Saunders, (2012), **pgs. 483–491 (Junior Residents Only)**.

Cordeiro PG, Henderson PW, Matros E, "A 20-Year Experience with 202 Segmental Mandibulectomy Defects: A Defect Classification System, Algorithm for Flap Selection, and Surgical Outcomes", *Plast Reconstr Surg.*, (2018);141(4):**571e–581e**.

Sinno S, Rodriguez ED, "Nuances and Pearls of the Free Fibula Osteoseptocutaneous Flap for Reconstruction of a High-Energy Ballistic Injury Mandible Defect", *Plast. Reconstr. Surg.*, (2016); 137(1):**280 Videos 1, 4, and 6 ONLY**.

Brown J.S., Ch. 42 "Iliac flap", Flaps and Reconstructive Surgery, Second ED, Wei FC and Mardini S, Elsevier Saunders, (2017); **pgs. 464–473**.

Largo RD, Garvey PB, "Updates in Head and Neck Reconstruction", *Plast. Reconstr. Surg.*, (2018); 141(2): **271e–273e, 279e–283e and Videos 2, 3 ONLY**.

Day KM, Kelley PK, Harshbarger RJ, "Advanced Three-Dimensional Technologies in Craniofacial Reconstruction", *Plast. Reconstr. Surg.*, (2021); 148(1):**94e–101e, Videos 1–3, Fig. 1 ONLY (Video 4 for gamers only)**.

Salgado CJ, Chim H, Mardini S, Wei F, Chapter 52: "Fibula Flap", Flaps and Reconstructive Surgery, Elsevier Saunders, (2017):**596–612 ONLY**.

Videos

Wei FC, Mardini S., "Ch. 19: Fibula flap for obliteration and osseous reconstruction of a persistent frontal basilar fracture infection associated with nasofrontal outflow tract obstruction", *Flaps and Reconstructive Surgery*, Elsevier Saunders, (2009): (**Minutes**: 17:40–31:10 ONLY).

Faculty Discussion and Study Guide

Editor's Note: Mandibular reconstruction is also included in Chap. 44.

Mandibular Defects

1. What is the method of classification of mandibular defects? (The simplest classification is anterior defects from, for example, canine or first bicuspid to the counterpart on the opposite side; lateral defects from a point anteriorly to the posterior dentition, for example, the molars; and posterior defects extending from a variable point in the posterior dentition and include a variable amount of the ascending ramus. With the exception of benign bone tumors, mandibular defects are attended by a component of loss of intraoral lining, skin coverage, or both. The addition of a letter "A" through "D" designates the soft-tissue defect: A—no defect; B—intraoral defect only; C—skin defect only; D—both. The classification adds a 1 or 2 to the IIB group, designating if two or three zones of intraoral structures that need to be reconstructed. See Fig. 37.1.)
2. The readings cite an opinion about bony reconstruction of the mandible versus a soft-tissue flap reconstruction with a reconstructive plate. What evidence is cited to support the position of bony reconstruction? (Reconstruction of both bony and the soft-tissue defect is preferred to that of soft-tissue reconstruction only plus a reconstruction plate for the mandible. The readings quoted a number of outcomes of plates only and soft-tissue-free flaps used for reconstruction with an unacceptable failure rate of non-union, extrusion, and necessity for secondary procedures.)
3. Each of the defects in Question 1 presents a set of reconstructive challenges. Describe. (Anterior defects may be

E. Luce, *A Curriculum for Plastic Surgery*, https://doi.org/10.1007/978-3-031-62087-4_37

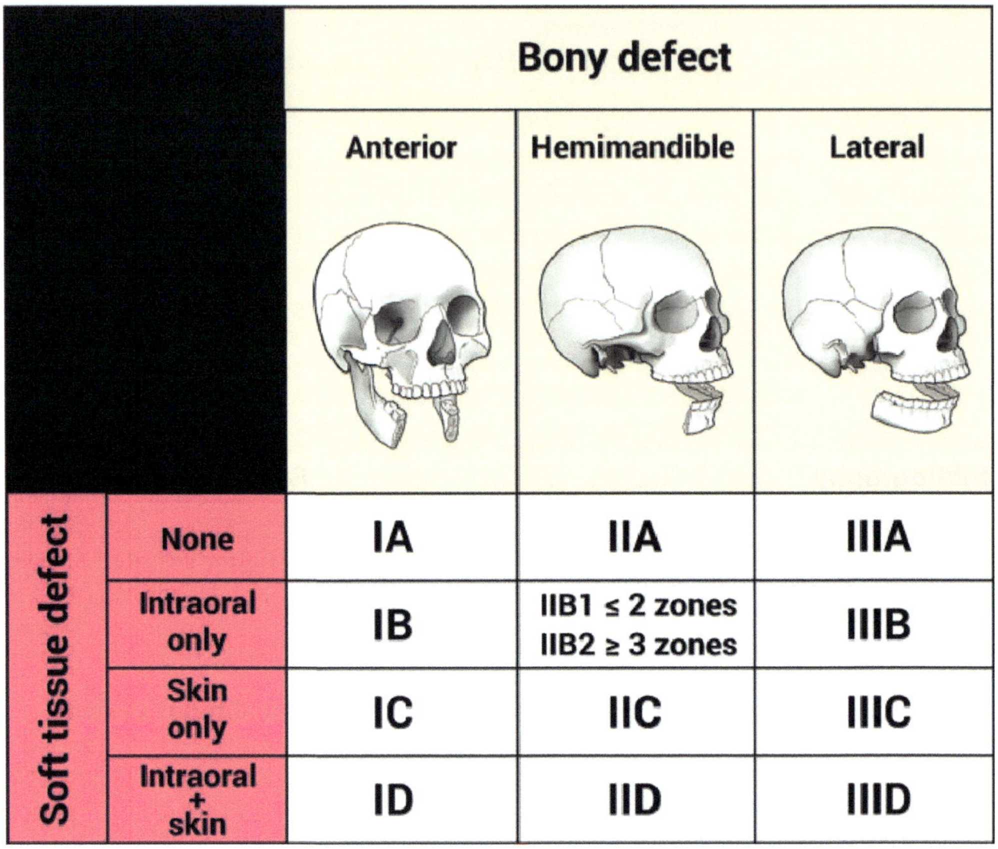

Fig. 37.1 Mandibulectomy defect classification system. (Cordeiro PG, et al., "A 20-Year Experience with 202 Segmental Mandibulectomy Defects: A Defect Classification System, Algorithm for Flap Selection, and Surgical Outcomes", *Plast Reconstr Surg.*, (2018);141(4):572e. (Reprinted with Permission))

the most demanding because of the necessity to maintain projection and support of the lower face. The potential for dental implants further emphasizes the necessity of bony reconstruction. The associated intraoral lining defect is common, although at least in the oncologic scenario, skin loss is considerably less common. In lateral defects in the absence of bony reconstruction, the posterior remnant, the ascending ramus, and angle will retract superiorly and medially. Again, in the cancer setting, an associated defect of the intraoral lining and, possibly, skin loss can be anticipated. Comprehensive reconstruction will dictate the placement of osseointegrated dental implants. A posterior defect from, for example, a retromolar trigone primary, usually spares the condyle and a variable amount of superior ascending ramus.)

(a) In some sets of circumstances, non-vascularized bone grafts may be an appropriate option. List. (Benign tumors, non-irradiated field, less than 6 cm. The critical defect size threshold may be considerably less in anterior defects.)

4. Discuss options and reconstruction of the mandible in association with oropharyngeal cancer from the aspects of the particular defect. The four possibilities are: (a) lateral segment with condyle intact; (b) hemimandible with anterior segment intact; (c) anterior segments only, the defect anterior to the first bicuspid bilaterally; and (d) subtotal mandibulectomy or anterior and hemimandible. ((a) Reconstruction plate only in those selected instances of patient intolerance of a microvascular procedure as a fibula-free flap; (b) fibula, iliac-free flap, and scapular-free flap; (c) fibula, iliac-free flap, and scapular-free flap; and (d) fibula. All will have soft-tissue considerations and the probability of an associated skin island.)

   (a) Some reconstruction defects will have a skin-soft tissue component. Discuss options. (Essentially, three options are available: fibula osteocutaneous, rectus abdominis, or two flaps of fibula and radial forearm. If the bone is not reconstructed in a lateral defect, IIIC in the classification, a scapular flap can address the associated skin-soft tissue deficit. The rectus with two skin islands is reserved for combined intraoral and skin defects. See Table 37.1.)

5. Describe the approach and key steps of the harvest of an iliac non-vascularized bone graft. (The anterior approach consists of an incision of 2 cm posterior to the anterior superior iliac spine and 1–2 cm inferior to the posterior iliac crest. The lateral cutaneous of the iliohypogastric nerve as well as the lateral femoral cutaneous nerve should be reflected anteriorly. The soft tissues and periosteum are stripped from the iliac bone medially which is harvested from the medial cortex including a cancellous component.)

Table 37.1 Relative strengths of the fibula, rectus abdominis, radial forearm, and scapula flaps

	Fibula	Rectus abdominis	Radial forearm (oc)	Scapula
Bone	+++	–	+	++
Skin (surface area)	++	+++	++	++
Soft tissue (volume)	++	+++	+	++
Pedicle (length)	+++	+++	+++	+
Ease of harvest	++	+++	+++	+

Editor's Note: The role of the osteocutaneous scapular or radial forearm flaps in mandibular reconstruction has been replaced by the fibula because of the lack of good bone stock in both, the necessity for position change in the former, and the frequency of fracture of the radius in the latter. The radial forearm-free flap is discussed in Chap. 38. Flaps derived from the scapular axis are discussed in Chap. 39.

Free Flaps

1. Describe the pertinent anatomy and briefly describe the harvest of the iliac-free flap. (The arterial supply is the endosteal perforating branches of the deep circumflex iliac artery, a branch of the lateral aspect of the external iliac or the common femoral deep to the inguinal ligament. The venous drainage is into the external iliac vein via the deep inferior epigastric and deep circumflex iliac veins. The ascending branch of the deep circumflex iliac perfuses the overlying internal oblique muscle but not the bone. The technique, if a skin island is included, consists of an obliquely oriented skin island from medial to lateral and inferior to superior that parallels the iliac crest from the anterior superior iliac spine posteriorly. The skin island continues on the same oblique axis while the iliac crest courses more posteriorly and transversely. Two-thirds of the skin island lies above the inguinal ligament and one-third below. Dissection of the deep circumflex iliac requires division of the external, internal oblique, and transversus muscles which will require repair after harvest of the flap. The lateral femoral cutaneous nerve, L2–3, lies just deep to the deep circumflex iliac artery as does the ilio-hypogastric and both must be preserved. The ilio-inguinal nerve, L1, is medial to the dissection.)
   (a) Advantages and disadvantages? (The principal advantage of the deep iliac bone flap is the harvest of substantial bone which can be contoured to parallel a reconstruction of the anterolateral mandible. If harvested from the ipsilateral side, the iliac flap is ideally utilized for a lateral mandibular defect which would require a single osteotomy, if any. Also, the bone stock is more than sufficient for osseointegrated implants. Simultaneous harvest is possible as a separate team. The principal disadvantages are the difficult dissection, a skin paddle that is bulky with limitation of mobility and independent orientation from the bone, and a significant incidence of donor-site problems of neuroma, hernia, and hematoma as well as disturbances of gait. In addition, the pedicle in comparison to the fibula is somewhat short. Some donor-site complications can be minimized by harvest of the medial or internal cortex only.)
   (b) Contrast with a groin flap in terms of blood supply and orientation of the skin island. (The groin flap arterial perfusion is via the superficial circumflex iliac artery, a branch of the common femoral. The axis is approximately 2 cm transversely inferior and parallel to the inguinal ligament, a skin island that lies more inferior to the iliac flap but some overlap exists. The groin flap is entirely below the iliac crest, but the iliac skin island in contrast is mostly above the crest, with some below.)
2. What is the anatomical relationship of the vascular pedicle of the fibula flap to the pertinent muscles of the mid-calf? (Peroneus longus and brevis in the lateral compartment, the flexor hallucis longus medial and posterior to the fibula, and the tibialis posterior, medial, and slightly anterior to the fibula.)
   (a) What two compartments does the posterior intermuscular septum separate? (Anteriorly, the lateral compartment; posteriorly, the superficial posterior compartment.)
3. The principal blood supply to the fibula flap is the peroneal vessels. What is the value of a CT angiogram or formal angiogram? (Of course, detection of any peripheral vascular disease but also determination of the presence or absence of peroneal magna or a single vessel leg that is present in 5–8% of the population.)
   (a) Approximate location of the nutrient artery. (Approximately 15 cm distal to the styloid of the fibula or 10 cm from the takeoff of the peroneal artery from the posterior tibial.)
4. What nerve(s) are principally at risk in the proximal dissection? (Common peroneal and more distally the superficial peroneal.)
   (a) What functional deficit would occur with an injury to the common peroneal nerve? (Foot drop from the loss, most importantly of the tibialis anterior but also

the extensor digitorum and extensor hallucis longus.)

5. How is the skin island perfused? (A high percentage of the perforators are septocutaneous rather than musculocutaneous. When septocutaneous, the vessels traverse the intermuscular septum between the lateral compartment and the superficial posterior compartment. If musculocutaneous, a cuff of flexor hallucis longus and soleus must be taken with the flap.)
   (a) Why is the skin island more reliable when placed distally rather than proximal? (The distribution of the perforators is more dense in the distal portion of the fibula.)
6. Describe the pertinent anatomy and briefly describe the technique of harvesting the fibula as a bone flap and as a composite flap. (The pertinent anatomy of the fibula-free flap is the location of the peroneal artery as it courses medial to the fibula in the posterior intermuscular septum between the tibialis posterior located anterior and medial and the flexor hallucis longus directly posterior. The posterior intermuscular septum lies at the posterior border of the fibula. The artery is accompanied by two venae comitantes and provides the principal endosteal blood supply through a nutrient artery approximately 15 cm from the head of the fibula. Other perforating vessels are segmental arterial branches that are primarily periosteal in location and nourish the underlying bone and adjacent muscle mass. At least 4 cm proximal and 6 cm of distal fibula must be preserved to minimize postoperative dysfunction.

   If a skin island is included, the design should be at the juncture of the middle and distal one-third. The skin island will be nourished by vessels that pass between the soleus muscle in the superficial posterior compartment and posterior to the septum and the peroneal brevis and longus laterally in the lateral muscle compartment. The initial incision is anterior over the fibula and the skin is elevated in a suprafascial plane off the peroneus longus and brevis. The posterior intermuscular septum is identified and the peroneal muscles are dissected free of the lateral surface of the fibula. The dissection continues with an incision of the anterior intermuscular septum to permit dissection of the extensor digitorum longus and extensor hallucis longus muscles free from the anterior aspect of the fibula. Inclusion of a cuff of the flexor hallucis longus and tibialis posterior can improve the reliability of the skin island, particularly if the skin perforators are primarily intermuscular rather than septocutaneous in nature although that is a minority of the instances. The posterior skin island incision is made and the dissection is performed suprafascial off the underlying peroneal muscles until the anterior edge of the soleus muscle where the fascia is then incised for a subfascial dissection. The posterior intermuscular septum is maintained intact and the septal vessels nourishing the skin island should be visualized. If the skin vessels appear primarily arising from the soleus muscle rather than the septum then dissection of that portion of the soleus muscle along those perforators until their origin from the peroneal vessels is encountered and preserved.

   Attention needs to be directed, particularly when a large skin island is harvested, to the identification and preservation of the superficial and common peroneal nerves.

   The final piece of dissection is done anteriorly with mobilization of the peroneal muscles of the anterior lateral fibula. Osteotomies are performed, and the proximal pedicle that consists of the peroneal branch of the posterior tibial artery just distal to the bifurcation is ligated as well as the distal peroneal vessels. The posterior interosseous membrane is incised, which later will be repaired in conjunction with the adjacent flexor hallucis longus and posterior tibialis. A cuff of flexor hallucis longus and tibialis posterior can be incorporated to ensure perfusion of the skin island, but the disadvantage is less flexibility of skin island location with respect to the bone and additional bulk.)
   (a) Advantages and disadvantages? (The fibula flap provides an excellent stock of bone which in most instances can be osteotomized to recreate the contour of the mandible or to create a "double-barrel" mandible reconstruction for increased vertical height. Additional advantages include the ability of a two-team approach and a long vascular pedicle. Disadvantages include the occasional lack of reliability of the skin component and some limitations of skin island mobility and orientation with respect to the bone. Large skin island harvest that requires skin grafting of the donor site can be a cosmetic concern, particularly in women. The pedicle length can be increased by a bone harvest design inferiorly, but may not incorporate the nutrient artery.)
7. Describe donor-site adverse side effects and complications. (All patients have some degree of gait disturbance at least temporarily and associated pain. If the flexor hallucis longus is not repaired properly at the time of closure or develops ischemic changes, a flexor contracture or diminished flexion of the big toe with a resultant gait disturbance can occur. Sensation is decreased over the distribution of the superficial peroneal nerve, primarily the dorsum of the foot.)

Technology

1. Contemporary mandibular reconstruction has evolved beyond the use of guesswork for the harvest of the donor

bone and inset into the recipient site as well as the use of reconstruction plates contoured in the Operating Room. Explain how computer-assisted design (CAD)/computer-assisted manufacture (CAM) may assist in reconstruction. (CAD refers to the use of imaging information obtained from thin-slice CT and 3D reformat manipulated with proprietary software. The technology enables the user at a computer workstation to engage in virtual surgical planning (VSP), including localization of osteotomies of the mandible and donor bone, positioning of the inset of the bone, and screw fixation points. The post-traumatic or post-resection images can be manipulated by virtual surgery to allow restoration of the absent or malpositioned bone segments. CAM is the use of the design data to generate stereolithographic models of the reconstructed mandible to subsequently manufacture customized, patient-specific cutting guides and reconstruction plates for concise osteotomies of both the mandible and donor bone, predominately the fibula. Dental occlusal information can be obtained in the traditional format from impressions of the patient and the stone models merged with the CT data or, alternatively, occlusal data derived with digital technology. Occlusal splints for use intraoperatively can be generated by either method. If high-resolution CT angiography is incorporated into the imaging process, a concise location of perforators is possible, judging the location of cutting jigs and osteotomies away from those points. Virtual surgical planning (VSP) is conducted in concert with the reconstructive surgeon and computer engineer. If an oncologic resection is involved with another service, the resection surgeon is included.)

2. Clearly, the implementation of CAD/CAM technology incurs a substantial cost. Give a perspective. (On the benefit side of the equation is the demonstrable decrease of operating and ischemia time. An additional benefit is an enhanced functional and aesthetic outcome. Although that benefit seems intuitive, the evidence is lacking at this juncture. There are several factors on the con or liability side of the equation. First, the resection, based on intraoperative findings, may be greater than anticipated. Second, additional imaging may be necessary. Third, although the technology permits precise dental rehabilitation, the cost of implants and prosthodontics frequently is not covered by insurance and is not implemented in many if not most patients. Finally, the overall expense of CAD/CAM technology is substantial, a time hiatus for the production of the patient-specific cutting guides and reconstruction plate is inevitable, and virtual surgical planning consumes additional time of the surgeon. As of this writing, a comprehensive cost-utility analysis has not been performed. The final concern is the unpredictability of soft-tissue movement, a variable that can impact the outcome.)

Video Notes

Fibula (Wei/Mardini)

General

Video 1

Good markings; video quality only fair, audio quality poor with long periods of silence.

Video 2

Suprafascial dissection anteriorly and subfascial posteriorly; landmark was the posterior intermuscular septum both anterior and posterior dissection.

Video 3

Dissection of the peroneal muscles of the lateral aspect of the fibula; small cuff of peroneal muscles included.

Video 4

Separation of the soleus from the posterior inferior fibula proximal with an osteotomy.

Video 5

Dissection of the pedicle distal to proximal.

Video 6

Repair of the flexor hallucis longus to the posterior tibia at the time of closure.

General

Video 1

Poor quality video, out of focus and overexposed but audio description *excellent*.

Case-Based Conference

Case 1: Draining Fistula

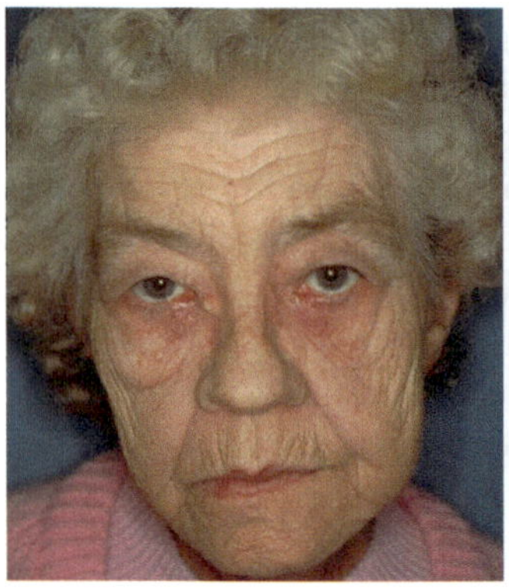
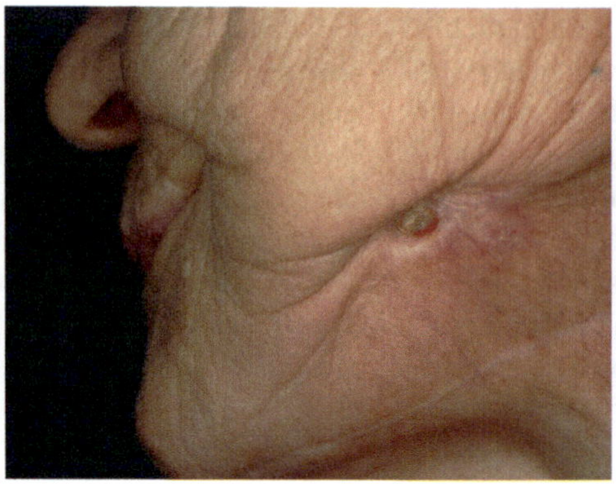
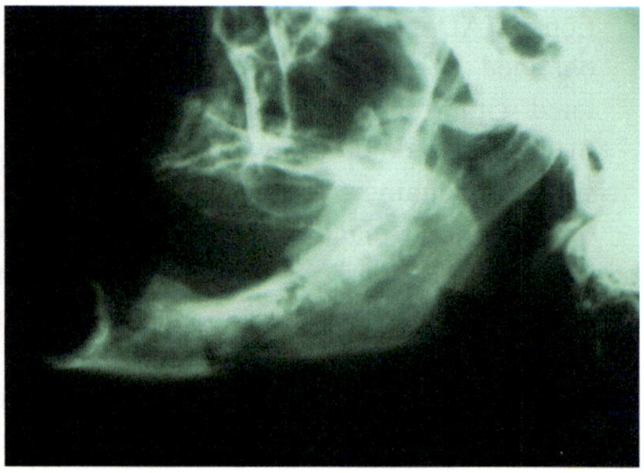

A 76-year-old woman who had an intraoral cancer resected with marginal mandibulectomy, neck dissection, and postoperative radiation 4 years ago. She has drained intermediately for the past 1 year. The interincisal maximal opening is 10 mm. Other than mild hypertension, she has no other medical problems.

1. Describe the slides and X-ray. Add a focused clinical examination.
    (a) Any tests indicated? The old path report revealed a squamous cell carcinoma of the lateral floor of the mouth, adequately excised, and negative neck nodes.
2. Give a differential diagnosis and assign probabilities to each item on your list. Give the pathophysiology and pathologic anatomy of your first choice.
3. Within the framework of your response to Question 2, your first choice, outline a treatment plan. Include a brief description of any operative procedures, if any, and perioperative care.

Case-Based Conference: Discussion

Case 1: Draining Fistula

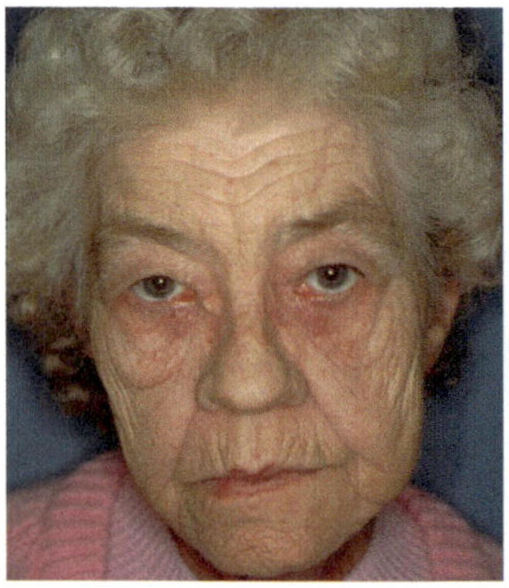
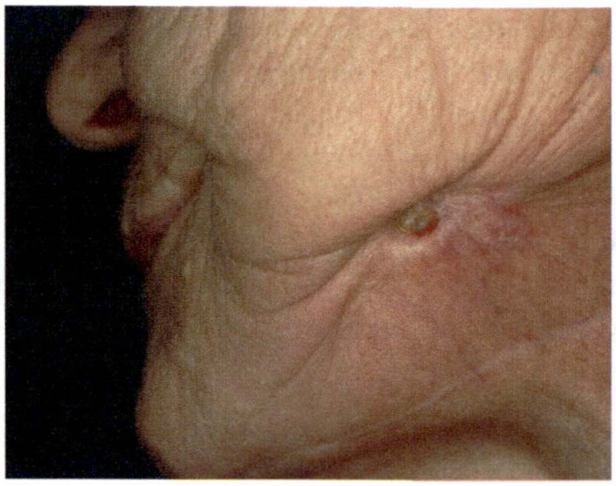
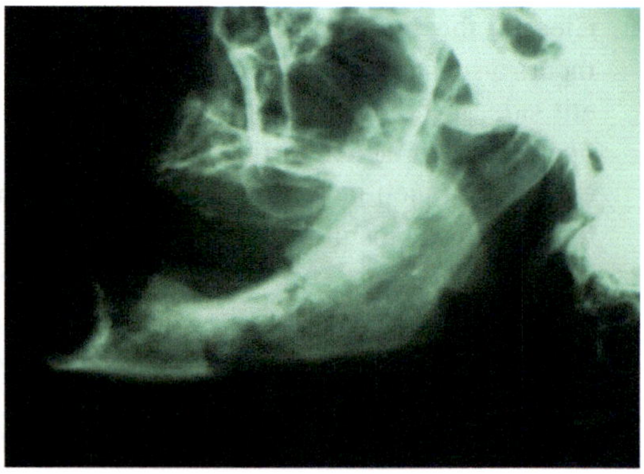

A 76-year-old woman who had an intraoral cancer resected with neck dissection and postoperative radiation 4 years ago. She has drained intermediately for the past 1 year. The interincisal maximal opening is 10 mm. Other than mild hypertension, she has no other medical problems.

1. Describe the slides and X-ray. Add a focused clinical examination. (Two clinical photos and a single X-ray are provided. The first photo is of an elderly woman with an appearance of the stated age or older. The view is a frontal full face from hairline to the chin but the neck is not visible. No deformity or asymmetry is evident, although the left side may be subtly more full or prominent. A festoon that is present on the right infraorbital area is not present on the left. The mouth is closed so the marked decrease in opening is not demonstrated. The second photo, a left lat-

eral view, depicts only a limited portion of the lower cheek and mandible from mid-nasal to chin and not the ear nor the neck. A long transverse mature scar is evident along the entire jawline. The most remarkable finding is a several millimeters to a centimeter circular ulcer several centimeters superior to the midpoint of the aforementioned scar. The ulcer is umbilicated, surrounded by contracted skin, particularly by folds medially and laterally. In addition, the skin inferior to the ulcer is marked by some mild erythema. The base of the ulcer is necrotic but without evident drainage.

The single X-ray provided is a lateral view of the mandible and maxilla. Several significant findings are present. Both the maxilla and mandible are edentulous with some bone resorption evident and a decrease in vertical height of the mandible. The anterior mandible is not visualized, perhaps secondary to an overexposure artifact. An area of 1–2 cm of radiolucency is seen inferior to the inferior border. The remaining mandible including about 2 cm of bone superior to the radiolucency does not appear grossly osteoporotic, but plane X-rays can be misleading.

The history component of the clinical examination will ascertain in addition to the information provided in the preamble, a determination of masticatory function immediately postoperatively, and the timeline of the onset and course of the trismus. Other historical information of value would be the periodic extrusion of small bone fragments, diet, and weight loss, and activities of daily living, particularly the elements that constitute an increase in the frailty index. Pain, if any, should be assessed, particularly throat or ear pain as well as the events, such as eating, that provoke drainage. The patient should be questioned about symptoms in the upper aerodigestive tract as dysphagia or hoarseness that may be a clue to the presence of a metachronous primary. The past medical history and review of systems should determine the presence of comorbidities, although the preamble states the patient is hypertensive only. A history of post-radiotherapy dental extractions should be pursued. Importantly, a social history should include tobacco and drug use. A rough estimate of the radiotherapy total dosage can be ascertained from the number of days per week and the total duration in weeks. At 5 days a week, the standard dosage is 10 Gy weekly.

The physical exam should focus on inspection, as much as possible because of the limited jaw opening, of the oral cavity including the lingual and buccal aspects of the left mandibular alveolar ridge and body to detect bone exposure. If the patient permits, bone stability is evaluated with bimanual manipulation of the mandible. The ipsilateral and contralateral neck is palpated for masses or lymphadenopathy as well as the skin-soft tissue in the area of the ulcer. Potential flap donor sites are examined as well.)

(a) Any tests indicated? The old path report revealed a squamous cell carcinoma of the lateral floor of mouth, adequately excised, and negative neck nodes. (CT imaging of the mandible, head and neck, and trunk will be necessary to determine the presence of osteoradionecrosis (ORN), bone invasion by tumor, a metachronous primary of the head and neck, or metastatic disease of the lung or liver. In anticipation of surgical management, a CT angiogram would be beneficial. Although some enthusiasm for imaging with positron-emission tomography (PET)/CT scan has appeared in the literature, the evidence is empirical at best and insurance may not provide coverage.

In addition to the path report, the operative note should be obtained and reviewed. Biopsy of the ulcer will be non-diagnostic and reveal acute and chronic inflammation only. See below.)

2. Give a differential diagnosis and assign probabilities to each item on your list. Give the pathophysiology and pathologic anatomy of your first choice. (Practically, only two diagnoses are probable, recurrent neoplasm with bony invasion or osteoradionecrosis (ORN). Given a hiatus of four years between treatment and current presentation and the duration, a year, of drainage, the more probable diagnosis is ORN. Nevertheless, the critical diagnosis to be considered in the development of a treatment plan is a recurrence or perhaps a new primary. Certainly, the area of radiolucency, although not inconsistent with ORN, could also represent a lytic lesion of neoplasm.

The pathophysiology and pathologic anatomy of osteoradionecrosis pivots on the damage inflicted on normal tissue as a side effect of the lethality to the cancer cells (see Chap. 3). Histologically, the lesion is one of an obliterative endarteritis of small vessels secondary to subintimal fibrosis. The result is a hypoxic environment, subject to impaired healing of trauma. As such, host predisposing factors include periodontal disease and caries, poorly fitting dentures, nutritional status, and tobacco abuse. Treatment variables include the total radiation dose particularly greater than 60–65 Gy and the use of older methods of radiotherapy. The use of intensity-modulated radiotherapy has reduced the incidence of ORN modestly in comparison to more traditional methods of radiotherapy. The interaction of these variables as well as an inciting event to initiate the occurrence and subsequent evolution of ORN are not well defined. Clearly, diminished vascularity sets the stage for a cycle of infection, fibrosis, and compromise of blood supply, all triggered by a mucosal injury or poor dental hygiene. Dental extractions in the irradiated mandible have also been implicated.

The other components of the pathological anatomy are the degree of bone involvement, the magnitude of mucosa and skin-soft tissue deficiency, if any, and the concomitant trismus. The operative report will provide clarification but if the intraoral defect was closed primarily, any resection treatment plan must include the contingency of a mucosal lining or coverage replacement. Trismus is the outcome of chronic pain, conversion to a non-chew diet, fibrosis, and further loss of masticatory function. As a result, weight loss and malnutrition become increasingly important elements of the clinical picture.)

3. Within the framework of your response to Question 2, your first choice, outline a treatment plan. Include a brief description of any operative procedures, if any, and perioperative care. (The CT imaging results will be crucial in the determination of the diagnosis including detection of any soft-tissue changes that are suspicious for neoplasm and the degree of bone involvement. A variety of staging systems have been offered, all of which would range in severity from involvement of the alveolus only to alveolus and mandible but still above the level of the inferior alveolar canal. All of the systems would assign an advanced stage to a patient with a skin fistula and exposed bone.

   Multi-detector thin-slice CT in axial and coronal views can establish with a reasonably high degree of certitude, the presence of sequestra or lytic bone changes indicative of the severity of the ORN.

   Management of more localized involvement limited to the alveolus can be accomplished with conservative measures of chlorhexidine mouthwashes, frequent outpatient local and limited debridement of necrotic bone, and tobacco cessation. The older literature trumpeted the efficacy of hyperbaric oxygen (HBO), but more recent studies have failed to demonstrate a benefit, particularly given the substantial cost. By using several pharmacologic agents including pentoxifylline combined with tocopherol, vitamin E, and clodronate, a bisphosphonate has been described and advocated but also lacks proof of benefit.

   With a high probability, the patient in this case under discussion will require surgical intervention with four objectives: A thorough intraoral exam under general anesthesia, resection of necrotic mandible, release of the trismus, and reconstruction. Optimization of the patient's nutritional status must be accomplished. Given the elective nature of the operative plan, preoperative nutrition indices can direct the aggressiveness and duration of nutritional intervention as well as the absolute necessity of cessation of tobacco use. General anesthesia should be administered via nasotracheal intubation. The procedural approach offers two options, of which, one is substantially more comprehensive. The less extensive would incorporate the old transverse jawline incision to raise a skin flap that would expose the mandibular body, a limited excision of the ulcer and the adjacent scarred skin, and debridement of bone. If the judgment that sufficient residual mandible 5 of 1.5 cm or more remains in continuity and the probability of a subsequent pathologic fracture is low, attention could be directed to the release of the masseter and internal pterygoid and primary closure of the skin. The opposite posterior muscles of mastication can be released transorally. A contingency plan should include the other option, a segmental resection, a high likelihood given the findings on X-ray alone, and a method of reconstruction of both bone and soft tissue. Segmental resection permits aggressive debridement to healthy bleeding bone. The skin-soft tissue needs are dictated by the necessity of a well-vascularized soft-tissue flap to drape the mandible in a tension-free closure. All four of the common vascularized bone transfers—iliac, radius, scapula, and fibula—have a potential cutaneous component. Of those four, harvest of the fibula is dominant in practice and the principal liability. Some limitation of orientation of skin island versus bone would not be a consideration in this case. The final consideration is that if the intraoral lining will also require augmentation, a determination will probably await an intraoperative decision. In elderly patients, an ample-sized nasolabial flap, 2.5–3.0 cm in width, can be rotated into a moderate defect, a likelihood in this case. A safe and prudent measure if segmental resection and free flap is mandated, is a conversion of endotracheal intubation to a formal tracheostomy at the same operative setting.).

Postoperative (8 Months)

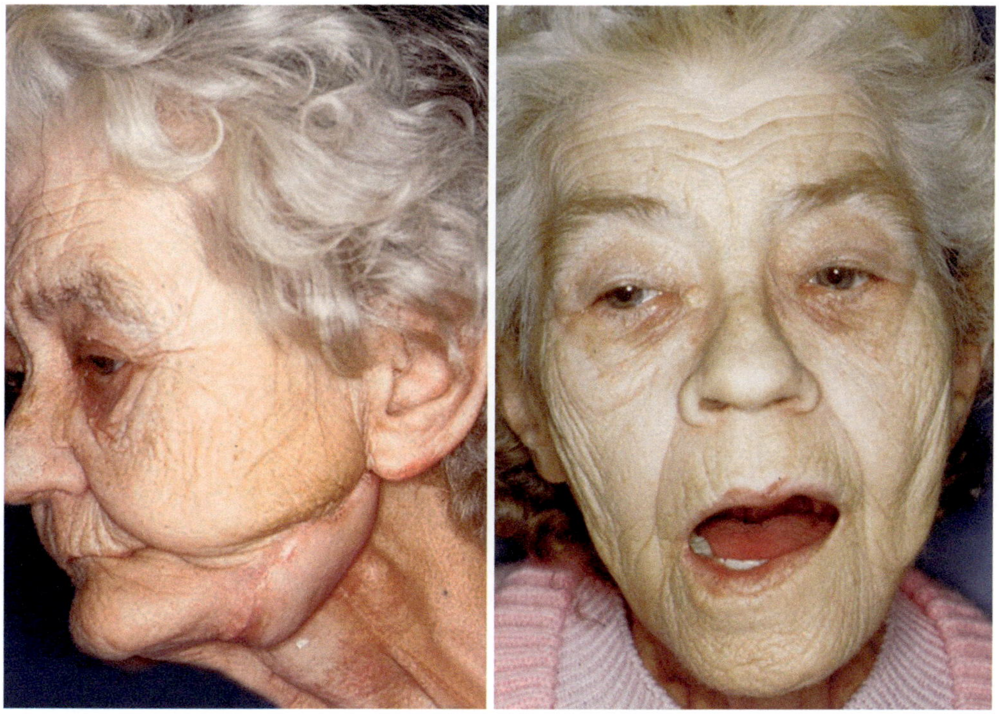

The two postoperative photos at 5 months include lateral and frontal views. The lateral view includes a well-healed skin paddle of a remote flap several centimeters in width in place over the course of the posterior mandibular body. In the final photo with the patient's mouth open, a full 2 cm of interincisal opening is evident. Dental rehabilitation is suggested by the presence of dentures. The lower lip on the left is asymmetrically elevated, indicative of a marginal mandibular nerve palsy.

Critique

The patient was reconstructed after segmental resection with a fibular osteocutaneous-free flap. Although the flap can have limited flexibility in orientation of the cutaneous versus the bone component, little flexibility would have been necessary in this defect. In the process of raising a cervical apron via the old transverse neck dissection incision, the presence of irradiated and fibrotic skin and soft tissue from the prior surgery, and prior radiotherapy placed the marginal mandibular nerve at risk.

In-Service Examination

1. The blood supply to the fibula osteocutaneous flap is:
   (a) Musculocutaneous perforators from the anterior tibialis
   (b) Musculocutaneous perforator from soleus and flexor hallucis brevis
   (c) Septocutaneous perforators from the peroneal artery
   (d) Septocutaneous and musculocutaneous perforators from the flexor hallucis longus
2. An inadvertent transection of the common peroneal nerve occurred during a fibula flap harvest. What are the anticipated motor and sensory deficits?
   (a) No sensory, weakness of flexion of the great toe
   (b) No sensory, weakness of extension of the great toe
   (c) Sensory loss of the dorsum of foot, weakness of both great toe and foot extension
   (d) Sensory loss of the first web space only, weakness of great toe extension, and foot dorsiflexion

38 Intraoral Defect Reconstruction

Bibliography

Cheng M.H., Ch. 12 "Oral cavity, tongue, and mandibular reconstructions", Neligan PC, Plastic Surgery, Elsevier 5th Edition, (2023), Volume 3: **pgs. 275 (Skip section on mandible reconstruction)**.

Stewart CE, Urken ML, Ch. 18 "Deltopectoral Flap" Flaps and Reconstructive Surgery, Wei FC and Mardini S, Elsevier Saunder, (2009); **pgs. 193–99 ONLY**.

Wei WI and Wai CY, Chapter 34 "Pectoralis major flap", Flaps and Reconstructive Surgery, Second Edition, Wei FC and Mardini S, Elsevier Saunders, (2017); pgs. **396–410 ONLY**.

Taghinia A.H., Upton J., Ch. 47 "Radial forearm flap", Flaps and Reconstructive Surgery, Second Edition, Wei FC and Mardini S, Elsevier Saunders, (2017); pgs. **525–534 ONLY**.

Moubayed SP, Rahal A, and Ayad T, "The submental island flap for soft-tissue head and neck reconstruction: Step-by-step video description and long-term results", *Plast. Reconstr. Surg.*, (2014); 133(3):**684–686. (Including Video)**.

Chang E.I., "Alternate Soft-Tissue Free Flaps for Head and Neck Reconstruction: The Next Generation of Workhorse Flaps", *Plast Reconstr Surg.*, (2023);**152(1):184, Pearls, Discussion, and Videos 1, 3, 4 ONLY**.

Mardini S, Chim H., Wei FC. Chapt. 59 "Anterolateral thigh flap", Wei FC and Mardini SL, Flaps and Reconstructive Surgery, Second Ed. Elsevier Inc., (2017); **pgs. 700–07**.

Mardini S, Lin LC, Moran SL, et al., "Anterolateral thigh flap" **Video**.

Videos (Videos Only)

Hallock, Geoffrey G.; Morris, Steven F., "Skin Grafts and Local Flaps", Geoffrey G. Hallock, *Plast. Reconstr. Surg.*, (Jan. 2011); 127:(1): 5e–22e. **(Only Video 3)** http://journals.lww.com/plasreconsurg/Pages/videogallery.aspx?videoId=64&autoPlay=true

Urken M, Buchbinder D, Wei FC, Dayan JH, "Video 1—Maxillary Reconstruction Using an Osteocutaneous Radial Forearm Flap—Part 2: Flap design and harvesting technique", *Plast. Reconstr. Surg.*, (March 2013); 131(3). p 411e–424e. https://journals.lww.com/plasreconsurg/pages/videogallery.aspx?autoPlay=false&videoId=332

Faculty Discussion and Study Guide

Anatomy—See Chap. 35.

Preoperative Evaluation

1. Outline the factors, not the anticipated defect, in the preoperative assessment of the oral cavity cancer patient as a candidate for reconstruction. (Nutritional and functional status, whether preoperative radiotherapy has been given or will be given post-operatively, the presence of significant comorbidities of pulmonary or cardiovascular disease.)
2. What measures may be necessary preoperatively in said patient? (If severely malnourished, or if a prolonged post-operative period of lack of oral alimentation is anticipated, placement of a gastrostomy or jejunostomy feeding tube may be necessary. A thin-slice CT will assist in the delineation of the extent of the tumor, although not definitively. CT scan of the neck can detect occult lymph node metastases. The CT scan can also be utilized for 3D reconstruction and virtual surgical planning. See Chap. 37. A preoperative angiogram is optional with the reconstructive surgeon. With sufficient resolution, a CT angiogram can replace traditional angiography.)
3. In general terms, not the specific area, describe the ideal option or options for the following defects: small mucosal, large mucosal, combined large mucosa and mandible, combined mucosa and mandible plus skin. (The small

E. Luce, *A Curriculum for Plastic Surgery*, https://doi.org/10.1007/978-3-031-62087-4_38

defect can be addressed with nasolabial or submental artery (SMA) flaps, large mucosa-only defect with a regional flap such as the pectoralis major, radial forearm, lateral arm, or a perforator flap of the profunda and medial sural arteries. A combined bone and mucosa reconstruction with a fibula osteocutaneous flap is most common. Massive defects involving oral cavity structures including bone and skin-soft tissue are a challenge, often requiring two flaps. Any number of notable exceptions and use of other flaps exist. The supraclavicular flap is discussed in Chap. 28.)

4. What is the functional disability for failure to or inadequately reconstruct the buccal cavity? (Trismus secondary to contraction fibrosis.)
   (a) What immediate adjacent structures may also be involved? (The buccal gingival sulcus, the oral commissure, the retromolar trigone, and cheek skin, all of which dictate a thin, pliable flap. In more extensive lesions that extend to the commissure, either the upper or lower lip or both may be involved. Because the combined mucosa, underlying structures, and skin is a relatively thin anatomic wall, skin involvement is not uncommon. Reconstruction will usually require a two-island flap.)
5. Consider the following defects and select the appropriate flap.
   (a) Buccal cavity alone (Radial forearm-free flap [RFFF]).
   (b) Buccal cavity and cheek or through-and-through defect (Radial forearm-free flap with two-skin islands if sufficient pedicle length is available *or* an anterolateral thigh (ALT) flap with two-skin islands, but in most patients, it would be bulky as would a pectoralis major flap of similar design.)
   (c) Buccal cavity with involvement of mandible or maxilla. (Defects that involve marginal mandibulectomy or a partial maxillectomy will require coverage of the exposed mandible or closure and obliteration of dead space created by the maxillectomy. Use of a myocutaneous alternative, the ALT with muscle, the vastus lateralis, is an appropriate option.)
6. What is a classification of tongue defects? (Hemiglossectomy or less than 50%, subtotal glossectomy or loss of entire mobile tongue, or total glossectomy.)
   (a) What are the functional demands for glossectomy defects? (Articulation, deglutition, and airway protection. The anterior tongue with the lips is important in articulation, although the loss can be substantially compensated in most patients. The anterior two-thirds of the tongue also plays a role in deglutition by propelling the food posteriorly into the oropharynx. The bulk of the base of the tongue assists in the closure of the oropharynx from the upper airway.)
7. Describe the optimal reconstruction for the following glossectomy defects. Assume no mandibular resection.
   (a) Hemiglossectomy? (If the defect is sufficiently lateralized, closure with the remaining tongue is an option in selected instances such as a T1 lesion. Otherwise, the radial forearm flap will provide pliability.)
   (b) Subtotal? (Since bulk and replacement components are required, either a pedicled pectoralis major or free ALT is appropriate, although the contemporary use of the ALT is more common.)
   (c) Total? (Defect requirements are bulk, replacement, and prevention of aspiration. An ALT flap, tailored to inset into the vallecula is the optimal free flap option. The pedicled pectoralis major is a regional flap option, but again the ALT is more commonly preferred.
   The sequelae in total glossectomy defects are, unfortunately, recurrent aspiration and ultimately tracheostomy or in extreme cases laryngectomy.)
8. What are the reconstructive needs of an anterior floor of mouth defect? (The anterior floor of mouth (FOM), provides the necessary mobility to the tongue, particularly the anterior tongue for both the propulsion of the food bolus posteriorly and in deglutition.)
9. Describe the appropriate flap for the following severity of defects of the anterior FOM:
   (a) A limited defect of mucosa only, less than 12 cm^2. (Bilateral nasolabial flaps, two stages as a local flap option. The submental artery flap is the regional option. Protection of the facial artery during the concomitant neck dissection is essential.)
   (b) A larger defect also involves adjacent ventral aspects of the tongue and tongue tip. (Radial forearm flap for thinness and pliability.)
   (c) A similar defect plus anterior mandible. (As discussed below, a fibula osteocutaneous flap provides mandibular and lining reconstruction.)
   (d) Retromolar trigone? (Defects of the retromolar trigone are somewhat unique. The mucosa is intimate to the underlying bone and a marginal mandibulectomy is usually necessary to obtain a clear margin. Frequently, the adjacent lateral tongue is involved. The reconstruction needs a thin, pliable fasciocutaneous flap such as the radial artery or perforator as the medial sural or profunda artery flap.)
   (e) Oropharynx? (Defects of the oropharynx such as the tonsillar fossa or lateral pharyngeal wall require some bulk, optimally filled with an anterolateral thigh (ALT) flap.)

Specific Flaps: Local and Regional

1. Describe the anatomy and design of the deltopectoral flap. Give some estimate of the utility value in head and neck reconstruction. (The deltopectoral flap is based on the perforators through the second and third intercostal space from the internal mammary vessels, which once they perforate, the fascia run transversely across the upper chest. The flap consists of skin, subcutaneous fat, and the underlying fascia because the vessels are suprafacial. The flap is thin and pliable, relatively easy to harvest, and of limited donor site morbidity in males. Nevertheless, in terms of intraoral reconstruction, the flap is of historical value. The principal utility value is coverage of a soft tissue defect in the neck.)
   (a) Disadvantages? (Perfusion of the soft tissue beyond the deltopectoral groove encroaches on the supraclavicular angiosome and further lateral, the posterior humeral circumflex angiosome, and as such, requires a preliminary delay; necessity of second stage for definitive inset.)
2. Describe the anatomy, design, and principal use and value of the pectoralis major flap. (The pectoralis major flap is a musculocutaneous unit based on the thoracoacromial vessels. The minor pedicles of the pectoralis major are the intercostal perforators medially and the lateral thoracic artery, both divided in the process of harvest of the flap. Although a sizable segment of the muscle must be included, the flap can be rotated on the pedicle pivot point which exits beneath the junction of the middle and lateral one-third of the clavicle. The topographical landmarks of the thoracoacromial artery exit from the axillary artery is a line drawn from the tip of the shoulder to the nipple. The skin island is designed medial to the nipple with the majority or all of the flap positioned on the inferior portion of the muscle which ends at the fifth rib. Any design of extension inferiorly to increase the length of rotation needs to consider a preliminary delay that incorporates ligation of the medial intercostal perforators. Once identified proximally, the thoracoacromial vascular pedicle can be dissected free of pectoralis major by decision of the clavicular portion of the muscle, a technique similar to the dissection of a perforator flap but in reverse. To do so will increase the rotation and flexibility of the flap by lengthening the pedicle. Care must be taken to ensure that the now-exposed pedicle is not kinked or compressed as the flap is rotated over the clavicle. The pectoralis major is the pedicled flap workhorse of head and neck reconstruction, but has been replaced, in part, by free flaps.)
   (a) Disadvantages? (The donor site is unsightly, the flap is bulky, and a second stage for division may be required, although the flap can be tunneled beneath intact neck skin as a single-stage procedure.)
   (b) Use? (The principal usage of the pectoralis major flap is a backup or "lifeboat" in situations of failure of the primary reconstruction. Closure of a pharyngocutaneous fistula and/or repair of a neck defect are two examples.)
3. Describe three local flaps. (Either unilateral or bilateral inferiorly-based nasolabial flaps can provide up to 10 cm^2 of tissue. They do require a second stage for retrieval and closure of the fistula. Tongue flaps have been described in the past but primarily are of historical interest since they can restrict the mobility of the anterior tongue. Lastly, the facial artery musculo-mucosal (FAMM) flap can be utilized but has been principally described for the closure of large palatal fistulas. Both the nasolabial and the FAMM flaps are based on the facial artery and are at substantial risk of necrosis if this structure was ligated in the performance of a concomitant neck dissection.)
4. What is the pertinent topographical anatomy of the submental artery (SMA) flap? (The flap is transversely oriented in the submental region with a maximum width of 5–6 cm and length of 10–12 cm to allow primary closure.)
5. What is the SMA flap's relationship with adjacent structures? (The flap consists of skin, fat, platysma, and the ipsilateral anterior belly of the digastric.)
6. What is the vascular anatomy of the SMA flap? (The SMA is a branch of the facial artery, coursing medially at the submandibular border, and terminates at the anterior belly of the digastric.)
7. Briefly, describe the key steps in elevation of the SMA flap. (The flap is outlined as described above and the ipsilateral inferior incision is accomplished to provide access for excision of the submandibular gland. Care is taken to avoid injury to the underlying lingual nerve and the facial vessels posterior. The submental branches of the facial vessels are identified. Further dissection is superficial to the mylohyoid. The anterior belly of the digastric is included by transection anteriorly at the mandible and inferiorly near the hyoid. Once the perforator is included, the superior incision of the skin island completes the dissection.)

Free Flaps

1. As discussed above, what defects are optimally managed by a radial forearm-free flap (RFFF)? (Floor of mouth, retromolar trigone, lateral tongue, buccal cavity—all defects that are optimally reconstructed with a thin, pliable flap.)
   (a) Appropriate preoperative assessment from the aspect of the donor site? (Performance of an Allen test to ensure that the hand is not radial artery dominant.)

2. Describe the pertinent anatomy and briefly describe the technique of harvesting the radial forearm flap, RFF. (The pertinent anatomy consists of the radial artery that courses between the brachioradialis and the flexor carpi radialis (FCR) in the proximal forearm within the intermuscular septum and is covered by the pronator teres. In the distal one-third or one-half of the forearm, the artery is only subfascial and is accompanied by the two venae comitantes and the cephalic vein. The technique consists of the performance of the proximal ulnar incision first. In the proximal forearm, the radial artery is deep to the pronator teres. A suprafascial dissection off the muscle bellies of the flexor digitorum sublimis distal to the pronator teres is performed leaving paratenon on the flexor carpi radialis and identification of the radial artery distally at the wrist. The dissection is switched to the radial side with retraction of the brachioradialis radially and identification of the superficial branch of the radial nerve and protection of the same. The intermuscular septum is divided deep to the overlying pedicle of the radial artery. A proximal or reversed radial forearm flap is almost always performed as a pedicle flap and differs principally in the wide fascial attachment that is necessary to ensure multiple distal perforators to the fascial plexus are preserved. The wide subfascial dissection of the proximal flap, distally based with a reversed pedicle, does not present a problem since a skin graft will take well over the muscle bellies. A suprafascial dissection is necessary distally until the septum is encountered to ensure paratenon on the flexor tendons, particularly the flexor carpi radialis, for a secure skin graft take. If the flap is to be employed as a free microvascular flap, the distal artery at the wrist is ligated first, the flap elevated dividing branches to the radial periosteum, and the proximal pedicle controlled last.)
   (a) What is the necessary maneuver to harvest an osteocutaneous flap? (The flexor pollicis longus is incised to leave a generous cuff of muscle on the volar aspect of the radius that will be incorporated with the skin flap.)
   (b) Advantages and disadvantages? (Principal advantages are the thinness and pliability of the flap as well as the consistent and long vascular pedicle if used as a free flap. Disadvantages: If used as an osteocutaneous flap, the bone stock is minimal with the hazard of fracture of the radius donor site; particularly donor site morbidity if the tendon of the flexor carpi radialis is exposed and cosmesis of the skin-grafted donor site.)
   (c) Venous drainage. (Venous is through the venae comitantes and, if incorporated, the cephalic vein.)
3. What is the difference between the dissection of a reverse, distal-based, and proximal-based radial forearm flap and why? (As outlined in the above question, a subfascial dissection proximally is performed more widely of a reversed radial forearm flap over the muscle bellies of the flexor carpi radialis and brachioradialis because of the greater space between perforators proximal as opposed to distally and the ease of skin graft take on the muscle bellies. Distally, in the most proximal-based and reverse distally based flaps, care should be taken to ensure the dissection is suprafascial to leave paratenon over the tendons, particularly the flexor carpi radialis. Of course, distally the dissection is deep or subfascial when intimate to the vessel and to facilitate the division of the intermuscular septum.)
4. What tendon can be incorporated? (Palmaris longus)
   (a) Nerve? (Lateral brachial cutaneous, the distal extension is the lateral cutaneous nerve of the forearm.)
5. What is the inferior cubital artery and its location? (The inferior cubital artery is a large proximal radial artery perforator, located at about 4 cm below the elbow flexion crease.)
6. Name two principal complications of the soft tissue radial forearm flap. (Neuroma of the superficial radial nerve, exposed tendon and loss of the flexor carpi radialis. To avoid poor graft, take with exposure and desiccation of the flexor carpi radialis (FCR) tendon, management has varied. The primary consideration is the preservation of paratenon and fascia over the tendons of both the FCR and the palmaris longus. One option is placement of Integra®, use of the portable negative pressure wound therapy device and delayed skin grafting.)
7. The anterolateral thigh (ALT) flap is actually, in most cases, a vastus lateralis flap. Why? (In a preponderance of cases, perhaps 87%, the perforators are musculocutaneous to the vastus lateralis, septocutaneous in the remainder.)
   (a) From what vessel? (The descending branch of the lateral femoral cutaneous. The latter exiting from the profundus about 3 cm below the inguinal ligament.)
   (b) What septum? (Intermuscular septum between vastus lateralis and rectus femoris medially.)
8. The principal perforators can be located where? (The midpoint of a vertical line from the anterior superior iliac spine to the lateral border of the patella. At that point inside a circle, 3 cm in radius usually in the inferior lateral quadrant, are the principal perforators to the flap. Because of some variability in the location of the perforator or perforators, identification should be accomplished with the Doppler.)
9. List the advantages and disadvantages of the ALT flap. (The advantages include a two-team approach, ample skin-soft tissue including two separate islands, bulk by the inclusion of the vastus lateralis and/or rectus

femoris, and long pedicle. Disadvantages include thickness, particularly in overweight or obese patients, and donor site cosmesis if a skin graft is necessary for closure.)

10. Briefly, describe the development and elevation of the ALT flap. (The medial incision is through the thigh fascia and a subfascial dissection is directed laterally over the rectus femoris into the lateral border and the intermuscular septum between that muscle and the vastus lateralis is visualized. Perforators may be seen at that point either coursing through the vastus lateralis or in the septum. The ascending branch of the lateral femoral cutaneous can be seen over the vastus lateralis and sending perforators to the skin. The flap is elevated from lateral to medial and the branches dissected off the surrounding tissue. If the flap is perfused by musculocutaneous perforators, intermuscular dissection through the vastus lateralis may be necessary, although a small cuff of muscle may be included.)
    (a) Contrast supra vs. subfascial dissection. (Suprafascial dissection enables the harvest of a thinner flap and sets the stage for defatting, if needed. Yet, the dissection is more tedious because of the necessity to identify both anteriorly and posteriorly the critical skin perforators. Subfascial dissection is more readily accomplished since it gains access to the septum that contains the descending branch quite readily and a "map" of the arterial anatomy is readily provided.)
    (b) What is the location of the pivot point for a pedicled ALT flap? (2 cm inferior to the inguinal ligament.)

Video Notes

Urken M, Buchbinder D, Wei FC, Dayan JH, "Video 1—Maxillary Reconstruction Using an Osteocutaneous Radial Forearm Flap—Part 2: Flap design and harvesting technique", *Plast. Reconstr. Surg.*, (March 2013); 131(3). p 411e–424e.

- Fair video, good narrative

Hallock, Geoffrey G.; Morris, Steven F., "Skin Grafts and Local Flaps", Geoffrey G. Hallock, *Plast. Reconstr. Surg.*, (Jan. 2011); 127:(1): 5e–22e. **(Only Video 3)**

- A slide presentation, but good quality and narrative

Case-Based Conference

Case 1: Oral Cavity Lesion

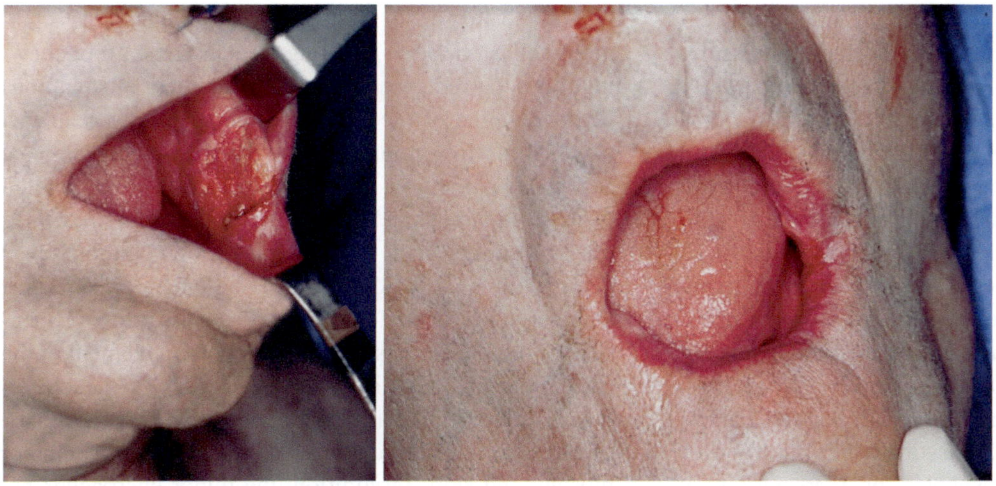

An 82-year-old snuff dipper woman with a 4–6-month history of an enlarging lesion as pictured. On examination, the cheek skin overlying the lesion is of limited mobility. The patient is in excellent health.

1. Describe the slide(s). Add a focused clinical examination including a physical. Limit your history to two or three pertinent questions.
    (a) Any tests indicated? Justify.
2. Describe the pathologic anatomy and add the most likely pathologic diagnosis.
3. Based on the response to Question 2, outline an oncologic and reconstructive plan.

Case-Based Conference: Discussion

Case 1: Oral Cavity Lesion

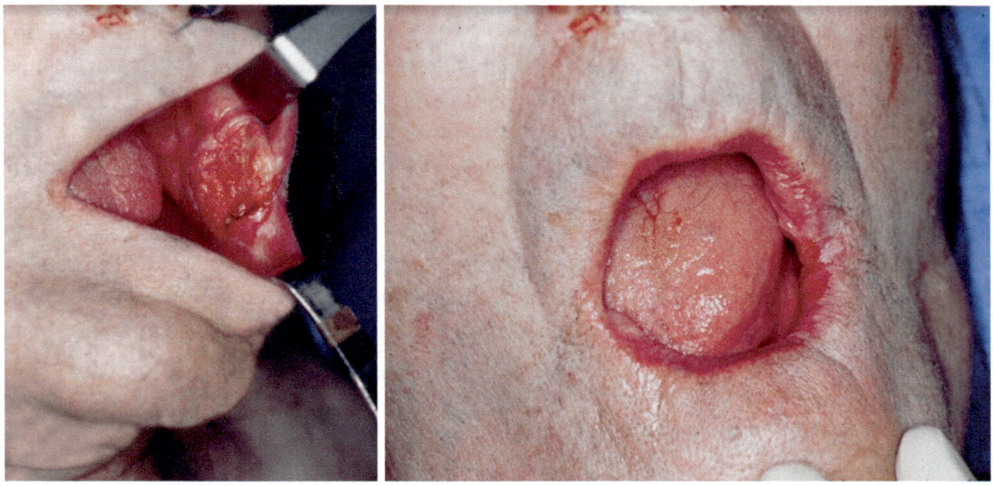

A 76-year-old snuff dipper woman with a 2–3-month history of an enlarging lesion as pictured. On examination, the cheek skin overlying the lesion is of limited mobility. The patient is in excellent health.

1. Describe the slide(s). (Intraoral view demonstrates a fungating lesion, apparently somewhat ulcerated with an overall verrucous appearance. The lesion which appears about 3 cm in diameter is located in the anterior buccal cavity, the anterior border just short of the commissure. Although the mandibular sulcus is visible and apparently not involved, the maxillary sulcus is not seen. The extraoral view demonstrates intact skin, commissure, and apparently a full oral excursion.) Add a focused clinical examination including a physical. Limit your history to two or three pertinent questions. (The history would focus on symptoms indicative of local spread, such as radiating facial pain over the distribution of the infraorbital nerve and trismus which would raise concerns about extension into the pterygoid fossa. Trismus could also be from tumor inflammation, although as mentioned the patient appears to open adequately. Questions eliciting the possible presence of otalgia, dysphagia, or hoarseness may point to a synchronous primary. Physical exam would focus on examination of the lymph node basins of the neck, particularly the submandibular and anterior cervical areas. An intraoral exam demonstrates the extent of tumor, involvement of maxillary and mandibular sulci, and posterior extension including Stensen's duct and pterygomandibular raphé. The preamble describes limited skin mobility, an important physical finding.)
   (a) Any tests indicated? Justify. (Clearly, a biopsy will be necessary but also a CT scan of the upper aerodigestive tract and chest as well as endoscopy of the oropharynx and larynx. A biopsy of the lesion can be accomplished in the same setting. Flexible endoscopy can be accomplished in the office as well as a biopsy. A CT scan of the head and neck and chest is indicated less for the extent of tumor in this case and more for the detection of a synchronous primary.)
2. Describe the pathologic anatomy and add the most likely pathologic diagnosis. (The probable diagnosis is squamous cell carcinoma. The long-term use of snuff or chewing tobacco predisposes to the development of squamous cell carcinoma of the oral cavity. A specific variant that occurs in this population is verrucous carcinoma. Verrucous carcinoma is an extremely well-differentiated form of squamous cell cancer with pushing rather infiltrating borders seen on histology often without even demonstrable invasion of the basement membrane. Clinically, verrucous carcinoma has a very low propensity for regional metastases. The important element of the pathologic anatomy is the cross-section of the cheek-buccal cavity in the area of the tumor. The layers consist of mucosa, buccinator space, buccal fat pad, buccinator muscle, and skin. In addition, the tumor encroaches but doesn't involve the oral commissure. The TNM, tumor size, nodal status, presence of metastases, stage is T2N0M0 or T4N0M0 if skin is involved.)
3. Based on the responses to Question 2, outline an oncologic and reconstructive plan. (Two theoretical scenarios; one, a diagnosis of a garden variety of squamous cell cancer, the other verrucous carcinoma. The diagnosis of verrucous carcinoma is important since the treatment plan would differ substantially. Neck dissection is not indicated in the treatment of a verrucous carcinoma nor is

radiotherapy since evidence exists that conversion to a more virulent form of squamous cell carcinoma is possible, although this aspect remains controversial. Resection would entail a minimal 1 cm mucosa margin and full-thickness excision including the overlying cheek and skin creating a through-and-through defect. In addition, a margin of the upper and lower lip, probably a minimum of 1.5 cm of each, will be excised. If the diagnosis is squamous cell and not verrucous variant carcinoma, a discontinuous or selective neck dissection should also be performed.

Reconstruction will need to address a full-thickness cheek defect of 4–5 cm in diameter. Although a two-skin paddle extended pectoralis major pedicle flap is an option, the bulk is considerable for the reconstitution of a thin, supple cheek. A microvascular free flap would also need to meet the same requirements. Of possible choices, the radial forearm-free flap would be optimal. Another option of a two-paddle skin island design is the anterolateral thigh (ALT) flap, particularly in an older, non-obese patient, but overall would not meet the criteria of thinness and pliability. Other free flaps available that permit the harvest of a double-skin island include the supraclavicular and superficial circumflex iliac perforator flaps. Both have a shorter pedicle than radial or ALT and the bridge will need to be de-epithelialized to ensure perfusion. Exposure of recipient vessels in the neck is facilitated by neck dissection in the instance of squamous cell cancer. In the case of a verrucous carcinoma, an exposure dissection will be necessary and, if enlarged, upper cervical nodes could be harvested as well. Hyperplastic cervical nodes are not uncommon in cases of verrucous carcinoma.

The resident should be able to describe the harvest of a radial forearm flap.)

Intraoperative

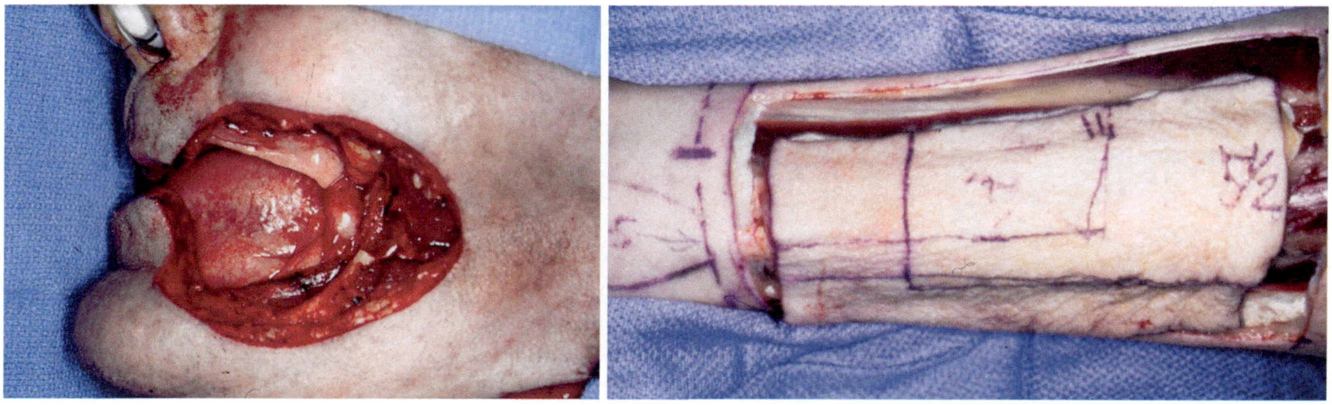

A single intraoperative view, lateral and limited to the lower face, illustrates the defect. What is visible is a full-thickness or through-and-through defect that includes skin-soft tissue of the commissure and 8 × 6 cm of the cheek. Intraorally, the buccal cavity lesion has been extirpated and the maxillary alveolus is visible and the mandible to the retromolar trigone. A single flap for reconstruction would mandate two separate skin islands and the radial forearm as a donor site has been marked.

Postoperative (2 and 8 Months)

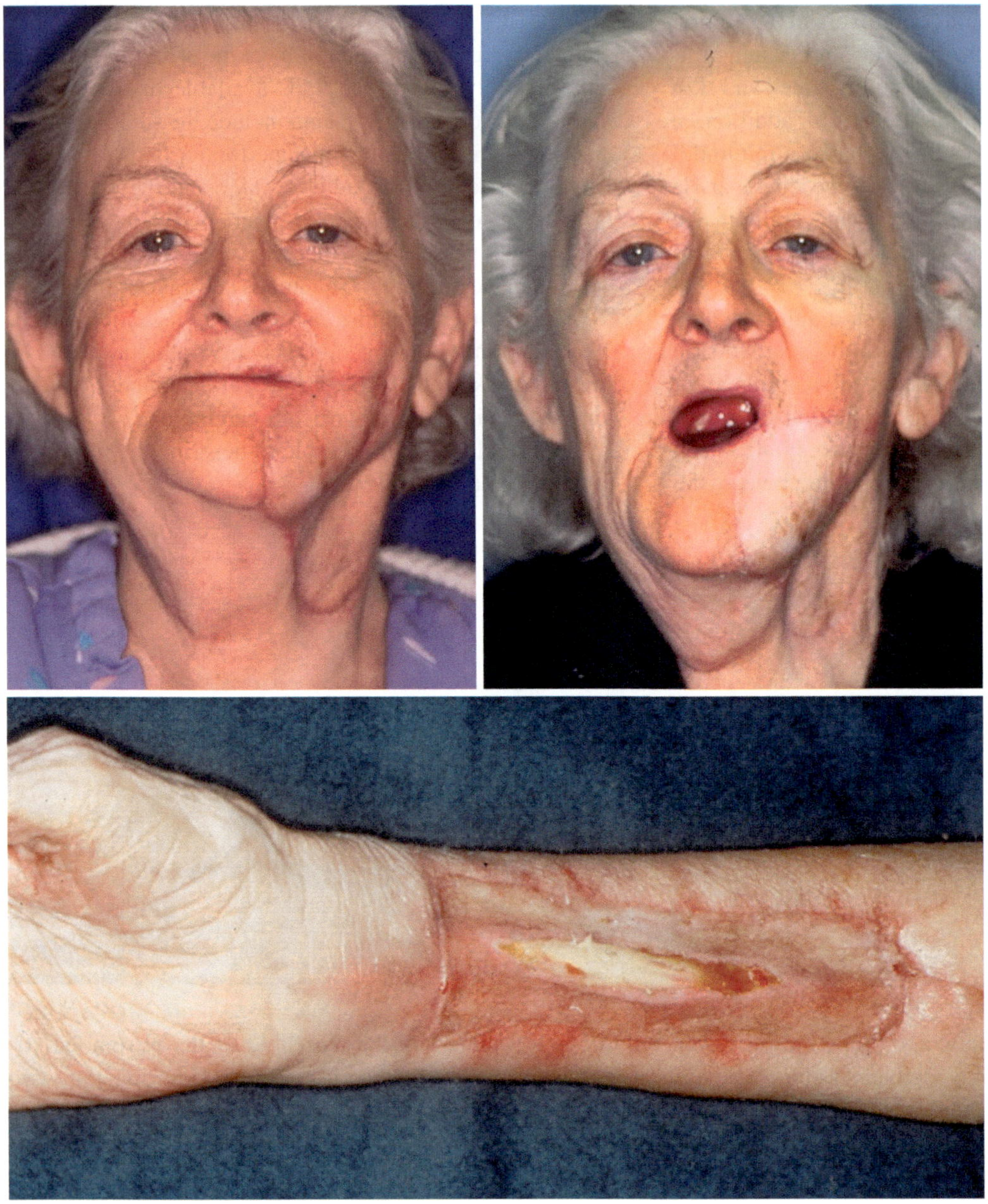

The postoperative photos represent the result at 2 and 8 months. In the former, the flap is well-healed and the patient is apparently on a postoperative diet. In the latter, 8 months, the color and hue difference between the forearm and cheek is more evident. The patient has a good oral opening.

The forearm donor site contains a large segment of the exposed tendon, probably the flexor carpi radialis at the 2-month hiatus. The potential for the occurrence of this complication is the principal drawback and liability of the radial forearm flap, a potential probably enhanced by the necessity to recruit most of the volar forearm for reconstruction. A variety of modalities have been employed in an effort to minimize the occurrence, including a suprafacial harvest in the distal forearm and the use of an acellular dermal matrix with the VAC, for coverage with a delayed application of a split-thickness skin graft. Exposure and eventual loss of the flexor carpi radialis is not an inconsequential complication, committing the patient to a period of dressing changes and loss of a major wrist flexor.

Critique

Another option could have been the supraclavicular perforator flap for coverage and a radial forearm for intraoral reconstruction. A considerably smaller skin island would have been required.

Case-Based Conference

Case 2: Ca of the Oropharynx

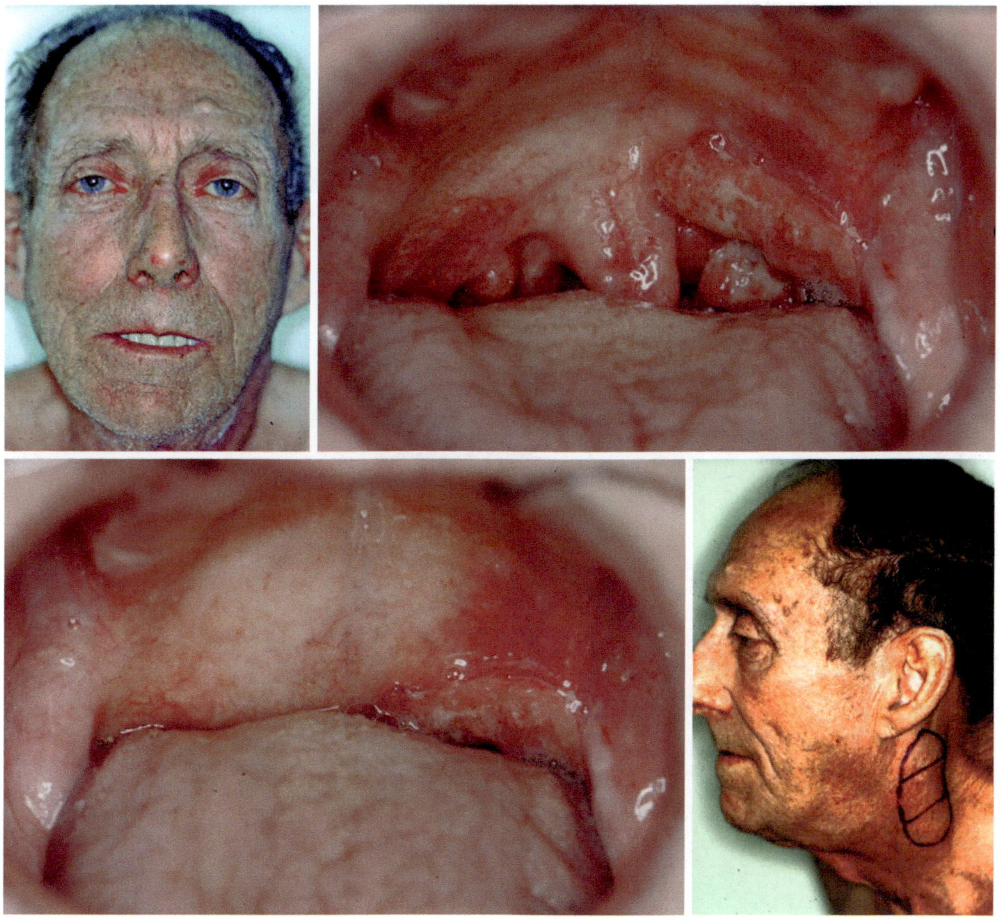

A 60-year-old male with a 6-month history of worsening dysphagia and otalgia. No significant medical problems and is a nonsmoker. Chemoradiation was aborted because of persistent toxicity.

1. Describe the slides. Add a focused clinical exam.
   (a) Any tests indicated? Justify.
2. Outline the pathologic anatomy.
3. Based on your response to Question 2, describe a management plan that encompasses the pre-, intra-, and postoperative periods.

Case-Based Conference: Discussion

Case 2: Ca of the Oropharynx

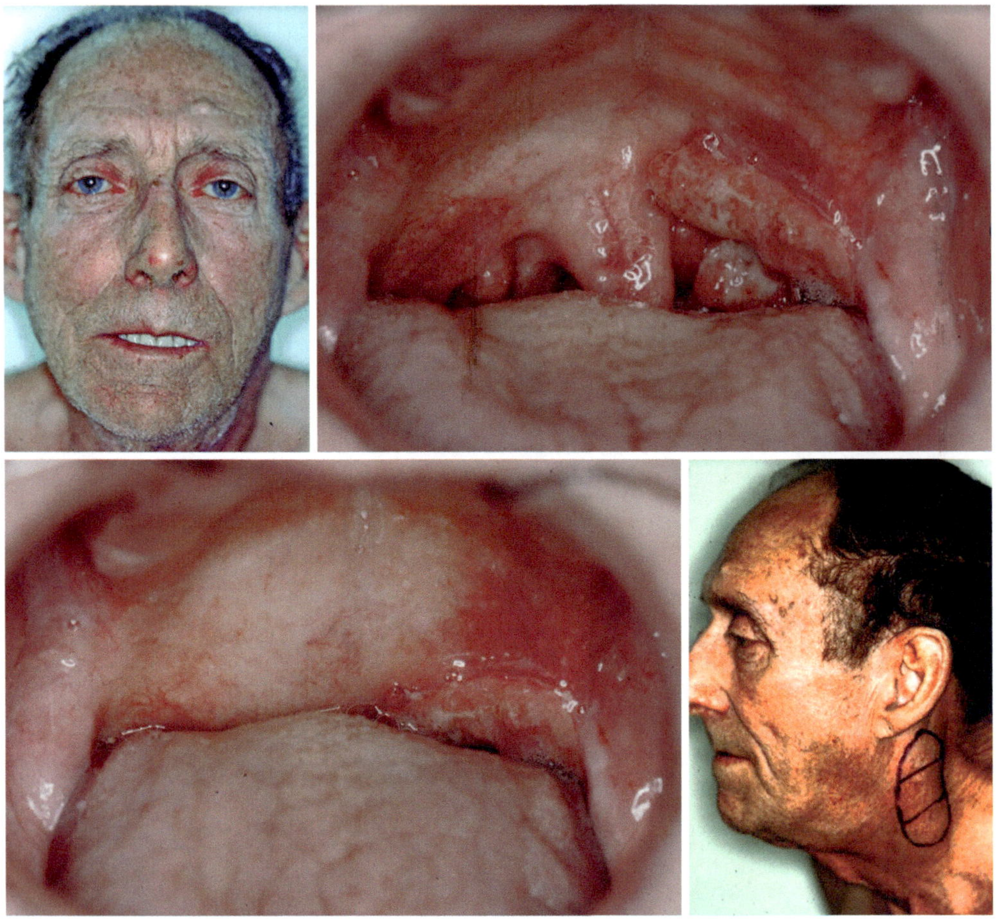

A 60-year-old male with a 6-month history of worsening dysphagia and otalgia. No significant medical problems and is a nonsmoker. Chemoradiation was aborted because of persistent toxicity.

1. Describe the slides. Add a focused clinical exam. (The four slides provided are a frontal and lateral view of the head and neck area of the patient as well as two intraoral views. The frontal view is of a white male who appears his stated age. The intraoral views demonstrate an exophytic mass that appears to arise from the left tonsillar fossa with involvement of the anterior tonsillar pillar and adjacent soft palate. The other intraoral areas of the lateral pharyngeal wall and base of tongue are not visible. The lateral head and neck view demonstrates the markings that appear to illustrate a large cervical mass perhaps 3 × 6 cm located superiorly at the apex of the confluence of the anterior and posterior cervical triangles. The patient's slides do not appear to depict a significant weight loss.

   The history centers on the possible systemic effects of a presumed oral neoplasm including weight loss, night sweats, pulmonary complaints, as well as the specifics of the dysphagia and otalgia: dysphagia for both solids and liquids, unilateral otalgia, and neck pain. Also important are complaints specific to the involvement of the fifth cranial nerve including trismus and facial pain. The circumstances of the failure of chemoradiation, particularly renal failure or diminished renal function, should be pursued in an estimate of the dose of radiotherapy administered. The physical exam would begin in the neck with palpation of the lymph node-bearing areas bilaterally, including the left supraclavicular fossa. The left neck mass is assessed for mobility and degree of firmness. A complete examination encompasses palpation of the axillae and abdomen including the liver. The intraoral exam attempts to define the extent of the tonsillar fossa tumor and an otoscopic exam to visualize the tympanic membrane on the left is important as well. The principal donor sites for flap reconstruction are examined: chest for a pectoralis major, abdomen for a rectus abdominis, thigh for anterolateral thigh (ALT), and, less likely, the arm for a radial forearm-free flap. Given the abortion of his neoadjuvant therapy, an important element of the overall assessment is the degree of cachexia induced by the chemoradiation.)

(a) Any tests indicated? Justify. (In the absence of a history of tobacco use, consideration should be given to a diagnosis of lymphoma or human papillomavirus (HPV)-related squamous cell carcinoma. The first is discussed below. Methods of molecular biology by a test of the p16 antigen have increased the detection of HPV substantially and may have some prognostic implications, particularly an enhanced response to neoadjuvant chemoradiation. A critical element of the assessment is imaging of the neck and the intraoral mass. Either with or without contrast, the scan should determine if the carotid is involved and the degree of involvement. Possible extension of the intraoral and tonsillar mass into the pterygoid space and base of tongue should be assessed. The CT scan can include the chest for detection of possible second primary or metastases. If a prior biopsy had not been accomplished, then the exam under anesthesia, biopsy, and laryngoscopy should be performed. As discussed below, a core needle biopsy of the neck mass would be advisable as well.)

2. Outline the pathologic anatomy. (The principal pathologic aspect of tonsillar lesions that impacts therapy is the extension of tumor into adjacent anatomic spaces. Extension deep or laterally can involve pterygoid muscles and superiorly the pterygoid fossa. Either can result in trismus because of involvement of the medial and lateral pterygoid musculature or perineural spread into the mandibular division of the trigeminal nerve. Spread of tumor posteriorly and superiorly into the fossa of Rosenmuller in the lateral nasopharynx can obstruct the orifice of the eustachian tube and produce otalgia and diminished hearing. Otalgia may also occur because of referred pain via the superior laryngeal nerve to the nerve of Arnold, a branch of the vagus. The presence of otalgia suggests involvement of the naso- and/or hypopharynx.

   The principal pathological anatomy of cervical metastatic disease is the involvement of the internal carotid. The size of the lymph node would be classified as either N2a (less than 6 cm) or N3, both of which are stage IV disease, regardless of the size or T stage of the primary. The cervical lymph node basin(s) involved are level II, III, and possibly IV.)

3. Based on your response to Question 2, describe a management plan that encompasses the pre-, intra-, and postoperative periods. (The first step in the management plan would be to establish or eliminate the possible diagnosis of lymphoma since 10–15% of primary neoplastic lesions of the tonsil may be lymphoma, a likelihood increased in this patient with a massive neck node as well as complete examination under anesthesia, examination under anesthesia (EUA), accompanied by direct laryngoscopy and biopsy of the primary. A portion of the biopsy should be submitted fresh in saline to aid the pathologist in distinguishing a diagnosis of lymphoma. The use of neoadjuvant therapy, a failure in this patient's scenario, to reduce the tumor load is beyond this discussion and given the N3 neck status postoperative or adjuvant chemoradiation would be a likely choice by some head and neck oncologists. The results of the CT scan will assist in guiding therapy.

   The surgical approach to resection would begin with a preliminary tracheostomy after prep and draping of the head and neck and chest. The patient will require a radical neck dissection, preservation of the internal jugular vein, dependent on tumor extent, and likely sacrifice of the spinal accessory nerve and sternocleidomastoid. The internal carotid is dissected sufficiently to minimize injury during the intraoral resection. Access to the intraoral excision, assuming a mandibular resection would not be necessary, would be a mandibular swing with a step-cut osteotomy at the midbody, incision on the lateral floor and mouth, and use of the tumor margin incisions on the soft palate, lateral tongue at the juncture of the mobile and base, and retromolar trigone tumor as further access for resection of the tumor. Most if not all of the lateral pharyngeal wall is the posterior limit, the deep or lateral margin dictated by tumor extent but in all likelihood the adjacent portion of the medial and lateral pterygoids.

   Reconstruction of the oropharyngeal defect, assuming mandibular preservation, could be accomplished with either a regional or a free flap. The regional flap of choice is a pectoralis major, perhaps with a preliminary delay at the time of the EUA, biopsy, and endoscopy. The principal negative of the pectoralis major flap is the bulk in the neck, less of an issue with loss of sternocleidomastoid, and atrophy will occur over months. The preferable free flap option is the anterolateral thigh (ALT) flap. The mandibular osteotomy is repaired with rigid fixation.

   Oral feedings begin at 7–10 days and the tracheostomy decannulation process begins as soon as feasible. Since the patient had extensive neck disease, postoperative radiotherapy is indicated and should be initiated after healing is evident and within the 6-week window of efficacy, possibly supplemented by concurrent chemotherapy.)

Postoperative (2 Months)

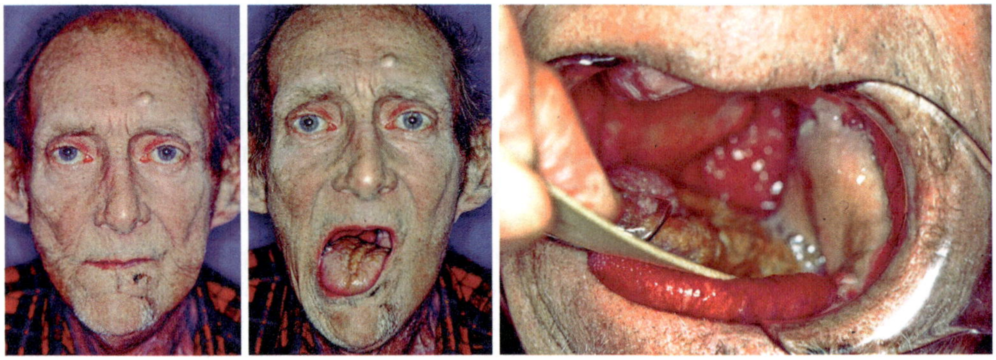

The three photos include a full-face view with the mouth closed and followed by the mouth open as well as an intraoral picture of the flap. The access for the resection was by a lip-splitting incision. No mandible was removed and reconstruction was accomplished with an extended pectoralis major flap, facilitated by a preliminary delay performed at the time of endoscopy. The improvement in perfusion enables the extension of the skin inferiorly over the rectus fascia. The skin island reconstructed the oropharyngeal defect and the oral cavity component of the retromolar trigone as well as the adjacent tongue. The patient demonstrates the mobility of the tongue enabled by the reconstruction.

Critique

The case is one of advanced, stage IV, oropharyngeal cancer that would dictate possible management with concurrent primary chemoradiation. The abortion of the therapeutic plan due to systemic toxicity presents the oncologic and reconstructive surgeons with a difficult task: extirpation of a large primary and extensive neck disease, followed by reconstruction. The option for reconstruction, a pedicled regional flap, may have hinged on the patient's preoperative frail condition. Free flaps as the radial forearm and ALT would have yielded an equally satisfactory result.

In-Service Examination

1. To increase the length of the pedicle of the ALT flap requires dissection beneath which muscle?
   (a) Sartorius
   (b) Rectus femoris
   (c) Tensofascia lata
   (d) Gracilis
2. The supraclavicular flap is perfused by what vessel?
   (a) Thoracoacromial
   (b) Thoracodorsal
   (c) Transverse cervical
   (d) Branch of the external carotid
3. Subtotal glossectomy defects with preservation of the base of the tongue are optimally reconstructed with which of the following flaps?
   (a) Pectoralis major muscle
   (b) Deltopectoral
   (c) Split-thickness skin graft
   (d) Rectus abdominis
4. In resection of the submandibular gland a nerve coursing superiorly is visualized. What is the nerve?
   (a) Lingual
   (b) Hypoglossal
   (c) Marginal mandibular
   (d) Vagus

39 Hypopharynx, Maxilla

Bibliography

Cordeiro PG and Chen CM, "A 15-year review of midface reconstruction after total and subtotal maxillectomy: Part I algorithm and outcomes", *Plast. Reconstr. Surg.*, (2012); 129(1):**124–136**.

Koshy JC and Hollier Jr. LH, "Discussion: A 15-year review of midface reconstruction after total and subtotal maxillectomy: Part I algorithm and outcomes", *Plast. Reconstr. Surg.*, (2012); 129(1):**137–138**.

Angrigiani C., Matthew M. Hanasono MM., Chapter 40 "Scapular and Parascapular Flaps", *Flaps and Reconstructive Surgery 2nd edition*, Wei F.C., Mardini S; Elsevier Saunders: **432–444**.

Cho N.J., Yu P., Ch. 13 "Hypopharyngeal, Esophageal, and Neck Reconstruction", Neligan PC, Plastic Surgery, Elsevier 5th Edition, (2023), Volume 3: **pgs. 302–335**.

Hanasono M.M., Cordeiro P.G., Ch. 9: "Midface Reconstruction" Neligan PC, Plastic Surgery, Elsevier 5th Edition, (2023), Volume 3: **pg. 217–228**.

Lee ZH., Cripps C., Rodriguez E., "Current Concepts in Maxillary Reconstruction" Plast Reconstr Surg., (2022); 150(1):**168e–175e**.

Supplemental

Cordeiro PG and Chen CM, "A 15-year review of midface reconstruction after total and subtotal maxillectomy: Part II. Technical Modifications to Maximize Aesthetic and Functional Outcomes", *Plast. Reconstr. Surg.*, (2012); 129(1):**139–147**.

Video

Tsao CK, "Anterolateral thigh flaps for reconstruction of head and neck upper and lower extremity defect", *Flaps and Reconstructive Surgery*, Wei F.C., Mardini S; Elsevier Saunders (2009).

Faculty Discussion and Study Guide

Anatomy, Classification of Maxillary Defects

Editor's Note: Maxillary reconstruction is also discussed in Chap. 42.

1. Outline the essential anatomy of the maxilla. (Consider the maxilla as a cube with six walls. The floor of the cube is the hard palate. The roof is the orbital floor. The four remaining walls are the anterior, lateral, posterior, and medial walls of the maxillary sinus. Importantly, the medial wall of the sinus is the lateral wall of the nasal cavity. The posterior wall is intimately related to the neurovascular structures such as the trigeminal nerve and the internal maxillary artery. The medial nasal wall has the apertures for the maxillary and fronto-ethmoid sinuses as well as the nasolacrimal duct. The maxilla is the site of the vertical naso-maxillary, zygomatico-maxillary, pterygo-maxillary buttresses. One of the transverse buttresses also courses through the maxilla.)
2. Outline a classification system for maxillectomy defects. (Type I is a partial maxillectomy, usually the anterior and medial walls as in a medial maxillectomy. Type II is a subtotal and consists of resection of the entire maxilla except for the orbital floor. Type IIa is a subtotal maxillectomy but less than one-half of the hard palate and Type IIb is greater than one-half. Type III is a total maxillectomy including the orbital floor and palate, namely, all six walls of the maxillary cube. Type IIIA the orbital contents are intact; Type IIIB involves orbital exenteration in conjunction with a total maxillectomy. In Type IV, the palate is intact, but in addition to resection of the remaining maxilla and an orbital exenteration, the dura and brain are exposed.)

E. Luce, *A Curriculum for Plastic Surgery*, https://doi.org/10.1007/978-3-031-62087-4_39

Reconstruction of Maxillectomy Defects

1. What are the essential goals of maxillary or midface reconstruction following oncologic resection? ((1) Wound closure with obliteration of the resultant defect. (2) Globe support or obliteration of the orbital cavity. (3) Maintain a barrier between nasal sinuses, nasopharynx, and the anterior cranial fossa. (4) Reconstruct facial width, height, and projection. (5) Reconstruct the palate.)
2. Briefly describe options in the reconstruction of Type I defects. (The flap choice will hinge more on the magnitude of the associated soft tissue resection including nose, cheek, and perhaps eyelids rather than the bone. A thin pliable flap such as the radial forearm-free flap is a good choice.)
3. Briefly describe options in the reconstruction of Type II or subtotal maxillectomy defects. (Assuming a radical maxillectomy with little or no skin resected, the reconstructive goals are primarily the bone. The simplest is a skin graft of the defect in combination with an obturator. If free tissue transfer is the option, a thin skin island will be necessary, and such as a Type IIA, sufficient hard palate should remain for dentures or obturator, and a radial forearm flap is a reasonable choice.

   Type IIB defects require bone as well as skin-soft tissue. A radial forearm osteocutaneous flap is an option as is a scapular osteocutaneous flap harvested with the two available skin islands and bone. The bone is sandwiched between the skin islands for reconstruction of the intraoral bony palate and lining for the nose.)
4. Briefly describe options in the reconstruction of Type III. (Since all six walls of the maxilla are resected for Type IIIA, intact orbital contents but no floor, bone graft support will be necessary as well as skin-soft tissue for the palate and maxillary defect. In the non-irradiated setting, a rectus flap plus non-vascularized bone grafts or titanium mesh is one choice as is a scapular osteocutaneous flap which would provide vascularized bone. In Type IIIB, maxillectomy, orbital exenteration, and the anterior cranial base may be exposed, particularly medially, and again a rectus abdominis-free flap with one or more skin islands is the choice.)
   (a) A method for orbital reconstruction in a Type IIIA reconstruction. (Nonvascularized bone, rib, cranial bone, or ilium is one option. Most of these patients will require postoperative radiotherapy, so a case can be established for the use of vascularized bone, the scapular flap. A case also could be established for an anterolateral thigh (ALT) with vastus lateralis muscle as an alternate option to the rectus abdominis advocated in the readings and the use of titanium mesh for support of the orbital contents.)
5. Briefly describe options in the reconstruction of Type IV. (Type IV reconstructive needs are not unlike Type IIIB and again a rectus flap with skin is one excellent option since what is needed is a soft tissue filler and skin. An anterolateral thigh flap (ALT) can also address the reconstructive needs satisfactorily. If the oncologic plan dictates a substantial portion of the medial wall of the orbit will be resected, a frontal craniotomy may be necessary to ensure protection of the intracranial contents during resection, particularly if the plan encompasses the superior medial wall which will potentially violate the anterior cranial fossa. In those instances, a pericranial flap can be utilized to assist in the construction of a barrier between the nasopharynx and intracranial space.)
6. In addition to the specific tissue needs for each type of defect, what other technical consideration influences the choice of flap? (The length of the vascular pedicle. Anastomosis will be necessary for the neck and shorter pedicles, such that the lateral arm may not reach from the apex of the defect to the neck. In the heavily irradiated neck, the vessels may need to extend to the contralateral neck or thyrocervical trunk. Both the ALT and rectus flaps have the potential for longer pedicles.)
7. What is the pertinent anatomy of the scapular flap? (The primary blood supply is the circumflex scapular artery that is derived from the subscapular artery or trunk that emerges from the third portion of the axillary artery. The subscapular branches into a descending thoracodorsal and a more transverse circumflex scapular artery that courses into the triangular space bounded superiorly by the teres minor, inferiorly by the teres major, and laterally by the posterior lateral surface of the long head of the triceps. The skin island is supplied by the two terminal branches, the scapular cutaneous or horizontal branch of the superficial circumflex scapular and a vertical branch of the superficial circumflex scapular or parascapular cutaneous artery. The scapular branch is more transverse in distribution, parallel to the spine of the scapula while the parascapular is a descending branch parallel to the lateral border of the scapula.)
8. What are the advantages and disadvantages of the scapular flap? (Pedicle length *if* dissected proximal and the caliber of the vessels are a distinct advantage. The ability to primarily close a substantial-size skin island up to 9 cm is advantageous as well. The ability to harvest the bone with a separate pedicle from that of the skin island allows for some flexibility in the third-dimensional placement of the skin island and bone for head and neck defects. The disadvantage is the positioning of the patient which in most instances prevents a two-team approach as well as the thickness of the flap in more obese individuals. The pedicle without dissection into the triangular space can be relatively, 5–6 cm, short.)

9. Briefly describe the harvest of a scapular cutaneous flap. (The exit of the circumflex scapular from the triangular space can perhaps be identified with a Doppler and if not, the space is situated at the lateral border of the scapula about one-third to two-fifths inferiorly on a line connecting the midpoint of the scapular spine to angle. The course of the cutaneous branch, as described above, is parallel to the spine of the scapula and represents the central axis of the flap. The initial incision is along the superior limb of the skin island and deepened to the aponeurosis of the infraspinatus, teres minor, and deltoid muscles. The exit of the circumflex scapular artery from the triangular space can be noted and the descending or vertical branch ligated unless a parascapular flap will be harvested as well. Dissection is taken more proximal on the circumflex scapular artery around the lateral border of the scapula until the infrascapular branch is encountered passing deep to the infraspinatus muscle which is ligated. The final step is the completion of the skin island and elevation of the flap on its pedicle. Dissection of the subscapular axis further proximal can be performed to lengthen the ultimate harvest of the pedicle but can be difficult in the small area proximal to the triangular space.)
10. Describe the modification of the scapular flap with harvest of scapular bone, the scapular osteocutaneous flap. (The harvest of the bone segment can be performed on the medial border of the scapula supplied by the transverse branch of the circumflex scapular artery or the scapular cutaneous artery, but a skin island is necessary to ensure perfusion to the bone and the dorsal scapular artery may be the primary blood supply. A separate segment of bone can be harvested from the inferior or lateral border of the scapula based on the parascapular cutaneous artery, but this requires some additional proximal dissection to ensure sufficient pedicle length because of a shorter pedicle, compared to the medial osseous flap. The lateral osteocutaneous flap is harvested from the inferior for the insertion of the long head of the triceps and preserves the tip or inferior angle of the scapula. In addition, the angle of the scapula should be kept intact to preserve the attachments of the rhomboids, teres major, and serratus anterior. As mentioned, the medial osseous flap requires a cutaneous component since the blood supply traverses the fascial and/or skin attachments. Also, the vertical height of the bone harvested is less than the lateral flap and the flexibility of orientation of the skin island from the bone component may be more limited.)
11. What are the key points in the development of an osteocutaneous scapular flap with harvest of the bone from the medial aspect of the scapula? (The lateral or distal aspect of the cutaneous flap needs to remain attached to the underlying scapula. Incisions are made through the infraspinatus muscle and periosteum to the lateral aspect of the segment of the medial scapula to be harvested with osteotomies at that point. The flap is elevated in the underlying or anterior attachments of serratus anterior and subscapularis muscles and then separated from the flap. A cuff of greater rhomboid muscle is released from its attachment on the medial border of the scapula but a small muscle cuff is left attached to the distal tip of the skin flap. The harvest of the osseous component should retain a small segment inferior to the spine as well as the inferior angle to allow reattachment to the greater rhomboid and serratus anterior. The lateral aspect of the scapula can be harvested up to 12 cm in length, preserving the tip and up to 2 cm inferior to the shoulder joint capsule. The infraspinatus muscle is elevated sufficiently to permit osteotomies and the teres minor superiorly and major inferiorly are released. The subscapularis is divided after the completion of the osteotomies. The teres muscles are reattached.)
12. What is the essential difference between the parascapular and scapular cutaneous flaps? (The essential difference is the blood supply. The arterial anatomy of the scapular flap, as described above, is the transverse or horizontal proximal branch from the superficial circumflex scapular artery and vein after exiting through the triangular space. The other terminal branch of the circumflex is the descending vertical portion or parascapular cutaneous artery. As a result, the axis of the blood supply to the parascapular flap is vertical in distribution rather than transverse as in the scapular flap. As mentioned previously, without proximal dissection, the pedicle is short and necessitates in some instances a separate transaxillary incision and approach, possibly a tedious dissection given the tight space and large neurovascular structures in the area.)
13. What is the treatment quandary in the use of vascularized bone-free flaps? (Essentially, no absolute ideal option exists. Harvest of the radius risk fracture of the donor bone as well as a quite limited amount of bone is available. The iliac is an ample amount of bone but is a difficult donor site, and usually can be osteotomized only once. The fibula, of course, is an excellent choice. Finally, the scapula requires position change and potentially a short pedicle.)

Reconstruction of the Hypopharynx

1. Describe the pertinent anatomy of the hypopharynx. (The hypopharynx extends from the oropharynx anterior and superior and the cervical esophagus inferiorly. The oropharynx is defined by the soft palate superiorly, the base

of tongue and lingual aspect of the epiglottis inferiorly, and the tonsillar fossa and lateral pharyngeal walls laterally. The posterior limit is the posterior pharyngeal wall ending at the level of the hyoid. The hypopharynx in turn is the pharynx inferior to the hyoid including the posterior pharyngeal wall at the level of the cricopharyngeus, the cervical esophagus further inferior, the pyriform sinuses laterally, and the common wall between the larynx and the hypopharynx as the anterior limit.)

2. Describe the classification system for hypopharyngeal defects. (Type I was less than 50% of the circumference. Type II was greater than 50% or even the entire circumference of the hypopharynx. Type III was extensive because of the involvement of adjacent structures, such as the nasopharynx, oropharynx, floor of mouth, or mandible.)
3. Preoperative evaluation of the patient with anticipated hypopharyngeal defect? (Prior or planned concomitant laryngectomy, prior irradiation, nutritional status and the possible necessity for enteral feedings, status of anterior neck skin, and flap donor site(s).)
   (a) Comment on each. (The principal impact of prior surgery, including a laryngectomy, and prior irradiation is the occurrence of the fibrosed or "frozen" neck with a significant increase in the incidence of wound complications and the paucity of recipient vessels. In addition, the anterior cervical skin may be heavily irradiated as well and require replacement. Because of the difficulty in oral alimentation, many patients are chronically malnourished. A concerted effort should be directed also toward the cessation of tobacco and alcohol use preoperatively. Flap options are discussed below.)
4. Outline options in the reconstruction of the hypopharynx and justify each. (Pedicled flaps including the pectoralis major, deltopectoral, and supraclavicular flaps have some significant limitations including the necessity for a longitudinal suture line in addition to a proximal and distal anastomosis. Partial defects that cannot be closed primarily can be reconstructed with a thin pliable flap such as radial forearm. For more extensive circumferential defects, the options that are available include a segment of jejunum, anterolateral thigh flap, rectus abdominis, and radial forearm flap.

   On balance, the ALT flap has emerged as a popular choice, although it may not be suitable for the obese patient. The free jejunum requires a laparotomy and an intestinal anastomosis with all the potential intraabdominal complications, and a rectus abdominis in many patients may be too bulky. The radial forearm-free flap has a significant incidence of pharyngocutaneous leak and fistula. The flap also must be wide, about 9 cm, for circumferential defects although the flap can be oriented transversely rather than longitudinally, proximal to distal in cases of shorter defects. Finally, no free muscle option is available in the radial forearm flap to achieve neck skin resurfacing if needed. Speech rehabilitation with tracheoesophageal puncture is more consistently successful with fascio-cutaneous flaps.)
5. What are the principal complications with respect to hypopharyngeal reconstruction? (Either anastomotic leak with pharyngocutaneous fistula or stenosis and stricture. As is the case with all buried free flaps, monitoring is an issue. Both the jejunum and ALT can be monitored with a segment of intestine or flap placed externally. Of course, any tubed flap for reconstruction of a defect requires both a proximal and distal anastomosis as with a jejunum but also a longitudinal suture line with a t-closure at both the proximal and distal end.)

Specific Flaps

1. Describe the pertinent neurovascular anatomy of the anterolateral thigh (ALT) flap. (The sensory innervation is provided by the lateral femoral cutaneous nerve or L2–L3 and the arterial supply by the descending branch of the lateral femoral circumflex artery, a branch of the profunda femoris artery.)
   (a) Describe the specifics of the descending branch of the lateral femoral circumflex. (After arising from the profunda, the lateral femoral circumflex artery courses deep to the rectus femoris and sartorius and branches into ascending, transverse, and descending portions. After arising from the lateral femoral circumflex, the descending branch travels inferiorly at the medial edge of the vastus lateralis. In one-third of the cases, the descending branch divides into a medial and lateral portion at about the midpoint of the femur with the medial coursing underneath the rectus femoris to supply the rectus femoris and the skin overlying the anteromedial thigh. The lateral branch of the descending artery travels deep to the rectus femoris to give rise to the perforators either through the vastus lateralis or the septum to supply the skin of the anterolateral thigh.)
2. Describe the topographic anatomy, namely the location, of the perforators for the ALT flap. (A line is drawn from the anterior superior iliac spine to the lateral border of the patella and at a halfway point, a circle of 3 cm radius incorporates the vast majority of the perforators. In particular, the inferior lateral quadrant of that circle contains the dominant perforators.)
   (a) What is the specific point to recall in terms of the course of the perforators? (Only in 10–15% of the cases are the perforators truly septocutaneous. The

remainder are intramuscular, the vastus lateralis muscle, which provide vascular supply of the overlying skin.)

3. What are the principal advantages and disadvantages of the ALT flap? (The advantages include a substantial size pedicle, the ability to harvest as a two-team approach with head and neck reconstruction, and the lack of a true donor site dysfunction. The disadvantages primarily include the necessity for a skin graft to the donor site if the skin island is large and a color mismatch for head and neck reconstruction. In the obese, the flap may be quite bulky.)
   (a) Specifically, what advantages does the ALT have over the jejunum and radial forearm for hypopharyngeal reconstruction? (Clearly, jejunum is a potentially more morbid donor site. Radial forearm flap provides no muscle, if needed, for coverage of vessels. Finally, the ALT not only has the ability to harvest muscle as a chimeric flap but also two large skin islands for both hypopharyngeal reconstruction and replacement of heavily irradiated neck skin as well. The two skin islands on the radial forearm flap would be too small to accomplish those goals and the harvest of a flap of sufficient size to reconstruct a 3 cm caliber lumen or a 9 cm wide flap inflicts a large donor site on the arm.)
4. Describe the harvest of the ALT flap. (Once the location of the perforators is identified with the use of the above description and a Doppler, the medial limb of the proposed skin island is incised and dissection carried beneath the fascia of the rectus femoris. Dissection is then taken laterally over the muscle with medial retraction until the intermuscular septum between rectus femoris and vastus lateralis is exposed and the descending branch of the lateral femoral circumflex artery can be visualized at that point. The lateral limb of the skin island is incised and dissection then proceeds medially. The next step is the intermuscular dissection, in the vast majority of cases, of the perforators free from the vastus lateralis muscle to their origin from the descending branch or, alternatively, harvest a cuff of muscle. The final part of the dissection is to release the descending branch from the surrounding septal attachments.)
   (a) Contrast supra vs. subfascial dissection. (Suprafascial dissection enables the harvest of a thinner flap and sets the stage for defatting if needed. Yet, the dissection is more tedious because of the necessity to identify both anteriorly and posteriorly the critical skin perforators. Subfascial dissection is more readily accomplished since it gains access to the septum that contains the descending branch and a "map" of the arterial anatomy is relatively quickly provided.)
   (b) What is the location of the pivot point for a pedicled ALT flap? (2 cm inferior to the inguinal ligament.)

Case-Based Conference

Case 1: Hypopharyngeal Stricture

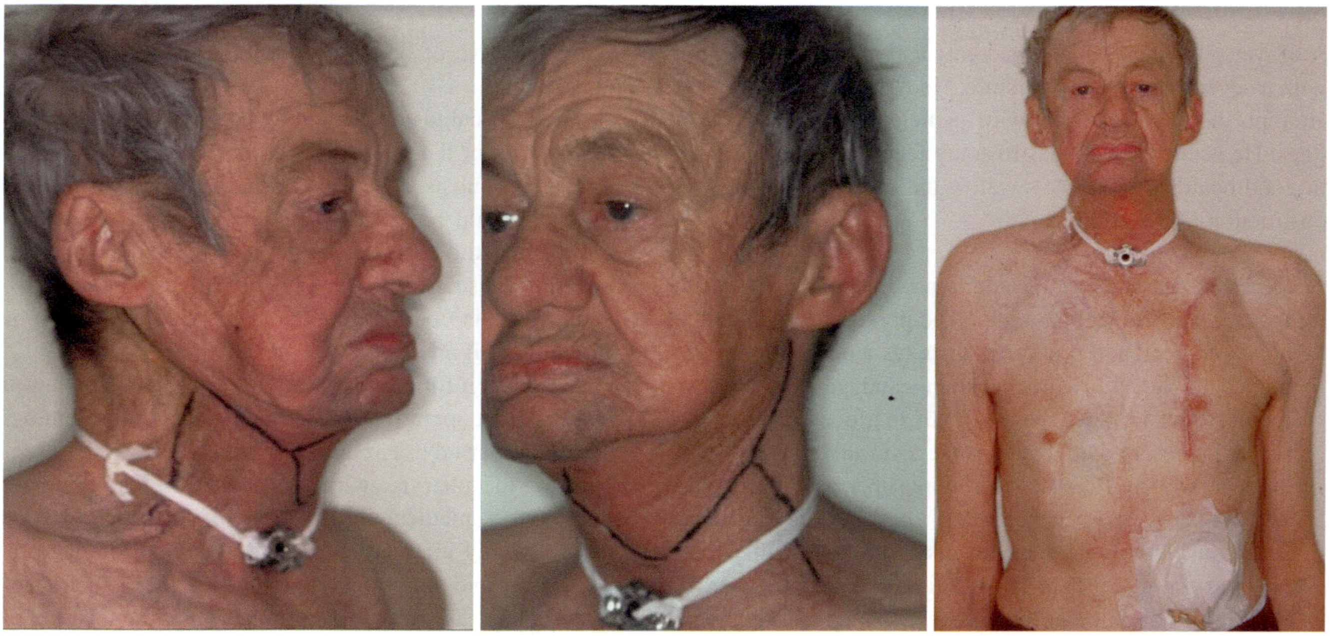

A 68-year-old s/p total laryngectomy and irradiation therapy with a severe pharyngeal stricture. He has had two previous attempts at reconstruction with pedicled pectoralis major flaps. He is currently on gastrostomy feedings but otherwise in good health. A contrast swallow indicates near-complete obstruction of the pharynx.

1. Describe the slides. Add additional information from a focused clinical examination.
   (a) Any tests indicated? Justify (as above).
2. Summarize the pathologic anatomy. Describe the likely contributing factors in the patient's case.
3. Outline a menu of options. Select your choice, justify, and describe. Be prepared to discuss the other options as well.

Case-Based Conference: Discussion

Case 1: Hypopharyngeal Stricture

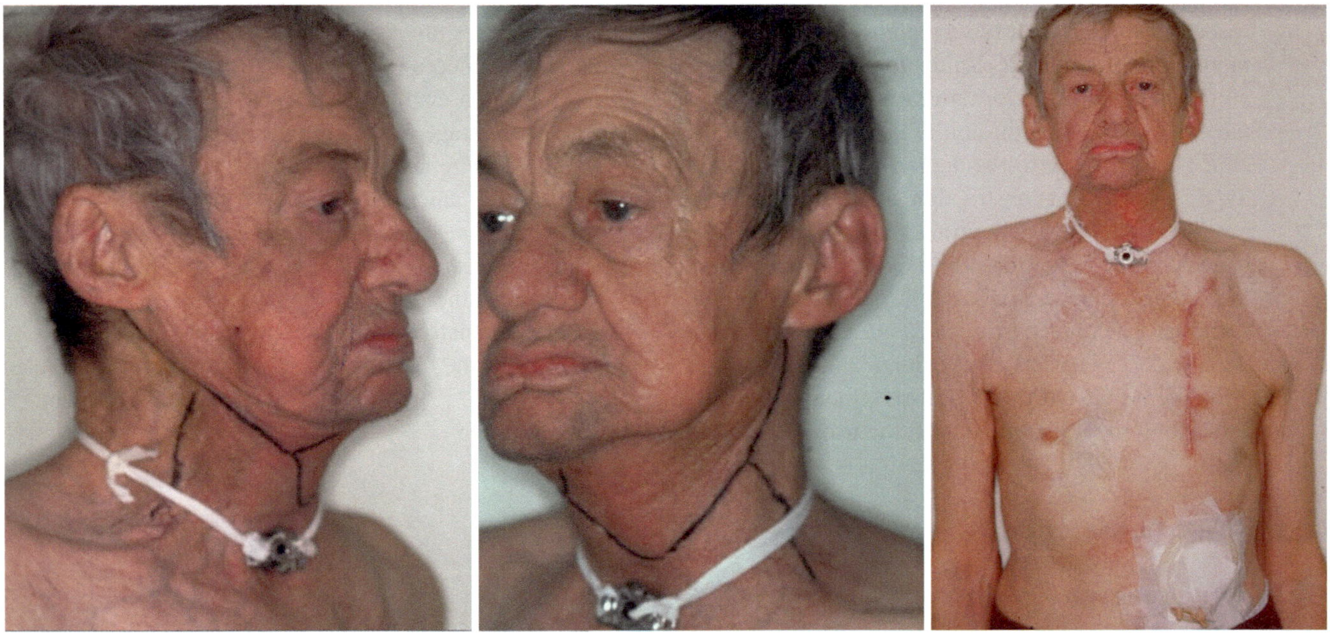

A 68-year-old s/p total laryngectomy and irradiation therapy with a severe pharyngeal stricture. He has had two previous attempts at reconstruction with pedicled pectoralis major flaps. He is currently on gastrostomy feedings but otherwise in good health. A contrast swallow indicates near-complete obstruction of the pharynx.

1. Describe the slides. Add additional information from a focused clinical examination. (The photo of the patient's head and neck and trunk demonstrates a male of normal, not cachexic with a tracheostomy and gastrostomy or jejunostomy in place. A skin graft that does not appear recent is present over the inferior chest wall and subcostal angle as well as a vertical scar more superiorly consistent with a history of a pec major flap. On the left is a vertical scar, considerably more recent, also consistent with a history of pect. major flap. The full face and neck view adds little information other than bronzed changes of the neck skin indicative of heavy irradiation. The patient has no facial edema.

   The medical history would focus, in this incidence, on the severity of the obstruction from the pharyngeal stricture and stenosis. The key questions to ascertain that severity would be: Can the patient swallow any liquids orally? In addition, is the patient able to handle and swallow his own secretions? The history of past nonoperative therapy of his obstruction should be pursued as well as weight loss, if any.

   Medical information that needs to be reviewed includes past operative notes. Presumably, the patient has had either partial or circumferential replacement of a segment of the pharynx with the pectoralis major flap or flaps. Other medical information of value would be a review of any imaging such as a computed tomography (CT) scan and a contrast swallow for the detection of recurrent disease and the determination of the location of the pharyngeal stricture. The preamble states the patient is in good health and does not appear malnourished but a nutrition profile would be advisable.

The physical exam would include palpation of the neck for any evidence of locoregional recurrence and an intraoral examination. Potential donor sites for esophageal reconstruction are examined including the abdomen and anterior thigh. An Allen's test is performed on the non-dominant arm.)

(a) Any tests indicated? Justify. (In addition, esophagoscopy under anesthesia with biopsy would be highly advisable)

2. Summarize the pathologic anatomy. Describe the likely contributing factors in the patient's case. (The inciting event was an initial suture line leak, perhaps abscess, and secondary healing that resulted in pharyngeal stenosis, a situation more commonly seen in laryngectomy patients who have been previously irradiated rather than postoperative irradiation. Regardless, in the setting of the occurrence of a salivary leak through a suture line or as a result of some element of minor flap necrosis, the proteolytic enzymes in saliva provide a scenario of chronic inflammation and secondary healing with the high possibility of stricture. The other consideration is a local recurrence of the cancer.)
3. Outline a menu of options. Select your choice, justify, and describe. Be prepared to discuss the other options as well. (Nonoperative management consists of bougie periodic dilatation of the stricture, a method that may be successful in mild to moderate strictures. The presence of irradiation does not set the stage for a favorable outcome of this option. Operative management requires an aggressive approach that entails excision of the contents of the anterior neck including remnants of any flap tissue from prior reconstructive efforts. Once complete, the anterior neck should be empty to the level of the prevertebral fascia. Hypopharyngeal-pharyngeal reconstruction will require free tissue transfer. Options include free jejunum, radial forearm, or anterolateral thigh (ALT) flap. Each has distinct advantages and disadvantages. The jejunum is placed in an antiperistaltic position, replacing like with like, and when spaculated, enables an optimal anastomosis to the wide aperture of the proximal hypopharyngeal inlet. The two disadvantages are the necessity of a laparotomy and small bowel anastomosis, as well as the heavy bowel secretions that may prevent a successful tracheopharyngeal (TP) puncture restoration of pharyngeal speech with a Blom-Singer prosthesis. The radial forearm-free flap also has a donor site deficit but is a thin fasciocutaneous flap that meets the needs for pharyngeal reconstruction but may require longer healing and NPO, no oral intake status. The ALT flap in a non-obese patient is the most recently described option that also permits, if cervical space permits, a harvest of muscle to reinforce either the suture line or coverage of the great vessels. If a thinned, suprafascial ALT flap is fashioned in the non-obese patient, the criteria of the desirable free tissue transfer for pharyngeal reconstruction can be met. In all three instances (jejunum, radial forearm, and ALT flaps), a small separate segment can be externalized as a monitor with the design of a separate skin island. Consideration should be given to whether replacement of a portion of the heavily irradiated cervical skin will be necessary. If so, the radial forearm probably will not have sufficient-sized flap harvest to both reconstruct the pharynx and provide coverage, and the jejunum, of course, will not have the capability to do so as well. The ALT flap, if planned carefully, could provide sufficient skin for coverage as well as pharyngeal reconstruction. In contrast to the jejunum, both the ALT and radial forearm flaps have a vertical suture line and both a proximal and distal "T" closure.)

Intraoperative

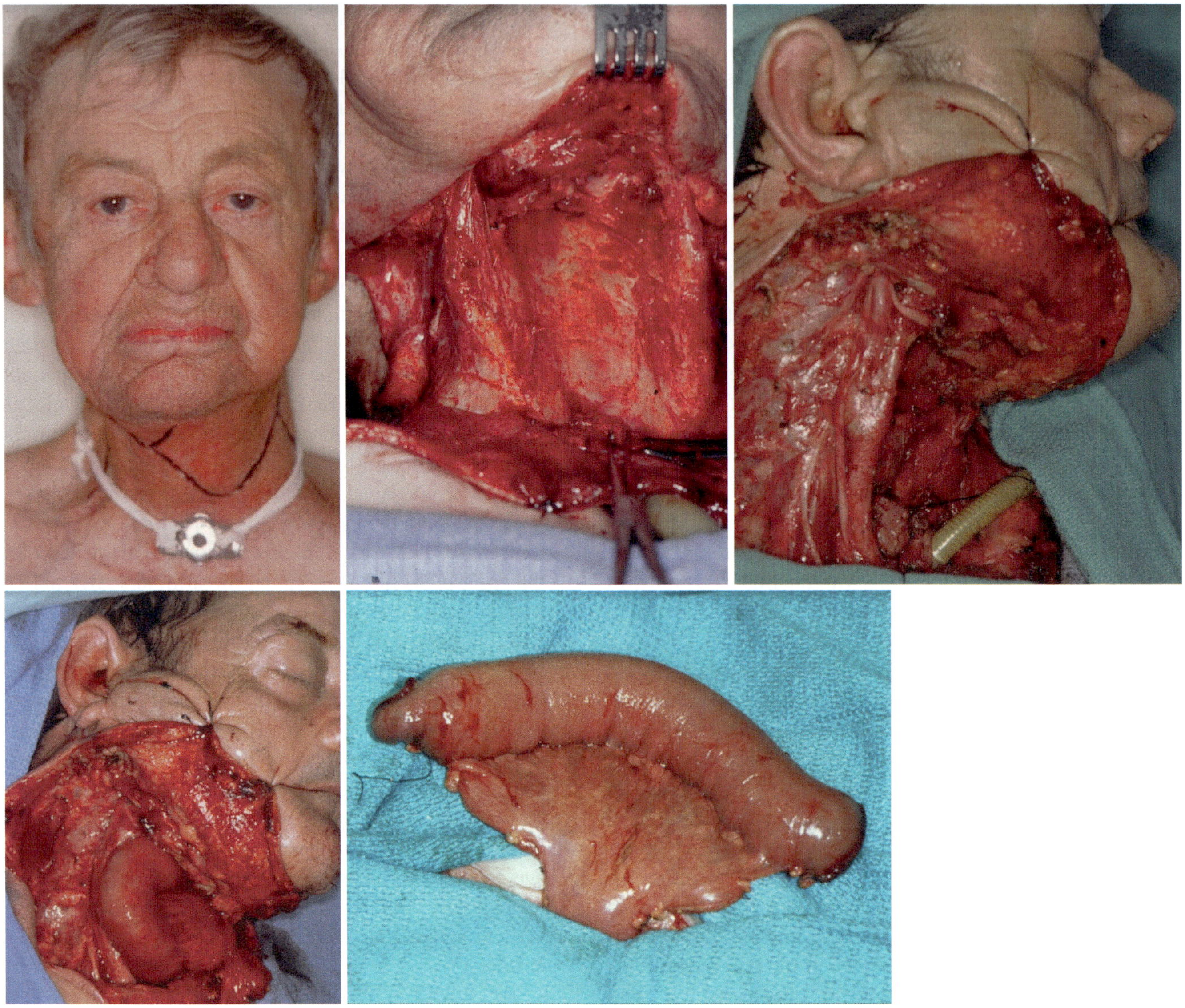

Two photos of the patient illustrate the design of the skin flaps for access, namely a cervical skin apron with short lateral incision extensions for additional exposure, if necessary. Post-resection the anterior neck compartment is empty and the prevertebral fascia posterior and the sternocleidomastoid muscles laterally are visualized. The Alice clamps are on the esophageal stump. On the right side, the carotid vessels and the hypoglossal nerve traversing over the external carotid are seen. In the second series of intraoperative photos, a loop of jejunum has been isolated and subsequently anastomosed to the hypopharynx proximal and the esophagus distally.

Postoperative

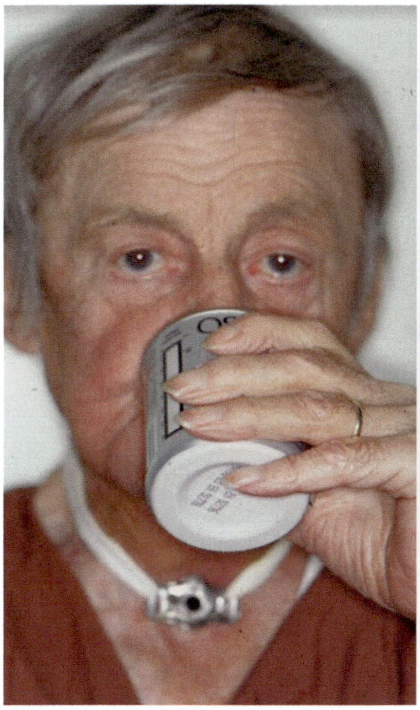

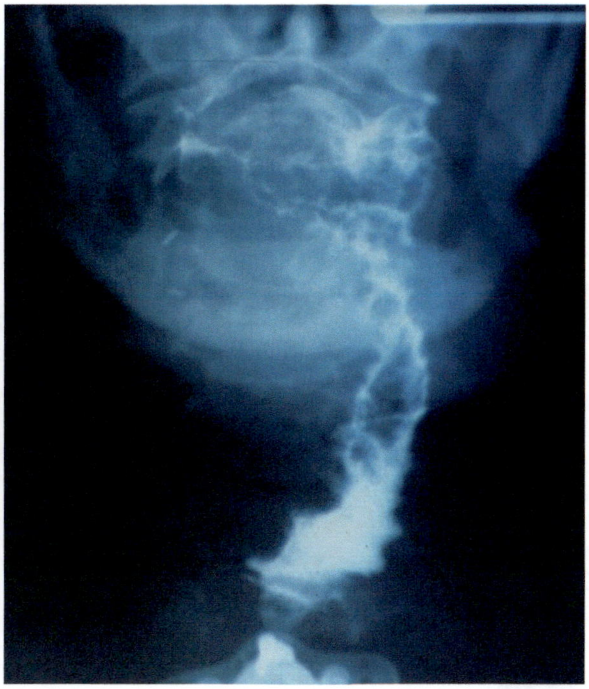

The patient is pictured drinking and a gastrografin swallow demonstrates a patent reconstruction and some peristaltic activity.

Critique

Some technical considerations are the provision of coverage or protection of the skeletonized carotid vessels. If possible, redundant mesentery can serve that role. The other consideration is the apparent redundancy of the jejunal loop interposition. If excessive, the redundancy can give rise to postoperative deglutition problems and should be revised.

Case-Based Conference

Case 2: Ca of the Maxilla

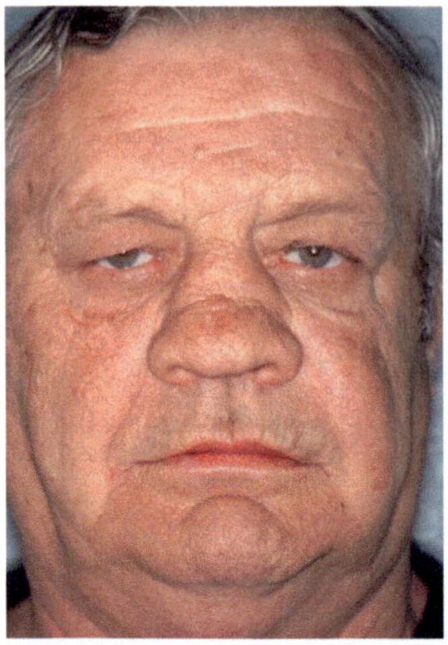
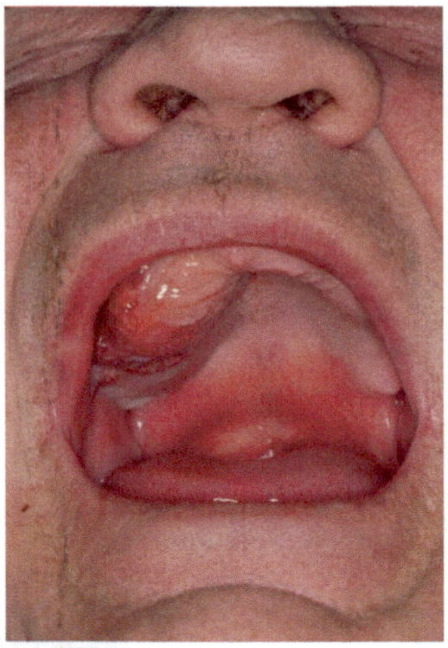
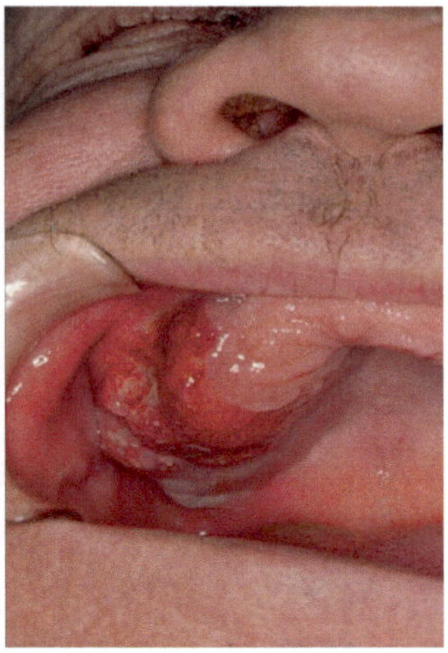
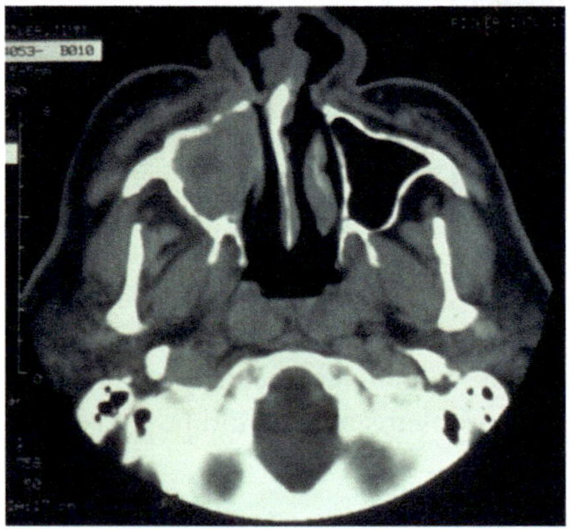

A 60-year-old otherwise healthy male with biopsy-proven moderately differentiated squamous cell cancer.

1. Describe the slide(s) provided and add a focused clinical examination. Interpret the CT scan.
   (a) Any tests indicated? Justify.
2. In anatomical terms describe the patient's tumor and give a likely resection scenario. Provide a classification for the anticipated defect.
3. Give a menu of reconstruction options, select yours, justify, and then describe. Be prepared to discuss the other options as well.

Case-Based Conference: Discussion

Case 2: Ca of the Maxilla

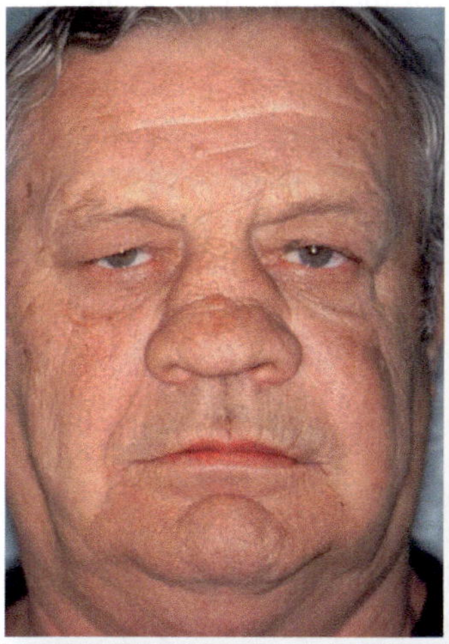
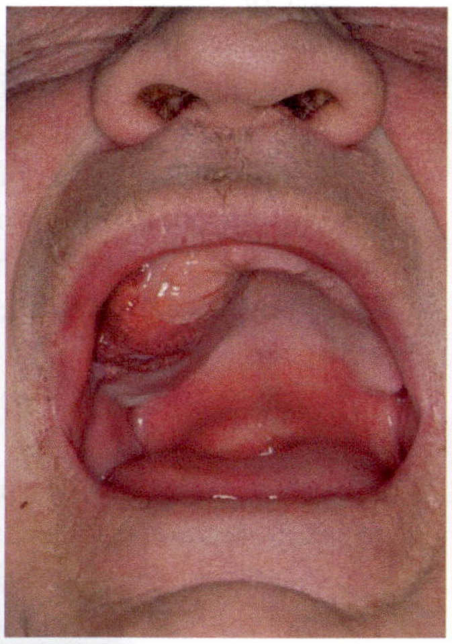
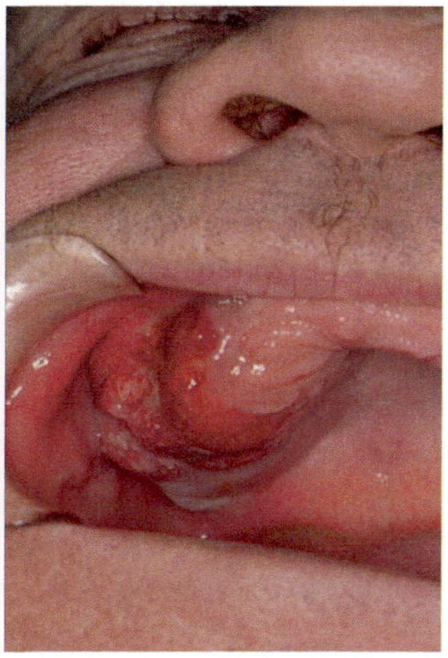
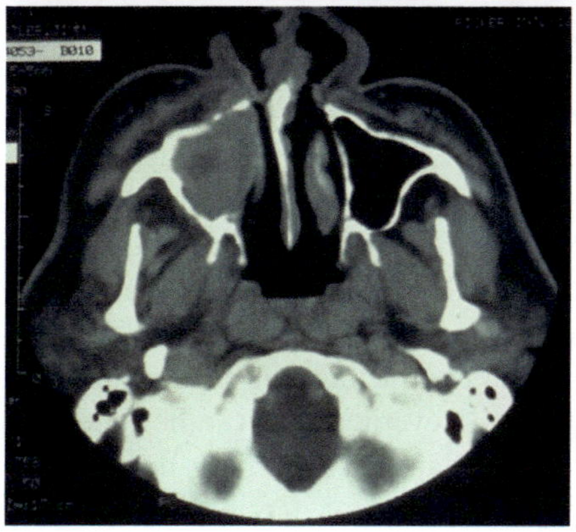

A 60-year-old otherwise healthy male with biopsy-proven moderately differentiated squamous cell cancer.

1. Describe the slide(s) provided and add a focused clinical examination. Interpret the CT scan. (Full-face photo demonstrates a heavy-set male who appears his stated age. No other obvious findings including no evidence of a bulge or deformity of the ipsilateral cheek. The intraoral photo without a retractor depicts a bulging mass with mostly intact mucosa of the hard palate and alveolar ridge, extending to the midline anteriorly. The lesion also extends into the lateral hard palate and appears to be approximately 3 cm in size. The second intraoral photo with a retractor in place demonstrates a lobulated mass with involvement of the maxillary buccal sulcus. Although no overt ulceration is seen, the overlying mucosa appears abnormal.

   Items of importance on medical history would be tobacco use (cigarettes or snuff/chewing tobacco) and symptoms such as numbness or radiating pain of the ipsilateral cheek or eye, and ocular symptoms such as double or impaired vision. The past medical history of operations or medical diagnoses is acquired as well as an estimate of overall physical conditioning and any weight loss. Physical examination would focus on a careful palpation of the lymph node-bearing areas of the neck, particularly the anterior cervical nodes, then an oral exam determining, as the photos depict, the degree of involvement superiorly into the maxillary sulcus and posteriorly into the lateral soft palate and retromolar trigone. Palpation with the examiner's fingers superiorly into the sulcus can perhaps determine the superior-anterior limit of the tumor. Sensation of the cheek and upper lip should be evaluated for possible involvement of the infraorbital nerve by extension from the anterior superior alveolar nerves. Ocular exam would determine any element of impaired vision or limitation of extraocular motion. Potential donor sites are examined and an Allen's test is performed on the non-dominant hand. An office endoscopy of the oropharynx, and if possible, the larynx for the presence of a synchronous primary would be important.)

(a) Any tests indicated? Justify. (The essential imaging is a CT scan of the head and neck and chest. The focus of the CT exam of the tumor is to determine the extent of involvement of the maxilla, in particular, does tumor involve the sinus, degree of involvement of the anterior wall, is the posterior wall involved? Does the tumor involve the floor of the orbit or even intraorbital? Images of the neck may detect lymphadenopathy or a synchronous primary. A chest CT to rule out the presence of lung primary is important as well. In the single slice of an axial CT scan, the right maxillary sinus is filled with fluid or mass. The lateral and posterior walls are intact but the medial anterior wall is not. The slice is relatively inferior at the level of the vomer.)

2. In anatomical terms describe the patient's tumor and give a likely resection scenario. Provide a classification for the anticipated defect. (Although the findings of the CT scan are not provided, the anticipated resection will be a subtotal maxillectomy. One perspective for classifying a subtotal maxillectomy is infrastructure or suprastructure; infrastructure referencing sacrifice of the hard palate, but not the orbit; suprastructure the reverse. The contemporary classification is by Cordeiro. Type I, a maxillary defect that involves one or two walls of the maxilla, most commonly a medial maxillectomy. Type II is a subtotal maxillectomy that involves resection of the maxilla but preservation of the orbital floor. Type IIA involves 50% or less of the hard palate and Type IIB greater than 50%. Type IIIA is a total maxillectomy including the orbital floor but preservation of the orbital contents, and Type IIIB is a concomitant orbital exenteration. Type IV is total maxillectomy, but resection of sufficient medial wall of the orbit exposes intracranial contents . The anticipated resection will be the ipsilateral alveolar ridge to 1–2 cm left of the midline anteriorly and about two-thirds of the hemi-hard palate perhaps sparing a posterior-medial ledge. The adjacent buccal mucosa will be resected but probably not Stensen's duct. Certainly, the anterior-medial maxillary wall, extending to the level of the infraorbital foramen and nerve will be resected but, in all likelihood, the floor of the orbit will be spared. This defect is a Cordeiro Type IIA or Type IIB, subtotal maxillectomy without the orbital floor and retention of either greater or lesser than 50% of the entire hard palate. The operative exposure is through a Weber–Ferguson, splitting the upper lip on a philtral column, continuing along the nasolabial fold, and then extending laterally and horizontally in a subciliary plane. In the absence of extension through the anterior wall or clinical bulging of the cheek, the odds are higher of an alveolar rather than a maxillary sinus origin. Nevertheless, substantial involvement of the sinus is probably likely with obstruction of the ostium beneath the middle turbinate and a secondarily fluid-filled sinus.)

3. Give a menu of reconstructive treatment options, select yours, justify, and then describe. Be prepared to discuss the other options as well. (The options available for reconstruction of a IIA defect range from simple to more complex; nothing, skin graft of the cheek flap and maxillary defect combined with an obturator for the palatal defect, temporalis muscle plus skin graft to cheek flap plus obturator, and, finally, free flap reconstruction without bone. Lacking any reconstruction, the cheek flap will contract substantially, the maxillary defect will continuously crust, and the maxillary defect and oral cavity will be one common space. Split-thickness skin grafting will avoid cheek soft tissue contracture but not collapse and loss of facial projection. Nevertheless, in some patients, a skin graft of the cheek flap and maxillary defect combined with a hard palate obturator may be a satisfactory option. Temporalis muscle does provide a space-filling reconstructive option, but the temporal hollow is a substantial deficit. The most sophisticated and optimal reconstruction is free muscle with recipient vessels in the neck either with or without bone. Since the palatal defect is less than 50%, an obturator would be quite satisfactory combined with a free muscle flap as a rectus or a deepithelialized anterolateral thigh flap for the soft tissue defect. If greater than 50%, dependent on the size of the residual palate, an ALT with a skin island intact is a reasonable choice.)

Intraoperative

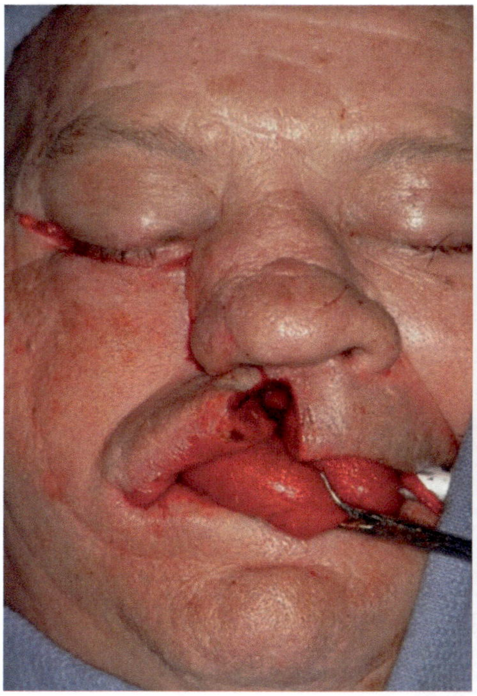

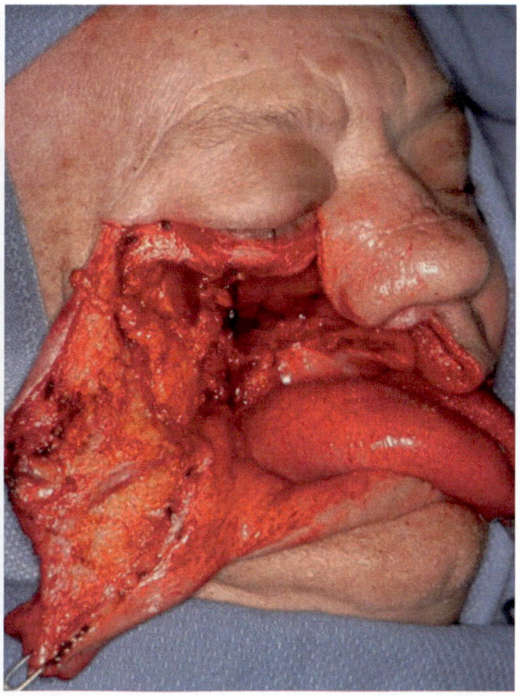

The two photos illustrate a Weber–Ferguson incision and an infrastructure maxillectomy. The Weber–Ferguson has been extended laterally with a lower lid subtarsal incision. The extent of the heart palate resection is not discernable.

Critique

Although the Weber–Ferguson incision parallels relaxed skin tension lines and delivers an aesthetically acceptable result, another operative result of an infrastructure maxillectomy is a facial degloving access, performed without external incisions. Exposure of the orbit is not optimal and assurance must be secured from the review of the CT scan of lack of any involvement of the orbit and floor.

Two additional cases are provided: a medial maxillectomy for lateral nasal wall tumor and a salivary gland tumor of the palate.

Medial Maxillectomy

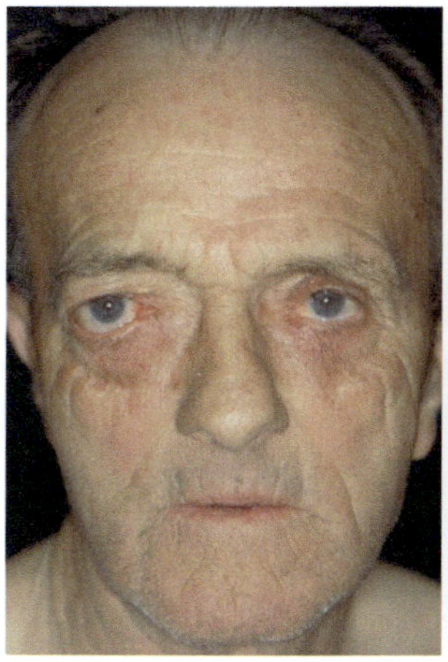

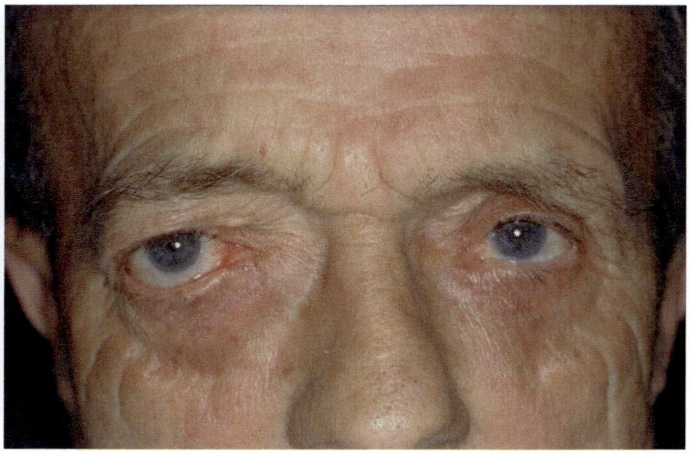

The indications for the performance of a medial maxillectomy are quite narrow, limited to unusual tumors of the lateral nasal wall and perhaps somewhat more frequently, nasal papilloma. Almost invariably, the nasolacrimal duct is transected but establishes a drainage into the anterior nasal cavity postoperatively. The inferior transverse osteotomy is at the level of the nasal floor and the superior osteotomy should be at the inferior medial orbital rim. More superior placement of that osteotomy will place the origin of the inferior oblique at risk as well as an encroachment of the medial orbital wall. The preoperative photos are of a 54-year-old male with a small carcinoma of the right lateral nasal wall. The photos demonstrate no obvious deformity other than scleral show and a mild ectropion of the right lower lid.

Intraoperative

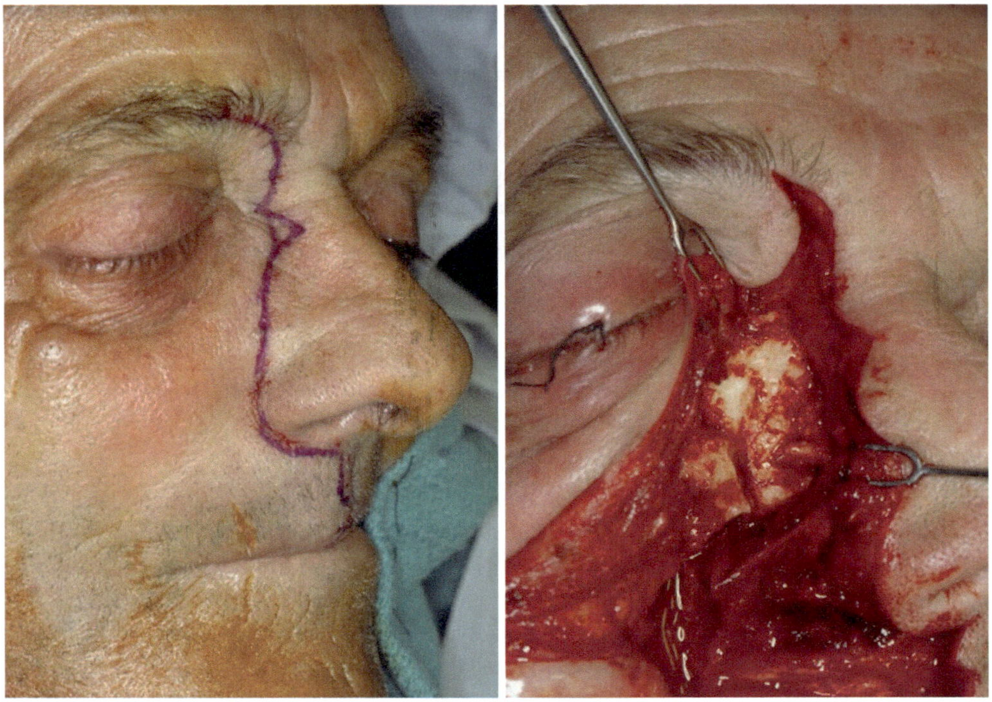

The intraoperative slides illustrate the markings for a Weber–Ferguson access incision and exposure.

Postoperative

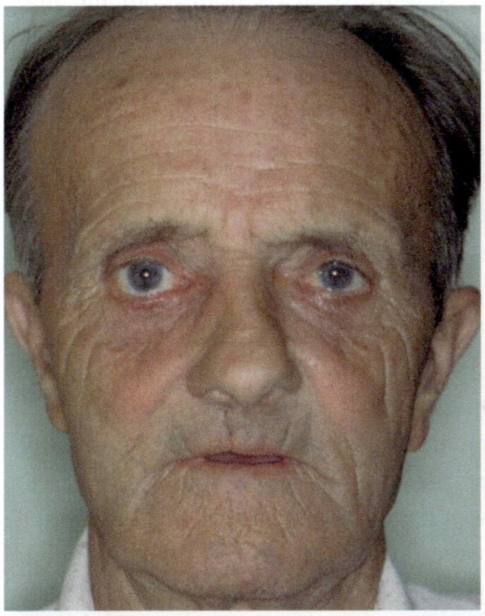
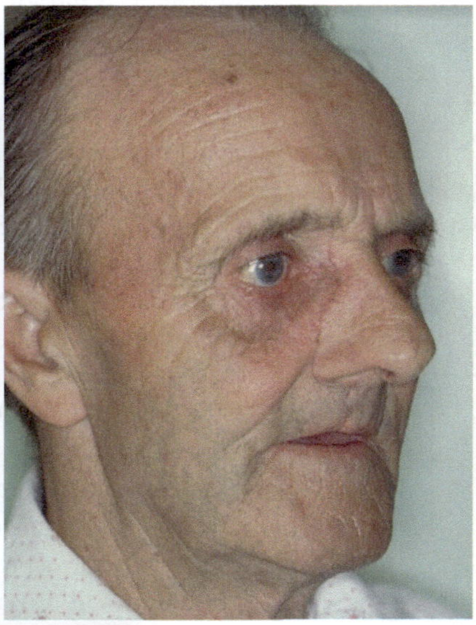
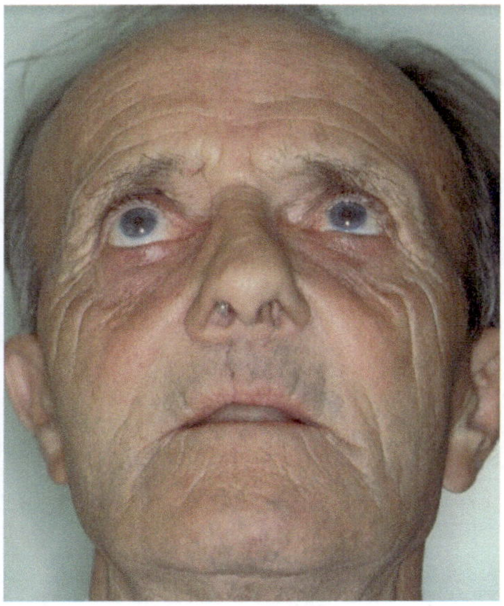
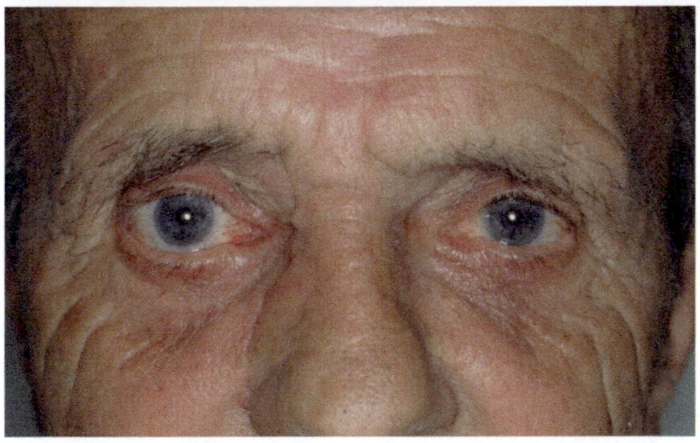

The postoperative photos are frontal, oblique, and submental vertex views of the midface. The incisional scars are not readily discernible and no deformities are evident.

Salivary Gland Tumor of the Palate

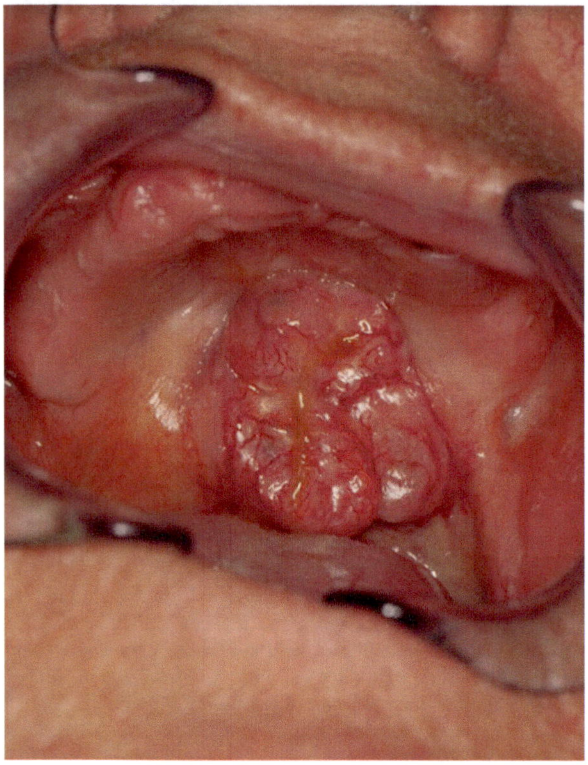

A 62-year-old male with a 2-year history of a mass growing in size. The intraoral view illustrates a multilobulated mass that occupies the central portion of the hard palate and onto the anterior soft palate. The alveolar ridge and adjacent hard palate are not involved. The patient is edentulous. The diagnosis is a benign mixed tumor of a minor salivary gland of the palate. Although adenoid cystic carcinoma is the most common pathologic diagnosis of tumors of the palatal salivary glands, benign mixed tumors can occur. In this case, a CT scan demonstrated erosion of the bone, and palatectomy was indicated. In the intraoral postoperative photo, the defect includes the central one-third to one-half of the hard and the entire soft palate. Operative reconstruction would be possible and would necessitate a microvascular option with a thin free flap as the choice, probably the radial forearm. Since the alveolar ridge and a substantial portion of the hard palate remain intact, a prosthetic nonoperative solution, a palatal obturator, will provide for closure of the nasal from the oral cavity. The design includes a pliable extension to simulate a soft palate on a more rigid hard palate prosthesis. No dentures were included.

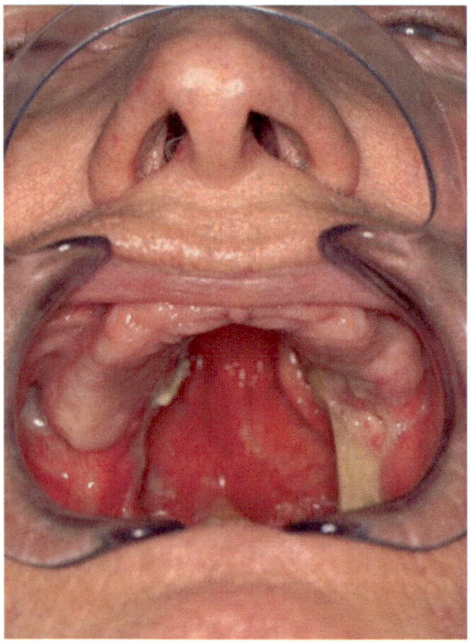

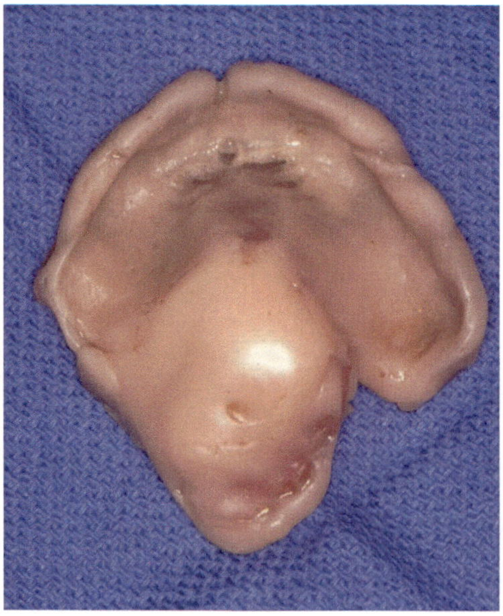

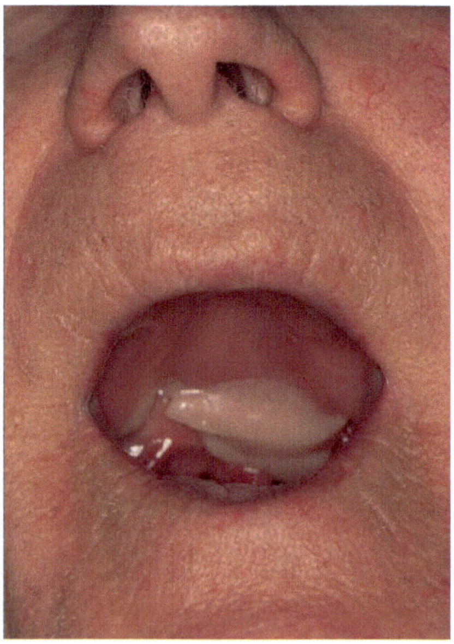

In-Service Examination

1. A Type IIA maxillary defect is:
   (a) Maxillectomy with resection of orbital floor, lateral maxillary wall
   (b) Maxillectomy with resection of less than one-half of the hard palate, preservation of orbital floor
   (c) Maxillectomy with resection of the orbital floor
   (d) Medial maxillectomy
2. The primary blood supply of the scapular flap emerges through the triangular space defined by what muscles?
   (a) Teres minor superior, teres major inferior, lateral head of the triceps laterally
   (b) Teres major superior, minor inferior, long head of the triceps laterally
   (c) Teres major superior, minor inferior, lateral head of the triceps laterally
   (d) Teres minor superior, major inferiorly, long head of the triceps lateral
3. The principal advantages of the ALT over jejunal-free flap besides donor site preference are:
   (a) Incidence of postoperative salivary leak is lower in use of the ALT
   (b) Tracheo-esophageal puncture for voice prosthesis is superior
   (c) Ease of monitoring
   (d) Ease of inset

40 Salivary Glands

Bibliography

Ellis, Harold. "Anatomy of the Salivary glands", Basic Science. **pp 569–572. (READ FIRST)**

Alvi, Aijaz MD, Myers, Eugene N. MD, et al. "Chapter 26: Malignant Tumors of the Salivary Glands." Cancer of the Head and Neck. Third Edition. **pp 525–527 (to Radiologic, etc.), 532–535 (to Staging to Acinic cell), pp 544–548 (to Cancer in Children).**

Granick, Mark S. and Hanna, Dwight C. III. Edited by Granick and Hanna. "Chapter 8: Surgical Management of Salivary Gland Disease." Management of Salivary Gland Lesions. **pp 145–148 (to Tumors), 163–165.**

Cheng S., et al., Ch. 8 "Overview of Head and Neck Soft Tissue and Bony Tumors", Neligan PC, Plastic Surgery, Elsevier 5th Edition, (2023), Volume 3: **pgs. 190–216 (Salivary Gland Tumors ONLY).**

Zhan KY, Khaja SF, Flack AB, Day TA, "Benign Parotid Tumors", *Otolaryngol Clin N Am*, (2016); 49:**333–337 ONLY.**

Tjoa T, Armstrong WB, "Chapter 37: Parotidectomy", in Operative Plastic Surgery, Second Edition, Gregory Evans, Oxford Press, (2019):**367 (Could not access online).**

Guntinas-Lichius O, Eisele DW, "Facial Nerve Monitoring", *Adv Otorhinolaryngol.*, (2016); 78:**46–51.**

Motz KM, Kim YJ, Auriculotemporal Syndrome (Frey Syndrome) *Otolaryngol Clin N Am*, (2016); 49:**501–506 ONLY.**

Videos

Ariyan S, "Superficial parotidectomy for primary tumor", (2013), Yale Med Video Sessions on Vimeo. Access at http://vimeo.com/71681521. (Accessed 6/24/2014) (not great, but good narrative.)

Faculty Discussion and Study Guide

Anatomy

> **Editor's Note**: Facial nerve, cranial nerve VII is also discussed in Chap. 45.

1. What is the embryological arch that derives the parotid? (Second or hyoid arch.)
2. Outline the type of secretion of each of the individual salivary glands. (Parotid serous, submandibular mixed mucous serous, lingual almost purely mucous.)
3. What is the relationship of the deep lobe of the parotid to the mandible? (The deep lobe hooks around the posterior aspect of the mandible and is medial or retromandibular in location.)
   (a) Relationship of the parotid to the retromandibular or posterior facial vein and internal jugular vein? (The posterior facial vein is on the posterior aspect of the parotid and the internal jugular vein is deep or medial and inferior to the parotid.)
   (b) Superficial temporal arteries and veins. (The superficial temporal vessels are on the medial aspect of the ascending ramus of the mandible and the deep lobe is lateral to the vessels.)
4. One of the readings relates that the superficial musculoaponeurotic system (SMAS) is continuous with the parotid-masseteric fascia. Is that your impression of the anatomy? (No. The two layers are distinct with the parotid-masseteric fascia deep to the SMAS.)
   (a) The submandibular gland relates to what nerve in the submandibular triangle? (Lingual nerve.)

E. Luce, *A Curriculum for Plastic Surgery*, https://doi.org/10.1007/978-3-031-62087-4_40

5. What sensory nerves are invariably sacrificed by a superficial parotidectomy and what are the sensory deficits? (Anterior branch of the greater auricular; loss of sensation over preauricular skin and a portion of the lobule; auriculotemporal with loss of sensation over the cheek and ear concha. See below.)
6. What are the branches of a facial nerve that arise *after* the nerve exits the stylomastoid foramen and *prior* to the branches to the mimetic muscles? (Branches to the posterior belly of the digastric, the stylohyoid, and the posterior auricular muscles, all supplied by the posterior auricular nerve.)
   (a) In the process of dissection several mm lateral to the facial nerve you encounter brisk arterial bleeding. What is the source? (The stylomastoid artery, a branch of the superficial temporal.)
7. Why would a laceration division of the mandibular or temporal branch of the facial nerve be more likely to result in a clinical deficit than an injury to the buccal or zygomatic branches? (In most of the six variants of the branching of the facial nerve, the mandibular and temporal branches tend to be an end distribution rather than interdivision branching, as is the case with the buccal and zygomatic portions.)
   (a) The buccal branch parallels what structure? (The parotid duct.)
8. What is the function and the importance of the auriculotemporal nerve? (The auriculotemporal nerve conducts the parasympathetic fibers to the parotid gland and when divided, it is responsible for the postoperative development of Frey's syndrome. See below for discussion.)
9. Discuss the course and exit of the parotid duct. (Stensen's duct arises from the anterior hilum of the gland, courses over the masseter muscle, hooks around the anterior edge of the muscle for a short distance, and then exits in the buccal cavity at the level of the maxillary second molar. The course of the most superficial location corresponds to the middle third of a line drawn from the tragus of the ear to the midportion of the philtrum of the upper lip.)
10. How would you use your knowledge of innervation of the submandibular gland to identify the lingual nerve? (Traction on the gland will reveal the parasympathetic branches to the submandibular gland, and the branches in turn arise from the lingual nerve through the submandibular ganglion. Inferior traction in this fashion pulls the lingual nerve into the field.)
    (a) What is the relationship of the submandibular gland to the posterior belly of the digastric muscle, mylohyoid? (The submandibular gland has a large superficial load and a smaller deep load. The posterior belly of the digastric lies inferior and medial to the submandibular gland. The anterior portion of the submandibular gland and certainly the course of the duct is deep and medial to the mylohyoid.)
11. True or False: The submandibular contains multiple lymph nodes. (No) Why? (Encapsulated prior to the development of the lymphatic system.)
12. Describe anatomically the course of Wharton's duct. (Exits from the anterior portion of the submandibular gland and courses in the submandibular triangle to pass beneath the posterior border of the mylohyoid muscle to exit intraorally just lateral to the lingual frenulum.)
13. Describe the anatomical boundaries of the buccal space. (Bounded medially and intraorally by the buccinator muscle and overlying mucosa. Bounded anteriorly or superficially by the mimetic muscles and posteriorly by the anterior edge of the masseter.)
14. Why does a tumor of the deep lobe of the parotid invariably present bulging into the lateral pharyngeal wall? (It is because the other three walls of the parapharyngeal space, occupied by the deep lobe of the parotid, are bounded by firm rigid structures: superiorly by the cranial base, laterally by the ascending ramus of the mandible, and posteriorly by the vertebrae and muscles. The only structures medially are the fibers of the superior pharyngeal constrictor. Consider the space as an inverted pyramid.)

Imaging and Workup

1. What are the key elements of a physical exam in a patient with a preauricular mass? (First, observe for facial movements and indications of a partial or complete facial nerve palsy. Second, palpate the mass for firmness and mobility as well as palpation of the neck for adenopathy. Examine the opposite parotid. Examine intraorally for trismus as evidence of pterygoid space involvement, as well as a medial bulge of the lateral posterior pharyngeal wall as an indication of parapharyngeal space extension. Palpate the lymph node-bearing areas of the neck including jugulodigastric.)
   (a) A patient with submandibular mass? (Examine bimanually externally and intraorally with the examining finger intraoral in the lateral floor of mouth. Palpate for cervical lymphadenopathy.)
2. What are some general precepts in imaging of the salivary glands? (In general, plain films are of little use except with the suspicion of a calculus. The decision between the choice of CT versus MRI is the same as elsewhere, namely, CT is useful in the vast majority of patients with contrast. Amalgams may create starburst effects that obscure the detail. MRI with contrast, and particularly with a high-resolution three-dimensional scan, may surpass CT scans in usefulness. Use of T_1 and

T_2-weighted images better define the margins of the tumor.)

(a) What are the imaging findings of benign or low-grade malignancy versus that of high-grade malignancy? (The findings are what one would anticipate intuitively, namely a pushing border in benign and low-grade malignancies and an infiltrating and poorly defined border with high-grade malignancies.)

3. What parotid tumor enhances with nuclear scanning with technetium? (Warthin's tumor or papillary cystadenoma lymphomatosum. Mostly of academic interest.)
4. What is the role of sialography? (Limited to trauma to the duct to outline stricture, obstruction, sialocele, and perhaps a better definition of Sjogren's syndrome.)
5. Discuss the role and shortcomings of fine needle aspiration (FNA). (It enables a tissue diagnosis to be made and gives information that can be communicated to the patient and family. Requires a skilled cytopathologist and may be nondiagnostic other than the presence of malignancy or not. In the appropriate setting, FNA has begun to play a more prominent role in the management of parotid tumors.)

   (a) Discuss the role of the frozen section. (Enables further treatment decisions to be made intraoperatively but requires considerable experience on the part of the pathologist and serious errors can be made as a result of a misdiagnosis.)

   (b) What is the preferable biopsy in a patient with a parotid mass? (Superficial parotidectomy.)
6. Outline TNM staging system in salivary gland tumors. (T_1 is less than 2 cm, T_2 2–4 cm, T_3 greater than 4 cm but less than 6 cm, T_4a is greater than 6 cm, T_4b invasion of adjacent structures, N is either the presence or absence of nodal metastases)

   (a) Other than the TNM staging what are the other prognostic factors in salivary gland tumors? (Presence of facial paralysis, histology, lymph node metastases, and perhaps pain.)

Pathology

1. What's a general rule with regard to comparable incidence of malignancy in the parotid, submandibular, lingual, and minor salivary glands? (Ascending incidence of malignancy in that order. Parotid about 20%, submandibular 40–50%, and lingual and minor salivary glands over 50%.)
2. Give the clinical and pathologic characteristics of a "benign mixed" tumor of the salivary glands. (Pleomorphic adenoma, or benign mixed tumor, histologically is composed of a stroma of connective tissue surrounding glandular/acinar epithelial cells. Seventy to eighty percent of benign tumors of the parotid are pleomorphic adenomas and compose a similar proportion of benign tumors of the submandibular gland and minor salivary glands, although benign tumors in the latter two are less common. The lesion is a firm, painless mass that compresses the adjacent salivary tissue, a "pseudocapsule," such that an adequate margin is necessary with extirpation. The tumor requires a superficial parotidectomy and for the submandibular gland, a total glandular excision. Enucleation has no role in the excision of any tumor of the parotid gland. In addition to placing the facial nerve potentially at risk, enucleation of pleomorphic adenoma entails a significant recurrence rate, a difficult management problem. Recurrences, although uncommon with adequate excision, are a difficult clinical problem and are attended by a high incidence of re-recurrence.)

   (a) What is the approximate risk of malignancy in benign mixed tumors? (7%)

   (b) What are the factors that can increase the risk of malignancy in benign mixed tumors? (Multiple recurrences, prolonged duration of presence perhaps 20 years or greater.)
3. What are the epidemiological characteristics of Warthin's tumor? Older white males who are smokers. Distinctly common in African Americans. 10% are bilateral in occurrence.)

   (a) Another term for Warthin's tumor? (Papillary cystadenoma lymphomatosum.)
4. Rank adenoid cystic carcinoma as a proportion of malignant tumors in the following: parotid, submandibular, and minor salivary glands. (Uncommon in the parotid, and proportionately more frequent and common in the submandibular and even more so in the minor salivary glands.)

   (a) What is the role of radical neck dissection in adenoid cystic carcinoma? (None, except for local control. Metastatic disease is most often hematogenous.)

   (b) What is the role of radiotherapy in adenoid cystic carcinoma? (Traditionally has been thought to have little role and a view that adenoid cystic carcinoma was radioresistant. The more current thought on the part of some head and neck surgeons is that radiation of adenoid cystic carcinoma may play a role in the control of local recurrence. One must recall in the decision process that local recurrence is quite high and the necessity for resection years later is not infrequent. Non-radiated tissues are more favorable for excision.)

   (c) Describe the clinical behavior of adenoid cystic carcinoma. (The tumor is slow growing, has a propensity for perineural spread, an extremely high incidence of local recurrence, eventual metastases, and a progressive decrease in survival in 5–10 and ultimately 20 years. Some correlation exists between histologic appearance and prognosis. A tubular or cribriform histologic pattern is more favorable than a solid or less differentiated.)

5. A patient with a 4 cm mass of submandibular gland has enlargement of the foramen ovale on CT scan. What is the probable diagnosis? (Adenoid cystic carcinoma—a cancer with a propensity for perineural involvement and proximal dissection along the lingual to the mandibular division of the trigeminal nerve, the latter exiting the cranial fossa through the foramen ovale.)
6. Give a classification system for mucoepidermoid carcinoma. Correlate the classification with histologic characteristics. (The most common classification is low grade and high grade with medium grade in between. The histologic characteristics of a low grade are much more differentiated with many more mucous-secreting cells than epidermoid cells. As the lesion becomes more high-grade the presence of mucous cells is more scant and epidermoid cells are much more common with poor differentiation.)
   (a) What is the role of radical neck dissection (RND) and selective neck dissection in mucoepidermoid carcinoma? (For high-grade lesions, an RND should be performed even in the N_0 neck. The most commonly modified neck dissection such as supraomohyoid is usually employed.)
   (b) What is the role of radiotherapy in mucoepidermoid carcinoma? (As mentioned above, in high-grade lesions, postoperative radiotherapy is beneficial.)

Treatment

1. Discuss anesthesia, draping, and incisions for parotid tumors. (General anesthesia with endotracheal tube. Draping consists of draping out the entire side of the face from the midline onward as well as the neck and upper chest. The incision for a superficial parotidectomy is a horseshoe incision that begins in the temporal scalp, extends in the preauricular region either behind or in front of the tragus, hooks gently underneath the earlobe over the mastoid, and then into the anterior neck in a cervical skin crease.)
2. Outline the steps in a superficial parotidectomy. (Briefly, use of the incision above, elevation of a subcutaneous facial and neck flap, identification of the facial nerve crancial nerve VII, see other questions, dissection of the superficial lobe from the facial nerve, hemostasis, drainage, and closure.)
3. Describe and compare antegrade and retrograde dissection of the facial nerve. (Retrograde consists of the identification of a peripheral branch usually over the course of the masseter and dissection back to the main trunk. Antegrade consists of identification of the facial nerve and then peripheral dissection, reflecting the gland free of the nerve. In most hands, antegrade is accomplished more readily than retrograde.)
4. Describe a technique for identification of the facial nerve. (Once the skin flaps are elevated with the incision as described above, initial dissection is the release of the fascia that extends from the posterior aspect of the parotid onto the external auditory canal. This fascia is thin and is readily released. The next point of release is the fascia extending onto the mastoid and overlapping onto the anterior border of the superior aspect of the sternocleidomastoid.

At this juncture, dissection can be taken along the external auditory canal until the tynpano-mastoid suture line and "tragal pointer" is palpated. Then, at least in this writer's hands, dissection shifts further inferiorly along the posterior superior aspect of the posterior belly of the digastric. This procedure will lead to a small neurovascular bundle that provides innervation to the posterior belly of the digastric and the stylohyoid. Following that branch superiorly for a distance of 1–2 cm will lead toward the facial nerve. Essentially, now the dissection is between two planes superior as outlined above and inferior over the posterior belly of the diagnostic. This maneuver essentially isolates the area of the facial nerve.)

5. Facial nerve electrophysiologic monitoring can replace or supplement visual monitoring during parotid dissection. What are the mechanics? (Electrodes are placed within the mimetic muscles and a recording of electromyography (EMG), activity including amplitude is recorded. Some familiarity with the technology is required that may assist in the prevention of nerve injury. Alternate approaches include visual monitoring and the intermittent use of the handheld nerve stimulator.)
6. What is Frey's syndrome? (Frey's syndrome or gustatory sweating is a result of transection of the sympathetic branches to the sweat glands in the process of elevation of the skin flaps and the subsequent parotidectomy. The other element that must be present is the division of the postganglionic parasympathetic branches of the auriculotemporal nerve that provide secretory innervation of the parotid gland. The stage is now set for misdirected nerves sprouting from the auriculotemporal branches to the sympathetic branches innervating the sweat glands. As a result, the stimulus of eating or mastication alone creates inappropriate sweating over the cheek and face, which in many patients can be quite troublesome. The traditional evaluation is the Minor Starch test, performed by iodine painted over the cheek, allowed to dry, and then coated with powdered starch. Once salivation is stimulated, the gustatory sweating will stain brown or purple.)

(a) What is the treatment? (Nonoperative management may be successful with scopolamine, an anticholinergic. A patient may find the side effects of the scopolamine, namely dry mouth, more troublesome than the gustatory sweating. More recent nonoperative treatment consists of periodic Botox injections. An operative approach is the elevation of the original skin flaps and placement of an intervening barrier such as Alloderm® or a flap of temporoparietal fascia. Transtympanic sectioning of Jacobsen's nerve, a branch of the glossopharyngeal that provides parasympathetic fibers to the auriculotemporal, has provided mixed results.)

7. Describe a technique of submandibular gland excision, including the important structures in the neighborhood. (A submandibular skin incision is performed with sufficient length to give exposure, division of the platysma and the facial artery and vein well below the ramus of the mandible. The vessels are then sutured upward onto the superior skin flaps to place superior traction on the mandibular branch of the facial nerve. The cervical fascia is then incised and the gland is identified, the stylohyoid and posterior belly of the digastric are retracted inferiorly, and dissection is accomplished about the gland inferiorly and then posteriorly. The gland is freed from beneath the mylohyoid and gently retracted to provide exposure of the lingual nerve by inferior traction on the gland, which will in turn pull the submaxillary ganglion and parasympathetic branches into the field, thus exposing the lingual nerve. Wharton's duct is then ligated and the gland is removed. The hypoglossal nerve is deep and anterior but could be injured by carelessness.)
8. What is the most likely tumor of the parotid in a patient with Sjoren's syndrome? (Lymphoma occurs 40 times more frequently than in the normal population.)

Benign Disease

1. Typically, salivary calculi are radio opaque or radio lucent? (Radio opaque, particularly in the parotid.)
2. What radiological modality would you order in Sjorgen's syndrome? (The earliest changes are normal. As the disease progresses, the gland becomes denser than normal on imaging with some element of enlargement. Further progression leads to a honeycomb appearance. Finally, in an occasional patient, cysts. The most definitive imaging is a CT sialogram. Diagnosis can be established by biopsy of a minor salivary gland in the lip.)
   (a) What is the typical patient profile in Sjorgen's syndrome? (A woman between 40 and 50 years in 90–95% of the cases.)
3. What is a ranula? What is a plunging ranula? (A ranula is an obstructed sublingual gland with cystic formation. A plunging ranula is due to rupture of the cyst and subsequent extravasation of salivary secretion and proteolytic enzymes that enable further dissection into the submandibular region and even into the neck.)
4. Briefly outline the medical and surgical treatment of acute suppurative parotitis. (Initial rehydration, oral feedings, improved oral hygiene, and intravenous antibiotics. Failure to improve within 72 h, increasing pain, septicemia, and development of an abscess mandate incision and drainage. The most common setting is an elderly, dehydrated, and often hospitalized patient.)
5. Review the therapy for acute sialadenitis. (Supportive therapy consists of gland massage, oral rinses, oral fluids, and oral antibiotics. Occasionally, cannulation of the duct with a lacrimal probe may be necessary. External incision and drainage are required for the development of fluctuance.)
6. Describe the surgical treatment of impacted stones in Stensen's duct. (Distally, large stones can be removed by gently dilating the orifice, incising the orifice with small scissors, and removing the stone with small forceps. When stones are large and more proximal, the preferred technique calls for opening and marsupialization of the distal duct. Most Stensen's duct calculi are distal, often just proximal to the orifice. Sialendoscopy may provide a less interventive method of management of salivary calculi.)

Case-Based Conference

Case 1: Cheek Mass

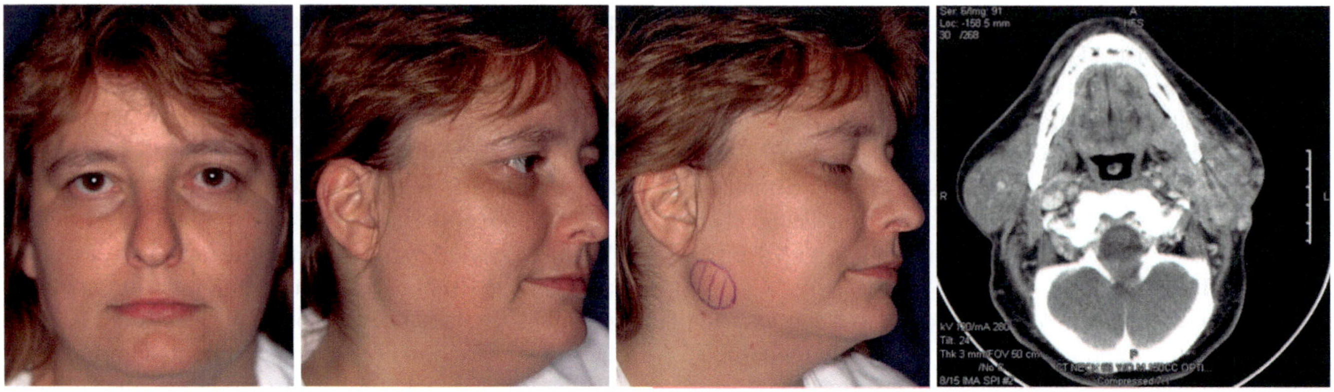

A 35-year-old woman with a 3-month history of a cheek "lump."

1. Describe the findings on the slide and add a clinical examination.
   (a) Interpret the CT scan provided and list additional slices of the CT scan of value.
   (b) Any tests indicated? Justify.
2. What is the differential diagnosis?
3. Prepare a treatment plan for three diagnoses given by your interrogator.
4. Manage the following complications:
   (a) Facial palsy evident immediately postoperative.
   (b) Positive deep margin on final pathology.
   (c) The patient complains of facial sweating while eating.

Case-Based Conference: Discussion

Case 1: Cheek Mass

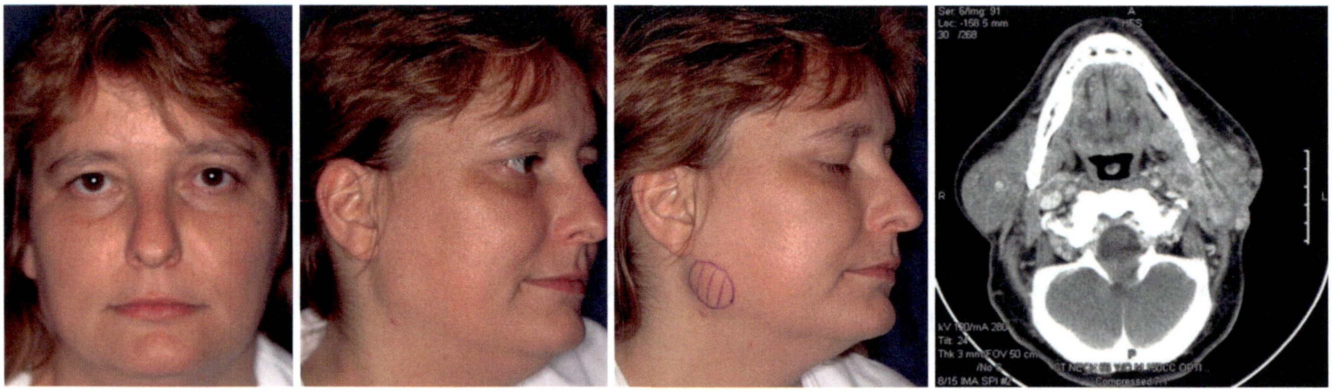

A 35-year-old woman with a 3-month history of a cheek "lump."

1. Describe the findings on the slide and add a clinical examination. (Three views are provided: a frontal and two right laterals. The frontal view demonstrates a woman of the stated age in facial repose without evidence of facial palsy, although she has a slight scleral show on the right with possible effacement of the right nasolabial fold. This view lacks a demonstration of facial animation. The first lateral view demonstrates a patient of mild obesity with a suggestion of some cheek fullness inferior and slightly anterior to the ear lobule. The third slide is the same view, lateral, but with markings indicative of a 2 cm mass. No skin changes or lesions are seen. A clinical examination would begin with a history if the mass has increased in size over the 3 months duration, facial twitching or pain, numbness, and scalp lesions. The history would move toward any constitutional symptoms of fever, night sweats, and weight loss, all perhaps worri-

some for the presence of lymphoma. Any symptoms such as fluctuating size of mass, tenderness, and pain with eating indicative of calculus disease and recurrent parotitis would open a particular workup pathway. The physical would begin with a facial exam to determine intact facial nerve function, examination of the scalp for any pigmented lesions as well as the upper eyelid and lip for lumps, and then palpation of the mass for degree of firmness and mobility. Examination of the lymph node-bearing areas of the neck, particularly zones II–IV is mandatory. Intraoral exam is important to eliminate the possibility of an intraoral primary as well as inspection of the lateral pharyngeal wall for any bulge indicative of deep parotid lobe involvement.)

   (a) Interpret the CT scan provided and list additional slices of the CT scan of value. (The CT scan demonstrates a homogeneous mass in the right parotid area overlying and lateral to the ascending mandibular ramus. Some parotid tissue appears compressed anterior and medial to the mass. Additional cuts of value would be an image of the facial nerve at the stylomastoid foramen as well as detection of any adenopathy in the neck.)
   (b) Any tests indicated? Justify. (As discussed above a CT scan has been obtained. An MRI would determine the composition of the mass, solid vs. cystic, as well as some indications of malignancy, well-defined vs. infiltrating border. The relationship of the mass to the trunk and branches of the facial nerve can be defined. Adenopathy in the neck can be detected as well. The other test possibility preoperatively is a fine needle aspirate. In some centers with the availability of an experienced cytopathologist, an FNA can provide some guidance in patient counseling.)

2. What is the differential diagnosis? (Since 80% of parotid tumors are benign and 80% of benign tumors are pleomorphic adenoma, the most likely diagnosis is a benign mixed tumor. The malignant diagnostic possibilities include oncocytoma, adenoid cystic, mucoepidermoid, and squamous cell carcinoma. Additional benign possibilities include Warthin's tumor. Warthin's tumor occurs predominantly in older white men and oncocytomas are usually seen in elderly patients. A single head and neck mass is unlikely an occurrence in lymphoma although if the patient has Sjogren's syndrome serious consideration should be given to that possibility.)
3. Prepare a treatment plan for three diagnoses given by your interrogator. (The three most likely diagnoses as listed above are pleomorphic adenoma, adenoid cystic, and mucoepidermoid. Regardless, the biopsy and operation of choice is a superficial parotidectomy. In the operating room, the entire head and neck and upper chest should be prepped and draped into the field. A preauricular incision extending into the temporal scalp and gently curving inferiorly, posteriorly, and then anteriorly following an upper cervical crease will provide exposure. Skin flaps are raised superficial to the superficial musculo-aponeurotic system (SMAS) and platysma, the fascia is reflected from the superior anterior border of the sternocleidomastoid, and the seventh nerve branch to the stylohyoid and/or the posterior belly of the digastric is identified. Dissection then shifts superiorly to release the fascia between the parotid and the external auditory canal, the parotid gently retracts anteriorly, and the avascular plane anterior to the external auditory canal is dissected. Use of the tympano-mastoid suture and the tragal pointer will assist in the dissection and exposure of the main trunk of the facial nerve. Further dissection will quickly expose the cervicofacial and temporo-facial trunk. Troublesome bleeding at this point is probably from the stylomastoid artery. Completion of the superficial parotidectomy is accomplished by careful exposure of the individual branches of the nerve in an antegrade fascia and ligation of the parotid duct. If the superficial parotidectomy appears to safely encompass the mass, the specimen is submitted for final pathology. Frozen section diagnosis certainly can be accomplished with confidence and the experience of the pathologist. A total parotidectomy with preservation of the facial nerve would be indicated if any concern exists of clearance of tumor or a frozen section diagnosis of malignancy. Sacrifice of cranial nerve VII is indicated in the presence of gross involvement of the nerve, but is otherwise preserved. If resection of the nerve is performed, immediate reconstruction should be performed with nerve grafts easily harvested from the branches of the cervical plexus. If the patient is elderly, a lateral tarsorrhaphy should also be performed. Some centers employ facial nerve monitoring and may be of value to those surgeons who perform an occasional superficial parotidectomy. Facial nerve monitoring is accomplished by placement of needle electrodes into the mimetic muscles and EMG activity including amplitude is recorded.

   Superficial parotidectomy will be sufficient if the diagnosis is pleomorphic adenoma, but less likely if the tumor is recurrent. Total parotidectomy is the operation of choice for adenoid cystic and mucoepidermoid carcinomas with a selected neck dissection added in instances of moderate and less differentiated mucoepidermoid tumors. Adenoid cystic carcinoma uncommonly spreads by regional recurrences but rather has a propensity for perineural spread, local recurrence, and, eventually, hematogenous dissemination.)
4. Manage the following complications:
   (a) Facial palsy evident immediately postoperative (At the completion of the parotidectomy, stimulation of

the main trunk with a handheld nerve stimulator will reassure that the nerve is intact and functioning. Palsy immediately postoperatively is probably a traction injury and should recover in 4–6 weeks.)

(b) Positive deep margin on final pathology (Regardless of the histologic diagnosis, if a superficial parotidectomy was performed, the patient should be returned to the OR for total parotidectomy and preservation of the facial nerve. If a total parotidectomy was performed, the next margin is the lateral pharyngeal wall, and, on balance, for a microscopically positive margin of a malignant primary, postoperative radiotherapy is probably the appropriate option.)

(c) The patient complains of facial sweating while eating. (The description is that of gustatory sweating or Frey's syndrome. Frey's syndrome is a result of the transection of the parasympathetic branches to the sweat glands in the process of elevation of the skin flaps and the subsequent parotidectomy. The other element that must be present is the division of the postganglionic parasympathetic branches of the auriculotemporal nerve that provide secretory innervation of the parotid gland. The stage is now set for misdirected nerves sprouting from the auriculotemporal branches to the sympathetic branches innervating the sweat glands. As a result, the stimulus of eating creates inappropriate sweating over the cheek and face, which in many patients can be quite troublesome. Nonoperative management may be successful with scopolamine, an anticholinergic. A patient may find the side effects of the scopolamine, namely dry mouth, more troublesome than the gustatory sweating. More recent nonoperative treatment consists of periodic Botox injections. An operative approach is an elevation of the original skin flaps and placement of an intervening barrier such as Alloderm® or a flap of temporoparietal fascia. Transtympanic sectioning of Jacobsen's nerve, a branch of the glossopharyngeal that provides parasympathetic fibers to the auriculotemporal, has provided mixed results.)

Intraoperative

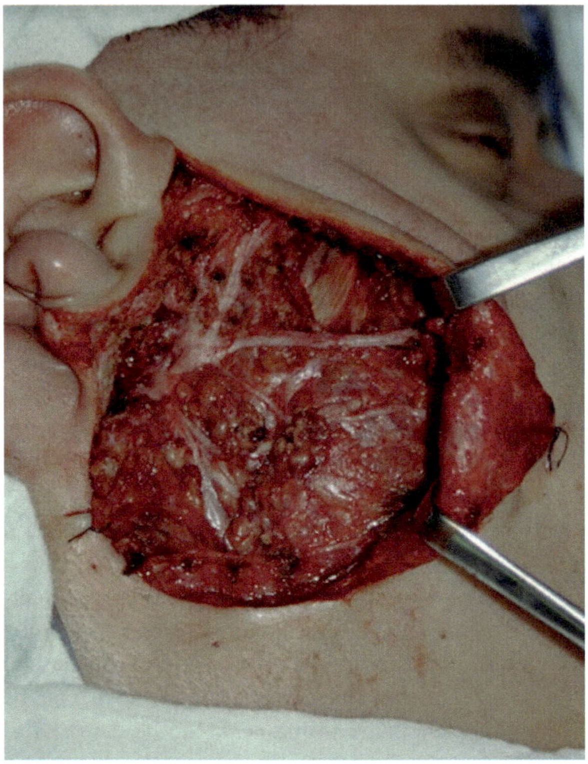

A single intraoperative photo is lateral with retraction of the skin flaps and exposure of the operative bed. The branches of the facial nerve are visible, although perhaps the lower trunks are not as distinct.

Postoperative (5 Days)

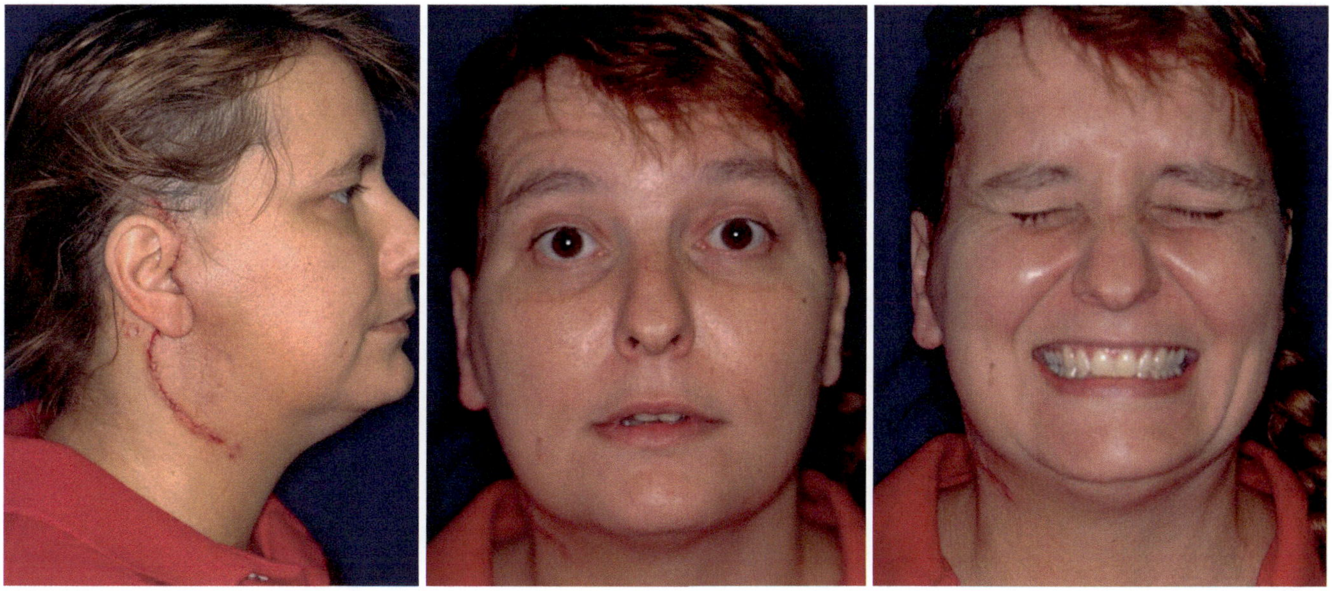

The patient at the time of suture removal. On lateral view, the use of a retrotragal approach conceals much of the preauricular incision. The incision after coursing posteriorly beneath the earlobe lies in an anterior cervical crease. The frontal views in repose and animation demonstrate full facial nerve function.

In-Service Examination

1. Frey's syndrome is the result of:
   (a) Aberrant sympathetic branches from the auriculotemporal nerve to the sweat glands
   (b) Aberrant sympathetic branches from the auriculotemporal nerve to the parotid gland
   (c) Aberrant parasympathetic branches from the auriculotemporal nerve to the sweat glands
   (d) Aberrant parasympathetic branches from the auriculotemporal nerve to the parotid gland
2. The ratio of benign to malignant tumors from highest to lowest:
   (a) Submandibular, parotid, minor salivary glands
   (b) Minor salivary, parotid, submandibular
   (c) Parotid, minor salivary, submandibular
   (d) Parotid, submandibular, minor salivary glands
3. The characteristics of Warthin's tumor include the following **EXCEPT**:
   (a) More common in African American
   (b) Occurs in the younger population
   (c) 10% bilateral
   (d) Enhances with technetium scans

Part V

Maxillofacial Trauma

41 Airway, Bleeding, Imaging, Clinical Examination

Bibliography

Perry, M. et al. "Emergency Care in Facial Trauma—A Maxillofacial and Ophthalmic Perspective." *Injury*, Elsevier Co. (2005); 36:**875–886**. (**pgs. 886–9 Inclusive** will be covered in General Principles part II) (Junior Residents).

Blanton MW and Marcus JR, Ch. 3: "Systematic Examination of Facial Trauma", Marcus JR. Essentials of Maxillofacial Trauma, Quality Medical Publishing, St. Louis, Missouri, (2012); **pg 35–43 ONLY**.

Schoemann M, Lee TC, Mukundan Jr. S., Ch. 5: "Radiographic Examination", Marcus JR. Essentials of Maxillofacial Trauma, Quality Medical Publishing, St. Louis, Missouri, (2012); **59–73**.

Luce, E. A. Edited by Mark M. Ravitch. "Maxillofacial Trauma", *Current Problems in Surgery: Maxillofacial Trauma*, (1984); 21(2):, **pp 8–11**.

Iarocci A.L., Winters R.D., "Laryngeal trauma: a review of current diagnostic and management strategies", *Current Opinion in Otolaryngology*, (2022); 30(4): **276–278 ONLY**.

Kellman MD, R. M. and Losquadro MD, W. D. "Comprehensive Airway Management of Patients with Maxillofacial Trauma." *Craniomaxillofacial Trauma & Reconstruction*, Manson MD, P. N., Thieme Medical Publishers, Inc. (2008) 1:**39–48**.

Luce EA and Alvarez SM., "Submental Intubation", *Plast. Reconstr. Surg. Glob. Open.*, (2018);6:**1–4**.

Cogbill MD, T. H., et al. "Management of Maxillofacial Injuries with Severe Oronasal Hemorrhage: A Multicenter Perspective." *The Journal of Trauma*. Lippincott Williams & Wilkins (2008) 65:**996–998**.

Morcos SS and Patel PK, "The Vocabulary of Dentofacial Deformities", *Clinics in Plastic Surgery*, (2007); 34(3):**589–94 ONLY**.

Gruss JS, "Complex Maxillary Fractures: Role of Buttress Reconstruction and Immediate Bone Grafts", *Plast Reconstr Surg.*, (1986); 78: **Figs. 1–3 ONLY**.

Faculty Discussion and Study Guide

Anatomy

The bony anatomy of the maxillofacial region will be discussed within each of the modules in maxillofacial trauma.

1. The principal blood supply to the scalp is (Anteriorly the supratrochlear and supraorbital arteries, terminal branches of the ophthalmic artery; laterally the superficial temporal artery; the posterior auricular; and posteriorly the occipital arteries.)
2. What is the major blood supply to the face? (Infraorbital, supraorbital, supratrochlear, facial, and superficial temporal.)
3. The principal motor innervation of the face is the facial cranial nerve, VII nerve. Give the two-dimensional anatomy of the temporal branch. (Located on a line approximately half a cm anterior and below the tragus to a point 1.5 cm lateral to the eyebrow. The depth location is discussed under the coronal approach.)
4. What is a rough guide for locating all three principal cutaneous branches of the trigeminal that provide sensation to the face, the supraorbital, the infraorbital, and the mental nerves? (Drop a vertical line through the mid pupil or medial limbus to the oral commissure. All three branches exit the bony skeleton on that line.)
5. Describe the three horizontal buttresses of the facial skeleton. (Superior is the cribriform plate and orbital roof; the middle buttress is the orbital rim and zygomatic arches; and the most inferior strut is the hard palate. Another view is the superior orbital rim through the glabella into the opposite superior orbital rim. Middle is a zygomatic arch into the inferior orbital rim and into the same structures on the contralateral side.)
   (a) What are the facial vertical supporting buttresses? (The nasomaxillary or medial buttress, the lateral buttress or the zygomatico-maxillary, and the posterior buttress or the pterygoid-maxillary buttress. The most

E. Luce, *A Curriculum for Plastic Surgery*, https://doi.org/10.1007/978-3-031-62087-4_41

medial or nasal maxillary extends from the anterior alveolar ridge superiorly along the lateral wall of the pyriform aperture and the nasal process of the maxilla to the frontal bone. The lateral or zygomatico-maxillary buttress courses from the lateral alveolar ridge to the anterior portion of the zygomatic arch and the lateral orbital rim. The posterior buttress attaches the maxilla posteriorly to the pterygoid plate of the sphenoid bone.)

6. List the names of the soft tissue relationships to the maxillary and mandibular dental arches. (The anterior teeth, incisors, and canines lateral surface are referred to as labial. The similar relationship in the posterior teeth, premolars, and molars is termed buccal. The inner aspect of all the maxillary teeth is termed palatal; the similar relationship in the mandibular teeth is termed lingual.)
7. Define mesial and distal. (The mesial direction is toward the midline, distal is away from the midline.)
8. Describe the numbering system for the secondary dentition. (Beginning with the right maxillary third molar, the 16 maxillary teeth are numbered from right to left with the left third molar, tooth number 16. The numbering system continues in a clockwise direction that begins with the left mandibular third molar tooth number 17 and continues about the dental arch until tooth number 32, the right mandibular third molar. Occlusal relationships will be covered in the mandibular fracture module.)

Airway

1. What pattern of facial fractures is most likely to produce upper airway obstruction? (Bilateral anterior mandible body, complex maxillary fractures.)
   (a) Why? (Loss of hyomandibular support for the base of tongue in the former, posterior displacement, or unstable maxilla in the latter.)
   (b) What can be done prior to endotracheal intubation, ET, to help reestablish the airway? (Since the problem is loss of anterior or hyomandibular support, placement of a 2° silk suture through the anterior tongue with traction to pull the base of the tongue free of the posterior pharynx and, of course, suctioning of blood and secretions can temporarily reestablish the airway until a definitive procedure is performed.)
   (c) What are the general guidelines for the obtunded patient? (Glasgow Coma Score is equal to or less than 8.)
2. What are the findings suggestive of laryngeal fracture? (Hoarseness, dysphagia, anterior cervical contusion, loss of the laryngeal prominence in males, crepitus. Patient demands to sit upright, drooling from secretions.)
   (a) How is the definitive diagnosis established? (CT scan.)
   (b) Emergent therapy? (Tracheostomy—avoid efforts at intubation.)
3. Discuss some options for the establishment of an airway in a nasotracheal trauma patient without "cleared" C-spines. (Inline stabilization of the head with direct endotracheal intubation, rapid sequence intubation, use of Bullard laryngoscope, nasotracheal intubation over a fiberoptic bronchoscope, use of the GlideScope, which is a video depiction of the anatomy obtained from the tip of the scope and displayed on a remote monitor, or simply direct laryngoscopy intubation.)
4. What is the principal concern with nasotracheal intubation in the presence of a Le Fort III fracture? (If a concomitant anterior fossa or skull base fracture exists, an endotracheal tube may be placed intracranially inadvertently. The most likely fracture location in those events is the cribriform plate.)
5. In a patient with significant nasoethmoid orbital fractures as well as fractures that dictate intermaxillary fixation, tracheostomy is one option for the airway. What are some other options? (Retromolar intubation, particularly in pediatric patients, submental intubation.)
6. Describe the method and possible complications of submental intubation. (The method consists of a skin incision, dissection through the mylohyoid, and transmucosally through the floor of the mouth. The endotracheal tube, previously placed orally, is then brought through the floor of the mouth and out of the incision. The potential complications are injury to the Wharton's duct, lingual nerve, and oral cutaneous fistula. Seemingly, a more advantageous route would be between the two anterior bellies of the digastric, avoiding the duct and lingual nerve.)

Editor's Note: Although the use of the laryngeal mask airway or LMA was described, it probably is an absolute last resort and a temporary measure only and should be avoided. Retrograde intubation by percutaneous placement through a large needle of an IV catheter and retrieval through the pharynx can be difficult and consume valuable time if unsuccessful.

Hemorrhage

1. Patients with severe, life-threatening bleeding are most likely to have what type of facial fracture? (Complex mid-face, such as LeFort II and III.)
2. Give a stepwise approach to severe intraoral and nasal hemorrhage in a facial fracture patient. (The key word is "severe." Less severe nasal hemorrhage alone should be addressed with anterior nasal packing as a first-line measure. Otherwise, posterior nasal packs followed by anterior nasal packing; if failure to control, then packing with gauze intraoral as well as into the maxillary sinuses if such is available. See editor's note.)
   (a) Nasal packing may present a problem in the presence of? (Disruption of the cribriform plate by nasoethmoid orbital fractures with extension into the fronto-basilar area.)
   (b) Describe the method of placement of posterior packs. (The papers describe placement of a Foley catheter, but perhaps a preferable technique is the placement of bilateral red rubber catheters, retrieval from the posterior pharynx, placement of a suture through the catheter attached to an antibiotic-soaked gauze and then pulling the catheter back out through the anterior nasal cavity thus, lodging the gauze in the posterior nasopharynx. Of course, a suture also needs to be placed on the gauze that can be brought out transorally for removal of the packs at a later date. Antibiotic-soaked gauze may be preferable from two aspects: One is better conformity to the posterior nasopharynx, and the other is to prevent infection as much as possible. One side effect or complication not discussed in the readings is the nasopulmonary reflex. Placement of posterior packs can precipitate pulmonary complications of pulmonary and systemic hypertension from the nasopulmonary reflex.)
3. What vessel(s) may be responsible for continuing hemorrhage despite placement of anterior/posterior nasal pack? (Internal maxillary, sphenopalatine)
   (a) Next step? (These vessels are best controlled by selective or super-selective arterial embolization by transarterial catheterization, bilateral if necessary.)
4. Transarterial embolization was the treatment in a multi-institutional study. The overwhelming majority of embolizations were of what vessel? (Internal maxillary)
   (a) Bleeding from what vessels cannot be treated or controlled with transarterial embolization? (Anterior and posterior ethmoid arteries. These vessels are derived from the ophthalmic artery and, in turn, from the internal carotid artery.)
5. What is the role of bilateral external carotid ligation? (None—ineffective because of the rich collateral flow and may prevent the performance of a subsequent transarterial embolization by angiography.)

Editor's Note: Not mentioned in the readings is control of severe arterial bleeding from the internal maxillary artery by transmaxillary sinus packing. Severe bleeding from the internal maxillary artery is almost always the result of comminuted maxillary fractures, including the posterior wall with laceration of the artery that lies just posterior to the maxillary sinus. In these instances, the comminution of the *anterior* wall will allow direct packing with roller gauze through the sinus and against the base of the skull to temporarily control arterial bleeding from the maxillary artery and subsequent transarterial embolization.

Evaluation

1. In the management of maxillofacial trauma, one needs to consider associated injuries. What is the frequency of intracranial or C-spine injuries in facial fracture patients? (Panfacial fractures, middle and lower or upper, middle, and lower, have an incidence of 18% and 13% intracranial or C-spine injury. Mandible fractures sustained in high-velocity circumstances have up to a 10% incidence of C-spine fractures. The occurrence of torso injuries in high-velocity MVA or pedestrian strikes is often occult and should be suspected.)
2. Assuming the primary survey is complete, what are the important elements of the initial history? (Mechanisms and circumstances of the injury, loss of consciousness, vision changes, perception of occlusion, pain with occlusion, and past medical history, including medications.)
3. Pertinent maxillofacial physical examination? (Inspection for obvious deformity of the periorbital region, presence of enophthalmos, and assessment of the transverse width of the face. Palpation begins in the superior third, forehead crepitus, the orbits for stepping off of the infraorbital rims, the maxilla for mobility, the mandible for occlusion, and any deviation with opening and closing. The next element is a more detailed examination with measurement of intercanthal distance for telecanthus, assessment of extraocular motion and pupillary reaction, vision evaluation by confrontation or Snellen card, nasal speculum exam, intraoral inspection for visible disrup-

tion of alveolar ridge indicative of mandibular fracture, loose or fractured teeth. Neurological assessment includes the facial nerve by facial expression and the three branches of the trigeminal by the status of sensation in the forehead, the medial cheek and upper lip, and the lower lip.)

Radiology

Editor's Note: Discussions of CT findings are also available in Chaps. 46–50.

1. What are the two principal disadvantages of the Panorex in mandible fractures? (The necessity for the patient to be in a sitting position and the blurring of the anterior symphyseal region due to overlap of the panoramic technique most commonly utilized in an outpatient setting.)
2. What particular maxillofacial fractures are optimally visualized with the following CT section: axial, coronal, sagittal? (Axial views depict the frontal sinus, lateral orbital wall, bony septum, mandible, zygomatic arch, medial-lateral wall of the maxilla, and nasal orbital ethmoid or NOE fractures. Coronal views are best for the orbital floor and medial wall, lateral orbital wall, bony septum, nasal orbital ethmoid, and NOE fractures. Sagittal views can be used to estimate the transverse dimension of orbital floor fractures and perhaps visualize the naso-frontal duct.)
   (a) Slice thickness? (To accomplish 3D reconstruction, thin, 1.0 mm slices are necessary.)
3. What is the role of 3D reconstruction? (Define the nature of the injury more clearly, a visual tool in the sense that combines the axial sagittal and coronal views and enables surgical planning at a workstation. The weakness is the lack of definition of orbital floor.)

The conference will consist of a review of the following in the facial trauma patient:

1. Systematic clinical examination
2. Reading of CT scans

Case-Based Conference

Case 1: Initial Care of the Maxillofacial Trauma Patient

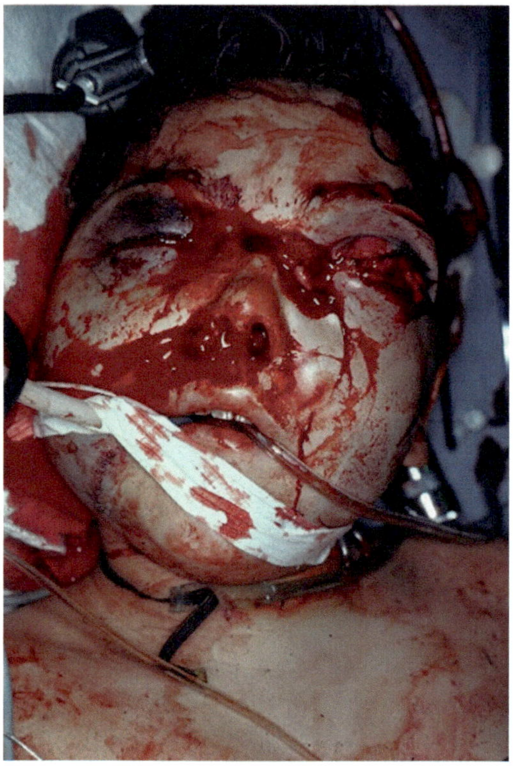

A 14-year-old who sustained primarily maxillofacial trauma in an MVA (no other injuries); clinically has a comminuted LeForte III fracture and is bleeding heavily from the mouth and nose that has required two units since arrival. He has been successfully intubated.

1. Describe an assessment with a clinical examination and initial treatment plan.

Case-Based Conference: Discussion

Case 1: Initial Care of the Maxillofacial Trauma Patient

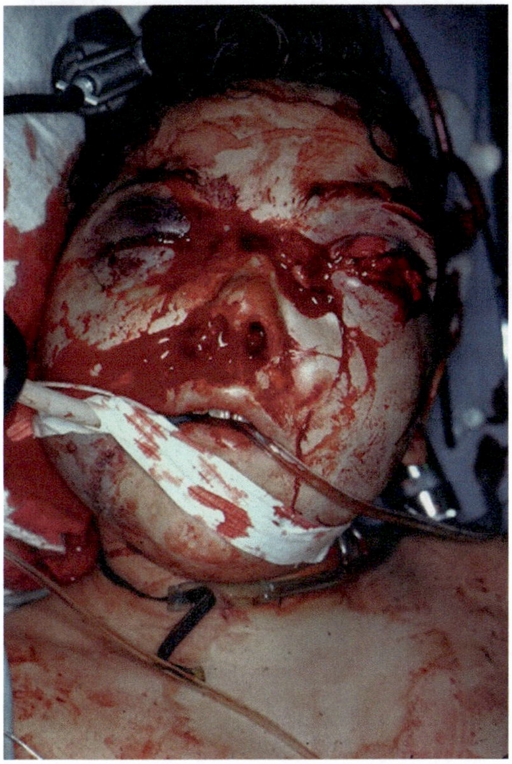

A 14-year-old who sustained primarily maxillofacial trauma in an MVA (no other injuries); clinically has a comminuted LeForte III fracture and is bleeding heavily from the mouth and nose that has required two units since arrival. He has been successfully intubated.

1. Describe an assessment with a clinical examination and initial treatment plan. (The initial airway management, although this patient has been intubated, would consist of suction, inline immobilization, and orotracheal intubation. A patient with a LeForte III fracture should not have a nasotracheal or blind nasotracheal intubation because of the possibility of intracranial misdirection of the endotracheal tube. The patient has *significant* bleeding. A number of sources are possible, but the most likely are lacerations of the internal maxillary artery, perhaps bilateral. Initial management after restoration of the airway should begin with the placement of anterior and posterior nasal packs. If bleeding continues, a not commonly described maneuver in patients with massive midface trauma and uncontrolled hemorrhage is packing the internal maxillary artery(s) *through* the maxillary sinuses against the posterior skull base. This packing can be accomplished with kerlix gauze, especially if the maxilla is comminuted, which is commonly the case in maxillofacial trauma patients with significant hemorrhage. One of the myths in the treatment of maxillofacial trauma is that significant bleeding can be successively controlled by the placement of the patient in intermaxillary fixation. Not only does that supposition not constitute good logic, but also valuable time will be consumed by doing so. If bleeding is controlled by this maneuver and certainly if uncontrolled, the court of final resort is selective embolization by interventional radiology. Unfortunately, the circumstances of this scenario, the necessity to transport to the radiology suite an actively bleeding patient who is on the cusp of becoming unstable, is more common than not.)

Case-Based Conference

Case 2: Initial Care of Facial Trauma

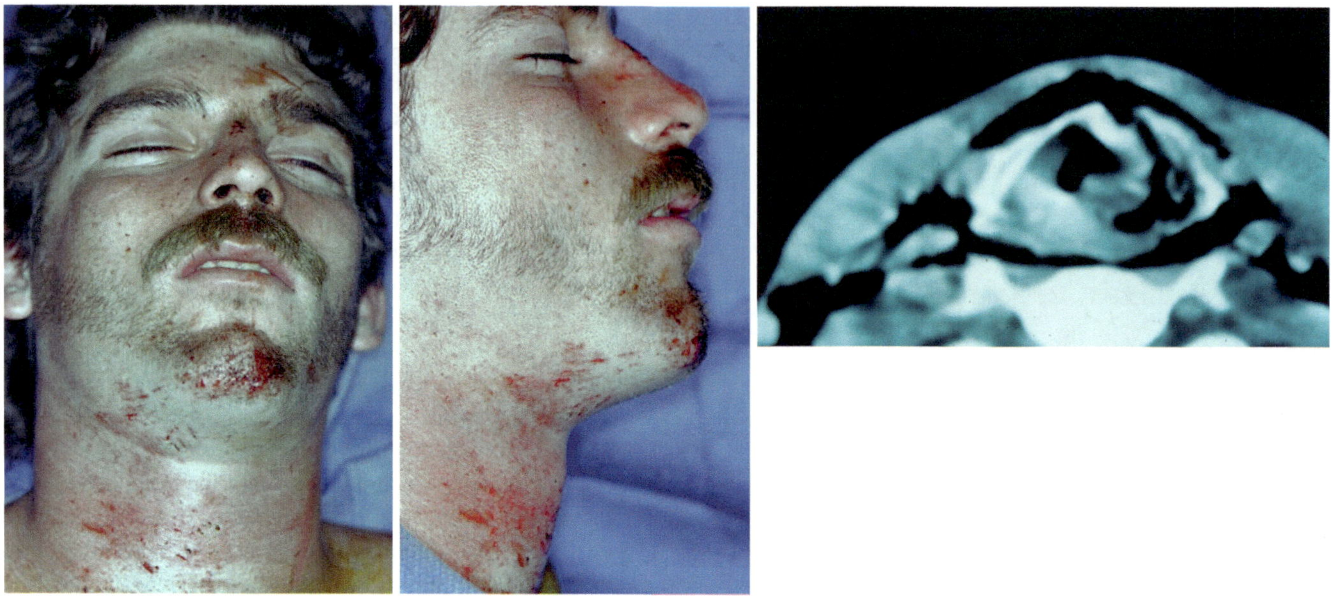

A 24-year-old unrestrained driver-occupant injured in an MVA. The patient complains of "inability to breathe." Attached is the CT scan.

1. Describe the slides, add a clinical examination and initial therapy, and give an assessment.
   (a) Now, read the CT scan. Any other tests? Assume the patient has no facial injuries and is alert.
2. Outline a treatment plan.

Case-Based Conference: Discussion

Case 2: Initial Care of Facial Trauma

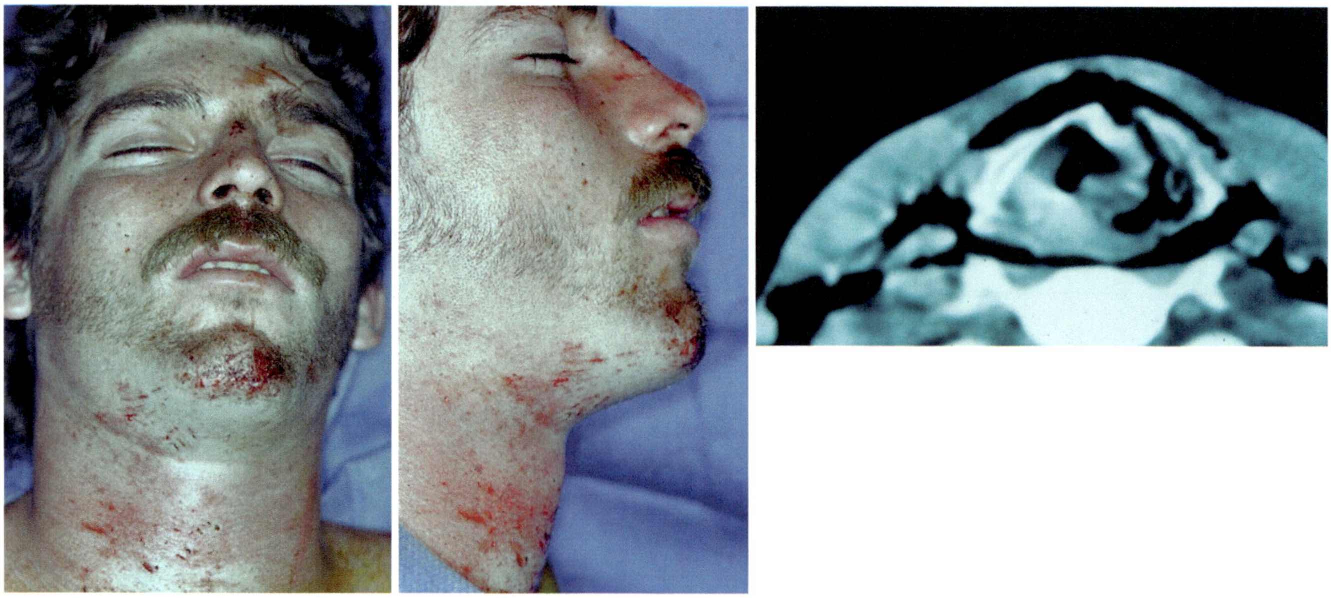

A 24-year-old unrestrained driver-occupant injured in an MVA. The patient complains of "inability to breathe." Attached is the CT scan.

1. Describe the slides, add a clinical examination and initial therapy, and give an assessment. (Two photos are available of the head and neck of a young male, a frontal and lateral view. A number of findings are evident, including areas of abrasion of the menton or tip of the chin, as well as the anterior lateral aspect of the right cervical region and the medial left eyebrow. The right lateral confirms these findings and further depicts that the area of abrasion of the right neck is more extensive than pictured on the frontal view. More subtle but equally significant on the lateral is the lack of thyroid prominence, normally present in a male. No periorbital ecchymosis or facial deformities are evident. The chin has normal projection without retrognathia.

The examination coincided with the initial treatment. With simultaneous immobilization of the head and neck, suction the oropharynx and posterior pharynx free of blood, teeth, debris, etc., and if necessary, pull the tongue forward. Although bilateral anterior mandibular body fractures can result in loss of hyomandibular support with upper airway obstruction, the setting is usually an elderly patient and/or the concomitant presence of a closed head injury. If these maneuvers fail to restore the airway, consider upper airway trauma as a laryngeal fracture. Does the patient have an inspiratory stridor? Can the patient talk, or is he profoundly hoarse? Palpation of the anterior neck in this patient with evidence of soft-tissue trauma may detect crepitus indicative of subcutaneous emphysema and perhaps pharyngeal laceration and/or laryngeal fracture. Perhaps, if the situation warrants and the patient is not in significant distress, a visualization of the glottis can be accomplished with a *single* attempt at laryngoscopy by an experienced individual. If not possible and/or blood, etc., obstructs the view, then a formal tracheostomy in the OR is indicated.)
   (a) Now, read the CT scan. Any other tests? Assume the patient has no facial injuries and is alert. (The single slice of an axial view is somewhat blurred but appears to be at the level of or just superior to the true vocal cords. Importantly, a paramedian fracture of the thyroid cartilage is visualized, as well as abundant areas of extralaryngeal air—all diagnostic of a laryngeal fracture. Of course, the patient needs C-spine films, CT of the head, and clearance of any visceral trauma by the trauma team.)
2. Outline a treatment plan. (This patient would benefit from immediate tracheostomy, the choice of setting would hinge on the degree of acuteness, either accomplished in the ER or the OR. Once in the OR, a complete laryngoscopy and pharyngoscopy needs to be accomplished *after* tracheostomy. Attempts at endotracheal intubation simply may consume the available reserves of time and patient stability and are not appropriate. Repair of the laryngeal fracture is a separate discussion.)

Intraoperative

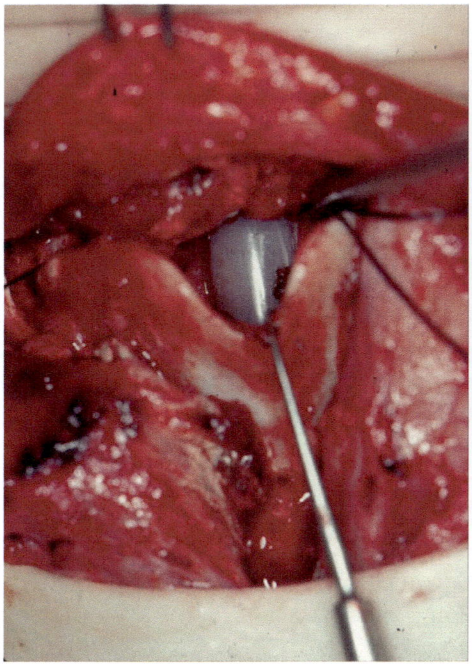

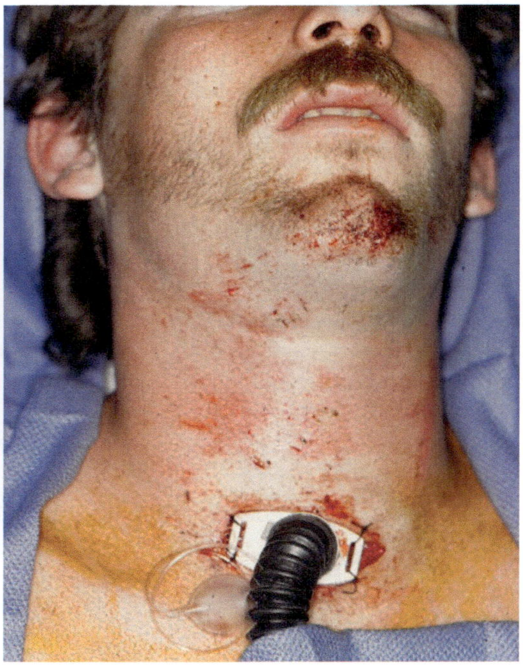

In the first slide, another case, the operative exploration for a suspected laryngeal injury, revealed complete disruption of the thyrohyoid membrane. Although the patient was successfully intubated for "shortness of breath," the endotracheal tube could have been easily misdirected through the disruption, necessitating an emergent tracheostomy under dire circumstances.

Postoperative (10 Days and 3 Months)

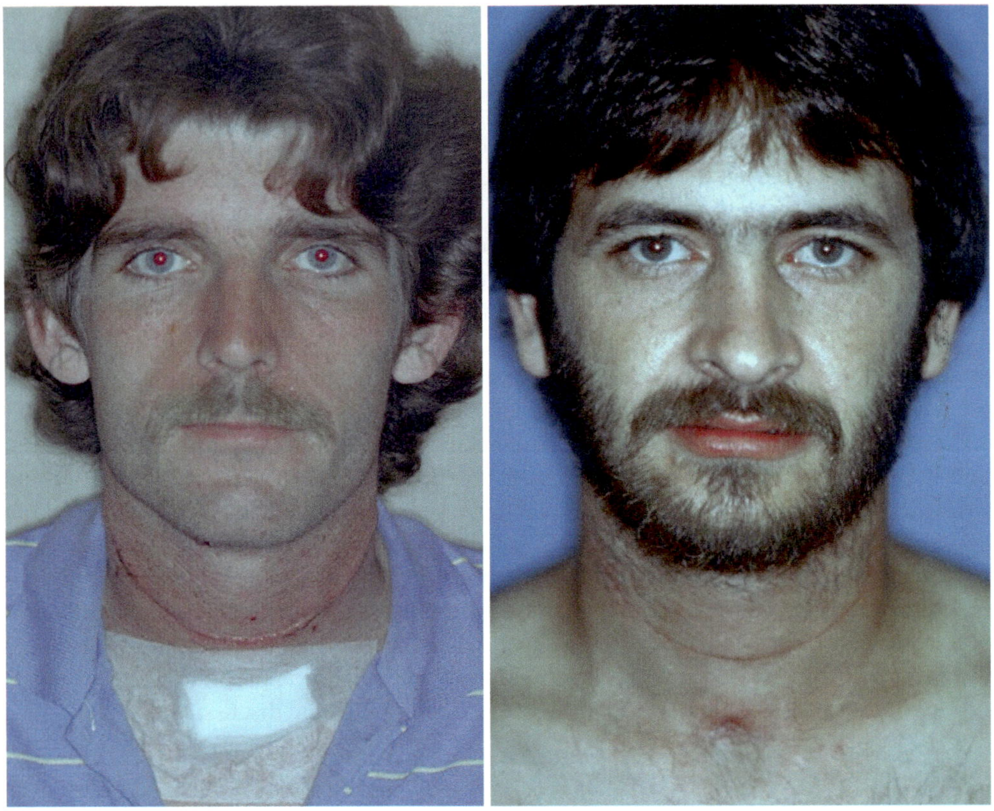

The patient, at 10 days postoperative, has been successfully decannulated, and 3 months later, the cervical access incision is less erythematous.

42 ORIF Principles, Operative Approaches, Optic Neuropathy

Bibliography

Soparkar CNS and Patrinely JR. "The Eye Examination in Facial Trauma for the Plastic Surgeon", *Plast. Reconstr. Surg.*, (2007) **49S–56S**.

Perry, M. et al. "Emergency Care in Facial Trauma—A Maxillofacial and Ophthalmic Perspective." *Injury*, Elsevier Co. (2005); 36:**886–92 ONLY**.

Wilcsek GA, Kazim M, Francis IC, et al., "Ch. 31 Acute Orbital Hemorrhage", Evaluation and Treatment of Orbital Fractures, Elsevier Inc., (2006): **pgs. 381–388**.

Chaon BC and Michael SL, "Is there treatment for traumatic optic neuropathy?" *Curr Opin Ophthalmol.* (2015), 26: **445–449**.

Ridgway EB, et al., "The Incidence of Lower Eyelid Malposition after Facial Fracture Repair: A Retrospective Study and Meta-Analysis Comparing Subtarsal, Subciliary, and Transconjunctival Incisions.", *Plast. Reconstr. Surg.*, (2009), 124(5):**1578–1586**.

Ellis III E and Zide MF, Chapter 3: "Transconjunctival Approaches", Surgical Approaches to the Facial Skeleton, Lippincott Williams & Wilkins, **pgs 38–50**.

Ellis III E and Zide MF, Chapter 6: "Coronal Approach", Surgical Approaches to the Facial Skeleton, Lippincott Williams & Wilkins, **pgs 65–86**.

Hadeed JG and Marcus JR, Chapter 6: "Internal Fixation Principles", Essentials of Craniofacial Trauma, Quality Medical Publishing, Inc., (2012); **pgs. 75–85**.

Niederhelman H and Shetty V, Chapter 4: "Principles and techniques of lag screw osteosynthesis", Yaremchuk MJ, Gruss JS, Manson PN, Rigid Fixation of the Craniomaxillofacial Skeleton, Butterworth-Heinemann, (1992); **pgs. 22–27**.

Videos

Sharabi SE, Koshy JC, Thornton JF, Hollier LH, "Facial fractures", *Plast. Reconstr. Surg.*, (2011); 127(2):**Video 1 ONLY**.

Faculty Discussion and Study Guide

Ocular Injuries

1. Describe the elements of the basic eye examination in the facial injury patient. (The eye exam should begin with an inspection for the detection of lid lacerations as well as pupil irregularity. The patient, if responsive, is queried about vision to confrontation. If the patient is unable to see a finger test, the next step is light perception. The extraocular muscles are assessed in four main directions: superior-inferior and medial-lateral. The pupillary reaction is judged both directly and consensually. If possible, the globe is gently palpated for tension.)
2. Explain the mechanisms that result in vision loss from intraorbital bleeding. (The fixed walls of the bony orbit create a compartment syndrome if bleeding occurs within the orbit. The increase in volume results in an increase in orbital pressure, culminating in obstruction of venous return. Similar to other compartment syndromes, a vicious cycle ensues with an unremitting increase in orbital pressure until occlusion of the central retinal artery, a branch of the ophthalmic, occurs. Experimental evidence would indicate that irreversible retinal injury occurs if the occlusion is longer than 90 min.)
3. What is the characteristic clinical picture in intraorbital bleeding or retro-orbital hematoma? (Severe pain, proptosis, dramatic loss of vision or light perception only, and if advanced, an afferent and efferent pupillary defect with ophthalmoplegia. On palpation, a firm to hard and non-ballotable globe.)
   (a) How might a fundus examination be helpful? (Detection of lack of retinal arteriole pulsations or even a pale optic disk.)
4. Outline a combination of medical and surgical therapies in the scenario of proptosis and diminished visual acuity either postoperatively or in the presence of orbital frac-

E. Luce, *A Curriculum for Plastic Surgery*, https://doi.org/10.1007/978-3-031-62087-4_42

tures. (Immediate measures should consist of intravenous mannitol, ocular Diamox drops, and a lateral canthotomy. If the clinical situation improves sufficiently to obtain a CT scan, the imaging can be helpful. Regardless, in all likelihood, more definitive surgical treatment will be necessary, which would consist of an operative orbital decompression by removal of the orbital floor, medial wall, and possibly lateral wall as well.)
   (a) What is the role of anterior chamber paracentesis? (None. The increased intraocular pressure may herniate the lens through the paracentesis site.)
   (b) Describe the technique of lateral canthotomy. (A transverse incision through the lateral commissure of the lateral canthus, conjunctiva, and skin to the lateral orbital rim is accomplished, essentially splitting the conjoint lateral canthal tendon horizontally. The upper and lower lid retinacula contributions are severed by the placement of the respective lid under tension and sharply incising along the bony rim, either inferiorly or superiorly. In the presence of a retro-orbital hematoma and increased intraocular pressure, the procedure should be viewed as a temporary measure only.)
5. Discuss the value of incision and drainage of an intraorbital hematoma. (Neither effective nor feasible. Bleeding into soft tissue and swollen, hemorrhagic orbital fat renders identification of a bleeding point extremely difficult, if not impossible. Definitive management is decompression by orbital enlargement.)
6. Traumatic optic neuropathy occurs both in closed-head injuries, particularly blunt trauma to the frontal bone without maxillofacial trauma, and in maxillofacial trauma without closed-head injuries. Motor function is intact so the efferent limb renders a positive consensual response. What is the hallmark clinical finding? (Afferent pupil defect and diminished or no vision. A test of perhaps more subtle optic nerve injury is red color saturation. The patient with an injured but still functioning optic nerve will, when confronted with a bright red object, relate a difference between the two eyes, the injured as more dull, less red. This clinical scenario is distinctly uncommon.)
   (a) What is the anatomic and functional pathology in traumatic optic neuropathy? (Direct penetration and transection of the optic nerve is possible, but because of the thick bony structure of the optic canal, such is quite rare. Much more common is stretch or traction injury with perhaps a secondary ischemic insult. The vasculature of the optic nerve consists of small pial vessels perfused by the ophthalmic artery as well as the central retinal artery, a branch of the ophthalmic. Edema from contusion or shearing at the junction of the fixed, intracanicular, and mobile, interorbital segments of the nerve can set the circumstances for an increase in pressure within the rigid bony confines of the intracanicular portion of the optic nerve and a secondary ischemic insult.)
   (b) Necessary diagnostic measures? (CT scan and fundoscopic exam for arterial occlusion or venous engorgement.)
   (c) Treatment? (Controversial: medical is high-dose steroids; surgical is decompression via transethmoidal or transcranial approach. The medical treatment with high-dose steroids clearly is attended by a significant incidence of complications, and the benefit is not readily demonstrable. The benefit of surgical decompression, even with an endoscopic transethmoidal and transnasal approach, is also not clearly demonstrable.)
   (d) What is the difference between the optic and the other cranial nerves in response to injury? (Cranial nerves II–XII are peripheral nerves and capable of regeneration. The optic nerve is a component of the central nervous system and cannot regenerate.)
   (e) What is the overall prognosis? (The overall prognosis is heterogeneous, composed of patients who begin with no vision or light perception, light perception only, and markedly diminished vision. As a total group, the permanent outcome viewed broadly is a complete or nearly complete recovery in one-third, no vision in one-third, and recovery with substantially diminished vision in the remainder.)
7. What is a hyphema? (Blood in either the anterior or posterior chamber.)
8. What are the findings on a penetrating injury of the globe that are of prognostic value? (Visual acuity that is light perception only, an afferent pupillary defect, and an injury in the more posterior or zone III of the globe all signal a poor prognosis.)
   (a) What is the initial treatment awaiting the arrival of an ophthalmologist? (Placement of a rigid shield over the eye to prevent inadvertent rubbing or pressure.)
9. An irregular or teardrop-shaped pupil may be indicative of what? (A penetrating injury of the anterior chamber. The teardrop shape is an incarcerated iris that has prolapsed and sealed the wound.)

Surgical Approaches

Editor's Note: Eyelid anatomy will be discussed in more detail in Chaps. 48 and 97.

1. What is the principal difference in terms of size and shape between the lower lid and upper lid tarsus or tarsal plate? (The upper lid tarsus vertical height in the midline

is about 10 mm, but the shape is as a half-moon with a sharply diminished vertical height more medially and laterally. The lower lid tarsus vertical height is 5–6 mm but maintains that height throughout most of the extent of the tarsus medially and laterally. Of course, in the coronal plane, both are gently curved to follow the configuration of the eyeball.)

2. What are the components of the orbicularis oculi? (A pretarsal, a preseptal, and an orbital portion. The pretarsal and preseptal portions contribute to the medial and lateral canthal tendons. The medial pretarsal and preseptal are the principal components of the lacrimal pump system. The orbital portion is principally responsible for the tight closure of the eye.)
3. Describe the difference between a subciliary and subtarsal transcutaneous approach to the inferior orbital rim in facial fracture repair. (Subciliary is 2–3 mm below the lash margin and is usually performed by direct incision with preservation and retention of the pretarsal portion of the orbicularis muscle on the tarsal plate and then the development of a skin-muscle flap. A subtarsal is an incision placed in a natural crease somewhat below the subciliary approach and also is performed by a skin muscle flap. Advocates of a subtarsal approach state a lower incidence of ectropion. The advocates of a subciliary approach favor the same for cosmetic reasons. See question and discussion below.)
4. Outline the two options in a transconjunctival approach. (The pertinent anatomy is the fusion of the orbital septum and the capsulopalpebral fascia, arising from the inferior rectus at 2 mm inferior to the tarsal plate. This conjoined tendon inserts into the inferior margin of the tarsal plate. A conjunctival incision made at the level of the inferior edge of the tarsal plate will access the rim and floor by a preseptal approach because of a conjoined septum at that point. A retroseptal approach is a conjunctival incision made several mm below the inferior edge of the tarsal plate and so posterior to the septum. Orbital fat will be within the plane of dissection.

A lateral canthotomy is often combined with a transconjunctival approach and requires meticulous repair. As outlined in the discussion of the paper on the comparison of lower eyelid complications regardless of the approach, suspension of the soft tissues to the malar eminence should be done routinely after a wide subperiosteal exposure of the infraorbital rim and zygoma.)

5. Describe the advantages, disadvantages, and performance of lateral canthotomy. (The advantage of the inclusion of a lateral canthotomy within the transconjunctival approach is the additional exposure. The principal disadvantage is the necessity of a meticulous repair, complicated by asymmetry, an unnatural appearance of the lateral canthus, and a lack of lid adherence to the globe.

   A lateral canthotomy is performed by an incision through skin, conjunctiva, and lateral canthal tendon at the lateral canthus or angle followed by outward traction on the lid and lysis of the lateral retinaculum.)
6. Describe a transconjunctival approach to the medial orbital wall. (A retrocaruncIar extension of a standard transconjunctival incision will provide access to the medial orbital wall. The incision is vertically oriented and placed posterior to the caruncle and the semilunar fold of the conjunctival. Initial dissection is directed posterior to the posterior lacrimal crest and posterior to Horner's muscle. The periorbita is incised, and subperiosteal dissection proceeds posteriorly for exposure of the medial orbital wall. The origin of the inferior rectus will be elevated with the subperiosteal dissection and does not need to be repositioned with closure.)
7. List the principal complication and the estimated frequency for the following three approaches to the infraorbital rim: transconjunctival access, subciliary, and subtarsal. (Principal complication in a transconjunctival is entropion; subciliary, ectropion; and subtarsal, hypertrophic scarring. The estimated incidence of entropion with transconjunctival is about 1.0%, hypertrophic scarring with subtarsal 3.5%, and ectropion with subciliary incisions 14%. Ectropion and scarring are likely to improve with conservative measures; entropion, although considerably lower in frequency, is unlikely to resolve spontaneously.)
8. The safe performance of a bicoronal incision and flap requires a knowledge of the anatomy of the frontal branch of the facial nerve. What is the relationship of the nerve to the following:

   Temporoparietal fascia? (Courses within or on the deep surface of the temporoparietal fascia.)

   Subaponeurotic space? (Subaponeurotic space is a loose areolar space beneath the temporoparietal fascia and, therefore, by definition, should be deep to the nerve but not sufficiently safe.)

   Superficial layer of the deep temporal fascia? (The superficial layer of the deep temporal fascia is the next layer deep to the subaponeurotic space, and beneath this layer is the recommended route.)

   (a) Describe the location of the superficial temporal fat pad and the importance of dissection of the bicoronal flap. (The superficial temporal fat pad lies between the superficial and the deep layer of the deep temporal fascia, directly superior and overlying the zygomatic arch. As described below, access by incision of the superficial layer of the deep temporal fascia will gain access to the superficial temporal fat pad, the zygomatic arch, and ensure that the frontal branch of the facial nerve is superficial to the plane of dissection.)

(b) Where is the middle temporal artery? (The artery can lie within the superficial temporal fat pad and can be lacerated.)

9. Where must you make the incision to gain access and dissect deep into the superficial layer of the deep temporal fascia? (The deep temporal fascia superiorly is a single layer overlying the temporalis muscle until proceeding from superior to inferior; the line of fusion is encountered at about the level of the superior orbital rim or to 4 cm superior to the palpated zygomatic arch. At that point, the deep temporal fascia splits into a superficial and deep layer, and the superficial layer of the deep temporal fascia must be incised to gain access to the zygomatic arch and optimally done 2 cm superior to the arch and as posterior as feasible. The deep layer of the deep temporal fascia courses posterior to the arch, and the superficial layer superficial to the arch.)
10. What are the components of the dissection of the flap further inferior? (If a pericranial flap is not necessary, a transverse periosteal incision is made about 2 cm superior to the superior orbital rim, and a subperiosteal dissection accomplished to the level of the supraorbital foramina, the supraorbital neurovascular bundles, possibly with an osteotomy, are dissected free of the bone. If additional exposure is necessary, the orbital roof periosteum is also dissected subperiosteal. A lateral extension can be performed by the continuance of the incisions inferiorly, either pre- or post-auricular.)

Reduction/Fixation

1. What are the stages of bone healing? (Similar to soft tissue wound healing, the initial stage is inflammatory with a cellular infiltrate of neutrophils, macrophages, as well as differentiated stem cells or osteoclasts and the presence of a hematoma. After an initial stage of several days, the reparative stage is heralded by the arrival of the osteo- and chondroblasts. Again, similar to the deposition of collagen in soft tissue wounds, bone deposition occurs in a somewhat disorganized pattern, as initially cartilage is replaced by woven bone. Grossly, this phase is recognized by the presence of a callus. Woven bone is converted to lamellar bone. The third stage, although a bright line demarcation does not exist, is signaled by the presence of trabecular bone, gradually remodeled into compact bone, imperceptible from native bone.)
2. Describe and contrast direct and indirect bone healing. (Direct or primary osseous healing occurs in the presence of precise, intimate contact of the two bone surfaces without intervening space or callus formation. Theoretically, direct or primary bone healing occurs with the implementation of rigid compressive fixation. Indirect healing is characterized by the stages described above. In reality, bone healing in rigid compression probably has an element of indirect healing.)
3. Internal fixation of facial fractures employs plates and screws. What measurement designates a plate system as 1.5 or 2.0? (The size of the screws in mm. Although standard and low profile plates are available and thicker instrumentation as reconstruction plates are utilized in mandibular fracture and reconstruction, the operative sets are organized by screw size.)
   (a) What are the principal characteristics of the screws used in the repair of facial fractures? (As discussed above, the outer diameter of the screw size and the nature of the screw. Pre-tapped or, more correctly, non-tapping screws have blunt tips and require prior use of a tap or tapping the hole before placement of the screw and are less commonly used in contemporary facial fracture management. Self-tapping screws are fluted and cut a thread during placement.)
4. What is the concept underlying lag screw osteosynthesis? (Lag screw osteosynthesis is based on the concept of torsion stress converted to compressive stress by a differential thread size between the proximal and distal fragment screw holes. By the passage of the screw through the larger proximal or gliding hole into the smaller drill hole of the distal fragment, the distal fragment is compressed into the proximal bone fragment.)
5. Describe the technique of lag screw synthesis. (The optimal fracture line for lag screw osteosynthesis permits the screw to bisect the fractured line at an angle of 90° or perpendicular. As described above, the technique requires a drilling of a larger proximal or gliding hole and a hole of smaller diameter in the distal fragment. Essentially, the glide hole diameter should equal the thread or outer diameter of the screw, and the distal or thread hole should correspond to the inner or core diameter. The initial hole is drilled with, for example, a 2.7 mm bit and then countersunk to recess the screwhead, and the distal hole is drilled with a smaller 2.0 bit. See Fig. 42.1.)

Fig. 42.1 Technique of lag screw fixation (Stern, Peter J., Chapter 8: "Fractures of the Metacarpals and Phalanges." Green MD, D. P., et al., Green's Operative Hand Surgery, (2011) 6th Edition; Churchill Livingstone, pgs. 250. (Reprinted with permission))

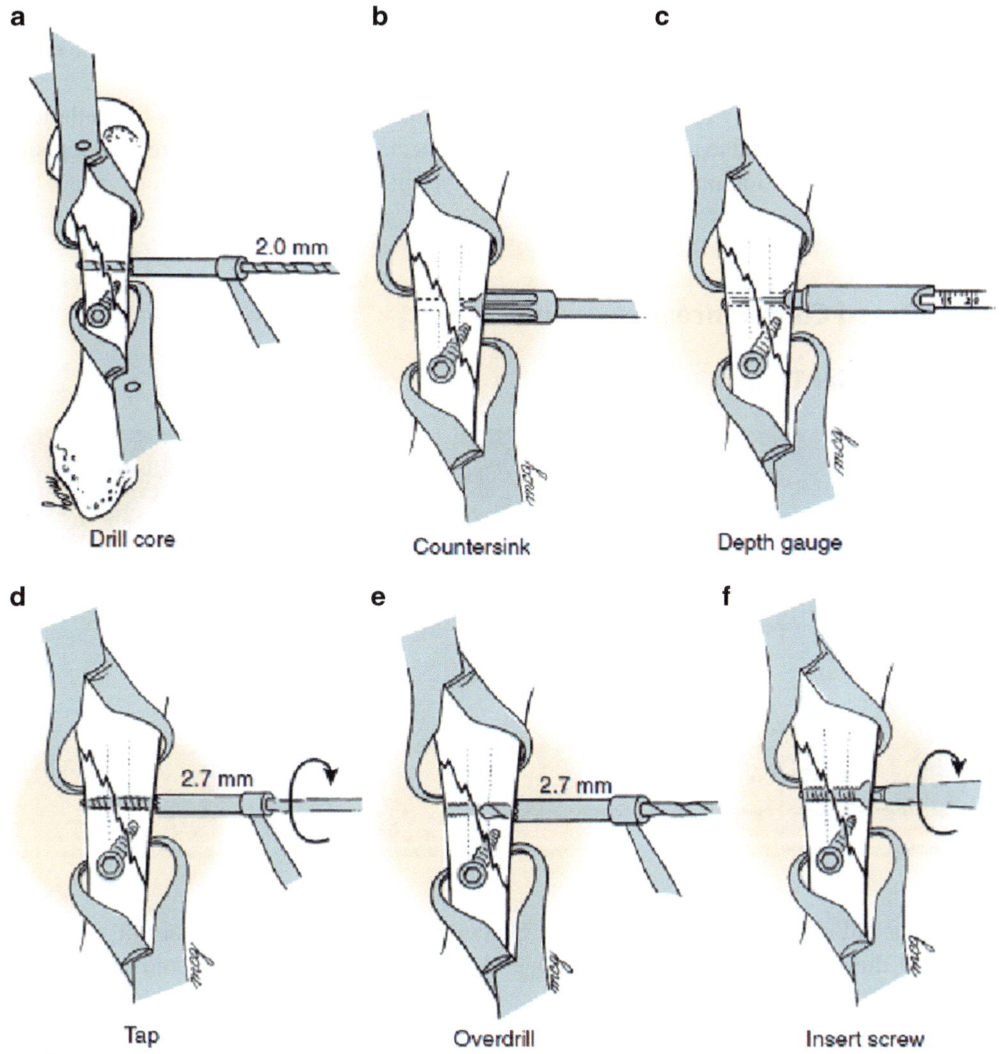

Case-Based Conference

Case 1: Ocular Trauma

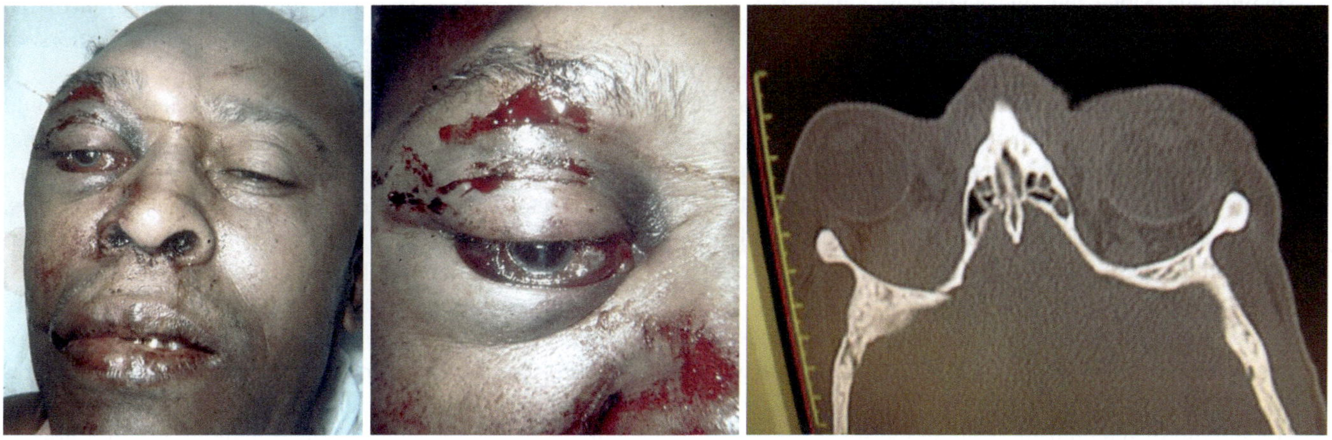

A 60-year-old male struck with a pool cue. He complains of pain and diminished vision in the right eye. Attached is a slice of the CT scan.

1. Describe the slide(s) and add a clinical examination. During your physical examination, the patient appears to have light perception only in the right eye, intact in the left eye.
   (a) Interpret the CT scan.
2. What's the most likely explanation(s) of the patient's problem?
   (a) What is the pathological anatomy?
3. Outline a treatment plan.

Case-Based Conference: Discussion

Case 1: Ocular Trauma

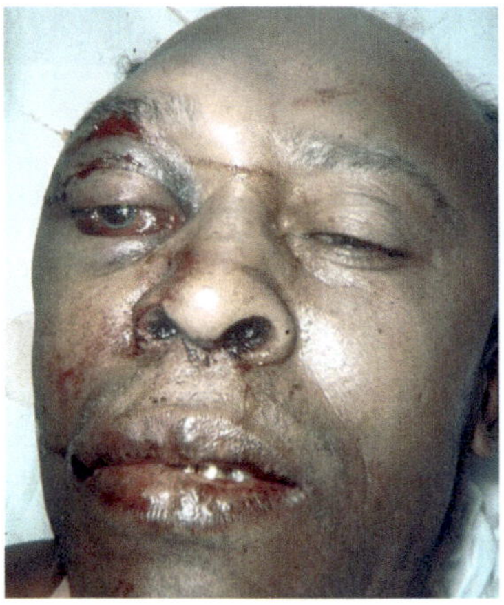
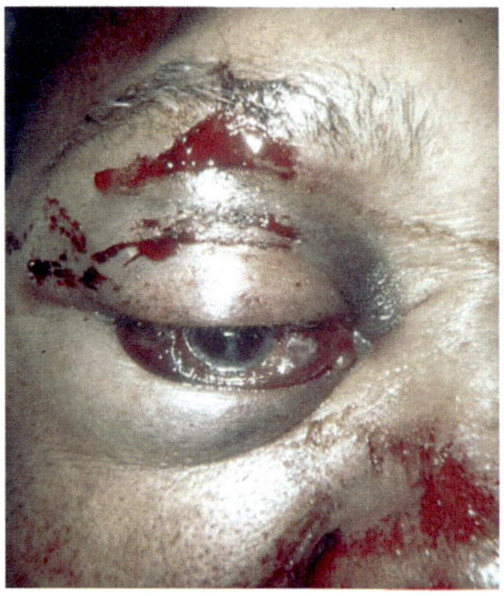
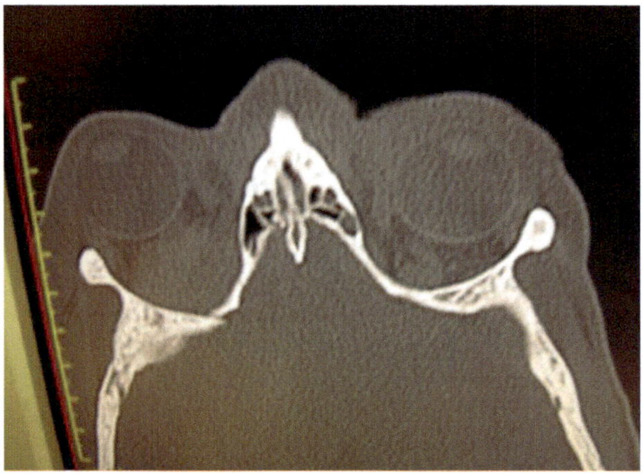

A 60-year-old male struck with a pool cue. He complains of pain and diminished vision in the right eye. Attached is a slice of the CT scan.

1. Describe the slide(s) and add a clinical examination. During your physical examination, the patient appears to have light perception only in the right eye, intact in the left eye. (Two clinical photos with signs of recent facial trauma. The most obvious findings are of the right eye, proptosis, substantial chemosis of the conjunctiva, and a swollen eye. Other findings evident are a probable transverse laceration of the infra brow upper eyelid area. Clotted blood is also visible in both nostrils. The entire right periorbital area appears edematous, as well as the upper and lower lips. The left eye is nearly closed, but no other significant findings are evident. The closeup photo is limited to the right periorbital region. The additional finding is an abnormality of the iris and pupil not clearly discernible. The proptosis is sufficiently severe the lash margin of the lower lid is not visible.

   The clinical exam would begin with brief questions about comorbidities and past eye pathology but would rapidly move toward ascertainment of vision. The critical component of the clinical examination is the assessment of the right eye. Evaluation of the vision consists of a finger count at a variety of distances. Although assessment by confrontation is only a gross estimation of visual capacity, if the finger count is correct at greater than 5 ft., the examiner can assume vision is grossly normal. If finger counting is not perceived or is indistinct at 12 in., the next step is the ability to perceive light. The ocular exam then progresses to pupillary reaction. Both direct and consensual pupil response is evaluated. Notation should be recorded as full, sluggish, or non-reactive. A careful inspection of the degree of distortion of the iris and pupil should be noted. The final step is an evaluation of the extraocular muscles by motion in the four vectors of superior-inferior and medial-lateral.

   The pupillary reaction is crucial: a nonresponse would confirm an afferent optic nerve lesion. If a consensual response is present, the status of the third nerve oculomotor is intact. If so, the function of the extraocular muscles, EOMs, are probably also intact. However, if ophthalmoplegia was evident on the exam, a consensual response is unlikely. A red object test would be redundant and only confirm the other obvious findings. An additional component of the examination could be measurements of intraocular pressures. This measurement can be difficult in the emergent setting, and the instrumentation is not always available. An elevated pressure just confirms the other aspects of the clinical picture. Of course, a relative difference in gross ocular pressure can be ascertained by palpation of the two eyes and a comparison of the same.)

   (a) Interpret the CT scan. (A single slice of an axial view of a CT scan with a bone window is provided. The image demonstrates moderate swelling of the right periorbital region. The most marked finding is a substantial collection in the posterior orbit, occupying perhaps a third of the orbital volume of this particular axial slice. The optic nerve is not visible.)

2. What is the most likely explanation(s) of the patient's problem? (A most likely diagnosis that explains the clinical presentation and CT scan finding it a large retro-orbital hematoma.)
   (a) What is the pathological anatomy? (The presence of the retro-orbital hematoma is a space-occupying mass within the rigid confines of the bony orbit. If sufficiently large, a series of pathophysiologic events consistent with a compartment syndrome, analogous to a compartment syndrome of the volar forearm, occurs. The increase in pressure within the bony orbit will occlude venous return, an event that alters the normal equilibrium of intravascular-interstitial fluid shifts with a resultant increase in egress of fluid from the intravascular to the interstitial space and a further increase in the compartment pressure. The increase in intraorbital pressure will also alter the normal fluid dynamics of the globe with a progressive increase in intraocular pressure and the adverse consequence of a diminution in perfusion. The cycle of an increase in intraorbital pressure, venous occlusion, further increase in the fluid shift into the interstitial space, and extravasation eventually culminates in arterial occlusion and an irreversible ischemic insult of the retina and optic nerve.)
3. Outline a treatment plan. (The clinical picture of an afferent pupillary defect, ophthalmoplegia, and proptosis combined with the CT findings of a retro-orbital hematoma, mandate immediate orbital decompression, again analogous to the performance of a fasciotomy in the instance of a volar forearm compartment syndrome. The management plan consists of the initiation of Diamox®, which can transiently diminish intraocular pressure as well as the performance of a lateral canthotomy. In the clinical setting of light perception only in a proptotic eye, those measures should be regarded as temporizing only until access to the operating room. The definitive treatment is to expand intraorbital volume. The bony confines of the orbit can be conceptualized as four walls, three of which are accessible to expansion. Access can be accomplished through an inferior marginotomy of the orbital rim with a blunt outfracture of both the floor and medial orbital wall. The third element, the lateral orbital wall, is thicker and may require more than a simple outfracture. Regardless, the conceptual approach is expansion or enlargement of the orbital cavity to decrease intraorbital pressure. Late reconstruction will be required to avoid the sequelae of enophthalmos.)

In-Service Examination

1. The components of the superior orbital fissure syndrome include the following **EXCEPT**:
   (a) Ptosis
   (b) Ophthalmoplegia
   (c) Blindness
   (d) Dilated unresponsive pupil
   (e) Absence of corneal reflex
2. A patient with a right optic nerve injury has what of the following pupillary reactions?
   (a) A nonreactive right pupil with direct light stimulation but an intact consensual response with light into the left pupil
   (b) Both pupils are nonreactive with light stimulation of the right eye
   (c) A nonreactive right pupil with light shone into the left eye
   (d) Both pupils are equally reactive, both direct and consensual, but the patient is blind in the right eye
3. A patient presents in the trauma bay after an MVA with a midface fracture, substantial bleeding, and hypotension. After a secure airway, the next initial step in control of the bleeding should be:
   (a) IMF
   (b) Interventional radiology for embolization
   (c) Anterior and posterior nasal packing
   (d) Operative intervention

43 Orbital Adnexal and Parotid Injury

Bibliography

Zide BM and Swift R, "How to block and tackle the face", *Plast Reconstr Surg.*, (1998); 101(3):**840–851**.

Tyers A.G., Ch. 18 "Eyelid and Lacrimal Injuries", Maxillofacial Trauma and Aesthetic Facial Reconstruction, Peter Ward Booth, Barry L. Eppley, and Rainer Schmelzeisen, (2012):**304–312, 320–322 ONLY**.

Jordan DR, Ch. 34: "Canalicular and Nasolacrimal Injuries Associated with Orbital Trauma", Evaluation and Treatment of Orbital Fractures, Elsevier, (2006); **pp. 409–421**.

Cho D.Y., Willborg B.E., Lu G.N., "Management of Traumatic Soft Tissue Injuries of the Face," *Semin Plast Surg.*, (2021);35:**229, 233–35 ONLY (Ear)**.

Chambers C.B., Moe K.S., "Periorbital Scar Correction", *Facial Plast Surg Clin N Am.*, (2017);25:25, **27–32 ONLY**.

Lewkowicz DMD, A. A., et al., "Traumatic Injuries to the Parotid Gland and Duct", *J. of Oral and Maxillofac Surg.*, (2002); 60:**676–680**.

Steinberg MJ, Herréra AF, "Management of Parotid Duct Injuries", *Oral and Maxillofacial Surgery*, (2005); 99(2): **136–141**.

Costan V.V., Dabija M.G., Ciofu M.L., et al., "A Functional Approach to Posttraumatic Salivary Fistula Treatment: The Use of Botulinum Toxin", *The Journal of Craniofacial Surgery*, (2019);30(3):**871–874**.

Faculty Discussion and Study Guide: Soft Tissue

Editor's Note: Post-traumatic optic neuropathy and retro-orbital hemorrhage are included in Chap. 42. Orbital and Periorbital anatomy is also discussed in considerably more detail in Chaps. 27 and 97.

Eyelid and Orbital Adnexal Injuries

1. The lateral canthal tendon inserts on what? (Whitnall's tubercle, located 5 mm posterior to the lateral orbital rim.)
2. Describe the components of the medial canthal tendon (The medial canthal tendon has both a posterior and anterior component as well as a muscular element. The anterior limb, which is thicker and more fibrous, inserts on the frontal process of the maxilla at the anterior lacrimal crest and passes anterior to the lacrimal sac. The posterior limb, thinner and filmier, runs posterior to the lacrimal sac and inserts on the posterior lacrimal crest. The muscular element is composed of preseptal orbicularis and is sufficiently specialized to be termed the Horner's muscle. Contraction of Horner's muscle during blinking aids in the lacrimal pump mechanism to squeeze tears from the palpebral sulcus into the canaliculi and eventually into the sac.)
   (a) What's the relationship of the levator aponeurosis to the medial and lateral canthal tendons? (The medial and lateral aponeurosis fans out and insert on the posterior aspect of the medial and lateral canthal tendons, respectively, as they insert onto the bone.)

E. Luce, *A Curriculum for Plastic Surgery*, https://doi.org/10.1007/978-3-031-62087-4_43

3. What anatomical structure separates the intra- from the extra-conal space? (Tenon's capsule, which encompasses and provides a sheath for the muscles of extraocular motion, terminating posteriorly at the annulus of Zenn.)
4. Describe the components of the lacrimal collecting system, including their length. (The upper and lower lid medially have a punctum with a short vertical 2 mm component that then drains into the superior and inferior canaliculus, respectively. The canaliculi run obliquely toward a common canaliculus and measure about 8–10 mm in length. The common canaliculus is about 3–5 mm and empties into the lacrimal sac. The vertical height of the lacrimal sac is 12–13 mm, which in turn drains inferiorly into the nasolacrimal duct. The length of the duct is 12–15 mm through bone and about a 5 mm meatus beneath the inferior turbinate or concha, known as the inferior meatus. The lacrimal sac lies directly posterior to the anterior limb of the medial canthal tendon, although the fundus of the sac bulges several millimeters superior to the superior limit of the tendon.)
5. How would you, theoretically, test the competency of the valve of Rosenmuller? (Blowing the nose with force will produce a puff of air in the corner of the eye. Air has refluxed up the nasolacrimal duct through the lacrimal sac and into the canaliculi because of an incompetent valve of Rosenmuller at the junction of the common canaliculus into the lacrimal sac.)
   (a) In contrast to the valve of Rosenmuller, where is the valve of Hosner? (At the aperture of the nasolacrimal duct in the nasal cavity.)
6. Briefly outline the clinical examination of the eye and orbital adnexa in a patient who has sustained a lid injury. (Observation estimates the extension of ecchymosis, bleeding confined to the preseptal area, will be more diffused and will extend beyond the bony limits of the orbit. In contrast, a postseptal hemorrhage is restricted to the origin-insertion of the orbital septum from the orbital bone. The visual acuity should be estimated with confrontation or finger counting. The pupillary response to a bright light should be estimated in both eyes with an anticipated direct and consensual response. Proptosis or enophthalmos should be detected. The globe should be gently palpated for an estimate of tension. Eye or globe vertical position should be estimated, and the levator function should be assessed. The extraocular muscle motion, EOMs, should also be evaluated.)

Editor's Note: The eye examination is also discussed in Chap. 42.

7. What wound finding in an upper lid laceration may signal injury of the levator? (Exposure of preaponeurotic fat, which means that the septum has been transected, and since the levator aponeurosis lies just posterior to the fat, the levator may be injured.)
8. Outline the technique of repair of a vertical lid laceration. (Skin, tarsal plate, and conjunctiva all must be repaired separately. The initial suture can be placed through the "gray line" to align the lid margin, the tarsal plate repaired with a 6° Vicryl, avoiding the conjunctiva and the skin closed with skin sutures. The conjunctiva is best closed with a running fast-absorbing suture. The suture in the "gray line" is a 6 or 7° silk to avoid irritation of the cornea that will occur with a monofilament suture such as nylon.)
9. What is the most common complication of a poorly repaired vertical lid laceration through both lamellae? (A notching defect due to poor alignment or failure to repair the tarsal plate.)
10. What is the definition of entropion and common presentation? (Entropion is the inward or posterior displacement of the lash margin and lower lid toward the globe. By definition, in the trauma setting, the etiology is posterior lamella, conjunctiva, deficiency, and/or scarring.)
    (a) Correction? (Release in the placement of a posterior lamella autologous graft. Several techniques are possible, including palatal mucoperiosteal grafts and buccal mucosa plus acellular dermal matrix grafts.)
11. What is the definition of ectropion and presentation? (Ectropion is an outward or anterior eversion of the lid margin with exposure of tarsal conjunctiva. In the trauma setting, the etiology is anterior lamella, skin orbicularis, and septum deficiency and scarring with perhaps associated age-related lid laxity.)
    (a) Correction? (Release including the septum and full-thickness skin grafting.)
12. A patient has sustained substantial acute traumatic loss of both eyelids. What temporary measures are available to protect the cornea? (If sufficient tissue is present, a temporary tarsorrhaphy. Otherwise, the construction of a chamber plus eye ointment prevents moisture and evaporation. One example is a careful seal of Opsite plus antibiotic ointment.)
13. Describe a technique for repair of a laceration of either the upper or lower canaliculus. (The simplest method is the Worst technique, which utilizes a silicone tubing threaded over a pigtail probe. Passage through the uninjured canaliculus into the lacrimal sac and back out the proximal end of the severed canaliculus will enable identification and intubation of the proximal end. The tubing can then be threaded through the distal end of the

severed canaliculus and out the punctum and tied with the end of the tubing from the uninjured canaliculus. This method has some disadvantages, including false passage and possible eventual loss of the intubation. The use of a rounded rather than a sharp probe will decrease the incidence of false passage. Other techniques involve bicanalicular intubation with the passage of the tubing through the sac, down the nasolacrimal duct, and into the nose. See below.)

14. What is the argument pro and con for the repair of both inferior and superior canicular systems if injured? (The principal argument in advocacy of repair of both is that in approximately one-half of the populous, one or the other of the two will be the dominating system, and failure to repair will result in at least mild or intermittent epiphora under circumstances of basal secretion. The epiphora can worsen in this group in situations of increased lacrimal production. The only con, which is not sufficiently persuasive, is the additional operative time and perhaps minimal, if any, increase in morbidity.)
15. Define the following: Worst probe, Veirs rod, Quickert probe, and Crawford intubation set. (The Worst pigtail probe is used as discussed above to intubate through an uninjured canaliculus to access the injured canaliculus; the Diers rod is a stainless steel rod passed through a canaliculus and subcutaneously through the skin; a Quickert probe is a stainless steel or silver rod that is used to intubate the system through the canaliculus, sac, the duct, and into the nose; the Crawford intubation set is a double-armed straight wire with a swedged on silicone tubing that permits intubation of *both* canaliculi and subsequently into the nose where the silicone tubing is tied and knotted intranasally.)
16. Although the readings appear to adopt a more aggressive approach, in general, what is the appropriate management of the nasolacrimal system in nasoethmoid orbital, NEO, and fractures? (Although the nasolacrimal system may be disrupted in a certain proportion of NEO fractures, most will improve without epiphora. The remainder, a minority, can be addressed with a DCR, dacryocystorhinostomy.)

Salivary Gland/Duct Injuries, External Ear

Editor's Note: The detailed anatomy of the parotid is also covered in Chap. 40.

1. A patient has sustained a vertical laceration of the preauricular cheek area. What structures might be injured? (Branches of the facial nerve, parotid gland, and/or duct.)
   (a) How do external landmarks assist you in your determination? (The readings divide the preauricular cheek area into three zones. A zone most posterior or directly preauricular which would more likely damage the parotid gland and not the duct; an area termed "B," which is the middle third and is most likely to injure the duct and/or the branches of the facial nerve; a "C" area which is anterior to the duct. That designation is enhanced by a topographic line drawn from the tragus of the ear to the mid portion of the philtrum upper lip. The middle third of this line, or "B," is directly over the masseter muscle and the parotid duct. The duct is superficial to the masseter muscle in this region and then hooks around the anterior edge of the masseter muscle to exit through the buccal fat pad and buccinator muscle in the oral cavity at the level of the maxillary second molar as Stensen's duct or papilla.)
2. In this same patient with a facial laceration, what is the management of an injury of the parotid gland? (Nothing particularly directed toward the gland but suturing of the laceration over a drain with the use of a postoperative compression head dressing and perhaps the administration of antisialogogues.)
3. From the topography of a cheek laceration, if you suspect a parotid duct injury, how can the diagnosis be established? (Identification and cannulation of the papilla of Stensen's duct at the level of the maxillary second molar with a small polyethylene or silicone catheter. Direct examination of the wound while the catheter is gently irrigated with 2–3 cc of saline. Methylene blue is not recommended because if a ductal injury does exist, staining of the tissues will occur.)
   (a) What nerve is most likely involved if the duct has been lacerated? (The buccal branch of the facial nerve.)
4. Is repair of a lacerated parotid duct indicated? If so, how? (Repair is indicated despite the controversy addressed in the readings. The duct is repaired with 6° Vicyrl or other absorbable sutures. This writer prefers not to use permanent sutures for repair. Once repaired, the wound is drained, compression dressing applied, and the catheter sutured intraorally. Maintenance of the catheter is recommended for 2–3 weeks.)
5. What are the two complications of parotid duct injury? How is it diagnosed? (Complications of an unrepaired parotid duct injury or, on occasion, a parotid gland

injury is either a salivary fistula or a sialocele, a collection of salivary fluid. The fluid from the fistula or aspirated from the sialocele will be extremely high in amylase content.)

   (a) Give methods of treatment for each with a comment on efficacy. (Both can be difficult to treat. Sialocele is best managed, in this author's opinion, by marsupialization. That procedure is accomplished by an intraoral incision with access to the sialocele and then a purse string suture around the edges to create an aperture, which is held open with a small mushroom catheter shortened and sutured intraorally for 2–3 weeks. A fistula is even more difficult to treat. One must ascertain the nature and severity of the distal duct stricture. One option is the excision of the fistula with an effort to direct the proximal stump intraorally, but that can be technically difficult and put branches of the facial nerve at risk. Historically, a number of therapeutic options have existed, including transtympanic neurectomy of Jacobsen's nerve, low dose radiation of 1500–1800 cGy, and superficial parotidectomy. All have had a low success rate except for parotidectomy, which can be technically quite difficult in the face of inflammation and scar and may place the branches of the facial nerve in jeopardy.)

6. Outline a non-surgical approach to the complications of sialocele and parotid fistula. (Some publications have described the use of an endoscopic approach, but the most commonly employed non-surgical method is the use of botulinum toxin injections. The method consists of injections within the parotid gland parenchyma, and a variety of dosages have been described. Clearly, given the duration of the pharmacological effect of botulinum toxin, repeated injections, in all likelihood, would be required. Some interest in the use of ultrasound-guided injections has also been described.)
7. Where is the submandibular duct most likely to be injured? (In the submandibular region, particularly in the presence of a laceration of the mylohyoid. The gland lies beneath the body of the mandible posteriorly, and the duct exits from the hilum and courses for a distance of about 4–5 cm in the submandibular region and subsequently deep to the mylohyoid to exit in the anterior floor of the mouth as Wharton's duct.)
   (a) What nerve can also be injured if the submandibular gland has been lacerated? (The lingual nerve runs directly superior to the gland.)
8. What is the appropriate management of a hematoma of the external ear? (Neither absence of treatment nor simple aspiration is not appropriate. The hematoma will be replaced by fibrous tissue that obliterated the normal contours of the underlying ear cartilage. A short incision over the hematoma within the curve of the antihelix, expression of the hematoma, and placement of bolsters with a compression head dressing to prevent reaccumulation.)

Facial Anesthetic Blocks

1. Describe the topographical location of the infraorbital foramen. (The foramen is approximately 5–7 mm below the palpable infraorbital rim on a vertical line from the medial limbus of the iris to the oral commissure.)
   (a) Blocking the infraorbital nerve will accomplish anesthesia in what areas? (Medial cheek, lateral nose, upper lip, and the teeth/gum from the central incisor through the premolars.)
2. Perform a block of the supraorbital nerve. (The foramen or notch for the nerve is on the same vertical line described in the prior questions. The lateral branch may not be accessed by a block directly on the rim, and additional infiltration superior for a 1 cm distance may be advisable.)
3. Describe a block of the mental nerve. (The mental nerve exits the mandible through the mental foramen at the level of the second premolar or bicuspid. The foramen is at the mid-height of the mandibular body, dependent on the patient's age and state of dentition. The nerve can be infiltrated intraorally through the buccal sulcus.)
4. Describe the location and block of the greater auricular nerve. (The nerve traverses the sternocleidomastoid from exit from the cervical plexus at the posterior border of the sternocleidomastoid about 6.5 cm below the external auditory canal termed Erb's point. The anterior and posterior border of the sternocleidomastoid should be ascertained, and then a vertical line 6.5 cm from the external auditory canal will cross the mid portion of the muscle. Infiltration of a 1–2 cm area at this juncture should be accomplished.)

Case-Based Conference

Case 1: Acute Eyelid Injury A

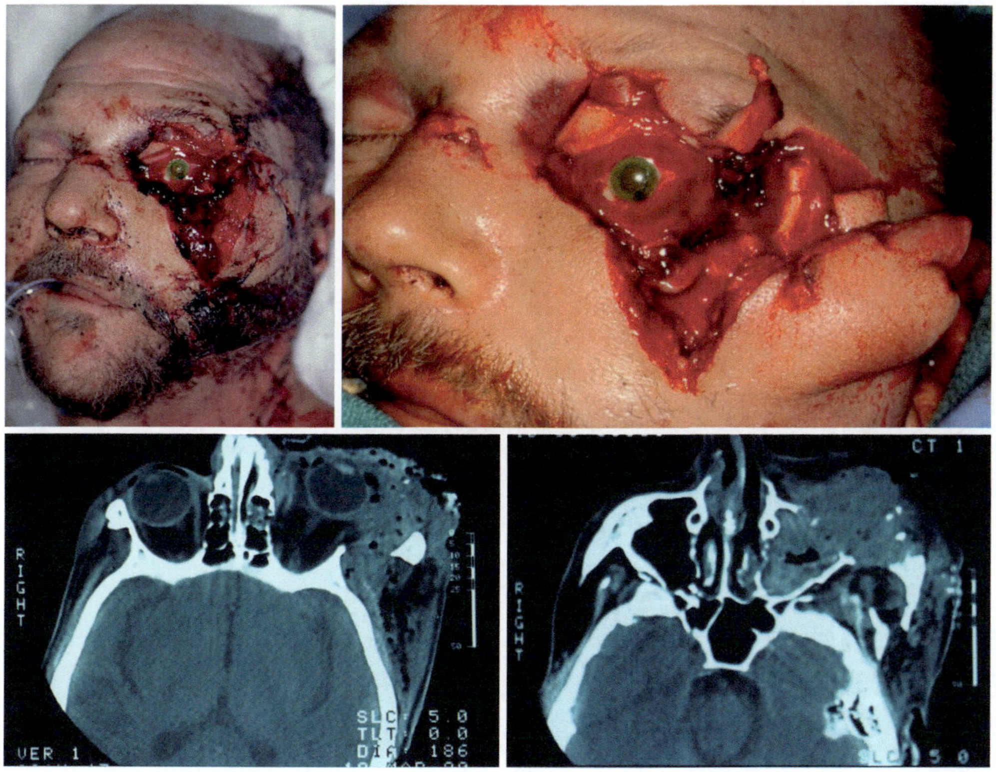

A 50-year-old MVA patient, cleared by the trauma team. Markedly diminished vision in the opposite eye from a prior injury.

1. Describe the slides. Add a focused clinical exam. Follow with the interpretation of the CT scan.
2. Summarize the treatment challenges posed by the patient.
3. Describe a treatment plan, including rationale and timing.

Case-Based Conference

Case 1: Acute Eyelid Injury B

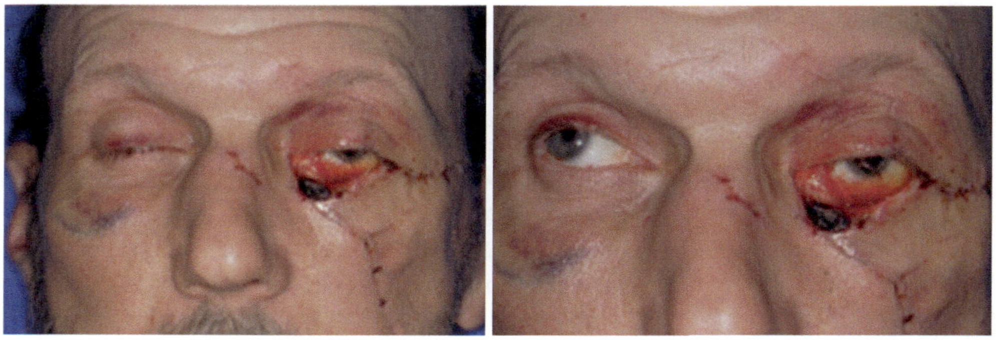

The patient, who smokes, at 2.5 weeks post-injury.

1. Describe the slides. Add the pertinent clinical exam.
2. Outline the pathologic anatomy.
3. Develop a treatment plan that addresses question 2.

Case-Based Conference: Discussion

Case 1: Acute Eyelid Injury A

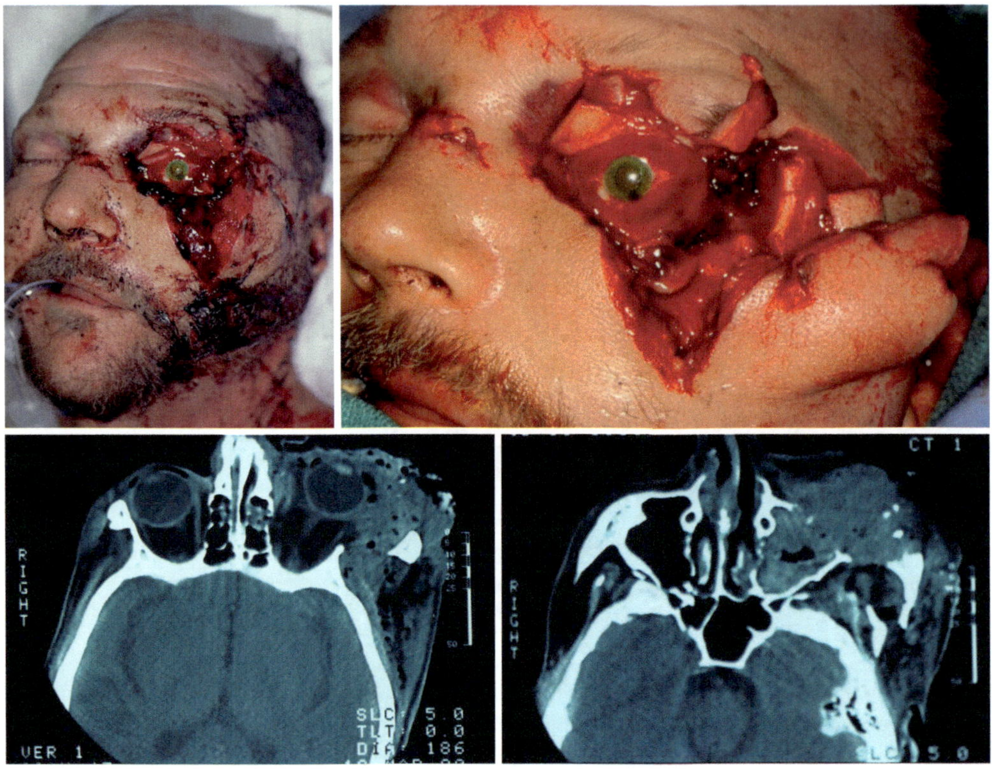

A 50-year-old MVA patient, cleared by the trauma team. Markedly diminished vision in the opposite eye from a prior injury.

1. Describe the slides. Add a focused clinical exam. Follow with the interpretation of the CT scan. (Three clinical slides are provided, and all are an oblique view. The first includes the full face of an intubated patient with extensive soft tissue injury of the left orbit and cheek. The globe is devoid of any visible soft tissue, with only the iris and a dilated pupil visible. No eyelid, upper or lower, is seen except for a medial segment of the upper lid or perhaps 1–1½ cm in size. The lateral and central cheek soft tissue has been avulsed and is pedicled laterally and inferiorly. The resultant defect created is filled with clotted blood. No other facial injuries are evident. The remaining two views are similar and include the orbit, cheek, and adjacent nose and upper lip. Some avulsed eyelid tissue with lashes can be detected laterally, probably the upper lid. The bulbar conjunctiva is still obscured by blood. Clotted blood is present lateral to the globe. The globe appears intact. A large fragment of bone, consistent in appearance with the lateral orbital rim, is present in the lateral portion of the wound. In an additional view, the skin and soft tissue flap is retracted laterally and adds no further information.

   The focused clinical exam would be limited since the patient is intubated and presumably under a general anesthetic in the operating room. If the patient was awake and able to cooperate, a short medical history would be of value to elicit the presence of any comorbidities. A physical exam would focus on the left eye and begin with a vision of confrontation or a Snellen card. Extraocular motions in all vectors need assessment, as well as pupillary reaction, both direct and consensually, particularly in the presence of a dilated pupil. Any exploration or manipulation of the wound would not be possible without general anesthesia. Early ophthalmologic involvement is essential to establish globe integrity, including measurement of intraocular pressure as well as a fundus examination.

   Two CT scans are provided. On the first, the cut appears to be at or just inferior to the inferior orbital rim. The cut depicts a fluid-filled maxillary sinus lacking an anterior wall, extending to and distending the area of the adjacent cheek. A large bone fragment is visible laterally, not consistent with the zygomatic arch. Small bone fragments are seen in the soft tissue, just inferior to the large bone fragment. On the remaining CT cut, the plane is superior through the midportion of the globe at the level of the lens. The globe appears intact, although prolapsed somewhat anteriorly. Multiple small pockets of air are visible in the soft tissue. No discernible lateral orbital wall or rim is visible. The medial orbital wall is intact.)

2. Summarize the treatment challenges posed by the patient. (The patient presents with a high-velocity/energy impact of the left orbit and cheek with an associated extensive soft tissue and bony injury. The soft tissue component includes avulsion and apparent loss of a substantial portion of both upper and lower eyelids and, possibly, loss of infraorbital skin/soft tissue. A fracture-avulsion of the zygoma has resulted in quite a substantial lateral displacement, including the lateral orbital wall, rim, and body, with probably associated bone loss. The globe appears intact, and presumably, vision is as well.).
3. Describe a treatment plan, including rationale and timing. (After evaluation, the next and urgent step is operation. In the OR, a complete assessment of the wound, an inventory of repair and reconstructive needs, and a wound toilet, including a conservative debridement, is accomplished. To begin, the obvious small bone fragments without periosteal attachments are debrided. The remaining zygomatic segments can be reduced through extensive lacerations and internal fixation performed with plates and screws. If a bone defect remains, particularly the orbital floor and/or lateral wall, that deficit dictates primary reconstruction with autogenous bone, split-rib grafts contoured to an orbital configuration. The soft tissue repair of the cheek flap is followed by the opposition of the skin and soft tissue, then a careful reconstitution of the eyelid fragments. If the eyelid loss and deficiency are sufficiently severe to raise a concern about corneal protection, consideration should be given to temporary tarsorrhaphy.)

Intraoperative

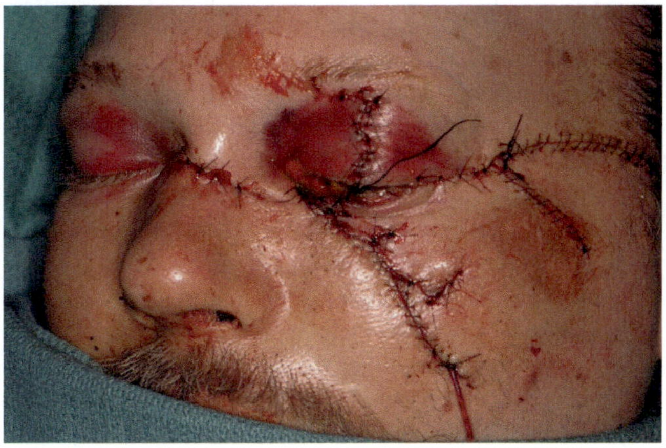

The wounds and tissue loss of the lower lid have been closed by the advancement of lateral cheek tissue, ala Mustarde flap, and a temporary tarsorrhaphy. The underlying zygomatic fracture has been reduced and plated. The upper lid is in a ptotic posture.

Case-Based Conference: Discussion

Case 1: Acute Eyelid Injury B

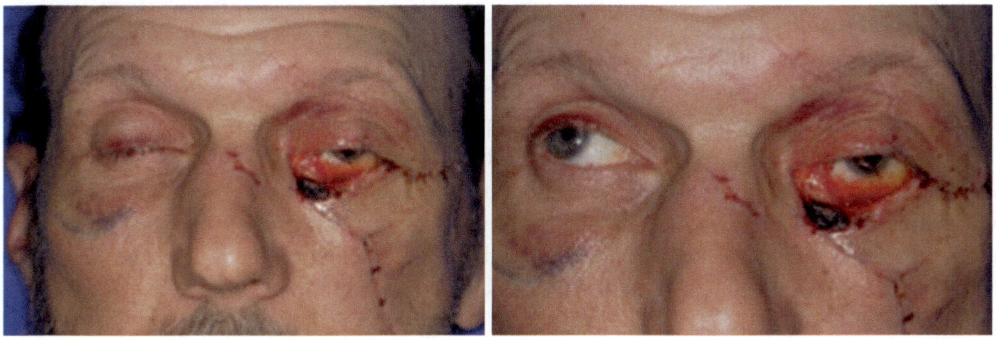

The patient, who smokes, at 2.5 weeks post-injury.

1. Describe the slides. Add the pertinent clinical exam. (Two photos are provided that include both orbits and the nose, one with the right eye open and the other with the eye closed. Within the view with the eye open, the right eye is either deviated or the patient is looking up and outward. The pupil is mid-position. Remarkable findings on the left are several: a missing entire medial one-third to one-half of the lower lid, replaced by an eschar of 1 × 1 cm in size with marked bulbar conjunctivitis and edema. The lateral one-half of the lower lid is present but lacks eyelashes, is oriented obliquely inferiorly, and is attached medially to the eschar. The edema of the medial conjunctiva is substantial and occupies and obliterates the entire medial canthus. No caruncle is visible. The upper lid and

lateral canthus appear intact, although the margin rests at mid-pupil. The pupil, in contrast to the right side, is dilated. The nasal dorsum is deviated to the right. Some residual ecchymosis exists in the right infraorbital region. The second photo, obtained with the right eyelid in closure, demonstrates little change of upper lid positioning in the left eye as well as the absence of any evidence of a Bell's phenomenon.)

2. Outline the pathologic anatomy. (The principal pathology is full-thickness loss of the medial one-half of the lower lid with contracture and inferior and lateral displacement of the remaining lower lid. Combined with an apparent immobile upper lid and absence of a Bell's phenomenon, corneal ulceration is a substantial risk, as manifested by the marked conjunctivitis. The status of the inferior canaliculus is unknown, and the punctum is absent. The patient certainly has epiphora secondary to the corneal exposure alone. The dilated pupil that was present at the time of injury is still evident, indicating traumatic mydriasis or an injury to either the afferent, efferent, or both components of the neural loop for pupillary reaction. Lid ptosis introduces concerns for either a levator injury or damage to the oculomotor nerve, although one would anticipate, in the absence of a direct globe injury, to detect myosis, not mydriasis. The deficiency includes full-thickness eyelid, but a deficit of the adjacent infraorbital skin exists as well.)
3. Develop a treatment plan that addresses question 2. (Some considerable degree of urgency exists because of the significant inflammation and edema of the conjunctiva, indicative of present or pending corneal ulceration. A variety of temporizing measures are available, including the placement of a chamber that maintains a constantly moist environment or simply the use of antibiotic ophthalmic ointment and eye patches. Definitive operative address will require excision of the eschar and an incision of the oblique laceration scar that courses inferiorly from the medial edge of the eschar. A progressive release of the contraction will be necessary until the lower lid remnant is restored to a transverse plane at the inferior limbus of the iris. To do so will define not only the lower lid defect but also the magnitude of the deficiency of the adjacent infraorbital skin. The lid component of the defect will consist of both posterior and anterior lamellae. Reconstruction of the posterior lamella could be accomplished with a mucoperiosteal graft harvested from the hard palate. Anterior lamella reconstruction will require a pedicle flap with three options available: two from the upper lid, a Hughes skin only, and a Trippier medially-based skin and perhaps orbicularis muscle. Both would be possible but probably not advisable in the presence of a damaged upper lid, particularly with a mid-lid laceration scar. Another option, more feasible, is a superiorly-based nasolabial flap rotated laterally to address both lid and cheek deficit. Since the patient has already sustained tissue loss in this region, in all likelihood, little lax skin exists to close the flap donor site, and a full-thickness skin graft will be necessary if this option is selected. A fourth option is a paramedian forehead flap, also to address both elements of the deficit. The flap will traverse uninvolved skin to reach the lid and cheek and will initially be bulkier than ultimately desired. Given the severity of the injury, the status of the left supratrochlear vessels should be determined with a Doppler examination.)

Intraoperative

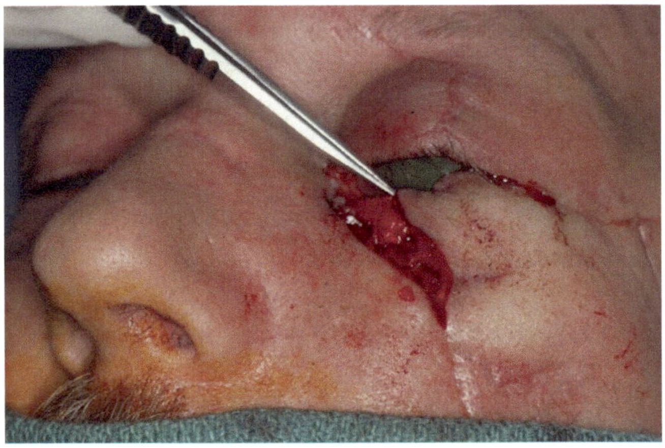

A single intraoperative photo illustrates the defect created by the release of the scar and reveals the deficit is not limited to the eyelid but also includes infraorbital skin and soft tissue. The other finding is one of blanching of the leading portion of the lateral flap, not local anesthetic-induced since the medial tissue is of normal skin tone.

Postoperative (5 Months)

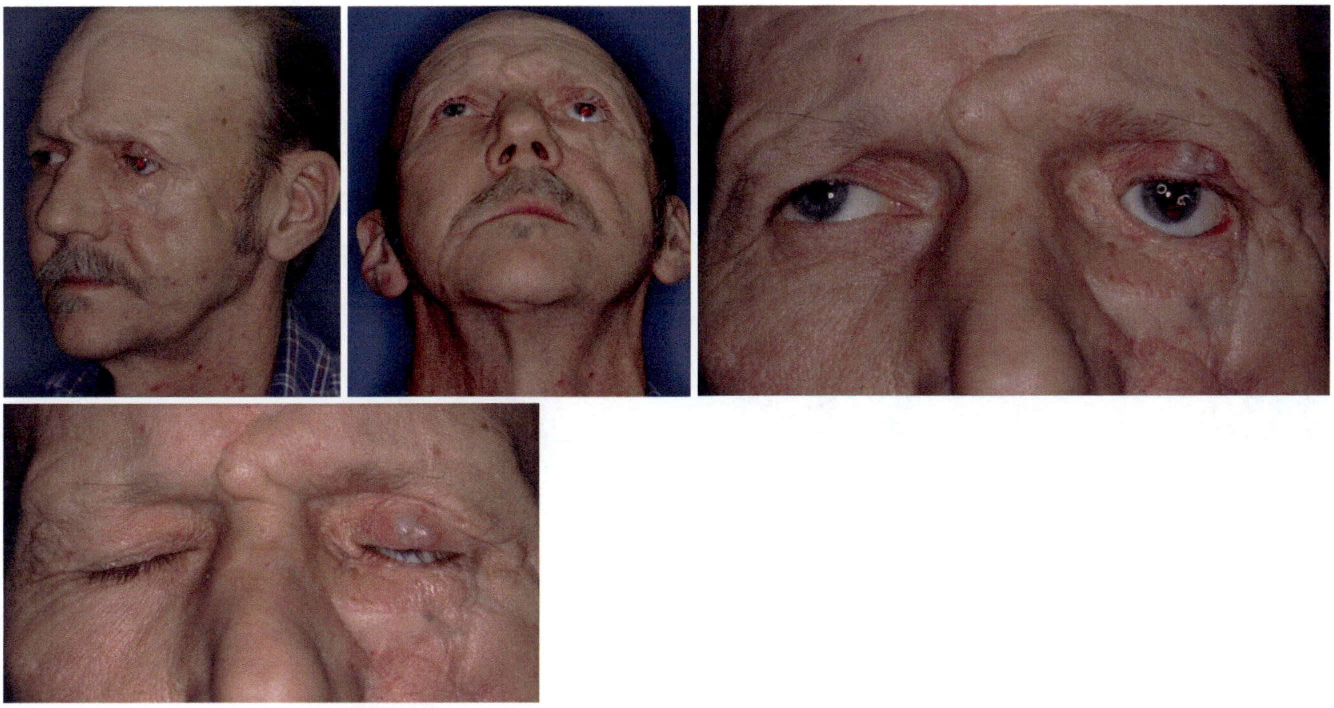

The four views provide different perspectives of the result. The most revelatory are the two close-ups of the midface. Considerable scleral show is evident with a threshold ectropion laterally. The closure of the lid is incomplete, but the cornea is covered. The stigmata of exposure conjunctivitis of scleral injection are absent. The aesthetic result is suboptimal.

Critique

Although, functionally, the outcome appears satisfactory, if the patient so desires, the appearance could be improved. In retrospect, a more extensive release would have permitted the advancement of the lid superiorly and the forehead flap, utilized to fill the additional deficit. The blanched skin demonstrates the inherent ischemia of the lateral flap, a consequence of injury and years of tobacco abuse.

Case-Based Conference

Case 2: Ectropion

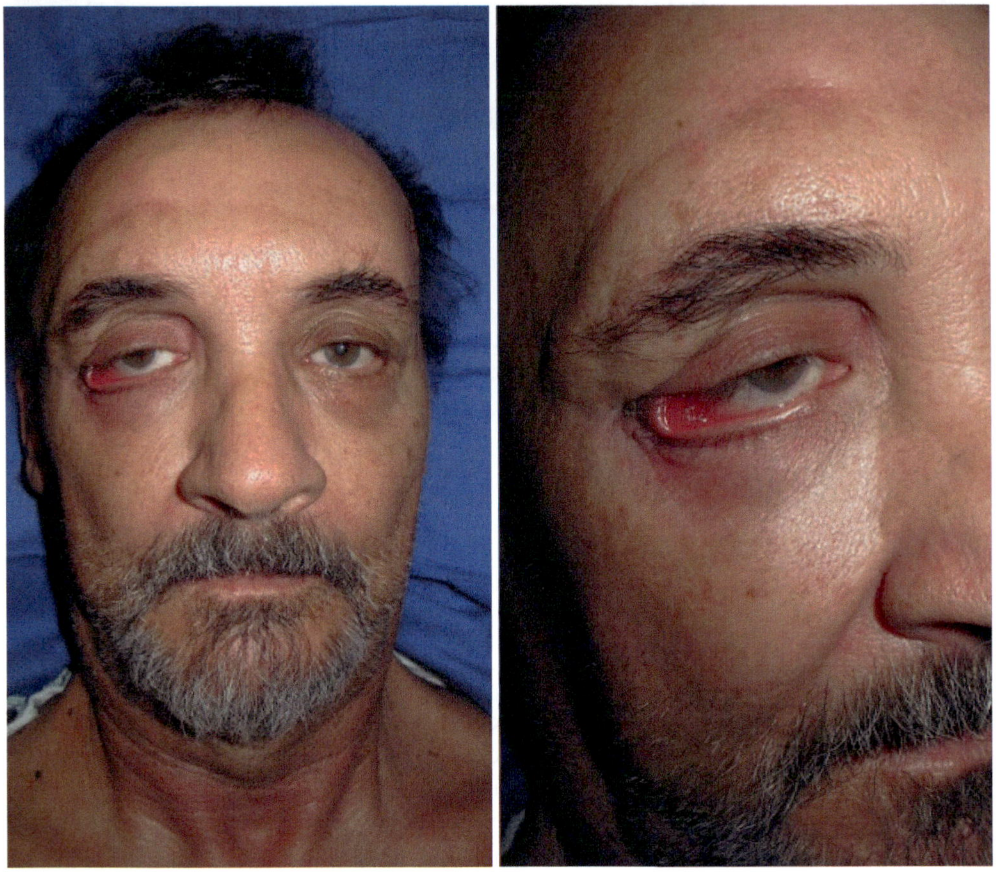

A 48-year-old 3 months status post eyelid injury.

1. Describe the slide(s). Add a focused history and physical examination.
   (a) Any tests indicated? Justify.
2. Outline the presenting pathologic anatomy and the probable explanation.
3. How would you persuade a reluctant patient to accept treatment or the sequelae of failure to do so?
4. List the treatment options, select your choice, and describe in detail, including post-operative care, if operation.

Case-Based Conference: Discussion

Case 2: Ectropion

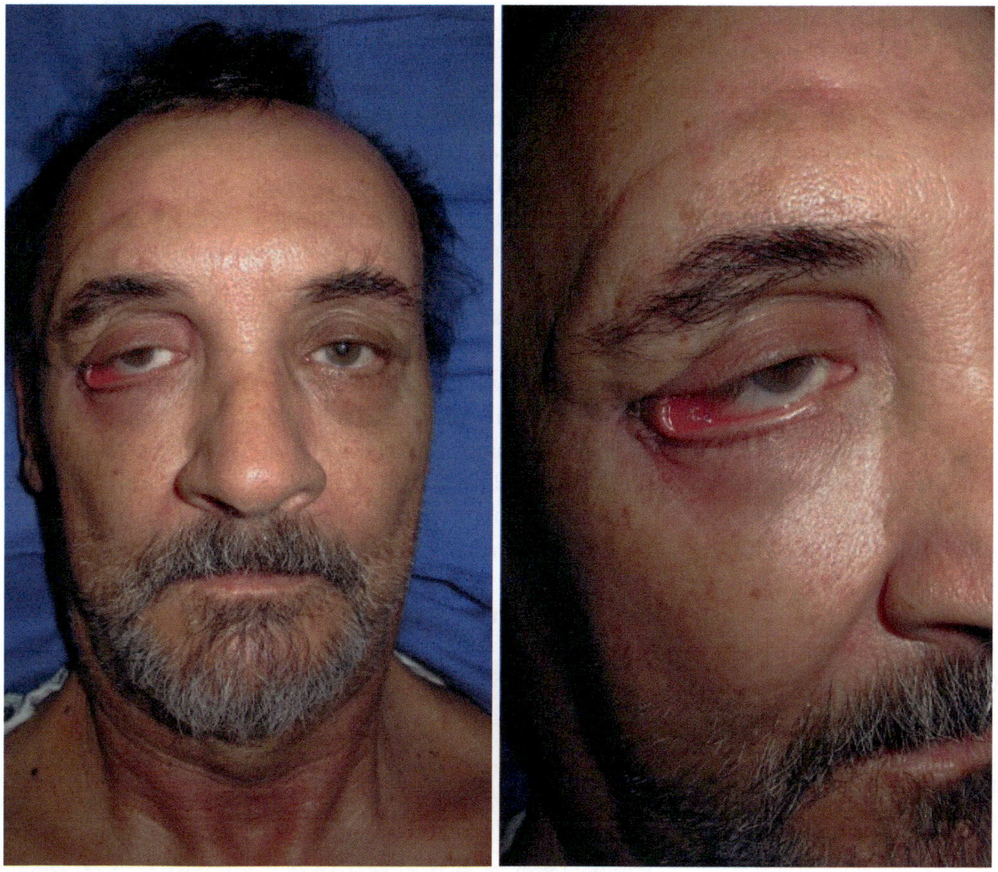

A 48-year-old 3 months status post eyelid injury.

1. Describe the slide(s). Add a focused history and physical examination. (Two slides are provided: one, a full-face frontal view, and second, a closeup of the right face only. Visible on the first slide is a male who appears his stated age with a significant ectropion of the right lateral lower eyelid. The ectropion has obliterated the visible eyelid skin, and the lash margin appears to abut on lateral cheek skin. A wide swath of lateral tarsal conjunctiva is visible. The upper eyelid has pathologic changes as well. The lid is pulled laterally and inferiorly with the lash margin at mid-pupil. In addition, the palpebral crease is displaced several millimeters superiorly with some superior orbital hollowing. The sclera demonstrates no evidence of bulbar conjunctivitis, and the tarsal conjunctiva does not appear inflamed. The brow is in a normal position. Assessment of the opposite or uninvolved eye and orbit reveals mild to moderate ptosis of approximately 2 mm with a lash margin at the superior edge of the pupil. Although the palpebral fold may be mildly elevated, the severity is not comparable to the opposite or left eye, and no hollowing is evident. The lower lid is in a normal position with no scleral show. No residual deformity of the right zygoma is evident.

   The history would have established the particulars of the injury, the details of the operation from the patient's understanding, the postoperative healing process if complicated, and the timing of the development of the ectropion. Ascertainment of the presence of any ocular symptoms such as photophobia, tearing, and morning crusting would be important to detect corneal irritation. Questions about adjunctive measures employed by the patient as a lubricant and nighttime taping would be helpful, as well as questions to the family about the posture of the globe in sleep. Other past medical history include general medical history, eye procedure, or operations. A physical exam would center on the tightness of the ectropion, eye closure, and the absence or the presence of the Bell phenomenon with attempted eye closure, as well as the severity, if any, of tarsal and bulbar conjunctivitis. Levator function is determined in both the left and right eye by blocking frontalis function and measuring the excursion of the upper lid lash margin from fully downward to full upward gaze. A similar assessment should be accomplished on the opposite eye. Visual assessment with a Snellen card completes the eye exam. Maxillofacial trauma evaluation for completeness purposes would include occlusion, oral opening, and infraorbital sensory nerve exam.)

(a) Any tests indicated? Justify. (The corneal should be tested with fluorescein eye drops and a Wood's light to detect epithelial loss and ulceration. A plain film would detect the presence of a fixation plate in the infraorbital rim in the area of the ectropion. Lacking other indications, CT imaging is probably not warranted.)

2. Outline the presenting pathologic anatomy and the probable explanation. (The pathologic anatomy is vertical shortening of the anterior lamella, the skin and orbicularis, and the middle lamella, the orbital septum. The posterior lamella is probably not involved. The pathologic process is scarring, secondary to the initial trauma and the retraction necessary through the subciliary incision for the ORIF of the zygoma. Constant retraction produces ischemia of the lower lid tissues, perhaps most significantly on the orbicularis, with secondary contraction of the skin. The tarsus prolapses anteriorly, and the conjunctiva is exposed with contraction of the septum secondarily as well. An infraorbital plate may contribute if the soft-tissue scars and adheres to the plate, perhaps the result of a subclinical infection. Subciliary incisions are at a higher risk for the occurrence of ectropion.

   The puzzling element is the presence of mild ptosis and the high palpebral fold. The mild ptosis on the left or uninvolved eye would indicate perhaps some involutional component, but the anatomic changes on the right are substantially more severe and introduce a concern for the presence of concomitant enophthalmos. The absence of any signs or findings of conjunctivitis or corneal ulcer defines the timing of an elective repair. The presence of positive fluorescein staining dictates a more urgent approach to operative address and correction of the ectropion.)
3. How would you persuade a reluctant patient to accept treatment or the sequelae of failure to do so? (Essentially, the objective indications, besides aesthetics, are the progression of signs and symptoms and the risk of corneal involvement, ulceration, and perforation.)
4. List the treatment options, select your choice, and describe in detail, including post-operative care, if operation. (The list of options is limited and centers on the release of a contracture. The release would require an incision through the scar of the prior subciliary incision, including the entire extent. The depth of release includes the underlying scarred orbicularis and, most importantly, a complete incision and release of the septum, signaled by the prolapse of intraorbital fat into the wound. A suture placed through the lash margin at the midpupillary line and retracted superiorly will help define the thoroughness of the release. Once released, the next decision is the removal of the infraorbital plate if present. Certainly, since 3 months have transpired, the plate could be removed safely. The subsequent decision is the necessity of a lateral canthal procedure. Any element of lid laxity would dictate a lateral canthalpexy, accomplished with a tarsal tuck or tarsal strip procedure. The skin deficit is addressed with a full-thickness skin graft, harvested from the post-auricular area and secured with a large bolster. No frost suture will be necessary since the bulk of the bolster will provide upper traction on the lower lid. The bolster remains in place for 1 week with the removal of both bolster and sutures at that junction.)

Intraoperative

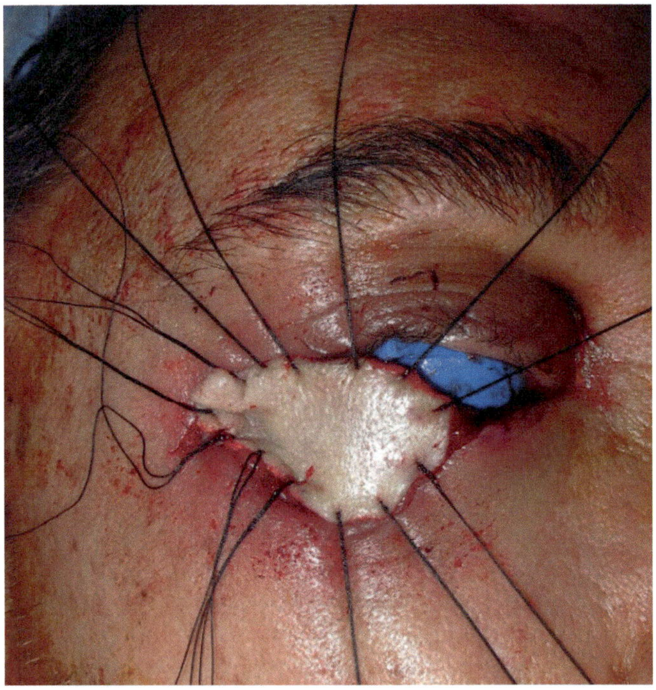

The complete release of only a moderately severe ectropion has created a skin deficit that requires a surprisingly large full-thickness skin graft of two centimeters harvested from a postauricular donor site. Even with aggressive thinning, postauricular skin remains thickened for a significant period postoperative.

Postoperative (2 Months)

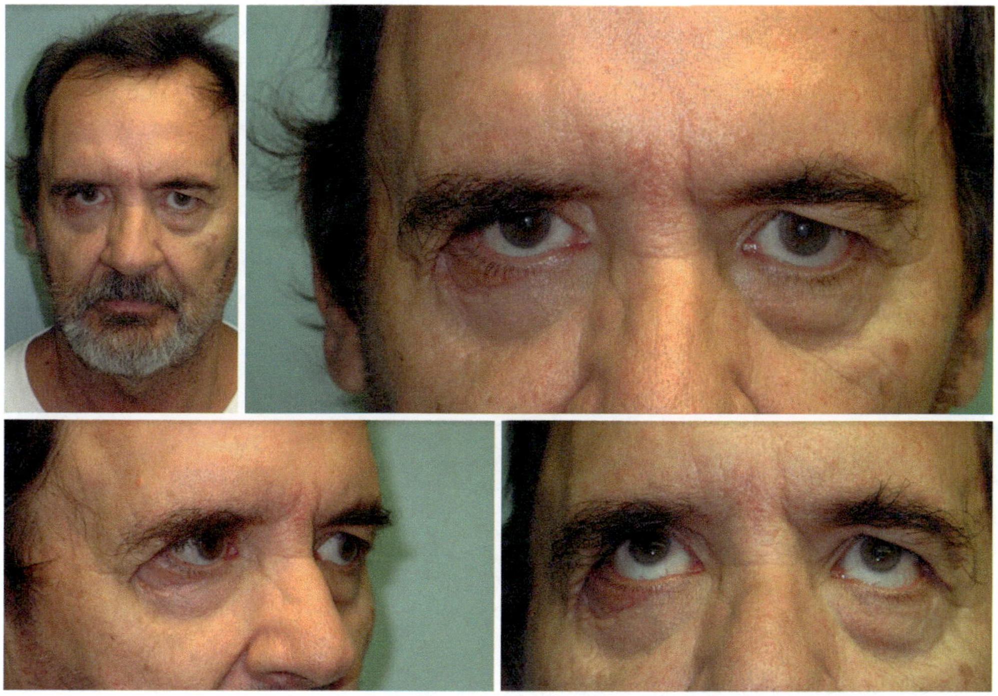

The ectropion has been corrected. In both central and upper gaze, 2 mm of scleral show is evident but also present on the left or uninvolved lid, reflective of bilateral tarsal laxity. Both upper lids have significant redundancy of skin and an element of brow ptosis, the left perhaps greater than the right.

Case-Based Conference

Case 3: Facial Laceration

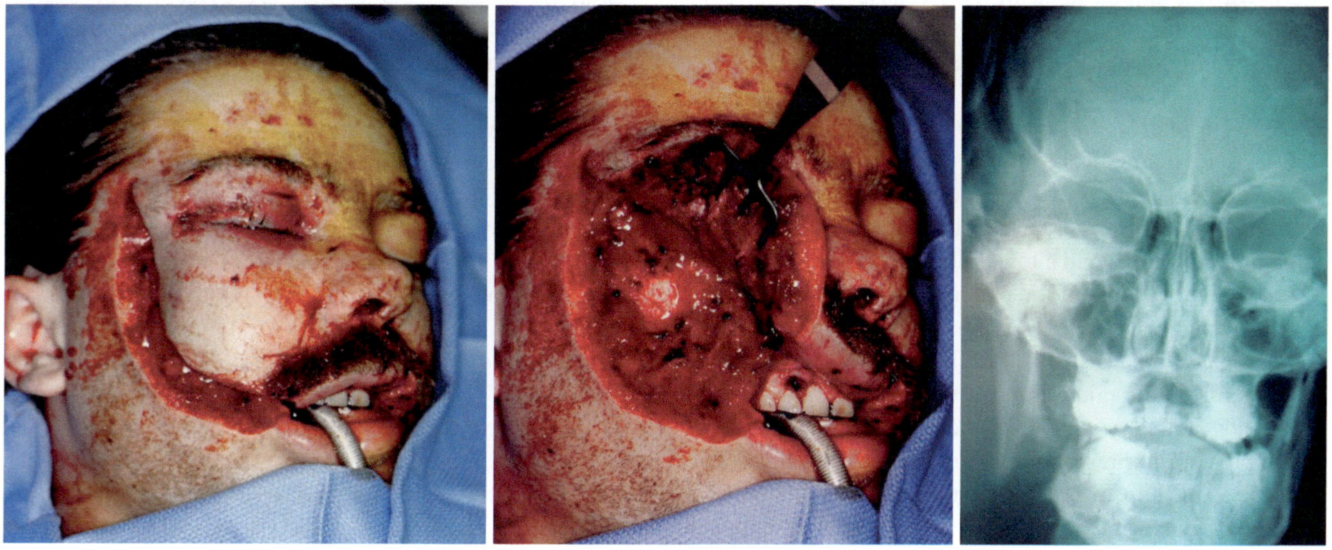

A 28-year-old injured in an MVA. Because of loss of consciousness, the patient was intubated at the accident scene but was readily responsive on arrival. No other injuries.

1. Describe the findings in the intraoperative slide(s). Describe your clinical examination prior to the OR.
   (a) Interpret the X-ray. The patient has a right zygoma fracture as well, but it will not be managed in this case. Pertinent to the mandible, what information should be obtained from the CT scan?
2. List and describe the possible pathology that will need to be addressed with the treatment plan.
3. Based on your response to question #2, outline a treatment plan, including sequence intraoperatively.

Case-Based Conference: Discussion

Case 3: Facial Laceration

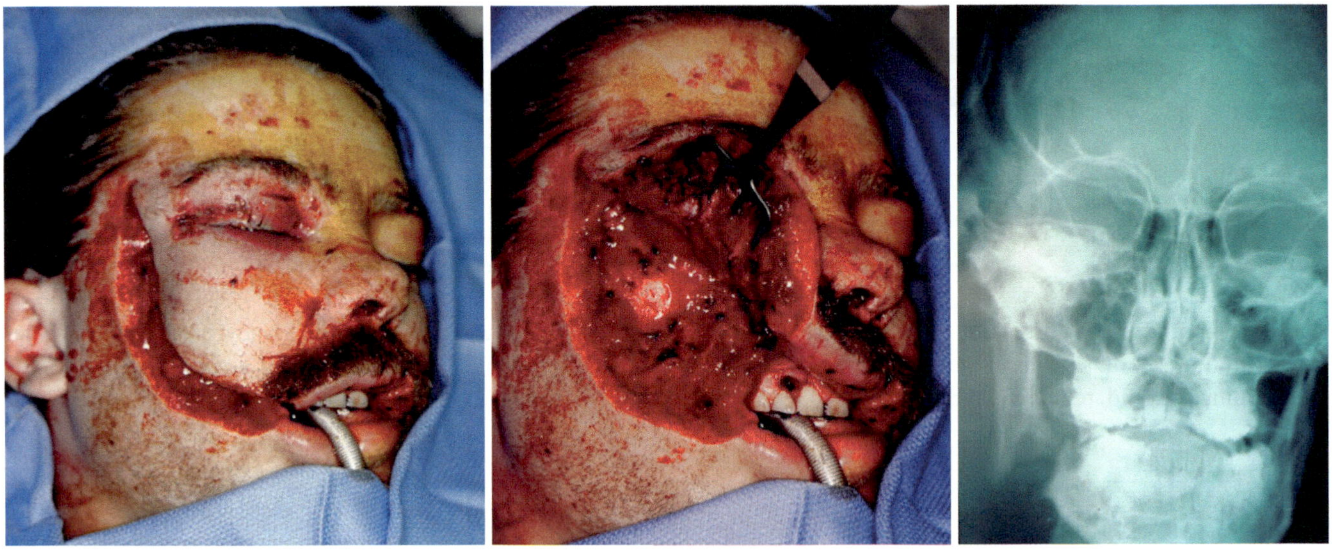

A 28-year-old injured in an MVA. Because of loss of consciousness, the patient was intubated at the accident scene but was readily responsive on arrival. No other injuries.

1. Describe the findings in the intraoperative slide(s). Describe your clinical examination prior to the OR. (Two clinical slides are provided—both described as intraoperative. The first is a full facial with the head turned slightly to the left and a towel-draped armored oral endotracheal tube evident. The patient, a male who appears to be stated age, has both eyes closed. The most remarkable finding is a large L-shaped laceration of the right face that begins from the mid-temple at the level of the brow and extends vertically in the mid-cheek several cm anterior to the preauricular region to a point on the same transverse plane as the upper lip. The extension horizontally courses through the right commissure. The resultant flap has retracted 1–2 cm, which strongly suggests the laceration is considerably deeper than the skin only. No other lacerations or gross deformities are evident. The second photo is the same perspective, a full facial with the head turned slightly to the left, but a four-pronged rake has retracted the cheek soft-tissue flap, exposing the underlying bed. The flap appears quite thick, thicker than skin alone. The combination of blood and lack of photo resolution does not permit discernment of individual structures within the wound bed, but exposed bone is not visualized. The lateral upper lip or commissure labial mucosa appears lacerated as well, although the posterior extent is not apparent. The underlying right maxillary alveolus and anterior dentition are exposed and appear intact.

   Since the preamble states that the patient was alert and oriented, a clinical examination, including a history, can be accomplished. Other than brief questions about the circumstances and loss of consciousness, the history would establish, if present, significant comorbidities, doubtful in this instance, medications and drug, tobacco, and alcohol use. Assuming no other injuries, the physical exam would focus on the face and, in particular, facial nerve function and the right eye. Vision to confrontation, pupillary reaction, and extraocular muscle function are all tested. The status of the frontal and zygomatic branches of the facial nerve is determined by the elevation of the brow and closure of the right eye by the patient. Exploration of the wound should not be attempted at this time.)

(a) Interpret the X-ray. The patient has a right zygoma fracture as well, but it will not be managed in this case. Pertinent to the mandible, what information should be obtained from the CT scan? (A single X-ray is provided, an A-P view that depicts a displaced right angle mandibular fracture. A fracture gap or displacement of at least a couple of cm is present. Grossly, the remaining mandible appears intact, and no other facial bone fractures are seen, although the area of the right zygoma is obscured by the artifact. The CT scan should detect associated mandibular fractures on the left and the status of both condyles. Although the management of the concomitant right zygoma fracture is not a component of the discussion of this case, the aspects of the CT scan pertinent to the zygoma fracture, e.g., the orbit, magnitude of displacement, etc., should also be determined.)

2. List and describe the possible pathology that will need to be addressed with the treatment plan. (Besides repair of the extensive facial laceration, consideration should be given to the necessity of repair of the parotid and facial nerve structures. The mid-portion of the laceration is anatomically in the vicinity of the parotid duct. The path of the duct lateral to the underlying masseter muscle can be outlined topographically on the normal face by a line drawn from the tragus of the ear to the philtrum of the upper lip. The transverse course of the parotid duct occupies the central one-third of said line. As such, the injury is probably anterior to the parotid gland proper. The other soft-tissue structure under consideration, the facial nerve in the area of the injury, has divided into five individual branches, of which three, frontal, zygomatic, and buccal, are at risk for transection in this injury. The mandibular fracture will require reduction and fixation, and consideration should be directed toward the method of exposure.)
3. Based on your response to question #2, outline a treatment plan, including sequence intraoperatively. (Unless the endotracheal tube can be moved into the left retromolar space, the airway will need to be exchanged to a left intranasal to facilitate placement of intermaxillary fixation. Once the airway is secured, the patient is placed into pre-injury occlusion with intermaxillary fixation.

The first step in the sequence of procedures after wound toilet and meticulous hemostasis, a careful and precise inspection of the wound bed and intraoral laceration is accomplished. If the normal course of the frontal branch into the right temple corresponds to a line drawn from the tragus to a point 1.5 cm lateral to the lateral extent of the brow, the most superior extent of the wound is at or just inferior to that point or line. If the preoperative examination determined injury, the proximal nerve should be identified and the distal nerve identified with a nerve stimulator, both tagged with a small suture. Repair should be deferred until the mandible is addressed. The zygomatic and buccal branches were certainly at risk for injury, and if the preoperative examination indicated a loss of continuity, some effort could be expended to locate them. Yet, evidence exists that spontaneous recovery of facial nerve injuries anterior to a vertical line at the lateral brow is likely, a fruitless search should not unduly prolong operating room time. The status of the parotid duct can be ascertained with an intraoral cannulation of Stensen's duct, the orifice located adjacent to the second maxillary molar. Cannulation is accomplished with a small intravenous catheter attached to a 3 cc syringe filled with saline. With direct inspection of the wound, the duct is gently irrigated, and extravasation is detected. The use of vital dyes, such as methylene blue, is not recommended since a positive test will stain the wound bed. If the duct has been injured, repair should be performed with small absorbable Vicryl®, interrupted sutures over a catheter that will be secured intraorally. The course of the buccal branch of the facial nerve is integral to and parallels the parotid duct, and if the duct is injured, the nerve can be identified and repaired as well.

Repair of the soft-tissue structures should be deferred once identified and tagged until the mandibular fracture is addressed because of the manipulation that will be required. Conceivably, the right angle fracture can be reduced in internal fixation placed to a combination of intraoral incisions and transcutaneous trocars. If not, and the likelihood of the necessity of an additional external approach is remote, a Risdon incision will provide exposure. The technical details of open reduction internal fixation of mandibular fractures are more fully discussed in Chap. 49.

Nerve repair is optimally performed under microscopic control. The final step is a precise repair of the facial laceration over a small drain and the application of a full head and neck dressing. The intermaxillary fixation should be maintained postoperatively.)

Postoperative (5 Months)

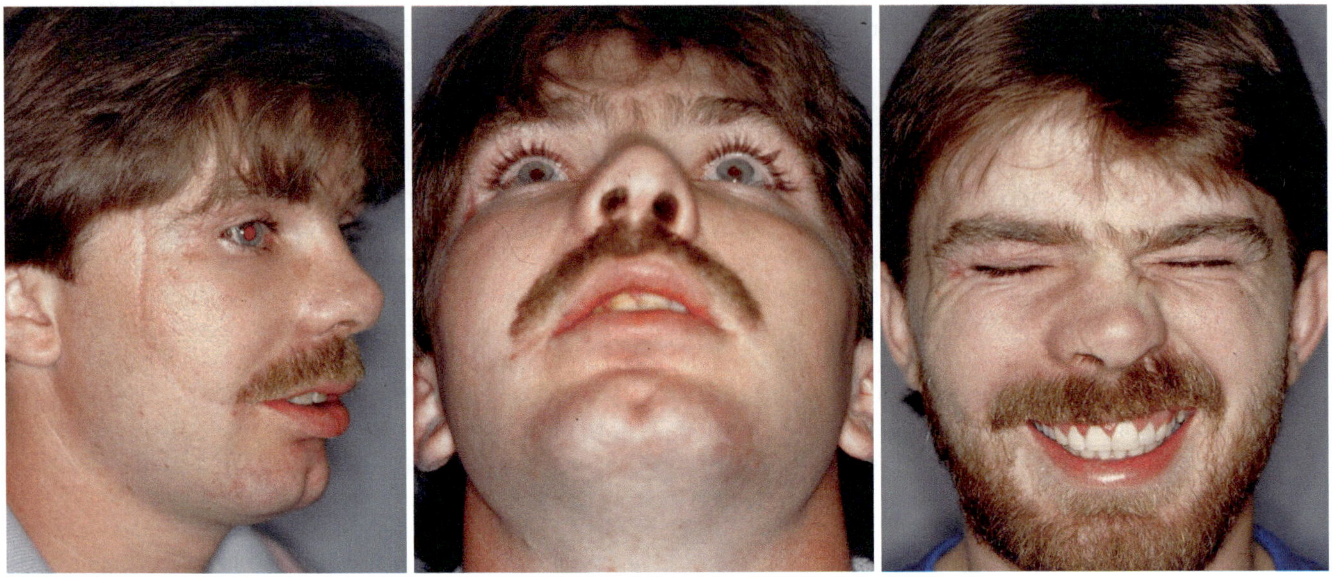

The three photos, lateral, submental vertex, and frontal, in full facial animation, demonstrate the status of the scar, restoration of malar prominence, occlusion, and facial nerve function.

In-Service Examination

1. The two valves in the lacrimal collecting system include:
   (a) Rosenmuller alone
   (b) Hosner alone
   (c) Rosenmüller and Hosner
   (d) Neither are the valves of the lacrimal collecting system
2. Transection of the parotid duct has a high probability of injury to which branch of the facial nerve?
   (a) Temporal
   (b) Zygomatic
   (c) Buccal
   (d) Marginal mandibular
   (e) None—no branches in close proximity
3. Erb's point for an anesthetic block of the greater auricular nerve is where?
   (a) On a vertical line 6.5 cm from the external auditory canal to the posterior border of the sternocleidomastoid
   (b) On a vertical line 8.5 cm from the external auditory canal to the posterior border of the sternocleidomastoid
   (c) On a vertical line 6.5 cm from the external auditory canal to the anterior border of the sternocleidomastoid
   (d) On a vertical line 8.5 cm from the external auditory canal to the anterior border of the sternocleidomastoid

Gunshot Wounds

44

Bibliography

Stefanopoulos PK, Filippakis K, Soupiou OT, et al. "Wound ballistics of firearm-related injuries—Part 1: Missile characteristics and mechanisms of soft tissue wounding" *Int J Oral Maxillofac Surg.*, (2014); 43:**1445–1449, 1453–54 (Shot-gun injuries) ONLY**.

Bluebond-Langner R, Baba R, Rodriguez E, "Gunshot Wounds to the Face", *Plastic Surgery Hyperguide*, (2009);**1–11**. http://www.plasticsurgery.hyperguides.com/tutorial.asp?tid=25006 **(OVERVIEW)**

Rodriguez ED, Bluebond-Langner R, Park JE, et al. "Preservation of Contour in Periorbital and Midfacial Craniofacial Microsurgery: Reconstruction of the Soft-Tissue Elements and Skeletal Buttresses", *Plast Reconstr Surg.*, (2008); 121:**1738–39, 1743–47**.

Borsuk DE, Christensen J, Dorafshar AH, et al. "Aesthetic Microvascular Periorbital Subunit Reconstruction: Beyond Primary Repair," *Plast Reconstr Surg.*, (2013); 131:**337, 340–47 Including Fig. 1**.

Rodriguez ED, Martin M, Bluebond-Langner R, et al. "Microsurgical Reconstruction of Posttraumatic High-Energy Maxillary Defects: Establishing the Effectiveness of Early Reconstruction," *Plast Reconstr Surg.*, (2007); 120:**103S–117S (Skip Results)**.

Schultz BD, Sosin M, Nam A, et al. "Classification of Mandible Defects and Algorithms for Microvascular Reconstruction," *Plast Reconstr Surg.*, (2015); 135:**743e–754e**.

Broyles JM, Abt NB, Shridharani SM, et al. "The Fusion of Craniofacial Reconstruction and Microsurgery: A Functional and Aesthetic Approach," *Plast Reconstr Surg.*, (2014); 134:**762–66 (to Lip Reconstruction) (Summary)**.

Supplemental

Clark MD, N., et al., "High-Energy Ballistic and Avulsive Facial Injuries," *Plast Reconstr Surg.*, (1996); 98(4):**583–601**.

Faculty Discussion and Study Guide

Wound Ballistics and Considerations

1. What is the physics or formula that expresses how a projectile inflicts damage in gunshot wounds, GSW? (Kinetic energy = $\frac{\text{Mass} \times \text{Velocity}}{2}$)
   (a) What is a high-velocity wound? (A wound produced by a projectile that has a muzzle velocity exiting from the weapon of at least 1000–1200 ft. per second.)
   (b) The readings describe handguns as having a limited capacity for avulsion or extensive injuries. If so, why does a 0.44 magnum handgun at close range produce substantial soft tissue and bony injury? (The muzzle velocity of any magnum handgun is considerably higher because of a much greater powder charge, and the mass of a 0.44 weapon is substantial as well. The heavier projectile and the velocity, although not high velocity, combine at close range to produce severe injury.)
   (c) Why does this formula not express the degree of tissue damage? (The formula quantifies kinetic energy. The magnitude of tissue damage is related to the efficiency of kinetic energy transfer to the tissues.)
   (d) Give some examples of other variables that may determine tissue damage besides $K = m \times v^2$. (With respect to the missile, the design of the bullet, shaped vs. round, the latter is more efficient in the transfer of energy but less efficient in velocity maintained in the passage from weapon muzzle to impact; whether the missile tumbles on passage through tissues which also transfers energy, and missile material whether soft or hard. Host factors include the type of tissue, for example, bone offers much higher resistance than fat and energy, so dissipation is much higher.)
2. What are the pertinent ballistics for shotgun wounds? (The tremendous wounding capabilities of shotguns are

E. Luce, *A Curriculum for Plastic Surgery*, https://doi.org/10.1007/978-3-031-62087-4_44

due to a combination of large mass, the shell and pellets, and a high muzzle velocity. Yet, the range is extremely limited because of the inefficient aerodynamics of the round pellet design that produces higher wind resistance and a rapid diminution in velocity as well as a nonrifled barrel. Other variables are the gauge of the weapon, the shot size, and the choke, if any.)

3. Describe the characteristics of the temporary and permanent cavities and the importance of each. (The permanent cavity is the actual track produced by the bullet, and the temporary cavity is the expansion of the tissues by the passage of the missile and represents the zone of injury. The cavity is considered temporary because after tissue expansion radially from the missile track, nearly instantaneous collapse occurs.)
4. How do the velocities of an individual GSW influence the management of that particular wound? (High velocity, high energy wounds require a serial approach to achieve definitive debridement of necrotic tissue. Both soft tissue and bone may be injured sufficiently that viability is lost, yet that status cannot be determined at perhaps the first or even the second debridement. Low velocity and low energy wounds, in contrast, can be debrided with definitive closure and bony reconstruction accomplished in the early postinjury phase.)
   (a) As the missile penetrates the tissues, what other characteristics besides mass and velocity may dictate the magnitude of the injury? (Chiefly, tumble, deformation, and fragmentation.)
5. What are the principal reasons for ultimate treatment failure and poor outcomes in high-velocity GSW of the face? ((a) Ongoing infection from inadequate debridement; (b) Delay in definitive reconstruction with progressive contracture of the soft-tissue envelope; (c) Inadequate restoration of skeletal support; (d) Persistent contamination from oral secretions because of inadequate restoration of lining leading to contracture and additional bone loss, including any bony reconstruction that might have been accomplished.)
6. Describe in general terms a management plan for high-energy GSW. (The first critical element is a careful physical examination and assessment of the type and magnitude of the injury that begins with the upper-one third, midface, and mandible and includes the three components of lining, skeleton, and soft tissue coverage. As outlined above, initial debridement with stabilization of facial and mandibular bone fragments and debridement and closure of soft tissue lacerations when possible. The patient is returned to the operating room every couple of days for wound exploration and additional debridement as needed. The goal is early definitive wound closure and skeletal stabilization before extensive fibrosis, scarring, and contracture of the soft tissue envelope can occur.)
   (a) What is a criterion based on the size of bone loss for free tissue transfer? (Bony-skeletal loss >5 cm and/or in the instance of associated insufficient soft-tissue coverage. Local flaps and non-vascularized bone grafts may be adequate in smaller defects.)
   (b) Critique the argument against the use of non-vascularized bone grafts in the reconstruction of complex gunshot wounds of the face. (The principal difficulties are the unpredictability of re-vascularization, particularly in the presence of extensive soft tissue injury, the unpredictability of the post-operative resorption, and the lack of suitability for osseointegrated implants, such as ocular, nasal, or dental.)
   (c) In facial injury with complex soft tissue and bony involvement, what is the argument against reconstruction with a soft tissue flap only? (Although initially successful, without underlying skeletal support, collapse, contracture, and deformity are inevitable.)
   (d) What wound objectives should a flap transfer accomplish? (Fill the dead space, close oral fistulas, reestablish the skeletal structure and maxillary buttresses, and reconstitute the soft tissue envelope.)
7. Other criteria for free tissue transfer? (The degree of mucosal lining and skin loss usually mandates against the use of local tissue for wound closure, so the implication is that of the necessity for free tissue transfer.)

Reconstruction of Facial Subunits

1. After division into low and high-velocity GSW, how can the location and magnitude of the wounds be further classified? (As the readings outlined, the four anatomical patterns were forehead and cranium ± orbit, orbit ± maxilla, central or midface, and mandible. The other aspect is how many of the three elements listed above are involved: skin soft tissue only, soft tissue + bone, or all three skin, bone, and lining.)
   (a) List the vertical and horizontal bony buttresses of the face. (Supraorbital rims or frontal bar as a superior third, inferior orbital rim, and malar eminences as the middle third, maxillary-alveolar arch as the inferior third. The mandible is considered separately and consists of the vertical pillars of the ascending ramus as one of the principles dictates the vertical height of the face and the body of the mandible as the most inferior horizontal buttress. See Fig. 44.1.)
2. Summarize the pros and cons of the two major options for the reconstruction of complex post-traumatic facial defects. (The deep circumflex iliac artery, DCIA, flap offers excellent bone stock of all of the osseous free

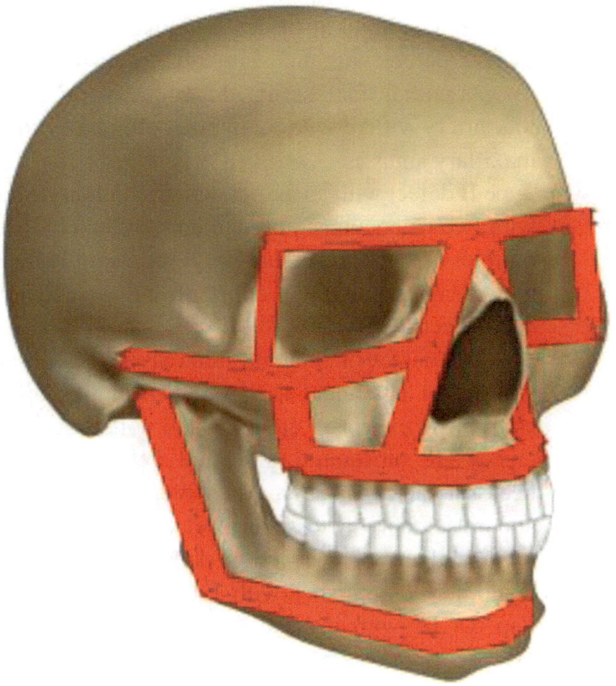

Fig. 44.1 Horizontal buttress of face

flaps, can be harvested in the supine position, a soft-tissue component is available with the inclusion of the portion of the inferior oblique, and a skin island can be incorporated. The disadvantages include the relatively short pedicle, frequently a tedious dissection, the lack of multiple perforators to permit osteotomies, and, in an obese patient, a thick skin island. The donor site may have significant morbidity. The fibula osteo- or osteocutaneous flap has a long pedicle, a segmental perforator vascular supply that permits multiple osteotomies, harvests possible in the supine position, and a skin island that can be positioned relatively independent of the bone segment.)

(a) Critique the use of the remaining two osseous free tissue options, the radial forearm and the scapular flap, in these scenarios. (The radial forearm free flap is an osteocutaneous reconstructive option of mostly historical interest secondary to the limited bone stock and donor site morbidity, including possible fracture of the residual radius. The scapular flap does offer two separate bone harvest sites with maximal flexibility of those two bone islands in positioning and space, as well as abundant skin-soft tissue. The drawbacks are the limited bone stock in comparison to the fibula and iliac flaps that may not be sufficient for dental implants, as well as the necessity for position change and a relatively short pedicle.)

Editor's Note: Although the readings are advocates of the use of the DCIA flap, in some instances, a double-barreled fibula may afford the same reconstructive efficacy without the disadvantages of the difficult donor site and harvest of a DCIA flap. Both are capable of placement of osseointegrated implants, even in a previously irradiated bed. The most recent enthusiasm is "jaw in a day," combining all the reconstruction, including the placement of implants in a single operative procedure.

3. What are the essential two pathways for reconstruction of the frontal cranium and supraorbital rim? (One approach is non-vascularized bone grafting and possibly local flaps. The other is the use of composite free tissue transfer, most notably the fibula as an osteocutaneous flap.)
4. What are the specific considerations in the reconstruction of composite periorbital defects? (The status of the periorbital soft tissue and adnexa, in particular the eyelids, globe intact or enucleation/exenteration, orbital bony defect, soft tissue volume requirements.)
5. Cite some examples of local soft tissue flaps that could be utilized for periorbital reconstruction. (Principally, forehead donor site and temporalis muscle to address a volume deficit.)
6. From the perspective of the use of an ocular prosthesis, why is bony orbital reconstruction with vascularized bone preferred over non-vascularized? (The ability to place bone-integrated anchors for the prosthesis.)
7. If necessary, what is the free flap of choice for composite periorbital reconstruction, and why? (The fibula osteocutaneous free flap has a lengthy pedicle and reliable skin paddle and can be osteotomized in multiple locations to provide a reconstruction of the buttress and the three dimensions of the periorbital regions.)
   (a) Is soft tissue reconstruction alone necessary? (Either a thin anterolateral thigh or radial/ulnar forearm flap. Certainly, a superficial circumflex iliac perforator flap would be an option.)
8. The readings propose a conceptual framework for the determination of the reconstructive needs for maxillary defects. What are the components? (Restoration of the orbital floor, reconstruction of the vertical buttresses, reconstruction of the vertical zygomatico- and nasomaxillary buttresses to link the orbital rims to the dental alveolar segment, reconstruction of the alveolar segment, restoration of malar projection and width.)
9. Based on the response to the above question, give a classification for post-traumatic maxillary defects. (Type I—Unilateral dentoalveolus or inferior partial maxillary

defect; Type II—Unilateral dentoalveolus extending to and loss of infraorbital rim; Type III—Bilateral Type I or dentoalveolus; Type IV—Bilateral Type II, namely, loss of infraorbital rim and probably nose in addition to bilateral dentoalveolus. The additional loss of the posterior maxilla and pterygoid plates is added as a plus or minus as well as an "a" or "b," the latter indicative of an associated skin deficit.)

(a) Why is the inclusion of the malar eminence, if involved, in the reconstructive plan crucial? (The malar eminence and the infraorbital rim are important to provide support for the orbital floor, to link bony support for the reconstructed alveolus, and to define the width and projection of the midface.)

10. What, in general, are the reconstructive goals? (Closure of mucosal defects, reconstitution of the horizontal and vertical buttresses, restoration of speech and deglutition, bony support for the globe, and dental processes.)
    (a) What walls of the maxilla must be reconstructed and why? (Superior, inferior, and anterior. Superior for support of the globe and ocular prosthesis, inferior for restoration of the palate and alveolus, and anterior for cheek and midface projection.)
11. What is the criticism of the use of soft tissue-only free flaps encasing non-vascularized bone grafts? (Eventual partial or total absorption that would require additional bone augmentation.)
12. Outline a reconstructive plan for the following: Assume a mucosal defect in all instances (see Fig. 44.2.)
    (a) Type I defect with no skin-soft tissue deficiency (Fibula with a small skin paddle or deep circumflex iliac artery with or without internal oblique to fill the maxillary sinus.)
    (b) Type II defect with an associated skin deficit (Fibula with two osteocutaneous segments created by osteotomies will be necessary to permit simultaneous bone reconstruction of the infraorbital rim and alveolar defect.)
    (c) Type III defect or bilateral dentoalveolar with and without an associated skin deficit (A similar option as Type II except if the skin and soft tissue deficiency are substantial, a second free flap may be necessary. Conceivably, since the infraorbital rim and presumably the osseous skeleton of the nose are intact and absent of coverage defect, reconstruction could be accomplished with a deep circumflex iliac flap, DCIA with internal oblique. If a substantial skin deficit exists, orienting the skin paddle independent of the bone can be problematic with the DCIA flap. The presence or absence of an intact pterygoid can play a role in the provision of a point of posterior bone fixation.)
    (d) Type IV (Virtually all Type IV defects, as well as the vast majority of Type III, represent massive midface injury and, in the case of Type IV, frequent

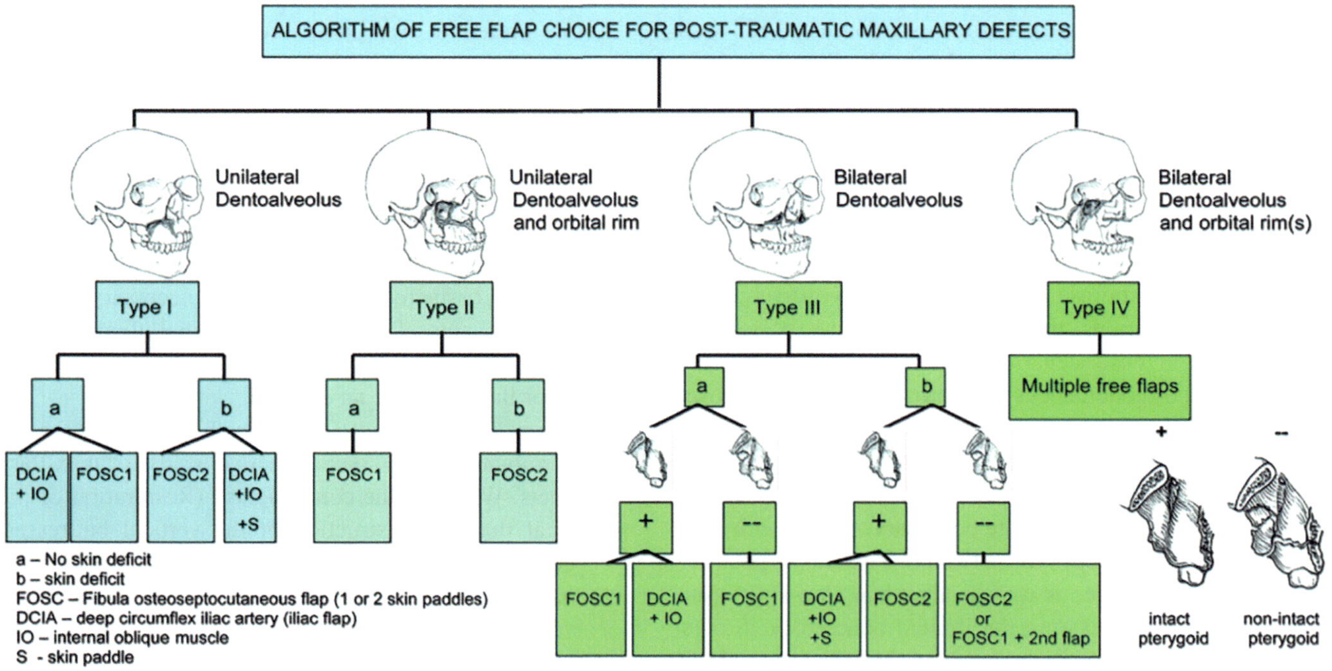

Fig. 44.2 Algorithm of free flap choice for posttraumatic maxillary defects. (Rodriguez E.D., Martin M., Bluebond-Langner R., et al., "Microsurgical Reconstruction of Posttraumatic High-Energy Maxillary Defects: Establishing the Effectiveness of Early Reconstruction", Plast Reconstr Surg., (2007);120(7):103S–117S. (Reprinted with Permission))

involvement of the globes as well. Type IV often requires multiple free flaps.)

13. What are the essential elements of preoperative planning in the address of late sequelae of inadequately or untreated complex gunshot wounds of the midface? (A clinical analysis of facial anthropometrics, CT including 3-D, dental impressions, virtual surgery modeling with the use of 3-D models. Consideration of potential donor sites. The use of CT-generated 3-D models of the defects has emerged as central to preoperative planning and performance of virtual surgery.)
14. What are the phases and timing of reconstruction of complex midface post-traumatic defects? (The first phase, accomplished within the weeks post-injury, is to restore the bony skeleton as well as plus-minus closure of mucosal defects and provision of soft tissue bulk. A later phase, perhaps weeks later, contours both bone and soft tissue as well as an address of nasal defects, possibly with forehead flap, and repositioning or reconstruction of eyelid defects. A late phase would include placement of dental implants and/or obturators, if necessary, and ocular prosthesis.)
15. Give a classification of mandibular defects. (Type 1 is a unilateral dentoalveolar defect, presumably segmental. Type 2 is a unilateral defect that extends posterior to the angle that does not cross the midline. Type 3 is a bilateral, anterior, and body defect that does not extend to either angle. Type 4 is a Type 3 plus involvement of one or both angles. The classification cited in readings also adds condylar involvement.)
    (a) Critique this classification. (Maybe oversimplified since it does not account for either initial intraoral lining or skin-soft tissue deficits. Also, the readings provide a subclassification hinging on the availability of ipsilateral recipient vasculature. Most head and neck reconstructive surgeons would avoid vein grafts if possible since the incorporation of the same results in a higher incidence of flap loss.)
16. Outline a suitable free flap for each of the following defects: (see Fig. 44.3.)

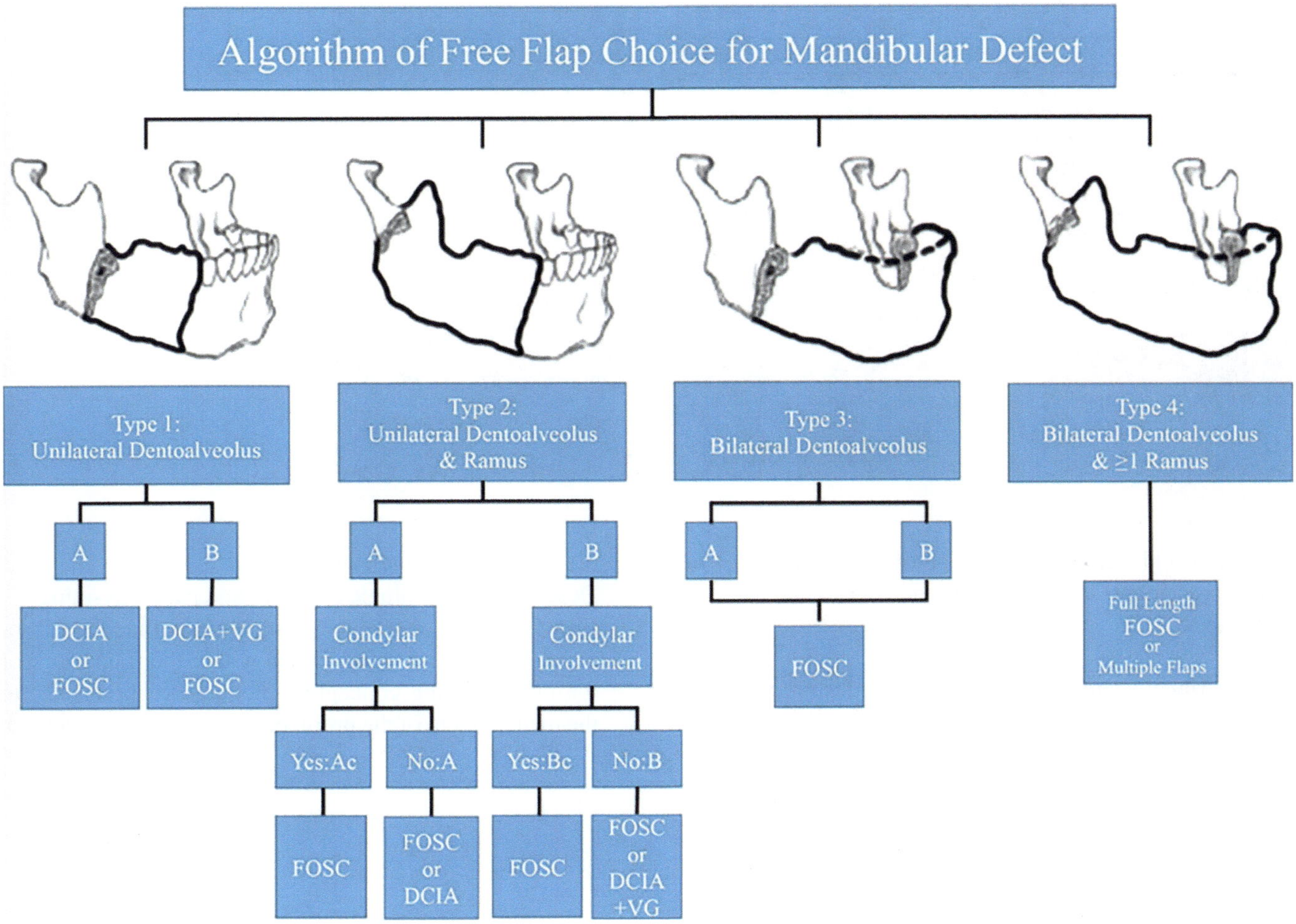

Fig. 44.3 Algorithm of free flap choice for mandibular defect. (Schultz BD, Sosin M, Nam A, et al. "Classification of Mandible Defects and Algorithms for Microvascular Reconstruction," *Plast. Reconstr. Surg.*, (2015); 135:743e. (Reprinted with Permission))

(a) Type 1 (Either DCIA or a fibula, dependent on the necessity of skin replacement and pedicle length.)
(b) Type 2 (Probably similar to Type 1 but more likely fibula since some contouring will be required as well as a skin island, although a DCIA can provide a skin island in obese patients that flap can be unacceptably thick.)
(c) Type 3 (Only a fibula will permit the multiple osteotomies necessary for this defect.)
(d) Type 4 (Type 4, and to a certain degree, Type 3, represent massive defects of the associated skin-soft tissue requirements and probably intraoral deficits as well. Multiple free tissue transfers will be necessary, including fibula.)

Editor's Note: Reconstruction of the mandible is also discussed in Chap. 37.

Case-Based Conference

Case 1: Gunshot Wound of the Face

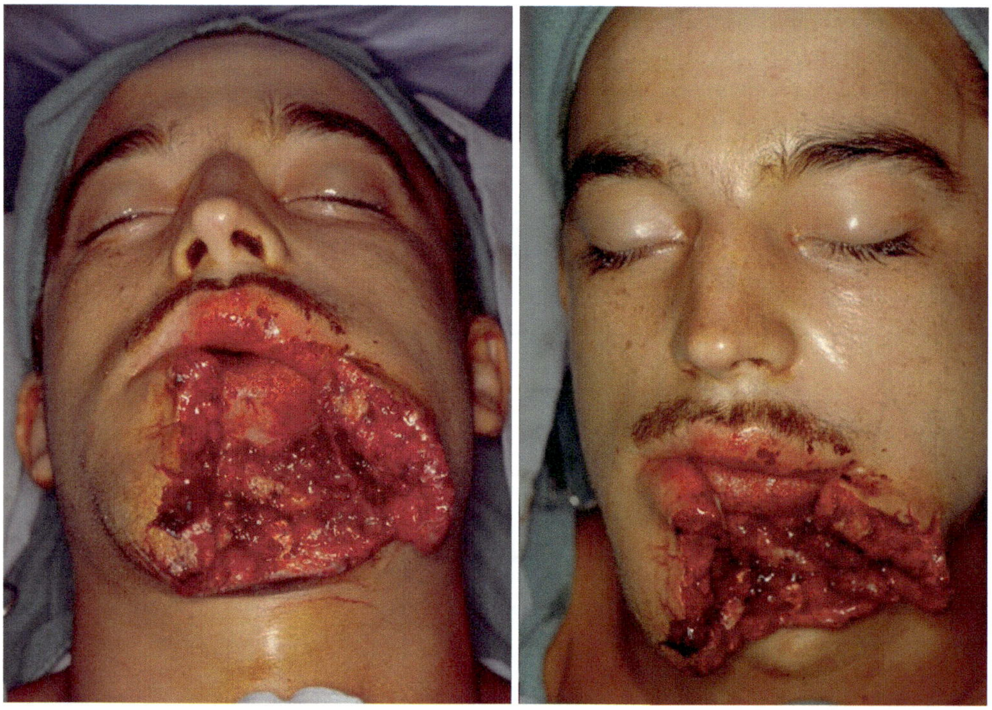

A 30-year-old who sustained a gunshot wound (rifle) in a hunting accident. The patient is in the ER and has been stabilized.

1. Describe the slide(s) and add an initial history and physical examination. Outline the initial management in the ER. Be brief.
   (a) Are any tests indicated?
2. Describe the pathologic anatomy and pathophysiology.
3. Based on the response to question #2, outline the subsequent management plan. Do so within the framework of the two opposing conceptual therapeutic approaches to the management of the problem, select yours, and defend.

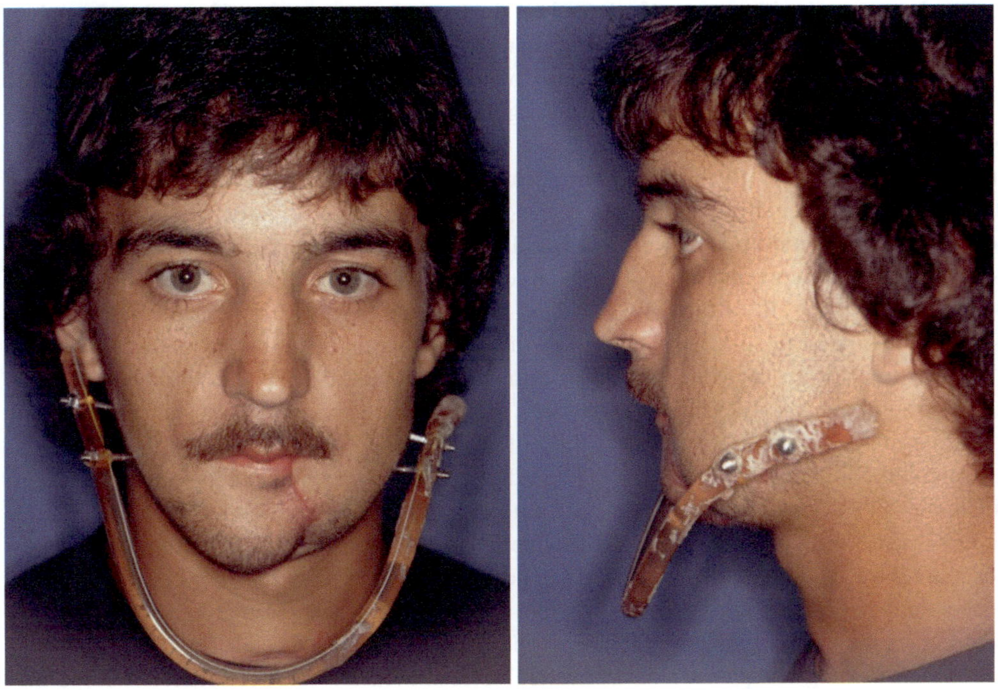

The patient was noncompliant with follow-up and returned 3 months post-injury.

1. Describe the two clinical photos.
2. What is the treatment plan at this juncture? What are the challenges posed by the hiatus between injury and the current presentation?

Case-Based Conference: Discussion

Case 1: Gunshot Wound of the Face

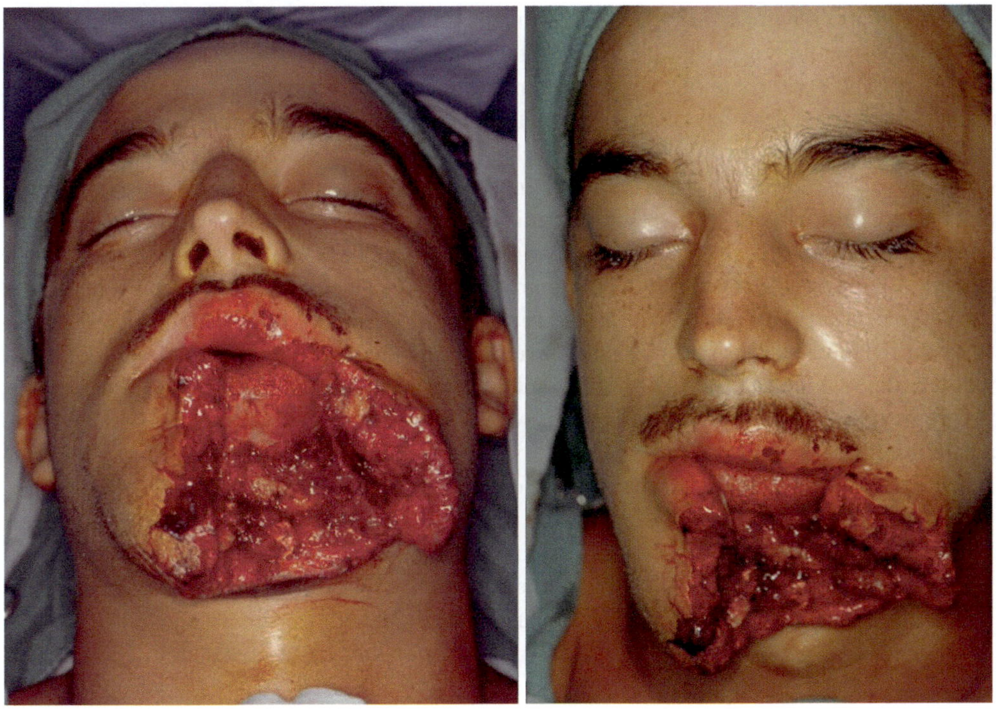

A 30-year-old who sustained a gunshot wound (rifle) in a hunting accident. The patient is in the ER and has been stabilized.

1. Describe the slide(s) and add an initial history and physical examination. Outline the initial management in the ER. Be brief. (The two slides are a full-face frontal-oblique view and a submental vertex. The frontal-oblique view demonstrates an extensive skin-soft tissue wound of the central and left lower lip and most, if not all, of the adjacent chin. The tongue is readily visible in the depths of the wound. In this view, no other injuries are evident. The patient appears to be under general anesthesia. The submental vertex again demonstrates a large skin-soft tissue wound of the entire central and left chin but also possible loss of the lower lip, including labial and adjacent floor of mouth mucosa, an intact tongue is again visualized. Importantly, no teeth or mandibles are seen in the wound and are absent. A tracheostomy has been placed.

   The initial history would center on the circumstances of the injury and the nature of the wounding weapon, a low or high-velocity rifle as a 0.22 caliber or, in contrast, a 30.06. A brief medical history would quickly establish the presence or absence of significant comorbidities. Of course, the initial physical examination is an assessment of the severity of the injury, including the degree of mandibular dentition and bone loss, as well as the status of the remaining teeth. An approximate amount of the chin soft tissue and lower lip loss is estimated. A secure airway should be established, perhaps by an endotracheal intubation initially, followed by a formal tracheostomy.)
   (a) Any tests indicated? (Although plain X-rays of the mandible would probably be adequate, a more comprehensive assessment of the status of the mandible can be obtained with CT imaging. The blunt force of the anterior and mandibular injury may also have fractured one or both condyles, an area not readily visualized on plain films.)
2. Describe the pathologic anatomy and pathophysiology. (The central element of the pathophysiology of this injury is the nature of the wounding agent. A hunting rifle is usually a high-velocity weapon with tremendous wounding capability. A high-velocity weapon fired at close range at the victim imparts a substantial amount of kinetic injury to the tissues. Avulsion injuries are sustained, in this case, by the soft tissues of the lip and chin, but also the resistance offered by hard tissues as the mandible results in a more efficient and complete transfer of the kinetic energy to the bone. The end result can be characterized by severe comminution, devitalized bone fragments, and segmental bone loss. The degree of devitalization may not be evident initially.)
3. Based on the response to question #2, outline the subsequent management plan. Do so within the framework of the two opposing conceptual therapeutic approaches to the management of the problem, select yours, and defend. (The two opposing therapeutic approaches are the more conventional treatment plan of serial debridement, primary closure of skin and soft tissues including mucosa, and stabilization of the remaining mandibular fragments either internally, perhaps with a reconstruction plate if sufficient soft tissue coverage is present, or externally with the use of an external fixation apparatus. A potential disadvantage of an internal reconstruction plate, particularly with a soft-tissue deficiency, is erosion and exposure of the plate.

   Regardless of which method is adopted, the patient is placed into proper occlusion with intermaxillary fixation. The benefits of the former are an assurance that the debridement is complete prior to the initiation of reconstruction. Since that assurance may require the expenditure of a number of weeks, in the absence of bony support, considerable contracture of the soft tissue envelope may occur, a contracture that may be difficult to reverse with secondary reconstruction. In contrast, the early implementation of skeletal reconstruction may be plagued by recurrent infection and bone resorption, a result of retained devascularized bone and soft tissue. Yet, the potential benefit is an address or minimization of the issue of soft-tissue contracture.

   The optimal approach to this patient's injury would be immediate operative debridement, probably primary closure of the skin, soft tissues, and intraoral mucosa. The latter, the mucosa defect, may require rotation of a local buccal mucosa flap. As discussed above, the mandibular fragments should be stabilized with an external fixation device or an internal reconstruction plate after placement of the patient in intermaxillary fixation. The patient would require close postoperative monitoring to ensure uneventful healing. Once that assurance was established, probably within the first 2 weeks post-operative, a definitive reconstruction of the bony and soft tissue defect should be accomplished. The selection of the appropriate option would hinge on the necessity to provide intraoral lining, skin envelope, and the magnitude of the bony defect. A mandibular defect of 3–4 cm could conceivably be reconstituted with non-vascularized bone and the skin envelope with a local flap. Larger bony defects will mandate the application of free tissue transfer as an osteocutaneous flap. An optimal donor site is the fibula osteocutaneous flap, an option that permits multiple osteotomies to configure the graft to the anterior arc parts of the mandible. A skin island harvested with the fibula and muscle could address any anterior soft tissue deficiency. The external fixation is maintained postoperatively until healing is assured, probably 3–6 months in the instance of nonvascularized bone grafts. If the lower lip was tight transversely because of lip deficiency, that defect should also be addressed but on a delayed basis with a lip-switch, an Abbé flap, or Karapandzic advancement flaps of the remaining lip segments.)

Intraoperative

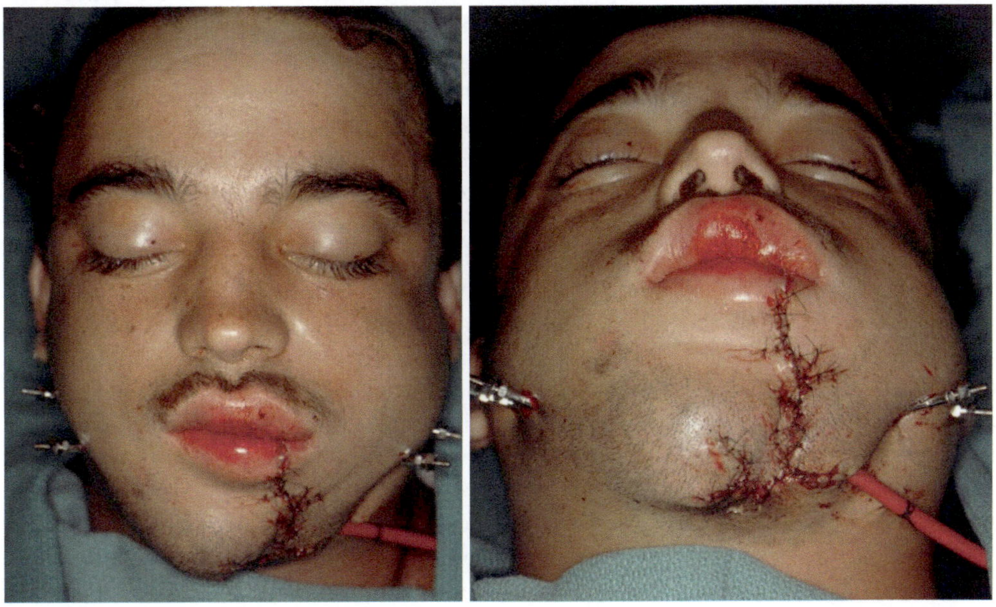

On the two views, a frontal and submental vertex, the lip and chin, have been primarily repaired, and the pins for an external fixation device are placed in the lateral mandibular segments. Considerable facial edema is present. Some tension of the inferior chin closure is evident.

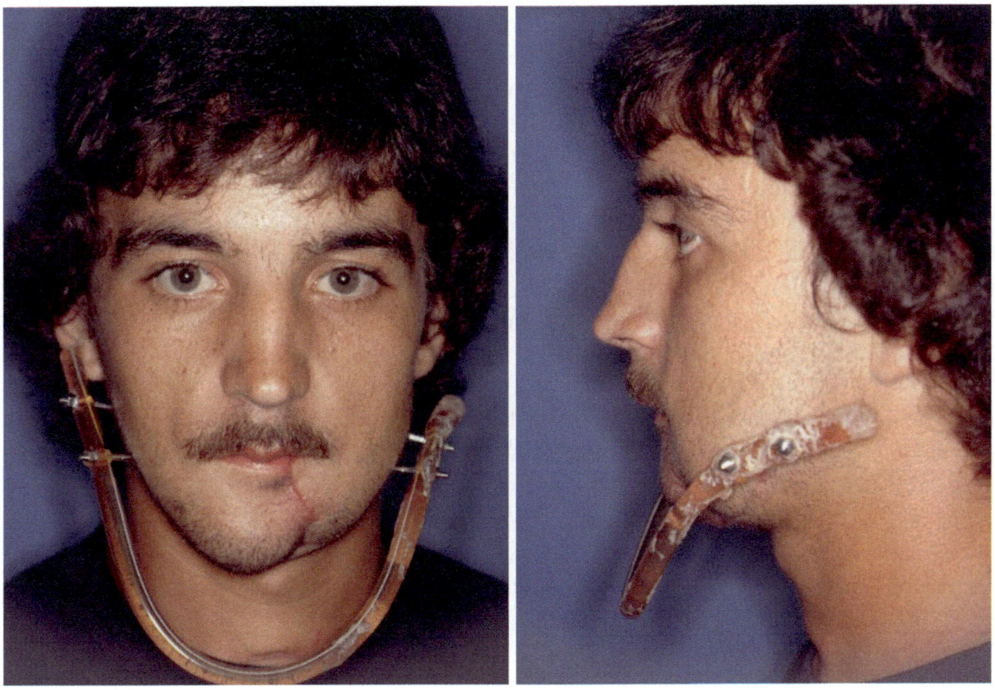

The patient was noncompliant with follow-up and returned 3 months post-injury.

1. Describe the two clinical photos. (The frontal view demonstrates a patient with external fixation pins in both lateral mandibles linked to an acrylic bar. The acrylic bar is directed so inferior that the entire face and neck are visible. The most apparent finding is a vertical scar that begins in the midportion of the left lower lip and extends below the chin. The appearance of the scar is consistent with the time hiatus. An additional finding is a contour deformity of the inferior border of the left lateral chin. A small transverse scar is present at the midline of the base of the neck, consistent with a history of tracheostomy. The principal finding of the lateral view is an element of retrognathia.
2. What is the treatment plan at this juncture? What are the challenges posed by the hiatus between injury and the current presentation? (A thorough clinical and imaging assessment at this stage is necessary for the development of a treatment plan. The clinical component is an evaluation of the intraoral tissues, including an estimation of adequacy to permit a mandibular bone graft or whether supplementation of lining is required. A similar evaluation of the skin-soft tissue envelope should be performed. The photos suggest a deficiency.

   To reconstitute mandibular continuity will require several treatment and operating steps. First, in preparation for a delayed bone graft, 3 months in this instance, the mandibular fragments will need to be repositioned in space. The left mandible segment, with loss of the anterior hyomandibular attachment, including the anterior belly of the digastric, geniohyoid, and mylohyoid, is retracted superiorly and medially from the unopposed vector of the masseter and pterygoid, respectively. The right mandible appears to have retained the anterior support. The above-mentioned findings, including the deficiency of skin envelope, a possible similar deficiency of intraoral lining, and the migratory malposition of the mandibular fragments, are all consequences of secondary contracture—liability of the delayed approach to reconstruction.

   The contemporary approach to mandibular reconstruction has been enabled by digital imaging with computer-assisted design and computer-assisted manufacture, CAD/CAM, of both assessment and the intraoperative application of the technology. Virtual surgical planning involves a variety of digital technology that has replaced the traditional and labor-intensive methods of acquisition of dental impressions, the use of the impressions to create casts, the use of an articulator and facebow to perform conventional virtual surgery, and, lastly, the creation of acrylic splints for intra- and post-operative use. Instead, thin-slice CT scans with a 3D component and manipulation of images replace the traditional method, and CAD/CAM technology-specific cutting guides are provided for precise osteotomies on native mandible and donor bone and the production of patient-specific reconstruction plates.

   Since a 3-month hiatus has passed since the primary repair and the current presentation, the left mandibular fragment may require some repositioning with an intraoral release. After repositioning, the leading edges of each fragment at the bony defect will require debridement with bone instruments and any fragments excised. The assumption in this instance is that both the lining and soft tissue envelope are sufficient for bone graft. If not, a contingency must be provided for one or both. Regardless, given a segmental mandible defect of this magnitude, probably a minimum of 4 cm, vascularized bone would be advisable with or without a skin island, as outlined above. Two possibilities exist: if vascularized bone is necessary, the two options are fibula or iliac. The fibula, the workhorse for mandibular reconstruction, offers the opportunity for osteotomies as well as an accompanying skin island. Iliac is less satisfactory from the standpoint of provision of soft tissue, but for a relatively straight defect that does not require osteotomies, it certainly is more than ample bone stock that would set the stage for osseointegrated dental implants if necessary. The use of the fibula in the double-barrel variation in the reconstruction of the vertical height of the mandible would facilitate the placement of osseointegrated implants. Finally, a nonvascularized bone graft is certainly an option if the defect is of limited size and the soft tissue envelope is satisfactory. Nonvascularized bone reconstitution of smaller mandibular segmental defects can be accomplished with cortical-cancellous blocks of autogenous bone. The other option is cancellous bone only, configured within an alloplastic tray, titanium or absorbable, and is probably of historical interest only. Regardless of the method of reconstruction, short-term intermaxillary fixation would be advisable to facilitate soft tissue healing. The external fixation will need to be retained until radiographic and clinical evidence of mandibular bone healing is evident. Clinical assessment would require removal of the external fixation bar, retention of the pins, and manipulation of the mandible to assess stability. If stable, the external fixation can be discontinued.)

Postoperative

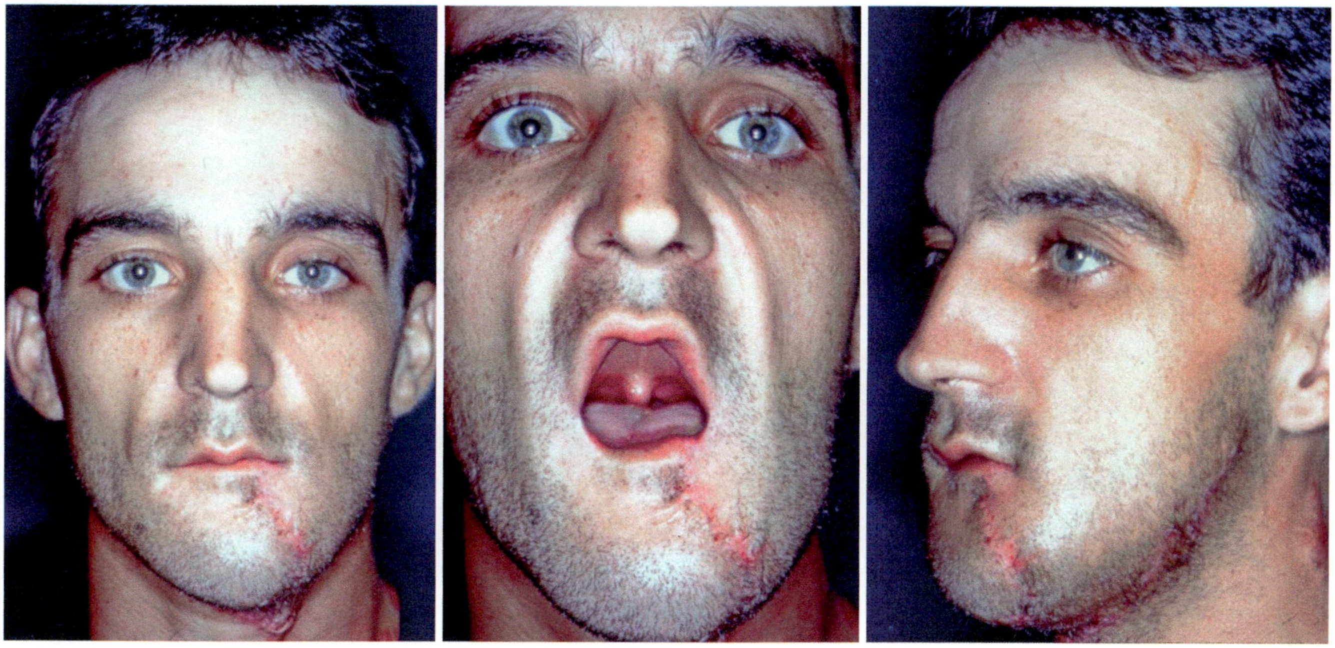

The three views depict the outcome of the soft tissue and, somewhat, the mandibular reconstruction. The lower lip is of normal configuration and transverse width, and the contour of the skin and soft tissue of the chin appear to be without tension. The patient has no evidence of microstomia. On the lateral view, excellent mental prominence and vertical height of the mandible are seen. An occlusal view would have been beneficial in judgment of the overall result. If anything, the mandible is perhaps excessively prominent. Over time, some resorption of the bone graft may occur.

In-Service Examination

1. The critical variables that determine the magnitude of injury from a rifle include the following **EXCEPT**:
   (a) Muzzle velocity
   (b) Mass of the missile
   (c) Design of the missile
   (d) Degree of resistance of the tissue struck by the missile
2. The degree of tissue damage in a shotgun wound is determined by the following variables **EXCEPT**:
   (a) The aerodynamic design of the pellets utilized
   (b) Distance
   (c) Amount of choke
   (d) Gauge

45 Facial Nerve

Bibliography

Roostaeian J, Rohrich RJ, Stuzin JM, "Anatomical Considerations to Prevent Facial Nerve Injury". *Plast Reconstr Surg.*, (2015); 135(5):**1318–1327**.

Granick, Mark S. and Hanna, Dwight C. III. Edited by Granick and Hanna. "Chapter 8: Surgical Management of Salivary Gland Disease." *Management of Salivary Gland Lesions*. **pp 192–193 (Figs. 10.5 and 10.6. ONLY)**.

Schliephake H, Hausamen JE, Chapter 21: "Facial Nerve Injuries", Peter Ward Booth, Barry L Eppley, Rainer Schmelzeisen, *Maxillofacial Trauma and Esthetic Facial Reconstruction*, Elsevier, (2003); **405–12 ONLY**.

Brown S, Isaacson B, Kutz W, et al., "Facial Nerve Trauma: Clinical Evaluation and Management Strategies", *Plast Reconstr Surg.*, (2019);143(5):**1498–1509 ONLY**.

Fattah A, Borschel GH, Manktelow RT, Bezuhly M, et al., "Facial palsy and reconstruction", *Plast Reconstr Surg.*, (2012); 129(2):**340e–350e (Videos 1, 2–Video 3 supplemental)**.

Garcia RM, Hadlock TA, Klebuc MJ, Simpson RL, et al., "Contemporary solutions for the treatment of facial nerve paralysis", *Plast Reconstr Surg.*, (2015); 135(6):**1025e–1044e (Videos are interesting but not necessarily informative)**.

Banks C.A., Jowett N., Iacolucci C., et al., "Five-Year Experience with Fifth-to-Seventh Nerve Transfer for Smile", *Plast Reconstr Surg.*, (2019);143:**1060e–61e, 1067e–70e ONLY**.

Stitik TP, Foye PM, Nadler SF, "Electromyography in Craniomaxillofacial Trauma", *Journal of Craniomaxillofacial Trauma*, (1999); 5(2):**39–43**.

Faculty Discussion and Study Guide

Neuroanatomy and Neurophysiology

Editor's Note: Neuroanatomy and neurophysiology are also included in Chaps. 73 and 74, including late problems.

1. In the embryology of the parotid gland and facial nerve, what is the important relationship and the interpretation of the same? (A superficial and deep lobe exists, but no natural tissue plane is present anatomically that facilitates dissection of the course of the facial nerve.)
2. What anatomic fact explains the occasional occurrence of facial nerve palsy with a difficult or forced delivery? (The subcutaneous and superficial course of the nerve after exit from the stylomastoid foramen in the neonate occurs because of the lack of development of the mastoid.)
3. The facial nerve has an extensive intrabony course. Where is the most likely site of injury in a transverse fracture of the temporal bone? (The horizontal portion of the nerve in the tympanic or more proximally in the petrous portion. The nerve can be injured in the vertical or mastoid portion during a mastoidectomy. See Figs. 45.1 and 45.2.)
   (a) If a patient with facial fractures who also has a fracture of the temporal bone presents with facial palsy, how can you determine the level of injury? (In all likelihood, the fracture is through the petrous or tympanic portion, so the greater petrosal nerve may or may not be injured since the geniculate ganglion is located in the labyrinth portion, proximal to the tympanic segment. The greater petrosal nerve supplies motor innervation to the lacrimal gland, and if intact, the performance of Schirmer's test can be

E. Luce, *A Curriculum for Plastic Surgery*, https://doi.org/10.1007/978-3-031-62087-4_45

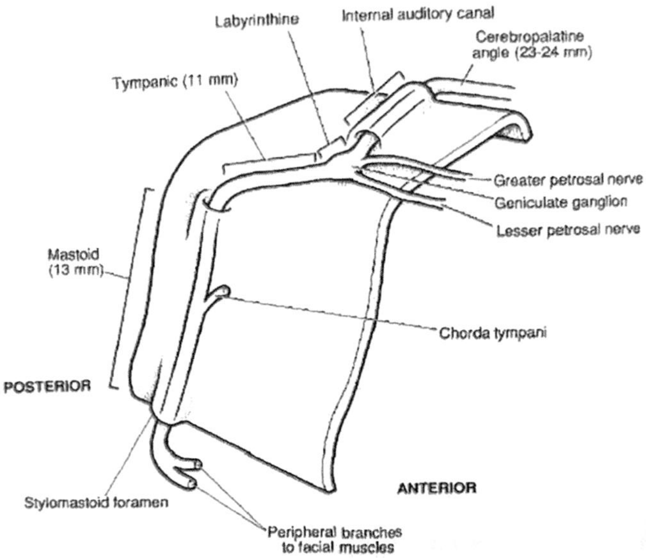

Fig. 45.1 Intratemporal path of the facial nerve and branches. (Granick, Mark S. and Hanna, Dwight C. III. Edited by Granick and Hanna. "Chapter 8: Surgical Management of Salivary Gland Disease," *Management of Salivary Gland Lesions*. pp. 192. (Reprinted with permission))

confirmatory. The high likelihood exists that the chorda tympani and stapedial nerve will not function. So, the tests of those branches are loss of taste on the anterior two-thirds of the tongue and high-frequency hearing loss. However, the stapedial branch is proximal to the chorda tympani and could be intact, yet the chorda tympani may not be functioning. Much of this discussion is academic since the findings will not impact management.)

4. What is the essential topography of the facial distribution of cranial nerve VII with respect to injury from a facial laceration? (The facial distribution of the five branches of the nerve can be simulated by the placement of the examiner's opposite hand and onto the injured side with digits spread, fingertips pointed anteriorly, and the thumb pointed inferiorly. To do so roughly duplicates the distribution of the branches of the nerve.)
   (a) What is the significance of a vertical laceration medial to the lateral canthus with respect to the facial nerve? (Operative repair is not necessary since spontaneous recovery is likely.)

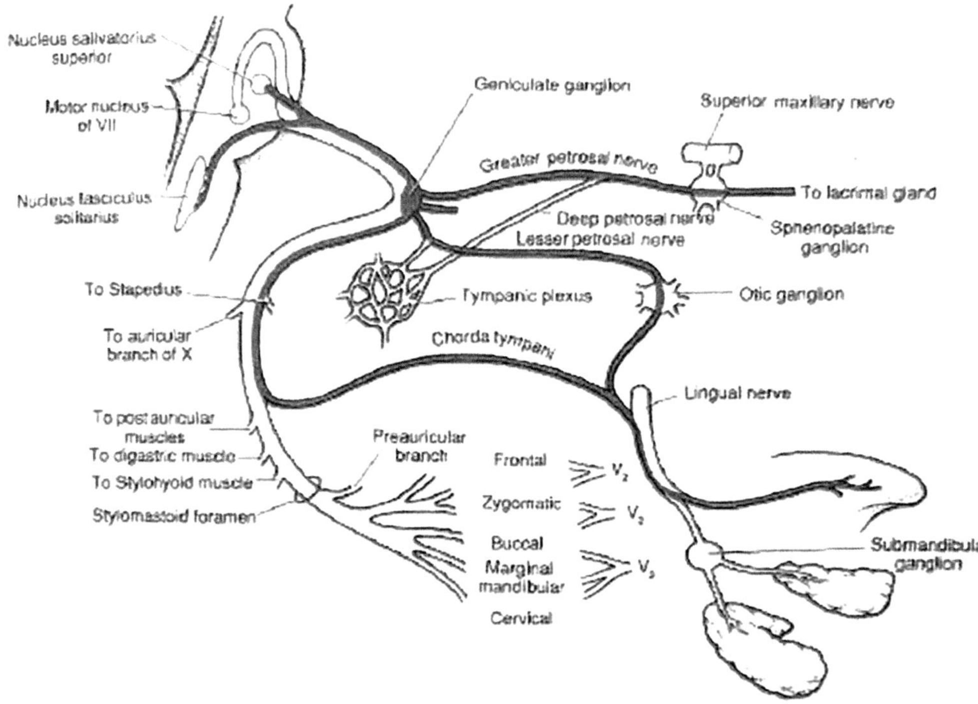

Fig. 45.2 Schematic diagram of intra- and extratemporal facial nerve. (Granick, Mark S. and Hanna, Dwight C. III. Edited by Granick and Hanna. "Chapter 8: Surgical Management of Salivary Gland Disease," *Management of Salivary Gland Lesions*. pp. 193. (Reprinted with permission))

5. Describe some absolute measurements and determination of the topography of the frontal or temporal branch of the facial nerve. (The classical description of the course of the nerve is a trajectory from 0.5 cm below the tragus to 1.5 cm superior to the lateral brow. The sentinel vein lies at the halfway point, about 7 mm, between the nerve and the lateral orbital rim.)
   (a) What is the relationship in the third dimension or depth? (As discussed in Chap. 42, the nerve is adjacent to the periosteum of the zygomatic arch and just deep to the temporoparietal fascia further superior but superficial to the superficial leaf of the deep temporal fascia, an important anatomical consideration in development of a bicoronal flap. More peripherally, the nerve enters the deep aspect of the frontalis muscle laterally.)
6. What is the most likely location of the marginal mandibular branch at the angle of the mandible? (Just posterior to the angle, the nerve courses over the posterior belly of the digastric muscle and, most commonly, directly over the angle. In one-third of the instances, the nerve will be 1 cm below.)
   (a) Relationship to the facial vessels? (Posterior to the facial vessels that cross the mandible about 3 cm anterior to the angle. Posterior to the vessels, the nerve will course on the inferior border, and anterior to the vessels will be found above the mandibular border.)
7. What are the factors that are responsible for a declining favorable outcome as the time hiatus increases between injury and nerve repair? (Increasing fibrosis of the distal axonal tubes, increasing fibrosis of the motor endplates, muscle fiber atrophy.)
   (a) Define the nerve cell body changes that occur with nerve injury and what determines the severity of those changes. (The magnitude of intracellular changes within the nerve cell body is directly dependent on the proximity of the injury or more proximal the more severe the nerve cell damage. The hypothesis is that the degree of axonal plasma that must be regenerated to complete re-innervation to the end organs, so the more proximal the lesion, the higher the possibility that from injury distalward, the cell body must produce greater amounts of axonal plasma and may be overwhelmed.)
   (b) Since denervated muscle will undergo fibrosis without re-innervation, what are the timelines to obtain muscle function? (Ideally accomplished within 3 months, still functional within a year, and irretrievably functionless after 3 years.)
8. You inadvertently transect a buccal branch of the facial nerve during a superficial parotidectomy. The next day, you cut the marginal mandibular branch during a facelift. Which patient is most likely to have normal function postoperatively? (The parotidectomy because of the cross-connections between the buccal and the zygomatic branches. In contrast, the marginal mandibular and temporal branches have a much lower frequency, 10–15%, crossover.)
9. You are referred a patient with a gradual onset of facial palsy and a diagnosis of Bell's palsy. What findings would indicate that the diagnosis may not be correct? (The speed of onset since Bell's palsy tends to be sudden onset, but tumor pressure is more gradual. The presence of other cranial nerve palsies is indicative of perhaps a nasopharyngeal tumor except the auditory cranial nerve VIII, which would be more consistent with a cerebellopontine angle lesion.)
10. Besides facial expression, what other functional complications can accompany complete facial nerve paralysis? (Eye irritation, obstructive nasal inspiration, oral incompetence, speech difficulties.)
11. Describe the muscle or muscles and specific function to test each of the five branches of the nerve. (Brow elevation—frontalis; eye closure—orbicularis oculi; smiling and grimacing—zygomaticus major and levator labii superioris; puckered lips—orbicularis oris; depressed lower lip—depressor labii inferioris; cervical contraction—platysma.)
12. Describe the performance of the following: Schirmer's test, maximal stimulation test, electroneurography, EMGs, and the value of each. (Schirmer's test is done with a filter paper strip placed in the eye with a minimal amount of mm of wetting secondary to tears as a division point between a positive and negative test. Maximal stimulation is an electrodiagnostic test that consists of stimulation of the proximal nerve with increasing amplitude of stimulation until either a response in the mimetic muscles is obtained or the patient has intolerable discomfort. Contraction of the facial muscles in the lower stimulus range would indicate a considerable amount of the nerve is intact; reaction in the higher ranges would indicate a much smaller proportion of the nerve is intact, but at least some conduction exists. The test will assist in the differentiation of neuropraxia, nerve fibers distal to the region that can still conduct an impulse, and axonotmesis, degeneration of the fibers that are now unable to conduct an impulse. Electroneurography measures the height of the muscle action potential, if present, and is designed to measure the strength of recovery. EMGs measure the activity of the facial muscles and consist of needle inser-

tion activity, fibrillation potentials if the muscle is denervated, and polyphasic motor potentials if re-innervation has begun. The presence of polyphasic motor potentials usually appears before clinical evidence. One can also follow the recovery of the nerve with this test.)

13. What is either the last intratemporal or first extracranial branch? (The branch to the posterior belly of the digastric muscle, followed by the branch to the stylohyoid.)
14. Describe the House-Brackmann scale. (The House-Brackmann scale was developed to assess the severity of facial nerve paresis or, conversely, the magnitude of recovery. The six levels of grades are from one, normal, to six, total paralysis. Grade two is a slight weakness only perceptible on close examination, five in contrast is only slight perceptible motion on effort. The remaining grades three and four consist of some motion in both but disfiguring asymmetry in grade four, despite normal symmetry at rest. A number of modifications or alternate grading systems have been proposed.)
15. Outline the significance of lid paralysis in facial nerve lesions and the examination and treatment of the same. (Examine the presence of Bell's phenomenon as a protective mechanism for the eye and the presence of keratoconjunctivitis as indicative of exposure to the cornea. The problem, at least in extratemporal lesions, is not tear production but rather lubrication of the cornea by an intact blink mechanism, as well as the possible problem of exposure and drying of the cornea during sleep. In fact, excessive tearing is common. Short-term measures consist of lubricant within the eye, taping the lower lid to avoid ectropion and scleral show, and finally, the necessity to perform a permanent lateral tarsorrhaphy.)

Repair, Reconstruction

1. Describe epineural, perineural, and interfascicular suture repair. (The terms apply to the particular structure that is sutured, such as the epineurium for epineural repair, usually done with a 7° suture; perineural or grouped fascicular repair is a bundle of fascicles sutured with the perineurium, and finally, the interfascicular repair is the suture of the individual fascicles with fine material. No study has demonstrated the superiority of one technique over the other, and the repair singly of each of multiple fascicles places a considerable burden of suture material within the body of the nerve.)
   (a) What other anatomic fact argues against microfascicular repair? (The interfascicular branching within the nerve is quite substantial.)
   (b) What is a readily available donor site for nerve grafting of the facial nerve? (Greater auricular or other branches of the cervical plexus, sural, medial antebrachial cutaneous.)
2. What types of nerve transfers can be performed, and what are the pros and cons? (A commonly performed and discussed is an end-to-side repair of the distal facial nerve stump into a partial proximal hypoglossal nerve stump. The disadvantage is the synkinesis and dyskinesis that can occur with such a transfer, as well as the extensive cortical reeducation to enable the patient to move the tongue to achieve motion of the face. In some patients, an intervening sural nerve graft may be necessary. Another application of hypoglossal transfer is as a "babysitter" procedure to maintain the integrity of the distal nerve stumps and facial muscles in preparation for cross-facial nerve grafting.

   Yet, other options exist, and the donor site deficit and dysarthria of the hypoglossal have rendered the choice remote. For example, if the duration since a proximal injury is limited, 2 years for some authors, 4 years for others, is the use of the masseteric nerve, a fifth to seven transfer. The advantages are more rapid neurotization, and the disadvantage is the use of a masticatory nerve for facial expression.

   A further modification is the employment of the masseter nerve as a "babysitter" in those instances when the subsequent reconstruction is accomplished with a cross-facial nerve graft.)
3. What are the indications for a cross-facial nerve graft? (Absence of the proximal trunk as in sacrifice with a cerebellopontine angle or parotid tumor are two examples. As discussed below, the hiatus between injury and reconstruction is the principal discriminatory factor in the options described.)
   (a) Describe the concept and technique of cross-face nerve grafting. (The concept is to transport axons of the desired portions of the facial nerve, buccal and zygomatic, from the normal contralateral side to the involved face to be utilized to reinnervate the injured branches, including the mandibular, as well, if possible. The buccal and zygomatic branches on the donor side are selected because the high incidence of interconnections between these branches will minimize the functional deficit. The donor nerves are anastomosed to a nerve graft, most commonly the sural nerve, and tunneled into the upper lip or opposite face. Several options exist, mostly dependent on the duration of the injury. The duration is critical since progressive fibrosis of the axonal tubes and motor

endplates occurs with time. The first option, if the facial nerve injury is relatively acute, is neurorrhaphy from the donor graft site on the contralateral side to the distal branches of the injured nerve, accomplished with a nerve graft, usually the sural as donor nerve as a single-stage procedure. Another option is also a cross-facial nerve graft with a hiatus of varying time, 6–12 months, to allow axonal sprouts from the distal stump of the facial nerve prior to neurorrhaphy to the distal branches of the injured nerve, namely, a two-stage procedure. A third option implemented when the duration from injury is a matter of years is the same procedure but a neurorrhaphy to the stump of a now neurotized free muscle transfer such as the gracilis. The choice of these options hinges quite substantially on the hiatus since injury and the mechanism of injury.)

4. Describe the concept and technique of revascularized muscle transfer for the paralyzed face. (The conceptual approach to free muscle transplantation is to replace the actions of the mimetic muscles in the lower and midface. A number of muscles have been studied and utilized, the most common choice being the gracilis. The origin is attached to the temporalis fascia or zygomatic arch. Points for attachment of the more distal muscle are determined by the placement of key sutures at several points, modiolus, upper and lower lip, and nasolabial fold. The potential vector of muscle pull is simulated by traction on the sutures. The microvascular anastomosis to either the facial or superficial temporal vessels is performed first, the muscles shortened and inset under slight tension, and either the ipsilateral masseteric nerve or cross-face nerve graft is attached to the obturator nerve. The disadvantage of the masseteric nerve option is the necessity of biting simultaneously with facial expression and the cortical reeducation to learn to do so. The disadvantage of cross-facial nerve graft is the two-stage procedure.)
5. Give a menu and briefly describe ancillary procedures for established facial nerve paralysis. (As mentioned above, particularly in the elderly, a permanent lateral tarsorrhaphy should be considered since a combined paralytic and senile ectropion can place the integrity of the cornea at significant risk. A gold weight can be placed in the upper lid for the lagophthalmos. Local muscle transfers to create some element of dynamic movement, such as transfer of the masseter or a portion of the temporalis, can provide some static and dynamic correction. These procedures are considered a second tier to the neurotized free muscle transfer. Finally, Botox injections can be used to address hyperkinesis, an isolated asymmetric action on the normal side.)
   (a) What are the disadvantages of a pedicled temporalis muscle transfer? (Can only be directed to the lower face, requires substantial cortical re-education since the muscle is innervated by cranial nerve V, and a bulge on contraction over the zygoma is frequently seen. The entire muscle can be transferred after release of the insertion on the coronoid and tunneled beneath the zygomatic arch. Often functions as a static sling.)

Scenarios

Editor's Note: No function is evident on clinical examination in any of the scenarios below.

1. A 20-year-old who has sustained an acute avulsive injury with a 3 cm segmental loss of the proximal facial nerve. (The soft tissue repair should be accomplished acutely, and the facial nerve should be explored in the same setting. Since the distal branches of the facial nerve are still reactive, identification is possible. The proximal stump is identified, and the gap is addressed with a nerve graft harvested from the greater auricular nerve. Although conduits have been utilized for defects of up to 2 cm in the upper extremity without grafts, that option is not appropriate in this scenario. The discussion of the use of conduits and allografts is in Chap. 73.)
2. A 40-year-old will require a total parotidectomy and facial nerve sacrifice. (The optimal management of this patient is immediate reconstruction of the deficit. Careful identification of the distal branches as well as a proximal facial nerve stump should be accomplished, as well as harvest of the greater auricular nerve for use as a graft. If an inadequate proximal stump is available, the additional length of the nerve can be obtained by drilling the temporal bone. The nerve graft created by the oncologic resection is bridged with an autologous nerve graft.)
3. A 30-year-old, 3 weeks postoperative, had an intracranial resection of the facial nerve for an acoustic neuroma. (No proximal nerve VII is available. To preserve the endoneurial tubes and motor end plates from the fibrosis of denervation, a "babysitter" procedure can be performed. The options are a partial hypoglossal or masseter nerve transfer to the main distal trunk of the facial nerve. The principal disadvantage of the former is the resultant dysarthria in some patients. The principal disadvantage of the latter is the necessity to invade the face, although some of that disadvantage can be mitigated by identification and tagging of the distal branches of VII in preparation for the next step.

The next step, optimally accomplished at the same operation as above, is cross-face nerve grafts. Once nerve regeneration has occurred through the nerve grafts to the involved side, 6–12 months, anastomosis to the distal branches of the injured nerve is accomplished.)

4. A 60-year-old's 2-year post-temporal bone fracture. (Testing would determine if function existed in the distal intratemporal branches, the chorda tympani, and stapedial and compared to baseline test results—if performed. Electrodiagnostic testing would also determine if any recovery was evident in the extracranial portion of the nerve. Assuming none, the critical time limit of two years implies extensive fibrosis of the distal endoneurial tubes and motor end plates has occurred. To achieve facial motion, a transplant will be necessary. A microvascular transplant most frequently used is the gracilis muscle, powered either by a previously performed cross-face nerve graft or by the masseter nerve. The principal disadvantage of the former is the necessity of a prior procedure and sacrifice of contralateral donor nerves. A disadvantage of the latter is the cortical re-education of conversion of chewing motion to that of mimetic function.)

Video Notes

From Garcia et al. PRS (2015)135:102

Video 1

Pre- and postoperative of the masseter nerve to distal facial (extratemporal) in a pediatric patient. The upper face of the patient is not visible.

Video 2

Pre- and postoperative of a pediatric patient with cross-facial nerve graft for eye closure. Eye closure is not evident, but good lower face function.

Video 3

Congenital facial palsy with temporalis transfer with pre- and postoperative views of an adult patient. A bulge is perceptible over the zygoma but overall good symmetry in a young adult patient.

Video 4

Not a nerve deficit. Add partial temporalis transfer to the upper lip.

Video 5

Intraoperative stimulation of the branches of the distal facial nerve in preparation for cross-face grafting.

Video 6

Intraoperative view of dissection of the recipient site.

Video 7

Intraoperative stimulation by the placement of retention sutures in preparation for a free muscle transfer.

Video 8

Dissection of the gracilis free muscle transfer.

Video 9

Postoperative cross-facial nerve grafts with a reasonably good symmetry.

Video 10

Postoperative cross-facial nerve grafts with a reasonably good symmetry.

Video 11

Somewhat older patient with pre- and postoperative views of a one-stage approach demonstrates that asymmetry persists at rest.

Video 12

Masseter transfer from the lower face with, again, some persistent asymmetry at rest.

Video 13

Moebius syndrome with free muscle transfer powered by the masseter nerve.

From Fattah *Plast. Reconstr. Surg.*, (2012); 129(2):**340e**

Video 1: 8 min and 15 s

- Cross-face facial nerve grafting
  1. Preparation of facial nerve branches on the uninjured side
  2. Harvest of the sural graft
  3. Placement of the sural graft in anastomosis
  4. Critique: acceptable resolution and excellent narrative

Video 2: 12 min and 30 s

1. Markings—excellent narrative of planning of vectors, placement of muscle transfer
2. Placement of traction sutures to mimic the pull of transplant
3. Dissection of the gracilis, inset, and completed vascular and nerve anastomosis
4. Summary of the steps in narrative

Video 3: 14 min

1. Mobius treated by single-stage gracilis, powered by the masseter nerve
2. Excellent narrative of marking and planning
3. Excellent result

1. Options (Acute)
   (a) Transected extra-temporal facial nerve
      • No gap → Primary anastomosis in first 48 h
      • Gap
         – Less than 2 cm → conduit ± autogenous nerve graft
         – >2 cm → autogenous nerve graft
         – Assumption: *not* a high-velocity blunt force, such as a gunshot wound; if so, consider tagging distal branches at exploration acutely
   (b) Transected intra-temporal with tumor resection (acute)
      • Nerve graft if proximal stump available
      • "Baby-sitter" with masseter nerve if proximal stump not available
2. Options (delayed)
   (a) Transected extra-temporal <6–9 months → repair as above
   (b) Transected extra-temporal ≥9–12 months → cross-face nerve graft as single-stage or 2-stage to distal branches
3. Options (late) **assumption**-motor endplates and distal axons fibrosed
   (a) Free muscle transfer powered by:
      • Masseter nerve
      • Cross-face nerve graft either as a single or 2-stage
   (b) Regional muscle transfer
      • Partial temporalis
      • Masseter to modiolus

Case-Based Conference

Case 1: Facial Paralysis

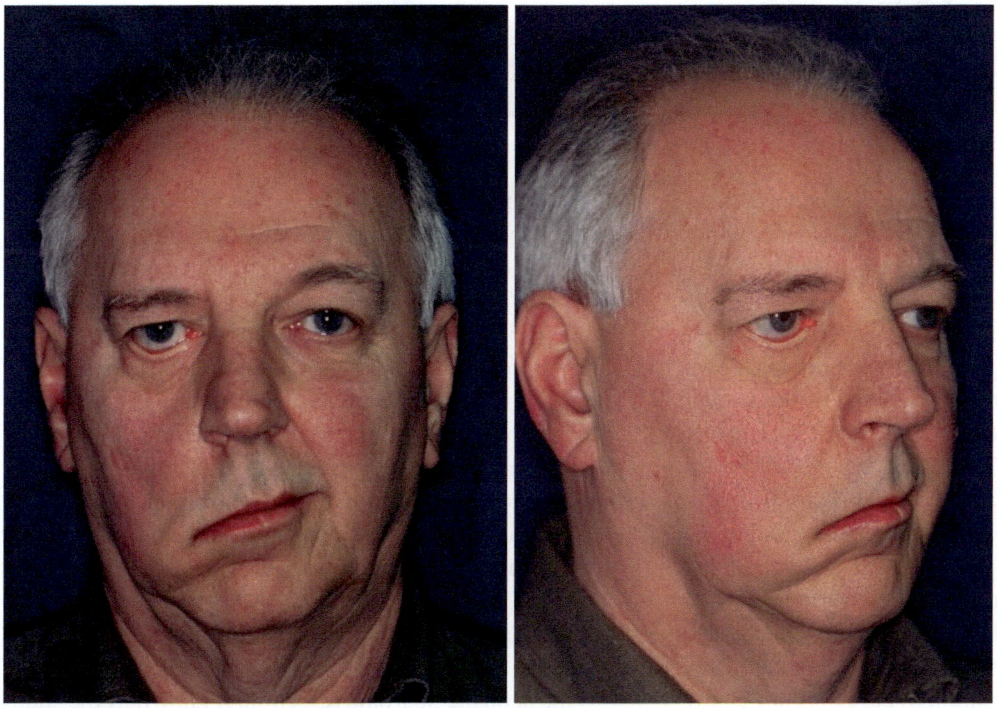

A 64-year-old male s/p 10 months resection of acoustic neuroma. The patient is tumor-free by a recent MRI and did not receive radiation therapy.

1. Describe the classic findings of facial nerve palsy exhibited in this patient and add a clinical examination.
   (a) Are any tests indicated?
2. Outline a treatment plan.
3. Describe a treatment plan for a 35-year-old patient.

Case-Based Conference: Discussion

Case 1: Facial Paralysis

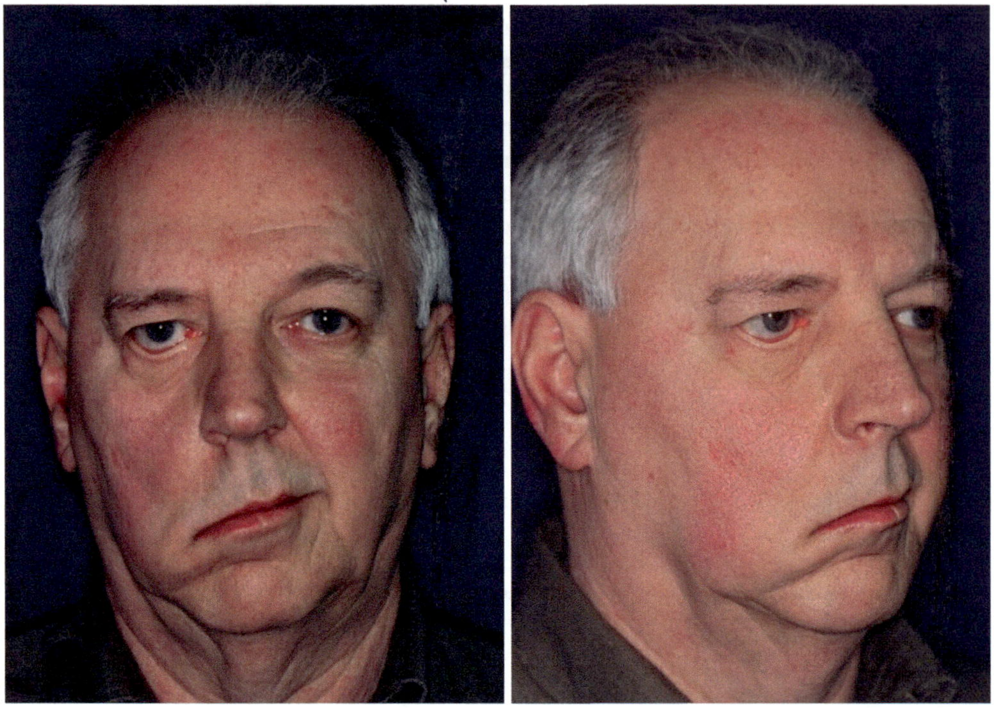

A 64-year-old male s/p 10 months resection of acoustic neuroma. The patient is tumor-free by a recent MRI and did not receive radiation therapy.

1. Describe the classic findings of facial nerve palsy exhibited in this patient and add a clinical examination. (Two photos provide a frontal and oblique view of the patient that depicts most of the aesthetic stigmata of a complete right facial nerve paralysis. Those findings include a sagging oral commissure, an effaced nasolabial fold, a paralytic ectropion with probably an age-related component as well, a combination of brow ptosis and redundant upper lid, and an asymmetrically smooth forehead. The other findings are an overall appearance of the stated age and a receding frontotemporal hairline. The oblique view adds little additional information. What is absent is any evidence of the adverse consequences of corneal exposure to keratoconjunctivitis. Also absent is evidence of oral incompetence manifest by a wet lower right lip.

   The clinical examination would elicit the symptoms of the complications of seventh nerve palsy, such as recurrent eye inflammation, oral incontinence, difficulty with the articulation of speech, and if the onset was delayed postoperatively or even present preoperatively. The impact of the patient's situation on activities of daily living should be determined as well. The past medical history ascertains the presence and severity of comorbidities, operations, and medications, including ophthalmologic. The physical exam determines if any element of voluntary activity is present, and an exam for keratoconjunctivitis would include perhaps fluorescein staining.)

   (a) Are any tests indicated? (Any information about the fate of the facial nerve intraoperatively at the time of the acoustic neuroma resection, if known. If the status of the nerve is uncertain, electroneurography and EMGs can be helpful. If the nerve is known to be transected, little information can be gained from electrodiagnostic tests. In instances of unknown status, the key question that will determine a treatment plan is whether the nerve is irreversibly injured. The extratemporal bone nerve can be assessed electrodiagnostically with evoked voltage potential, if present, or the provocation of facial twitching and the degree of necessary stimulation. To obtain such is compared to the normal side. In the absence of any activity in the extratemporal portion, the intratemporal branches can be tested: the first branch, the greater petrosal, by a test of lacrimation as the Schirmer's test; the next branch, the stapedial, can be evaluated with an audiologic exam; the third, the chorda tympani, supplies taste to the anterior tongue.

The above discussion, though, is largely academic from two viewpoints. The first is that unless some electrodiagnostic evidence of recovery is evident, the hiatus in this age of a patient signals little probability of spontaneous recovery. Second, in all likelihood, in a patient of this age, operative intervention in the form of a neurotization procedure such as a cross-facial nerve graft, discussed below, or even masseter motor nerve transfer to the facial branches, is probably not indicated.)

2. Outline a treatment plan. (Although the efficacy of cross-facial nerve grafts and free muscle transfer in the elderly has been debated, probably the appropriate approach to this individual case is a temporalis myoplasty for the lower face and local procedures for the upper. The conventional method of the use of the temporalis muscle as a dynamic transfer is to harvest from the temporalis fossa using a supraperiosteal extension and then reflect a portion of the muscle, usually anterior, over the arch of the zygoma and subcutaneously to the lips and modiolus. The more contemporary method of the use of the temporalis is termed temporalis myoplasty and is performed through a coronal incision and release from the coronoid process of the tendon of insertion and passage beneath the zygomatic arch through the buccal space to the upper lip and commissure. The temporalis tendon is employed for the repair, and the muscle is limited to the anterior portion. Occasionally, the arch is osteotomized. Patients, by cortical re-education, learn to trigger the trigeminal, the innervation of the temporalis as a muscle of mastication, to enable contraction. The myoplasty modification avoids the potential prominence created by the muscle reflection over the zygomatic arch as well as temporal hollowing by the loss of the muscle from the fossa. Salutary procedures for the upper face include permanent tarsorrhaphy, if needed, for cornea protection, direct brow lift for ptosis, and possibly placement of upper lid gold weights.)
3. Describe a treatment plan for a 35-year-old patient. (To complete the discussion, in a younger patient in a similar clinical scenario, the treatment plan would consist of either a single- or two-stage approach, both achieved with microvascular transfer of muscle flaps, usually the gracilis. Other muscles described include the pectoralis minor and serratus anterior. The donor nerve in the gracilis is innervated by the obturator nerve. In single-stage reconstruction, the obturator is powered by the motor nerve to the masseter. With two-stage reconstruction, cross-face nerve grafts are employed by identification of branches of the facial nerve on the uninvolved side, usually buccal and zygomatic, that provide the donor nerves to be anastomosed to the cross-face nerve grafts, usually the sural. The grafts are tunneled across the upper lip to lie in the subcutaneous tissue on the paralyzed side in anticipation of the eventual provision of power to the obturator nerve of the gracilis.

The other aspect of rehabilitation of facial paralysis is the concept of a "babysitter" procedure. Since the time interval for axonal growth at an inch a month from the donor branches of the uninjured facial nerve to the distal end of the cross-face nerve grafts is approximately 9 months minimum and an additional several months to continue growth into the obturator nerve to arrive at the motor end plates of the muscle, concerns arise about progressive fibrosis of the axonal tubes as well as the motor end plates. In the past, the "babysitter" procedure was performed with a hemi-hypoglossal nerve transfer, which has been replaced by the availability of the motor nerve to the masseter. The babysitter procedure is optimally applied to patients with an irreversible, more proximal nerve injury to preserve the structure and function of distal facial nerve branches in anticipation of eventual anastomosis of the cross-face nerve grafts.)

Case-Based Conference

Case 2: Facial Paralysis

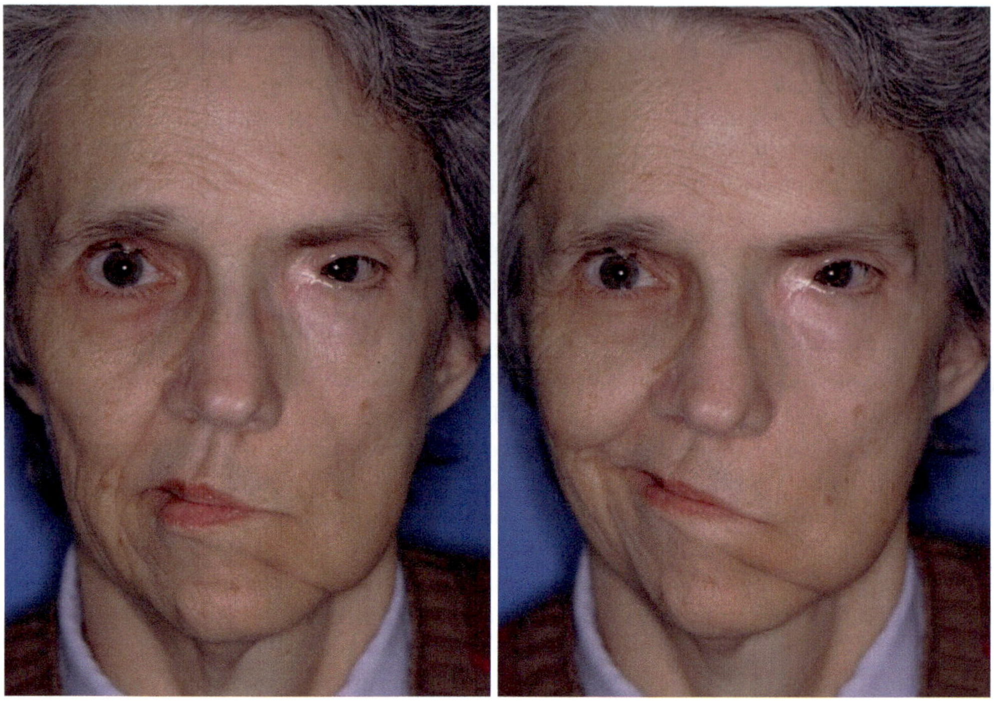

A 65-year-old s/p 2 years after resection of acoustic neuroma and performance of a medial tarsorrhaphy. The patient is tumor-free by a recent MRI and did not receive radiation therapy.

1. Describe what you see on the slide(s) and add a focused history and physical examination to yield the information you need to outline her treatment plan.
   (a) Are any tests indicated? Justify.
2. How does this injury differ from a facial nerve injury in parotid surgery, and how would you apply that difference in terms of this particular case with the EMG?
   (a) Additional tests?
   (b) Why might this patient be more at risk for keratitis than a patient who suffered facial nerve injury during a parotidectomy?
3. What is the pathologic anatomy?
4. Give a treatment plan if the scenario is 7 months post-injury.
5. In the current scenario, what would be the most comprehensive approach, and what are the pros and cons? What would be the components of an alternate treatment plan?

Case-Based Conference: Discussion

Case 2: Facial Paralysis

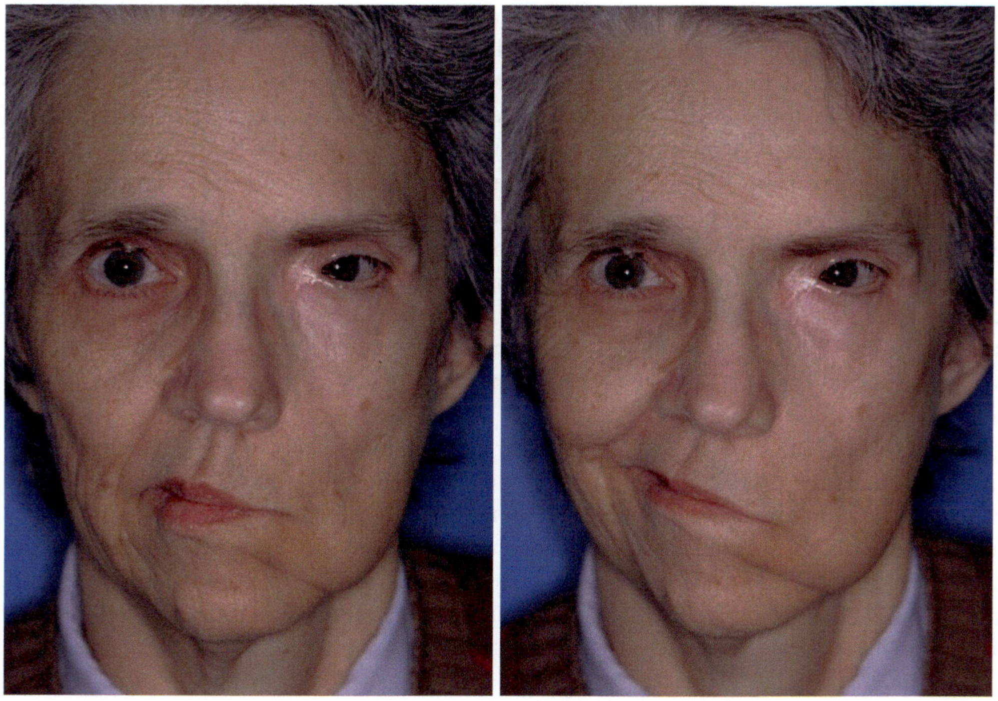

A 65-year-old s/p 2 years after resection of acoustic neuroma and performance of a medial tarsorrhaphy. The patient is tumor-free by a recent MRI and did not receive radiation therapy.

1. Describe what you see on the slide(s) and add a focused history and physical examination to yield the information you need to outline her treatment plan. (The photos demonstrate the patient's face in partial and full animation. Present are all the stigmata of complete left facial palsy: brow ptosis and a smooth forehead without frontalis creases, effaced nasolabial fold, and a sagging oral commissure. All of these findings are accentuated in full animation. Evident also is a left medial tarsorrhaphy.

   The clinical examination would begin with questions about recurrent eye inflammation and oral incontinence and then queries if the patient had evidence of facial palsy immediately postoperative. Some estimate of the level of fitness/frailty should be accomplished by questions about activities of daily living. Past medical history for comorbidities and social history for tobacco and drug use would be important. The physical examination essentially focuses on the eye for any evidence of keratoconjunctivitis and the presence of a Bell's phenomenon.)
   (a) Are any tests indicated? Justify. (If the status of the nerve is uncertain, electroneurography and EMGs are indicated. Evidence, if any, of an evoked action potential, evidence of fibrillation activity in the facial muscles, or a totally silent EMG can be helpful. If the nerve is known to be transected or resected with the tumor, little information could be gained from EMGs.)
2. How does this injury differ from a facial nerve injury in parotid surgery, and how would you apply that difference in terms of this particular case with the EMG? (The parotid injury is, of course, extratemporal, and the facial nerve was injured in the case scenario with the cranial procedure medial to the internal auditory meatus. As such, the intratemporal bone branches can be assessed: the greater petrosal, the first branch, by a test of lacrimation such as the Schirmer's test; the next branch, the stapedial, can be evaluated with an audiologic exam; the third, chorda tympani, supplies taste to the anterior tongue. The function of any or all of these branches, if the status of the nerve is unknown, can indicate recovery.)
   (a) Additional tests? (If any doubt exists, the eye should be examined with fluorescein to determine the presence of exposure keratitis.)
   (b) Why might this patient be more at risk for keratitis than a patient who suffered facial nerve injury during a parotidectomy? (The combination of paralysis of the orbicularis and the absence of or markedly diminished lacrimation.)

3. What is the pathologic anatomy? (Complete loss of mimetic function from a complete intracranial facial nerve lesion.)
4. Give a treatment plan if the scenario is 7 months post-injury. (The plan would hinge on a totally different pathophysiology than the representative case. The physiology of peripheral nerve injury in this instance, an injury 7 months ago, is that irreversible damage to the motor end-plates and axonal conduits has not occurred yet. A hemi-hypoglossal nerve transfer to the facial nerve is possible but is probably of historical interest only. A simple one-stage approach is the transfer of a motor nerve, the innervation of the masseter, to the proximal stump of the facial nerve. That option often results in mass actions and a relatively low patient satisfaction index. The problem with direct nerve transfers is that often facial symmetry is restored at rest if the duration, including the 6 or more months necessary for peripheral regeneration, sums to less than 2 years post-injury, yet synkinesis is still a usual occurrence. Although direct motor transfer would preserve the distal axons and the motor end plates and could function as such as a "babysitter procedure". A more comprehensive treatment plan would be a cross-face nerve graft. Cross-face nerve grafting is accomplished by identification of the buccal and zygomatic branches of the facial nerve on the contralateral side as donors, anastomosis to a harvested autologous sural nerve that is tunneled via the upper lip to the opposite side. After a hiatus of several months, a muscle, most commonly the gracilis, is designed and tailored to provide dynamic contraction and mimic the actions of the functional musculature of the mouth. The gracilis is powered by anastomosis of the sural to the obturator nerve.

   To provide an objective yardstick of the results, the House-Brackman scale of six levels of severity of the facial nerve injury can be utilized or, more contemporaneously, the use of 3D video.)
5. In the current scenario, what would be the most comprehensive approach, and what are the pros and cons? What would be the components of an alternate treatment plan? (The most comprehensive approach to this patient would be a two-stage plan with a preliminary cross-facial nerve grafting followed at about 9 months by free gracilis muscle microvascular transfer with anastomosis of the cross-facial nerve graft to the obturator nerve of the gracilis as described above. The pros are the possible restoration of voluntary mimetic muscle function of sufficient strength to enable a satisfactory cosmetic and functional result. The principal con is the progressive obliteration over time of the distal axonal pathways and fibrosis of the motor end plates. Since the patient is two years post-injury and an additional 15–18 months for innervation to be complete, the probabilities of a successful outcome are not great.

   An alternate treatment plan would be directed toward a symptomatic approach, driven by a careful and detailed consultation with the patient. Although the patient does not seem to have exposure keratitis and has a long-standing medial tarsorrhaphy, in a similar scenario, another initial option would be lubrication with taping/patching at night time: a lateral horizontal lid shortening procedure such as a Kuhnt-Zymanoski canthoplasty or permanent tarsorrhaphy. Lid loading, either alone or in combination with the above procedures, can be performed with the placement of a gold wafer within the upper eyelid. The lower face paralysis could benefit from a regional muscle transfer as a digastric for the lower lip ± a transfer of the masseter as well. The temporalis can be used as a segmental transfer in either a dynamic or static, dynamic preferred, for the lower face. Mini-temporalis can also be utilized for eyelid closure, but frequently, muscle transfers either to the eye or to the mouth are performed as a secondary or adjunct procedure in those patients with incomplete recovery.)

Intraoperative

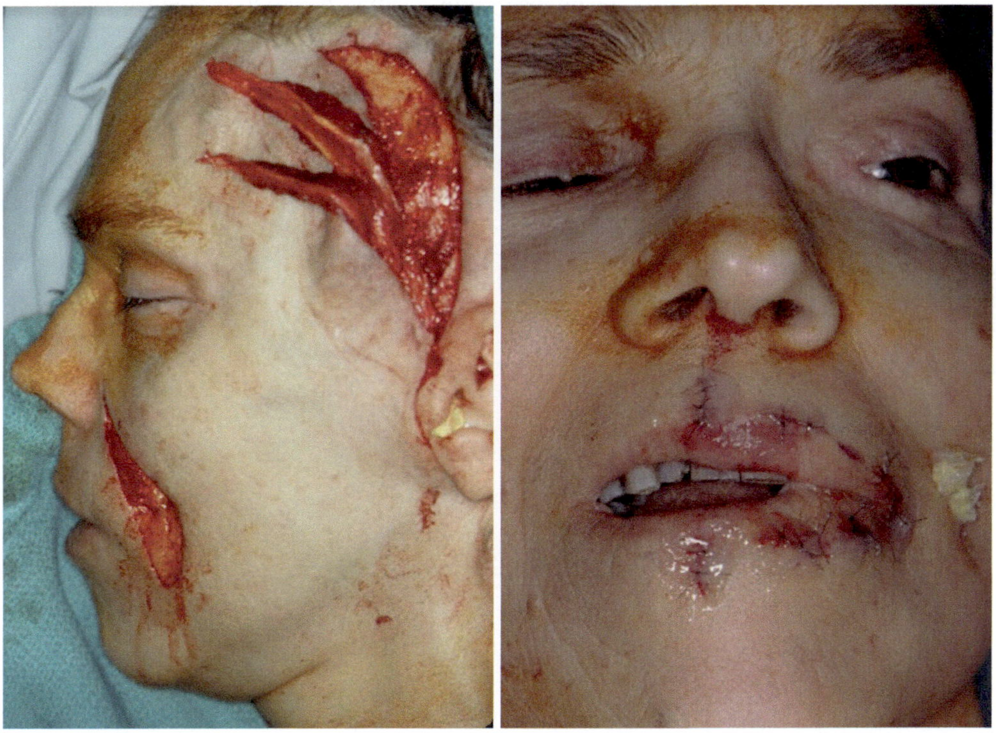

A temporalis dynamic transfer has been selected and divided into three mini temporalis transfers to both the upper and lower lip. The second photo depicts the patient after completion of the transfer with a transcutaneous bolster in place.

Postoperative (6 Months)

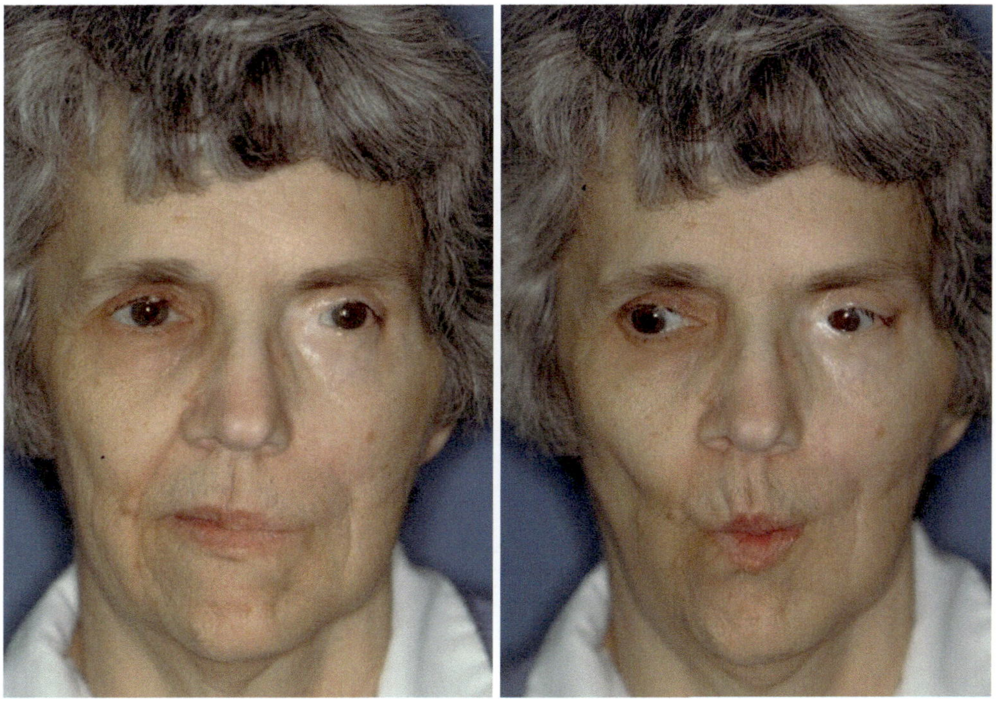

Two photos are provided that illustrate the patient postoperatively in repose and with voluntary pursing of the mouth.

In-Service Examination

1. An injury to the facial nerve during mastoidectomy, in addition to facial palsy, will produce the following deficits:
   (a) Loss of lacrimation, lingual taste, and high-frequency hearing loss
   (b) Loss of lingual taste
   (c) Loss of lacrimation
   (d) Loss of lacrimation, lingual taste, and vertigo
2. Resection of the proximal facial nerve during parotidectomy is optimally managed by:
   (a) Immediate autologous nerve graft
   (b) Delayed autologous nerve graft
   (c) Immediate masseteric motor nerve transfer
   (d) Delayed masseteric motor nerve transfer
   (e) Immediate cross-facial nerve grafting
3. The maximal hiatus between injury and primary repair in facial nerve injury before irreversible changes in the distal nerve and motor end plates is:
   (a) 3 months
   (b) 6 months
   (c) 12 months
   (d) 24 months

46 Upper One-Third Fractures

Bibliography

Sharabi SE, Koshy JC, Thornton JF, Hollier LH, "Facial fractures", *Plast Reconstr Surg.*, (2011); 127(2):**25e–34e and Videos 6, 7 ONLY (For junior residents)**

Ricketts S, Gill HS, Fialkov JA, et al., "Facial fractures", *Plast Reconstr Surg.*, (2016); 137(2):**424–26e and Video 1 and 2 ONLY. (For junior residents)**

Manolodis S and Hollier Jr LH, "Management of Frontal Sinus Fractures", *Plast Reconstr Surg.*, (2007); 120(7) Supplement 2:**32S–46S. (Overview)**

Sawatari Y and Caceres J, Ch. 43 "Frontal Sinus Fractures", Current Therapy in Oral and Maxillofacial Surgery, *Saunders*, (2011); pgs. **346–353.**

Jain SA, Manchio JV, Weinzweig J, "Role of the Sagittal View of Computed Tomography in Evaluation of the Nasofrontal Ducts in Frontal Sinus Fractures", *The Journal of Craniofacial Surgery*, (2010); 21(6): **1672–1673 (Discussion only).**

Cole P, Kaufman Y, Momoh A, et al., "Techniques in Frontal Sinus Fracture Repair", *Plast Reconstr Surg.*, (2009); 123(5):**1578–1579 (Video).**

Chen TM, Wang HJ, Chen SL, et al. "Reconstruction of Post-traumatic Frontal-Bone Depression Using Hydroxyapatite Cement", *Annals of Plastic Surgery.* (2004) 52:**303–308.**

Manson PN and Iliff NT, Chapter 116 "Fractures of the Orbital Roof." Hornblass, A. Oculoplastic Orbital and Reconstructive Surgery. Williams & Wilkins, (1990), **pp 1139–1150.**

Coon D, Yuan N, Jones D, Howell LK, et al., "Defining pediatric orbital roof fractures: Patterns, sequelae, and indications for operation", *Plast Reconstr Surg.*, (2014); 134(3):**442e–448e.**

Cayli, SR, Kocak A, Alkan A, et al. "Intraorbital Encephalocele: An Important Complication of Orbital Roof Fractures in Pediatric Patients", *Pediatric Neurosurgery.* (2003) 39:**240–245.**

Gebran SG, Lopez J, Wasicek PJ, et al., "Surgical Treatment and Visual Outcomes of Adult Orbital Roof Fractures", *Plast Reconstr Surg.*, (2021); 147(1):**82e–83e, 89e–92e.**

Abu-Ghname A, Banuelos J, Oliver JD, et al., "Outcomes and Complications of Pediatric Cranioplasty: A Systematic Review", *Plast Reconstr Surg.*, (2019); 144(3):**440e–42e (Discussion).**

Piazza M, Grady MS, "Cranioplasty", *Neurosurg Clin N Am*, (2017); 28:**257 (Table 1 ONLY).**

Brichacek M, Antonyshyn O, Edwards G, et al., "Decision-Making in Adult Cranial Vault Reconstruction", *Plast Reconstr Surg.*, (2021); 148(1):**109e–118e including videos.**

Videos

Chaudhry O, Isakson M, Franklin A, et al., "Facial Fractures Pearls and Perspectives", *Plast Reconstr Surg.,* (2018); 141(5):**742e Video 5 ONLY.**

Sharabi SE, Koshy JC, Thornton JF, Hollier LH, "Facial fractures", *Plast Reconstr Surg.*, (2011); 127(2):**25e Video 7 ONLY.**

Faculty Discussion and Study Guide

Frontal Sinus: Anatomy, Epidemiology

1. What is the age of initiation of pneumatization of the frontal sinus? (Age 2 but radiographically age 8.)
   (a) Adult size? (12–15 year old)
   (b) Frequency of congenitally absent? (4%)
2. Draw a schematic or graphic representation of the anatomical relationships between the frontal sinus, orbital regions, ethmoids, nasopharynx, and anterior fossa (see Fig. 46.1).
3. What is the importance of the presence of a frontal bone fracture and the frontal sinus? (A frontal bone fracture, by

E. Luce, *A Curriculum for Plastic Surgery*, https://doi.org/10.1007/978-3-031-62087-4_46

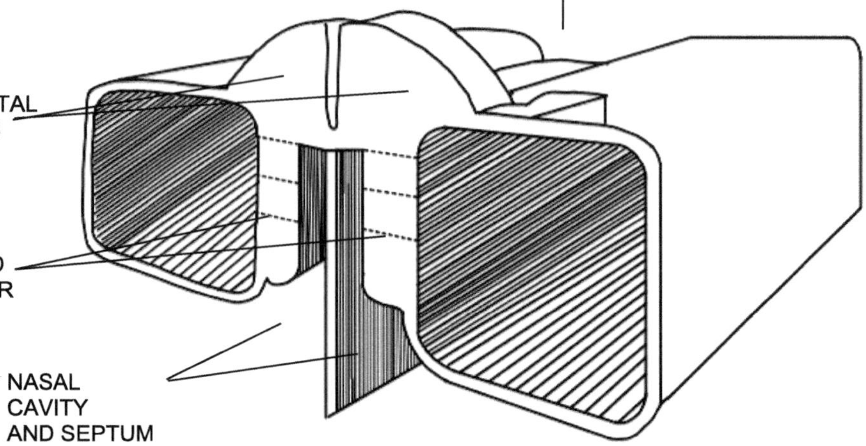

Fig. 46.1 Diagrammatic representation of the relationship of the nasal ethmoid orbital region to the frontal sinuses and anterior cranial fossa

definition, involves both tables. If the fracture line extends into the frontal sinus, the posterior wall is involved.)

4. Discuss the anatomy and normal variance of the frontonasal duct. (Lies in the posterior medial portion of the sinus, lined with pseudostratified columnar respiratory epithelium, and drains into the anterior portion of the middle meatus. An ostium only exists instead of a duct in about a third of the cases, and drainage through anterior ethmoid air cells in perhaps another one-third.)
   (a) Into what part of the nasal cavity does the duct drain? (Technically, beneath the most anterior portion of the middle meatus. Actually, the ostium of the duct is superior and anterior to the most anterior portion of the middle meatus.)
5. What are the foramina of Breschet? (Mucosa-lined dehiscences of the bone that allow venous drainage through the posterior wall of the sinus into the extradural space.)
   (a) Significance? (A potential route for the spread of infection into the intracranial space that can lead to meningitis and even epidural, subdural, and cerebral abscesses.)
6. Epidemiology: What are the type and frequency of associated head and neck injuries in frontal sinus fractures? (A high incidence of nasoethmoid orbital, NEO, and orbital fractures, forehead lacerations, and intracranial injury such as cerebral contusion.)
7. How does the epidemiology of associated injuries differ in the pediatric population between the frontal sinus and orbital roof fractures? (Orbital roof fractures can frequently, perhaps evenly commonly, for an uncommon fracture, occur with relatively minor trauma such as a fall. In contrast, frontal sinus fractures in children are the result of a tremendous frontal impact force. Also, obviously, the average age for frontal sinus fracture in children is considerably older than orbital roof fractures.)

Evaluation, Management

1. Given the overall perspective of why optimal management of frontal sinus fractures is crucial. (Inappropriate or inadequate treatment can result in not only cosmetic deformity but also acute meningitis, intracranial abscess, and the chronic complication of mucopyocele and osteomyelitis.)
2. What are the clinical findings in frontal sinus fractures? (Few. Edema may obscure depression-deformity and cerebrospinal fluid, CSF, and rhinorrhea may be concealed by mucus and clotted blood or drainage posteriorly into the posterior pharynx.)
3. Associated ocular injuries are considerably more frequent in frontal sinus fractures. What associated fracture should heighten suspicion of the same? (Extension of the frontal sinus fracture into the orbital roof or superior orbital rim.)
4. Rather than focus on classification, what are the three principal factors that dictate management? (Fracture location and displacement for which the anterior table is an aesthetic consideration; involvement of the central nervous system, CNS, which is determined by posterior wall fracture and displacement; and finally, the involvement of the drainage system, the nasofrontal duct, which can be responsible for both early and late complications.)
   (a) What can be a source of CSF rhinorrhea besides the posterior wall of the frontal sinus? (A fracture through the cribriform plate, which may or may not be evident on a CT scan. However, one should assume the source of the CSF leak is a dural tear behind a posterior wall fracture, if present.)

5. What associated facial fracture in conjunction with a frontal sinus fracture increases the probability of nasofrontal duct involvement? (NEO)
   (a) Why? (Extension of the fractures into the anterior ethmoid air cells may involve the nasofrontal duct.)
6. What is the laboratory confirmation of CSF rhinorrhea? (Beta-2 transferrin)
   (a) A bedside test? (Filter paper halo test. Not particularly sensitive or specific.)
   (b) What is the logistical problem with beta-2 transferrin? (Usually, the test requires a distant laboratory assessment, which may require anywhere from 3–5 days.)
7. Discuss the important findings of the CT scan. (Determine the magnitude of anterior table fracture and degree of displacement, if the posterior table is fractured and displaced, the presence of associated NEO, nasoethmoid orbital fractures, the presence of pneumocephalus, and the presence of a fluid-filled sinus.)
   (a) What single view may be of assistance in the determination of the patency of the nasofrontal duct? (Sagittal. Frequently, the sagittal view will not be sufficiently definitive to determine the status of the duct.)
8. List surgical incisions for the management of frontal sinus fractures and describe the optimal choice. (Incisions that have been utilized include access through extensive forehead lacerations and transverse incisions through frown lines and, historically, a bilateral supra brow incision. The latter two are of historical interest only and are not utilized for a number of reasons, including the division of the supratrochlear and supraorbital nerves with resultant anesthesia superior to the incision. The most optimal approach is a bicoronal flap.)
   (a) Briefly describe the elevation of a bicoronal flap. (The design of the initial incision varies among surgeons, but the initial dissection is subgaleal and supraperiosteal until 2–3 cm superior to the superior orbital rim and then becomes subperiosteal unless a pericranial flap is planned. See below. The frontal branch of the facial nerve must be protected as the dissection progresses inferiorly and temporally. That protection is accomplished by utilizing the split of the deep temporal fascia into a superficial and deep portion approximately 3 cm or so superior to the zygomatic arch. By incision of the superficial portion, one accesses the superficial temporal fat pad and continues the dissection further inferiorly. The nerve is now superficial to the plane of dissection.)
9. How would you gain access to a frontal sinus for inspection of duct patency, repair, etc., if not possible through the fracture? (One must be able to define the location of the proposed sinusotomy through intact bone at the periphery of the sinus. The extent of the sinus can be mapped topographically on the anterior wall by one of two methods: One, a Caldwell view obtained at a 6 ft distance, which is then life-size or 1:1, and a template fashioned from the x-ray, sterilized, and utilized intraoperative to define the extent of the sinus on the cranial bone. Digitally, the view can be printed and subsequently sterilized. A second method is to illuminate the interior of the sinus by a nasal endoscope passed into the sinus from an endonasal approach. The latter requires intranasal cocaine to constrict the mucus membranes and passage of the endoscope at least into the anterior ethmoid air cells in order to illuminate the sinus. That maneuver can be technically difficult for the novice.)
10. Describe the technique of obliteration. (All sinus mucosa must be eradicated usually with a fine burr as well as periosteal elevators, small picks, curettes, ect; the plugging of the nasofrontal duct with temporalis muscle or fascia; the filling of the sinus with either corticocancellous bone or abdominal fat. This reviewer prefers the former since much of the fat, as in fat grafting elsewhere, will disappear. No role exists for the of alloplastic materials. That repair can be reinforced with a pericranial flap or, if more bulk is needed, a galeal frontalis flap. The latter can create a soft tissue contour defect of the bicoronal scalp flap and the forehead. The nasofrontal duct must be plugged with temporalis fascia, muscle, or bone to prevent communication between the obliterated sinus and the nasopharynx. The use of a pericranial flap needs to be anticipated since the standard periosteal incision 2–3 cm superior to the superior orbital rim will devascularize the flap.)
11. Describe the technique of cranialization. (Cranialization is essentially the removal of the posterior wall to allow the frontal lobes and dura to expand into the space previously occupied by the sinus and is done in conjunction with a craniotomy for repair of dural tears. The posterior wall bone is simply excised and removed. Some writers have described the removal of the posterior wall through the frontal sinus alone. Clearly, if the indications are present for removal of the posterior wall, such as CSF leak and dural tears, the conventional approach would be a craniotomy. A pericranial or galeal frontalis flap, as outlined above, is usually added. To gain access to the sinus for the flap, a small bone gap is left inferiorly just above the orbital bar much as a letter into a mailbox.)
12. Differentiate and describe a pericranial and a galeal-frontalis flap. (Although these terms are used interchangeably, a strict anatomical definition would entail a pericranial flap as composed of periosteum only at least inferiorly. Characteristically, this is accomplished by a periosteal incision at a variable point superior, dependent on the length needed, to the bicoronal skin incision

through the periosteum and subperiosteal dissection to preserve a flap of periosteum or pericranium. Galeal-frontalis flaps are inferiorly based soft tissue flaps raised from the deep surface of the bicoronal flap and are based on the supraorbital and/or supratrochlear vessels. The drawback of a pericranial flap is the thin and somewhat flimsy nature of the tissue; a galeal-frontalis flap certainly will be thick and well-vascularized but may create a vertical soft tissue deformity of the forehead.)

13. What is spontaneous osteoneogenesis? (The technique of obliteration of a sinus by the methods outlined above, except the sinuses remain empty and, presumably, will fill with new bone. Although that occurs in experimental animals, such has not been demonstrated in humans and is probably not a recommended technique.)
14. The endoscopic approach to frontal sinus injuries is described in some of the readings. Outline the pros and cons. (Actually, two different routes of the endoscopic approach are described, one from a subcutaneous scalp approach and the other endonasal. The latter has been described much more commonly for the management of frontal sinusitis. The pros are obviously the lack of an external incision. The cons are substantial. First, considerable expertise is required; second, no port exists for operating instruments, so the method is primarily inspection only, and third, usually not mentioned, is a necessity for internal ethmoidectomy for adequate access. As a result, the endoscopic approach to frontal sinus fractures has not gained widespread acceptance and cannot be regarded as a conventional approach to these injuries. One possibility is a displaced anterior table and a non-obstructed sinus. A scalp incision for port access could be utilized, and a small direct incision for reduction and plate placement.)
15. Manage the following problems:
    (a) A closed linear nondisplaced fracture of the anterior wall with an air-fluid level. (Observe; repeat CT scan 4–6 weeks? Endoscopic assessment of the nasofrontal duct.)
    (b) An open overlying laceration anterior wall fracture with little displacement. (Operative management with irrigation of the wound and sinus with determination of nasofrontal duct patency. Determination of nasofrontal duct patency by irrigation of the duct with methylene blue with concomitant Q-tips or cottonoid patties placed intranasally in the region of the nasal frontal duct ostium. Prior vasoconstriction of the mucosa with 4% cocaine can be helpful.)
    (c) A displaced fracture of the anterior wall. (Operative repair with a bicoronal approach with ORIF and intraoperative assessment of duct patency.)
    (d) A fracture of the anterior wall with a concomitant NEO or medial superior orbital rim fracture. (Repair and probable obliteration because, in all likelihood, the nasofrontal duct is obstructed.)
    (e) Comminuted fracture of the anterior wall with bone loss. (Repair with split cranial bone grafts; determine ductal patency. If the duct is patent, nothing else; if obstructed, then obliteration. Small defects, even in the presence of comminution, can be managed with the use of titanium mesh.)
16. Fracture of the anterior and posterior table. (Exploration: determine if CSF leak is present through the posterior table; if not, assure patency of the nasofrontal duct as above and repair the anterior table. If dural tears and CSF leaks are evident, repair with craniotomy will probably be necessary.)
    (a) Posterior table fracture with disruption, dural tear, and CSF leak on exploration. (Needs a bifrontal craniotomy and cranialization of the sinus by excision of the posterior wall with burring of the mucosa of the anterior wall and base of the sinus; plugging nasofrontal duct +/− pericranial flap.)
17. Complications: In general terms, what are the early versus the late complications? (The early complications are related to intracranial infections such as meningitis and epidural abscess, etc.; late complications are either mucopyocele secondary to an obstructed injured frontal sinus or deformities of the forehead region. The mucosa of an obstructed frontal sinus or any of the paranasal sinuses will continue to secrete mucus and form a mucocele. Bacterial colonization from the nasal cavity will create a mucopyocele, capable of osteomyelitis and destruction of adjacent bone, including the ethmoid and posterior wall of the frontal sinus.)
18. Briefly discuss the management of the late complications of frontal sinus fractures: mucopyocele and forehead contour deformities. (The treatment of mucopyocele hinges on the extent of the disease process. A common thread through the variety of procedures available consists of excision of all osteomyelitis bone and either obliteration of the sinus or, in cases of intracranial involvement, cranialization of the sinus with soft tissue closure of any communication with the nasal cavity, usually with a galeal-frontalis flap. The late treatment of contour deformities is most commonly accomplished by a bicoronal flap with a variety of filler materials. Frequently utilized filler materials are the two commercially available varieties of hydroxyapatite paste that serve as bone conduction.)

Caveats

1. CSF rhinorrhea may not be from the sinus but may be the result of a cribriform plate fracture.
2. Obliteration is best performed with cancellous bone plus autogenous bone paste. Fat is not a particularly good

choice since only about 20% of the original volume may persist. The process of neo-osteogenesis as an appropriate option is highly questionable.
3. Alloplastic materials are not suitable for obliteration.
4. A galeal-frontalis flap is not necessary in primary cases and does leave a contour deformity of the forehead.
5. Associated naso-orbital ethmoid and complex midface fractures in conjunction with frontal sinus fractures represent a higher energy injury, more likelihood of a CSF leak, probable involvement and obstruction of the nasofrontal duct, and a more aggressive approach.
6. Undisplaced frontal sinus fractures and CSF leaks in the absence of other facial fractures, a distinctly uncommon combination, may be treated with bedrest for a week since 80% of such CSF leaks will resolve spontaneously. "Prophylactic" antibiotics are not indicated.

Orbital Roof Fractures, Skull Fractures

Editor's Note: The optic nerve and muscle involvement are discussed in the Orbital Fracture module VE.

1. What are the principal bony components of the orbital roof? (Lesser and greater wing of the sphenoid posteriorly; orbital plate of the frontal bone anteriorly and actually most of the roof)
2. Differentiate direct and indirect orbital roof fractures and describe the treatment implications. (Direct orbital roof fractures are very frequently associated with supraorbital ridge, frontal bone, and frontal sinus injuries, all of which will need repair. Indirect roof fractures are secondary to a direct impact force to the frontal bone/supraorbital ridge area with buckling that will produce fractures of the thin orbital roof, but the ridge and frontal bone remain intact and are subsequently more frequent in the pediatric population. If indirect fractures are asymptomatic and frequently are, treatment other than observation is usually not necessary.)
3. What are the clinical findings that are relatively specific to the supraorbital ridge/roof fractures? (One of the most accurate findings is secondary to the downward displacement of the rim and orbital roof fragments that produce a characteristic downward and forward position of the globe. That displacement may be sufficiently severe as to produce proptosis.)
4. Contrast the adult and pediatric orbital roof fracture populations. (The incidence and severity of associated intracranial injury is much higher than in the adult population.)
5. What are the important CT findings? (Degree of displacement of the roof, the magnitude of the diastasis in the pediatric population, particularly if greater than 2 mm; the presence of intracranial contents in the superior orbit; frontal bone fracture extending into the roof, orbital emphysema, pneumocephalus. As discussed below, the size of any bony defect can be measured in both the coronal and sagittal views.)
   (a) What is the importance of pediatric orbital roof fractures in the determination of the magnitude of the diastasis of the fracture fragments? (Fracture fragments with a diastasis of more than 2 or 3 mm have a propensity toward the development of a late, greater 30 days traumatic intraorbital encephalocele, particularly in the presence of contused brain parenchyma.)
6. Discuss blow-in and blow-out, or "up," orbital roof fractures. (Blow-in is the collapse of the orbital roof into the orbital space. Blow-out is an expansion of the orbital roof into the intracranial space.)
   (a) How do the mechanics of injury differ between the two? (Blow-in fractures are distinctly more common, and the mechanics are direct impact injury with associated fractures of the frontal bone and supraorbital ridge with extension into the orbital roof. Blow-out fractures, much less common, occur probably as a direct blow to the orbital contents with the extension of that force into the roof, similar to that mechanism of orbital floor fractures. The mechanics and injury are a clue to the considerably higher incidence of ocular injury in blow-out fracture than blow-in, although they are frequent in both.)
   (b) What are the clinical findings of each? (Blow-in may result in proptosis, dystopia, ptosis, and ocular motility problems. Blow-out may result in enophthalmos, dystopia, and ocular motility problems. Both may be complicated by CSF leak.)
7. What are the possible ocular motility problems? More specifically, what extraocular muscles may be involved? (Superior oblique and superior rectus.)
   (a) What are the findings in each? (The findings depend on whether the principal problem is entrapment or dysfunction, so an important muscle is the superior rectus, if entrapped, the patient will have difficulty looking downward on the involved side. If dysfunctional, the patient will have difficulty in looking upward. If a concomitant orbital floor fracture is present, the clinical picture can mimic entrapment of the inferior rectus.)

(b) What other ocular motility problems? (Involvement of the superior division of cranial nerve III can lead to ptosis and +/– pupillary changes. Levator palsy may be present.)
(c) Other ocular problems? (Optical nerve injury)
(d) What is the typical globe displacement in orbital roof fractures? (Downward and laterally as well as proptosis.)

8. What complication may present at 2–3 weeks, and how should the patient be worked up? (Pulsating exophthalmos and the workup indicated is MRI)
   (a) What can present a similar picture? (Carotid-cavernous sinus fistula)
9. What are the indications for operative repair in the pediatric orbital roof fracture population? (In addition to the finding of a diastasis of greater than 2–3 mm, the other indications are ocular motility issues, proptosis, exophthalmos, and perhaps a bony defect greater than 2 cm^2. Only a minority of patients will require operative interventions, and the majority will have non-displaced or minimally displaced fractures.)
10. What are the indications for operative repair of the adult orbital roof fracture patient? (Similar to pediatric patients, most adults with orbital roof fractures can be managed conservatively. The presence of globe displacement, ocular motility problems, and bony defects greater than 4 cm^2 are indications for operative interventions.)
11. Discuss and contrast the operative management of blow-in and blow-out fractures. (Blow-in possibly can be approached through a subcranial route with reduction and titanium mesh repair. Blow-out usually means an intracranial approach with either titanium mesh or, preferably, autogenous bone grafts harvested from the craniotomy bone plate.)

Cranioplasty

1. The available materials for reconstructive cranioplasty include autogenous and alloplastic. List. (Autogenous is available as fresh bone harvested from the usual donor site as calverial, rib, and iliac and "banked" craniectomy bone flaps. The last is usually the result of an acute decompressive craniectomy; the bone flap is stored, usually by freezing. Alloplastic materials include polymethylmethacrylate, PMMA, hydroxyapatite, HA, polyetheretherketone, PEEK, and titanium.)
   (a) Give a brief description of the alloplastic materials, including properties relative to bone growth. (None except HA have any capability to induce bone growth. HA has limited osteoinductive properties, and edge adherence occurs with PMMA.)
2. Give the pros and cons of each of the five available materials for cranioplasty. (Fresh bone for large defects requires the harvest of substantial amounts of autogenous bone with the potential morbidity of the donor site. Banked craniectomy bone flaps appear to have a substantial late infection rate; nevertheless, the principal advantage is the ideal in situ fit for the defect. HA has some osteoconductive capability, but that property is limited by defect size. In addition, HA is somewhat brittle and can be subject to fracture in vivo. PMMA has perhaps the highest infection rate, particularly in long-term follow-up, which may be the result of minimal contamination yet the formation of a biofilm. PMMA is readily available, relatively economical, and can be molded. The intraoperative disadvantage is an exothermic reaction during the admixture of the substances. PEEK is the most recent alloplastic material described and can be customized with the use of CAD/CAM. As an inert material, PEEK may also have a somewhat higher infection rate. Last, titanium mesh has been utilized and may have the overall lowest infection rate among the alloplastic materials.)

Video Notes

Sharabi SE, Koshy JC, Thornton JF, Hollier LH, "Facial fractures," *PRS*, (2011); 127(2):25e.

Video 6

A brief video of the assessment of frontal sinus fractures

Video 7

Operative video of a bicoronal flap with obliteration

Critique: A narrator disparages the evaluation of nasofrontal duct patency. Relies on neo-osteogenesis instead of filling the obliterated cavity with autogenous material.

Ricketts S, Gill HS, Fialkov JA, et al., "Facial fractures," *Plast. Recon. Surg.*, (2016); 137(2):424e.

Video 1

Slide presentation of bicoronal flap as well as buccal peroral approach to zygoma

Video 2

Slide presentation (short) of the basics of the frontal sinus assessment—similar to the video in Sharabi

Chaudhry O, Isakson M, Franklin A, et al., "Facial Fractures Pearls and Perspectives," *Plast. Reconstr. Surg.*, (2018); 141(5):172e.

Video 5

Slide Presentation-A child with pulsating exophthalmos with vertical dystopia

1. A bony defect of the orbital roof was repaired.

Brichacek M, Antonyshyn O, Edwards G, et al., "Decision-Making in Adult Cranial Vault Reconstruction", *Plast. Reconstr. Surg.*, (2021); 148(1):109e.

Video 1: Approximately 5 min

1. Acrylic cranioplasty with CAD/CAM; simulation to determine if skin-soft tissue is sufficient.
2. Acrylic poured and molded in OR!!
3. Galeal scoring of the raised flap.

Video 2: 4.5 min

1. Use of titanium when ultimate defect size is unknown, such as time, osteomyelitis, osteoradionecrosis, mucopyocoele, etc.
2. Use CAD/CAM proprietary "molding and forming tool" (Calavera surgical design) for use in the OR.
3. Fibrous dysplasia case- frontotemporal; simulated defect; modeled the titanium plate intraoperatively.

Video 3: 4 min 40 s

1. Use of autogenous bone, and the specific indications were potential contamination by paranasal sinuses; defects not precisely determined preoperatively.
2. Structural integrity is the use of cortical bone and the space-filling use of cancellous bone.

Video 4: Hostile environment; 6.5 min

1. Examples: radiation; multiple prior surgeries; infection; composite defects including cranial base; potential dead space; soft tissue deficit
2. Approach is staged- the first stage addresses the primary risk factor
3. Second stage is then acrylic cranioplasty designed in the OR, although it could have been prior to CAD/CAM

Case-Based Conference

Case 1: Orbital Roof

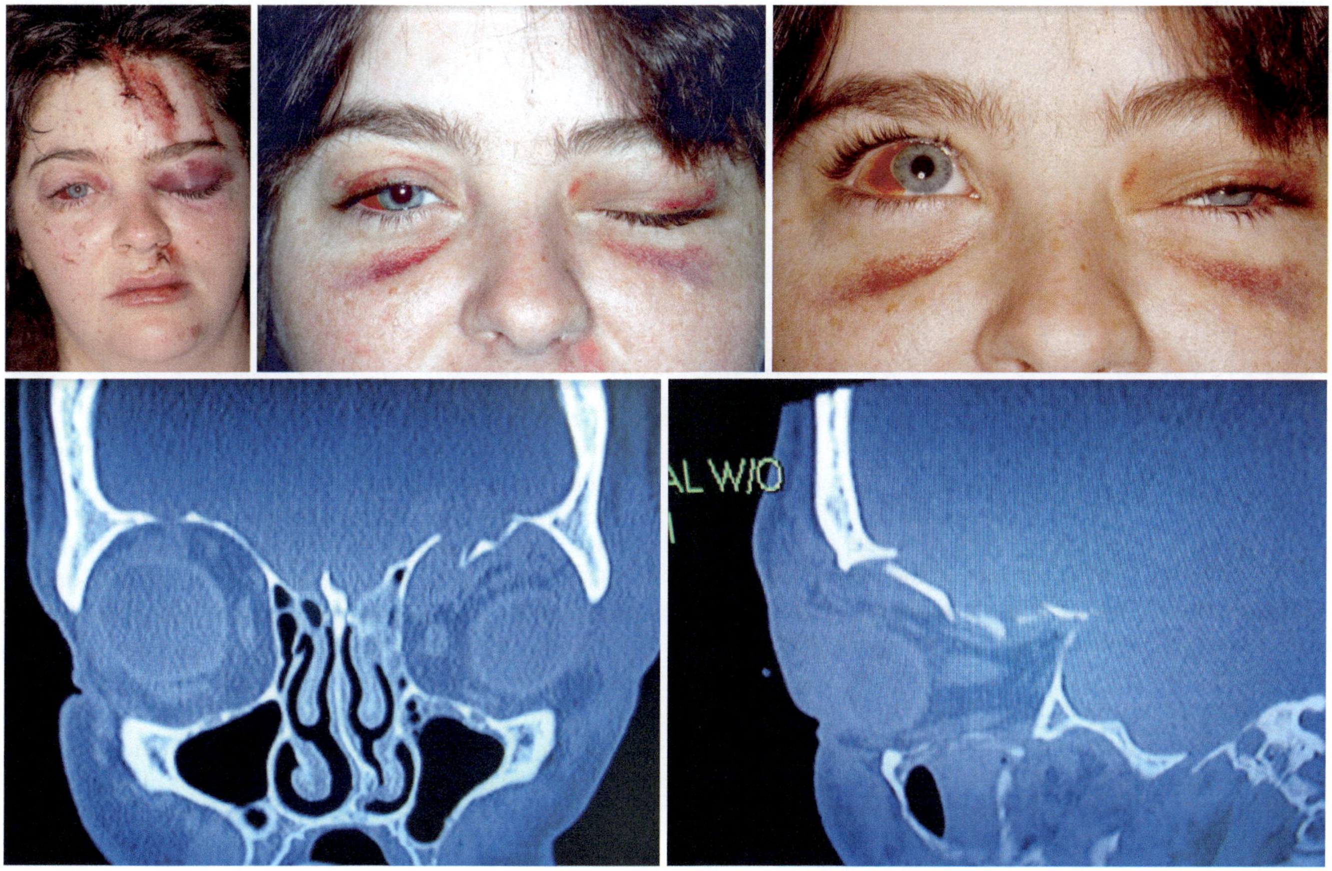

22-year-old injured in an MVA. The first photo is 18 h post-injury. Photos 2 and 3 are 10 days.

1. Describe the findings in the slide(s) and add a focused clinical exam. The patient is alert and oriented. Describe the CT slices provided.

2. What additional slices, if any, would be of value in your treatment plan?
3. What is the pathologic anatomy, and what aspects of the pathology dictate the treatment plan?
4. Develop a treatment plan.

Case-Based Conference: Discussion

Case 1: Orbital Roof

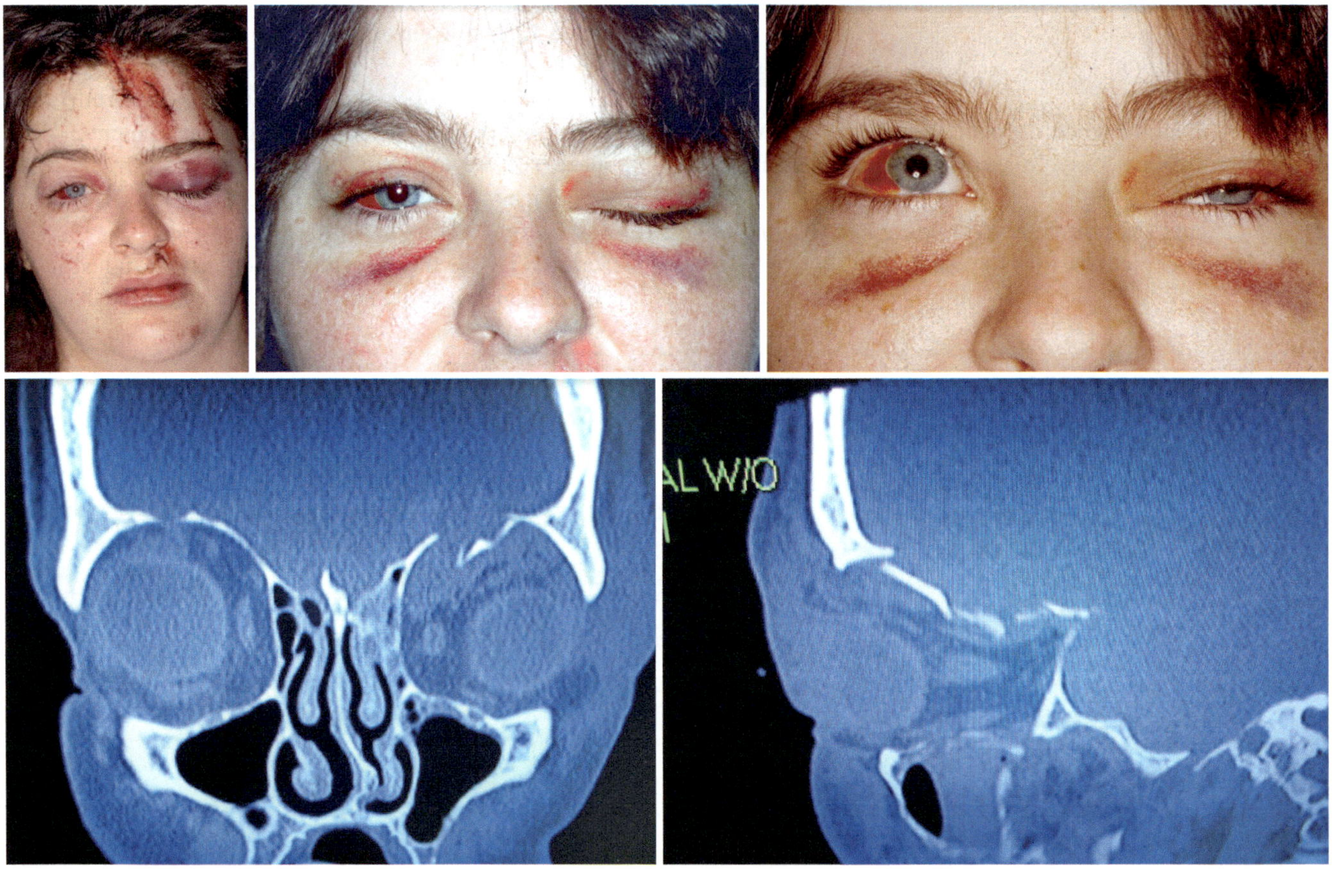

22-year-old injured in an MVA. The first photo is 18 h post-injury. Photos 2 and 3 are at 10 days.

1. Describe the findings in the slide(s) and add a focused clinical exam. The patient is alert and oriented. Describe the CT slices provided. (The first photo, 18 h post-injury, depicts a full facial frontal view of a young woman. The forehead has two vertical lacerations, just off midline, beginning at the frontal hairline and extending for approximately 3 cm inferiorly-recently sutured. An additional vertical laceration of similar length is present in the mid-left forehead. The left forehead has broad areas of contusion consistent with blunt force. The remarkable finding is the left periorbital region, marked by a diffusely ecchymotic upper eyelid, the superior limit of the ecchymosis is the infrabrow region. The lid is completely closed, and no ecchymosis is seen in the visible infraorbital area. The right orbital region has a small, mild ecchymosis in the medial upper lid. The right pupil is mildly constricted. The only remarkable finding is a bulbar conjunctival hematoma limited to the lateral sclera. A small sutured laceration is present in the superior aspect of the left upper lip. No deformity of the lip, asymmetry of the face, or telecanthus is evident.

   Photo 2, at 2 weeks post-injury, is a close-up limited to the orbit, nose, and upper lip. The ecchymotic areas, particularly in the left upper lid, are resolving. The left eye is closed, and the right upper lid is now ptotic in this view. The lash margin is about a mm below the superior limbus of the pupil. The pupil is constricted in mid-position. In photo 3, the right upper lid is fully elevated, and the eye is looking in an upward gaze. In the left eye, in contrast, the lid is markedly ptotic, the lash margin at mid-pupil, and the gaze is central.

The preamble states the patient is alert and oriented, so the first specific questions after circumstances of injury and co-morbidities, doubtful in this instance and assuming the patient has been cleared by the trauma team, are centered on the ocular and periorbital area such as pain and subjective vision changes in either eye. Any change, improvement, or deterioration during the 2 weeks post-injury of lid ptosis, pain, or vision changes should be elicited. The physical exam would include, as with any facial trauma patient, palpation of each facial third, including a careful palpation of the left supraorbital region and assessment of the integrity of the bony forehead. Evaluation of facial nerve function is included, as well as sensation over the distribution of the left supraorbital and supratrochlear nerves. The exam will then center on the evaluation of vision by confrontation with finger counting at 3 ft, pupillary reaction, and extraocular motions in each quadrant of each eye. The upper lid levator function, if any, is measured in the left eye. The patient would benefit from a formal retinal and ophthalmologic exam. Of course, optimal medical care would have mandated at the time of the injury the performance and documentation of a complete maxillofacial and ocular examination.)

Describe the CT slices provided (The coronal view demonstrates pathology in the left orbit. The slices provided depict a roof fracture with a "blow-in" component with some degree of comminution. The degree of inferior displacement is substantial, probably 7–8 mm. The soft tissue is abnormal as well, with a soft tissue density in the superior orbit occupying the superior one-third and confluent with the roof. A discrete soft tissue density, discernible separate and superior to the globe, is also seen in the same area as the superior rectus. Another similar-size soft tissue density is apparent medial to the globe, probably the medial rectus. Although the two orbits are not exactly at the same level, the left globe appears displaced inferiorly. The other CT slice is a sagittal view that also demonstrates an extensively comminuted orbital roof fracture. The soft tissue density seen on the coronal view appears to be primarily anterior, at least on the slice provided. Thickening of the entire superior periorbital region is evident. The level of the slice appears to be mid-globe, although the lens is not seen. A sagittal soft tissue density consistent with the inferior rectus is pictured, as well as a soft tissue structure consistent with the optic nerve. The superior rectus is not visualized on this slice.)

2. What additional slices, if any, would be of value in your treatment plan? (The importance of the CT scan is to establish the presence of a concomitant fracture of the frontal sinus or the frontal bone.)
3. What is the pathologic anatomy, and what aspects of the pathology dictate the treatment plan? (The patient has apparently sustained a frontal and forehead impact force, perhaps primarily on the left. The scans would rule out frontal sinus or frontal bone fracture, although the latter is quite common. The primary pathology is a left orbital roof fracture, and assuming the absence of a concomitant sinus injury, the treatment plan should be directed toward the orbital roof. A characteristic of this patient's fracture is one of extensive comminution and an inferior or inward displacement with a substantial associated soft tissue collection, consistent with either an intraorbital hematoma or perhaps a cerebrospinal fluid accumulation. On the sagittal view, the soft tissue density appears to involve the superior rectus. The clinical photos depict lid ptosis and loss of upward gaze on the left, indicative of impairment of levator function as well as compromise of the superior rectus. The former, levator dysfunction, may be secondary to the space-occupying soft tissue density of the anterior/superior orbit. The latter, superior rectus dysfunction, is either the result of entrapment by the roof fracture or by a direct nerve injury. The pathology that dictates the treatment plan includes the significant inward depression of roof bone fragments, the loss of superior rectus function, the possibility of dural injury and cerebrospinal fluid leak, and the prolapse of intracranial contents into the superior orbit.)
4. Develop a treatment plan. (The patient apparently has not improved over the 10 days subsequent to the injury. The appropriate treatment plan is the operative repair of the orbital roof. Given the CT and clinical findings at 18 h, certainly, an argument can be established for repair at that juncture. Nevertheless, the treatment plan at this juncture dictates a frontal craniotomy and repair of small dural leaks by neurosurgery. The bony fragments of the orbital roof are elevated and reconstructed with mini plates. If supplementary bone grafts are necessary, the frontal bone plate can be split and harvested.

Postoperatively, a pupillary response is checked in the postoperative recovery room. Although orbital roof fractures of a limited extent can, in a certain set of circumstances, be approached extracranially through an infra brow or upper lid incision, most particularly with the necessity to ascertain the presence of dural injury, roof fractures do not lend themselves to an extracranial approach. Significant dural disruption can set the stage for late encephalocele, more common perhaps in the pediatric setting but described in adult patients as well. To accomplish the goals of repair will require an intracranial approach and a frontal craniotomy. With an extradural elevation of the frontal lobe, the orbital roof is exposed, bone fragments debrided, the dura inspected, and evacuation of an intraorbital hematoma, if present, is accomplished. No attempt at incision and drainage of the fluid collection, probably blood, present in the intraconal fat. The larger bone fragments are elevated, and fixation is obtained with low-profile mini plates. Reconstruction of the roof may be necessary and can be accomplished with alloplastic material such as a titanium plate or the use of autologous bone, combined with the open reduction internal fixation of the native bone fragments. The autologous bone can be harvested from split calvarial bone grafts harvested from the craniotomy bone plate, and the dura is repaired either with resuture or alloplastic dura patch. The outcomes of the ocular findings in orbital roof fractures are guarded, dependent on the magnitude of the associated direct nerve and muscle injury.)

Postoperative (2 Months)

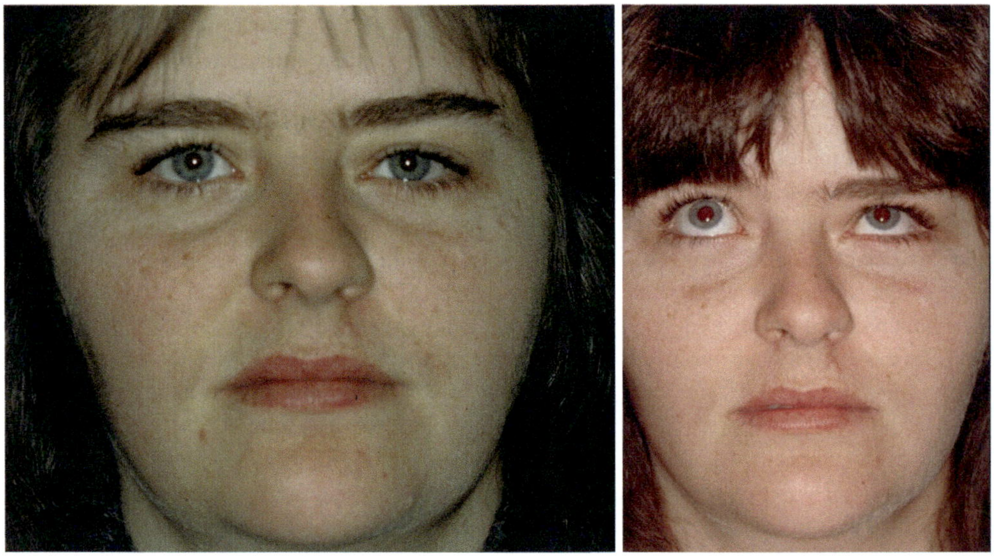

Postoperatively, upward gaze has been restored, and no enophthalmos or exophthalmos is present. A suggestion of vertical dystopia is depicted.

Case-Based Conference

Case 2: Frontal Sinus Injury

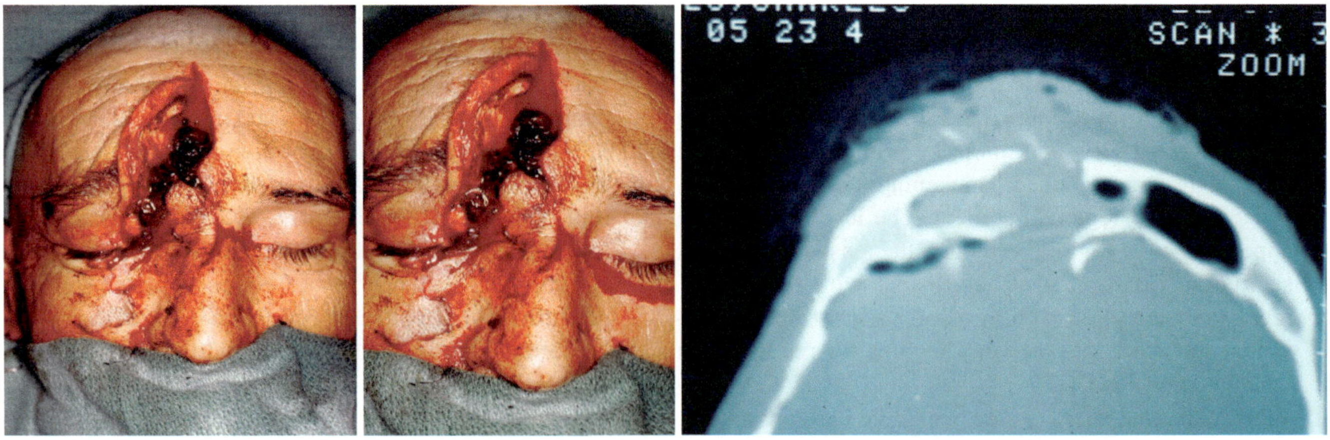

38-year-old. Injured in an industrial accident, unconscious and intubated.

1. Describe the clinical slide prior to the review of the CT scan findings. Add a physical examination.
   (a) Review the CT scan findings. Any additional slices that would be of value to you in devising a treatment plan?
   (b) Any other tests indicated? Justify.
2. Briefly outline the pathologic anatomy of this patient and how that pathology will determine your treatment plan. Consider in your description additional CT findings perhaps not evident on the slice provided. Outline your treatment plan in general and then give specifics, including incisions and a sequence of procedural steps.

Case-Based Conference: Discussion

Case 2: Frontal Sinus Injury

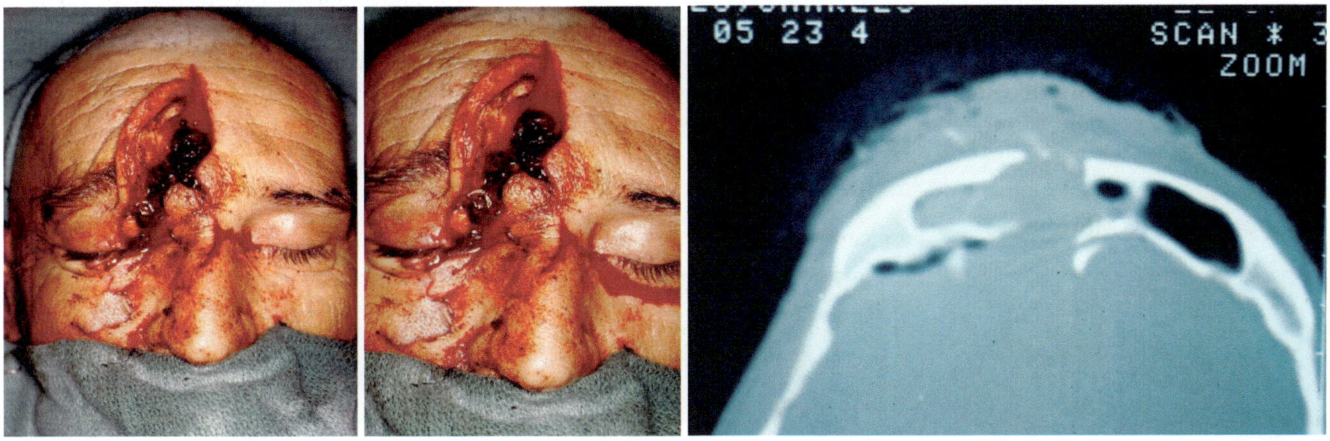

38-year-old. Injured in an industrial accident, unconscious and intubated.

1. Describe the clinical slide prior to the review of the CT scan findings. Add a physical examination. (The slide depicts an unconscious patient who is probably intubated with the most dramatic finding of a large vertical laceration of the forehead. The laceration extends from the frontal hairline through the medial right brow, upper eyelid, and to the lash margin. In the forehead component of the wound, bone is exposed on the right, and within the interior of the wound is dark, gelatinous material consistent with clotted blood. At the inferior extent, the upper eyelid, is a lobule of fat, probably intraorbital. The lids in both eyes are closed. No other deformities or findings are evident.

   Assuming the patient has been cleared by the trauma team, the principal objective of the physical examination is an assessment of the right globe for enophthalmos, exophthalmos, and pupillary reaction. The facial examination is completed, including detection of telecanthus of the right orbit, cerebrospinal fluid rhinorrhea within the right nares, occlusion, and the stability of the maxilla and the mandible.)
   (a) Review the CT scan findings. Any additional slices that would be of value to you in devising a treatment plan? (A single axial slice approximately at the level of the mid-sinus illustrates gross disruption of both anterior and posterior walls with a fluid-filled right frontal sinus. A bony defect of 2 cm of both the anterior and posterior walls is evident, as well as two small bone fragments intracranial. A small area of pneumocephalus is present behind the right lateral posterior wall. The left sinus is fully aerated.

       The remainder of the CT axial and coronal cuts need to be read to determine the status of the orbital roofs and the remainder of the maxillofacial area. Neurosurgical assessment of intracranial contents on the CT scan is essential.)
   (b) Any other tests indicated? Justify. (As described above, since a potential injury to the right globe may exist, an ophthalmologic consult is appropriate.)
2. Briefly outline the pathologic anatomy of this patient and how that pathology will determine your treatment plan. Consider in your description additional CT findings perhaps not evident on the slice provided. (The impact force must have been substantial, with considerable kinetic energy transferred as the wounding agent. A number of

assumptions can be established that include probable bone loss, dural tears and disruption, involvement of the right orbital roof with fracture and a consequent "blow in" compression of the globe, and involvement of the muscles of extraocular motion, particularly the superior rectus. Given the high velocity, extension into the medial orbital wall is a distinct possibility as a nasoethmoid orbital fracture with disruption of the medial canthus.)

3. Outline your treatment plan in general and then give specifics, including incisions and a sequence of procedural steps. (The above knowns and assumptions drive the development of the treatment plan. A bicoronal flap will provide access for a formal craniotomy. In raising the bicoronal flap, consideration must be given to a parallel harvest of an inferiorly-based pericranial flap. Once neurosurgery has completed the debridement of the frontal lobe, if necessary, and dural repair, any associated naso-orbital ethmoid, NOE, and/or roof fractures are addressed and repaired. Because of disruption, the posterior wall will be excised, and cranialization of the sinus to allow the brain to expand and fill the space. To separate the intracranial from the extracranial space, the nasofrontal duct should be plugged after stripping the sinus mucosa from the floor and anterior wall. The duct can be plugged with the pericranial flap passed via the supraorbital craniotomy osteotomy site or with cancellous bone chips harvested from the frontal craniotomy bone plate. In a similar manner, any anterior bone deficit can be reconstructed with autogenous grafts obtained by splitting the bone plate.)

Postoperative (6 Months)

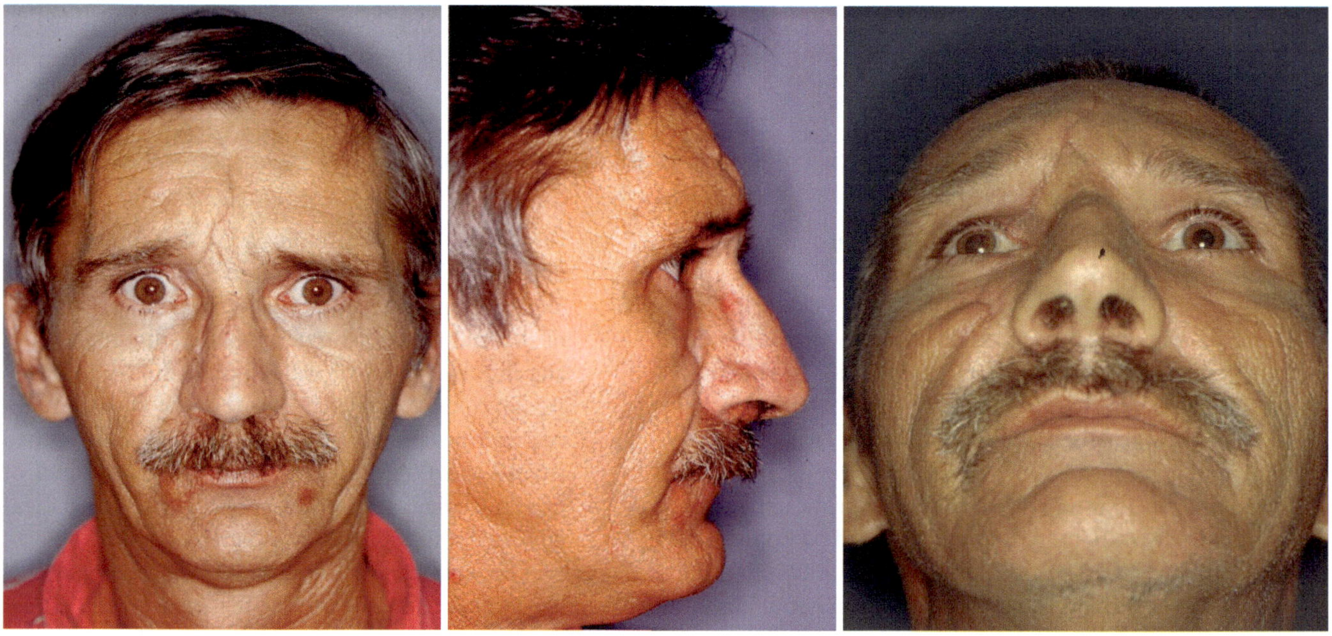

The three postoperative photos, frontal and lateral, demonstrate restoration of the normal convex forehead contour and no evidence of enophthalmos of the right eye.

Case-Based Conference

Case 3: Frontal Sinus Fracture

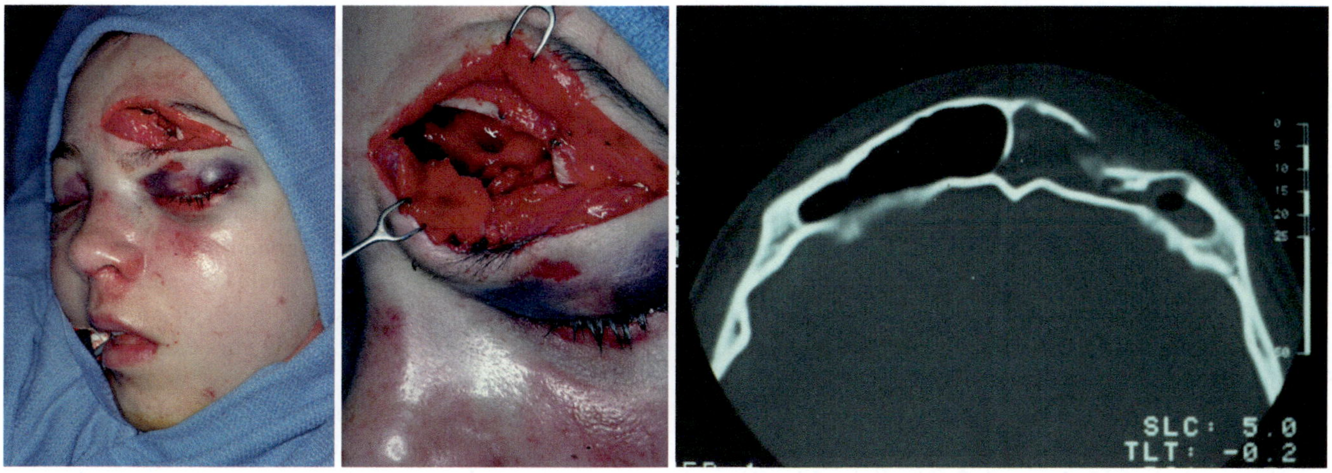

A 24-year-old woman involved in an MVA. The patient arrived slightly obtunded but oriented to time and place and cleared by the trauma team.

1. Describe the findings in the slide(s) and add a focused clinical exam. Describe the CT slice provided.
   (a) Interpret the CT scan.
2. Describe the pathologic anatomy.
3. Develop a treatment plan.

Case-Based Conference: Discussion

Case 4: Frontal Sinus Fracture

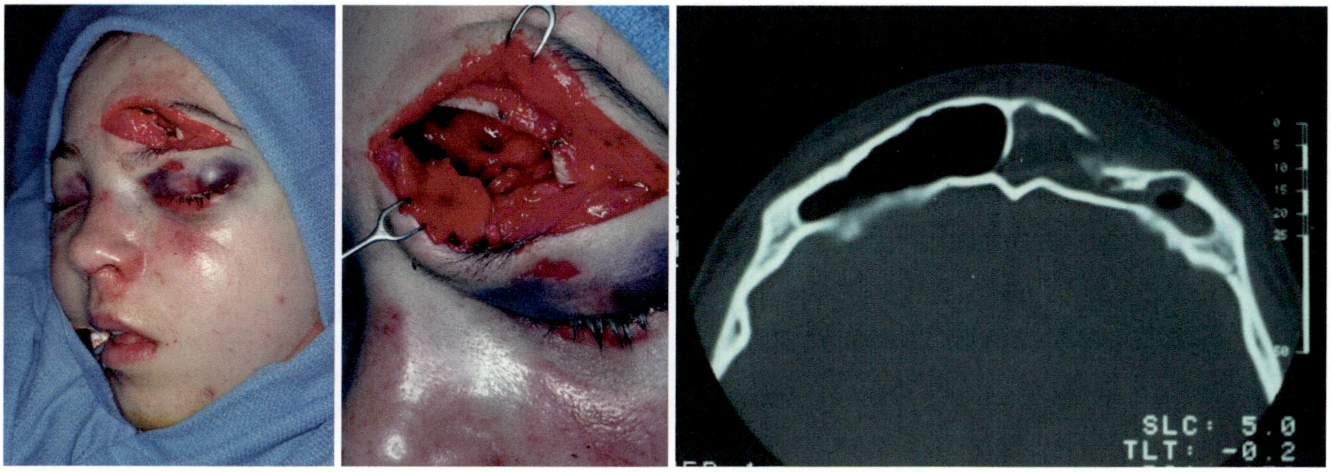

A 24-year-old woman involved in an MVA. The patient arrived slightly obtunded but oriented to time and place and cleared by the trauma team.

1. Describe the findings in the slide(s) and add a focused clinical exam. Describe the CT slice provided. (The two photos provided are a full-face oblique view of the left side, followed by more close-ups from the same perspective. The patient is intubated, and both eyes are closed. The particular findings depicted are an extensive laceration through the left brow extending transversely from the midline of the inferior forehead into the infrabrow area and terminating at the level of the lateral canthus in the infrabrow skin. Visualized in the full-face view but apparent in more detail on the close-up are fractures and disruption of the underlying bone. The anterior wall, presumably of the frontal sinus cavity, is depicted. Since the laceration divides the brow at the junction of the medial and central thirds, the lateral brow is retracted superiorly. Ecchymosis of the entire upper lid is also evident, which is limited to the lid and infrabrow. A suggestion of ecchymosis in the opposite lids is present, although that area is mostly obscured. Some minimal bruising of the infraorbital region is evident on the left.

   The clinical examination includes a short history of circumstances, any important past medical history, and social history- all if available. The physical, hopefully completed prior to intubation, primarily focuses on a maxillofacial exam that includes palpation, assessment of occlusion, any abnormal motion of the maxilla and/or mandible, and sensation over the distribution of the branches of the trigeminal nerve. A crucial component is the examination of the eye that would include vision to confrontation, evaluation of extraocular muscle motion, levator function, and pupillary reaction. Even if intubated and not able to respond, pupillary reactions can be tested. No attempts should be made to probe the wound.)

   (a) Interpret the CT scan. (A single slice is provided-approximately at mid-forehead. The frontal sinus is quite large, extending from one frontotemporal suture line to the other, almost consistent with hypersinus. The pathologic findings are several and include a fractured and depressed anterior wall of the left sinus, confirmed on the scan. Fluid fills the left sinus as well, although the right side is fully aerated, indicative of a well-developed intersinus septum. Of course, inspection of the remaining CT scan axial, coronal, and, if performed, sagittal views is mandatory. With respect to the sinus, the additional information obtained could impact the treatment plan. The two critical variables in fractures of the frontal sinus, in addition to the displacement of the anterior wall, are the involvement of the nasofrontal duct and associated fractures of the posterior wall. The latter is readily discernible on the routine axial slices of the scan. The former, the duct, is not. Some enthusiasm and experience have been published regarding the use of the sagittal view to assess the patency of the nasofrontal duct, but unfortunately, the sensitivity of that examination is low. The inconsistency may be derived from the variability in the anatomy of the drainage system, including a well-formed tract, an ostium only, and a pathway through the anterior ethmoid air cells. The imaging information would include if the fracture has extended into the ethmoid, anterior ethmoid air cells, and findings indicative of possible involvement of the nasofrontal duct as well as the medial orbital wall. The remaining maxillofacial slides of the zygomatic orbital, maxillary, and mandibular elements of the facial skeleton are evaluated for associated injuries. The underlying assumption is that the patient's C-spine and intracranial imaging are negative for injury.

   The principal other "test" to consider is an ophthalmology consultation. A low threshold for the consult should exist in the presence of periorbital injury. The ophthalmologist can determine intraocular pressure and perform retinoscopy to a degree of expertise beyond the maxillofacial surgeon.)

2. Describe the pathologic anatomy. (The evident pathologic anatomy is a depressed fracture of the anterior wall of the left fluid-filled frontal sinus. The status of the posterior wall is unknown but can be determined from the CT scan. The status of the nasofrontal duct is also unknown but may not be ascertained from imaging alone.)
3. Develop a treatment plan. (An operative treatment plan should be developed to address the three critical elements of a frontal sinus fracture: the status of the anterior and posterior walls and the nasofrontal duct. The remainder of this discussion will assume the posterior wall is intact. If not, and if any degree of uncertainty exists about the integrity of the dura and certainly in the presence of significant disruption of the posterior wall, a frontal craniotomy is indicated. The incision selected will hinge on the exposure obtained through the existing laceration. Regardless, the patient should be prepped and draped for the execution of a bicoronal approach should the exposure through the laceration prove inadequate. To do so prepares for the unlikely contingency of the discovery of unanticipated injury to the posterior wall as well as the capacity to harvest cranial bone if grafts are required for a bone defect of the anterior wall. Regardless of the approach, the first objective is an exploration of the sinus and the removal of bone fragments and clotted blood. The next step is a determination of the patency of the duct. That determination can be accomplished with a 3 cc syringe with an attached flexible intravenous catheter. The catheter is used to gently irrigate with saline the duct in the location of the medial inferior portion of the sinus. Vasoconstriction of the mucosa of the left nasal cavity is

obtained with cottonoid pledgets soaked in a vasoconstrictive agent. The pledget remains in place after a similar injection with 3 cc of methylene blue. A waiting period of 15–30 min is necessary before the pledgets are inspected for the presence of methylene blue. During the hiatus, an assessment of the anterior wall will be done to ascertain if sufficient native bone is available for reconstruction or if additional bone will be harvested, as right calvarial grafts will also be needed.

After an adequate wait, the pledgets are removed, and in the absence of any evidence of methylene blue stain, the nasofrontal duct is assumed to be non-patent. If so, obliteration of the sinus must be performed since obstruction of the duct will lead to the eventual occurrence of mucopyocele, an infectious, insidious, but progressive destruction of the sinus and adjacent structures, including the possibility of extension intracranially. Obliteration is a process of several steps, including stripping of all sinus mucosa, burring of all bony surfaces with a fine burr, and plugging of the duct with autogenous material, either bone chips or temporalis muscle plus fascia. If a bicoronal approach was utilized, a pericranial flap could be inserted into the duct and the floor. In a minority of patients, the intersinus septum is sufficiently well developed to effectively partition the frontal sinus into two distinctly separate compartments. On a CT scan, this patient's right sinus is fully aerated, not involved with the fracture, and can probably be left untreated.

The reconstruction of the anterior wall, with or sans bone grafts, is done with mini plates and screws. Some expressions of an opinion that the sinus can be left unobliterated and will eventually self-obliterate have been offered, but substantial evidence to support that hypothesis does not exist.

Although the final step in what was perhaps a lengthy operation, careful attention and detail should be directed toward a scrupulous repair of the brow, even a minor misalignment will be obvious postoperatively. The patient should be informed about the permanent loss of sensation over the forehead and anterior scalp unless identification and repair of the supraorbital nerves was performed, probably unlikely.)

Postoperative (1 Month)

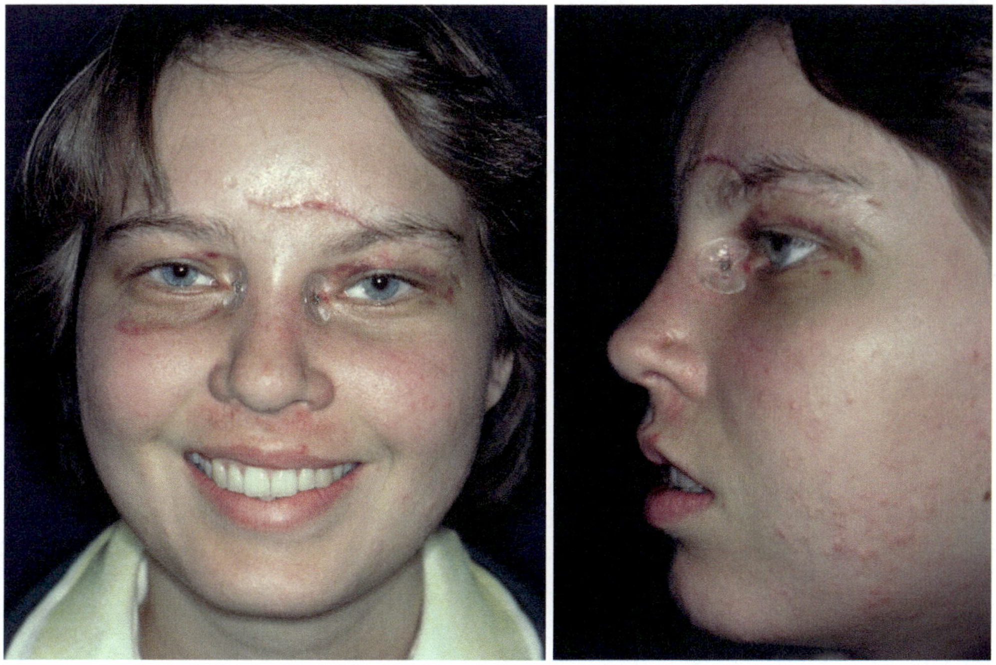

The two postoperative photos, frontal and left lateral, depict full restoration of the forehead, anterior frontal sinus wall, and contour. External nasal buttons are in place, indicative of probable transnasal wiring, representative of a left NEO fracture.

Case-Based Conference

Case 4: Cranioplasty

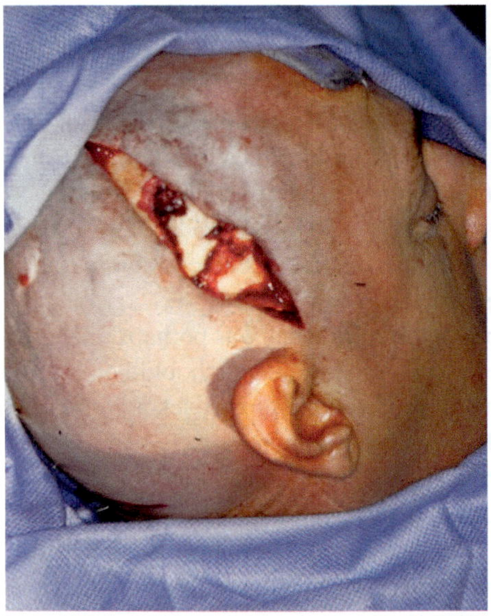
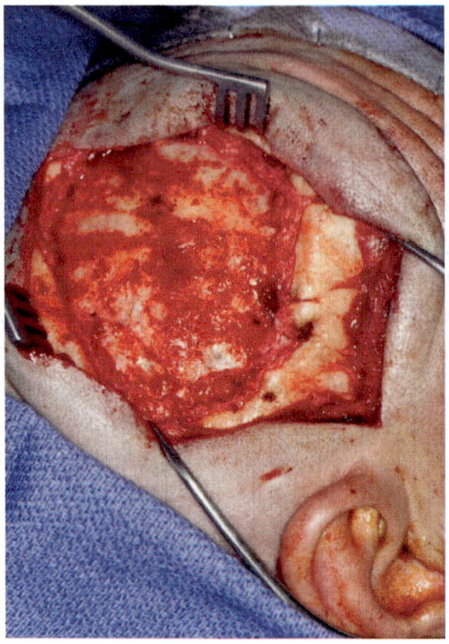
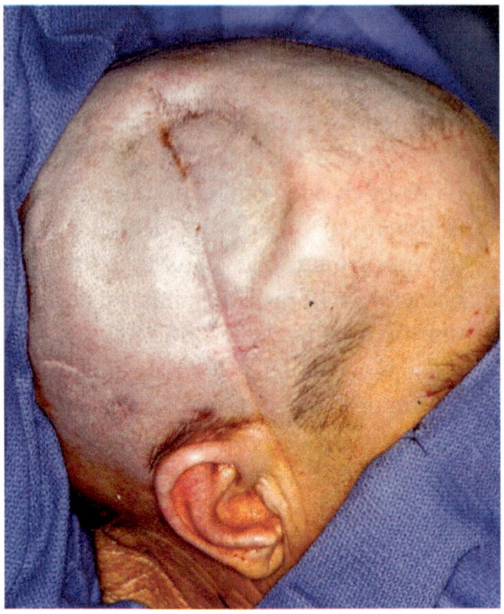
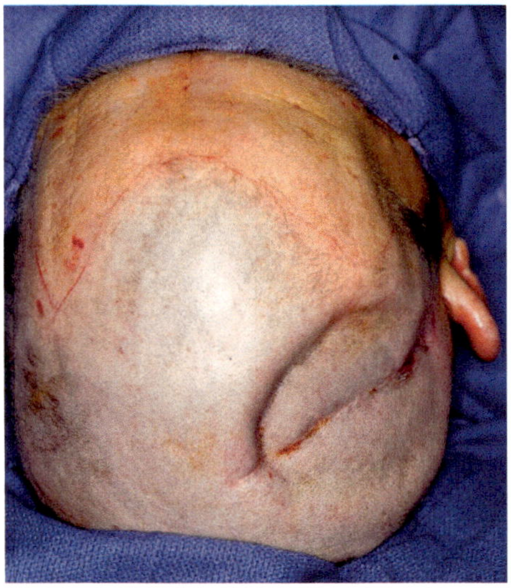

A 50-year-old male who has an infected depressed skull fracture. The first two slides demonstrate the debridement. He presents 3 months postoperative with a skull defect that measures 8 × 7 cm and is otherwise in excellent health. Photos of the original debridement are available.

1. Briefly describe the defect illustrated on the slides and add a focused clinical examination.
   (a) Any imaging indicated? Justify.
2. Summarize the pathologic anatomy.
3. Describe reconstruction. When addressing the bony defect, give a menu of options, give the pros and cons of each, and select one with justification.

Case-Based Conference: Discussion

Case 4: Cranioplasty

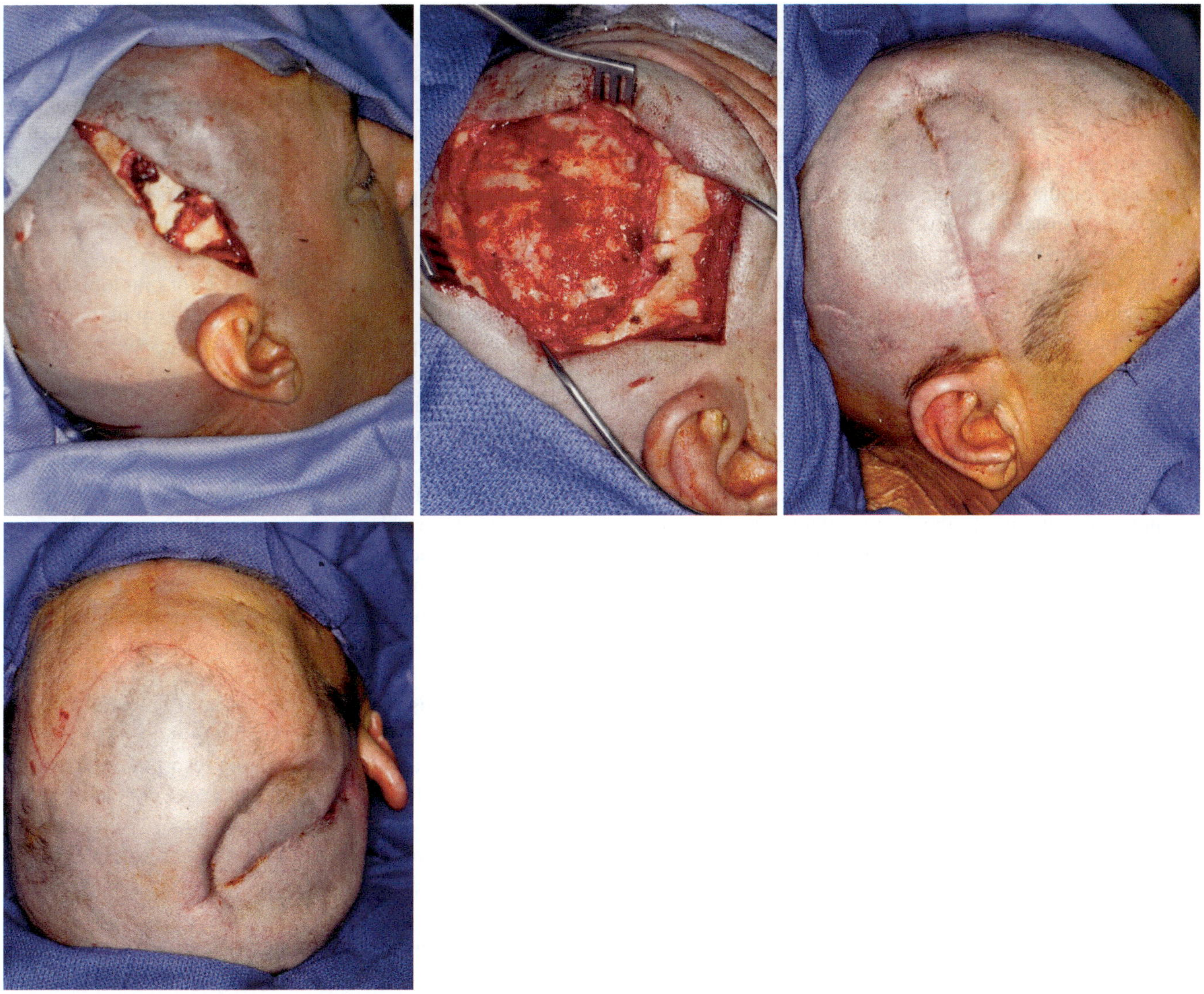

A 50-year-old male who has an infected craniotomy for a depressed skull fracture. He presents 3 months post-operative with a skull defect that measures 8 × 7 cm and is otherwise in excellent health. Photos of the original debridement are available.

1. Briefly describe the defect illustrated on the slides and add a focused clinical examination. (The two debridement slides of a lateral view limited to the skull illustrate a linear incision of 12 cm in length from the superior edge of the preauricular region superiorly into the temporal scalp with an exposed skull with probable fracture lines and soft tissue of indeterminate nature. The subsequent slide after debridement with the skin-soft tissue retracted depicts a large bony defect and apparently dura with bleeding or granulation tissue. Some chronic granulation tissue is present on the visible bony edges inferiorly. The next two slides are also intraoperative, at 3 months, and are from two different perspectives, lateral and from above, illustrating a well-healed incision that bisects the bony defect. The bony defect is substantial, probably 7.0–8.0 cm, circular in nature, and readily seen through the soft tissue contour defect. The skin and soft tissue have adhered to the underlying dura to produce a concave configuration. No other scalp scars are perceptible. The frontal hairline is mostly receding bitemporally.

The original and any subsequent op notes should be reviewed, and the interval history should be elicited for any wound drainage or infection. Review of past microbiology cultures and results are also reviewed. The history would also establish smoking, occupational status, and a review of systems for cardiopulmonary status. Discussions with the neurosurgeon will clarify the patient's status with respect to the original diagnosis. The patient's desires will be discussed in the consultative phase, question three. The physical examination of the head and neck centers on the assessment of the quality of the scalp soft tissue, superficial temporal artery pulse, and examination for potential bone donor sites.)

(a) Any imaging indicated? Justify. (The essential test is imaging to detect the presence of residual osteomyelitis. MRI is superior to CT in accuracy in terms of sensitivity and specificity.)

2. Summarize the pathology anatomy. (The patient has sustained a full-thickness bony loss of approximately 55–65 cm square without obvious skin-soft tissue loss and an intact dura. The soft tissue cover, however, has an incision that bisects the bony defect. The underlying causation was infection osteomyelitis. A more subtle deficit is the relative loss of skin and soft tissue envelope, secondary to contraction over time. One of the cardinal principles in facial reconstruction of complex defects is the inevitable contraction of the soft tissue envelope in the absence of underlying skeletal reconstruction and support. That principle applies to the skull as well.)
3. Describe reconstruction. When addressing the bony defect, give a menu of options, give the pros and cons of each, and select one with justification. (The two components of the reconstructive needs are the skin-soft tissue and the bony defect. Although a soft tissue deficiency is not evident, once the normal convexity of the skull is restored by reconstitution of the skull defect, unless addressed, the skin envelope will be insufficient. As discussed above, in the absence of underlying bony support, the skin-soft tissue, over time, will relentlessly contract as has occurred in this patient, as exemplified by the concave contour of the defect. The most straightforward approach would be a scalp rotational flap, but it would require a skin graft to the donor site. A prior expansion of the adjacent skin would dictate a two-stage treatment plan and a necessary hiatus to accomplish the expansion and the inherent risk of expander exposure-extrusion. Since the anticipated tissue coverage requirement is not massive, the optimal option is local tissue rearrangement as a Z-plasty, incorporating as the central limb the old incisional scar.

Reconstruction of the bony defect or cranioplasty can be performed with alloplastic or autogenous materials. The first group, alloplastic, has two classes of options: one, bone substitutes such as calcium hydroxyapatite, and second, rigid biomaterials. The other rigid options are titanium mesh and complex polymers such as methyl methacrylate or polyethylene ketones, PEEK, both with a limitation of infection and exposure in long-term follow-up. Bone substitutes are usually composed of, as mentioned above, calcium hydroxyapatite that permits bony ingrowth. The rate-limiting factor of the degree of bone ingrowth is the size of the bone defect, and defects greater than 5.0 cm in diameter will probably ossify incompletely.

Autogenous bone options are split calvarial rib and iliac. All have donor site side effects and potential complications. In addition, some bone resorption may occur in long-term follow-up. Lacking stress or load-bearing, bone grafts are susceptible to resorption, Wolff's law. In the skull or forehead, the resorption can result in a "washboard" effect as the process produces space between the grafts.

This patient was managed with split-rib autogenous bone and a large Z-plasty incorporating the prior incisional scar.)

Intraoperative

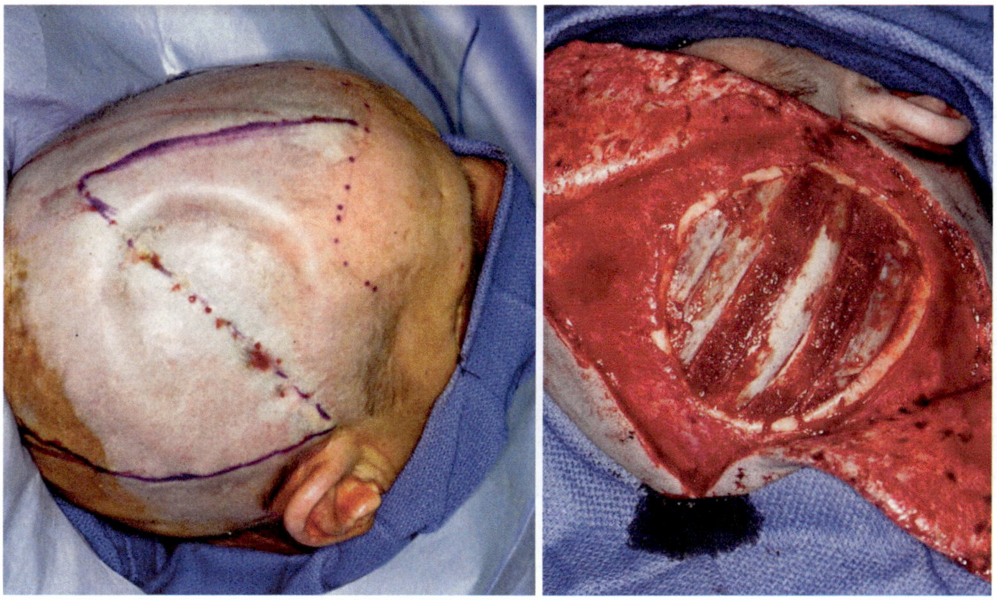

A large Z-plasty with 60° angles has been drawn, the medial or superior limb in the midline and the inferior limb transverse at the level of the superior ear. The central limb was incorporated into the old incision. In photo 2, split ribs have reconstructed the defect.

Postoperative (3 Months)

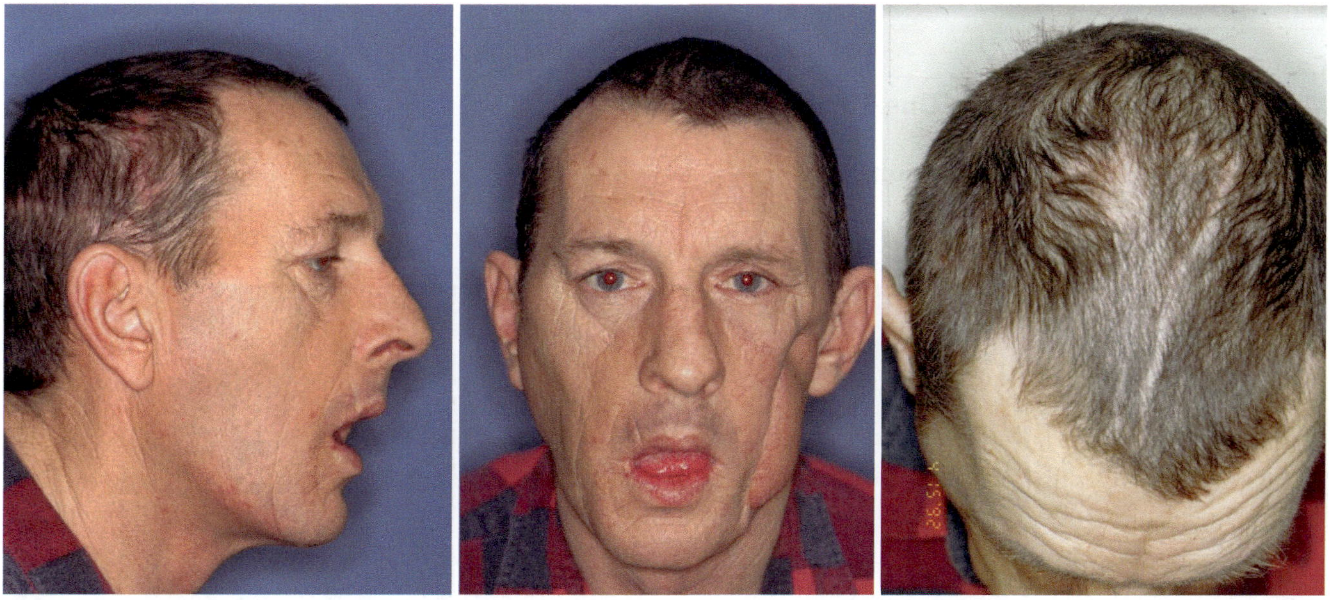

In three views, lateral, frontal, and above, the patient has excellent restoration of contour and sufficient hair growth to conceal incisional scars.

Case-Based Conference

Case 5: Infected Cranioplasty

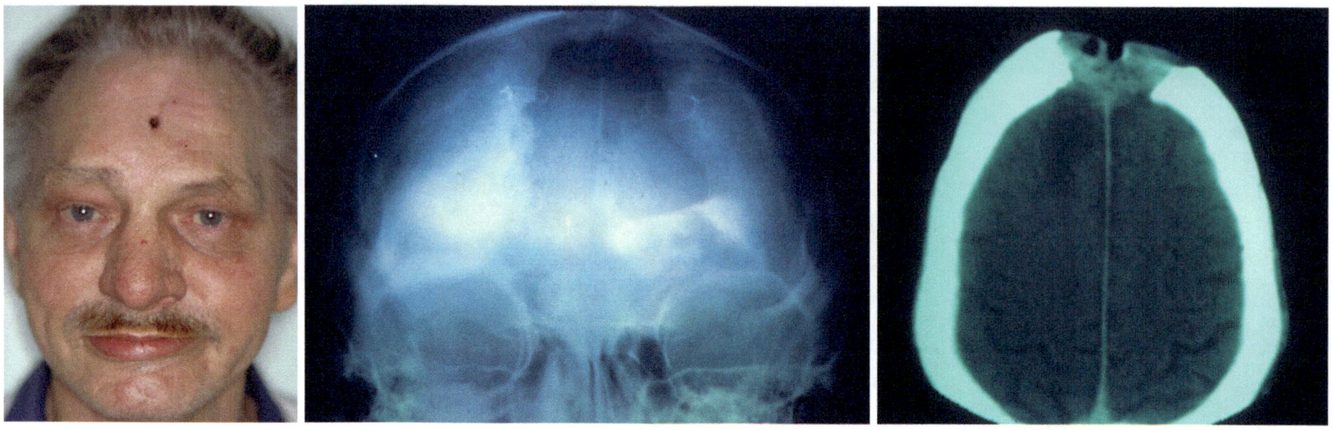

A 50-year-old male sustained a "skull fracture" in an MVA with subsequent emergent management 7 years ago. Subsequently, it was reconstructed with "plastic." He has had intermittent purulent drainage from a forehead wound and nose for the past 4 months.

1. Describe the photo, the x-ray, and the single CT slice. Add a focused clinical examination.
   (a) Any tests indicated? Justify. What additional slices of the CT scan will be of benefit in the outline of a treatment plan?
2. Describe the pathologic anatomy and pathophysiology.
3. Outline a treatment plan. Begin with a menu of options, select yours, and describe.

Maxillofacial Trauma: Upper One-Third

Case-Based Conference: Discussion

Case 5: Infected Cranioplasty

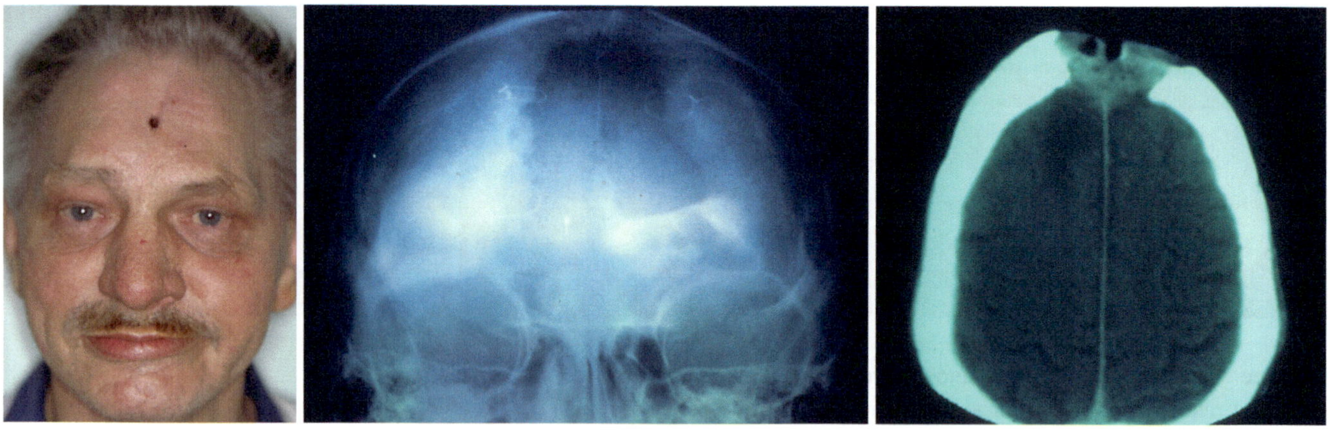

A 50-year-old male sustained a "skull fracture" in an MVA with subsequent emergent management 7 years ago. Subsequently, it was reconstructed with "plastic." He has had intermittent purulent drainage from a forehead wound and nose for the past 4 months.

1. Describe the photo, the x-ray, and the single CT slice. Add a focused clinical examination. (The single clinical photo is a full-face frontal view of a male who appears the stated age. In the mid-forehead in the midline is a 2 mm circular black encrusted area. No purulence is visible. No deformity of the frontal, adjacent temporal, or supraorbital bones is evident. No facial or orbital deformity is pictured, nor are forehead scars visible, although the photo is slightly blurry.

   An x-ray is provided with an A-P view of the skull and orbits. The most pronounced finding is a large central frontal radiolucent defect, trapezoid in shape and extending centrally from the supraorbital ridges throughout the extent of the frontal bone. Two small wire fragments are seen at the mid portion of the edge of the defect on the left and right side. The edges of the defect are irregular and poorly defined. No air-fluid level is discernible.

   A single axial CT slice depicts the full-thickness defect of the frontal bone as well as a U-shaped soft tissue depression centrally. Two separate radiolucencies are present within the said soft tissue defect consistent with gas bubbles. No other bony abnormalities are present. No lesions are seen in the parenchyma of the brain.

   The history component would attempt to accrue additional information regarding the circumstances surrounding the management of the patient at the time of the accident, including other injuries sustained, the number of operations and intervening hiatus, and, if possible, more specifics about the reconstruction. The details of the drainage should be gathered, including frequency and other associated symptoms such as fever, chills, and headache. If recent treatments such as antibiotics have been administered, the details should be established. The past medical history is completed to establish comorbidities, if any, and a social history of tobacco, alcohol, or drug abuse. The physical exam should include a general neurologic assessment of cognitive function and a vision exam. The forehead and supraorbital ridge should be palpated for deformity or any unstable or mobile bone fragments. The scalp and forehead are inspected as well for incisional or posttraumatic scars. A nasal speculum examination completes the physical, although potential bone donor sites are inspected.)

   (a) Any tests indicated? Justify. What additional slices of the CT scan will be of benefit in the outline of a treatment plan? (An effort to secure past medical records would be of value. If purulence can be expressed through the forehead sinus tract, cultures can be obtained. The remaining CT scans are examined for evidence of fluid collection, either epidural or subdural. The bony structures surrounding the area of the radiolucency, the anterior ethmoid, and the cribriform plate are inspected for irregularity suggestive of osteomyelitis. The sequential axial cuts are viewed for evidence of the collapse of skin and soft tissue directly onto the dura.)

2. Describe the pathologic anatomy and pathophysiology. (The presumptive diagnosis is an infected alloplastic implant. The pathophysiology is not complex- alloplastic material used to reconstruct cranial defects is commonly employed, including PEEK, titanium, and, historically, methyl methacrylate. In general, alloplastic materials in contact with contamination by the sinuses or the nasopharynx via an open nasofrontal duct are doomed to infection and secondary complications. The infection, in this instance, is chronic and possibly secondary septic complications, including purulent collections, abscess in the epidural or subdural spaces, as well as osteomyelitis of adjacent skull and/or ethmoid sinuses, which is clearly possible. In this particular case scenario, periodic decompression of the purulence through the nasopharynx and nasal cavity probably prevented accumulation in the form of an abscess. The offending organisms are usually the upper respiratory tract, the nasopharynx, or the paranasal sinuses in origin. The other possibility is a CSF leak, unlikely given the duration without episodes of meningitis and/or sepsis.)

3. Outline a treatment plan. Begin with a menu of options, select yours, and describe. (A number of treatment decisions need to be established and include access, disposition by removal of a particular foreign body, mode and material of reconstruction of the resultant defect, ascertainment of the status of adjacent bone, and stages if more than a single procedure. The single photo is somewhat indistinct, but a suggestion is present of a depressed forehead vertical scar coursing in the midline superiorly from the sinus tract. That impression is supported by the CT findings. Regardless, access is via a bicoronal incision with particular care directed toward dissection in the area of the defect. Conceivably, particularly if suggested on the CT scan, the soft tissue envelope can be adhered to the dura, and caution is required in the dissection. The offending alloplastic material should be easily removed, as well as any interosseous wires. The following step is a careful debridement of the underlying bed of the infected and necrotic material overlying the dura, as well as curettage and rongeuring of the adjacent bone to the bleeding vital cranium. Attention must be directed toward the anterior central portion of the anterior fossa to identify communication with the nasopharynx. Once determined, debridement of all soft tissue and mucosa, as well as osteomyelitic bone, is accomplished.

   At this stage, a decision must be reached if immediate or delayed second-stage reconstruction should be performed. Each has benefits and liabilities. The reconstruction at the time of wound toilet is subject to an increased potential for re-infection and loss of the reconstruction. A delayed approach is more prudent but requires dissection of the fibrotic skin envelope free of the dura with the risk of dural tears and CSF leak. The optimal material for bone reconstruction is autologous bone, replacing "like with like." Potential donor sites include cranial, rib, and iliac. Cranial bone is the most accessible through the bicoronal incision and is usually an imperceptible donor site, but the bone is somewhat difficult to contour a large convex-concave defect. Split rib grafts are easily contoured, but the donor site has the possibility of complications and results in a visible incisional scar. The cancellous bone should be harvested to pack into and seal any communication with the nasopharynx.

Culture-specific perioperative antibiotics are administered, and drains are placed for postoperative suction beneath and superficial to the reconstruction. Postoperative patient instructions include avoidance of nose blowing.)

Intraoperative

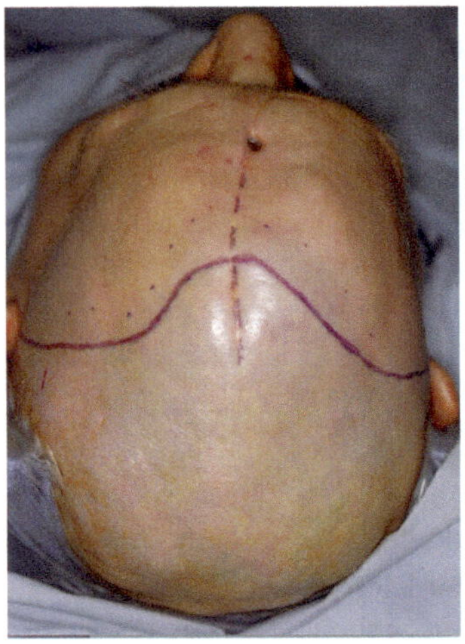

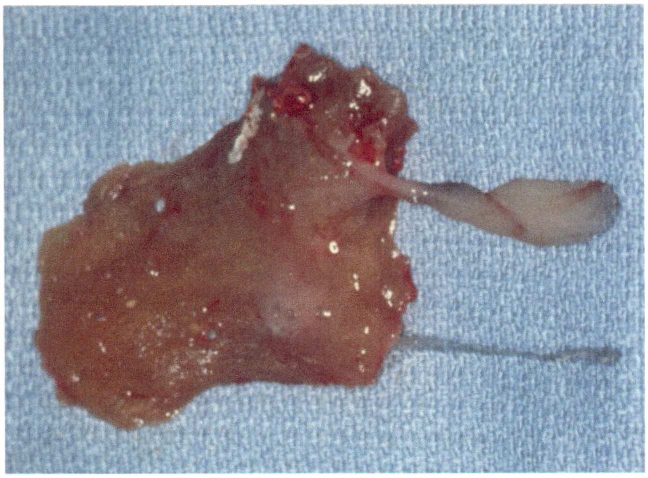

The initial photo illustrates the bicoronal incision with a vertical dotted line over the old scar. The second is of the purulent alloplastic material.

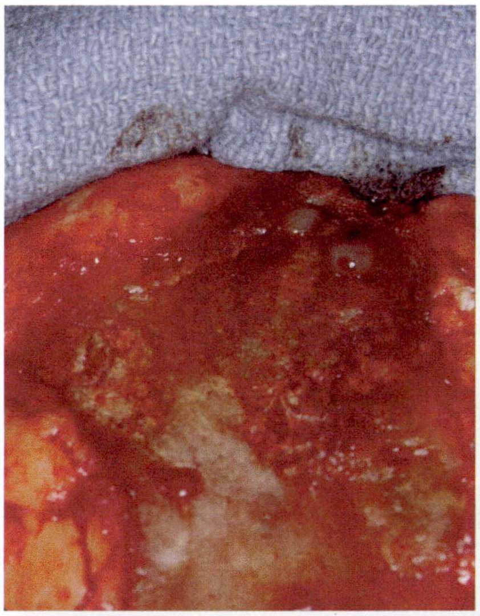
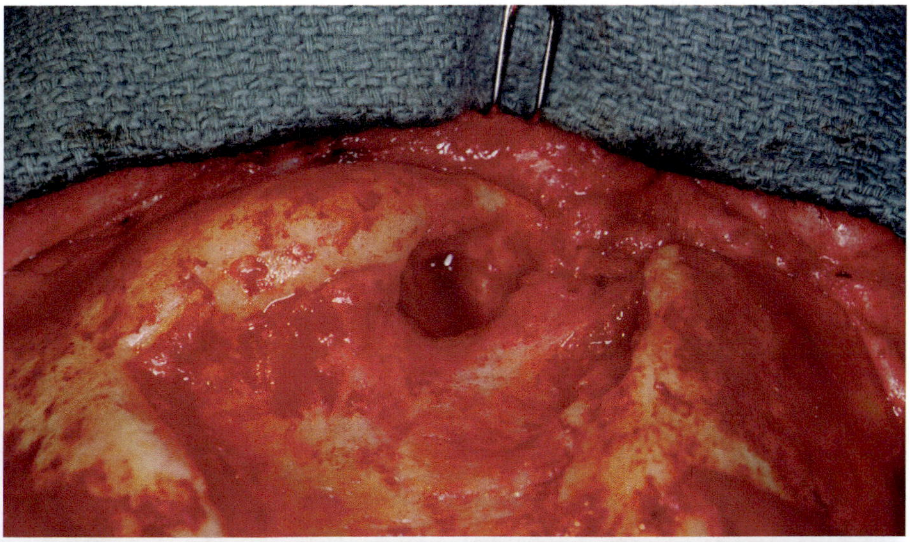
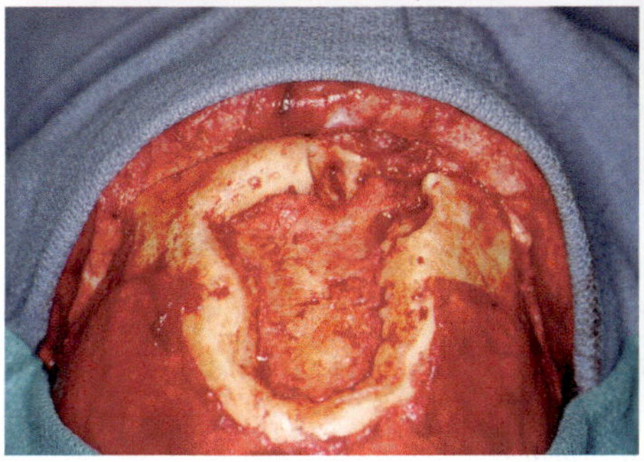
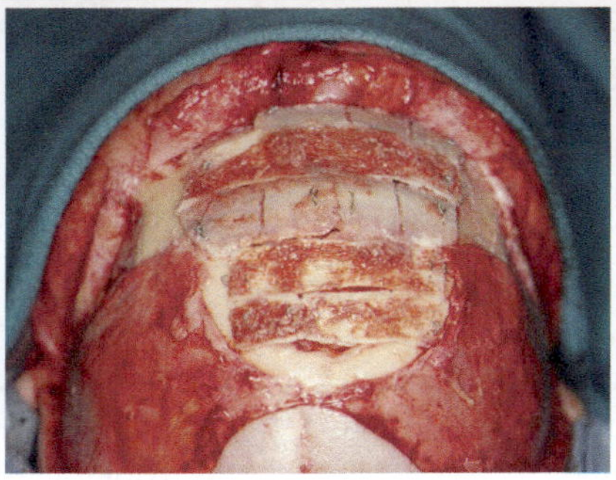
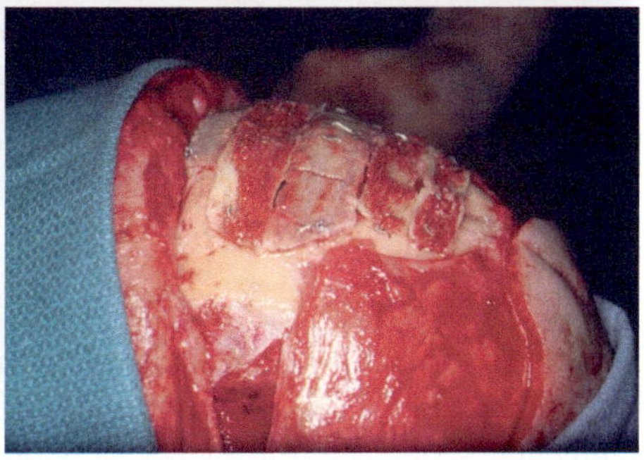

The following photos, including a close-up, depict the underlying bed and purulence anteriorly in the region of communication with the forehead sinus tract. The fifth photo is of the communication with the nasopharynx after removal of the purulence and debridement. The final pre-reconstruction photo is of the operative site after the completion of the wound toilet. In the two reconstruction photos, split rib grafts have been contoured and designed to be fixed securely into the defect with plates and screws.

Postoperative (6 Weeks)

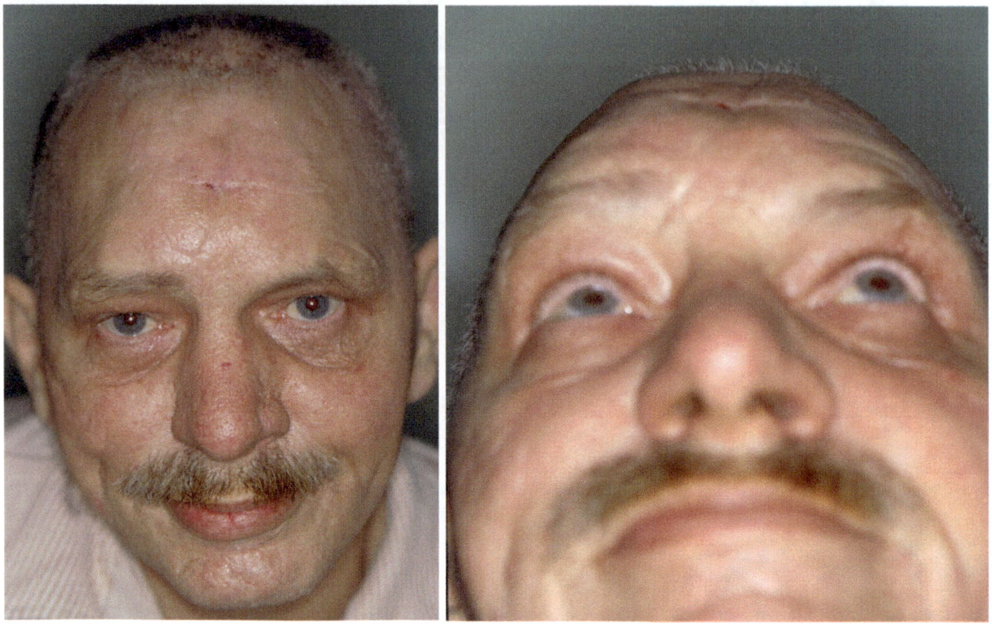

A postoperative full-face frontal view demonstrates excellent contour and shape. The site of the fistula has healed. A submental vertex confirms the above findings.

Critique

A single-stage reconstructive option was selected in this instance. At this early stage, 6 weeks, the patient has a successful outcome. The passage of several months will be necessary to ensure that infectious complications do not occur. Also, autologous bone, when grafted into recipient sites without load or stress as the forehead, is subject to partial resorption, which can detract from the final aesthetic result.

An alternate reconstructive method would be the use of titanium mesh either alone or in combination with a particulate cancellous bone. The use of titanium mesh has emerged as an option in cranioplasty but has been associated with exposure and extrusion in some instances.

In-Service Examination

1. The usual anatomic site for drainage from the nasofrontal duct is:
   (a) Anterior ethmoid air cells
   (b) Anterior middle meatus
   (c) Anterior inferior matus
   (d) Lacrimal fossa
2. The laboratory confirmation of CSF rhinorrhea is a positive:
   (a) Alpha-ketoglutarate
   (b) Matrix metalloproteinase
   (c) Beta-transferrin
   (d) Glucose content
3. Failure to fully eradicate all frontal sinus mucosa in obliteration will result in what complication?
   (a) Meningoencephalocele
   (b) Chronic sinusitis
   (c) Mucopyocele
   (d) CSF leak
4. The appropriate option in the address of a frontal sinus fracture with comminuted anterior and posterior wall fractures include:
   (a) ORIF both walls
   (b) ORIF both walls and autogenous bone graft
   (c) Cranialization, ORIF anterior wall
   (d) Ablation
   (e) Obliteration

47 Maxillary, Nasoethmoid, Orbital, Nasal Fractures

Bibliography

Luce, EA, "Developing Concepts and Treatment of Complex Maxillary Fractures" Advances in Craniomaxillofacial Fracture Management, *Clinics in Plastic Surgery*, (1992); 19:**125–131 (Background).**

Gruss JS, "Complex Maxillary Fractures: Role of Buttress Reconstruction and Immediate Bone Grafts", *Plast Reconstr Surg.*, (1986); 78:9–22. **Figs. 1 and 3 ONLY.**

Ricketts S, Gill HS, Fialkov JA, et al., "Facial fractures", *Plast Reconstr Surg.*, (2016); 137(2):**426e–432e, 439e, 442e, Figs. 18 and 19, and Video 3, 4, 8 for the Junior Residents ONLY (Exposure, evaluation of LeFort).**

Low C, "Sequencing of Panfacial Fractures", Plastic Surgery Hyperguide, www.plasticsurgery.hyperguides.com

Hendrickson M, et al, "Palatal Fractures: Classification, Patterns, and Treatment with Rigid Internal Fixation", *Plast Reconstr Surg.*, (1998); 101(2):**319–332.**

Leipziger LS and Manson PN, "Nasoethmoid Orbital Fractures", *Clinics in Plastic Surgery*, (1992); 19(1): **167–193.**

Engelstad M. "Chapter 42: Naso-Orbito-Ethmoid Fractures", Current Therapy in Oral and Maxillofacial Surgery, (2012);**pg. 341 ONLY**

Potter JK, et al. "Aesthetic Management of the Nasal Component of Naso-Orbital Ethmoid Fractures", *Plast Reconstr Surg.*, (2006); 117:**10e–18e.**

Higuera S, Lee EI, Cole P, et al., "Nasal Trauma and the Deviated Nose", *Plast Reconstr Surg.*, (2007); 120(7):**64S–70S.**

Chaudhry O, Isakson M, Franklin A, et al., "Facial Fractures Pearls and Perspectives", *Plast Reconstr Surg.,* (2018); 141(5):**742e Video 3 ONLY.**

Supplemental Reading for Junior Residents

Fraioli RE, Branstetter BF, and Deleyiannis FWB, "Facial Fractures: Beyond Le Fort", *Otolaryngol Clin N Am.*, (2008); 41: **61–65, 69–74 ONLY.**

Beumer HW and Puscas L, Chapter 13: "Nasal and Septal Injuries", Essentials of Craniomaxillofacial Trauma, Quality Medical Publishing, (2012); **pgs. 189–200.**

Faculty Discussion and Study Guide

Anatomy, Evaluation

1. What were Milton Adams's contributions to the management of midface fractures? (Dr. Adams, from Memphis, described the use of internal fixation of facial fractures rather than the use of external devices that was the vogue at the time. Paradoxically, he advocated craniofacial suspension for maxillary fractures.)
   (a) What are the sequelae of an untreated or inadequately treated maxillary fracture? (Midface retrusion and anterior open bite.)
2. Describe in detail the three vertical buttresses of the face. (The principal vertical buttresses are the naso-maxillary, zygomatico-maxillary, and the pterygoid maxillary. The naso-maxillary courses from the canine superiorly, lateral to the pyriform aperture to the nasal bones and medial-orbital rim region and to the frontal cranial base; the zygomatico-maxillary progresses up from the area of the premolars across the face of the zygoma anteriorly and malar body into the lateral orbital rim and the zygomatic process of the frontal bone; the pterygoid-maxillary, the most postero-lateral, courses upward from the region of the second molar into the skull base. In addition, what is frequently overlooked is the role of the mandible, namely, the vertical ramus and condyle as the fourth vertical buttress of the face.)
3. What are the bones that comprise the nasoethmoid orbital NEO area? (Nasal, ethmoid, lacrimal, frontal, maxillary, and by stretch, the lesser wing of the sphenoid.)

E. Luce, *A Curriculum for Plastic Surgery*, https://doi.org/10.1007/978-3-031-62087-4_47

(a) What are the elements of the ethmoid bone as they relate to NEO fractures? (The perpendicular plate, cribriform plate, anterior ethmoid air cells.)
(b) How does the maxilla relate to the NEO area? (The nasal process of the maxilla is the foundation of and posterior to the nasal bone.)

4. What structures encompass the anterior 3/4 of the medial wall of the orbit? (Nasal process of the maxilla, lacrimal bone, ethmoid air cells.)
5. List the pertinent bones and describe the bony anatomy of the nasoethmoid-orbital regions. (Frontal process of the maxilla, maxillary process of the frontal bone, nasal bones, ethmoid and lacrimal bones, ethmoid plate of the septum, floor of the frontal sinus(es), and the cribriform plate. The thicker bone of the frontal process of the maxilla and the thicker bone of the maxillary process of the frontal bone contribute primarily to the superior portion of the nasomaxillary buttress.)
   (a) Describe how the maxilla is the central pillar of the midface. (The maxilla links the two zygomatic-orbital regions and bears two of the three transverse buttresses, the middle from the zygomatic arch to the infraorbital rim to the frontal process of the maxilla and the inferior buttresses at the level of the alveolus to below the pyriform fossa. Vertically, the maxilla bears each of the three vertical buttresses that link the occlusal plane inferiorly to the cranial base superior.)
   (b) Diagram and label the interorbital space, including the lateral walls, center, lower, and ceiling. (Interorbital space is that space between the medial walls of the two orbits and is partitioned by the septum, principally the ethmoid plate of the septum. The lateral wall is composed of lacrimal bone anteriorly and the ethmoid bones more posterior. The roof is the cribriform plate. Of course, the interorbital space is also the superior aspect of the anterior nasal cavity.)
6. The prior question described two of the four coronal or horizontal buttresses of the face. What are the remaining two? (The most superior consists of the superior orbital rim, the maxillary process of the frontal bone, and the opposite superior orbital rim. The most inferior buttress is the infra-alveolar plane of the mandible.)
   (a) Describe a sagittal buttress of the midface. (The only sagittal buttress is the vomer and ethmoid bone, as well as the cartilaginous septum. The vomer is a thick bone, difficult to fracture, but the ethmoid is not. As described in the NEO submodule, fractures and telescoping of the ethmoid plate are quite common in midface fractures, and overall, the facial sagittal buttress is weak, which explains why retro-displacement of the maxilla is common. See below. See Fig. 47.1.)

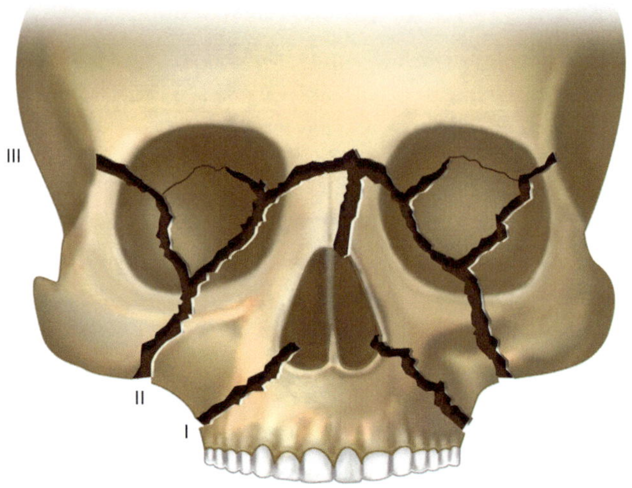

Fig. 47.1 LeFort fracture

7. Outline the specific direction(s) of LeFort fractures. (LeFort I is a transverse fracture above the maxillary alveolar plane extending through the vomer; a LeFort II or pyramidal fracture line is through the zygomatico-maxillary buttress, medial orbital wall across the nasal bones or nasal frontal suture line. In the sagittal plane, the fracture line is through the septum at the level of the ethmoid and posterior vomer; LeFort III or craniofacial dysfunction is essentially a fracture that dissociates the facial bones from the cranial base and extends through the arch, lateral orbital rim, lateral orbital wall, floor, and medial orbital wall through the nasal bones and/or nasal frontal suture line. In the sagittal plane, a LeFort III is high on the septum through the ethmoid and may involve the cribriform plate, hence the occurrence of CSF rhinorrhea.)
8. What functional role does the medial canthal tendon, MCT, play? (Medial canthal tendon or ligament is the confluence of the upper and lower lid tarsus and the associated orbicularis muscle. The MCT, as described, inserts with both a posterior and anterior limb into the anterior and posterior lacrimal crest, respectively.)
9. Describe the three-dimensional anatomy of the medial canthal region lateral to medial, beginning with the skin and ending with the interior of the nasal cavity. (Skin, subcutaneous tissue, anterior limb of the medial canthal tendon, lacrimal sac, posterior limb of the medial canthal tendon, specialized aspect of the pretarsal portion of the orbicularis or Horner's muscle, lacrimal bone/fossa, nasal mucosa. As mentioned above, the ethmoid bone with the contained air cells lying posterior to the lacrimal bone.)

10. Discuss the anatomy of the lacrimal duct system and how it relates to NEO fractures. (The lacrimal sac drains transversely and inferiorly into the nasal lacrimal duct, which courses through the ethmoid region, inferior orbital rim, and into the nasal cavity underneath the middle meatus. The ductal system and/or the sac can be disrupted by NEO fractures).
11. Give the normal intercanthal distance. (See Fig. 47.2.) (32 mm, slightly more in men with some normal variance)
    (a) Differentiate among epicanthus, telecanthus, and exorbitism. (Epicanthus is soft tissue or skin widening only due to epicanthal skin folds located anterior to the medial canthus. Telecanthus is widening the intercanthal distance. Exorbitism is a widening of the interorbital distance, most commonly seen in congenital conditions such as hypertelorism.)
12. Outline the physical examination of the patient with complex maxillary fractures. (Observation can establish a diagnosis: Patients with complex maxillary or mid-face fractures can have an absence of facial projection, diminished facial height, and increased facial width. The occlusal pattern should be examined, and the maxilla manipulated for abnormal mobility and the level, low or high, of the transverse component of the mobility. The infraorbital rims are palpated for a bony step-off. The intraoral cavity is examined for possible lacerations of the palate. Examine for CSF leak and, of course, an ocular exam. The CNS and ocular considerations are more comprehensively addressed in Chap. 42.)
    (a) What is the most common malocclusion pattern in mid-face fractures? (Class III and anterior open bite as a result of maxillary retrusion and cephalic rotation.)
13. What fracture lines must exist to establish a diagnosis of NEO fracture? (The four components, namely, lateral nasal, nasal maxillary buttress, inferior orbital rim, and frontomaxillary suture line at the frontal process of the maxilla and the maxillary process of the frontal bone. The fracture lines are transverse and inferior from the piriform aperture through the infraorbital rim, the frontal process of the maxilla articulation with the nasal bones vertically and anteriorly, the frontal process of the maxilla articulation with the frontal bone transversely and superiorly, and through the ethmoid bones vertically and posterior.)
    (a) What we, as clinicians, refer to as the central fragment is called what by anatomists? (Frontal process of the maxilla.)
14. What are the physical findings of a NEO fracture? (Flattened nasal dorsum, upturned nasal tip even telescoped and foreshortened, little septal support on digital pressure of the nasal tip, telecanthus, or a widened intercanthal distance. Examination for mobility is often limited due to patient pain. Lateral traction on the medial lower eyelid will result in displacement and loss of the normal concave configuration of the medial canthal area if the medial canthal tendon has been disrupted vs. adherence if not. An eyelid traction test consists of lateral traction on the lower lid and observation of the medial canthal dimple. In the presence of disruption of the medial canthal ligament, the lower eyelid orbicularis will pull the soft tissues of the medial canthus laterally.)
15. What are the other elements of a focused physical examination of a NEO patient? (The facial appearance is described in the above question; observe for CSF rhinorrhea; determine maxillary mobility; place digital pressure on the dorsal septum to determine integrity; test the EOMs pupillary reaction, do eyelid traction test.)
16. What are the physical findings in an untreated or inadequately treated NEO fracture? (Telecanthus, enophthalmos, epicanthal folds, depressed nasal dorsum.)

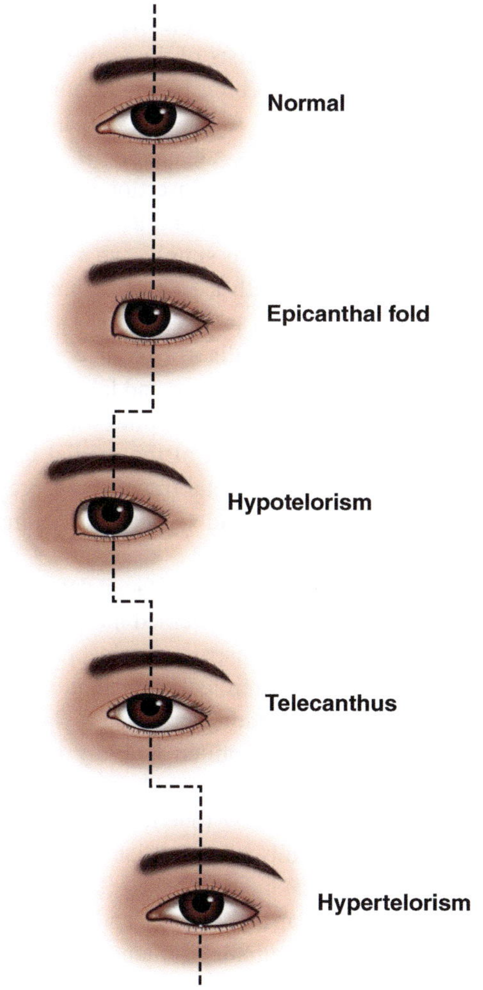

Fig. 47.2 Alterations of orbital soft tissue or bone

Treatment: Maxillary Fractures

1. In broad and general terms, what are the goals and steps in the management of complex midface fractures? (Restoration of facial projection, width, and height. Application of IMF, incisions, sequencing, internal fixation plus/minus primary bone grafts, decisions with respect to release of IMF, soft tissue repair.)
   (a) What anesthesia considerations exist? (The selection of the anesthesia route is determined by the potential presence of skull base involvement in LeFort III fractures. An awake nasal fiberoptic intubation, submental intubation, or tracheostomy may be required.)
   (b) What are the considerations for the release or not of IMF? (Consideration for maintenance postoperatively would be the presence of palatal fractures and/or a badly comminuted maxilla. Considerations for immediate release postoperatively of IMF would be concerns about the pulmonary and/or nutritional status of the patient.)
2. Describe the incisions available for ORIF of complex maxillary or mid-face fractures. (Bicoronal, a variety of lower lid incision options, lateral upper lid incision, labial sulcus.)
3. Give an approach to sequencing of complex mid-facial fractures. (Disimpaction of the maxilla as necessary, the establishment of normal or preinjury occlusion with the institution of IMF; mandibular body fractures, if present, should be plated at this juncture; explore all fracture lines with the use of incisions as outlined above, reduce and plate the zygomatic arches and frontozygomatic suture line, add internal fixation at the frontal-nasal suture line disruption; plate the infraorbital rim and treat the floor and wall defects, if any, as necessary; repair the NEO component including the medial canthal tendon with transcutaneous wiring or plating; application of a primary cantilever bone graft to the nose; plate the maxillary buttresses intraorally, and finally soft tissue suspension with canthopexy techniques. Essentially, by the use of thick cortical bone or the superior and inferior buttresses, frontal bone, and mandible, respectively, and reduction and fixation of the zygomatic orbital component, the complex midface fractures have been essentially reduced to that of a LeFort I. The final stage is the repair of the buttresses linking the now stable upper midface to the maxillary-alveolar ridge.)
   (a) In addition to the provision of a stable base, what other role does the mandible play in the reconstruction of complex midface fractures? (An intact condyle-vertical ramus sets the vertical height of the face.)
   (b) In a similar vein, what is the role of the zygomatic arches? (To establish, once reduced, the transverse facial width.)
4. What are the general and specific indications for ORIF of concomitant condylar fractures from the standpoint of associated mid-face trauma? (If bilateral condylar fractures are present, in this writer's opinion, and four or more buttresses are disrupted, then one or both condyles should be open, reduced, and plated to restore the ramus-condyle buttress and set the vertical facial height.)
5. What are some specific indications for the construction and use of an acrylic occlusal splint or wafer? (A preinjury malocclusion, particularly an anterior open bite, an edentulous or partially edentulous patient where dentures are not available, presence of palatal fractures, combined maxillary and mandible fractures.)

Treatment: NEO Fractures

1. Of the several available, describe a classification system. (See Fig. 47.3.) (Hinges on the size of the central fragment bearing the insertion of the medial canthal tendon: I, If a single segment exists of the entire medial orbital rim; II, if the medial orbital rim is fractured in one or more places but a large fragment exists and the medial canthal tendon remains attached; III, comminution including a disruption of the insertion of the tendon.)
   (a) A considerably more complex classification has been described. More simply, what are some fractures associated with a NEO fracture? (Maxillary, medial orbital wall, and nasoseptal.)
   (b) Explain. (The maxilla, of course, is intimately related to the more superior and lateral nasoethmoid orbital region. The medial orbital wall is involved in the ethmoid component of the medial orbital wall. Similarly, the nasal septal fracture is represented by an injury to the ethmoid vertical plate component of the septum.)
2. What are the three components of facial deformity in NEO fractures? (Telecanthus or increased intercanthal distance, depressed nasal dorsum, narrowed palpebral fissure.)
   (a) What is the anatomical explanation for each? (Medial canthal tendon attachment to lacrimal bones is disrupted and so pulled laterally by the orbicularis; telescoping of the nasal bones into the ethmoid area; loss of transverse tone/length of orbicularis).
3. Outline the advisability of immediate treatment of NEO fractures during the acute phase. (Delayed treatment allows secondary scarring, fibrosis, and contracture of the soft tissue envelope with the resultant difficulty in restitution of a narrow and normal intercanthal distance.)

Fig. 47.3 NEO fractures classification system

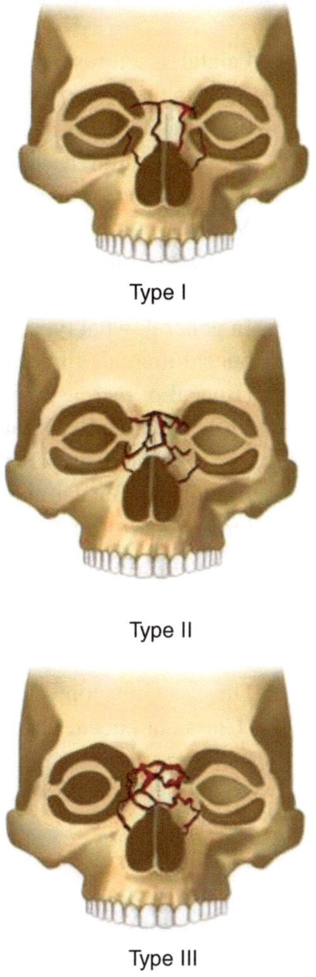

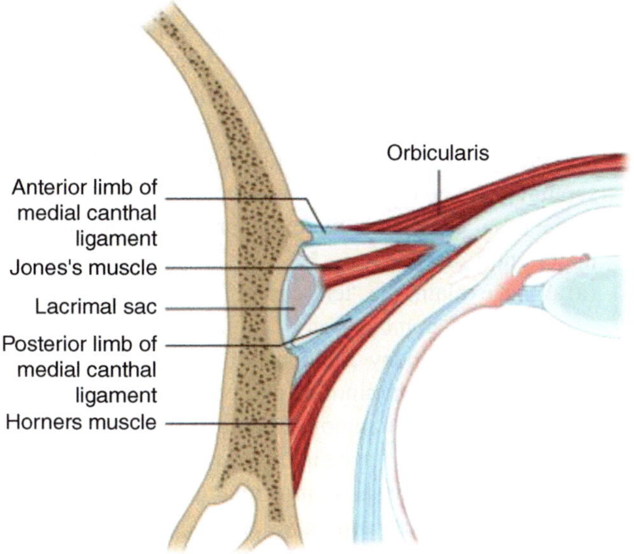

4. Outline a treatment plan, including preferred incision(s), steps and sequence, and overall guiding principles. (Bicoronal flap is usually necessary to repair NEO fractures. A small "w" shaped local medial canthal incision can be done to facilitate transnasal wiring. Subtarsal incisions are necessary in the majority of cases, as well as intraoral buccal degloving incisions for reduction and fixation of the maxillary component. The guiding principles are complete exposure of all fracture lines, reduction of fractured fragments, rigid internal fixation, and reattachment of medial canthal tendon if necessary. The steps after wide exposure are reduction of the fracture fragments with fixation at the nasal frontal and nasal maxillary suture lines from above through the bicoronal incision, reduction of the fracture fragment containing the medial canthal tendon with transnasal wiring, and fixation of the associated maxillary fragments including the nasal maxillary buttress through the buccal incision; the harvest of cranial bone grafts as necessary for bone grafting of the medial orbital wall as necessary; dorsal cantilevered bone graft for nasal dorsal support and possibly a columellar bone graft linked to the cantilevered bone graft for tip support; reduction of the septum with the placement of sutures at the anterior nasal spine and possibly the use of Doyle splints.)
   (a) What is the usual/finding, if any, with respect to residual bone attachment of the medial canthal tendon, MCT, in displaced NEO fractures? (In 90%, a fragment or larger piece of bone will be attached to the MCT.)
5. What's the general rule that guides the placement of the anchor wire and medial-canthal tendon wire? (Transnasal drill holes are made posterior and superior, and the medial canthal tendon with its usual associated bony fragment is secured to the opposite side, sometimes with the use of a bone graft for a bolster or tied to a screw. Associated fractures of the medial rim are addressed with mini-plates, avoiding thick plates in the medial-canthal region because of the thin skin coverage and associated obliteration of delicate soft tissue landmarks.)

6. What are the issues associated with medial orbital wall fractures? (The occurrence of enophthalmos, if not addressed, and the necessity to explore the medial orbital wall and repair with bone grafts or titanium mesh as indicated)
7. What is the role of the septum in the structural support in the three vaults of the nose? Explain. (In the lower vault, the septum plays a crucial role in tip support by its relationship and support of the lower lateral cartilages as well as the soft tissues of the tip of the nose. In the middle vault, the septum provides support for the upper lateral cartilages and the dorsum. In the upper third, the septum plays no critical role in support but rather relates to the nasal bones, which are the primary support in the upper one-third.)
   (a) What explains the "telescoping" of the nose seen clinically? (A combination of multiple fracture lines of the ethmoid bony component of the nasal septum as well as the comminution and posterior displacement of multiple cartilaginous fragments of the septum.)
8. What are the four principles of reconstitution/reconstruction of the nasal component of NEO fractures? Describe. (The four principles are the role of the nasal pyramid in dorsal support, tip projection and support, the septum as a potential obstruction of the nasal passageway, and augmentation of the lateral nasal wall.)
9. What is the relationship between the perceived intercanthal distance and nasal dorsal height? (Increased dorsal height gives the perception that intercanthal distance has narrowed, an important aspect of the perception of the intercanthal distance in NEO fractures.)
   (a) How is the first principle accomplished? (A dorsal cantilevered graft for stabilization of the bony nasal pyramid and dorsal septal support.)
   (b) How accomplished is the second principle? (Columellar graft as a strut linked to the cantilever bone graft.)
   (c) How accomplished is the third aspect? (Reduction of the nasal septum, sutured inferiorly and anteriorly at the spine. Possible stabilization with Doyle splints.)
   (d) The fourth principle? (Augmentation of the lateral nasal wall is controversial and probably rarely indicated.)
10. What are the possible associated acute complications of NEO fractures? (CSF rhinorrhea from a cribriform plate fracture, possible frontal sinus fracture-related complications, or epiphora from disruption of the lacrimal duct system.)
11. How often is the nasolacrimal system injured in NEO fractures? (20%)
   (a) How often is repair necessary? (5–10%)
   (b) What and when? (DCR; at least 3 months after injury)

Palatal Fractures

1. Palatal fractures are relatively uncommon. In general, what is the pattern, without particular focus on the numbers, of palatal fractures and frequency? (Most common are parasagittal, least common are transverse. Other types include anterior alveolar, posterior-lateral, and complex).
2. Most common associated facial fractures? (All will have LeFort I, one half have mandible fractures, one half LeFort II or III fractures.)
3. In general, what type of displacement of the transverse or buccal/lingual direction occurs in palatal fractures? (Buccal or increase width of the maxilla.)
4. More specifically, what is the direction of displacement in non-impacted parasagittal fractures? Posterior lateral fractures? (Buccal-anterior in parasagittal fractures; posterior superior in posterior lateral fractures.)
5. What are the important buttresses in a fractured palate/maxilla? (Alveolar, the palatal vault in a transverse direction; nasal-maxillary, zygomatico-maxillary, in either maxilla.)
6. Discuss incisions for exposure to palatal fractures. (Classical buccal vestibule, paramedian for the hard palate, elevation of a cleft palate-type flap for posterior lateral; at least theoretically transnasal, although not practical.)
7. Discuss the modalities available and the sequencing of palatal fractures. (Modalities consist of arch bars, internal fixation of the alveolar ridge and buttresses, rigid fixation of the vault, occlusal splint, and IMF.)
   (a) Apply those principles to a parasagittal fracture or a Type III. (Apply arch bars with an anterior arch bar crossing or perhaps cut at the alveolar fracture line; perform ORIF of the palatal vault as well as the alveolar ridge; add internal fixation of the nasal-maxillary buttress or additional fractured buttresses, and keep in IMF for 3 weeks. Apply IMF before buttress fixation.)
   (b) A fracture through the incisors consisting of an alveolar segment or a Type I or II. (Arch bars with wire ligature to adjacent stable teeth +/− occlusal splint but certainly IMF.)
   (c) Lateral fracture of the alveolar ridge at the canine with the extension of the fracture line through the posterior border of the lateral aspect of the hard palate, or Type IV (Arch bars, ORIF at the alveolar ridge and buttress, add IMF.)
8. You elect to manage a parasagittal fracture of the palate with arch bars and internal fixation with plates and screws across the alveolar fracture line only, what problem might you create, and how would you address it? (The tendency for the posterior aspect of the fracture line on the hard palate to splay open; treat with plates and screws in the

palatal vault posteriorly as a tension band or use of an occlusal splint. Avoid the splint if IMF establishes correct occlusion.)

9. In what type of palatal fracture is a prefabricated occlusal splint mandatory? (Complex palatal fractures with multiple segments.)

Naso-septal Fractures (Junior Residents)

1. Describe the anatomical relationship between the nasal bones or bony pyramids and the three components of the septum: ethmoid, vomer, and cartilage plate. (Viewed in the sagittal section, the nasal pyramid sits on the ethmoid component of the septum. The remaining portion of the nasal dorsum inferior to the bony pyramid consists of the cartilaginous portion of the septum. The cartilaginous septum sits on the bony vomer, which is the inferior-posterior component of the septum. One useful visual picture is the cartilage plate sitting as a quadrangle on the inferior-posterior vomer and on the anterior-superior ethmoid.)
2. Describe an appropriate timing for operative management of an acute naso-septal fracture. (Little argument can be made for an acute reduction because of the associated swelling and difficulty in determining adequate reduction. A 3–5-day period to allow resolution of the edema and elective scheduling is preferred. After 2 weeks, the reduction can be quite difficult because of the initiation of bony healing.)
3. Briefly describe the steps in the closed reduction of a naso-septal fracture. (Adequate anesthesia-either conscious sedation with local anesthetic block and intranasal cocaine or general anesthesia but usually with an intranasal vaso-constricting agent. Next, digital manipulation with one hand with perhaps a butter knife or Asch forceps placed intranasally. Once the bony pyramid is reduced, a nasal speculum exam should determine if the nasal septum, if displaced, has been reduced into the vomerine groove.)
   (a) What are the indications for an open approach? (A comminuted sepal fracture might, quite infrequently, require an open approach for reduction of the fragments and replacement of Doyle splints. Bony osteotomies in the acute or subacute stage are not indicated.)

Video Notes

Ricketts S, "Facial fractures," *Plast. Reconstr. Surg.*, (2016); 137(2):426e.

Video 3: NEO assessment (Slide presentation)

1. Review of telecanthus measurement encephalo rhinorrhea
2. Types of NEO fractures, including a 3D demonstration
3. Nasal involvement

Video 4: Operative exposure

1. Lower lid subtarsal and trans conjunctival, both pre- and post-septal

Video 8: Midface (Slide presentation)

1. Review of horizontal and vertical buttresses
2. Review of LeFort patterns
3. Review of palatal fracture types
4. Physical exam findings
5. Clinical examples

Chaudhry O, "Facial Fractures Pearls and Perspectives," *Plast. Reconstr. Surg.*, (2018); 141(5):742e.

Video 3: Endoscopic view of transnasal wiring

Case-Based Conference

Case 1: Midface Fractures

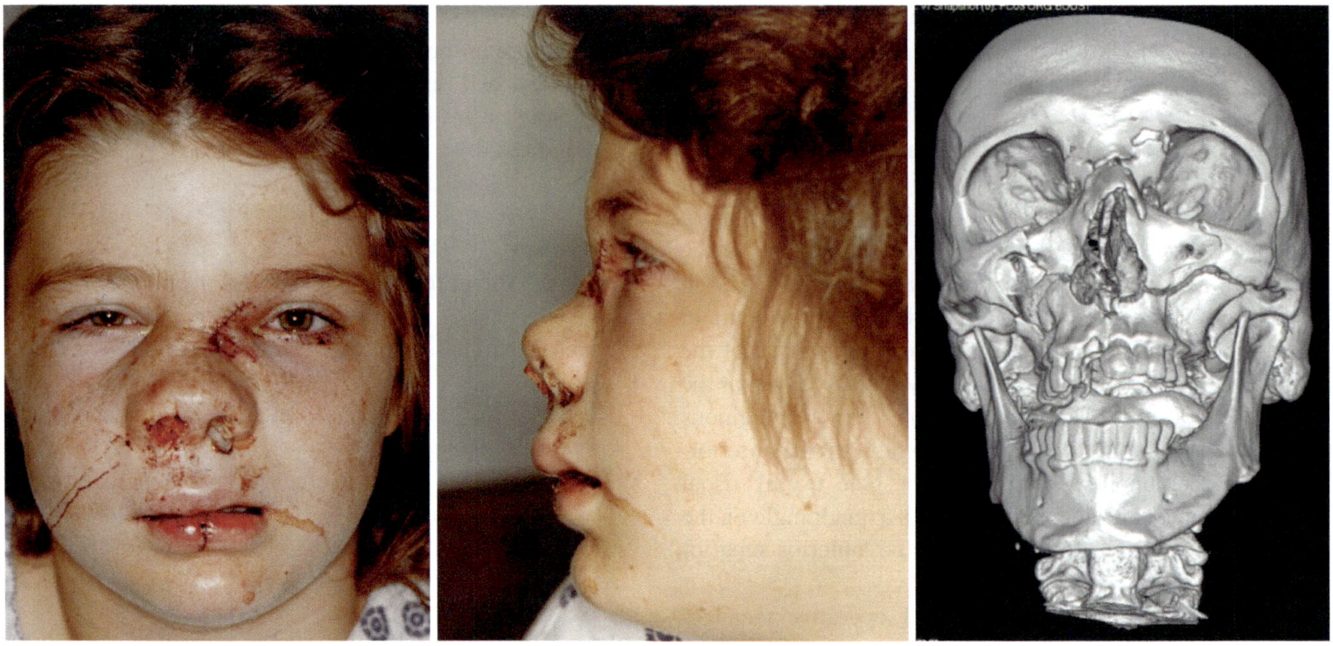

An 18-year-old was injured in an MVA 24 h ago. Slightly obtunded.

1. Describe the slide(s) and add a focused history and physical exam. Now, describe the findings on the 3D CT.
   (a) In addition to the 3D CT scan provided, any other tests indicated? Justify.
   (b) What views/slides on the CT scan, in addition to the 3D CT, would be of value in the derivation of a treatment plan? Be specific.
2. Are any immediate treatment measures indicated?
3. What is the pathologic anatomy of this injury?
4. Outline a treatment plan, including incisions, sequence, etc.
5. Assuming complete correction of the deformity, what are other potential late complications?

Case-Based Conference: Discussion

Case 1: Midface Fractures

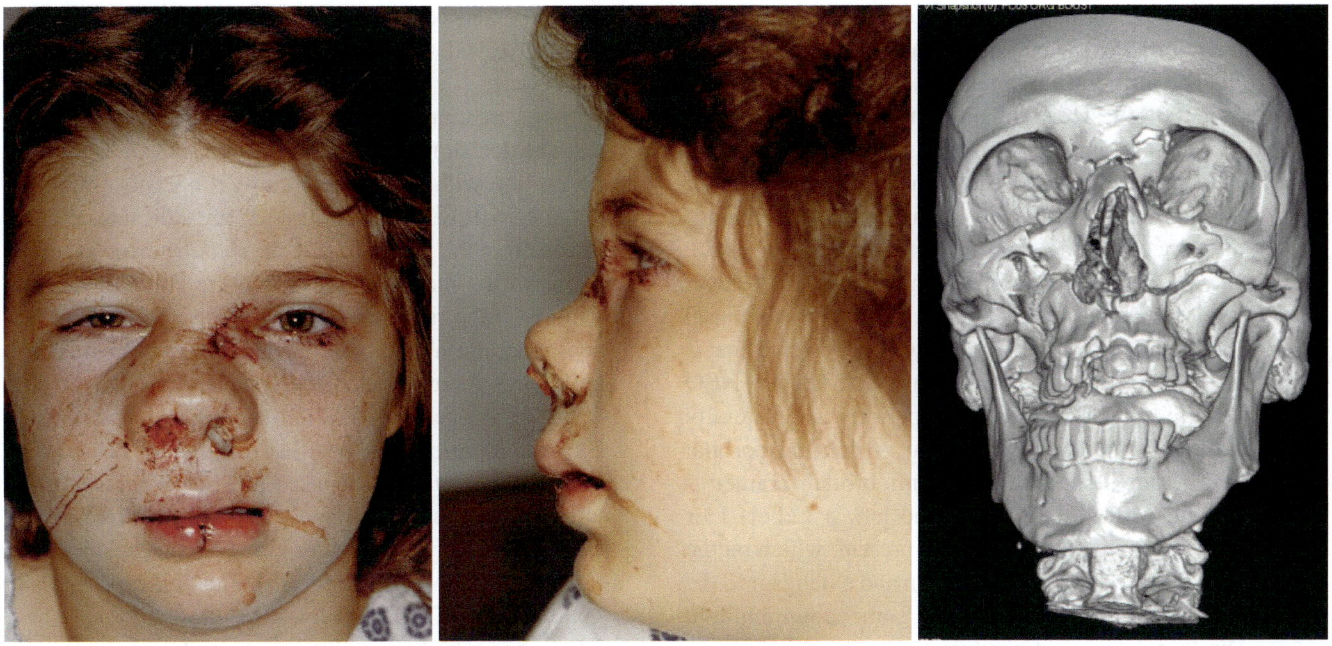

An 18-year-old injured in an MVA 24 h ago. Slightly obtunded.

1. Describe the slide(s) and add a focused history and physical exam. Now, describe the findings on the 3D CT. (Young woman with closed facial trauma. The anterior-posterior view demonstrates a widened intercanthal distance, bilateral nasal packing in place, with little blood evident in both nostrils. An upturned tip is readily evident, and the dorsum is deviated to the right with a lack of left medial canthal definition and increased intercanthal distance on the left. The palpebral distance on the right appears narrowed, and a left medial canthus laceration has been repaired. No enophthalmos is evident. Other findings include a sutured vertical midline lower lip laceration. The extreme lateral edge of the face on the right has not been included in the photo, but the transverse facial width appears to have decreased and increased on the left. No other deformities or lacerations are evident. The lateral view demonstrates a marked depression of the nasal dorsum with telescoping of the nose. Some elements of retrognathia are also evident. The CT demonstrates a left nasoethmoid orbital, NEO, fracture with a rotated nasal dorsum and an apparent overlap with a possibly medially displaced left maxillary fragment. A right infraorbital rim fracture at the level of the infraorbital foramen is present. The left NEO fracture appears to extend superiorly and laterally into the medial supraorbital rim. More inferiorly, a LeFort I or transverse maxillary fracture is present, which on the right extends into the infraorbital rim fracture with some comminution. A fracture line is evident in the alveolar ridge between the right medial and lateral incisor. In summary, the CT scan demonstrates a left nasoethmoid orbital fracture, a LeFort I transverse maxillary, and probably a unilateral right LeFort II fracture. The 3D scan is suggestive of an alveolar fracture anteriorly on the right. The principal history questions would ascertain orientation to time and place and any symptoms that may have developed in the post-injury period with nasal packing in place over the 24 h. Of course, the patient should have been cleared by the trauma team, and if transferred from another facility, a similar assurance is mandatory. A past medical history, including any preinjury orthodontics and social history, completes the historical portion of the clinical examination. The vital signs, including temperature, are reviewed. With nasal packing in place and given the patient's pattern of injury—see below—concern about the presence of a CSF leak and with nasal packing, a potential for the occurrence of early meningitis. On a physical exam, intercanthal distances should be measured from the midline of the nose and compared to normal. A traction test could be performed on the left lower eyelid, but it should be negative since the scans appear to represent a

Markowitz I nasoethmoid orbital fracture pattern. An eye exam, including vision to confrontation, pupil reaction, and extraocular motion, should be performed. Sensation over the infraorbital nerve is tested bilaterally. The intraoral exam is performed for the detection of lacerations, and the mobility of the maxillary fragments is determined as well. The intraoral examination should also include an assessment of the status of dentition and detection of any hard palatal laceration.)

(a) In addition to the 3D CT scan provided, any other tests indicated? Justify. (An ophthalmology consult if any concerns arise from the screening ocular exam. The CT 3D reconstruction demonstrates a left nasoethmoid orbital, NEO, fracture with a rotated nasal dorsum and apparent overlap with a possibly medially displaced left maxillary fragment. The left NEO fracture appears to extend superiorly and laterally into the medial supraorbital rim. A right infraorbital rim fracture at the level of the infraorbital foramen is present. More inferiorly on the left, a LeFort I or transverse maxillary fracture is present, which on the right is more superior in location and extends into the infraorbital rim fracture with some comminution. The fronto-zygomatic suture lines are intact bilaterally. Some bowing of the left zygomatic arch is present.)

(b) What views/slides on the CT scan, in addition to the 3D CT, would be of value in the derivation of a treatment plan? Be specific. (Axial slices more superior than the midorbit for determination of the size of nasoethmoid orbital fragment on the left; slices through the medial orbital wall for evidence of disruption of the ethmoid component of the medial orbital wall. Axial slices through the nasal septum for degree of displacement, if any; coronal views for determination of the integrity of the cribriform plate as well as the orbital floor bilaterally.)

2. Are any immediate treatment measures indicated? (Removal of the nasal packing and determination of the presence of a CSF rhinorrhea. In instances of complex midface fractures, the possibility of CSF rhinorrhea exists, which, if nasal packing is placed, may result in retrograde bacterial contamination and meningitis, as discussed above.)
3. What is the pathologic anatomy of this injury? (Clinically, the nose is telescoped posteriorly and superiorly, the inferior maxillary or occlusal fragment in the presence of a LeFort I fracture is probably mobile. In addition, that fragment is further split into two right and left fragments by the longitudinal palatal split. A fracture of the nasoethmoid orbital region, namely, a fracture fragment that involves nasal bones, ethmoid, and the orbit. In this case, the left nasal bones, left infraorbital rim, the ethmoid perpendicular plate, probably the left medial orbital wall and the nasofrontal suture line are all involved. These findings are consistent with a left nasoethmoid orbital and central maxillary fracture. The nose is telescoped posteriorly and superiorly, and possibly a fracture of the cribriform plate with a CSF leak is present. The maxilla may or may not be mobile.)
4. Outline a treatment plan, including incisions, sequence, etc. (The decision on the airway for anesthesia is made in conjunction with anesthesia. Many, if not most, anesthesiologists will be reluctant to perform right nasotracheal intubation in the presence of CSF rhinorrhea or even in a patient with a maxillary-NEO fracture. If so, placement of the ET tube retromolar, submental intubation, or tracheostomy are all options dependent on individual circumstances. As mentioned, the first priority is the removal of the nasal packing. If CSF rhinorrhea is present, an observation period with bed rest is indicated. The operative management would consist of a set of incisions that include a transbuccal sulcus for exposure of the LeFort I fracture line, a right transconjunctival for repair of the infraorbital rim, and a bicoronal flap for exposure and repair of the NEO fracture lines.

Following intubation, disimpaction of the central maxillary fragment, displaced and impacted superiorly and posteriorly, may be necessary with a reduction process prior to plate fixation. This impaction is accomplished with the Rowe disimpaction forceps after cocaine vasoconstriction of the intranasal mucosa. Centralization of the septum is accomplished at the same time. The patient is placed into occlusion and intermaxillary fixation. Attention is now directed towards the inferior maxilla. If no splints have been constructed on an articulator with a cast model or generated digitally, then the longitudinal palatal fracture is stabilized with plates and screws. The now single maxillary fragment is related to the mandible and secured with IMF with interdental wires. The mandibular arch bar can be placed at the initiation of the case. Finally, the LeFort I fracture lines across the nasal maxillary buttress are secured with plates and screws.

Reduction and repair of the nasoethmoid orbital fracture can be performed through the bicoronal incision with a "C" plate extending from the superior orbital rim to the medial infraorbital rim. The other approach available to repair NEO fractures, perhaps particularly applicable to a unilateral pattern, is transnasal wiring. Using either a wire-passing drill bit or with an 18 G spinal needle as a twist drill, the medial canthal fragment is secured with a 3° permanent suture passed in a mattress fashion to the opposite side. Placement of the suture as posterior and superior as possible is crucial. All maxillary fracture lines and the right infraorbital fracture are plated. In some instances, the use of intercanthal external sutures, tied over bolsters or buttons, removed at 2 weeks postoperative, may help prevent the development of soft tissue edema, which may be slow to resolve. The right infraorbital rim is plated after reduction of the maxilla, and all midface reduction should be accomplished prior to internal fixation.)

5. Assuming complete correction of the deformity, what are other potential late complications? (Given the pattern of fractures, the possible late complications include epiphora, nasoseptal deviation with nasal respiratory obstruction, malocclusion, and residual nasal aesthetic issues.)

Postoperative (3 Months)

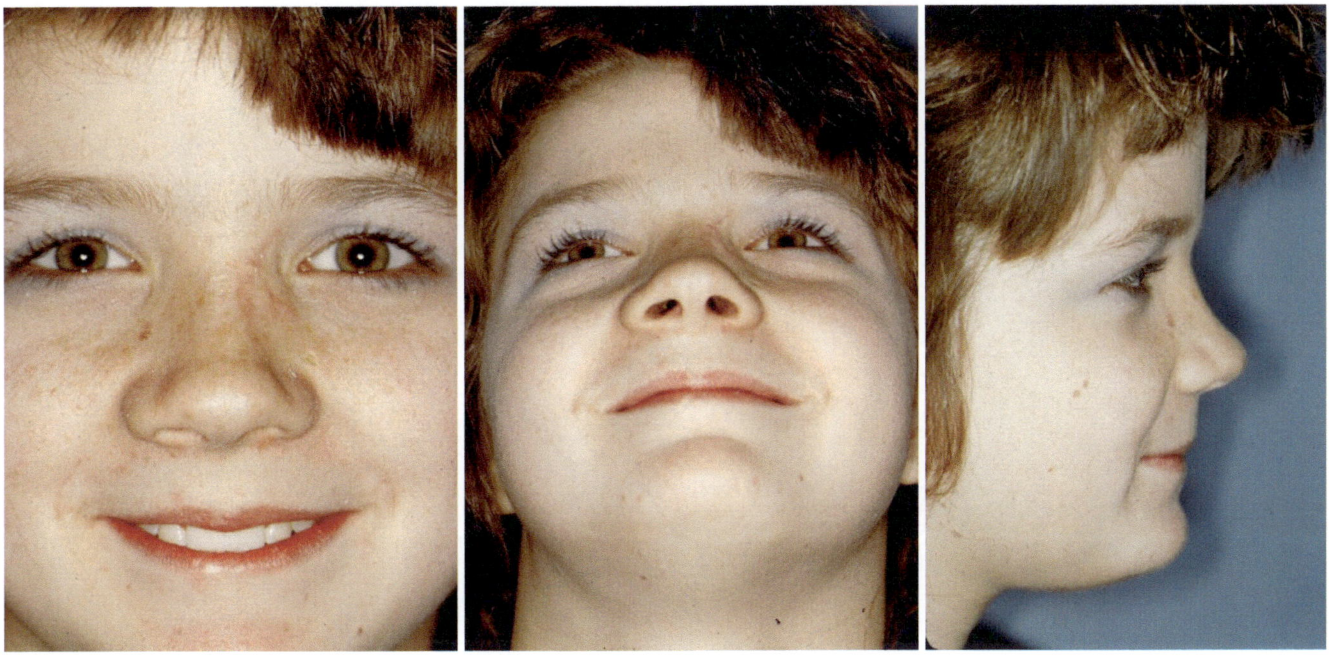

The three photos, frontal, submental vertex, and right lateral illustrate several findings: some probable residual telecanthus, symmetrical, and within the realm of aesthetically normal. The configuration of the nasal tip and dorsum has been restored to normal, and on lateral view, the prior retrognathia is absent. On the submental vertex, the tip prominence is reduced, and the alar bases are splayed and widened. The occlusion cannot be assessed on these photos.

Critique

Although a dorsal cantilever bone graft was performed, the postoperative appearance would suggest that perhaps a columellar strut graft should have been added.

In-Service Examination

1. The following bones comprise the medial orbital wall **EXCEPT:**
   (a) Lesser wing of the sphenoid
   (b) Zygoma
   (c) Maxilla
   (d) Ethmoid
2. The bone or structure involved in all LeFort facial fractures is:
   (a) Zomer
   (b) Orbital floor
   (c) Pterygoid
   (d) Zygoma
3. The correct vector to repair the medial canthal tendon in transnasal canthopexy is:
   (a) Anterior, inferior
   (b) Anterior, superior
   (c) Posterior, inferior
   (d) Posterior, superior

48 Zygoma, Orbit

Bibliography

Jelks G and Zide B, Chapter 1: "Bones, Vessels, and Nerves", Surgical Anatomy of the Orbit, Raven Press, New York (2006); **pp 1–16.**

Wilson S and Ellis III E, "Surgical Approaches to the Infraorbital Rim and Orbital Floor: The Case for the Subtarsal Approach", Clinical Controversies in Oral and Maxillofacial Surgery: Part One, *J Oral Maxillofac Surg*, (2006); 64:**104–107.**

Kusbner GM, "Surgical Approaches to the Infraorbital Rim and Floor: The Case for the Transconjunctival Approach", Clinical Controversies in Oral Maxillofacial Surgery: Part Two, *J Oral Maxillofac Surg*, (2006); 64:**108–110 (See supplement).**

Kelley P, Hopper R, and Gruss J, "Evaluation and Treatment of Zygomatic Fractures", *Plast Reconstr Surg.*, (2007); 120: **pp 5S–15S.**

Ricketts S, Gill HS, Fialkov JA, et. al., "Facial Fractures", *Plast Reconstr Surg.*, (2016); 137: **432e, Videos 4, 5 and 7, Figs. 11 and 15 ONLY**.

Chang A, et al, Chapter 6: "Orbital Floor Fractures", Evaluation and Treatment of Orbital Fractures, Holck DE and Ng JD, Elsevier Sanders, (2005); **pp 93–100, Table 1.**

Blaydon SM, et al, Chapter 7: "Medial Orbital Wall Fractures", Evaluation and Treatment of Orbital Fractures, Holck DE and Ng JD, Elsevier Sanders, (2005); **pp 103–116 ONLY.**

Manson PN, Clifford CM, Iliff NT, et al., "Mechanisms of Global Support and Posttraumatic Enophthalmos", *Plast Reconstr Surg.*, (1986); 77(2):**201–202 ONLY.**

Grant MP, Iliff NT, Manson PN, Chapter 48: "Reconstruction of Orbital Defects", Operative Plastic Surgery, Evans, G. R., McGraw-Hill Medical Publishing Co., (2005); **pp 563–568.**

Supplemental Reading for Junior Integrated Residents

Fraioli RE, Branstetter BF, and Deleyiannis FWB, "Facial Fractures: Beyond Le Fort", *Otolaryngol Clin N Am.*, (2008); 41: 65–69.

DeSerres J.J., Budning A., Antonyshyn O.M., "Current Management of Late Posttraumatic Enophthalmos", *Plast Reconstr Surg.*, (2022);150(4):**888e–890, 899e, Videos 1 and 4.**

Faculty Discussion and Study Guide

Anatomy

1. What muscles originate from the zygoma? (Masseter, zygomaticus major and minor. The temporalis fascia relates to the zygomatic arch but originates from the temporal bone.)
2. The zygoma articulates with what four bones and where? (Frontal at the frontal process, the greater wing of the sphenoid within the orbit, the maxilla anteriorly, and the temporal bone at the arch.)
3. The zygoma is described as a "quadrapod." What are the legs and the base? (The base is the lateral orbital wall, and the four legs are the inferior orbital rim, lateral orbital rim, zygomatico-maxillary buttress, and the arch-consider the suture lines when answering this question. Two fixation points to the cranium and two to the maxilla exist.)
   (a) What's the vertical and transverse buttress of the zygoma? (Vertically, the zygomatico maxillary buttress and fronto-zygomatic or lateral orbital rim; transverse is the frontal process of the maxilla, the inferior orbital rim, the malar portion of the zygoma, and the zygomatic arch.)

E. Luce, *A Curriculum for Plastic Surgery*, https://doi.org/10.1007/978-3-031-62087-4_48

4. The readings describe the term zygomatic "arch" as a misnomer. Why? (The arch is only curved the most anteriorly and most posteriorly; otherwise, it is straight in the A-P direction.)
5. What are the principal components of the orbital floor, lateral wall, medial wall, and "posterior" wall? (Floor is maxillary and zygomatic, medial wall lacrimal and ethmoid, lateral wall is sphenoid and zygomatic, a critical suture line to judge adequate reduction, and posterior wall is mostly sphenoid.)
   (a) What is the configuration of the orbital floor from the inferior orbital rim posteriorly? (Initially and anteriorly, the floor is somewhat concave. So, if the surgeon is standing from the head of the table, the initial dissection posterior to the rim is inferior by 5–8 mm. The floor then slants more superiorly and becomes somewhat convex at a 25–30° angle. The medial orbital wall slants slightly laterally from anterior to posterior. More importantly, the inferior one-half of the medial orbital wall bulges moderately into the orbital space in transition to the floor, often referred to as the inferior medial bulge.)
   (b) The principal bony components of the orbit include the zygoma, frontal, maxilla, lacrimal, ethmoid, and sphenoid. What is the seventh bone and minor contribution? (The orbital plate of the palatine)
   (c) Define the location and the importance of the lamina papyracea. (The lamina papyracea is an eggshell-thin bone of the medial orbital wall posterior to the posterior lacrimal crest. The ethmoid air cells or sinus are medial to the lamina papyracea. This area is often involved in medial orbital wall fractures.)
6. What is the importance of the anterior ethmoidal foramen and the posterior ethmoidal foramen? (The importance is twofold: The foramina lies at the junction of the frontal bone and the ethmoid bone in the medial orbital wall and serves as a marker between extracranial and intracranial cavities. The foramina also provides a guide to the depth of the orbit in the dissection of the medial orbital wall.)
7. What is the distance from the anterior lacrimal crest to the anterior ethmoid foramen (AEF), the anterior ethmoid foramen to the posterior ethmoid foramen (PEF), and the posterior ethmoid foramen to the optic canal? (24 mm from the anterior lacrimal crest to the AEF, 12 mm from the AEF to the PEF, and 6 mm from the PEF to the optic canal)
   (a) Any discussion of measurements within the bony orbit must include:
      - Distance from the bony rim to the apex or optic foramen (45 mm, less in women versus men)
      - "Safe" dissection distances (30+ mm medially and superiorly, 35–40 mm more inferiorly, 40 mm laterally)
      - What defines "safe"? (The presence within the posterior orbit of the annulus of Zenn.)
   (b) True or false: Safe dissection can be done on the medial orbital wall to a depth of 40 mm from the anterior lacrimal crest. (False. The annulus of Zenn sits just anterior to the posterior ethmoidal foramen or approximately 35 mm posterior to the orbital rim.)
8. What is Whitnall's tubercle, where is it, and what is attached to it? (Whitnall's tubercle is a bony prominence at the lateral canthus within the orbit at the lateral orbital rim about 7–10 mm inferior to the fronto-zygomatic suture line and 5–7 mm posterior to the lateral orbital rim. The following structures are inserted on Whitnall's tubercle: the levator lateral expansion, Whitnall's ligament, and the superior and inferior retinaculum of the lateral canthal tendon, as well as an extension of Lockwood's ligament.)
9. How would you map out the location of the infraorbital foramen to perform an infraorbital nerve block percutaneously? (With the visual axis at neutral, drop a vertical line parallel to the medial limbus, palpate the rim on the line, and the foramen lies 5–8 mm inferiorly.)
   (a) Supraorbital block? (Same guideline except slightly medially)
10. The superior and inferior orbital fissures are primarily structures of which orbital wall? (Lateral. The superior fissure is located at the junction between the medial lesser and lateral greater wings of the sphenoid, with the two configured into a reversed L in the right orbit with the optic canal sitting medial to the "knuckle" of the L.)
11. The bony orbit is often described as a cone with the optic foramen and nerve at the apex. Is that an anatomically correct analogy? (No. With some minor variations, perhaps the bony orbit is a cone, but the optic foramen is located at the posterior limit of the medial wall.)
   (a) What bone contains the optic foramen? (The optic foramen is within the lesser wing of the sphenoid.)
12. What structures exit through the inferior orbital fissure? (Maxillary division of cranial nerve V, infraorbital artery, the inferior ophthalmic vein, and branches of sphenopalatine ganglion. The zygomatico-facial and zygomatico-temporal branches exit the maxillary division prior to the entrance into the infra-orbital canal.)
   (a) Through what foramen does the maxillary division enter the orbit? (Rotundum, situated between the confluence of the superior orbital and inferior orbital fissure.)
13. What structures exit the superior orbital fissure within the annulus of Zenn? (Cranial nerve III, oculomotor, VI, abducens, as well as the nasociliary nerve, ophthalmic vein, and all the EOM except the inferior oblique.)
   (a) Outside the annulus of Zenn? (Cranial nerve IV or trochlear, lacrimal, and frontal nerves.)

14. Anatomy of the ligamentous sling and intramuscular cone fat? (Lockwood's in the upper lid and Whitnall's ligament in the lower lid. The intermuscular cone fat is contained in Tenon's capsule that surrounds the extraocular muscles and the remainder of the intramuscular structures.)
    (a) Name the inferior and the superior transverse globe supporting ligaments. (Lockwood for the lower lid and Whitnall's for the upper lid)
    (b) What are the two muscles of extraocular motion, superior and inferior, that give rise to the capsulopalpebral fascia inferiorly and the fascia of the levator superiorly? (Inferior rectus and superior rectus, respectively.)
15. A patient with orbital fractures has profuse hemorrhage from the anterior and posterior ethmoidal arteries. The first-year plastic resident suggests selective embolization. What is your decision? (Ethmoidal arteries are branches of the ophthalmic artery, which in turn is a branch of the internal carotid artery, a contraindication for selective embolization.)

Diagnosis, Examination

1. What are the pertinent physical exam findings in a zygomatic fracture? (Periorbital ecchymosis, trismus, malar flattening, decreased sensation over the infraorbital nerve, palpable step-off at the infraorbital rim, inferior displacement of the lateral palpebral fissure or loss of the upward slant, diplopia, limitation of upward gaze.)
    (a) Explain the etiology of trismus and inferior displacement of the palpebral fissure. (Trismus is most commonly from blood in the masseter muscle, but impingement of the coronoid process by a medially displaced arch fracture can be a cause; the normal upward cant of the lateral canthus of 2 mm is displaced inferiorly by the depression of the malar eminence and the attached lateral canthal tendon).
2. What are the principal secondary deformities seen in an unreduced zygoma fracture? (Malar flattening or lack of cheek projection, increased transverse facial width, probably vertical dystopia, and quite possibly enophthalmos.)
3. Why might the detection of enophthalmos be difficult acutely? (Edema and minor hemorrhage of the soft tissues of the orbit can produce a relative proptosis.)
    (a) What are the hallmark findings in enophthalmos? (Decrease in the anterior projection of the globe, accentuation or deepening of the upper eyelid palpebral sulcus, narrow palpebral fissure.)
    (b) What is an objective method of measuring exophthalmos? (Hertel exophthalmometry.)
4. Describe and explain the physical findings in the superior orbital fissure, SOF, syndrome (The findings are secondary to involvement of the major nerves within the superior orbital fissure, abducens, oculomotor, trochlear, and frontal or supraorbital branch of the trigeminal. Slight proptosis, ptosis of the upper lid, ophthalmoplegia, dilated non-reactive pupil either directly or consensually, intact consensual response in the opposite pupil, loss of sensation over the ipsilateral forehead. A slight proptosis and ophthalmoplegia are both secondary to loss of tone and paralysis of muscles of extraocular motion that hold the globe in the normal situation modestly posterior. Ptosis of the lid and loss of pupillary response is the absence of sympathetic innervation via the oculomotor nerve. Loss of sensation is secondary to injury of the ophthalmic division of the trigeminal. A collateral finding is anesthesia of the cornea and loss of ipsilateral lacrimal gland function, both the result of the injury to cranial nerve V.)
    (a) Diagnosis of orbital apex? (Same as above, plus blindness and non-reactive pupil. Direct and consensual and absence of consensual response in the opposite pupil.)
    (b) Diagnosis in the unconscious, intubated patient (Only pupils are available, so the findings in SOF: consensual response in the opposite pupil; orbital apex: neither a consensual nor a direct response in the ipsilateral pupil; if optic nerve only: consensual response intact by stimulation of the opposite pupil, a finding in optic neuropathy.)

Treatment

1. What underlies the concept of early, within 2 weeks of injury, open reduction internal fixation of zygomatic fractures? (Late corrections of the resultant facial deformity are quite difficult and frequently incomplete or unsuccessful due to secondary soft-tissue contraction.)
2. What incisions are available for ORIF of the zygoma? (Eyelid, either transconjunctival or transcutaneous, the lateral portion of an upper blepharoplasty incision, and the upper buccal sulcus. A bicoronal approach is reserved for complex fractures that require exposure of the arch.)
    (a) Variations of a transcutaneous incision? (Subciliary, subtarsal, and rim incision.)
    (b) Advantages and disadvantages of each. (A subciliary incision is a hidden scar more than the other two but at the expense of an increased incidence of ectropion, considerably higher than a subtarsal or rim incision. Subtarsal incision minimizes the risk of ectropion but may be a more modestly visible scar, particularly in young patients. Rim incision is

of historical interest only and, although it allows direct access to the rim, is at the expense of a visible and possibly contracted scar.)

3. Discuss the anatomy and technique of the transconjunctival incision, including the types. (Two choices, retroseptal versus preseptal. The key point is that the incision at the inferior border of the tarsus will divide the conjoined portion of the anterior leaf of the septum and the posterior capsulopalpebral fascia and thus gain access to the preseptal space. A conjunctival incision below the inferior border of the tarsus will divide just the posterior limb or capsulopalpebral fascia and thus be placed retroseptal or within the orbital fat.)
   (a) What can further enhance the exposure in a transconjunctival incision? (Lateral canthotomy.)
   (b) Give the pros and cons of a transconjunctival approach. (The obvious pro is the lack of a visible scar as well as a considerably lower incidence of ectropion compared to either the subciliary or subtarsal approach. The principal con is the learning curve as well as the 2% incidence of entropion, a less familiar complication to many plastic surgeons to treat. In addition, if a lateral canthotomy is performed, reconstitution of the lateral canthal ligament may produce asymmetry.)
4. What is the single most persuasive argument that would mandate the internal fixation of a zygoma, openly reduced into good alignment? (The chronic inferior pull of the masseter muscle.)
5. Describe the critical points of fracture in a zygoma and explain the relative importance of each in terms of a. reduction and b. fixation. (The most important points of determination of reduction are as follows in a hierarchy: lateral orbital wall or the zygomatico-sphenoid suture line, inferior orbital rim, zygomatic arch, probably zygomatico-maxillary buttress equivalent, and finally the zygomatico-frontal suture line. The hierarchy for fixation would be zygomatico-frontal suture line, zygomatico-maxillary buttress, zygomatic arch, and inferior orbital rim. Fixation of the zygomatico-sphenoid suture line is not possible except in rare instances of an associated sphenoid fracture, and the zygomatic arch is infrequently subject to ORIF. Three-point fixation, namely, the zygomatic-frontal suture, the zygomatic-maxillary buttress, and the infraorbital rim, is the optimal and common method.)
   (a) What is the role of the zygomatic arch in the reduction of zygomatic fractures? (Important to reduce and possibly fix to set the transverse width and projection of the midface.)
6. Describe techniques for reduction. (A Carol-Gerard screw placed into the body of the malar bone and/or bone hook used in a similar fashion percutaneously with anterior traction; Caldwell-Luc reduction through the maxillary sinus with placement of a blunt instrument such as a urethral sound posterior to the body of the zygoma.)
7. Discuss plate size vs. location in internal fixation. (Larger plates, perhaps 2.0 mm, are necessary at the buttress, and smaller 1.3 or 1.5 mm plates are placed on the infraorbital rim and the fronto-zygomatic suture line. Larger plates, particularly at the fronto-zygomatic suture line, may be palpable.)
8. Transfacial K-wires, intraosseous wire fixation, and external pin fixation play what role in the management of zygomatic fractures? (Historical interest only)
   (a) Comment on the use of intra-maxillary sinus packing. (Again, of historical interest. A risk of blindness exists)
9. Discuss the anatomy and technique of two different approaches to an isolated zygomatic arch fracture. (The Gillies approach is an incision in the temporal scalp with dissection beneath the deep temporal fascia to access medial to the zygomatic arch and is a good approach for reduction of a medially impacted arch as well as medial and posterior or clockwise rotation of the zygoma. The Keen approach is intraoral, more direct than Gillies, and can also be used to reduce the arch as well as rotate the body of the zygoma, although it is less efficient mechanically to rotate than through the maxillary sinus.)
   (a) Define the indications for an open approach to the zygomatic arch. (Lateral displacement, segmental fractures, telescoping, and comminution with the necessity of open reduction internal fixation, ORIF. The most common scenario is one of the associated complex midface fractures, including nasoethmoid orbital. An open approach will require a bicoronal flap.)
   (b) What are two complications of a bicoronal flap? (First, paralysis of the frontal branch of the facial nerve. If mobilization of the temporalis muscle out of the temporal fossa is necessary for a lateral sphenoid fracture, quite uncommon, possible temporal hollowing may be a sequela.)
10. What is particularly important about the presence of concomitant nasoethmoid orbital, NEO, fractures unilateral to a zygomatic fracture? (May, particularly if displaced posteriorly, provide misleading information about the adequacy of reduction if the lateral edge of the NEO fracture at the inferior orbital rim is used as a guide.)
11. How should the soft tissue be managed following ORIF of zygomatic fractures? (Because of the extensive subperiosteal dissection, the soft tissue should be resuspended to the body of the zygoma. In particular, in the area of the lateral canthus, the soft tissues should be replaced/resuspended with sutures placed through the periosteum and the soft tissues and then through a bone hole in the zygoma or lateral orbital rim.)

Orbital Component of Zygomatico-orbital Fractures

1. What is the basic pathology of orbital floor fractures that is responsible for surgical indications? (Herniation +/– entrapment of orbital content, usually septum, fat, and uncommonly the inferior rectus muscle into the fracture line and the maxillary sinus, acute enophthalmos.)
   (a) What are the two explanations of the pathomechanics? (One is a direct impact on the globe, which in turn is displaced and fractures the orbital floor and medial orbital wall. The other possible explanation is a buckling due to a direct impact on the body of the zygoma, which also, in turn, fractures the floor.)
2. Discuss your examination of a patient with orbital floor fracture(s). (Examine for extraocular motion, particularly upward gaze, the reactivity of the pupil, test visual acuity, and the presence of diplopia. Perform a forced duction test, but requires maximum patient cooperation. Obtain CT scan, retinal exam, Hertel exophthalmometry, and intraocular pressure if possible.)
3. A therapeutic enigma exists with the patient with a moderate-size medial orbital floor defect, no dystopia or limitation in ocular motility, and mild proptosis. What is it? (Mild proptosis can be the result of edema of the soft tissues that can conceal an underlying enophthalmos that may become evident with a resolution of the edema.)
4. Summarize recommendations for observation vs. immediate repair vs. delayed repair. (If a patient has good motility and no enophthalmos, then observation would be indicated. Diplopia and CT evidence of herniated tissue, a positive force duction test, and acute enophthalmos all mandate immediate repair. A defect greater than 2 cm^2 in an asymptomatic patient should be repaired. If a co-existent medial wall fracture is present contiguous with the floor fracture, the possibility of fat herniation is increased. An area of controversy is the asymptomatic patient with a floor defect of 1–1.5 cm^2, but a defect greater than this dimension should be repaired, and lesser defects in conjunction with medial wall defects. One must consider the basic work performed by Manson and his colleagues on mechanisms of global support and post-traumatic enophthalmos.)
5. In follow up to the question above, discuss timing, early or late surgical intervention in orbital floor and wall fractures with the benefits and risks of each. (Early surgical intervention can be done acutely in a scar-free dissection plane. However, some patients may not have ultimately required surgery. Late timing sorts out the patients who do and do not require surgery but, unfortunately, must be performed within an environment of scar fibrosis with frequently a less than optimal outcome.)
6. Describe a clinical scenario when exploration and reduction are urgent. (In the pediatric patient who presents with an orbital floor fracture, perhaps a trap door picture on the CT scan and associated bradycardia, nausea and vomiting, and marked restriction in vertical gaze. These patients are at substantial risk for ischemic fibrosis of the entrapped inferior rectus.)
7. What is the potential significance of a medial orbital wall fracture? (Entrapment with involvement of the medial rectus, although actual muscle entrapment is uncommon. As mentioned above, a concomitant medial wall fracture can certainly contribute to the occurrence of enophthalmos in the presence of an orbital floor fracture.)
8. Medial orbital wall fractures that produce limitation of motion in extraocular muscles will be manifest as: (Limitation of adduction and, to some degree, abduction, dependent on the site of entrapment of the medial rectus.)
9. Describe the trans-or retrocaruncular approach to the medial orbital wall. (A transconjunctival incision is extended medially and superiorly just behind the caruncle with the Colorado tip monopolar cautery. Once the conjunctiva has been divided, Stevens tenotomy scissors are used to dissect medially and slightly posteriorly to access the bony orbital wall and, in particular, the posterior lacrimal crest. That aperture is widened, and then a Joseph elevator is used to continue the dissection subperiosteally. If additional exposure is necessary, the bony origin of the inferior oblique can be subperiosteally dissected and is commonly performed.)

Mechanisms of Global Support in Post-traumatic Enophthalmos

1. Blepharoplasty with removal of fat does not produce enophthalmos because: (No increase in bony orbital volume, no disruption of the ligamentous support, extraconal fat is anterior.)
2. What is the normal approximate orbital volume? (28 cc in women, 30 cc in males.)
3. Briefly review the components of the ligament sling support of the globe. (Medial and lateral canthal ligaments and check ligaments. Superior lid sling: Whitnall's ligament, condensation of the levator and superior rectus fascia, Tenon's capsule. Inferior lid sling: Lockwood's ligament and extension of the inferior rectus and capsulopalpebral fascia; Tenon's capsule.)
4. Where in the orbit is a bone defect most critical? (Posterior to the equator of the globe.)
5. What role does late scar contracture play in the development of enophthalmos? (When an orbital defect is present, soft tissue will contract into the defect, in essence pulling the globe, dependent on the location of the defect, posteriorly and inferiorly.)

6. The reading provided a study performed to attain a better knowledge of the pathologic anatomy of enophthalmos. What are some of the prevailing theories? (Fat atrophy, descent of fat into a wall or floor defect, increase in size of the bony orbit, loss of ligamentous support, scar contracture.)
7. Cadaver work can produce enophthalmos by a variety of methods. Discuss. (Removal of the orbital floor alone did not produce enophthalmos, nor did removal of extraconal fat. What is necessary is a bony defect, namely an increase in intraorbital volume, disruption of ligamentous support, and loss of intraconal fat.)
8. The readings discuss some of the anatomical features and volume relationships. Outline. (Overall volume is 30 cc., and a 10% change will cause noticeable enophthalmos; one cubic cm increase in volume will lead to one mm enophthalmos, and 3 mm is the upper limit before enophthalmos is obvious, so a volume increase greater than 3 cm^3 or 10–13% will be clinically apparent.)
9. Discuss the late correction of enophthalmos. (The globe has fallen posteriorly and inferiorly, so bone grafts or alloplastic material must be placed posterior to the equator of the globe. Also, the volume needs to be sufficiently corrected, as outlined above. A complete and difficult dissection of the scarred orbital contents from the bony defect will be necessary.)

Video Notes Videos from Sharabi PRS (2011) 127: 27e videos 3–4

Video 3

Rudiments of ophthalmologic exam and also assessment of zygoma fractures.

Rating 6.5/10

Video 4

ORIF zygoma fracture-good narrative, video suboptimal. Video resolution over-exposed from headlight, surgeon's hands in view, etc. Rating 6.0/10, Narrative 8.5/10.

Case-Based Conference

Case 1: Facial Fracture

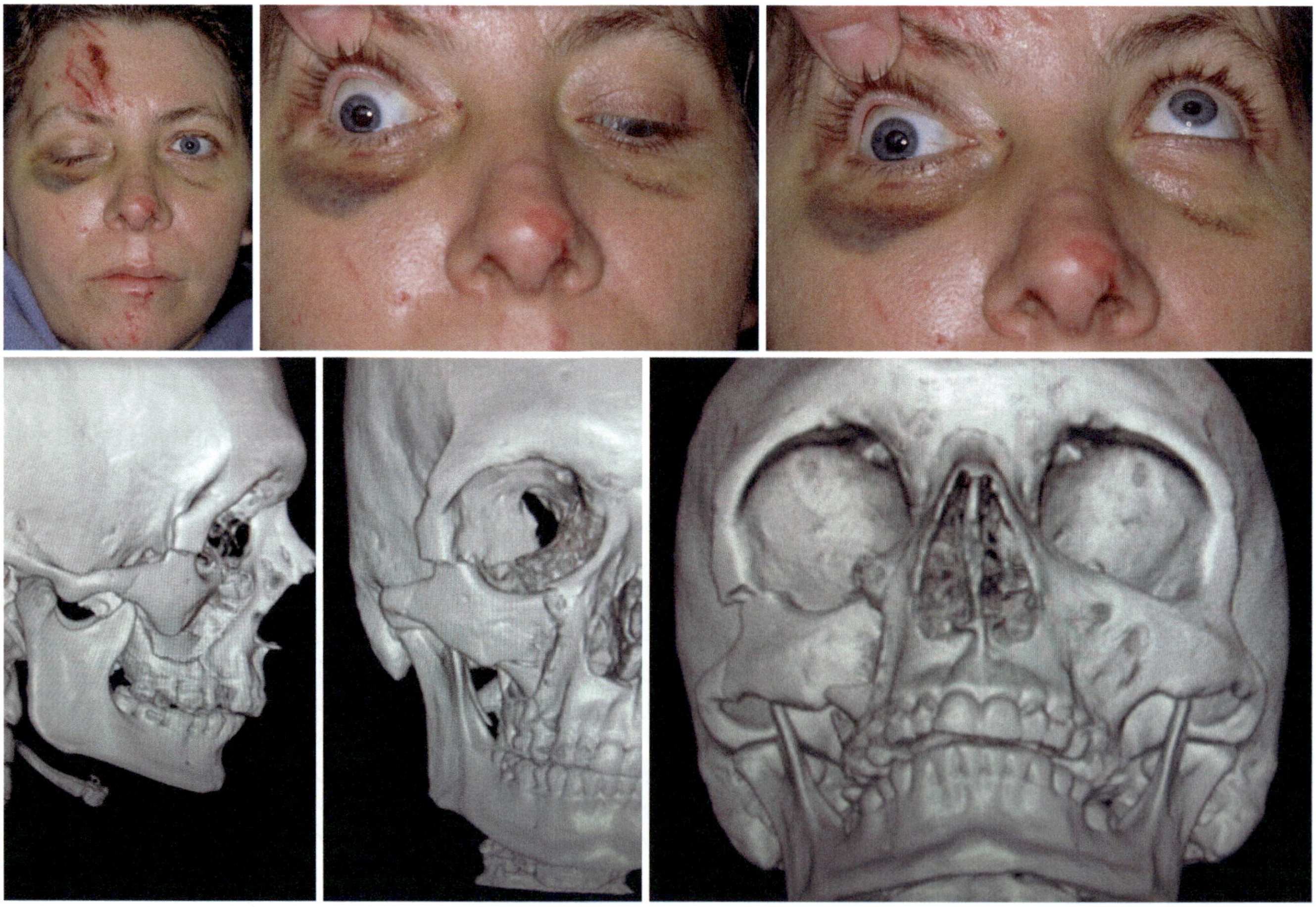

A 34-year-old woman was injured in an MVA 5 days ago.

1. Describe what you see on the slide and add any additional findings you would seek on a clinical exam.
2. Interpret the eye exam findings.
   (a) Read the 3D CT scan. Any additional imaging findings that you would consider essential for the development of a treatment plan?
3. Discuss the pathomechanics in the type of facial fracture under discussion. Describe the pathologic anatomy of her clinical findings.
4. Outline an operative plan, including set up, anesthesia, incisions, and steps or sequence.
5. List two or three undesirable sequelae in order of frequency of occurrence and explain why such might occur.

Case-Based Conference: Discussion

Case 1: Facial Fracture

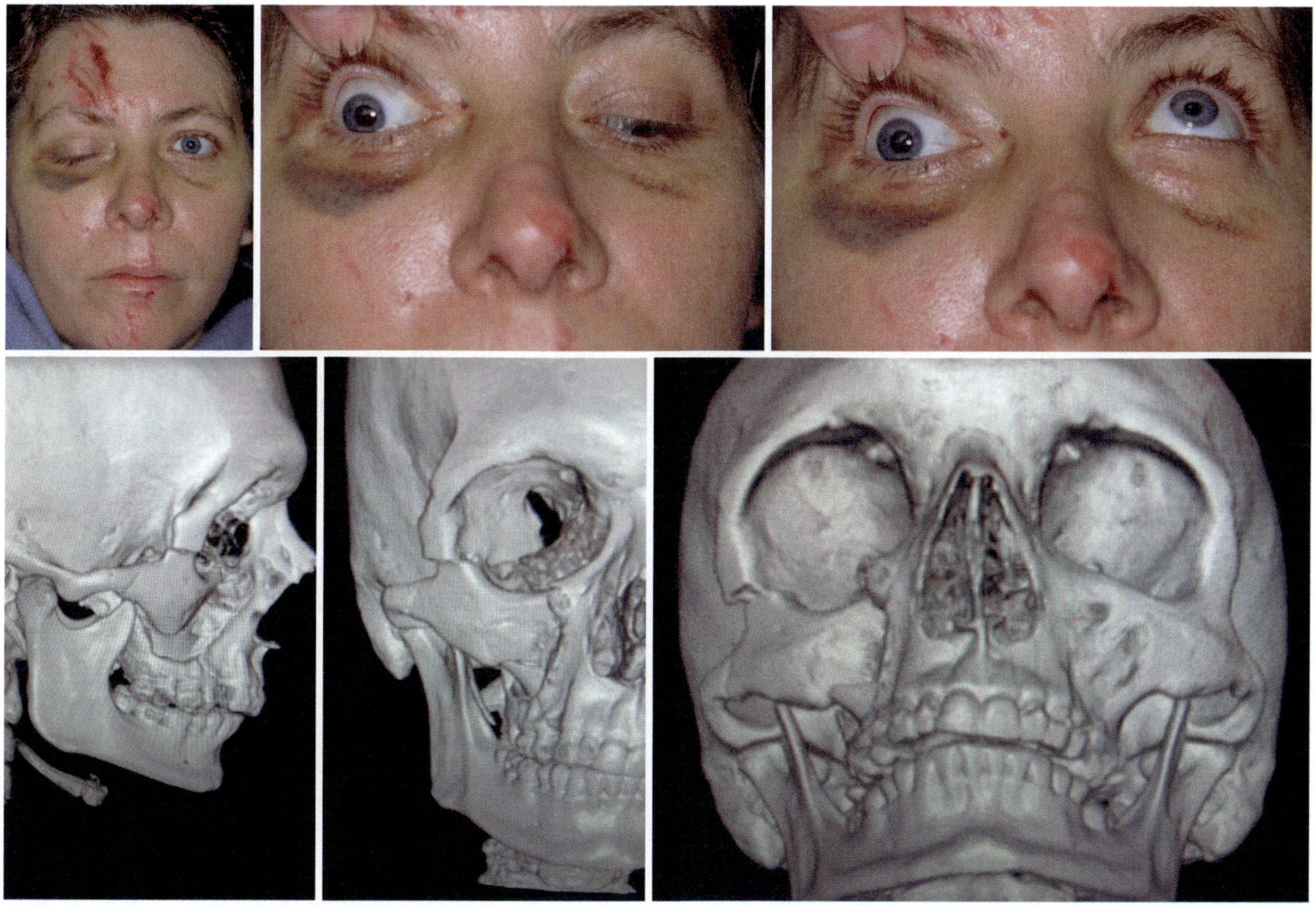

A 34-year-old woman was injured in an MVA 5 days ago.

1. Describe what you see on the slide and add any additional findings you would seek on a clinical exam. (A series of three clinical slides are provided. The first, a full facial view, demonstrates a woman with superficial abrasions of the forehead, a right infraorbital ecchymosis, and a right complete ptosis of the upper eyelid. The left periorbital area has a mild ecchymosis in the infraorbital region. In both instances, the inferior extent of the ecchymosis is limited by the arcus marginalis at the infraorbital rim. The right transverse facial width appears moderately decreased. The second slide is limited to the orbital-midface region and demonstrates the upward gaze of the left eye, the right upper lid manually held upward by a finger, and the right eye in a central to slightly lateral

gaze. The right pupil appears mid-position, the left mildly constricted. In the third slide, the left eye is in a downward gaze, and the right remains in the same position as the second slide.

The history would attempt to elicit those symptoms in a facial fracture patient: complaints of trismus, malocclusion, facial numbness, and those specific to the right orbit, namely, vision loss, diplopia, and pain. The physical exam would focus on the eye for intact vision, pupillary response, extraocular motion, and the presence of proptosis or enophthalmos. In addition to the examination in the frontal view for asymmetry, the patient is viewed from the submental vertex. Any alteration in the normal medial to lateral canthal tilt of +2 mm is noted, as well as any decrease in sensation of the distribution of the infraorbital and supraorbital nerves. Of course, a thorough assessment for the presence of other associated facial fractures (NEO, maxillary, mandibular) should be completed.)

2. Interpret the eye exam findings. (The right eye findings of ptosis, ophthalmoplegia, and, probably, a nonreactive pupil sum to a diagnosis of superior orbital fissure syndrome. The atypical finding is that of a slightly laterally deviated eye rather than a central ophthalmoplegic position that might indicate the presence of an intact abducens nerve innervating the lateral rectus. The classic superior orbital fissure syndrome, though, is a neuropathy of all three nerves of extraocular muscles as well as an ipsilateral forehead numbness secondary to involvement of the superior orbital and superior trochlear nerves.)
   (a) Read the 3D CT scan. Any additional imaging findings that you would consider essential for the development of a treatment plan? (Three 3D views are provided that demonstrate a significantly displaced zygomatic complex fracture, impacted posteriorly, medially, and probably inferiorly. The medial fracture line appears to be located at the zygomatico-maxillary suture line rather than more laterally at the infraorbital foramen, although that point is not well-defined. The lateral orbital rim is fractured considerably inferior to the zygomatico-frontal suture line, and the third fracture line appears to be the zygomatico-maxillary buttress. The two 3D slices provided do not detail the arch, so this particular axial view would be helpful, although, in comparison to the opposite or left side, the arch does not appear involved. The 3D also does not provide detail in regards to the orbital floor, and the coronal and sagittal cuts would need to be reviewed.)
3. Discuss the pathomechanics in the type of facial fracture under discussion. Describe the pathologic anatomy of her clinical findings. (The supraorbital fissure, an aperture linking the lesser and greater wing of the sphenoid, is the passageway for the three cranial nerves to the muscles of extraocular motion, including the oculomotor, trochlear, and abducens, the nasociliary nerve for corneal sensation, and the supraorbital and supratrochlear for forehead sensation. Loss of pupillary constriction is secondary to loss of parasympathetic fibers conducted in the oculomotor nerve, but a consensual response in the opposite pupil should be intact if the ipsilateral optic nerve is uninjured. If the ipsilateral optic nerve is also involved, the findings of above plus blindness are termed the orbital apex syndrome. The impact force appears directly anterior and perhaps somewhat medial. The principal distracting force is the chronic inferior pull of the masseter, originating on the body of the zygoma.)
4. Outline an operative plan, including set up, anesthesia, incisions, and steps or sequence. (The appropriate instrumentation and plating system should be available. Endotracheal anesthesia peroral route would be satisfactory. Corneal shields are placed. Management of the zygomatico-orbital component of the facial fractures requires addressing the displacement by reduction and fixation of the body and exploration and possible repair of the orbital floor and medial wall. The choice of incisions is an extension of an upper lid blepharoplasty combined with either a subtarsal or transconjunctival-retroseptal lower lid approach, and a transbuccal access. All three incisions are completed with a subperiosteal dissection exposure of the floor, regardless of CT scan findings. Using both a transmaxillary sinus and retro zygomatic approach, the zygoma is disimpacted, utilizing a broad periosteal elevator or male urethral sound. The orbital floor should be directly visualized during reduction. Adequacy of reduction is judged by a restoration of alignment at the fronto-zygomatic suture line, the infraorbital rim, and most importantly, by alignment of the greater wing of the sphenoid with the zygoma at the zygomatico-sphenoid suture line on the lateral orbital wall. Fixation is accomplished in three locations: the zygomatico-frontal fracture line with a 1.5 plate, the infraorbital rim with a 1.0 or 1.3 plate, and the zygomatico-maxillary buttress with a 2.0 plate. The floor must be explored regardless of the findings of the CT scan. As described above, the floor should be exposed early to visualize during any transantral reduction. Once the zygoma is reduced, the floor is scrupulously examined for disruption and magnitude of the same. If an orbital floor defect exists, a decision must be reached about autogenous or alloplastic implantation. The criteria are those of a floor defect of greater than 50% or 2 cm^2. The lower end of that spectrum of defects can be addressed with a bone graft from the anterior maxillary sinus wall or larger grafts with alloplastic implants such as porous polyethylene or titanium plates. The final step, if extensive degloving of the soft tissues has been necessary, is a soft tissue canthopexy to the zygomatic periosteum.)

5. List two or three undesirable sequelae in order of frequency of occurrence and explain why such might occur. (Although the frequency of occurrence differs from published series to published series, the two major complications or undesirable sequelae are enophthalmos and facial asymmetry from loss of facial projection and inappropriate transverse facial widening on the involved side. Enophthalmos is the result of expansion of the bony orbital volume either as a result of inadequate reduction of the zygomatic complex, inadequate correction of the floor component, or an overlooked medial orbital wall fracture. Loss of facial projection is secondary to incomplete reduction. Correction of late secondary deformities can be quite challenging.)

Case-Based Conference

Case 2: Facial Fractures

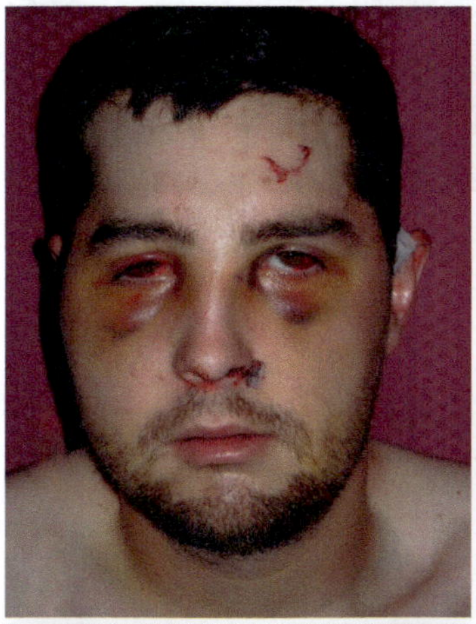
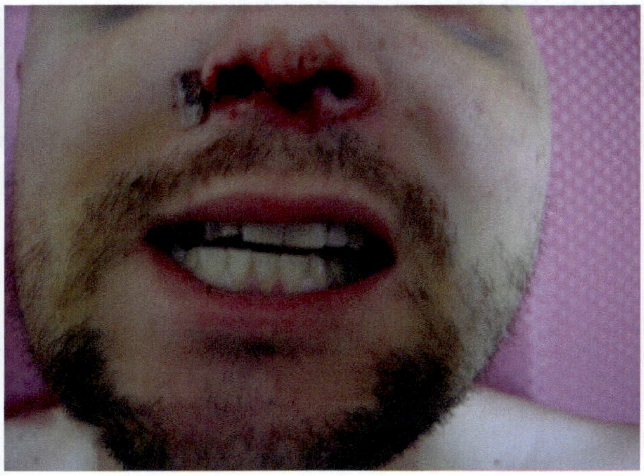
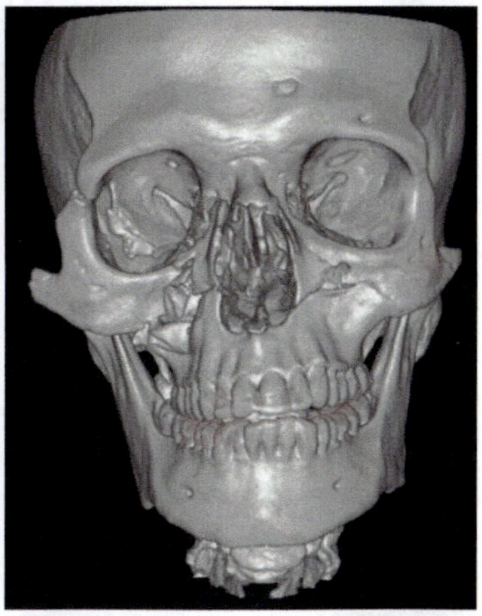
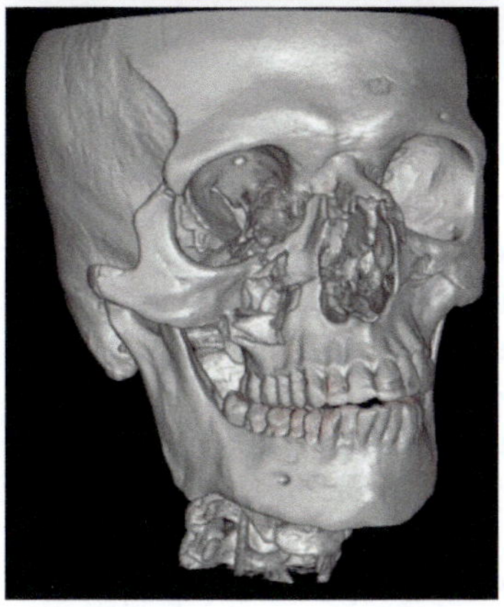

A 34-year-old male was injured in an MVA 72 h ago. No other injuries.

1. Describe what you see on the slide(s) and add any additional findings you would seek on a clinical exam. The closeup photo was obtained during a request to "put your teeth together." What other views would you have desired?
   (a) Read the 3D CT scan. Any additional imaging findings that you would consider essential for the development of a treatment plan?
2. Discuss the pathomechanics in the type of facial fracture under discussion. Describe the pathologic anatomy of the clinical findings in this patient.
3. Outline an operative plan, including operating room setup, anesthesia, incisions, and steps or sequence.
   (a) How would you determine the adequacy of the reduction of the fractures?
4. List two or three undesirable sequelae in order of frequency of occurrence and explain why such might occur.

Case-Based Conference: Discussion

Case 2: Facial Fractures

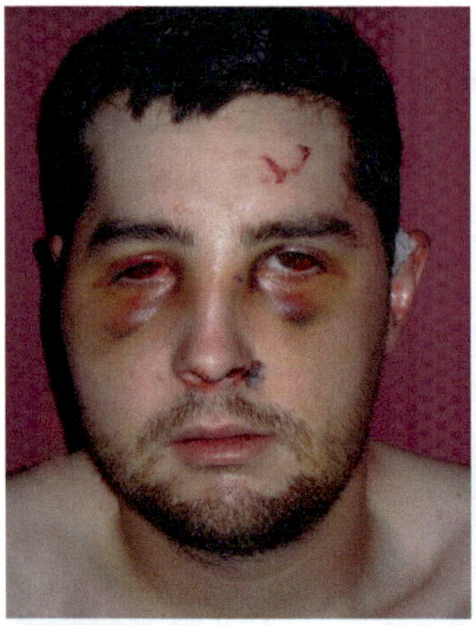
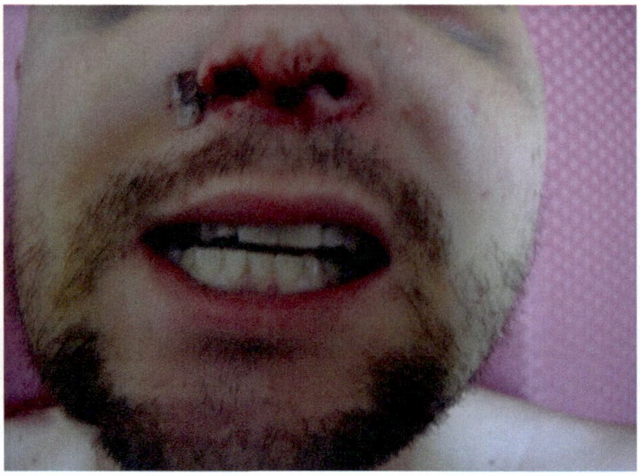
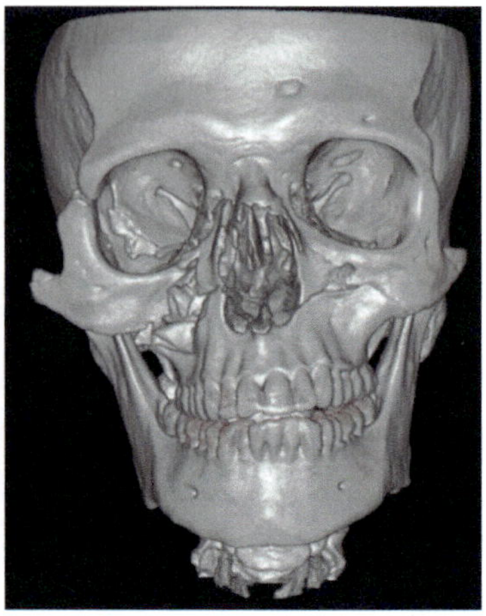
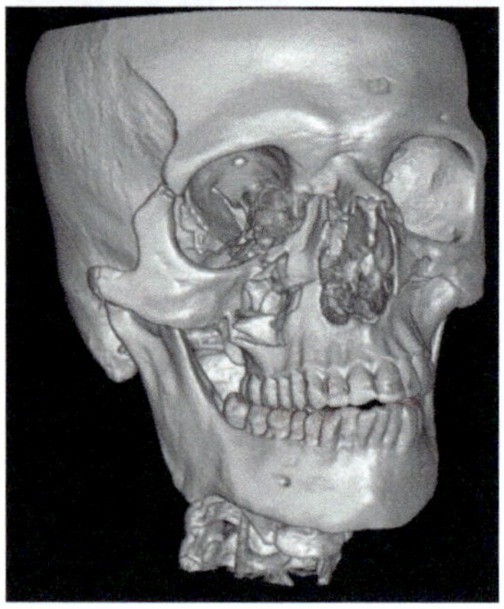

A 34-year-old male was injured in an MVA 72 h ago. No other injuries.

1. Describe what you see on the slide(s) and add any additional findings you would seek on a clinical exam. The closeup photo was obtained during a request to "put your teeth together." What other views would you have desired? (The first clinical slide provided depicts a full frontal view of the head and neck of a facial trauma patient. A 2 cm abrasion is present on the right forehead. Both orbital areas are marked by periorbital ecchymosis, including the medial canthal region. Both upper lids are ptotic, with the lash margin at the superior pupillary limbus. Chemosis of both sclerae is also present. By inspection, some element of telecanthus or widening of the intercanthal distance of the medial canthus appears to exist. The nasal dorsum is not deviated or depressed. A clearly evident inferior displacement or reversal of the normal positive lateral canthal tilt on the right is apparent. The transverse facial width on the right appears to have increased. A small amount of blood is present in the right nostril. No deformity is apparent in the lower one-third of the face. The second slide is of the lower one-half of the face and depicts incomplete closure into occlusion and a probable left buccal posterior cross-bite and right lingual. The patient appears to have full dentition. An additional view from the submental vertex perspective would provide information about the loss of projection of the malar eminence.

   The clinical exam would ascertain the presence or absence of the complications of his injuries, questions about nasal drainage, vision changes, and perception of bite abnormality, all of which would steer the subsequent physical examination. Circumstances of the injury and past medical and social history are obtained as well. Vision assessment by confrontation or Snellen card, pupillary response, and evaluation of the extraocular muscles are all important components of the eye exam. The unilateral intercanthal distance from the midline of the glabella to the medial canthus is measured and compared to normal. Lateral retraction is performed on the lower lid to ascertain, if present, loss of medial canthal tendon attachment. The occlusion is examined with gentle traction of the lips and commissures with the examiner's gloved fingers. Both infraorbital rims are palpated for a bony step-off. Sensation over the distribution of the infraorbital nerve is examined with particular emphasis on the right. As a final maneuver, the incisors are grasped by the examiner's thumb and fingers, and mobility of the maxilla is evaluated.)

(a) Read the 3D CT scan. Any additional imaging findings that you would consider essential for the development of a treatment plan? (Two views of the 3D reconstruction are provided. One is a direct anterior-posterior view, and the other is a right oblique. The most remarkable finding is a severely displaced right zygomatic fracture. Fracture lines are evident at the fronto-zygomatic, zygomatico-maxillary, zygomatico-temporal, as well as the zygomaticomaxillary buttress. The buttress appears comminuted. On both views, the zygoma is badly displaced and rotated counterclockwise, with the medial segment impacted posterior and the arch component rotated laterally. The 3D CT has additional findings: a fracture line is visualized at the nasal process of the maxilla on the right, a probable fracture of the right anterior medial orbital wall, which combined with a transverse fracture of the mid-portion of the inferior maxillary buttress strongly implies a right nasoethmoid orbital, NEO, fracture. An incomplete transverse fracture line is also seen in the left maxilla. No evidence of a mandibular or frontal sinus fracture exists on the 3D CT views. The two 3D views would not be sufficient to develop a treatment plan. A review of the coronal cuts would be imperative to assess the orbital floors and right medial orbital wall. Axial views will assist in the evaluation of the zygomatic arch displacement and the configuration of the right medial orbital wall, as well as the involvement and status of the septum. Viewed from the perspective of the patient's malocclusion and left crossbite, critical to the development of the treatment plan is the delineation of the associated maxillary fractures.)

2. Discuss the pathomechanics in the type of facial fracture under discussion. Describe the pathologic anatomy of the clinical findings in this patient. (The summary of the clinical and image findings are that of a posterior impacted and clockwise rotated right zygomatic fracture with a laterally-splayed zygomatic arch and a comminuted zygomatico-maxillary buttress. The other pathology is a probable right nasoethmoid orbital and a probable high LeFort I transverse maxillary fracture. A right anterior and lateral impact force was responsible for the overall fracture pattern.)
3. Outline an operative plan, including operating room setup, anesthesia, incisions, and steps or sequence. (No suggestion exists of extension of the fractures into the cranial base, although that possibility should be excluded on review of the individual CT slices; thus, nasotracheal intubation can be accomplished. Instrumentation will include Rowe disimpaction forceps. The choice of operative incisions should consider a bicoronal, a choice that would hinge on the configuration of the zygomatic arch and the right NEO fractures. Corneal shields are placed. Cocaine or other vasoconstrictive agent is placed intranasally; arch bars are secured on the maxilla and mandible, and, if necessary, disimpaction forceps are utilized to reduce the maxilla. That eventuality is unlikely since the LeFort fracture is unilateral. Other incisions are an extension of an upper lid blepharoplasty, either a subtarsal or transconjunctival-retroseptal lower lid approach, and transbuccal access. Given the severity of the displacement of the zygoma, a transcutaneous approach via a subtarsal fold incision is advisable. The maxillary fracture should be reduced, and the patient should be placed into intermaxillary fixation.)

(a) How would you determine the adequacy of the reduction of the fractures? (The NEO fracture is assessed and dependent upon the clinical determination of the intercanthal distance, perhaps a reduction of the right NEO fragment, which appears to be Type I with transnasal wiring to the opposite or left uninvolved side. Management of the zygomatico orbital component of the facial fractures requires the address of the displacement by reduction and fixation of the body and exploration and possible repair of the orbital floor and medial wall. The choice of incisions is an extension of an upper lid blepharoplasty, either a subtarsal or transconjunctival-retroseptal lower lid approach, and transbuccal access. All three incisions are completed with a subperiosteal dissection exposure of the floor, regardless of CT scan findings. Using both a transmaxillary sinus and retro zygomatic approach, the zygoma is disimpacted, utilizing a broad periosteal elevator or male urethral sound. The orbital floor should be directly visualized during reduction. Adequacy of reduction is judged by a restoration of alignment at the fronto-zygomatic suture line, the infraorbital rim, and most importantly, a correct alignment of the greater wing of the sphenoid with the zygoma at the zygomatico-sphenoid suture line on the lateral orbital wall. Fixation is accomplished in three locations: the zygomatico-frontal fracture line with a 1.5 plate, the infraorbital rim with a 1.0 or 1.3 plate, and the zygomatico-maxillary buttress with a 2.0 plate. As described above, the floor should be exposed early to visualize during any transantral reduction. Once the zygoma is reduced, the floor is scrupulously examined for disruption and magnitude of the same.

Finally, with an operative approach that consists of "top-down" first, the LeFort 1 component is plated, which will enable early release of intermaxillary fixation.)

4. List two or three undesirable sequelae in order of frequency of occurrence and explain why such might occur. (The definition of undesirable sequelae would be, for example, the development of chronic recurrent dacrocystorhinitis as a result of interruption of the nasolacrimal duct drainage system. Although the frequency of occurrence differs from published series to published series,

the two major complications or undesirable sequelae of zygoma fractures are enophthalmos and facial asymmetry from loss of facial projection and inappropriate transverse facial widening on the involved side. Enophthalmos is the result of expansion of the bony orbital volume either as a result of inadequate reduction of the zygomatic complex, inadequate correction of the floor component, or an overlooked medial orbital wall fracture. Loss of facial projection is secondary to incomplete reduction. Correction of late secondary deformities can be quite challenging. All are probably equally infrequent in occurrence.)

Case-Based Conference

Case 3: Orbital Floor Fracture

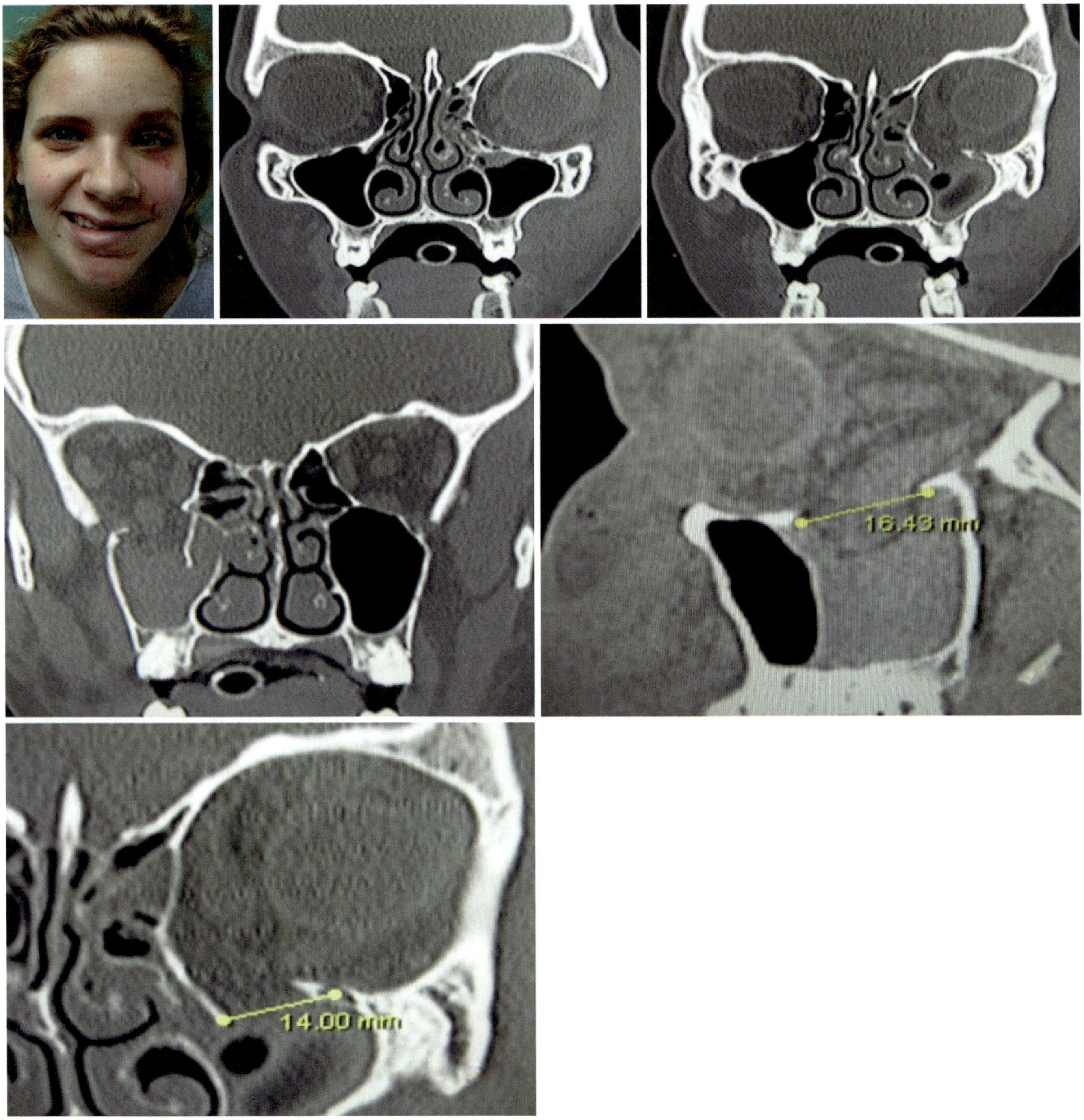

A 25-year-old referred 5 days after a motor vehicle accident. No other injuries.

1. Describe the slides and add a focused clinical examination. Now, review the CT findings.
   (a) Are any tests indicated? Justify.
   (b) What additional CT images, if any, would assist in the development of a treatment plan?
2. Summarize the pathologic anatomy and pathophysiology.
3. Based on the response to question two, outline a treatment plan and describe it in detail.

Case-Based Conference: Discussion

Case 3: Orbital Floor Fracture

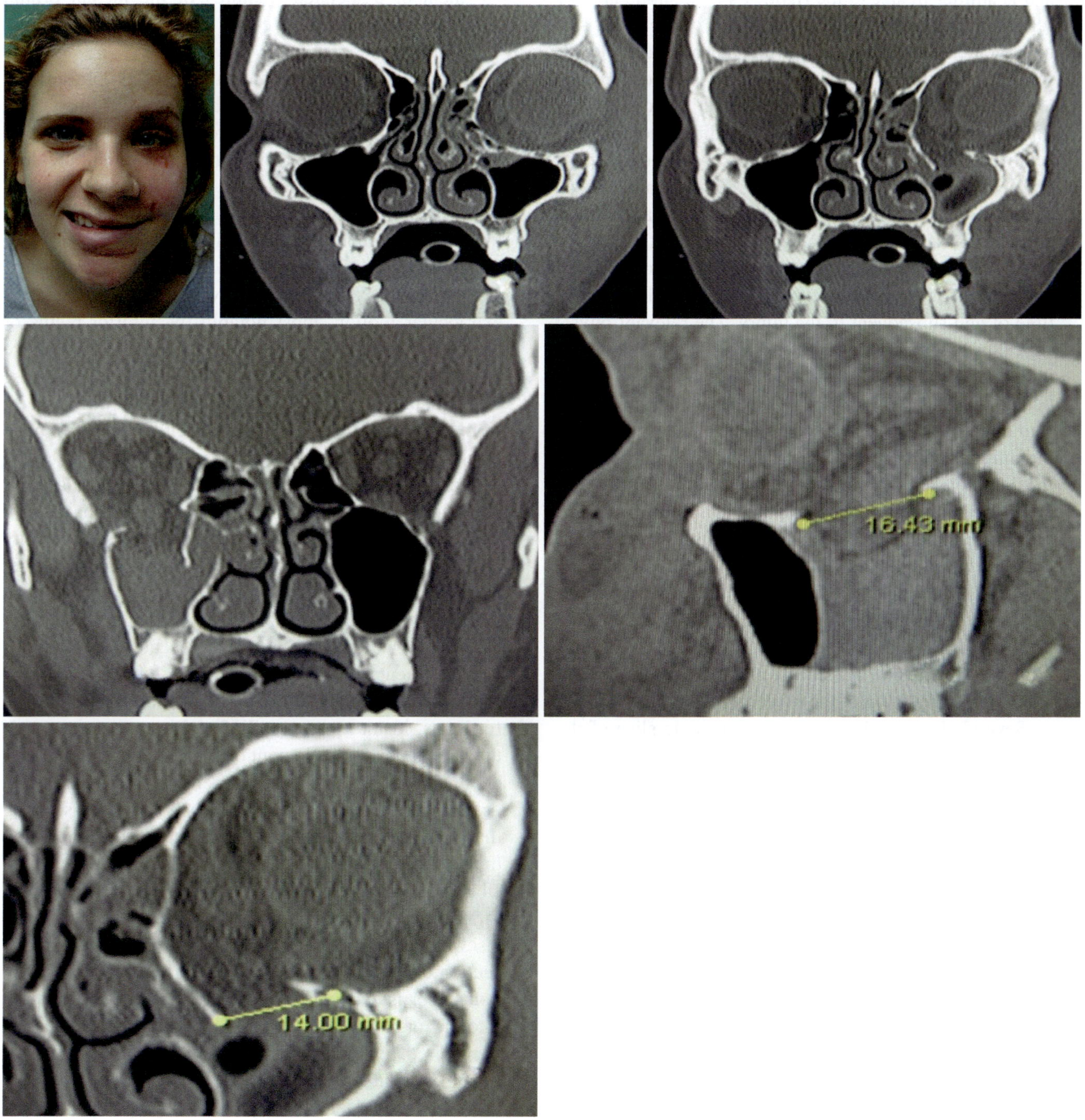

A 25-year-old referred 5 days after a motor vehicle accident. No other injuries.

1. Describe the slides and add a focused clinical examination. Now, review the CT findings. (The single photo is of a young woman with several findings. Two small, superficial abrasions of the cheek, two or three skin sutures in the most lateral left ala, and an oblique 4–5 cm healing laceration extending from the lower lip vermilion on the right to the most lateral extent of the submental crease on the left. The remarkable findings, though, are the absence of significant periorbital ecchymosis, scleral show, proptosis, and enophthalmos. The left pupil is at mid position and is similar in size to the right. A small, subtle area of scleral injection is present at the limbus of the left iris at nine o'clock. More of the upper lid and palpebral fold are visualized on the left, but the right brow is lower, perhaps a result of voluntary or reflexive action. Although these findings may represent a subtle, subthreshold form of acute enophthalmos, they are more likely a photographic artifact. The left lateral canthal tilt is positive, and no evidence is seen, at least in this view, of malar flattening or alteration of transverse facial width.

   The clinical exam begins with questions about the circumstances of the injury and medical care rendered at the time of and subsequent to the injury. The relevant physical exam focuses on the eyes and face. The ocular exam includes evaluation of vision to confrontation, the extraocular muscles with particular attention focused on all four directions of gaze, and complaints of diplopia during the muscle motility test. The sensation is examined over the distribution of the infraorbital nerve. The infraorbital and lateral orbital rims are palpated for a bony step-off. Of course, the stability of the maxilla and mandible are addressed, and an intraoral examination is completed.

   Performance of forced duction testing, the traction of the globe by grasping conjunctiva soft tissue and passively rotating the eye upward, is best reserved after induction of general anesthesia and performed initially and at the completion of the procedure.

   Several slices of the coronal and a single slice of the sagittal view provide some information. The coronal slices illustrate different orbital depths, including anterior, mid-globe, and more posterior at the muscular cone. Significant findings are an intact floor anteriorly and an aerated maxillary sinus, a disrupted floor and resultant defect at mid-globe, and a complete disruption with a trapdoor fracture at the muscular cone of the orbit with fluid in the sinus. The most posterior coronal slice would appear to illustrate the inferior rectus within the fracture defect. The two other CT slices are a sagittal and an additional coronal view, and a measurement of the floor defects has been performed. The dimensions of the aforementioned floor defect at mid-globe are 14 and 16.4 mm on the sagittal view. The sagittal slice appears approximately at or close to mid-orbit.)

   (a) Are any tests indicated? Justify. (If any concerns arise from the results of the ocular exam, an ophthalmology consult is indicated. Many maxillofacial surgeons consider a consultation in the presence of any orbital or adnexal injury as appropriate to ascertain the possible presence of traumatic glaucoma, retinal detachment, or other injuries.)
   (b) What additional CT images, if any, would assist in the development of a treatment plan? (All images should be reviewed for evidence of muscular entrapment or associated fractures of the medial orbital wall, both of which could influence the treatment plan.)
2. Summarize the pathologic anatomy and pathophysiology. (The patient has sustained an orbital blowout fracture on the left. The pathomechanics are an increase in intraorbital pressure from blunt force trauma with that pressure imparted to the thin orbital floor. Another possible mechanism is a buckling of the infraorbital rim and zygoma from impact, rebound, and fracture of the floor as a result. Regardless, the clinical sequelae are related to the expansion of orbital volume and/or involvement of muscles of extraocular motion, most notably the inferior rectus or orbital fat by the bony fragments. The latter can produce enophthalmos with loss of globe protrusion and a decrease in the palpebral aperture, and the former motility defects from entrapment and/or direct muscular injury by bone fragments.)
3. Based on the response to question two, outline a treatment plan and describe it in detail. (An additional benefit of an eye consultation is the expertise to measure motility disorders, if present, in prism diopters. The clinical picture, to a large extent, will drive the treatment plan. Although considerable debate exists about absolute indications for exploration and repair, acute enophthalmos and persistent motility disorders with demonstrable disruption of floor integrity, all represent important findings for many, if not most, maxillofacial trauma surgeons. If the patient has some element of significant motility disorder and given the CT findings, operative intervention is in order. A further delay will produce fibrosis and scarring that increases the difficulty of the procedure, including the reduction of prolapsed intraorbital structures and possibly a less predictable result. A detailed description of the technical aspects of the operative repair can be found elsewhere, but the essential points are a subperiosteal dissection of the floor, continued posteriorly until an intact bony floor is encountered. Orbital contents, if prolapsed into the maxillary sinus, are reduced, and the floor defect is repaired. An additional decision is the nature of the repair material since a selection from a variety of materials is available that include porous polyethylene as a common choice or fenestrated titanium plates.

In pediatric patients, the phenomenon of a narrow trapdoor fracture with entrapment of muscle can present with a vasovagal picture as a result of the oculocardiac reflex. That clinical presentation is an urgent indication for operative intervention. Some maxillofacial surgeons subscribe to the necessity of autogenous bone.

The asymptomatic patient presents a clinical conundrum. The relative value of any prophylactic operation is predicated on the prevention of the development of late enophthalmos. A number of predictable CT variables have been presented to provide a guideline for the decision process, most commonly a quantification of the magnitude of the defect greater than 50% or 2 cm^2 of the orbital floor. The location of the defect may be significant as well, posterior of a greater concern.

In the case example, the asymptomatic patient's bony defect is 1.4 × 1.6 cm or 2.25 cm^2, at or slightly above the theoretical threshold. In addition, the defect appears to be, in part, retrobulbar, a more critical area in the potential for the occurrence of late enophthalmos. Given the posterior extent of the fracture defect, if undertaken, exposure and repair would be a challenging task.

Postoperative (6 Weeks)

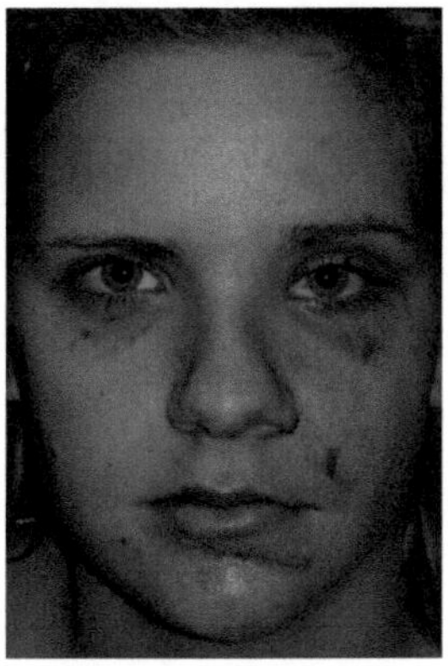

The patient was managed nonoperatively and remained asymptomatic. The findings are unchanged from the acute injury photo. A slight discoloration of the left infraorbital area with a healing chin laceration is evident. As in the prior photo, the left brow is more elevated than the right. No enophthalmos is present, although the hiatus post-injury is relatively early. A subtle suggestion of a vertical dystopia of the left medial canthus is pictured, also present in the 5-day post-injury photo. The patient appears to have sustained an injury to the buccal and perhaps mandibular branches of the facial nerve.

In-Service Examination

1. All of the following structures insert on Whitnall's tubercle **EXCEPT:**
   (a) Lockwood's ligament
   (b) Whitnall's ligament
   (c) Orbicularis
   (d) Expansion of the levator aponeurosis
2. The following structures exit the superior orbital fissure **EXCEPT:**
   (a) Oculomotor nerve
   (b) Nasociliary nerve
   (c) Lacrimal nerve
   (d) Maxillary division of the trigeminal nerve
   (e) Trochlear nerve
3. The capsulopalpebral fascia arises from what structure?
   (a) Arcus marginalis
   (b) Inferior rectus muscle
   (c) Orbital septum
   (d) Lockwood's ligament
4. Adequate reduction of a displaced zygomatic fracture is optimally judged where?
   (a) Lateral orbital wall
   (b) Orbital floor
   (c) Frontozygomatic suture
   (d) Zygomaticomaxillary buttress
   (e) Inferior orbital rim

49 Mandible (Anatomy, Examination, Treatment: General Principles, Reduction/Fixation)

Bibliography

Note: Skip sections on Condylar Fractures.

Clark N, Chapter 35: "Mandibular Fractures", Plastic, Maxillofacial and Reconstructive Surgery, Georgiade, G. S. et al., Williams & Wilkins Third Edition, (1997); **pp 379–84, 390–93 ONLY.**

Stacey D, Doyle J, Mount DL, et al. "Management of Mandible Fractures", *Plast Reconstr Surg.*, (2006); 117:**48e–55e.**

Ellis E, Miles B, "Fractures of the Mandible: A Technical Perspective", *Plast Reconstr Surg.*, (2007); 120(7): **76S–89S.**

Ricketts S, Gill HS, Fialkov JA, et al., "Facial fractures", *Plast Reconstr Surg.*, (2016); 137(2):**440e, Video 9, 10 ONLY**.

Pickrell BB and Hollier LH, "Evidence-Based Medicine: Mandible Fractures", *Plast Reconstr Surg.*, (2017);140:**192e–197e, Video 2, 3 ONLY**.

Hadeed JG and Marcus JR, Chapter 6: "Internal Fixation Principles", Essentials of Craniomaxillofacial Trauma, Quality Medical Publishing, (2012); pgs. **75–85.**

Blitz M, Notarnicola K, "Closed Reduction of the Mandibular Fracture", *Atlas of the Oral and Maxillofacial Surgery Clinics of North America*, (2009); 17: **3–7 ONLY.**

Lazow SK, Tarlo I, "Mandible Fracture; Transoral 2.0-mm Locking Miniplate plus 1 Week Maxillomandibular Fixation", *Atlas of the Oral and Maxillofacial Surgery Clinics of North America*, (2009); 17: **27–28 ONLY.**

Faculty Discussion and Study Guide

Anatomy

> **Editor's Note:** The elements of occlusion, cephalometrics, and dental vocabulary are included in Chap. 18.

1. Give the origin, insertion, and action of the following posterior muscles of mastication: masseter, temporalis, medial pterygoid, lateral pterygoid. (Masseter muscle originates on the zygoma and runs posteriorly and inferiorly to insert along the buccal aspect of the angle, inferior ascending ramus, and inferior border of the body; temporalis originates in the temporal fossa of the temporal bone and inserts on the coronoid process; medial pterygoid originates from the pterygoid plates and posterior wall or tuber of the maxilla and inserts on the lingual aspect of the mandible. The combination of the masseter and internal pterygoid form a muscular sling. The two heads of the lateral pterygoid muscle, inferior and superior belly, run posteriorly and superiorly to insert on the condyle and capsule. The superior belly originates from the sphenoid bone and inserts on the capsule and disc; the inferior belly originates from the lateral pterygoid plate and inserts on the fossa of the condyle and joint capsule. The masseter acts to close the mandible powerfully, as does the temporalis, but the temporalis also retracts the mandible. The medial pterygoid also closes the mandible and, when unopposed, distracts the mandible to the opposite side, as does the unopposed inferior belly of the lateral pterygoid. The course of the inferior belly is from anterior, the origin on the lateral pterygoid plates, to a posterior insertion on the condyle. The superior belly of the pterygoid acts to stabilize the articular disc, and the inferior belly assists in opening the mouth and protrudes the mandible when acting bilaterally but deviates to the opposite side if acting unilaterally.)
2. What are the muscles, including the origin and insertion of the anterior mandible? (The principal anterior muscles are the anterior and posterior belly of the digastric, the mylohyoid, and the geniohyoid, all of which act to open the mouth or mandible. The difference in innervation of these muscles is interesting because the posterior belly of the digastric is innervated by cranial nerve VII, the anterior belly by cranial nerve V while the mylohyoid is

E. Luce, *A Curriculum for Plastic Surgery*, https://doi.org/10.1007/978-3-031-62087-4_49

innervated by V, but the geniohyoid by cranial nerve *XII*, the hypoglossal. The mylohyoid and geniohyoid act to open the mandible, as does the digastric. The three muscles are considered the suprahyoid mandibular depressors and also retractors.)

3. What are the principal nerves with respect to mandibular fractures? (The inferior alveolar nerve, as a branch of the mandibular division of cranial nerve V, enters the mandible on the lingual aspect of the ascending ramus and traverses the body to exit at the mental foramen. The other nerves of interest are the branches of the mandibular division of the trigeminal that innervate the temporalis, masseter, and the two pterygoid muscles, as well as the facial. The latter is at risk in a transcutaneous approach.)
   (a) If you administer bilateral inferior alveolar nerve blocks, the patient should be advised not to eat or drink for 3 h. Why? (Lidocaine can diffuse more proximally into the main trunk of the mandibular division and block the lingual nerve bilateral as well as the branches of IX.)
4. With respect to the mechanical forces acting upon the fracture line, what forces are exerted at the dental-alveolar line and what at the inferior border? (Tension at the tooth line, which acts to distract the fracture fragments, and compression at the inferior mandibular border, which tends to compress the fragments, in general. These forces dictate the necessity of placement of a plate at the inferior border and a smaller plate more superior that will act as a tension band or neutralization of the distracting forces at the dental-mandibular line by an arch bar. These generalities may not apply in the parasymphyseal and symphyseal region.)
   (a) What are the forces exerted on the buccal and lingual aspect of the mandible? (The masticatory forces produce compression on the buccal aspect and tension or potentially a distracting force on the lingual aspect. Slight overbending of the plate to fit against the convex buccal surface of the mandible will neutralize the tension forces on the lingual aspect.)
5. Describe primary and secondary bone healing. (Secondary bone healing is the classical model of bone healing, which consists of an inflammatory stage with round cell infiltrate, vascularization followed by deposition of cartilage, and then bone deposition on the cartilaginous framework, presumably by osteoblasts. Primary bone healing occurs when compression of the viable bone on either side of the fracture reduces the gap to nil with good bone apposition. The intervening stage of callus does not occur but rather directs bone-to-bone healing. The sequence for all secondary bone healing is inflammation or formation of granulation tissue, followed by the deposition of fibrous tissue, cartilage formation, and disorganized bone. The bone deposition is initially woven, ultimately lamellar, and finally, remodeled. The hallmark finding in secondary bone healing is the presence of callus. The implication also is that if a bone gap, even as little as a few millimeters, exists at the time of reduction of a fracture, secondary bone healing, not primary, will occur.)
6. Define by direction of the fracture, favorable and unfavorable fractures of the angle of the mandible. (In the coronal plane, if the direction of the fracture line from buccal to lingual is posterior to anterior, the fracture is unfavorable because of the pull of the medial pterygoids, and to a lesser degree, the lateral pterygoids will tend to pull the fractured fragment out of reduction. When viewed in the sagittal plane, if the fracture line courses from superior to inferior in a posterior to anterior direction, the fracture is favorable since contraction of the masseter and pterygoid muscles will tend to pull the fracture into reduction. This distinction is somewhat irrelevant in the contemporary era of open reduction internal fixation.)
   (a) Describe the probable displacement of a left parasymphyseal fracture, a segmental body fracture. (A parasymphyseal fracture on the left will allow unopposed contraction of the mylohyoid with a resultant lingual and posterior displacement of the proximal fragment. The right side, containing the symphyseal area, will have some but less lingual displacement. A segmental body fracture such as an ipsilateral angle and parasymphyseal fracture permits unopposed retraction of the ipsilateral mylohyoid with the resultant lingual displacement of the segment.)
   (b) Describe the displacement of a bilateral midbody fracture. (The distracting forces on the posterior mandible, distal to the fracture line, will produce a widening of the gonial angle and inferior and posterior displacement of the anterior segment.)
7. An Angle class 1 occlusion is what? (By definition, the mandibular teeth are slightly anterior to the maxillary teeth so the mesiobuccal, anterior and outside, cusp of the maxillary first molar fits into the mesiobuccal groove of the mandibular first molar and the maxillary canine fits over the groove between the mandibular canine and first premolar.)
   (a) An Angle class II? III? (In a class II occlusion the maxilla is anterior so the mesiobuccal cusp of the maxilla is distal or anterior to the buccal groove of the mandibular first molar. An example would be the distobuccal cusp of the maxillary first molar, which

sits in the buccal groove of the mandibular first molar. In class III, the mandible is anterior, so the mesiobuccal cusp of the maxillary first molar sits distal or posterior to the buccal groove of the mandibular first molar.

8. You have performed a transbuccal reduction and fixation of an angle fracture with an intraoral incision, and the plate is easily placed at the mid portion instead of the inferior border of the mandible. Advisable? (No. The screws will be placed into the canal and pathway of the inferior alveolar nerve. Also, it ignores the necessity to place the plate as inferior as possible as well as a tension band superior.)
   (a) The inferior alveolar canal is more lingual or buccal? More inferior or superior? (The canal is more buccal and inferior.)

Examination, Diagnosis

1. Give the specifics of a clinical exam. (Ask the patient about whether the occlusion is "normal" or not, the mechanism of injury, exam for the presence of condylar heads palpable in the external auditory canal, limitation of mandibular opening or trismus, the intraoral exam for lacerations, broken teeth, etc., the occlusal pattern on closing; sensory disturbances in the distribution of the mental nerve in the lower lip and adjacent alveolus.)
2. What is the most likely scenario for a patient with a mandible fracture who presents with airway obstruction from the fracture? (Bilateral anterior body fractures. With that pattern of fractures, the hyomandibular support mechanism for the base of the tongue is lost because of posterior displacement of the anterior mandibular fragment and airway occlusion at the level of the oropharynx by the base of the tongue. Treatment consists of pulling the tongue forward. The most likely setting is an elderly edentulous patient, and the airway is restored by grasping the tongue and pulling the anterior combined with suctioning of the oropharynx.)
3. A patient with a clinical suspicion of a mandibular fracture has no neurologic indications for a CT scan. What are the plain X-ray techniques to image the mandible? (Panorex, AP, lateral, and oblique mandible films, as well as possibly a Towne's view. Nevertheless, a CT scan including 3D reconstruction is more comprehensive, and plain X-rays are mostly of historical interest.)
   (a) Briefly describe the Panorex and its pros and cons. (The Panorex is a panoramic view of the mandible from most posterior to the symphyseal region. The film is obtained with a patient in a sitting position in a dental chair, and the X-ray machine performs a half circle around the patient to form the image. The pros are visualization of all of the mandibles, including the condyle, on a single view. A panorex may also detect small areas of dental infection, such as a periapical abscess or unerupted third molar, perhaps in an angle fracture line. The disadvantages are the overlap in the symphyseal region and the inability to detect symphyseal and parasymphyseal fractures in many cases, as well as the single view of the condyle. Additionally, the other potential disadvantages are the necessity for the patient to be alert and in a sitting position, often not possible in the trauma setting.)

Treatment: General Principles

1. What are the variables in mandible fractures? (Site, degree of fragmentation or comminution, line of direction of fracture with respect to the masticatory forces, state of a dentition or lack of same including if teeth in the fracture line, age of the patient, open fracture or not, soft tissue status, duration since the injury.)
2. What is the timing issue in treatment? (Particularly in open fractures, contamination with virulent oral organisms can lead to established soft tissue and bone infection in a relatively short period of time. Although some controversy exists, patients benefit from preoperative antibiotics and early reduction, 24–36 h after injury, and fixation.)
3. What are the evidence and indications for, or not, the use of antibiotics in mandible fractures? (No evidence that antibiotics are a benefit in "uncomplicated fractures." Perhaps the use of clindamycin or Flagyl in complicated fractures. Clearly, no evidence for use post-operatively.)
4. Define the following: Ivy loops bridle wires. (Bridle wires are the technique of ligating the teeth on either side of a fracture for temporary fixation. Ivy loops are a technique for maxillo-mandibular fixation with the use of wire only rather than arch bars.)
5. Describe the technique for splint construction. (The essentials of splint construction consist of the necessity to take dental impressions with the use of impression trays and dental alginate, the creation of a stone model of the dental arches with the use of the impressions as a mold, and sometimes the use of an articulator with the stone models cut or "model surgery" to correct for the malocclusion in the models as a result of fracture frag-

ment displacement. Finally, the construction of a wafer or occlusal splint with the use of the models as molds for the same. The use of digitally-derived imaging, termed computer-assisted design/computer-assisted manufacture or CAD/CAM, has replaced most of the above steps.)

6. What are the indications for open reduction and internal fixation in mandible fractures? (Frequently, this is a judgment call, but some guiding principles are: unfavorable fracture line, displaced on CT scan such as parasymphyseal, elderly edentulous patients, soft tissue injury and/or loss, noncompliant patient.)
7. What is the Risdon incision? (A gentle curving incision beginning posterior to the vertical ramus continues into a relaxed skin tension line of the neck and sufficiently far anteriorly to turn a soft tissue flap for exposure of the ascending ramus and the posterior portion of the mandibular body.)
   (a) Describe the transbuccal trocar approach to angle fractures. (Actually, combined intraoral with limited transcutaneous incisions for trochar insertion to permit drill and screw placement. The principal limitation is access to the most inferior aspect of the mandible.)
8. You plan a Risdon incision for an open reduction, internal fixation, or ORIF, of a body fracture. Where is the marginal mandibular nerve? (Coursing across the angle in 80% of the cases, in the remaining 20%, 1 cm below. The anterior portion of the nerve actually crosses the body of the mandible at approximately mid-body or at the facial vessels.)
   (a) What incision, approach, and possible complications are involved in open access to a condyle? (A preauricular incision, often combined with a Risdon incision, is required for exposure of the condyle. The Risdon incision is used for the placement of an interosseous wire and downward traction of the mandible to facilitate exposure of the condyle. The temporal branch and temporofacial trunk of the facial nerve are at risk. The other possible complication is devascularization of the condylar head as a result of the operative manipulation.)
9. Give some indications for the removal of teeth in the fractured mandible. (If the tooth is in the fracture line and two-thirds or more of the socket is disrupted; fractured tooth; premolars or molars with either the root or roots disrupted from the socket in the fracture line; partially erupted third molar in the fracture line; the presence of an apical abscess or significant periodontal disease; full thickness mucosal wound of the lingual or buccal cortex of the root of the tooth.)

Reduction/Fixation

1. Give the principal elements of the historical evolution of management of mandibular fractures of the past 30–40 years. (With the advent of open reduction in the mid-twentieth century, internal fixation for mandibular fractures was accomplished with interosseous, IO, wires used for fixation. In Switzerland, extrapolation from the management of internal fixation of extremity fractures to the mandible was advocated by the AO or AO/ASIF group, consisting of the principles of rigid compression fixation to obtain direct bone healing. As outlined in the questions below, enthusiasm waned because of the reasons listed. Currently, probably most maxillofacial trauma surgeons favor noncompression. One widely adopted compromise is the use of 2.0 or 2.3 plates with locking screws, but also with some potential disadvantages.)
2. What role do arch bars with interdental ligatures play in mandibular fractures besides intermaxillary fixation or IMF? (The arch bars serve as a tension band to prevent splaying of the fracture fragments at the alveolar margin and allow for the use of postoperative traction with elastics for rehabilitation.)
   (a) What are some of the caveats in the placement and use of arch bars? (Do not include the anterior teeth incisors because the risk of extraction is particularly high with placement of elastics anterior. If absolutely necessary, as in some alveolar fractures, interdental wires can be placed if two incisors are included in a figure-of-eight fashion.)
   (b) How can arch bars be applied to a mandible with edentulous segments? (Circummandibular wires.)
3. List and discuss the two possible sites of distraction that may occur with rigid plate fixation and why. (Superiorly at the alveolar border and the lingual aspect of the mandible. The superior border distraction occurs because of the tensile forces and can be prevented with a tension band, applied either as a separate smaller unicortical plate or by an arch bar. Lingual distraction occurs because of the application of a straight plate to the curved convexity of the mandible and can be prevented by slight overbending of the plate.)
4. Outline the types of fixation plate materials. (Stainless steel, vitallium, and titanium. Stainless steel is usually a chrome alloy and is rarely, if ever, utilized currently. Vitallium was the first material utilized by European craniofacial surgeons for its low reactivity and high strength. Currently, titanium is overwhelmingly, perhaps exclusively, the most commonly utilized material in maxillofacial plates and screws.)

5. What are the advantages of rigid internal fixation? (The advantages are to allow a primary bone union with the formation of little callus since micromotion is minimized. If so, prolonged maxillo-mandibular fixation is not necessary, at least from the aspect of bone healing, since the mechanical load is borne entirely by the hardware. Larger bone plates, such as a reconstruction plate, are substantially stronger than mini plates, and the share of the load is shifted toward the hardware and less load-bearing by the bone. In reality, contemporary rigid fixation is noncompressive, and as such, some micromotion and an element of secondary bone healing must occur.)
6. A more radical form of rigid internal fixation is a rigid internal fixation with compression. How is that accomplished, and what are the disadvantages? (Compression occurs by the use of a glide plane for the screw that advances the fracture fragment as the screw is tightened. The potential problem is foreshortened bone with any degree of comminution of the fracture and overriding or telescoping of the fracture fragments in oblique fractures.)
7. Other disadvantages of rigid compression methods for mandibular fractures are: (1. Stress shielding not only at the fracture site but on adjacent normal bone may create relative osteoporosis. 2. More periosteal stripping is necessary, for example, reconstruction plates for the mandible and the resultant increase in ischemia. 3. Even with perfect reduction, the compression pressure between the fractured bone ends will lead to bone resorption, and some element of reduction will be lost. In addition, the complex curvature of the mandible does not lend well to the use of straight-line compression. True rigid dynamic compression, DCP, prevents the use of postoperative elastics for minor adjustments in occlusion. Finally, the screws were non-fluted and required tapping after placement of drill holes. Because of these reasons, the use of compression fixation plates in mandibular fractures has been abandoned.)
8. Describe the lag screw in terms of definition as a technique and as a type of screw. (A lag screw is a screw that is threaded on the distal one-half only, with the proximal half of the screw smooth with a core diameter. A single drill hole is placed through the proximal and distal fragments with the use of a drill bit that is the same size as the core diameter of the screw, but the non-threaded proximal portion of the screw does not engage the proximal bone or cortex. The lag screw technique consists of two different size drill holes. The proximal hole is larger or overdrilled to the same caliber as the thread of the screw, and the distal hole is drilled at the same diameter as the core diameter of the screw. For example, with the utilization of a 2.0 screw, the proximal hole, termed the glide hole, is drilled out 2.3 mm, and the distal hole, termed the pilot hole, is drilled to 2.0. A 2.0 mm screw is then used, which is not engaged until the distal fragment is encountered. The process compresses the proximal bone fragment against the distal fragment.)
   (a) Describe the fracture line that is conducive to a lag screw technique. (An oblique fracture such that the screws can be placed nearly perpendicular to the fracture line. Two screws are necessary to prevent rotation of the fragments around a single screw.)
9. What is a compromise, i.e., define rigid noncompressive fixation? (Rigid noncompressive fixation is accomplished by the use of plates and screws but without compression. Depending on the size of the hardware, rigidity of fixation is still obtained, but no compressive element exists and represents the current method for internal fixation.)
   (a) Express this compromise in terms of load-sharing vs. load-bearing. (A larger fixation appliance, such as a reconstruction bar with three screws on either side of the fracture, represents a load-bearing fixation. Smaller plates, certainly with a Champy approach as described below, represent load-sharing fixation because both the bone and the hardware share in the compressive and tension loads.)
   (b) Discuss the design and conceptual approach of locking plates. (Locking plates are designed with threads within the screw holes of the plate. That property permits the screw to be locked to the plate and then into the bone rather than the plate "adapting" to the underlying contour of the bone. Although somewhat more expensive when utilized, many have adopted the locking variety of reconstruction plates.)
10. Discuss the advantages and disadvantages of the Champy technique. (The advantages are that almost exclusively, the mini plates can be placed transorally and are unicortical and neutralize tension forces to permit compression with mastication. Namely, the conceptual approach is to use the normal muscular forces. The disadvantages are that the principle of the Champy technique is to identify lines of tension within the mandible at the site of the fracture and utilize those tension-compressive forces in the maintenance of fracture reduction, but the exact location of those forces may be difficult to ascertain. One final advantage is the ability to use light elastics for minor adjustments in the occlusion postoperative.)

11. What are the indications for continued IMF immediately after ORIF? (Concomitant subcondylar fracture; a single plate inferiorly has been used, and the arch bar needs to be retained as a tension band; presence of comminuted fractures, possible use of elastics postoperative.)
12. Outline the conundrum in comminuted mandible fractures. (The difficulty in comminuted mandible fractures is to achieve enough fixation yet not further embarrass the blood supply to the healing fragments and bones. Two opposing schools of thought exist: One is a large reconstruction plate that spans the comminuted gap. The advantage is more than adequate fixation, but the disadvantage is the necessity for considerable periosteal stripping as well as stress-shielding of the fragments. The other approach is the use of multiple small mini plates from fragment to fragment. The advantage is less devascularization, and the disadvantage is less rigidity of the fixation. If a significant defect greater than 5 mm exists after debridement, some consideration should be given to the primary bone graft with autogenous cancellous bone. The other option is the application of external fixation.)
13. In the edentulous mandible, what is the minimal vertical height or degree of atrophy when management becomes problematic? (15–20 mm).
    (a) What are the options? (Conservative treatment with Gunning splints and IMF or the patient's dentures plus IMF; internal fixation with a reconstruction plate; titanium crib plus autogenous bone graft. Simple fractures can be frequently managed with a blenderized diet only.)
14. What are the indications for the application of external fixation? (Loss of soft tissue coverage, segmental bone loss, the most common scenario is a high-velocity gunshot wound. Another indication is the occurrence of an infected and or nonunion. See complications, Chap. 50)

Video Notes

PRS (2016) 137: 440e–441e. Videos 9, 10.

Video 9: 3′30″

1. The video is a slide presentation and is devoted to the assessment of the mandible fracture patient.
    (a) Examine the mouth for lacerations, broken and missing teeth, and overall dentition status, as well as the sensation of the distribution of the mental nerve.
    (b) Value of panorex for ascertainment of dental abscesses impacted third molar.

Video 10: 5′ 20″

1. A continuation of the slide presentation of the slide presentation from Video 9.
    (a) Discussion of load-sharing vs. load-bearing. Load-bearing usually has three screws on either side of the fracture in larger plates, while load-sharing often is monocortical screws and plates.
    (b) In the use of a load-bearing plate, consider primary bone graft in mandible infections.
    (c) Emphasize that edentulous mandibles require load-bearing reconstruction plates of the entire mandible.

PRS (2017) 140: 192e–200e. Videos 2, 3.

Video 2: 3′45″

1. ORIF of parasymphyseal fracture.
    (a) Advocates are opening the fracture prior to the application of IMF with "gross reduction."
    (b) Despite arch bars placed a tension band with monocortical screws; used a 2.4 plate inferior.
2. Percutaneous ORIF of angle fracture with the use of trocars. Video quality overall was 7–8.

Case-Based Conference

Case 1: Mandible Fracture

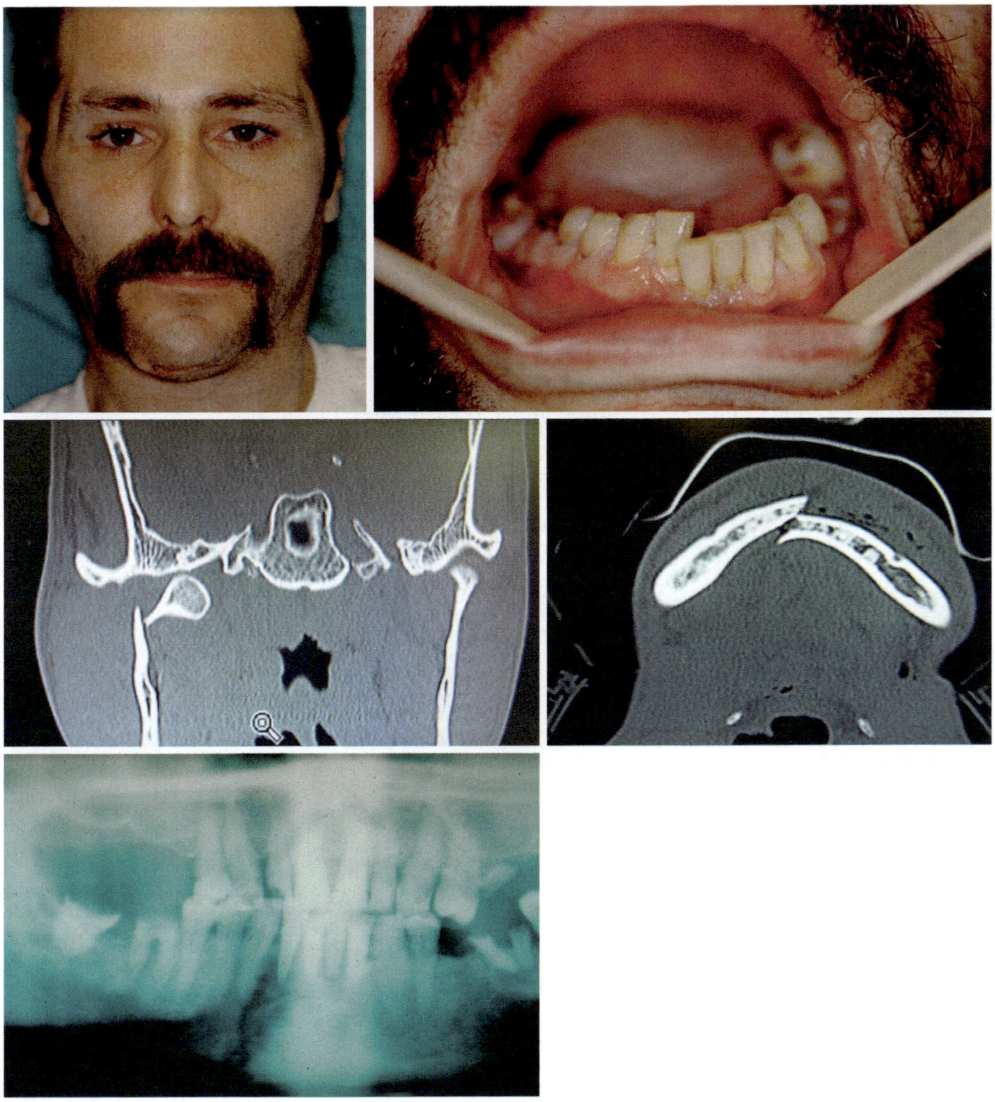

A 39-year-old with blunt trauma to the mandible. No medical problems and no other injuries.

1. Describe the clinical slides and add an exam prior to interpretation of the Panorex and CT scan.
   (a) What other relevant information would you derive from the CT scan?
2. List the challenges the patient's fractures pose for successful management. Use the pathologic anatomy to explain.

Outline a treatment plan in the context of your response to Q2. Include the postoperative management.

Case-Based Conference: Discussion

Case 1: Mandible Fracture

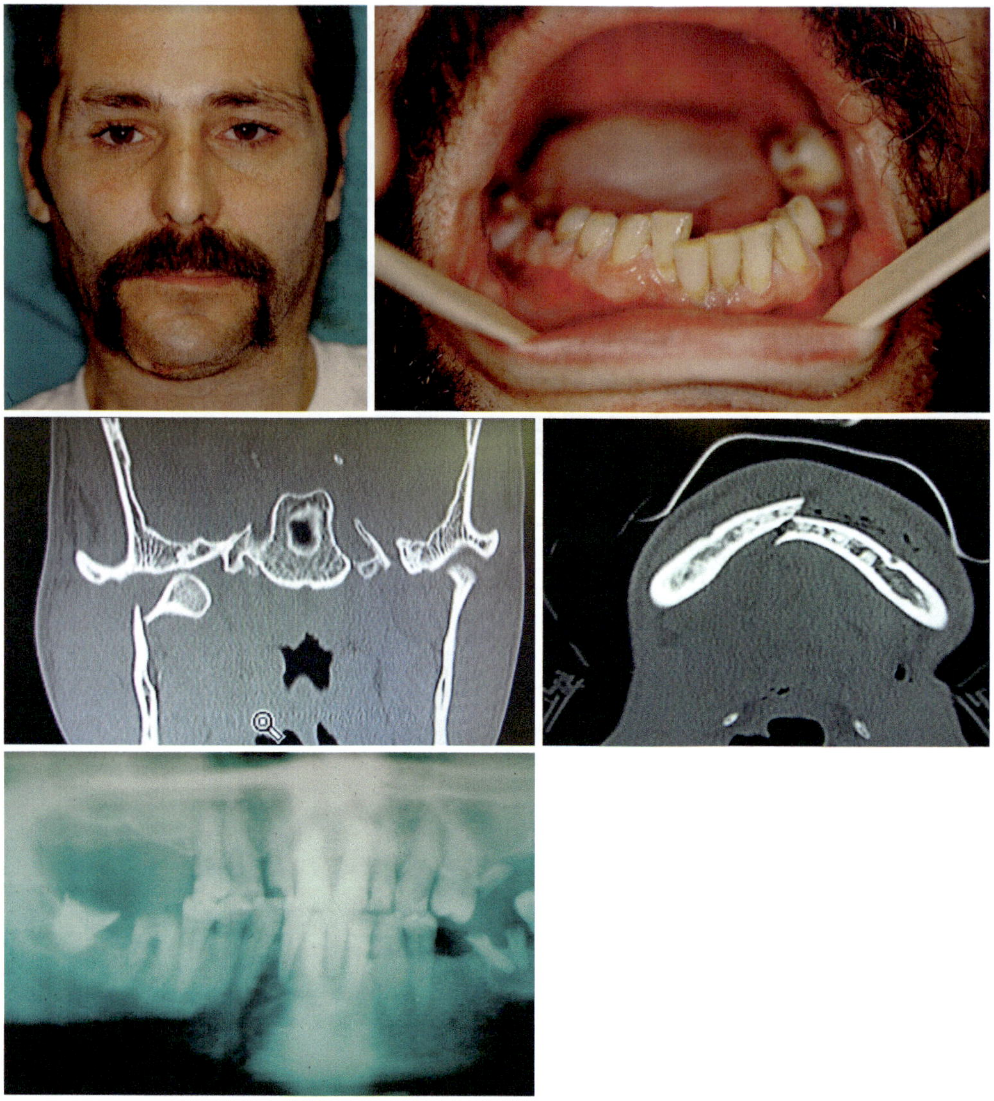

A 39-year-old with blunt trauma to the mandible. No medical problems and no other injuries.

1. Describe the clinical slides and add an exam prior to interpretation of the Panorex and CT scan. (Two clinical slides, a Panorex, and two slices of a coronal and axial view CT scan are provided. The first clinical slide is a full-frontal view of the head and neck of a male who appears the stated age. No swelling, ecchymosis, or facial deformity is visualized. Some subtle asymmetry of the anterior chin is evident. Also, an oblique scar or recently healed laceration is present at the most inferior aspect of the submental mandible. The second clinical view is intraoral and demonstrates a step-off between the right central and lateral mandibular incisor, consistent with a fracture, although no laceration of the alveolar gingiva can be seen. The proximal or posterior right mandibular segment is tilted lingual significantly. Evident also is multiple missing posterior mandibular teeth posterior to the first bicuspid on the left other than a single molar and proximal to the second bicuspid on the right. No gross caries of the remaining dentition, but some gum recession is also present. The maxillary dentition is not seen in the photo.

   The history portion of the clinical exam establishes, as stated in the preamble, that the absence of any complaints suggestive of other injuries and past medical history should be pursued, including orthognathic surgery or orthodontics. The hiatus since injury is established and, although obvious, other questions center on complaints relative to the mandibular fractures, including any bleeding from the ear or intraoral drainage. The physical exam should ascertain the state of dentition mandibular excursion, including the location of pain precipitated and sensation over the distribution of both mental nerves. A useful maneuver is for the examiner to place index fingertips in both external auditory canals and request the patient to open and close. Normally, the condylar heads can be palpated with opening, but the exam can be limited by the inability of the patient to open sufficiently.

The imaging provided included a Panorex, a single coronal cut at the level of the temporomandibular joint, and an axial view. The Panorex demonstrates a parasymphyseal fracture on the right. Because of the overlap anteriorly normally produced by the panoramic nature of the film, blurring of some of the incisors has occurred. The missing posterior mandibular dentition is apparent, as well as a similar finding in the maxillary dentition. A single right molar is missing the crown. The maxillary dentition is missing all bicuspids and molars on the right and molars on the left. A single coronal view on the CT scan demonstrates a subcondylar fracture on the right with medial displacement of the condylar head completely out of the temporal fossa of the temporomandibular joint. The opposite condyle is intact. The axial view illustrates a fracture of the parasymphyseal fracture of the right mandible.)

(a) What other relevant information would you derive from the CT scan? (Besides the presence of the fractures, the pattern and degree of comminution, if any, of the right parasymphyseal fracture.)

2. List the challenges the patient's fractures pose for successful management. Use the pathologic anatomy to explain. (Several challenges in this clinical scenario pose an obstacle to a successful result and include the displacement forces of the muscles of mastication, the status of the detention, the addition of a displaced subcondylar fracture, the delay in management, and the circumstances of the injury that imply a possible issue with patient compliance.

The lingual displacement of the right posterior or proximal fragment is the result of the unopposed pull of the mylohyoid, released by the fracture from the restraining force of the anterior muscles of the hyoid-mandibular complex. In addition, the pterygoid-masseteric sling composed of the masseter and medial pterygoid enveloping the lateral and medial aspect of the ascending ramus, respectively, will mutually act to displace the posterior body superiorly and medially. Although historically, the superior-inferior direction of the fracture determined a favorable vs. unfavorable configuration, in the era of rigid fixation, that factor is probably not relevant. The status of the dentition is relevant, though, because of the absence of posterior stops molars, which would be of value in the application of intermaxillary fixation and the implementation of arch bars and elastics for postoperative rehabilitation. The last point, the use of arch bars and elastics, is particularly cogent because of the associated displaced subcondylar fracture. See below. A substitute for the traditional arch bar secured with interdental wires is a "hybrid" bar placed on both maxilla and mandible and secured with interosseous screws. Flanges are present that enable the application of intermaxillary fixation. The final factor, patient compliance, is a specter provoked by the circumstances of the injury, the delay between injury and presentation, and the patient's dentition that appears to reflect a chronic lack of dental hygiene. All of these potentially adverse and detrimental factors must be addressed in the development of the patient's treatment plan.)

3. Outline a treatment plan in the context of your response to Q2. Include the postoperative management. (The treatment plan must include the contingencies outlined in the prior question. Without an arch bar, unless an additional hardware modality such as the hybrid described above is available, intermaxillary fixation, IMF, will not be feasible. One option could be possible if splints, both maxillary and mandibular, were fabricated and incorporated an arch bar. The maxillary splint could be secured with intraosseous screws and the mandibular with circummandibular wires. To achieve optimal occlusion, an occlusal splint for placement of the patient in IMF could be fabricated, all of which require dental impressions and the generation of models digitally. Regardless, once the patient was secured in occlusion and IMF, the parasymphyseal fracture will require open reduction and internal fixation through an intraoral approach with a 4- or 6-hole plate placed inferior on the mandibular body. The arch bar would serve as a tension band to prevent splaying at the alveolar borders. Overbending of the plate will assist in compression of the lingual cortex. The treatment enigma is the displaced condylar fracture in the setting of a possible noncompliant patient. Patient counseling is essential to emphasize the importance of retention of IMF in the postoperative period, followed in 7–10 days by conversion to elastics, strategically placed to advantage masticatory forces to reduce the subcondylar fracture.)

In-Service Examination

1. The principal vector of the lateral pterygoid muscle:
   (a) Medial, downward, and posterior
   (b) Medial, downward, and anterior
   (c) Lateral, downward, and anterior
   (d) Lateral, upward, and anterior
2. Angle classification is dictated by the position of what teeth?
   (a) Lateral incisors
   (b) Canines
   (c) First and second premolars
   (d) First molar
3. The exit of the mental nerve at the mental foramen is located where?
   (a) Inferior to the lateral incisors
   (b) Inferior to the canines
   (c) Inferior to the first premolar
   (d) Inferior to the second premolar
   (e) Inferior to the first molar

50 Condylar, Pediatric Fractures, Complications

Bibliography

Stacey D, Doyle J, Mount DL, et al. "Management of Mandible Fractures," *Plast Reconstr Surg.*, (2006); 117:**55e–57e ONLY.**

Pickrell BB and Hollier LH, "Evidence-Based Medicine: Mandible Fractures," *Plast Reconstr Surg.*, (2017);140:**196e–197e ONLY.**

Smartt JM, Low DW, and Bartlett SP, "The Pediatric Mandible: II. Management of Traumatic Injury or Fracture," *Plast Reconstr Surg.*, (2005); 116:**28e–39e.**

Alpert, B., "Management of the Complications of Mandibular Fracture Treatment." Operative Techniques in Plastic and Reconstructive Surgery, Culbertson Jr., J. H. et al., W.B. Saunders Co. (1998); 5:**325–333.**

Mehra P, Heukelom EV, Cottrell DA, "Rigid Internal Fixation of Infected Mandibular Fractures," *J. Oral. Maxillofac. Surg.* (2009); 67:**1046–51.**

Ostrander BT, Wang HD, Cusano A, et al., "Contemporary Management of Mandibular Fracture Nonunion-A Retrospective Review and Treatment Algorithm," *J Oral Maxillofac. Surg.*, (2018); 76:**1479–80, 1482–92.**

Kazi AA, Lee TS, Vincent A, et al., "The Role of External Fixation in Trauma and Reconstruction of the Mandible in the Age of Rigid Fixation," *Facial Plast. Surg.*, (2019); 35:**614–622.**

"Xternal Fixator", *KLS Martin,* (2009); 3.1(98): **1–15.**

Braidy H.F., Ziccardi V.B., "External fixation for mandible fractures," *Atlas Oral Maxillofac Surg Clin North Am.* (2009); 17(1):**49–52 ONLY.**

Faculty Discussion and Study Guide

Condylar Fractures

1. Outline a classification system of condylar fractures that enables the description of the important characteristics. (Level of fracture or anatomical site, relationship of the fragments to each other, relationship of the condylar head to the fossa.)
   (a) Give details. (Site: head, neck, or subcondylar; relationship of fragments: the condylar fragment, if dislocated, is either medial or lateral to the fossa.)
   (b) How does the medial or lateral displacement of the condylar head impact the treatment plan? (Most commonly, over 95% of the fragment is displaced medially because of the tough, fibrous nature of the lateral capsule as well as the anterior and medial traction of the inferior belly of the lateral pterygoid. If displaced laterally, the implication is that the condylar head has been displaced through the fibrous lateral capsule, which would preclude closed reduction.)
2. Discuss the pathologic anatomy and treatment of intracapsular condylar fractures. (The problem is comminution and extreme difficulty with any type of internal fixation. Because of the nature of the injury, the desire would be to mobilize the patient to avoid fibrosis and ankylosis of the temporomandibular joint, the TMJ, so intermaxillary fixation, IMF, for 7–10 days with guiding elastics for an additional 2 weeks.)
   (a) What are the long-term outcomes frequently complicated by? (Osteoarthritis of the TMJ)
3. A patient with a left condylar fracture has an open bite on the right, and the chin deviates to the left when opening, explain. (The open bite is because of premature closure on the left or injured side as a result of vertical overriding of the superior and inferior fragments. The chin deviates to the left because of the unopposed action of the right lateral pterygoid muscle, particularly the inferior belly.)
4. Outline the pros and cons of operative versus conservative therapy of extracapsular condylar fractures. (Operative treatment assures anatomic reduction and fixation but at the price of an incisional scar and, more worrisome, the potential for facial nerve injury as well as devascularization of the condylar head. Conservative management avoids those problems but at the potential

E. Luce, *A Curriculum for Plastic Surgery*, https://doi.org/10.1007/978-3-031-62087-4_50

expense of inadequate reduction and late TMJ problems. The topic is one of ongoing discussion.)

(a) What are the absolute indications for ORIF of condylar fractures? (Displacement of the condylar head into the temporal fossa, probably quite rare, lateral rather than medial dislocation, a low subcondylar fracture-dislocation, bilateral fracture-dislocation that fails to reduce and/or persistence of an anterior open bite or premature posterior closure after 2 weeks of IMF and elastics, bilateral fracture-dislocation in association with complex maxillary fractures. A relative indication would be severe angulation in combination with dislocation of the condylar head from the fossa.)

(b) What are the relative indications for ORIF of the condyle? (Unilateral or bilateral where IMF and elastics are not possible either because of patient compliance or coexisting medical problems; bilateral in the edentulous patient and splints are not available.)

5. Discuss the conservative management of condylar fractures. (If no malocclusion exists, liquid-soft diet only with periodic reassessment; if malocclusion exists, reduction into proper occlusion, then 7–10 days of wire IMF followed by guiding elastics with periodic reassessment and progressive release and removal of elastic IMF.)

Management of Pediatric Fractures

1. What are some of the major and unique considerations in the treatment of pediatric mandible fractures? (A significant implication is the rate of bone healing in children, which results in shorter periods of immobilization, 2–3 weeks, to achieve union. Rapid remodeling of fracture sites also implies a less exact opposition of bone surfaces is required. In the same vein, a potential adverse effect exists on growth and development with surgical intervention. An additional consideration is the configuration of the primary or deciduous teeth.)

   (a) What is the configuration of the deciduous or primary teeth that becomes problematic with IMF? (Conical shape with a wider neck than the occlusal surface, narrowed body; potential for extraction with the force generation by IMF; potential for damage of the secondary tooth buds from the screws with the application of the hybrid arch bar.)

2. What are some measures that can be utilized to overcome these limitations? (Use of occlusal splints plus circummandibular wires. The splints are composed of acrylic and can be fashioned in the OR or, in more complex fractures, constructed in the dental lab.)

   (a) Describe the technique of circummandibular wires. (Use of a spinal needle to pass the wire from intraorally to externally and then return to the intraoral cavity and ligature about the arch bar. At least one and perhaps two on each side are required, and a small stab incision is made at the skin to allow the wire to be advanced up against the inferior border of the mandible. Avoidance of the mental nerve at the first deciduous molar or second permanent bicuspid is important.)

   (b) What is the technique to secure the maxillary arch bar? (Use of an intraosseous hole just lateral to the piriform aperture, and the drop wire spans to the maxillary arch bar. Another technique is a drop wire from the superior lateral orbital rim subcutaneously to the lateral aspect of the maxillary arch bar. This option requires a small incision at the superior orbital rim.)

3. What are the indications for consideration of ORIF of pediatric condylar fractures? (Low subcondylar fracture with significant displacement in a child older than 10 years. In reality, virtually all condylar fractures in young children can be managed conservatively, and the vast majority of preadolescent patients as well. See Fig. 50.1.)

4. Besides condylar fractures, what other type of mandibular fracture in a child might require ORIF and why? (Angle fractures, which are posterior to the dentition and therefore difficult to control during healing. If the child is less than 3–5 years old, closed reduction with occlusal splints, circummandibular wires, and drop wires to the maxillary arch bar. Even older children, 5–12 years old, usually can be managed conservatively.)

5. If internal fixation is necessary, what are the recommendations? (Because of concerns of injury to the permanent tooth buds, use the plate on the most inferior border of the mandible with monocortical screws, use small 1.3 and 1.5 mm plates, and consider resorbable hardware. In older children older than 12 years of age, bicortical screws may be utilized because the space between the secondary tooth buds and the inferior border is sufficiently large.)

6. Describe the pros and cons of bioabsorbable plates. (Since the plates will resorb with time, the risk of growth restriction, possible with nonresorbable plates, does not exist. The disadvantages include the necessity for larger plates and screws to achieve the same rigidity of fixation of a smaller permanent plate and the occurrence of an occasional sterile abscess as a complication of the resorption process. If nonresorbable plates are utilized in a growing child, later removal should be planned.)

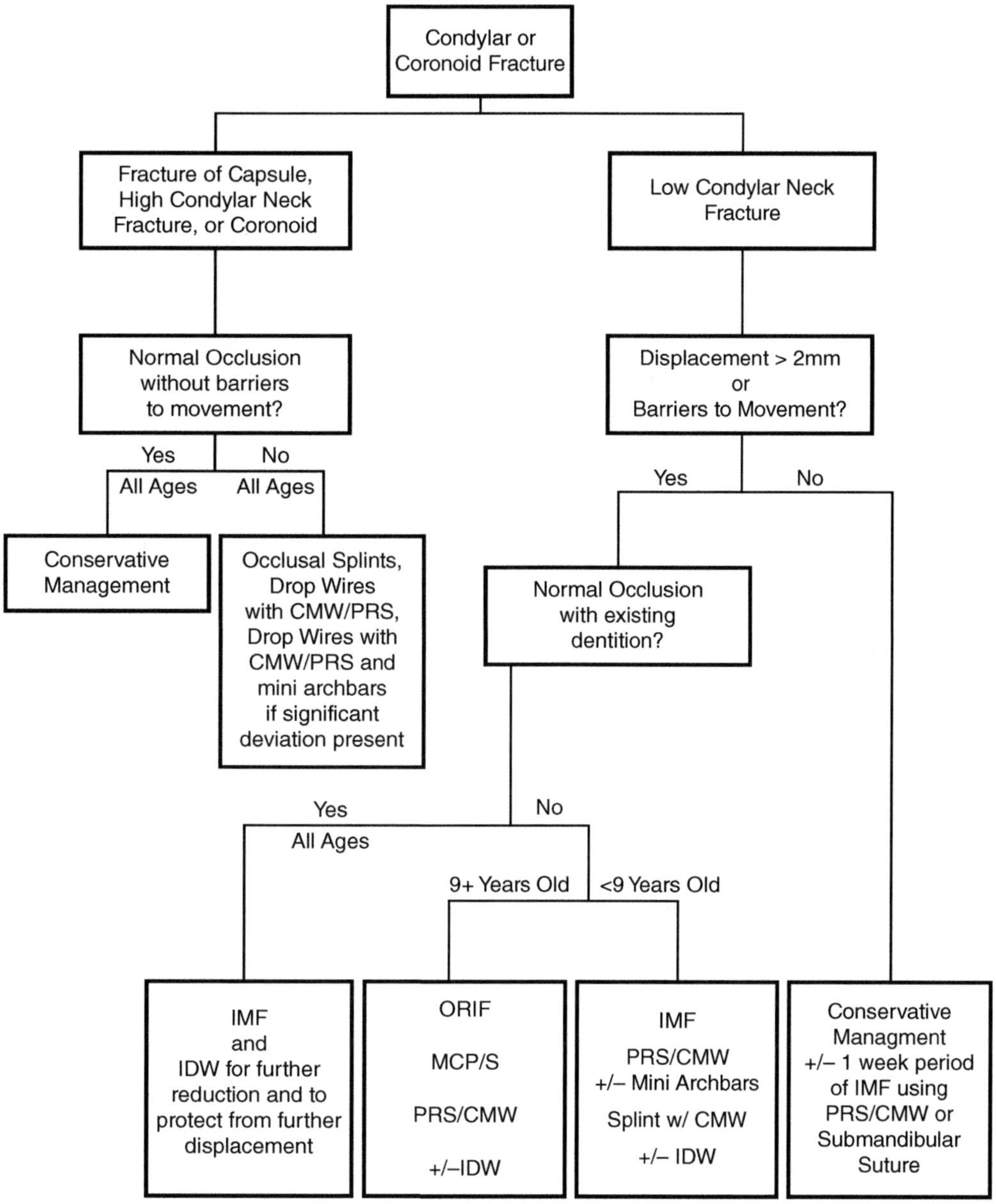

Fig. 50.1 Algorithm for management of pediatric condylar or coronoid fractures. (Smartt JM, Low DW, and Bartlett SP, "The Pediatric Mandible: II. Management of Traumatic Injury or Fracture," *Plast. Reconstr. Surg.*, (2005); 116:38e. (Reprinted with Permission))

Dental Trauma, Complications

1. Although complex classifications of dental trauma are available, logically and stepping away from the issue of management of a tooth or teeth in the fracture line, what are the three general possibilities of injury pertinent to management in maxillofacial trauma? (Is the tooth completely avulsed or still in the socket but loose, or not loose but tender to tapping or percussion.)
   (a) Discuss the management of each. (Tenderness to direct percussion requires no immediate treatment. A loose or subluxated tooth is managed with splinting, accomplished with the placement of a segmental arch bar incorporating two teeth on either side of the injured tooth and securing the tooth to the arch bar with a 28 G wire placed perpendicular to the interdental wires. An avulsed tooth is repositioned in the socket after gentle irrigation and splinted, similar to the technique described above, and maintained for 2 weeks. Teeth that have been avulsed longer than 1 h are unlikely to survive.)
2. A patient with midface fractures also has a fractured tooth. What are the important injury variables? (Does the fracture involve enamel alone, limited to enamel and dentin, or involve the enamel, dentin, cementum, and possibly the pulp.)

3. Extrusion of teeth can occur with IMF. In what set of circumstances and what teeth is the risk higher? (Pediatric fractures particularly less than the age of eight or nine. The incisors, if individually ligated and placed in elastics, can be extruded at least partially, and that hazard is increased in the pediatric patient. Another technique, such as Figure-of-eight, should be utilized if the incisors must be incorporated in the arc bar.)
4. The most common cause of infection and nonunion of mandible fractures is: (Inadequate fracture stabilization, which leads to increased micro- or even macromotion at the fracture line, which, in turn, creates increased inflammation and perhaps additional necrotic material, including bone and then secondary microbial infection. Besides necrotic bone, devitalized and/or carious teeth can provide a nidus. Multiple technical reasons may be responsible.)
5. Describe the usual presentation of an infected mandible postoperatively. (Swelling, pain, possibly extraoral or intraoral drainage.)
6. How might the timing of the postoperative presentation affect management? (Early postoperative presentation, less than 3 weeks, may represent a wound infection only, such as an infected hematoma or seroma. That scenario implies a probable intraoral incision for drainage and perhaps less exposure. Late presentations, greater than 6–8 weeks, will require greater exposure with probable bone debridement and an external incision such as a Risdon. The management of the intermediate timing group will be on an individual or a case-by-case basis.)
7. After incision and drainage, what is the appropriate management of an infected body fracture? (After drainage and exposure of the fracture site, an assessment of the hardware is mandatory. If loose, the plates and screws are removed. If the hardware is still intact and not loose, particularly in the early postoperative period, drainage and antibiotics can be employed with continuance of IMF for 2–3 weeks. Once the hardware is removed and the bone is debrided, a decision must be made whether the rigid internal fixation with a reconstruction plate or a standard 2.0 or 2.3 plate would be advantageous vs. the placement of an external fixation appliance. The above maneuvers assume that the patient has been placed into intermaxillary fixation, IMF. If the bone debridement is relatively small with only 2–3 mm of gap, a reconstruction plate may be satisfactory. An additional option is the use of autogenous cancellous bone graft in combination with the fixation plate, an additional option that seems counterintuitive, but a successful experience has been published. The emphasis is on adequate debridement of devitalized and osteomyelitic bone and rigid internal fixation with a multiple-hole plate, possibly a reconstruction plate, but the disadvantage is the necessity of extensive soft tissue stripping. The other option is the use of an external fixator with the disadvantage of the resultant pin scarring and the patient inconvenience, but if a significant bone gap exists, that option should be employed. IMF should be continued for 7–10 days postoperatively.)
8. The line between nonunion and infected nonunion is blurred. List the factors that might favor a single-stage approach and describe them. (The traditional management is two-stage, with drainage, bone debridement, and application of external fixation. A single-stage approach is a debridement, cancellous bone grafting, and rigid fixation with either a multi-hole reconstruction plate or a shorter, standard 2.3 plate. See above. The former requires greater periosteal stripping, the latter perhaps less rigid fixation.)
9. Describe the technique of application of external fixation. (The patient is placed into occlusion with intermaxillary fixation. The location of the pins is determined on the inferior aspect of the mandible to avoid injury to the inferior alveolar or mental nerve. Percutaneous drill holes are placed, followed by threaded pins, two on either side of the fracture or segmental loss. The pins are placed a minimum of 1–2 cm from the fracture(s) or segment loss and connected with a prebent titanium rod, or the rod is bent to fit. An alternate technique is a two-step process with the fixation provided by an acrylic splint poured into a tray available with the system and allowed to harden and subsequent removal of the tray. Yet, another and perhaps most economical is the placement of a small-bore chest tube over the inner set of pin screws, filling the tube with liquid acrylic, and tightening the outer set of screws over the chest tube.)
10. Complications of external fixation? (The technical error of failure to restore premorbid occlusion with the placement of intermaxillary fixation. Pin tract infection can occur with loosening of the pins and loss of occlusion. Diligent pin care by the patient is a necessity.)
11. The principal cause of late malocclusion in a patient managed with ORIF is usually technical. What are the treatment alternatives for late malocclusion in a stable, healed fracture? (Minor malocclusion can perhaps be managed with orthodontics. Many, if not most, will require orthognathic surgery.)
12. How would you advise a patient with a mid-body fracture with preoperative lip/gingiva numbness about the prospects for recovery? (Actually, it's quite good if followed for 1 year. The emphasis is on the detection preoperatively of an inferior alveolar nerve injury and counseling the patient.)
13. A patient with a mandibular mid-body fracture is missing the canine, and the first premolar in the area of the fracture is easily placed into occlusion under general anesthesia and prior to the placement of arch bars. Yet,

once arch bars are wired into place, restoration of pre-injury occlusion with IMF is not possible. Why? (The length of the mandibular arch, "circumference," has been shortened because of the missing teeth. The management is to cut the arch bar into two segments, one posterior to the fracture line and the other on the remaining portion of the circumference of the mandible, and replace the patient with proper occlusion and intermaxillary fixation.)

14. You have performed open reduction internal fixation of a Le Forte II maxillary fracture and an angle and symphysis fracture of the mandible. The patient at the end of the procedure is in satisfactory maxillary, mandibular fixation, IMF, with arch bars and wires. In the clinic, 1 week postoperatively, with the release of the IMF, the patient slips severely out of occlusion. What is the explanation? (The maxilla was not satisfactorily disimpacted and is displaced posteriorly with respect to the cranial base. As a result, the mandible has related temporarily to the maxilla because of the mobility of the TMJ, but with the release of the IMF, the muscles of mastication pull the mandible and the TMJ into a "normal" position. Treatment is reoperation, disimpaction of the maxilla, and replacement into IMF.)

Case-Based Conference

Case 1: Mandible Fracture

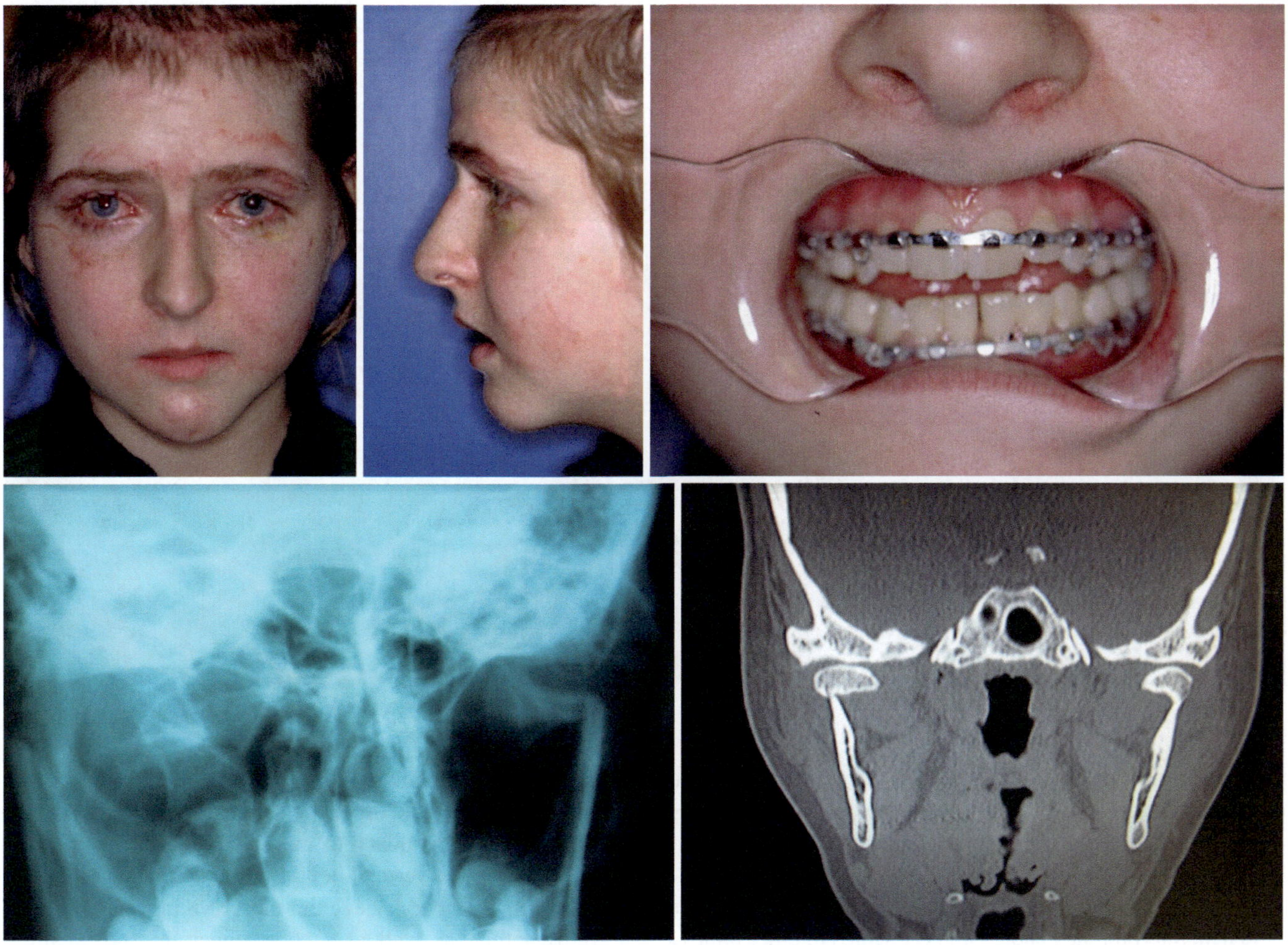

A 20-year-old two and a half weeks after management with closed reduction and IMF. Arrives at the consultation with a Panorex and CT scan from her dentist's office.

1. Interpret the clinical slides. Add a focused clinical exam. Then, interpret the Panorex and CT scan. No other injuries, excellent health.
   (a) Any additional studies? If so, why?
2. What is the pathologic anatomy of this injury?
3. What are the likely outcomes of inadequate treatment?
4. Outline your treatment and describe it in detail.

Case-Based Conference: Discussion

Case 1: Mandible Fracture

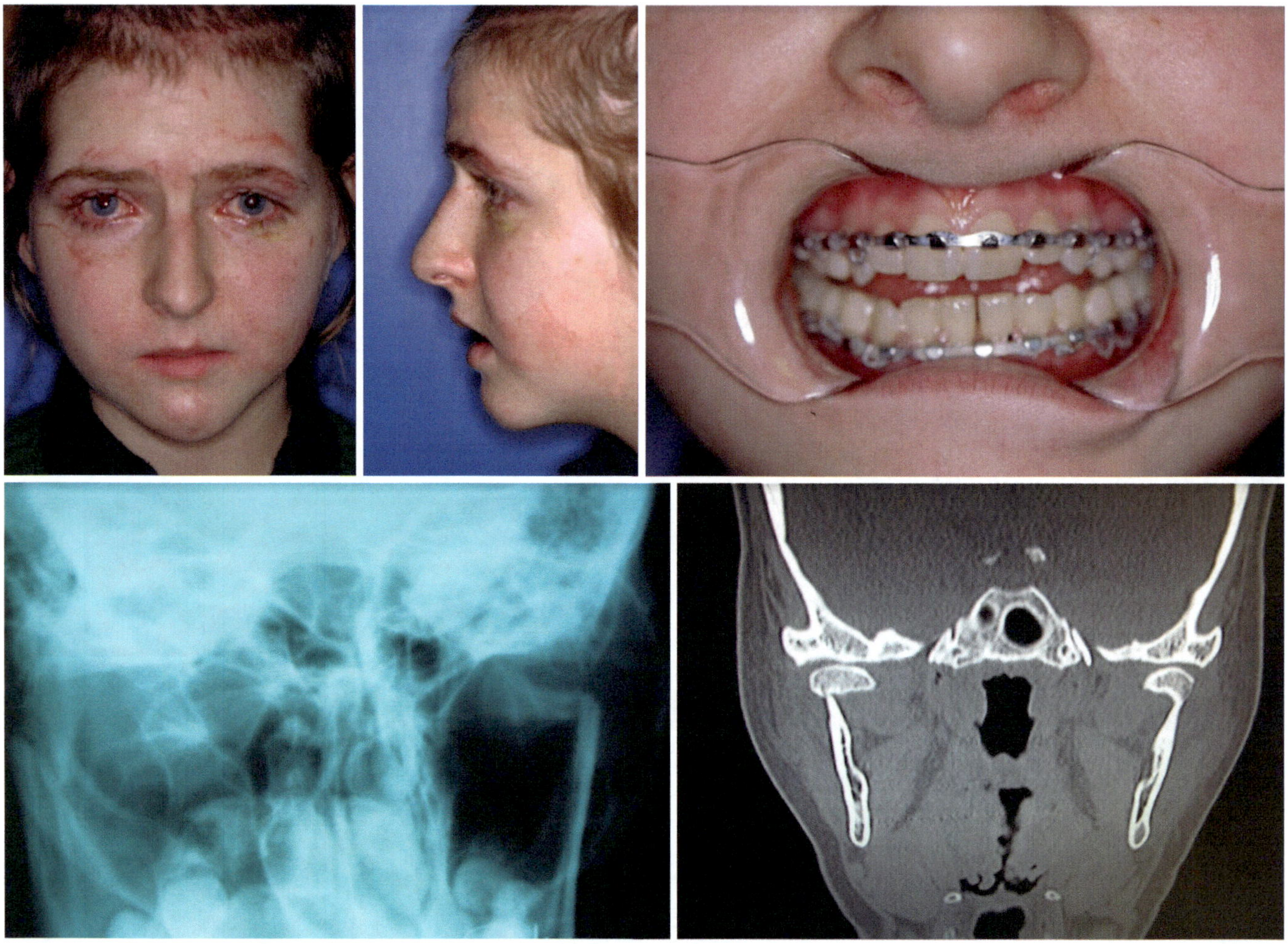

A 20-year-old two and a half weeks after management with closed reduction and IMF. Arrives at the consultation with a Panorex and CT scan from her dentist's office.

1. Interpret the clinical slides. Add a focused clinical exam. Then, interpret the Panorex and CT scan. No other injuries, excellent health. (The frontal view demonstrates a young woman with a few superficial abrasions on her face. No facial deformity is evident other than facial proportions that reveal a proportionately diminished lower one-third. The normal facial proportions are those of an equal distance of the glabella to the subnasale as that distance from the subnasale to the tip of the chin. Although some distortion may be secondary to the lens length utilized in the photograph, the vertical height of the chin appears diminished. In the lateral view, the most striking finding is the retrognathia, as well as a short upper lip and, again, a diminished vertical height of the chin. An intraoral occlusal view is available that appears to demonstrate a significant anterior open bite that extends from the visible first molar to the opposite first molar, as well as, perhaps, a congenital retraction of the maxillary lateral incisors bilaterally.

The history would center on the prior treatment. Namely, was the patient taken to the operating room in an attempt at closed reduction and application of arch bars and intermaxillary fixation? Was the patient converted from IMF wires to elastics, and if so, how long ago? Any preexistent orthodontic treatment or malocclusion? The physical exam would focus on wear facets that may indicate a preexistent over or underbite, although the image would suggest neither is the case. The condylar head can be palpated with the examiner's finger placed in the external auditory canal while the patient opens and closes. This exam may indicate whether the condylar head is palpable on the right or not. The mandibular excursion should also be determined. An intraoral examination for the detection of any lacerations indicative of any other mandibular fractures should be performed. The Panorex demonstrates a condylar neck fracture on the left with a 90° medial displacement of the condylar head. On the right, a neck or subcondylar fracture is present with overriding. The film is indistinct, and a judgment about the condylar head dislocation is not possible. A single slice of a coronal view CT scan demonstrates bilateral condylar fractures displaced and angled medially. The level of the fracture is quite superior, and a question arises if the right condylar head is no longer related to the neck.)

(a) Any additional studies? If so, why? (The remaining CT images are reviewed for a better delineation of the characteristics of the fractures on CT, which would be appropriate, particularly a determination of the displacement, if any, of the right condylar head.)

2. What is the pathologic anatomy of this injury? (Patient must have sustained blunt trauma to the chin with bilateral condylar neck fractures. She apparently has failed closed reduction and attempted rehabilitation with elastics. The principal pathology is a severe medial dislocation of the left condylar fracture and overriding with displacement on the right. The left is fractured and displaced. Both of those fractures permit shortening of the vertical ramus of the mandible bilaterally under the influence of the pterygoid-masseteric sling with the resultant premature posterior closure and creation of an anterior open bite and retrognathia. The primary dislocating force on the condylar head is the lateral pterygoid muscle, mostly the inferior belly. Since the muscle belly courses from the pterygoid plate and the face of the sphenoid from anterior to posterior and medial to lateral, the dislocating force retracts the mandibular head medially and anteriorly. The subcondylar neck fracture on the opposite or right side mitigates the use of an intact vertical ramus as a lever force for the use of elastics to gradually reduce the left condylar fracture.)
3. What are the likely outcomes of inadequate treatment? (Unless restoration of the vertical height is accomplished, a persistent anterior open bite will occur.)
4. Outline your treatment and describe it in detail. (Given the degree of dislocation, an alternative is open reduction and fixation of the right side. Because of the above pathophysiology, an open reduction and internal fixation of the left condyle is indicated. Once skeletal stability is achieved on the left, postoperative elastics can be utilized to restore the right subcondylar fracture.

Open reduction and internal fixation require a preauricular approach combined with a submandibular incision. If a preauricular incision is utilized for direct exposure from a lateral route to the condylar neck and head, the submandibular incision is utilized for inferior traction of the ramus by means of a bone clamp or an interosseous wire. The principal hazard with the open exposure of the condyle is injury to branches of the facial nerve. This potential complication can be minimized in a couple of ways. One is the exposure of the main trunk of the nerve as in the initial steps of the superficial parotidectomy with dissection of the temporofacial trunk and then isolation of the temporal branch with retraction anteriorly out of harm's way. Another option is a direct incision just anterior to the external auditory canal through the deep temporal fascia and temporalis muscle. The condylar head will be hidden beneath the zygomatic arch, and inferior retraction of the mandible will be necessary. The final step, if necessary, in the exposure is the incision of the temporomandibular joint capsule. An option is the use of an endoscopic approach for reduction and plating. This discussion assumes the operator is not conversant with an endoscopic option. Occasionally, with the attempts at operative reduction, the entire condylar head will come free of the fossa and will then need to be plated on the inferior ramus and relocated into the fossa. Postoperatively, elastics are utilized to reduce the right subcondylar fracture.

Regardless, the outcome of operative and nonoperative treatment of severe bilateral condylar fractures is a certain proportion of the patients who sustain long-term TMJ arthritis.)

Intraoperative

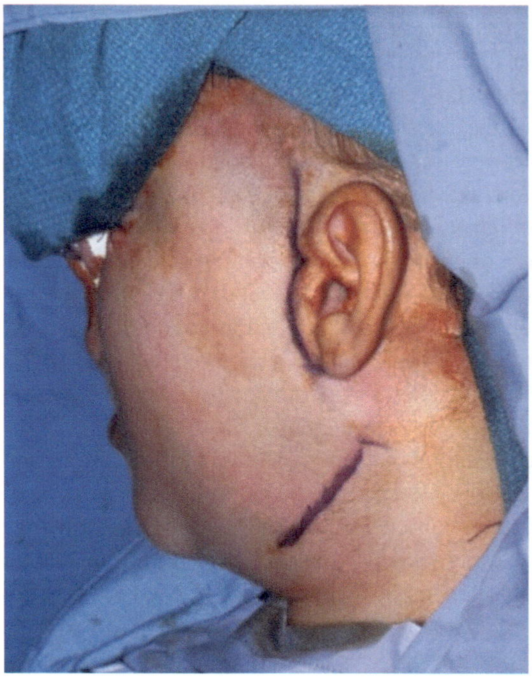

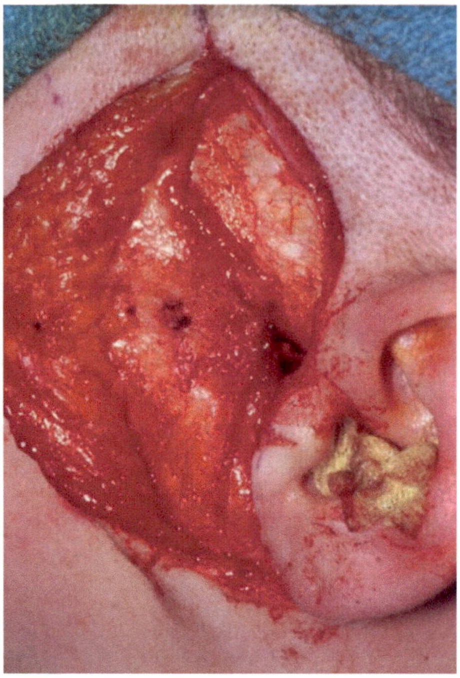

The first of two photos illustrate a pretragal preauricular and submandibular incisions. Retrotragal is preferred. The second photo depicts exposure prior to the incision of the deep temporal fascia.

Postoperative (2 Months)

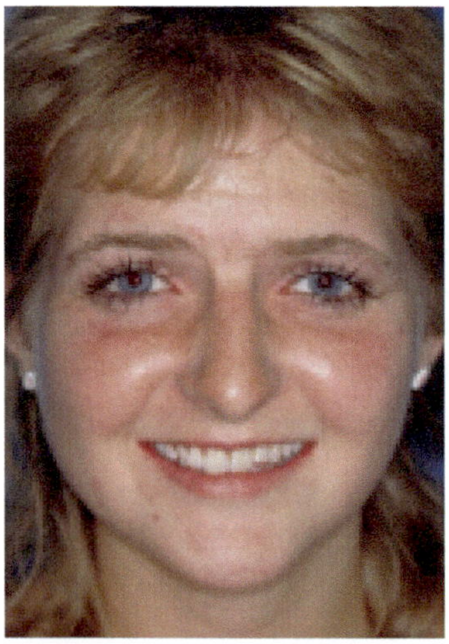

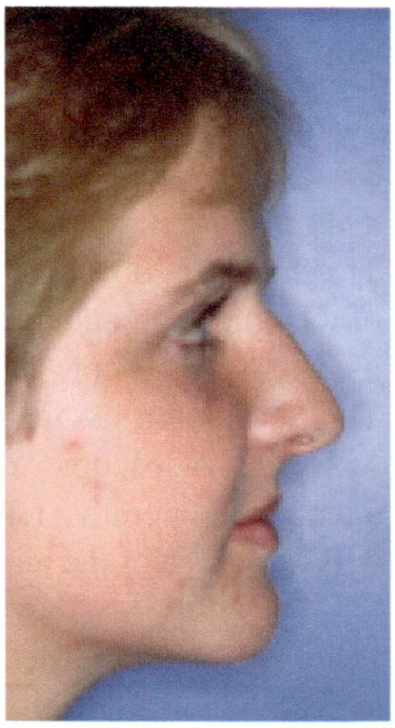

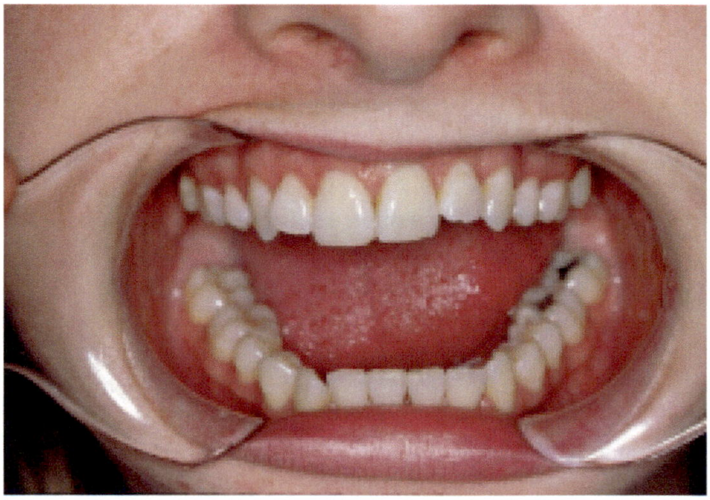

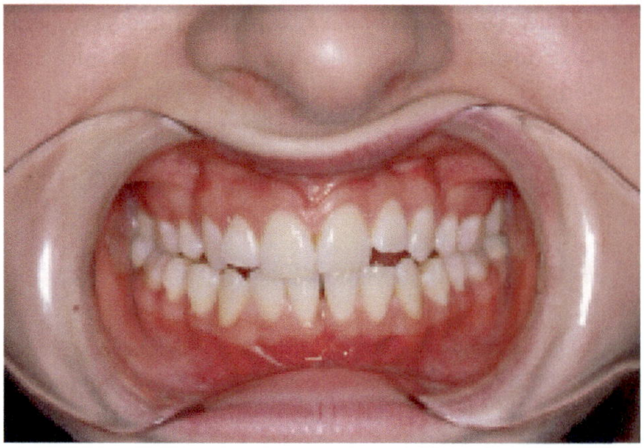

The two facial views are frontal and right lateral. Normal facial proportions and chin prominence have been restored, and the retrognathia is absent. Interincisal distance or opening is excellent, as is the occlusion. The retraction of the lateral maxillary incisors is still observed.

Case-Based Conference

Case 2: Infected Mandibular Fracture

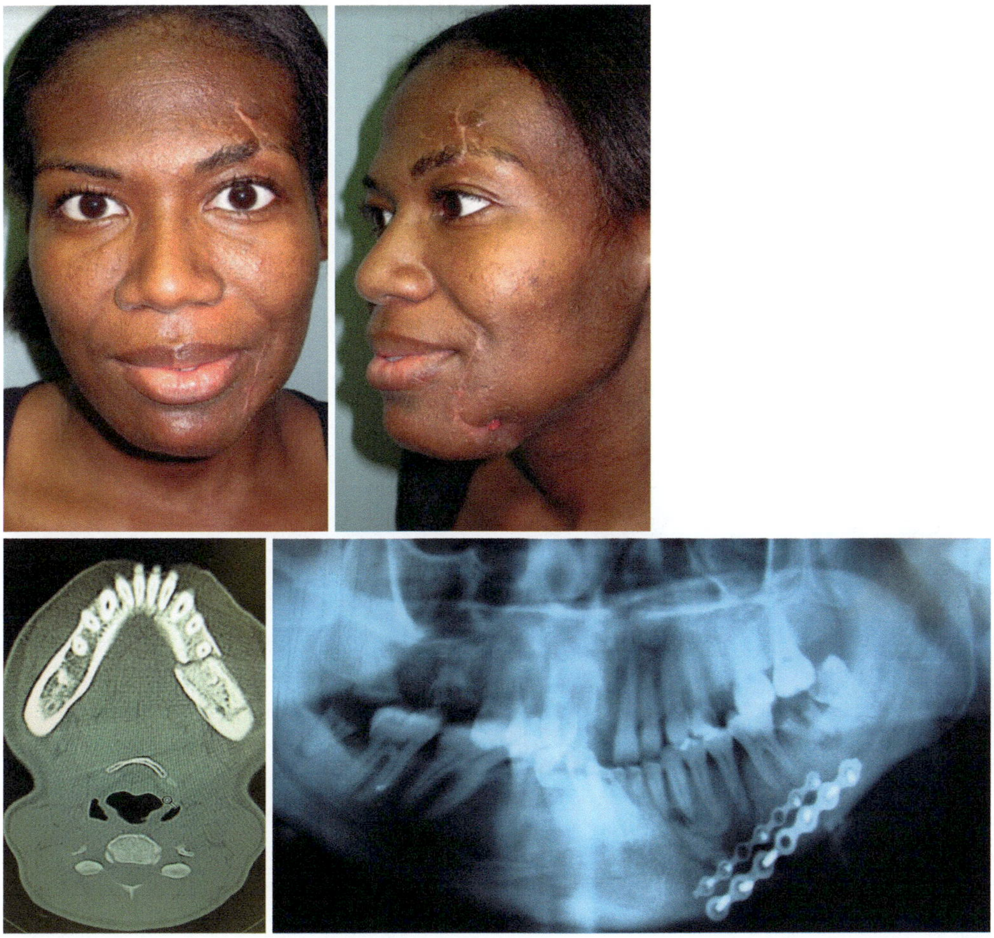

A 30-year-old 2 months postoperative from open reduction, internal fixation of a left mandibular body sustained in an assault. Two-week history of facial swelling followed by drainage. No other injuries. A Panorex was obtained in the clinic. The preoperative CT scan is available.

1. Describe the slides and add a clinical examination.
   (a) Interpret the postoperative Panorex and preoperative CT scan. Add and justify any additional tests.
2. What is the pathologic anatomy and pathophysiology of your presumptive diagnosis? Other or alternate diagnoses under consideration?
3. Give a menu of treatment options. Select yours and justify.

Case-Based Conference: Discussion

Case 2: Infected Mandibular Fracture

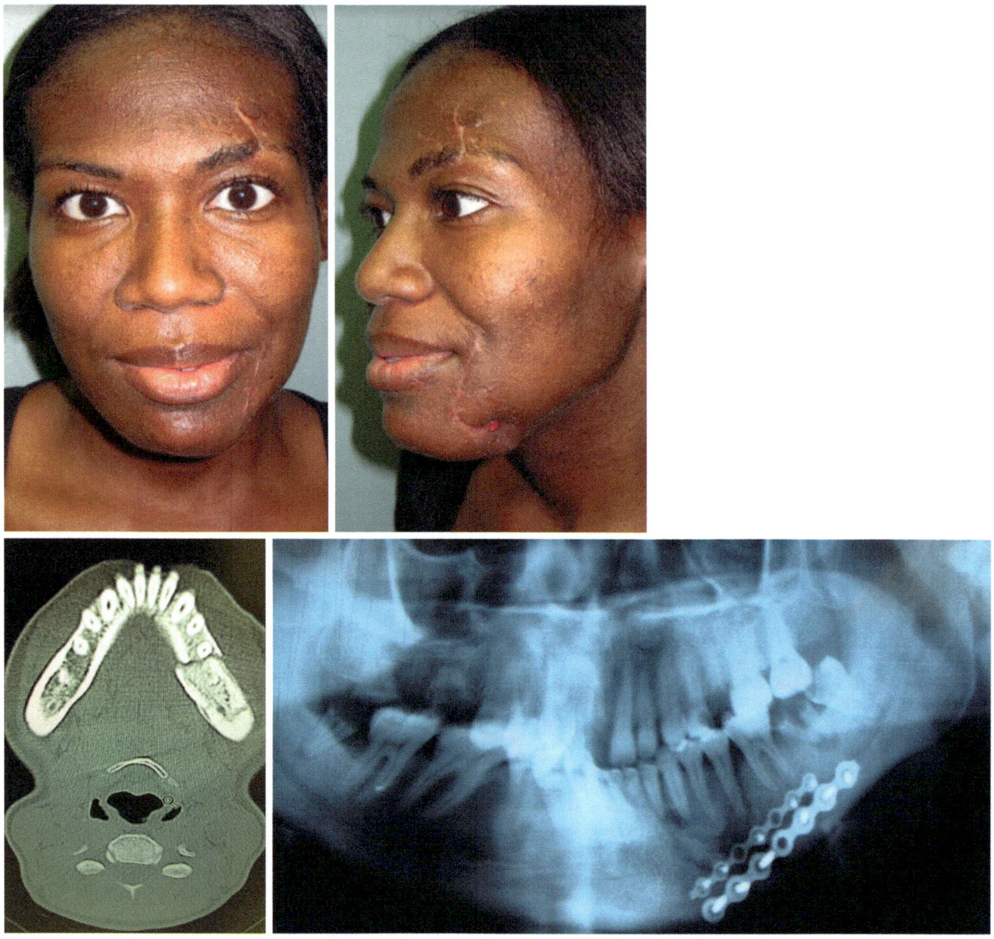

A 30-year-old 2 months postoperative from open reduction, internal fixation of a left mandibular body sustained in an assault. Two-week history of facial swelling followed by drainage. No other injuries. A Panorex was obtained in the clinic. The preoperative CT scan is available.

1. Describe the slides and add a clinical examination. (Two clinical photos are provided. The first is a full-face frontal view of the head and neck of a woman with a slight smile, but the dentition is not visible. A healed laceration scar is visible through the left mid-eyebrow with some modest superior retraction. Another 3 cm vertical probable laceration scar is present just lateral to the left commissure. No obvious swelling or deformity is present. The left oblique view yields some significant findings. The vertical scar is in the form of a reverse "J," at the termination of which is a several-millimeter area of granulation tissue. That point lies directly over the anterior body of the mandible, and some umbilication exists of the soft tissue surrounding the granulation tissue. No evidence of an external incision is present, and no other deformities are evident.

   The clinical exam would begin with a history of treatment and symptom milestones. A minimal number of questions regarding the assault would be followed by details of the hiatus between injury and repair, a single operative procedure, or if reoperation was necessary and perceived occlusion immediately postoperative. Additional questions about the ability to eat and the nature of the diet are advanced. The subsequent history should focus on postoperative management, including duration of intermaxillary fixation IMF, followed by queries dictated toward the determination of the onset of current symptoms of swelling and pain and subsequent drainage and include if any intraoral drainage is present. The presence of systemic symptoms of fever and chills should also be ascertained. The patient should also be asked about perceptions of current occlusion. The ability to open, chew, and the pain with mastication is determined. The history is complete with the pursuit of possible preexisting comorbidities and medications. The physical exam centers on the head and neck and includes gentle palpation of the left-sided facial swelling, but no effort to determine the false motion or crepitus of the mandible is attempted. Assessment of sensation over the distribution of the left mental, inferior alveolar nerve of the lower lip is completed. The patient should be requested to open to whatever degree possible and close with the lips gently retracted by the examiner and, in doing so, assess occlusion. The left buccal cavity is inspected for residual sutures, evidence of an intraoral approach as well as possible exposed hardware. The cheek can be gently pressed to elicit possible intraoral drainage. A routine complete physical exam is performed.)

(a) Interpret the postoperative Panorex and preoperative CT scan. Add and justify any additional tests. (A Panorex illustrates some findings. Two plates are present in the mid-body of the left mandible. The first is at the inferior border with three screws, proximal and distal to the fracture line. A smaller, also seven-hole plate, is more superior, at approximately mid-height. Two screws are proximal and distal, with a single screw in the middle hole. The inferior plate appears to be a 2.0, the mid-body perhaps a 1.5 plate. A distinct and considerable-sized area of radiolucency is present from the roots of two teeth to the inferior border of the mandible. A full set of teeth is present except a molar that appears to have lost a crown. Absent is any evidence of tooth fragments or bony sequestrum in the area of the fracture, but the film quality is not superb.

    A CT scan at this juncture is mandatory to further delineate the wound circumstances in the region of the fracture, the radiolucency, and the nature of the bone immediately adjacent. Routine lab work is probably indicated.)

2. What is the pathologic anatomy and pathophysiology of your presumptive diagnosis? Other or alternate diagnoses under consideration? (The pathologic anatomy of this scenario is an infected mandible body fracture, perhaps complicated by osteomyelitis. The pathophysiology is the genesis of infection of mandible fractures in general and factors specific to this patient. The proven pertinent variables that predispose to postoperative infection and nonunion are tobacco and substance abuse and the severity of the fracture. The latter, severity, is assessed by location, degree of comminution, degree of soft tissue injury, and mechanism as assault versus higher velocity motor vehicular accident or gunshot wound. High-velocity fractures are at increased risk for complications of infected nonunion, but otherwise, the mechanism in this clinical scenario was low velocity and unlikely comminuted. An additional factor is the state of the dentition and the presence of caries and periodontal disease. Factors not significant include the use of antibiotics postoperative, and the hiatus between injury and repair is inconclusive as a predictive variable. The known treatment factors may be significant. The adequacy of reduction is but one of a number of technical particulars that can play a role in predisposition to infection, all of which, in this case, of course, are unknown. The role of the degree of magnitude of inappropriate motion, termed macromotion, is also unknown. In the era of rigid but not compressive fixation, some element of micromotion is appropriate, desirable, and facilitates bone healing. Excessive motion disrupts the normal cascade of cartilage deposition and callus formation, lamellar, and eventually woven bone formation, all elements of stable healing. Excessive motion predisposes to inflammation and infection. IMF is necessary to achieve the first stages of healing but should be discontinued and elastics initiated to minimize the secondary iatrogenic issues of temporomandibular joint dysfunction. To do so relies on the security of the internal fixation.)

3. Give a menu of treatment options. Select yours and justify. (The menu of treatment options begins with a selection of approaches, intra-or extraoral incisions. The decision would hinge somewhat on CT scan findings, including the magnitude of the diastasis presence or not of isolated bone fragments, but in all likelihood, an extraoral Risdon incision will provide the necessary exposure for thorough evaluation and treatment. If an intraoral incision has been dehisced, the inclination would be toward an intraoral approach solely, but the difficulty is adequate exposure, particularly of the inferior aspect of the angle. Assuming an extraoral incision, the fracture and plate are exposed to the anterior and posterior limits of the extent of the plates. In this instance, the plate and screws are removed, and nonviable bone on either edge of the fracture is debrided. Clearly, devitalized, loose, and/or grossly carious teeth should be removed, including, in this instance, the first molar. The sinus tract should be excised at either orifice, intraoral, or cutaneous, and thorough curettage should be accomplished. At this junction, the treatment options diverge. Available are three alternatives, all after adequate debridement: one, the most traditional, is drainage and the placement of an external fixation device with the prior placement of IMF to secure correct occlusion. After satisfactory soft tissue healing and a time interval of approximately 3 months, a second-stage autogenous bone graft, followed by retention of the external fixation for a variable period, is dictated by the presence of a healed and stable fracture. Second, again after bone debridement and plate fixation are removed, a reconstruction or locking plate is applied with two to three screws on either fragment, IMF is maintained for a

short period postoperative, and fracture healing over time is anticipated. The employment of this option mandates that following debridement, little or no bone gap exists, an unlikely outcome in this scenario. Third, an autogenous cancellous bone graft is added to the second option, packed into the fracture site. Each technique has proponents. Application of the external fixation requires less periosteal stripping as is necessary for reconstruction plate and screw placement, but the inconvenience and appearance of the apparatus is a distinct drawback. The use of the reconstruction or locking plate burdens the wound with a considerable amount of hardware and implies no bone defect. The third option, bone grafting in the presence of established infection, appears counterintuitive and has the attendant necessity of the graft donor site. Nevertheless, as experience has accrued, considerable enthusiasm has been established for the combination of rigid fixation and concomitant cancellous bone grafts.)

Postoperative (1 Month)

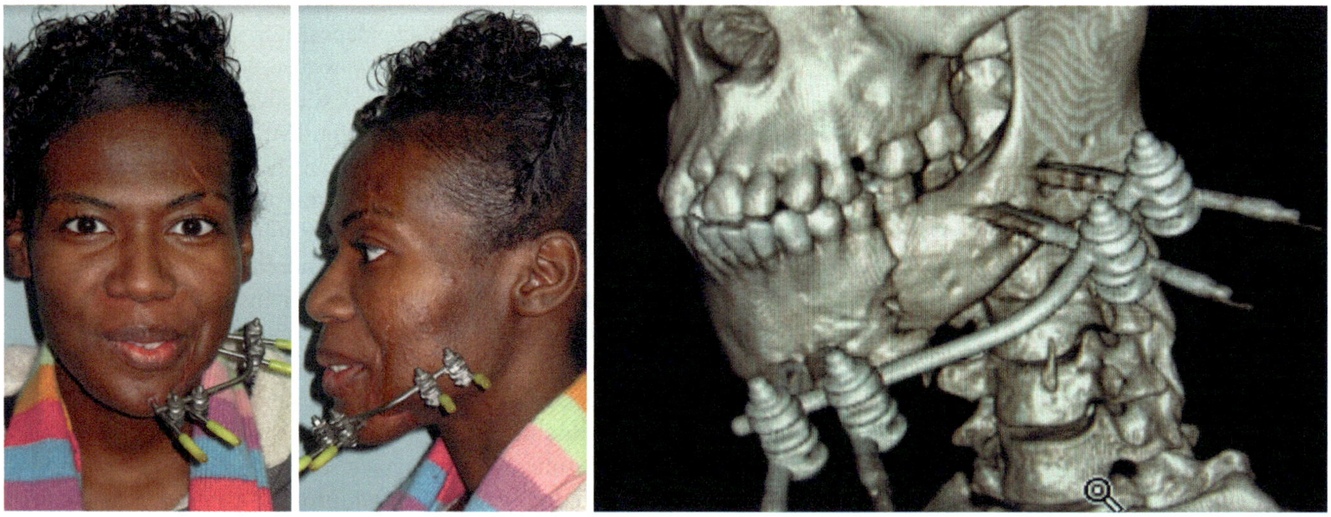

Two views are provided: frontal and lateral. In each, the patient has an external fixation device in place with two pins, both proximal and distal to the fracture site. The occlusion is not visible.

A single CT image is a 3D reconstruction. The two fracture fragments of the body are in close apposition and reduction without a gap.

The patient progressed to healing and stability with satisfactory occlusion without the necessity of an interval bone graft.

Critique

The CT scan and clinical course suggest the patient could have been managed with a reconstruction plate alone.

In-Service Examination

1. The proportions of lateral or medial displacement in condylar neck fractures are:
   (a) Equal distribution
   (b) Much greater medial
   (c) Much greater lateral
   (d) Neither—a much greater proportion posteriorly
2. A dentate patient sustains an intracapsular fracture of the condyle. Appropriate therapy?
   (a) Soft diet only
   (b) Closed reduction and IMF
   (c) IMF plus ORIF
   (d) IMF, ORIF, and prosthetic replacement
3. The clinical picture of a patient with a left condylar fracture with malocclusion is:
   (a) Open posterior bite on the right, chin deviation to the right
   (b) Open posterior bite on the right, chin deviation to the left
   (c) Open posterior bite on the left, chin deviation to the right
   (d) Open posterior bite on the left, chin deviation to the left

Part VI

Trunk, Lower Extremity, and Perineum

51 Trauma: Principles and Coverage

Bibliography

Lee, Z., Daar, D.A., Yu, J.W., Kaoutzanis, et al., "Updates in Traumatic Lower Extremity Free Flap Reconstruction", *Plast Reconstr Surg.*, (2023);152(5):**913e–916e ONLY (Overview).**

Colohan S and Saint-Cyr M, "Chapter 2: Management of lower extremity trauma", Plastic Surgery 3rd Edition, Neligan P.C., (2013); 4:**66 (Treatment)-87 and Table 2.4.**

Olson S.A., Glasgow R.R., "Acute Compartment Syndrome in Lower Extremity Musculoskeletal Trauma", *J Am Acad Orthop Surg*, (2005); 13(7):**436–44.**

Hollock GG, "Evidence-based medicine: Lower extremity acute trauma", *Plast Reconstr Surg.*, (2013); 132(6):**1733–1735 ONLY.**

Lachica, RD. "Evidence-Based Medicine: Management of Acute Lower Extremity Trauma", *Plast Reconstr Surg.*, (2017); 139(1):**287e–299e, including Video 1 and 2.**

Glass GE, Pearse MF, & Nanchahal J., "Improving lower limb salvage following fractures with vascular injury: a systematic review and new management algorithm" *Journal of Plastic, Reconstructive & Aesthetic Surgery,* (2009); 62:**Fig. 1, Discussion, pgs. 574–78 ONLY.**

DeFranzo, A.J., et al. "The Use of Vacuum-Assisted Closure Therapy for the Treatment of Lower-Extremity Wounds with Exposed Bone", *Plast Reconstr Surg.,* (2001); 108:**1184–1191.**

Cierny, G. "Surgical Treatment of Osteomyelitis", *Plast Reconstr Surg.* (2011); 127: **190S–202S.**

Mohan AT, Sur YJ, Zhu L, et al., "The Concepts of Propeller, Perforator, Keystone, and Other Local Flaps and Their Role in the Evolution of Reconstruction", *Plast Reconstr Surg.*, (2016);138(4):**710e, 715e–721e including Video 1, 2, and 8.**

Supplemental

Engel H, Lin CH, Wei FC, "Role of Microsurgery in Lower Extremity Reconstruction", *Plast Reconstr Surg.*, (2011); 127(1S): **228S–235S ONLY.**

Faculty Discussion and Study Guide

Anatomy

Editor's Note: Anatomy of the thigh is discussed in conjunction with harvest of the ALT flap in Chaps. 37 and 38 and later in this module in Chap. 52. The anatomy of the lower leg is also discussed in harvest of the fibula in Chap. 36.

1. Name three muscles of the anterior compartment of the leg. (Tibialis anterior, extensor hallucis longus, extensor digitorum longus.)
   (a) Innervation and action? (Innervation of all three is the deep peroneal nerve. The tibialis anterior dorsiflexes and inverts the foot. The extensor hallucis longus and extensor digitorum longus dorsiflex the large toe and remaining toes, respectively. Function of the common peroneal nerve can easily be assessed by the ability to dorsiflex the large toe against resistance.)
   (b) Lateral compartment? (Peroneus brevis and longus.)
2. The posterior compartment is divided into a superficial and deep portion. What are the principal muscles in the deep compartment? Superficial compartment? (The superficial compartment consists of the medial and lateral head of the gastrocnemius and more superficially the compartment consists of the soleus muscle. The deep compartment contains the flexor hallucis longus intimate to the tibia, the tibialis posterior, posterior to the interosseous membrane, flexor digitorum longus posterior to the tibia.)
   (a) Innervation to the gastrocnemius? Vascular supply? (Innervation is via the tibial nerve, the vascular supply is the medial and lateral sural arteries. The func-

E. Luce, *A Curriculum for Plastic Surgery*, https://doi.org/10.1007/978-3-031-62087-4_51

tion of the gastrocnemius in conjunction with the soleus is the plantar flexion of the foot.)

   (b) What is the blood supply to the soleus? (The lateral hemi soleus is vascularized by the peroneal artery, the medial by the posterior tibial, both branches of the popliteal.)

3. What if the difference in terms of reconstructive capabilities between the lateral and medial heads of the gastrocnemius? (The lateral head is substantially smaller in bulk and the common peroneal nerve is at risk, located between the origin of the muscle and the insertion of the biceps femoris, the lateral hamstring. The nerve courses lateral and just superficial to the neck of the fibula.)
   (a) What portion of the soleus may be of value in reconstruction and why? (The middle third of the medial or hemi soleus remains more muscular than tendinous further distally in the gastrocnemius and can be rotated for coverage of smaller tibial defects.)
4. You are dissecting via the intermuscular septum between the posterior and lateral compartment to access the proximal fibula and you visualize a muscle in the lateral compartment. What is the muscle? (Peroneus longus, the sole occupant of the proximal lateral compartment.)
5. You elect to obtain additional bulk with a free fibula flap but not the soleus but rather the immediately adjacent muscle in the deep posterior compartment. What dysfunction can you expect postoperatively from the harvest of that muscle? (The muscle is the flexor hallucis longus. The patient will be unable to flex the large toe, a potential problem with gait.)
6. The only continuation of the femoral nerve distally is sensory in nature. What and where is the nerve? (The nerve is the saphenous coursing longitudinally and medially nearly to the ankle. The most important nerve found medially and distal is the posterior tibial, providing sensation to the plantar aspect of the foot.)

Limb Salvage vs. Amputation

1. Describe the Gustilo classification. (Type I and II are essentially open fractures with small 1 cm or longer lacerations but without extensive soft tissue damage. Type III are extensive soft tissue damage and/or higher velocity GSW fractures as well as fractures that are older than 8 h before initial management.)
   (a) What are the type III subtypes? (A, B, and C. Type A is high-energy trauma but with adequate periosteum over the fracture, an extremely uncommon type of injury. Type B is extensive soft tissue loss usually with massive contamination. Type C is B plus an arterial injury requiring repair but without respect to the degree of soft tissue injury.)
   (b) Does the Gustilo classification apply to plastic surgery reconstruction? (Not really. The plastic surgery reconstruction is indicated overwhelmingly in those patients with type III A, B, and C. As mentioned, type A is distinctly uncommon.)
2. Are guidelines available for directing treatment for salvage or amputation? If so, describe in general and critique. (Injury scores for the lower extremity have been described that have the *potential* for prediction of amputation and include the variables of age, magnitude of bone and soft tissue loss, coexisting nerve injury, shock, and lag time operation.)
3. Describe the components of the MESS and compare and contrast with other extremity injury severity scales. (MESS: skeletal/soft tissue injury, ischemia, shock. The problem with all the extremity injury severity scores is their inaccuracy. If any one scoring system may be more accurate than the others, it would be the MESI system.)
   (a) Outline the MESI classification. (The MESI classification includes the overall Injury Severity Score, the mechanism of both soft tissue and bone injury with a quantification of the amount of bone loss, the nature of nerve and vascular injury if present, age, shock, and lag time to operation.)
4. Why might the results of the Leap study be quoted to you more often than other studies? (Multi-institutional study, namely eight institutions participated in the study.)
5. From your summary perception of this group of readings, give your rankings from the highest to the lowest as a predictive determinant of amputation outcome: (a) presence of shock, (b) warm ischemia time greater than 6 h, (c) fracture pattern or severity, (d) transection of the sciatic nerve (b, d, c, a.)
6. Compare the relative difficulty of injury severity scores in the lower versus the upper extremity. (More difficulties in the upper extremity—although difficult in both.)
   (a) Why? (Neurovascular repairs have a higher success rate in the upper extremity, bone shortening is possible, stability and weight bearing are the primary outcome measures in the lower extremity versus active prehensile and grasping functions in the upper extremity, higher success with a prosthesis in the lower extremity.)
7. Give an overall global view of the conclusions and summary of this topic. (Psychological and social factors become extremely important in the decision tree of amputation versus reconstruction. Additional factors include the tremendously higher cost of primary limb salvage including a necessity of multiple operative procedures, the societal cost of failure to return to gainful employment, and long-term chronic disability of patients with successful limb salvage.)

8. The reading by Dagum performed a retrospective chart review and then administered prospectively an evaluation of the overall health status and specific dysfunction in a group of severe lower extremity injuries. In essence, what were the results? (Most patients were successfully salvaged, with 9 of 55 patients having primary amputations. The limb was salvaged in approximately 90% of the remaining patients. Testing indicated that the physical outcomes score regardless whether the leg was salvaged or amputated was lower than many serious medical illnesses, suggesting that severe lower extremity trauma impairs health quite severely. The medical score was the same as a healthy population, which indicated the disability is primarily physical and not psychological. Over 90% of the patients preferred to keep the reconstructed or salvaged leg rather than an amputation. The evolution and enhancement of imaging with CTA has replaced conventional angiography in many relative indications.)
9. In summary, what are the indications to consider primary amputation? (The patient in poor health, segmental tibial defects greater than 5–6 cm in combination with other extremity injuries, ischemia time longer than 6 h, and severance of the posterior tibial or sciatic nerves, although an insensate foot or even transection of the posterior tibial nerve is no longer considered an absolute indication. Ischemia time is also relative because the magnitude of the combined soft tissue/bone injury as well as the mechanism of injury, e.g. crush, should be considered.)
10. What are the relative and absolute indications for vascular imaging? (An absolute indication is the absence of markedly diminished pulses, recipient vessels intended to supply a free flap and a relative indication is a high-energy mechanism such as a pedestrian injury.)

Management of Acute Trauma

1. Define "zone of injury"? (Refers to the inflammatory response of traumatized soft tissue of the lower extremity that extends beyond the visible gross wound and results in perivascular changes in the blood vessels.)
2. Does the use of negative wound therapy, VAC, extend the "golden period" for flap coverage to longer than 7 days? (Probably not. Although some substantial controversy persists in this arena, as described in the readings a series of patients managed in that fashion, namely deferral for closure longer than a week with the use of the VAC, had a significant increase in infection and amputation risk.)
3. A IIIC injury presents some injury-specific considerations. Comment on the following: role of angiography, role of vascular shunts, prophylactic fasciotomy. (A critical factor is the duration of ischemia time. Formal angiography delays revascularization and on-table angiography is utilized in instances of possible multi-level injury. Another option is a CT angiogram but only if the patient requires a CT for other injuries. The use of shunts is a valuable adjunct to address ischemia time. Prophylactic fasciotomy has relative indications but should be readily applied in instances of ischemia time longer than 2–3 h. The potential detrimental effect is exposure to fractures.)
   (a) Fixation vs. vascular repair done primarily? (Each has benefits and liabilities. Fixation initially enables a stable platform for the vascular repair but prolongs ischemia time. Vascular repair first followed by fixation minimizes ischemia time but the repair is at risk during skeletal fixation. An option to address the conundrum is the use of shunts during skeletal fixation.)
4. List and describe the important timelines in plastic surgical management of complex lower extremity trauma. (As outlined by the readings plastic surgeon Godina advocated, based on the pathophysiology of high-energy trauma, the necessity for radical debridement and early tissue coverage within the first 72 h. Other authors have advocated either coverage within the first 6 days or deferred until after 6 weeks. Again, as outlined by the readings, acute coverage by day 5–7 is generally accepted as a good prognosis in complex lower extremity trauma. Open fractures with loss of soft tissue coverage left uncovered for longer periods of time have a higher risk of osteomyelitis and nonunion. Although not completely defined, the use of negative pressure wound therapy probably has not altered those timelines since the problem is colonization of the bone. Finally, a limited number of studies have reported a relatively low infection rate with wound coverage extending to day 15 after injury.)
   (a) Define an emergency free flap. (Flap done within 24 h after injury and/or primary debridement.)
   (b) Alternate viewpoint? (Serial debridement and coverage 7–14 days.)
   (c) Recommendation of the readings? (5–7 days.)
5. Define the goals of initial management including "washout" of complex lower extremity wounds. (The basic surgical principles of wound management are not different in lower extremity trauma and include thorough debridement, achievement and maintenance of fracture stability, and repeated procedures in the operating room as necessary. What is particularly important is removal of free fragments of bone without vascular or periosteal attachment.)
6. According to the readings, what two key factors should be considered for the selection of closure with a free flap? (The presence of an exposed vital structure and the risk of infection. A vital structure such as an artery/vein,

major nerve, joint surface, tendons, or extensive areas of bone denuded of periosteum that may set the stage for infection. The readings discussed as the risk of infection escalates, a choice of a free flap for primary closure becomes less appropriate.)

7. What are the requirements for the use of non-vascularized bone grafts for a large extremity defect? (The bed must be clean and well vascularized and the defect ≤5 cm in length.)
8. General guidelines on use of local flaps versus free flaps. (Indications for free flap include soft tissue defect greater than 25 cm^2, lower one third of the leg. With the advent of reverse sural flaps and the use of Integra, these indications have been modified. See other included readings in this module.)
9. Discuss options for local flaps for proximal one-third leg coverage including anatomy, blood supply, pros and cons. (The workhorse flap is the medial head of the gastrocnemius. The blood supply is from the medial branch of the sural artery arising inferior to the origin of the muscle from the medial femoral condyle. The lateral head is used less often because of concerns about injury to the common peroneal nerve as well as the length of the flap. The pros of the gastrocnemius are the use of a local muscle only and if the remaining head is retained the functional deficit is relatively small. The cons are the use of a flap potentially in the zone of injury.)
10. Discuss options for local flaps for coverage of the middle one-third of the leg including anatomy, blood supply, pros and cons. (The soleus supplied by the posterior tibial artery in the medial belly and the peroneal artery for the lateral belly. Muscle rises from the posterior aspect of the fibula and the middle one-third of the tibia. The pros are as listed for the gastrocnemius, namely, the use of a local muscle flap. The cons are that of a flap in the zone of injury and particularly if the injury is located further inferiorly, the muscle may be of inadequate length to cover the fracture.)
11. Discuss the relationship between the use of the Ilizarov technique and free tissue transfer in the injured extremity. (Microsurgery can be combined with the Ilizarov procedure, both acutely to permit coverage of the soft tissue defect and chronically such as the situation of malunion. In essence, free flaps for the injured lower extremity should be coordinated with the orthopedist.
    (a) What are some of the problems with the Ilizarov device? (Pain, daily adjustments, pin tract infections, and neuropathies.)
12. Describe types of situations when the Ilizarov technique is utilized. (The device can be used as an external fixator alone or in combination with a distraction osteogenesis to close with a distraction time table a bone defect. The last use is immediate bone shortening, cortectomy, and subsequent distraction for a bone defect.)
13. What is the appropriate management of the injured leg with a 7 cm bony defect and small soft tissue defect? (Free tissue transfer of vascularized bone with a small skin island if necessary. The defect is too great for either a non-vascularized bone graft or probably the Ilizarov technique.)
14. Briefly describe the appropriateness of open wound management of bone defects and healing by secondary intention. (Of historical interest, only since a chronic wound will result with granulation tissue and even if healed will be inadequate coverage. The same comments could apply to the Papineau technique or open cancellous bone grafting.)
15. The readings present a large number of lower extremity wounds managed with vacuum-assisted closure, VAC, therapy and had some very good outcomes. What are some of the caveats? (A complete debridement is necessary which could be accomplished with one-half of the group. The other half required multiple debridements in the operating room. The VAC needs to be changed every 48 h, according to the authors. 70 of 75 wounds were closed with skin grafts, five patients had a musculocutaneous or fasciocutaneous flap. If hardware is exposed, VAC is an option in selected cases of small areas and if instituted *before* infection supervenes.)

Compartment Syndrome

1. What is the common denomination in all compartment syndromes regardless of etiology? (Elevation of tissue pressures higher than capillary perfusion pressure.)
2. Describe the pathophysiology of a compartment syndrome that occurs in a lower extremity successfully revascularized after 8 h of femoral arterial occlusion. (Revascularization of the ischemic tissues results in transudation of large amounts of fluids and possibly protein because of loss of integrity of the vascular system basement membrane. The transudation of fluid and protein into the interstitial compartment raises interstitial fluid pressures to the point of occlusion of the capillaries. Occlusion of the capillaries leads to further transudation of fluid and protein that exacerbates these problems and increases interstitial pressure to the point of occlusion of the venules. Further increasing local interstitial tissue and elevated venous pressure will eventually occlude arteriole nutritional blood flow.)
3. How would you examine for an acute anterior compartment syndrome of the leg? (Anticipate motor deficits of the extensor hallucis longus, anterior tibialis, decrease in sensation over the first web space.)

   (a) Posterior compartment? (Decrease in plantar flexion, pain on passive extension of the large toe.)
   (b) Other findings? (Direct measurement of tissue pressures may yield interstitial tissue pressures of >30 mmHg as a threshold for many practitioners and 40 mm as an absolute indication for fasciotomy.)
4. What are the time limits for ischemia of muscles and nerves? (The readings discuss 4 h before muscle damage occurs and 8 h for irreversible muscle damage. Actually, using sophisticated muscle histological analysis, functional damage can be demonstrated after 2 h of tourniquet time.)
5. What are the indications for fasciotomy? (If a patient has clinical findings highly suspicious for compartment syndrome, then fasciotomy needs to be performed. If tissue pressures are measured and are equal to or greater than 40 mm, immediate fasciotomy is also indicated. Tissue pressures of 30 mm that persist over repeated measurements are also an indication for fasciotomy.)
   (a) Is arteriography indicated in the acute compartment syndrome? (No)
6. Briefly describe fasciotomy of the lower leg from the perspective of incisions and compartments to be decompressed. (The four compartments are the anterior just lateral to the length of the tibia, the lateral compartment lateral to the fibula, and the superficial and deep posterior compartments. Two longitudinal incisions are employed that include a lateral one a finger breaths anterior to the palpable fibula and an additional incisions 2 cm medial to the medial edge of the tibia. Particular caution in performance of the lateral incision is to ensure the superior limit is 3 cm below the head of the fibula to avoid injury to the peroneal nerve. The medial incision should avoid transection of the greater saphenous vein.

The intermuscular septum between the anterior and lateral compartments is released as is the septum between the superficial and deep posterior compartments. The latter is accomplished by release of the muscle fibers of the soleus and gastrocnemius from the tibia.)

Osteomyelitis

1. What is the blood supply to long bones? (A nutrient artery that supplies the marrow cavity and inner cortex; periosteal vessels that perfuse the outer cortex and metaphyseal and epiphyseal vessels that traverse the cortices and anastomose with the nutrient artery.)
2. Describe Cierny classification of adult chronic osteomyelitis. (See Fig. 51.1.) (I Medullary; II superficial; III localized; IV diffuse. The difference between superficial and localized is periosteal involvement only vs. a full-thickness defect in the cortex, see figure 159-2. The Cierny classification also allows for characterization of the host as either A, B, or C with a B host affected by one or more compromising factors and C as a patient severely compromised.)
3. What is the value of a bone scan in the diagnosis of osteomyelitis? (Can be highly sensitive and can detect infection as early as 2 weeks. Unfortunately, false positives are common.)
   (a) What other imaging modality might be more useful? (MRI with T1 and T2 signals.)
   (b) What is the "gold standard"? (Bone biopsy.)
4. Give the general basic sequence of management of stage III and IV extremity osteomyelitis? (Wide debridement, hardware removal if necessary, management of the osseous dead space with antibiotic beads, possible soft tissue coverage with local or more likely free tissue transfer, external fixation of the long bones with external fixation, soft tissue coverage may be deferred until after an interim period of antibiotic beads and external fixation. Finally, 6 weeks of postoperative antibiotics.)
   (a) The readings describe an debridement approach to osteomyelitis. (Adequate debridement requires excision of the involved soft tissue and bone. The readings suggest an oncologic approach to bone to ensure excision of all involved bone with pin point bleeding as the end point.)
5. What is the role of antibiotic beads? (Antibiotic beads are a mixture of methacrylate and antibiotics, usually gentamicin. The bead pouch is placed when immediate reconstruction is not possible and also serves as a filler for the dead space.)
   (a) Systemic antibiotics? (Usually for a week if the wound is clean, but 6 weeks is the general indication in the treatment of osteomyelitis.)
6. One technique for combined soft tissue-bone defects is a delayed approach incorporating the use of antibiotic beads. Describe. (The technique utilizes a combination of radical debridement and the use of antibiotic spacers. The soft tissue is addressed with a soft tissue flap, free or vascularized combined with placement of an antibiotic polymethylmethacrylate spacer. A final stage occurs 6–8 weeks later with removal of the spacer and placement of cancellous bone grafts.)

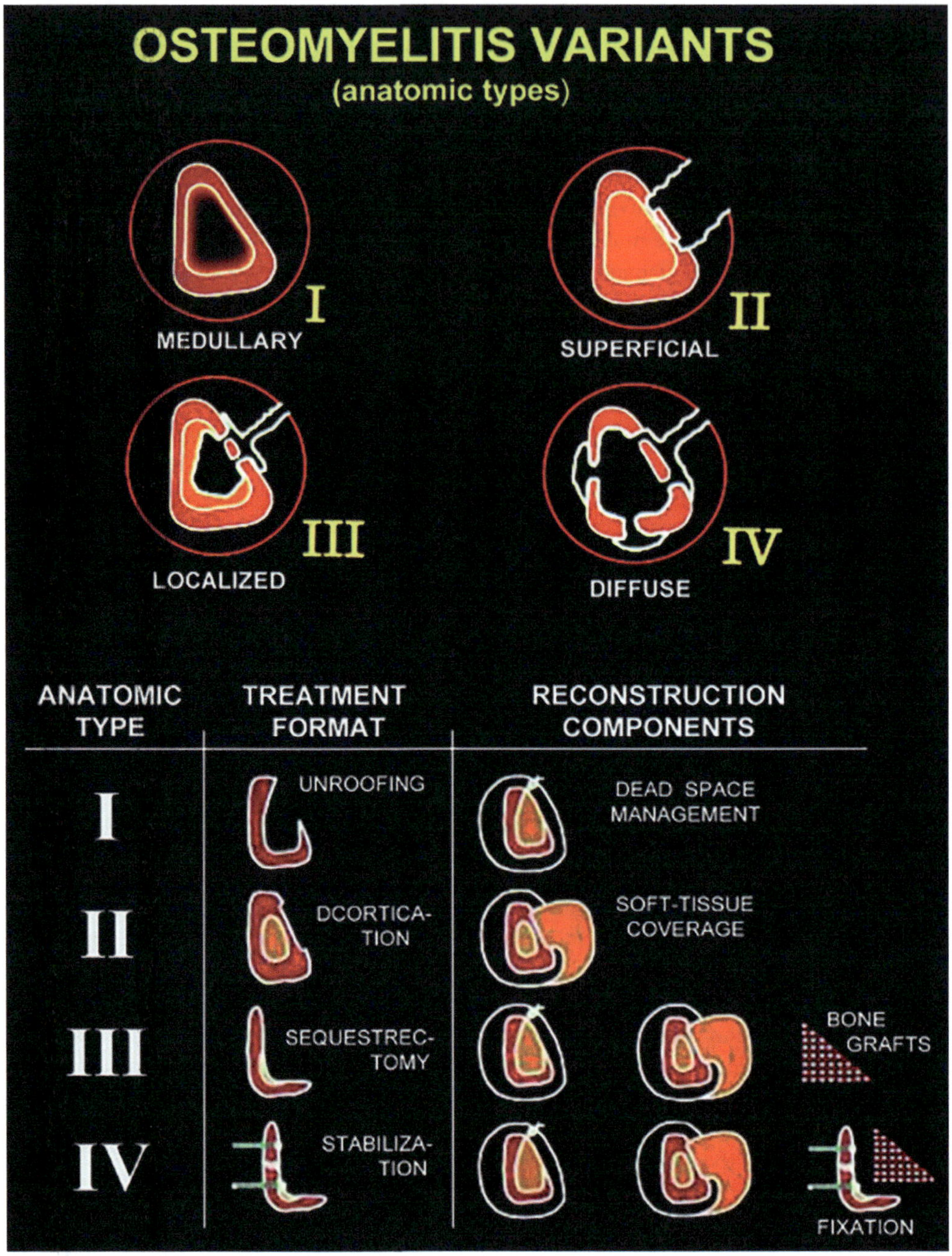

Fig. 51.1 Types of osteomyelitis and treatment. (Cierny G. "Surgical Treatment of Osteomyelitis", *Plast. Reconstr. Surg.* (2011); 127(1S): 190S–204S. (Reprinted with Permission))

(a) Critique. (Multiple stages are necessary, the use of non-vascularized bone, the initial defect could have been addressed with an osteocutaneous free flap.)

7. What are the principal advantages and disadvantages of antibiotic cement beads? (Principal advantages are the ability to deliver high concentrations of antibiotics locally, not possible with systemic therapy. The principal disadvantages are the necessity for a second operation for removal of the beads and the concern that antibiotic resistance may occur due to the prolonged release of antibiotics at subtherapeutic levels. Of course, the cement does not participate in bone healing but is used for dead space management only.)

Case-Based Conference

Case 1: Lower Extremity Trauma

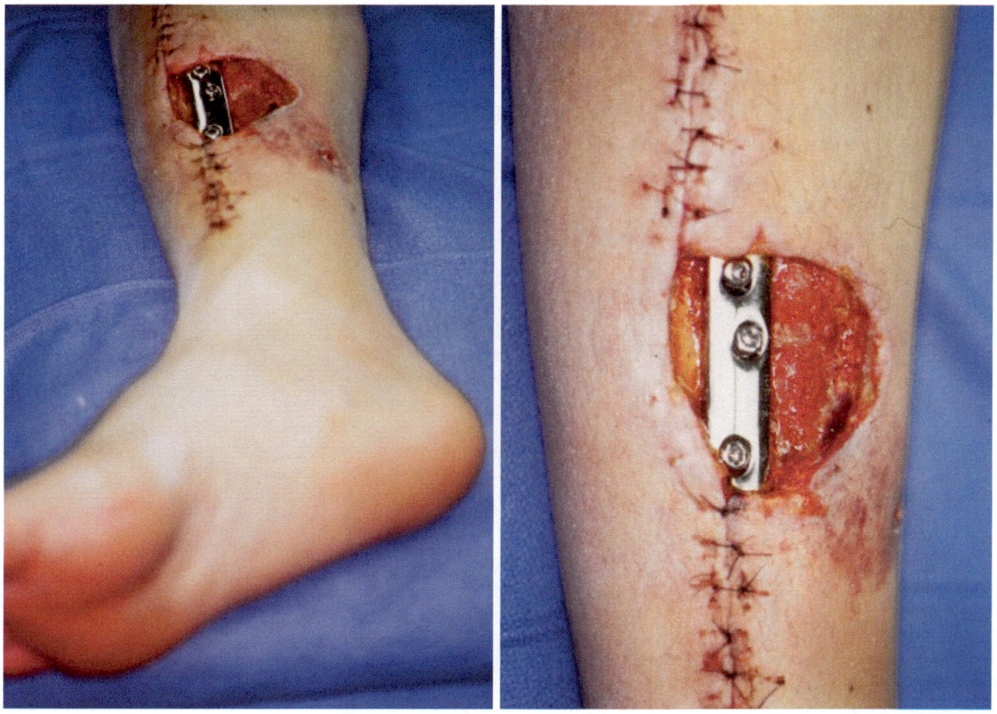

A 28-year-old smoker who sustained a tibial fracture 4 weeks ago managed elsewhere with a plate and primary closure of his traumatic laceration. Returned to the operating room 2 weeks post injury because of dehiscence and "local advancement flaps" closure followed by further skin necrosis and wound breakdown.

1. Describe the slides and add a focused clinical examination. X-rays reveal a transverse fracture with good alignment and reduction.
   (a) Any further tests indicated? Justify.
2. Summarize the clinical situation depicted by this scenario. Was the patient's orthopedic management contemporary?
3. Based on your response to question two, outline a treatment plan. Include management of the bone, soft tissue, and sequence of steps required.

Case-Based Conference: Discussion

Case 1: Lower Extremity Trauma

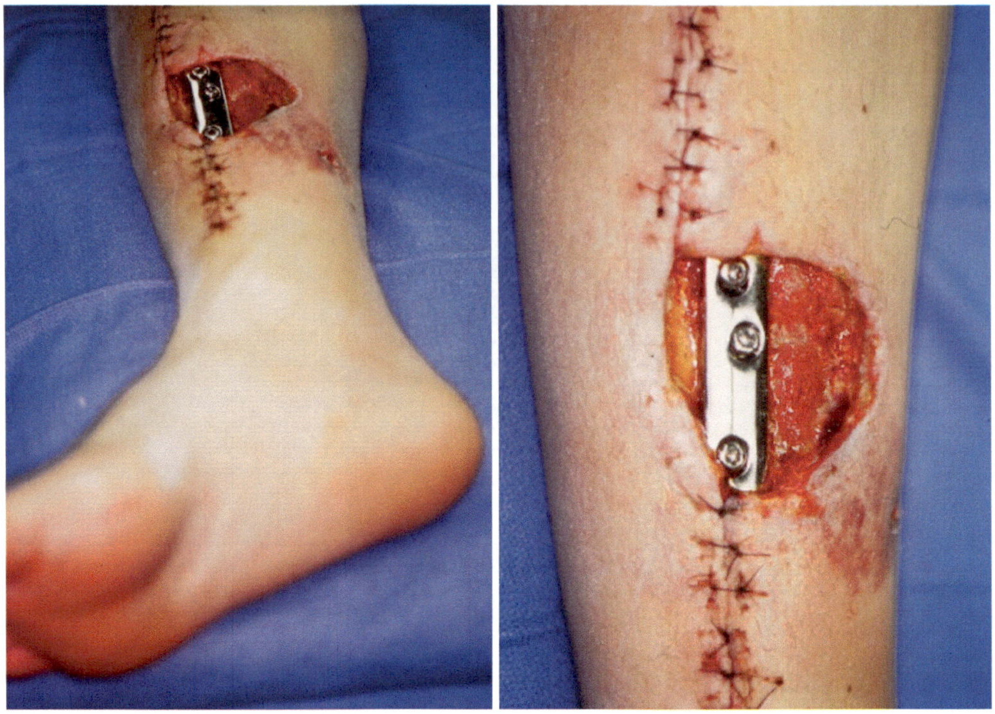

A 28-year-old smoker who sustained a tibial fracture 4 weeks ago managed elsewhere with a plate and primary closure of his traumatic laceration. Returned to the operating room 2 weeks post injury because of dehiscence and "local advancement flaps" closure followed by further skin necrosis and wound breakdown.

1. Describe the slides and add a focused clinical examination. X-rays reveal a transverse fracture with good alignment and reduction. (Two slides are provided of the medial aspect of the patient's leg and foot, probably from mid-calf. The central finding is a sutured vertical laceration or incision that extends from a point about 2–3 cm superior to the medial malleolus to above the limits of the photo. The laceration-incision parallels the medial aspect of the tibia. In the midportion of the distal third of the leg is an open wound of 4 × 3 cm. In the middle of the wound is an exposed fixation plate. No erythema is present either in the incision or outside of the wound. A triangular-shaped area of intact skin with a sharply demarcated, slightly violaceous skin changes abutting the wound at 4 o'clock is present. The area is approximately 1–2 cm in dimensions. The tissue within the open wound is red with no visible bone posterior to the plate. The closeup photo of the wound yields some information. Either bone or fat is present anterior to the plate. Posterior to the plate is tissue, presumably muscle with perhaps early granulation tissue. Of concern is a small area of dark tissue resembling eschar at the edge of the wound, immediately adjacent to the aforementioned violaceous skin. Again, no purulence or erythema is present. No other wounds or deformities are visualized.

   The clinical examination will need to determine several medical history items including the circumstances of the injury to judge the energy forces involved e.g. a struck pedestrian versus a fall from a ladder. The initial management including other injuries, if any, and if a soft tissue wound was present at the time of injury. Questions about the initial and subsequent orthopedic treatment and the postoperative course would follow. Those questions would determine the hiatus between injury and initial wound management and definitive treatment, open reduction internal fixation. The timeline of the wound breakdown or dehiscence and current wound treatment would be helpful. To ascertain if an element of infection was involved, questions about erythema and/or purulence would signal an affirmative. The patient's postoperative course from the perspective of rehabilitation including weight-bearing completes the Present Illness. The Past Medical and Social History are pursued including the magnitude of the patient's tobacco use, other substance abuse, and vocation.

The physical exam includes palpation of the pedal pulses, sensation of the foot, most notably the plantar aspect and examination of possible flap donor sites.)

(a) Any further tests indicated? Justify. (Of course, review of the injury x-ray is highly advisable. Imaging to diagnose osteomyelitis will probably be negative at this juncture. In anticipation of flap coverage, imaging of the vessels of the injured extremity is a requisite. CT angiography has evolved in sophistication and resolution in many centers to replace formal angiography. A few utilize Doppler ultrasound.)

2. Summarize the clinical situation depicted by this scenario. Was the patient's orthopedic management contemporary? (The known information that constitutes the clinical scenario is an exposed but apparently intact plate, exposed for an unknown duration. The wound closure sustained necrosis and may have an additional small area of ischemia—all occurrences in a smoker. What is unknown is the nature of the fracture, and if early osteomyelitis has begun within, particularly the fixation screws. Obviously, what is also unknown is the thoroughness of the initial wound management and the delay, if any, in treatment. Judged by the clinical setting, an alternate and more optimal approach even if a concomitant small wound was present at the initial management, would have been placement of an intramedullary rod.)
3. Based on your response to question two, outline a treatment plan. Include management of the bone, soft tissue, and sequence of steps required. (Of the unknowns listed above, the most critical is the question of osteomyelitis within the screw tracks to a degree that, if the screws are retained, will become established and result in an infection within the bone and failure of the reconstructive plan.

The treatment includes two components: management of the bone and provision of soft tissue coverage. The soft tissue component remains the constant throughout the various bone management options, debridement and coverage with a free flap. Given the appearance of the wound and absence of evidence of active infection or necrosis, wound toilet and coverage could be performed as a single-stage coincident with the orthopedic management. The orthopedic possibilities include retention of the current fixation alone, removal of the plates and screws and placement of an intramedullary rod, and removal of the current internal and replacement with external fixation. Clearly, if no loosening of the screws or plates is determined, the simplest measure is to maintain the fixation. If the decision is established to remove based on findings indicative or heightened suspicion of infection, an intramedullary rod would not be appropriate. The use of an external fixation device would then be required. Any number of other options or treatments have been established of either historical interest only or of completely unsubstantiated efficacy.

Regardless, the considerations of flap coverage is ascendancy of the rungs of the reconstructive ladder. Because of the perspective of the photo, exact proximal–distal location is not discernible but probably the wound exists at the junction of the mid- and distal one-third of the leg. Available, in general, pedicle flap choices include hemisoleus muscle and posterior tibial perforator.

The injury and incision will eliminate the posterior tibial perforator as a pedicle possibility. The medial hemisoleus, proximally based, is most commonly employed in small defects of the middle third and the principal question is if sufficient length will be available to close the wound in question without tension. The vascular supply is segmental with a more dominant pedicle derived from the posterior tibial and a middle or distal branch from the peroneal artery. Access is through a medial incision at the posterior edge of the tibia but the present sutured vertical incision could provide exposure with retraction. Otherwise, a transverse extension superiorly may be necessary. The muscle is bluntly dissected from the overlying gastrocnemius and medially and anteriorly from the flexor digitorum longus. The invagination or septum divides the medial from the lateral head and the contribution to the Achilles tendon is divided as far distally as feasible. Dissection of the tibial origin may be necessary in this instance.

Free flap choices are multiple. Size is not a consideration but, in some circumstances, probably not this case, length of the pedicle may play a more dominant role. Flaps that meet the criteria of small size, primary closure of the donor site, and minimal bulk include the superficial circumflex iliac perforator, supraclavicular artery, and anterior-lateral thigh, the last the work horse in lower extremity coverage. Overshadowing the necessity of tissue transfer as part of the wound management is the patient's tobacco habit.

> **Editor's Note:** The resident, after selection of their preferred option, should be able to describe the major steps in the harvest of their flap of choice.

An intraoperative decision may necessitate conversion of the reconstruction plan to the selection of a free flap. Both the patient preoperatively and the operating room team intraoperatively should be so prepared.

In-Service Examination

1. The deep peroneal nerve provides innervation to the following muscles **EXCEPT**:
   (a) Tibialis anterior
   (b) Peroneus longus
   (c) Extensor hallucis longus
   (d) Extensor digitorum longus
2. A 35-year-old struck pedestrian presents with open tibia-fibula fractures of the proximal one-third with a 6 × 6 cm skin and soft tissue and a 5 cm tibial defect. No other injuries. Appropriate management is as follows:
   (a) External fixation, antibiotic beads, a latissimus dorsi free flap
   (b) External fixation, antibiotic beads, and VAC
   (c) External fixation, antibiotic beads, VAC plus open cancellous bone graft
   (d) VAC only for 10 days with a delayed reconstruction
3. The common peroneal nerve is injured in harvest of a fibular flap. Anticipated motor and sensory deficits:
   (a) Loss of foot plantar flexion and loss of sensation of the lateral leg
   (b) Loss of foot dorsiflexion and sensation to the lateral leg
   (c) Loss of foot plantar flexion and sensation of the medial leg
   (d) Loss of foot dorsiflexion and sensation of the medial leg

Foot Reconstruction, Oncologic Defects Reconstruction, Specific Flaps

52

Bibliography

Colen LB, Uroskie T, "Chapter 160: Foot reconstruction", Plastic Surgery, Mathes, (2013); 6: **Figs. 160–1, 3–6, 8, 9 Only**

Hallock, GG. "Evidence-Based Medicine: Lower Extremity Acute Trauma" *Plast. Reconstr. Surg.*, (2013); 132(6):**1737. (Figure 3 ONLY)**

Deldar R. et al., Chapter 8: "Foot Reconstruction", Neligan PC, Plastic Surgery, Elsevier 5th Edition, (2023), Volume 4: **pgs 228–264.**

Crowe CS, Cho AY, Kneib CJ, et al., "Strategies for Reconstruction of the Plantar Surface of the Foot: A Systematic Review of the Literature", *Plast. Reconstr. Surg.*, (2019); 143(4):**1239, Fig. 6 ONLY**.

Giessler GA and Sauerbier M, "Chapter 4: Lower extremity sarcoma reconstruction", Neligan PC, Plastic Surgery 3rd Edition (2013); 4:**101–112.**

Walton RL, Beahm EK, Maguire KE, et al., "Reconstruction of the lower extremity after ablative resection for cancer", Ariyan S, Surgical Oncology Clinics of North America, (1997); **133–39 ONLY.**

Kovach SJ and Levin LS, "Chapter 7: Skeletal reconstruction", Neligan PC., Elsevier Saunders, Plastic Surgery, Vol. 4, (2013); **pp. 173–181, 183–184.**

Chen CM, Disa JJ, Lee HY, et al., "Reconstruction of extremity long bone defects after sarcoma resection with vascularized fibula flaps: A 10-year review", *Plast. Reconstr. Surg.*, (2007); 119(3):**Intro, Discussion, 915, 920–27 ONLY**

Hallock, GG; Morris, SF. "Skin Grafts and Local Flaps" *Plast. Reconstr. Surg.*, (2011); 127(1):**13e-19e ONLY, including Videos 7, 9, 10, 11, 12.**

Faculty Discussion and Study Guide

Foot Reconstruction—Anatomy

1. The principal blood supply to the dorsum of the foot is the anterior tibial artery and to the plantar aspect is the posterior tibial artery. Provide additional detail. (The anterior tibial artery continues as the dorsalis pedis which provides the arcuate vessel, analogous to the carpal arch in the hand, which in turn provides the dorsal metatarsal arteries 1–5. The first dorsal metatarsal artery also at the first web space branches the deep plantar artery, an anastomosis with the plantar arch and plantar metatarsal arteries. The other notable more proximal branches are the two medial tarsal arteries and the lateral tarsal artery. The posterior tibial artery supplies both the medial and lateral plantar arteries, both branch proximally in the proximal medial hindfoot. The ankle vascular anatomy is discussed below.)
   (a) What is the principal anastomotic relationship between the dorsalis pedis and the posterior tibial arteries? (In the first web space, the deep plantar branch of the dorsalis pedis artery dorsally anastomoses with either a medial extension of the lateral plantar or the medial plantar artery directly also a branch from the posterior tibial. The digital branches of the arcuate artery of the dorsalis pedis also anastomose with the digital branches of the medial plantar artery.)
2. Briefly describe the anastomotic arterial relationship around the lateral ankle. (The dorsalis pedis artery is a continuation of the anterior tibial and is the principal contribution to the medial malleolar arteries as well as the medial tarsal arteries. Laterally, the lateral tarsal artery as well as the lateral malleolar artery branches of the dorsalis pedis anastomose with the perforating branches of the peroneal artery, the principal arterial source for the distally based sural flap.)

E. Luce, *A Curriculum for Plastic Surgery*, https://doi.org/10.1007/978-3-031-62087-4_52

3. You plan an innervated first web space flap for thumb coverage. What nerve must be harvested for anastomosis to a thumb digital nerve? (The distal or sensory portion of the deep peroneal nerve.)
4. In the central plantar aspect of the foot, what is the most superficial muscle group? Where are the long flexor tendons? (The central superficial group just beneath the plantar fascia is the short flexors, flexor digitorum brevis, of the toes. On the medial and lateral aspect of the foot, respectively, lie the abductor of the big toe and the little toe, the abductor hallucis brevis and digiti minimi, respectively. The tendons of the long flexors of the toe lie in the second layer together with the lumbricals beneath the short flexors. Whether one encounters muscle bellies of the short flexors and the abductors or the tendons of the same is determined by whether the compartments are accessed posteriorly, the muscle bellies, or distally, the tendons.)
5. Essentially, the vast majority of the innervation and arterial supply to the compartments of the plantar aspect of the foot stem from: (Posterior tibial artery and nerve via the medial and lateral plantar arteries and nerves.)
6. What are the zones of the foot as they relate to coverage and reconstruction? (Zone 1 are the toes, zone 2 the plantar aspect of the metatarsal heads, zone 3 the dorsum of the foot, zone 4 the instep, zone 5 the plantar aspect of the heel or calcaneus, and zone 6 the lateral and medial aspects of the ankle.)
7. Essentially, the angiosomes of the plantar aspect are perfused by the medial and lateral plantar arteries. What supplies what? (The instep is supplied by the medial plantar, the remaining plantar aspect by the lateral plantar. The toes have multiple contributions by both anterior and posterior tibial vessels, the posterior heel by the posterior tibial and peroneal, the latter via the lateral calcaneal.)
8. The principal innervation of the foot is via the posterior tibia and common peroneal nerves except for what? (The saphenous as a terminal branch of the femoral nerve provides sensation to the medial and dorsal-medial foot and the sural nerve to the lateral aspect of the ankle and foot.)
   (a) Sensation to the dorsum of the toes is from what nerves? (Branches of the deep peroneal.)
   (b) Sensation to the plantar aspect of the foot and toes is provided by what nerves? (The lateral and medial plantar nerves, the terminal branches of the posterior tibia.)
9. What are the essential or minimal prerequisites or requirements for weight-bearing and unsupported, no cane or crutches, ambulation? (Plantar sensibility, stable knee extension, a limb length discrepancy of less than 2–3 cm.)
10. What are the five phases of gait analysis? (Initial heel contact or heel strike, early mid stance when the weight is distributed in the posterior portion of the midfoot, late mid stance when weight is now distributed toward the anterior portion of the mid foot, toe off or weight distribution onto principally the first and fifth metatarsal heads, and finally mid swing phase when the foot is off weighted and the entire lower extremity is swung forward for the next step.)
11. Discuss the comorbidities that can adversely affect management of foot and leg wounds. (The principal comorbidities to consider are diabetes and vasculopathy, often linked. The culprit is diabetic neuropathy that culminates in plantar ulcers. Vasculopathy in the form of microangiopathy also plays a role as can, independently, major vessel occlusion.)

Foot Reconstruction—Clinical

1. Describe the vascular assessment in a patent with a foot ulcer. (Clinical exam of pedal pulses and sensation, Doppler in the absence of palpable pulses, ankle–brachial indices, Doppler ultrasound and pulse volume, perhaps angiography.)
2. Malperforans diabetic plantar ulcers at the first and second web space are due to occlusion of what vessel? (Deep plantar artery branch of the dorsalis pedis.)
   (a) The chief contributor to the plantar arterial arch in most patients is: (Deep plantar branch of the dorsalis pedis artery entering the plantar aspect though the first web space.)
   (b) What are the specific issues with diabetic foot ulcers? (Diabetics are susceptible to development of chronic ulcerations of the plantar aspect of the foot. The pathogenesis is a combination of diabetic neuropathy and small vessel vascular disease including microvascular. The abnormal pressure distribution and diminished sensation culminates in chronic ulcerations that are recalcitrant to therapy. Prophylaxis is important by assiduous foot care. Treatment is wound care with periodic conservative debridement and dressing. Use of platelet-derived and transforming growth factors applied topically have had some success in healing.)
3. What are the flap reconstructive options for the following small anatomic defects?
   (a) Anterior ankle? (A extensor digitorum brevis, EDB, muscle flap, perfused by the lateral tarsal branch of the dorsalis pedis artery or the lateral calcaneal flap.)
   (b) Plantar forefoot, zone 2? (Local flaps, as rotational, V-Y etc. are possible with quite small defects. Larger defects will require a free flap.)

(c) Plantar instep? (Again, small defects can be closed with small rotational or V-Y advancement flaps.)
(d) Plantar hindfoot or heel? (A critical area—three local muscle flaps are available: flexor hallucis brevis, FHB, abductor hallucis brevis, AbHB, and abductor digiti minimi, AbDM. The FDB is the central muscle and the most superficial layer of the plantar foot, perfused principally by the lateral plantar artery, rotated posteriorly for plantar hindfoot defects. AbHB and AbDM are also the medial and lateral components of the superficial layer and can be rotated posteriorly, based on the medial and lateral arteries, respectively. A fasciocutaneous option is the medial plantar artery flap, harvest of the skin and plantar fascia of the instep, pedicled on the medial plantar artery. Even with proximal dissection, though, the pedicle is relatively short. All of these choices are suitable for quite small defects only, a narrow band of the spectrum of soft tissue wounds of the foot.)

4. What is the challenge posed by the use of free flaps to reconstruct plantar defects? (By definition, free flaps are insensate and are to some degree bulky. In addition, the low tolerance to shear forces are a result of loss of the plantar fascia.)
   (a) How is flap choice dictated by these challenges? (Muscle flaps soley are favored with the use of split-thickness skin graft rather than fascio- or musculocutaneous of the muscle. An equally desirable option is the use of thin perforator flaps such as the anterior lateral thigh, especially in a thin patient or the gracilis muscle only. The choice is highly variable with the defect and patient. No flap fulfills all criteria.)

Reconstruction of Bony Oncologic Defects

Editor's Note: The general pathology and oncologic management is discussed in Chap. 34.

1. Give the epidemiology of the most common bone malignancy. (Osteogenic sarcoma occurs most commonly in adolescents, more frequently in males and in the distal femur and proximal tibia.)
2. What are the prognostic factors in soft tissue sarcomas? (Size namely >5 cm, grade, and deep or superficial location.)
3. Give some general guidelines about biopsy of soft tissue sarcomas. (Only masses smaller than 3–5 cm and superficial in location should have an excisional biopsy. The incision should parallel the long axis of the limb. Larger masses should be approached with either a core needle or incisional biopsy.)
4. What are some general guidelines for resection of soft tissue sarcomas? (Elliptical resection of 4–5 cm. Skin–soft tissue margins and 2 cm. deep. A cuff of 2–3 cm. of soft tissue about the tumor is also important.)
   (a) Management of regional lymph nodes? (Mostly none. Exceptions are tumors such as rhabdomyosarcoma or angiosarcomas that have a predilection for lymphatic spread.)
5. Briefly describe the evolution and current conceptual approach to the oncologic management of extremity sarcomas. (Historically, amputation was the primary surgical treatment that evolved to compartmental resection based on the observation that soft tissue sarcomas spread along tissue planes within the confines of the particular extremity compartment. More recently, wide local excision coupled with the aggressive use of chemotherapy and external radiation as well as, in certain circumstances, brachytherapy. The survival rates compare favorably to methods described above.)
6. What is the essential reconstructive challenge presented by limb-sparing oncologic resection of long bone tumors? (Essentially, the reconstruction of an intercalary defect with allograft bone even if covered with adequate soft-tissue is the high rate of bony malunion, infection, and even limb loss with the complication rate approaching 50%. Complications also postpone the resumption of adjuvant chemotherapy or radiotherapy. See below.)
7. Intercalary defects refer to the diaphyseal portion of long bones. What are the options in reconstruction of such defects and the pros and cons? (An older option is the use of tissue bank allograft bone with local flap coverage. The pros of this option are obviously the absence of a donor site. The cons are the necessity to heal by creeping substitution, often complicated as referenced in a prior question by a complication rate of 50%. The other option, as the readings describe, is the use of a vascularized free fibular graft with or without accompanying soft tissue. The pros are much more rapid healing and restoration of function. The cons are the necessity for a donor site. Current practice favors the option of vascularized bone.)
8. Briefly describe the Capanna technique for long bone defects. (The Capanna method employs both an allograft and vascularized fibula, the latter encased in the allograft. The approach provides stability via the allograft and long-term bony union by the vascularized fibula.)

Specific Flaps

ALT

1. What are some of the advantages listed for the ALT flap? (Long pedicle, potentially hidden donor site, two team dissection, potential for supra-thin flap.)
   (a) What is a supra-thin flap anatomically? (Subdermal plane with fascia not harvested.)
2. What nerve courses with the artery? (Motor branch of the femoral nerve to the vastus lateralis.)
   (a) What is the principal artery? (The descending branch of the lateral circumflex femoral artery.)
   (b) What is the ratio of musculocutaneous to septocutaneous perforators? (About 85–87% musculocutaneous, 13–15% septocutaneous.)
   (c) How can the flap be rendered sensate? (Include the anterior branch of the lateral femoral cutaneous nerve.)
3. Describe mapping out the flap. (Draw a line from the anterior superior iliac spine to the lateral border of the patella, draw a 3 cm radius circle at the midpoint and the vessels are in the inferior lateral quadrant of the circle. Put two-thirds of the oval skin island anterior to the line.)
4. The readings advise minimizing the donor site morbidity. (Only a small cuff of vastus lateralis is necessary. Preserve the motor nerve to the vastus lateralis.)
5. Briefly describe the harvest of the flap. (The ALT flap can be performed either as a suprafascial or subfascial flap. A suprafascial flap requires a perforator dissection through the fascia of the dominant skin vessels. A subfascial dissection begins with a medial skin incision along the longitudinal portion of the flap and then dissection through the fascia exposing the rectus femoris muscle which is retracted medially with exposure of the source vessel. Dissection from that point proceeds laterally until the septum of the rectus femoris from the vastus lateralis is visualized. The descending branch of the lateral circumflex femoral artery then is exposed coursing over the vastus lateralis. At this point, the vessels can be seen either perforating the vastus lateralis muscle as musculocutaneous or within the septum as septocutaneous.

The lateral incision is made and dissection taken medially towards the medial plane. The main vascular pedicle courses beneath the rectus femoris muscle from lateral to medial.)

Distal-Based Sural Flap

1. Describe the vascular anatomy of the sural fasciocutaneous flap. (The superficial sural artery, a branch of the superficial femoral or popliteal artery, with two accompanying veins and the lesser saphenous vein is the principal superiorly based blood supply. The flap, raised in a reverse or distal manner, is based on perforators from the peroneal artery that emerge about 5 cm superior to the lateral malleolus. Occasionally, the lateral tarsal artery, a branch of the anterior tibial artery may form a vascular connection with the branches from the peroneal artery.)
   (a) What is the venous drainage of a reverse sural flap? (The venae comitantes as well as incorporating the lesser saphenous vein.)
2. Describe the sural artery. (Actually, the sural artery of interest is the median superficial sural artery although a lateral superficial sural artery is present about 80% of the time. The origin of the sural artery is *usually* from the popliteal. The course of the artery distally is parallel to that of the sural nerve.)
3. Describe the anatomy of the medial cutaneous sural nerve. (The sural nerve or medial sural cutaneous nerve arises from the tibial nerve and actually forms a union with the lateral sural cutaneous nerve, a branch of the peroneal. Regardless, the nerve exits the deep compartment between the heads of the gastrocnemius and courses in a subfascial location until far distally. Distally, the nerve courses between the lateral aspect of the Achilles tendon and the lateral malleolus and then passes posterior to the malleolus into the lateral foot and is a potential donor for autologous nerve grafts.)
4. What is the usual, average, size? (6 × 8 cm)
   (a) What is the key structure to be included to ensure good venous drainage? (Lesser saphenous vein.)
   (b) What is the key structure to be avoided in the superior dissection? (Common peroneal nerve best identified by identification of the cutaneous branch or the lateral sural cutaneous nerve.)
5. Describe the flap elevation (The island is drawn approximately between the heads of the gastrocnemius. The superior or proximal portion of the flap should be incised first and then dissection deep and in the midline beneath the fascia of the gastrocnemius to identify the sural artery and sural cutaneous nerve. Fascia should be included as well as the neurovascular, sural, pedicle. The flap is elevated on a distal pedicle to a point about 5 cm superior to the lateral ankle. The perforators should be located exactly with a Doppler.)
6. Describe a method of delay. (Several variations exist, but the critical point in any flap delay is to ligate the collateral supply which in the case of a reversed sural flap would be the median superficial sural artery superiorly. The proximal, ultimately on rotation the distal 1/3 of the flap, can be incised, the fascia incised, the sural artery, nerve, and vein identified and ligated with a transfer performed 1–2 weeks later.)
7. Discuss the necrosis rate as revealed by the review of the literature and contrast with the readings of a single-

institutional experience. (Review of the literature yielded a partial and complete necrosis rate of something in the neighborhood of 15–18%. The institutional experience with 70 flaps was partial or complete flap necrosis in 36% with 17% with partial and 19% with complete necrosis. When the authors examined patients without any medical problems, the necrosis rate was about 11%.)

Gastrocnemius Flap

1. Outline the vascular supply to the medial gastrocnemius flap including name, location, and origin. (The vascular supply to the medial gastrocnemius flap is the medial sural artery, which arises from the popliteal artery slightly proximal to the knee joint. Other important arteries include the medial and lateral inferior genicular arteries. Both the medial and lateral sural arteries penetrate the deep, proximal, and medial aspect of the muscle for the lateral flap and the lateral aspect of the medial gastrocnemius flap.)
2. Outline the nerve supply to the medial gastrocnemius flap. (The medial sural motor nerve, a branch of the tibial nerve which in turn is the distal continuation of the sciatic nerve.)
3. What is the origin of the medial gastrocnemius; lateral gastrocnemius? (The medial and lateral gastrocnemius arises from the medial and lateral condyle of the distal femur, respectively.)
   (a) Arc of rotation. (The lateral head has somewhat less of an arc of rotation because of the smaller muscle belly and the more proximal musculotendinous junction. The medial head can cover the proximal one-third of the tibia as well as the infrapatellar region and quite possibly the anterior knee particularly if the origin is divided from the medial condyle of the femur. The latter maneuver, division of the origin, is more technically difficult because of the superior take off of the vascular supply from the popliteal artery. One must retract the medial hamstrings medially and access the origin *above* the medial sural artery.)
4. What is one potential hazard seen with the lateral gastrocnemius flap and not the medial? (The proximity of the common peroneal nerve.)
5. Outline the incisions for development of a medial gastrocnemius muscle flap. (Incision is about 2 cm. posterior to the medial border of the tibia. The crural fascia is divided. The first muscle encountered is actually the soleus and some additional posterior dissection for a cm or two will identify the anterior edge of the medial head of the gastrocnemius.)
   (a) How would that incision be modified to divide the origin? (The incision needs to be then tapered superiorly and posteriorly.)

Soleus Flap

1. What is the anatomical location of the soleus flap? (In the calf within the superficial posterior compartment, deep or anterior to the gastrocnemius.)
2. Describe the blood supply. (The soleus is a bipennate or, similar to the gastrocnemius, two heads each with a separate vascular supply. The medial head is perfused by the posterior tibial artery, the lateral head by the peroneal, both branches of the popliteal.)
3. What is the origin of the soleus and what is a comparison to the gastrocnemius? (The origin is almost entirely from the proximal fibula so blood supply and innervation is more distally located than the gastrocnemius. Also, the ratio of muscle/tendon is greater than the gastrocnemius. To continue with the comparison, the dissection is more tedious, the arc of rotation more distal, and if utilized for tibial defects requires a longer arc than a medial gastrocnemius flap.)
4. Describe harvest. (If possible, use of the medial head only will minimize dysfunction. An incision 2 cm. medial to the tibia and distal will enable identification of the medial aspect of the Achilles and proximal dissection to identify the soleus contribution. The soleus is reflected from the overlying gastrocnemius, the median raphe between the two heads of the soleus also identified and dissection proximal until adequate rotation is obtained.)

Integra® (This Material Is also Covered I. G. in Basic Principles—Biomaterials)

1. The composition of Integra® is: (Shark ground substance, bovine collagen, and silicone sheeting.)
   (a) Bilaminar refers to? (The silicone sheeting.)
2. Discuss the use and rationale for meshing Integra® and the use of the VAC. (The empiric evidence is that a mesh of the Integra® hastens vascularization from the underlying bed which seems intuitively correct. The VAC has been employed also to shorten the hiatus between application and removal of the silicone layer and placement of a split-thickness skin graft.)
3. The timing of the second stage, removal of the silicone layer and skin grafting, coincides with what phenomenon within the Integra®? (Revascularization. Considerable differences of opinion exist between the classical 4 weeks and a more contemporary 2 weeks in timing before removal of the silicone sheet and placement of a skin-graft.)
   (a) Signaled by what color change in the Integra®? (Actually, a development of a pale yellow from pink.)

Case-Based Conference

Case 1: Soft-Tissue Loss, Foot

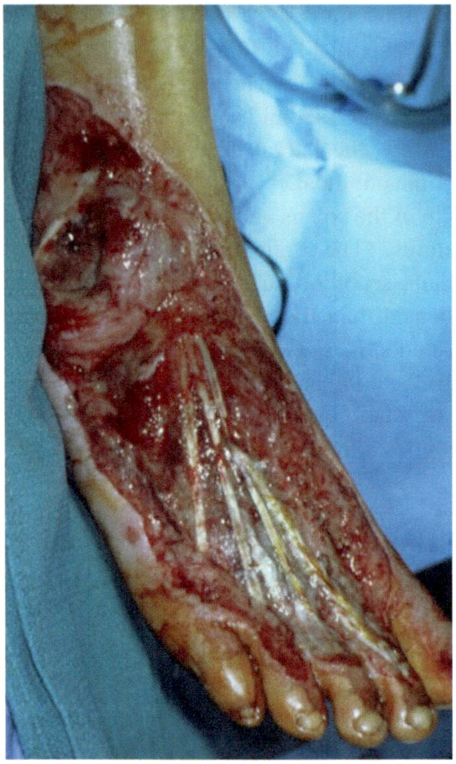

A 42-year-old male in good health sustained avulsion injury of the right foot in an industrial accident 4 days ago. X-rays reveal no fracture.

1. Describe the slides. Add a pertinent history and physical exam.
   (a) Any additional tests indicated? Justify.
2. Describe the injury in anatomical and functional terms. Does the circumstances of injury influence your treatment plan?
3. List options for reconstruction with pros and cons, select yours and describe.

Case-Based Conference: Discussion

Case 1: Soft-Tissue Loss, Foot

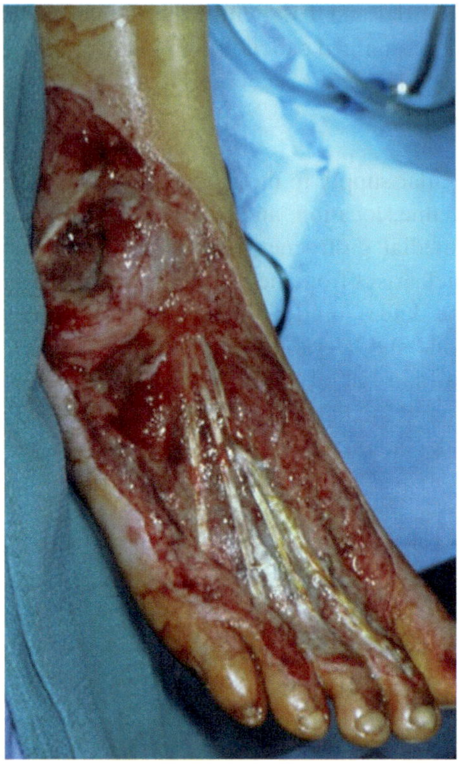

A 42 year-old male in good health sustained an avulsive injury of the right foot in an industrial accident 4 days ago. X-rays reveal no fracture.

1. Describe the slides. Add a pertinent history and physical exam. Any additional tests indicated? Justify. (A single view is available of the foot, ankle, and distal one–fourth of the leg. An extensive soft-tissue injury is evident of the entire dorsum extending distally onto the second and third toes at least to the PIP joint. Proximally, the soft-tissue loss involves the ankle dorsally and laterally, the posterior extent is not evident. The wound continues proximal to involve the antero-lateral aspect of the most distal leg. The plantar aspect of the foot appears intact.

   The dominant finding is exposure of the toe extensor mechanism to toes 2–5. That exposure extends from the base of the toes to the level of the ankle. The extensor mechanism of the large toe is not exposed. The other notable finding is the area of the distal fibula at or just proximal to the ankle joint. An area approximately 2 × 2 cm appears to be exposed, eburnated bone.

The clinical exam would begin with a history of the circumstances of injury if a crushing component particularly if a sharp element was also involved. The second question would ensure that the patient has been cleared of the presence of other injuries by the trauma team, if involved, although highly unlikely since the patient is 4 days post injury. If the current contact represents the initial exposure to the patient, 4 days post injury, what has been the wound care since injury? The exam would focus on the wound, in particular the absence of paratenon overlying the extensor mechanism and the nature of the soft-tissue coverage in the vicinity of the distal fibula, described above and not well visualized in the photo. In addition, the wound should be inspected carefully for the presence of an exposed anterior tibial tendon and functional assessment by active dorsiflexion of the ankle. Palpation for the presence of an intact dorsalis pedis artery as well as the posterior tibial would provide a vascular assessment. Sensation on the plantar aspect of the foot would ensure that the posterior tibial nerve is intact as well. Finally, probing of the lateral or talo-fibular joint in the area of the apparent exposed bone would complete the wound assessment. The other aspects of the physical exam would consist of assessment of the potential donor sites for provision of definitive coverage.)

   (a) Any additional tests indicated? Justify. (With negative x-rays, further characterization of the wound alone by imaging is probably not necessary but may be indicated for reconstructive planning—see below.)

2. Describe the injury in anatomical and functional terms. Does the circumstances of injury influence your treatment plan? (The primary influence is the degree of contusive injury. If the crushed-contusive component is significant, serial inspection and debridement in the Operating Room, perhaps on multiple occasions would play a vital role in wound management. The presence of an intact extensor mechanism would signal the injury is primarily avulsive in nature which in turn would imply the potential for early wound closure. What is crucial in the anatomical analysis of the defect is the structures exposed that necessitate coverage and what local structures are not exposed. Briefly, neither the short nor the long extensor of the large toe is evident in the wound, a key finding given the importance of these structures in ambulation and balance. The other dorsal structure, apparently intact, is the extensor retinaculum, a key structure to prevent bowstringing of the extensor mechanism. The peroneal tendons on the lateral aspect of the foot appear to be covered as well. A finding of concern is the possible exposure of the talo-fibular joint that would deserve investigation as outlined in the physical examination. In summary, the wound closure/reconstructive challenge is posed by the presence of exposed extensor tendons and probably an open talo-fibular joint.)
3. List options for reconstruction with pros and cons, select yours and describe. (Once assurance that the wound is clean, probably shortly since a hiatus of 4 days between injury and the present posed by the scenario, definitive closure should be accomplished. Given the characteristics of the wound, exposed extensor mechanism, and possible open ankle joint, flap coverage is indicated. No regional flap of sufficient size is feasible and indications are appropriate for free flap coverage. In preparation, a CT angiogram may be of value, although if a dorsalis pedis artery is readily palpable, a microvascular anastomosis further proximal to the anterior tibial artery as a recipient vessel is entirely feasible. Lacking a palpable pedal pulse, dorsalis pedis or posterior tibial, then imaging assessment of the vascular anatomy is essential.

   The next step is the assessment and selection of the donor sites. The reconstructive requirements are those of relatively thin coverage either a fasciocutaneous flap or muscle and split-thickness skin grafts. Fasciocutaneous flaps of the dimensions required without the necessity of intraoperative position change would include the radial forearm but the donor site is probably not justifiable. Muscle flaps include an antero-lateral thigh, serratus, and rectus abdominis. Of those three, the anterolateral thigh, ALT, is an option unless the patient is obese. The serratus, lower slips, does not provide sufficient muscle for the wound requirements. The rectus abdominis enables harvest in a supine position, is an acceptable donor site deficit, and is of sufficient volume for coverage of the wound in a young male. The latissimus is the workhorse for coverage of large defects but does require a position change. On balance, the selection of the latissimus plus split-thickness skin graft is certainly an appropriate option. The latissimus provides the volume required and will shrink in bulk with time. Once wound stability has been accomplished postoperatively, active therapy to enhance foot dorsiflexion and avoidance of equinus deformity would be essential to an optimal outcome.)

Postoperative (2 Weeks and 10 Months)

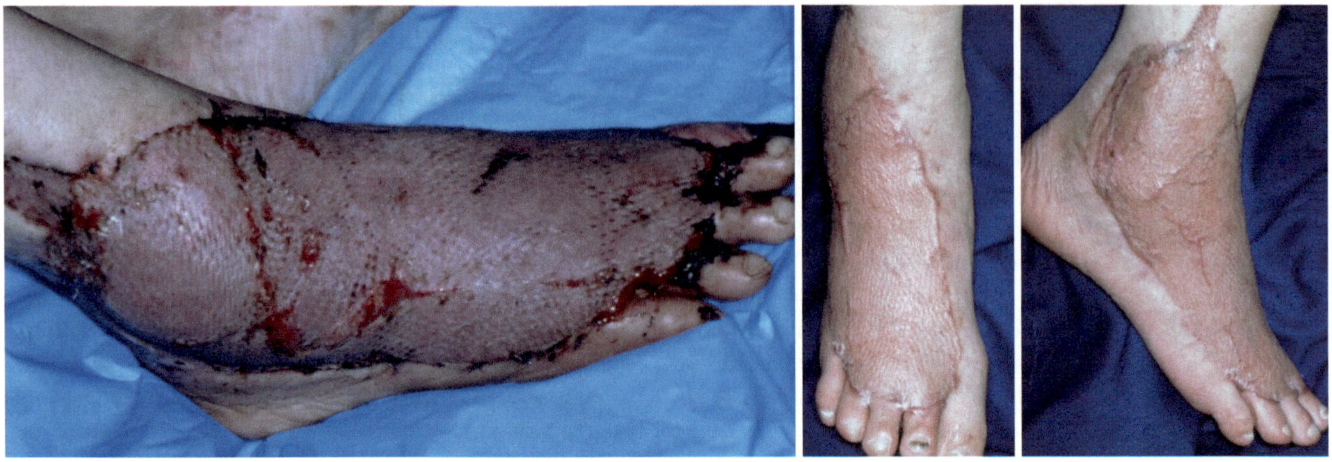

At 2 weeks, the split-thickness skin graft has adhered and taken with the exception of some areas at the periphery of crusting and a small area lateral. The bulk of the muscle is substantial at this early stage.

At 10 months, the muscle has atrophied and a flat and convex contour of the foot has been restored.

Critique

Perhaps an alternate approach would have been application of Integra®, maintenance of 2 weeks with negative wound pressure therapy, and then delayed split-thickness skin grafting. The difficulty with this option is the possible partial loss of Integra® and/or skin graft, desiccation, and loss of the extensor tendons.

In-Service Examination

1. An innervated first web space flap of the foot is planned for thumb coverage. The principal artery and nerve supply is:
   (a) Medial tarsal artery, distal sural nerve
   (b) Medial tarsal artery, distal deep peroneal nerve
   (c) Deep plantar branch dorsalis pedis, distal sural nerve
   (d) Deep plantar branch dorsalis pedis, distal deep peroneal nerve
2. In design of an ALT flap, the perforators can be located in what portion of a 3 cm oval at the midpoint of a line drawn from:
   (a) The anterior superior iliac spine to the medial border of the perforator, perforators in the superior medial quadrant of the circle
   (b) The anterior superior iliac spine to the medial border of the patella, perforators in the inferior lateral quadrant of the circle
   (c) Anterior superior iliac spine to lateral border of the patella, perforators in the inferior lateral quadrant of the oval
   (d) Anterior superior iliac spine to the lateral border of the patella, perforators in the superior medial portion of the circle
3. The optimal flap for coverage of a 3 cm calcaneal wound is perfused by:
   (a) Sural artery
   (b) Medial plantar artery
   (c) Lateral calcaneal artery
   (d) Lateral plantar artery

Complex Groin Wounds, Lymphedema

53

Bibliography

Meland NB, Arnold PG, Pairolero PC, et al, "Muscle-flap coverage for infected peripheral vascular prostheses", *Plast Reconstr Surg.*, (1994); 93(5):**1003 ONLY.**

Alkon JD, Smith A, Losee JE, et al, "Management of complex groin wounds: Preferred use of the rectus femoris muscle flap", *Plast Reconstr Surg.*, (2005); 115(3):**776–783.**

Sumpio BE, Allie DE, Horvath KA, et al., "Role of Negative Pressure Wound Therapy in Treating Peripheral Vascular Graft Infections", *Vascular*, (2008); 16(4): **194–199**

(Overview) Kung TA, Champaneria MC, Maki JH, et al, "Current Concepts in the Surgical Management of Lymphedema", *Plast Reconstr Surg.*, (2017); 139(4): **1003e–1013e and Videos 1, 2.**

(Overview) Schaverien M.V., Coroneos C.J., "Surgical Treatment of Lymphedema", *Plast Reconstr Surg.*, (2019);144(3):**738–39, 741–45 ONLY.**

Chang DW, Masia J, Garza R, et al, "Lymphedema: Surgical and medical therapy", *Plast Reconstr Surg.*, (2016); 138(3S):**209S–213S and Video of ICG**.

Weinstein B, Le NK, Robertson E, et al., "Reverse Lymphatic Mapping and Immediate Microsurgical Lymphatic Reconstruction Reduces Early Risk of Breast Cancer–Related Lymphedema", *Plast Reconstr Surg.*, (2022);149(5):**1066–1068 ONLY.**

Akita S, Nakamura R, Yamamoto N, et al, "Early detection of lymphatic disorder and treatment for lymphedema following breast cancer", *Plast Reconstr Surg.*, (2016); 138(2):**192e, Fig. 2 ONLY.**

Cheng MH, Chen SC, Henry SL, et al, "Vascularized groin lymph node flap transfer for postmastectomy upper limb lymphedema: Flap anatomy, recipient sites, and outcomes", *Plast Reconstr Surg.*, (2013); 131(6):**1288–90, 1295–96, Fig. 13.**

Tourani SS, Taylor GI, Ashton MW, "Vascularized lymph node transfer: A review of the current evidence", *Plast Reconstr Surg.*, (2016); 137(3):**987–991 ONLY.**

Greene A, "Diagnosis and management of obesity-induced lymphedema", *Plast Reconstr Surg.*, (2016); 138(1):**111e–118e.**

Mohan AT, Sur YJ, Zhu L, et al., "The Concepts of Propeller, Perforator, Keystone, and Other Local Flaps and Their Role in the Evolution of Reconstruction", *Plast Reconstr Surg.*, (2016);138(4):**710e, Video 6 ONLY.**

Faculty Discussion and Study Guide

Complex Groin Wounds

1. Describe a classification of infected arterial grafts. (The simplest and established classification of infected arterial grafts is the Szilagi of Grade 1—superficial infection of skin only; Grade 2—an infection that extends into subcutaneous tissue but not to the graft and; Grade 3 infection involving the graft. Further modification divides Grade 3 into Stage I, no additional complications other than the infection; Stage II "minor complications" such as trickle bleeding; Stage III "major complications" of systemic sepsis, recurrent and/or massive bleeding, and thrombosis of the graft. Clearly, overlap exists particularly in Stage II and III and trickle bleeding may be a herald, a harbinger of substantial hemorrhage.)
2. What are the preoperative and postoperative risk factors for the occurrence of infected groin wounds in elective vascular surgery? (The patient risk factors are prior groin surgery, obesity, and diabetes. The intraoperative risks are duration of surgery and use of alloplastic graft material vs. autogenous vein grafts. The postoperative risk factors are the occurrence of hematoma or lymphocele/fistula.)
3. Given the presence of an infected groin wound that extends to a prosthetic graft, what are the treatment options? Provide a continuum of treatment options. (To some degree the selection of an option will hinge on severity. The traditional or historical option was incision and drainage, periodic dressing changes, and wound irrigation. This protocol was attended by a high incidence of

E. Luce, *A Curriculum for Plastic Surgery*, https://doi.org/10.1007/978-3-031-62087-4_53

graft rupture and/or amputation. Superficial wound infections without exposure of the graft could be managed. Plastic surgeons are not usually involved with superficial wound infections. Regardless, the more severe option is excision of the graft and extra-anatomic bypass. Graft preservation can be accomplished with incision, debridement, and utilization of negative wound pressure therapy, NWPT, with periodic VAC changes. The third option is incision, debridement, and rotation of a muscle flap with or without split-thickness skin graft for wound closure. Of course, any number of variations and combinations exist with these options. See next question.)

4. Critique the use of NWPT in infected groin wounds for vascular surgery. (As mentioned above, the institution of NWPT by VAC is an option in this scenario. Aggressive debridement, IV antibiotics, and close observation are prerequisites. Contraindications would be late, >30 days postoperative, graft infections or Grade 3 with bleeding. The late or chronic presentation of infected groin wounds with a draining sinus probably represents a graft infection that would be a poor candidate for management by VAC alone as is infection with pseudomonas. The optimal setting would be an early postoperative wound infection, particularly without graft exposure. The risk, particularly with prolonged therapy, is significant, perhaps even torrential hemorrhage from a ruptured arterial graft. The blended approach is debridement, application of a wound VAC as a bridge to definitive closure with a muscle flap.)
5. What are the arguments for and against the use of muscle flaps in the management of complex groin wounds? (The use of muscle flaps have emerged as the pre-eminent treatment option in management of complex groin wounds from the complications of vascular surgery. The benefits include bulk to address dead space concerns as well as well-vascularized tissue rotated into perhaps an inherently ischemic wound. Ample evidence exists from the classic studies that muscle, if well-vascularized, has intrinsic bactericidal properties. The liabilities relate to the additional operative site and the functional loss, if any, from sacrifice of the donor muscle.)
6. Describe blood supply and the pros and cons of the various muscles that have been proposed for the treatment of complex groin wounds. (The three regional muscles that have been utilized are the sartorius, rectus femoris, and gracilis. The possible fourth is the rectus abdominis, although probably should be considered a last resort option because of the arterial supply, the deep inferior epigastric, is a branch of the external iliac that may be involved by peripheral vascular disease and the rotation point is at a distance from the groin. The sartorius is easily accessible but has two significant disadvantages: One, a segmental blood supply and two, a blood supply derived principally from the superficial femoral artery which is usually occluded by peripheral vascular disease. The sartorius has been principally utilized as a prophylactic muscle flap in high risk groin surgery. The gracilis is perfused by the medial circumflex femoral, a branch of the profunda, almost always patent. The disadvantages are insufficient bulk in some instances and the necessity to undermine medial thigh skin to rotate the flap into the groin which can result in delayed healing and skin necrosis. The rectus femoris is perfused by the lateral circumflex femoral, also a branch of the profunda with a dominant proximal pedicle readily visualized and has bulk as a component of the quadriceps. Harvest and rotation is easily accomplished either with a subcutaneous tunnel or an extension of the donor incision. The disadvantage is loss of 10–15° of terminal extension of the knee. At the level of the suprapatellar tendon and above, two to three sutures of 2° Prolene should be utilized to suture the medial and lateral vastus together.)
7. Describe the technique including landmarks. (A line is dropped from the anterior superior iliac spine to mid patella and the rectus femoris lies along that line with the blood supply entering about 8–10 cm distal to the pubis. The incision is made on that same line, the rectus femoris identified, and the length necessary determines the length of the incision. The muscle is divided just distal to the musculotendinous junction, the minor vascular pedicle from the superficial femoral artery is ligated, the muscle mobilized and brought into the groin defect. The readings suggested tunneling but others prefer a direct incision to avoid tension or compression of the flap. The muscle is then skin grafted. The vastus medialis and lateralis are plicated in the suprapatellar region with large, 2°, Prolene sutures.)
   (a) Vascular supply (The principal blood supply to rectus femoris as a Type II flap, is the transverse branch of the lateral femoral circumflex.)

Lymphedema

1. What is the normal physiology of lymphatic circulation? (Lymph fluid is protein-rich and a primary function is the transport of large molecular proteins including albumin centrally into the venous circulation. Diffusion from the capillary system of said proteins occurs as obligatory transport with fluids from the capillary pressure. Transport from the interstitium into the lymphatic system is crucial to maintain oncotic pressure equilibrium with the diffusion or hydrostatic pressure of the capillaries.)

2. Give a classification system of lymphedema. (Lymphedema is either primary or secondary. Primary lymphedema is idiopathic and further subclassified into congenital termed Milroy's disease with a probable genetic component present at birth or onset before 2 years of age. Praecox onset typically is in adolescence and tarda, onset after age 35. Secondary lymphedema is secondary to oncologic surgery of the groin or axillary lymph node-bearing basins, mastectomy, or pelvic surgery. Secondary lymphedema can also occur as a result of filarial infestation by Wucheri bancrofti of inguinal lymphatics in undeveloped countries.)
   (a) What are the risk factors for the development of lymphedema after axillary regional lymph node dissection? (ten or greater lymph nodes excised, post-operative radiation therapy, possibly adjuvant chemotherapy, obesity.)
3. Outline the pathophysiology in natural history of lymphedema (The sentinel cause of secondary lymphedema is obstruction of the proximal lymphatic collecting system. The etiology in primary lymphedema is the absence of development of the lymphatic system in the hypoplastic forms, although an element of proximal obstruction may exist in primary lymphedema also since the lymphatics in the distal extremity may actually be hyperplastic. The late onset or the tarda forms have never been fully understood since they are idiopathic in etiology as well. Regardless, onset of limb swelling is accompanied by soft, pitting edema. The edema is driven by an increase in colloid pressure within the interstitium secondary to accumulation of protein macromolecules. This event is followed by fat deposition and an inflammatory component. With worsening lymphatic function further swelling results in thick, fibrotic, non-pitting edema.)
   (a) In addition to the above physiologic explanation, what other events may worsen lymphedema? (Primarily, skin infections with secondary cellulitis which probably result in further fibrotic obstruction of remaining lymphatics.)
4. List a categorization of severity of lymphedema. (See Table 53.1.) (Stage I is potentially reversible and characterized by soft, pitting edema that resolves with elevation and compression therapy. Stage II only partially responds and edema is not pitting. Stage III is elephantiasis with thickened, fibrotic skin and soft tissues, irreversible with conservative therapy.)
5. Describe methods and diagnostic workup of the patient with a swollen lower extremity patient. (Accurate diagnosis of the presence and type of lymphedema is of paramount importance since one clinic estimated that 25% of the patients referred with the diagnosis of lymphedema had a different diagnosis such as congestive heart failure or venous thrombosis. A careful history and physical examination will help differentiate causes of extremity edema.

   Further testing is indicated beyond an ultrasound of the deep venous system. In the past, the use of lymphangiography by the injection of oil-based contrast medium is largely of historical interest. The imaging method most readily available with the best sensitivity and specificity is lymphoscintigraphy by the use of Tc-99m injected in the distal extremity. The benefits of lymphoscintigraphy is that an assessment of the rate of lymphatic transport can be accomplished. The disadvantage or liability is relatively poor resolution. Since the resolution is suboptimal and the information derived is the point of obstruction and characteristics of the pre-obstruction lymphatics, but can aid somewhat in planning.

   MRI, combined with a water-based contrast medium and indocyanine green lymphography, imaging performed by a laser-assisted infrared camera, can determine the character of the lymphatics by the absence or presence of fluorescence in lymphatic channels and grade the severity. The principal limitation of ICG lymphography is a penetration of only 1–2 cm. Nevertheless, ICG lymphography has emerged as an important diagnostic and therapeutic tool in the treatment of lymphedema. The advantages of MRI with contrast is the good resolution and the ability to determine the presence and number of functioning lymphatics. The advantage of ICG lymphography is the identification of patent subder-

Table 53.1 Lymphedema stages

ISL stage (20)	Campisi stage (22)	Clinical features
0 or Ia	1A	No edema in the presence of likely lymphatic dysfunction (e.g., after surgery), no difference in volume/consistency between limbs
I	1B	Mid edema—reversible with appropriate positioning of limb
	2	Persistent edema—partially reversible with appropriate positioning of limb
II	3	Persistent edema—continually becomes more severe, recurrent acute lymphangitis
	4	Fibrotic lymphedema with lymphostatic warts, column shapes limb
III	5	Elephantiasis with severe limb deformation, scleroindurative pachydermatis, widespread lymphostatic warts

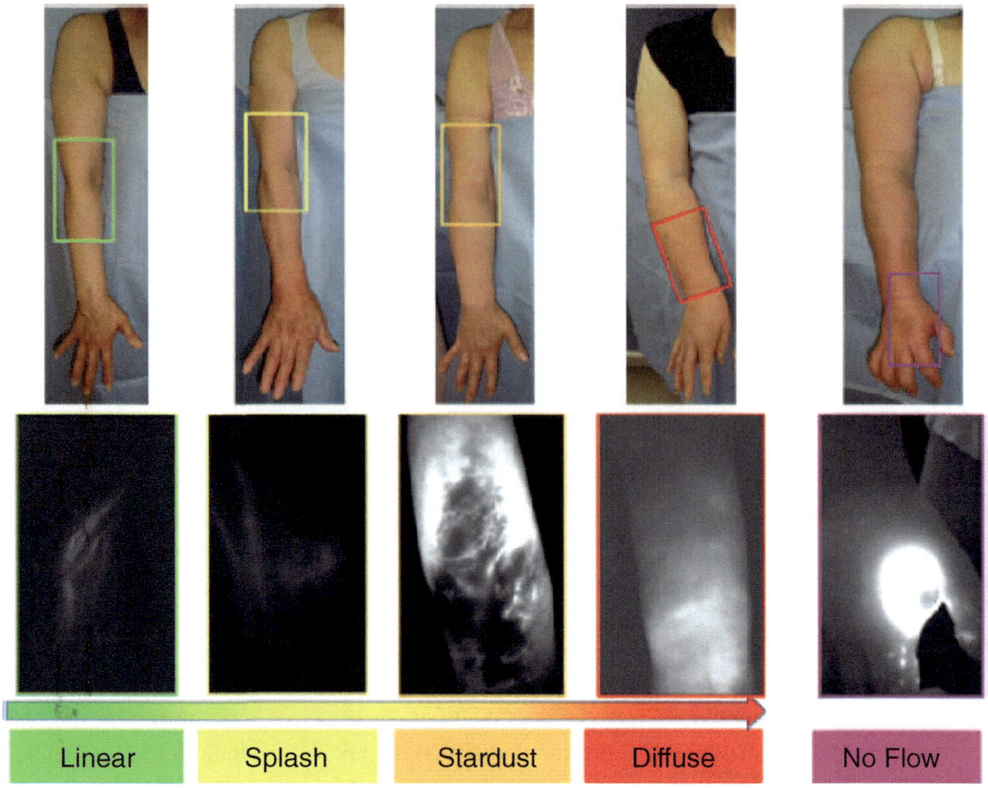

Fig. 53.1 Patterns of lymphedema flow by indocyanine green imaging. (Akita S, Nakamura R, Yamamoto N, et al, "Early detection of lymphatic disorder and treatment for lymphedema following breast cancer", *Plast. Recon. Surg.*, (2016); 138(2):194e. (Reprinted with Permission))

mal lymphatics for lymphaticovenous anastomosis. The disadvantage as stated above is limited penetration. See Fig. 53.1.)

(a) How can ICG lymphangiography stage disease in lymphedema? (A linear pattern would indicate normal flow; splash is early obstruction while a star dust pattern is more severe or progressive disease. Finally, diffuse is the most severe form of the disease and no flow is apparent. All of these patterns are those of dermal backflow indicative, with the exception of linear, of some element of obstruction.)

6. Pediatric patients may be misdiagnosed as primary lymphedema. What are some findings on clinical examination that may indicate another diagnosis? (Skin color or stains, limb overgrowth, bone hypertrophy, sparing of foot and lower leg, in the absence of pitting edema, at least in early childhood are indications of an alternate diagnosis. MRI may detect involvement of muscle or the presence of macro- or micro-cystic changes of lymphangioma. The definitive test is lymphoscintigraphy.)
7. Describe conservative or non-surgical approaches to the management of lymphedema and the selection of patients for said management. (The success of conservative therapy hinges on implementation at an early stage of the disease. Compressive decongestive therapy consists of the use of manual decompressive massage and the use of compression garments and elevation. Conservative therapy requires a substantial investment of time and effort to be successful and if aborted lymphedema will promptly recur and progress.)
   (a) How would one estimate the success with conservative therapy? (Obviously a diminution in the magnitude of the edema. Objective evidence is circumference measurements performed periodically at fixed points on the extremity.)
   (b) Discuss the evidence for the value of avoidance for venipuncture and blood pressure measurements in the lymphedematous upper extremity. (Little.)
8. Give a list of surgical options for the management of lymphedema. (Measures that are probably of historical interest only consist of excision of the skin soft tissue to the level of the muscular fascia and application of skin grafts, known as the Charles procedure. In addition to the deformity inflicted, long-term follow-up indicates the development of progressive verrucous changes in the skin grafts. Probably this method is reserved for advanced disease with severe hyperkeratosis, drainage, and repeated infections, namely stage III. The other methods employed are liposuction, vascularized lymph node transfer, and lymphaticovenous anastomosis.)
   (a) Why would an excisional procedure, as Charles, be employed in a patient with advanced disease? (The soft tissue volume excess, fibrosis, and lipodystrophy will not be responsive to physiologic operations.)

9. Critique the efficacy of liposuction in management of lymphedema. (Utilization of liposuction in lymphedema is somewhat controversial. In early stages of the disease, some reduction of girth can be obtained with longitudinal liposuction. The liability is the potential for destruction of the remaining lymphatics as well as the complications of liposuction as seroma and hematoma. Regardless, the patients are still committed to universal use of compression garments postoperatively.)
10. List two procedures that can be considered "physiologic" and the conceptual basis for utilization in the treatment of lymphedema? (Two "physiologic" procedures are those of vascularized lymph node transfer, VLNT, and lymphaticovenous anastomosis. Two theories exist particularly in the instance of vascularized lymph node transfer. The first is that VLNT functions as a pump by the absorption of lymph fluid into the nodes and subsequent transport to venous circulation via native anastomoses. The second mechanism is possible lymphangiogenesis by the stimulation of the development of lymphatic connections between the VLNT and the recipient site into which VLNT has been placed. A possible role is the presence of vascular endothelial growth factors, VEGF, that reside in the lymph nodes. The excision of scar tissue and placement of healthy, vascularized tissue may also provide benefit.)
11. What are available donor sites for vascularized lymph node transfer, VLNT? (Most commonly the groin, followed by supraclavicular and thoracic donor sites. Omentum has been utilized in the past as well.)
12. An option in post-mastectomy lymphedema is vascularized lymph node transfer, VLNT. What are the indications and options for the same. (VLNT can be offered to patients with Stage two disease, no local recurrence, and total obstruction on technetium 99 or ICG lymphoscintigraphy. As with other techniques more consistent improvement is seen in earlier stages or severity of the disease. The options are recipient site, wrist or elbow.)
    (a) What are the difficulties with the axilla as the recipient site? (The dissection of suitable recipient vessels and scarred, postoperative field, often with prior irradiation. The gravity effect appears most beneficial in the wrist rather than the elbow or axilla. Cosmesis is better in the elbow than the wrist.)
13. Briefly describe the technique, for example the groin, including the vascular pedicle. (The vascular pedicle is the superficial circumflex iliac, the vascular supply of the groin flap as well. An obliquely oriented skin island is raised with inclusion of the superficial only groin nodes and restriction of the harvest to the more laterally based nodes. The superficial circumflex iliac is identified lateral to the sartorius and the composite flap transferred to the recipient site. If placed anatomically, wide excision of scar, for example in the axilla, is necessary as well as the identification of the planned recipient vessels.)
14. What is the concept of the performance of lymphaticovenous anastomosis coincident with lymph node dissection. (With current oncologic approach, the patient selection for regional lymph node dissection with SLN biopsy, those patients that ultimately require regional lymph node dissection, RLND, are at significant risk for the development of postoperative lymphedema, particularly if postoperative radiotherapy is administered. The performance of lymphaticovenous anastomosis at the same setting has the potential to significantly reduce the incidence and occurrence of lymphedema.)
    (a) What are the logistical issues with doing so? (The reconstructive surgeon usually is scrubbed in the operating room with the oncologist who is in the process of performing the lymph node dissection in order to identify lymphatic channels to be utilized in the lymphaticovenous anastomosis.)
15. Briefly describe the performance of lymphaticovenous anastomosis. (Lymphaticovenous anastomosis or bypass is accomplished with supra microsurgery since the vessels are 0.3–0.8 mm in caliber. ICG is utilized by injection into the dermis of the distal extremity and lymphatics identified with a laser-assisted infrared beam. Confirmation of the presence of lymphatics is performed with both isosulfan blue and ICG. Multiple anastomoses are usually performed.)
    (a) What are the ingredients for success? (Earlier stage of disease, identifiable functioning lymphatics, and a small recipient vein with lower intraluminal pressures. Vessels located deeper within subcutaneous tissues cannot yet be identified with the ICG technology.)
16. Briefly discuss the clinical findings in obesity-induced lymphedema. (The lymphedema is always bilateral and since the most important risk factor is obesity patients with a BMI of 50 or higher by implication are obesity induced. The history can be helpful if a patient is either normal or moderately overweight as a young adult and that progressive weight gain was accompanied by eventual lower extremity leg swelling. Physical examination in obesity lymphedema will reveal relatively normal-appearing skin as opposed to the pitting or non-pitting fibrotic soft tissue of the primary or secondary lymphedema patient.)
    (a) Differentiate lipedema from obesity-induced lymphedema. (Mostly girls or young women and perhaps with a familial component. The lipedema is a lipodystrophy that disproportionately affects the lower extremities. The trunk and upper extremities either are not obese or mildly so.)

17. What test or imaging will differentiate obesity-induced lymphedema? (Lymphoscintigraphy is highly sensitive and specific.)
18. Outline the steps in management of the patient with obesity-induced lymphedema. (The key is the treatment of obesity. Since the vast majority of these patients have a BMI of 50 or higher, referral for bariatric weight loss is appropriate since conservative measures of diet and exercise are highly unlikely to be successful. With substantial weight reduction with bariatric surgery, excision of excess skin–soft tissue can be performed on an elective basis.)

Case-Based Conference

Case 1: Radiotherapy Ulcer

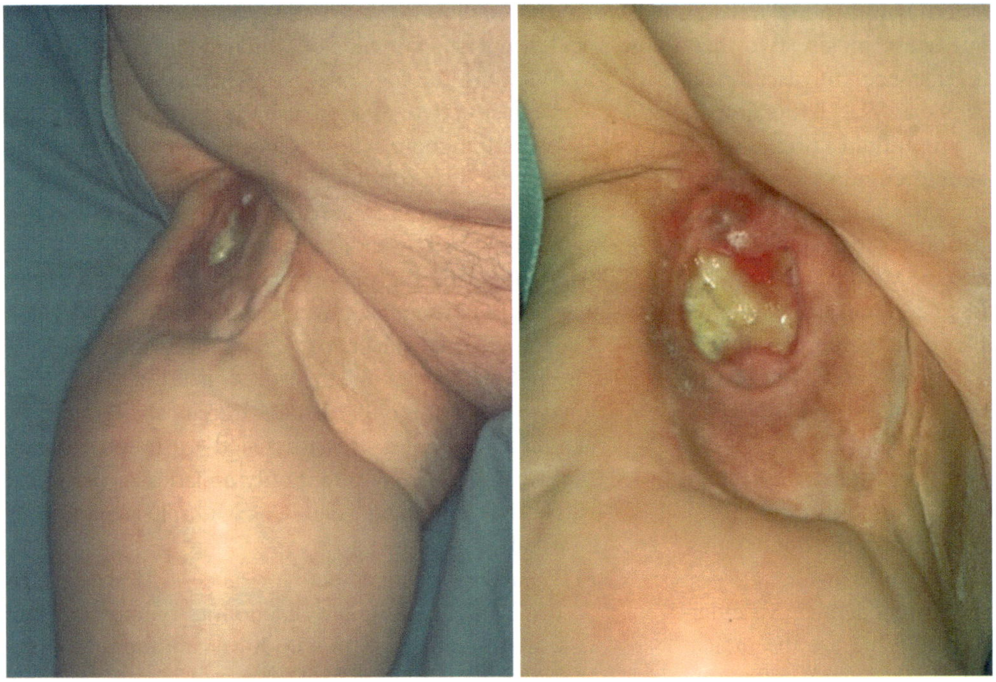

A 72-year-old woman who 3 years ago had a fibrosarcoma resected from the proximal right thigh, skin-grafted, and received postoperative radiotherapy. Has developed an ulcer over the past 6–8 months without healing. The patient is otherwise in excellent health.

1. Describe the slide(s). Abdomen is at the top. Add a focused clinical exam.
   (a) Tests? What and why?
2. Outline the pathophysiology of the problem and the specific anatomic pathology.
3. Within the context of the response to question 2, outline a treatment plan. If an operation is included, describe and draw incisions.

Case-Based Conference: Discussion

Case 1: Radiotherapy Ulcer

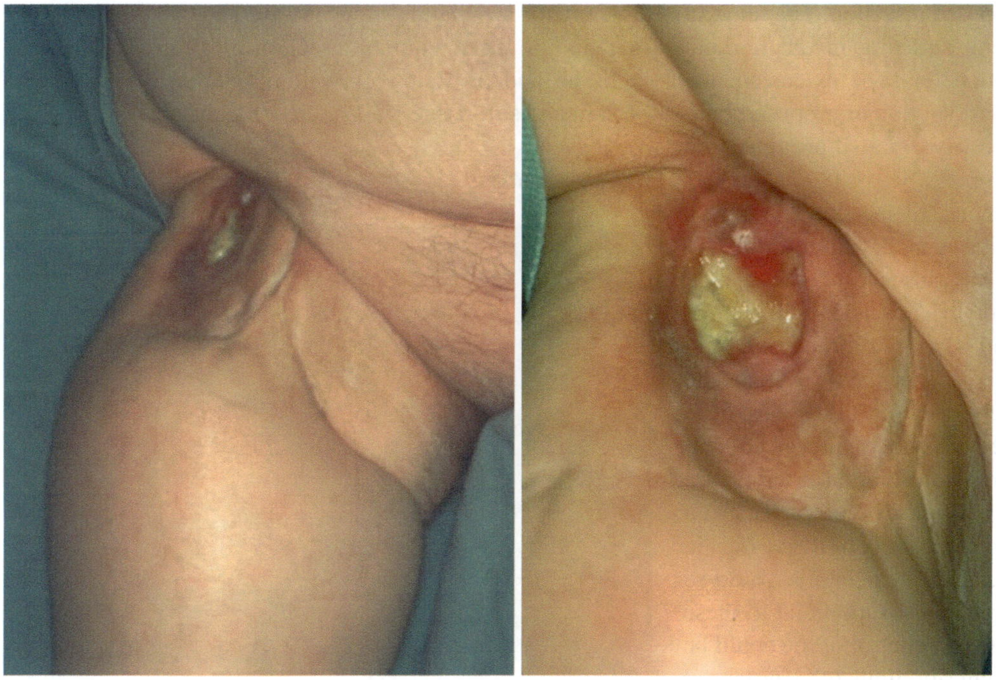

A 72-year-old woman who 3 years ago had a fibrosarcoma resected from the proximal right thigh, skin-grafted, and received postoperative radiotherapy. Has developed an ulcer over the past 6–8 months without healing. The patient is otherwise in excellent health.

1. Describe the slide(s). Abdomen is at the top. Add a focused clinical exam. (Visible in the central-lateral portion of the proximal, anterior, and lateral thigh, approximately at the level of the inguinal ligament is an ulcer 4 × 2 cm with a necrotic base and a zone of violaceous skin changes is perceptible, mostly inferior. The surrounding soft tissue is a healed skin graft consistent with her history. Some element of contraction of the adjacent soft tissue is present. The indentation of the thigh and the contour of the skin graft suggests the prior resection had a component of substantial thickness. The closeup view appears to suggest some rolled or elevated edges of the ulcer but adds little other information. The pertinent history consists of a review of the original pathology including the adequacy of resection and margins. Since postoperative radiotherapy was indicated, the tumor was either relatively high-grade and/or a size of greater than 3 cm and/or close margins. Given the probable proximity of the primary to the contents of the femoral triangle, a review of the operative note may indicate that nerve and vessel preservation resulted in a close deep margin. In addition, if the radiotherapy consult is available that information should be obtained. Other historical information of value would be swelling of the extremity, weakness of knee extension, radiating pain, or constitutional symptoms. An important historical item is the occurrence of any bleeding episodes. The physical exam would center on the character of the ulcer, motor function of the quadriceps muscles innervated by the femoral nerve, and the presence of palpable adenopathy.)
   (a) Tests? What and why? (Imaging, MRI, would determine to some degree the depth and extension of the ulcer. A biopsy would probably be nonproductive but, if performed, should encompass adjacent non-ulcerated tissue. The MRI should be extended to include a scan of the abdomen/pelvis. Use of contrast dye can also ascertain the proximity of the femoral vessels to the lesion.)
2. Outline the pathophysiology of the problem and the specific anatomic pathology. (The differential diagnosis is principally two—recurrent fibrosarcoma and radiation ulcer. If imaging indicates infiltration into the deeper soft tissues, considerations should be given to recurrent disease. Of course, absence of the same does not rule out that possibility. Regardless of diagnosis, tumor recurrence, or radiation ulcer, wide local excision will be

required and definitive full-thickness wound closure reconstruction necessary.

The specific anatomic pathology is the proximity of the contents of the femoral canal, in particular, the femoral artery and vein to the proposed resection. The femoral nerve lies as the most lateral structure in the femoral canal and provides innervation for knee extension, the nerve is at risk as well. A consideration of proposed incisions should include the necessity of initial proximal and distal control of the vessels.)

3. Within the context of the response to question 2, outline a treatment plan. If an operation is included, describe and draw incisions. (Assuming the absence of widespread infiltration on imaging, a wide local excision will be necessary, including ulcer, old skin graft, and adjacent abdominal thigh and soft tissue, necessary even in the presence of benign disease since this tissue has been heavily irradiated. Since inevitably the major groin neurovascular structures, the common femoral artery, vein, and nerve will be involved and must be protected from the resection, proximal and distal control of the vessels in the early stages of the procedure is mandatory. To do so will permit dissection of a plane just superficial to these structures. Proximal exposure and control of the could be accomplished through the inferior limb of a proposed TRAM flap. The resultant defect will require flap coverage since the base of the defect, despite the resection, will also be irradiated tissue not likely to sustain a skin graft. Available regional pedicle flaps are all based on the iliac-femoral system. Those options from the profunda femoral include the tensor fascia lata, perfused by the transverse branch of the lateral circumflex femoral, LCF, the rectus femoris, perfused by the descending branch of the LCF, the ALT or anterolateral thigh flap perfused by the descending branch of the LCF, and the gracilis, perfused by the medial circumflex femoral. A flap option, perfused by a branch of the external iliac, the deep inferior epigastric artery, is a variation of the TRAM flap. Some consideration should be given to the magnitude of the skin–soft tissue requirements and the reliability of the skin island. Although the lateral thigh cannot be adequately visualized, either the blood supply to or the tensor fascia lata flap itself could be involved. The gracilis may not provide sufficient skin–soft tissue and the skin island is not consistently reliable. The rectus femoris as a myocutaneous flap is a possibility dependent on the requirements of the defect. An option that will provide ample skin–soft tissue as well as well-vascularized muscle to fill the resultant dead space is a transverse rectus abdominis muscle, TRAM, flap, utilized in this instance.

In summary, this is a radiation ulcer status postresection of a sarcoma and postoperative radiotherapy. The postoperative hiatus, 3 years, indicates that recurrent disease is a remote possibility and the period of time is too short for a radiation-induced sarcoma. The diagnosis of radiation ulcer requires resection of all heavily radiated tissue and provision of well-vascularized non-radiated skin and soft tissue.)

Intraoperative

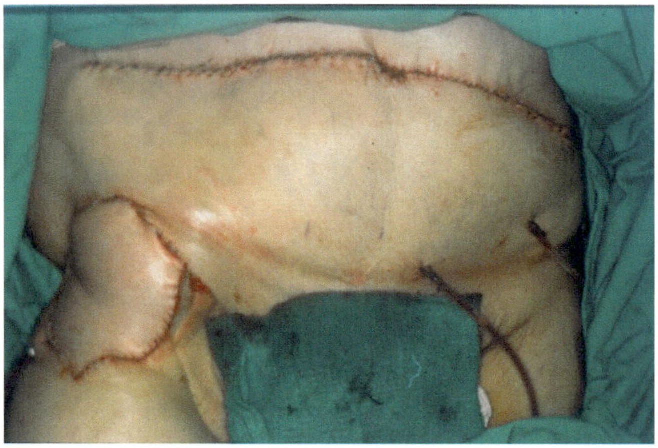

Intraoperatively, a rectus abdominis flap harvested in a transverse fashion has been utilized for wound closure. Clearly, only one-half, the ipsilateral portion, has been performed.

Postoperative (4 Months)

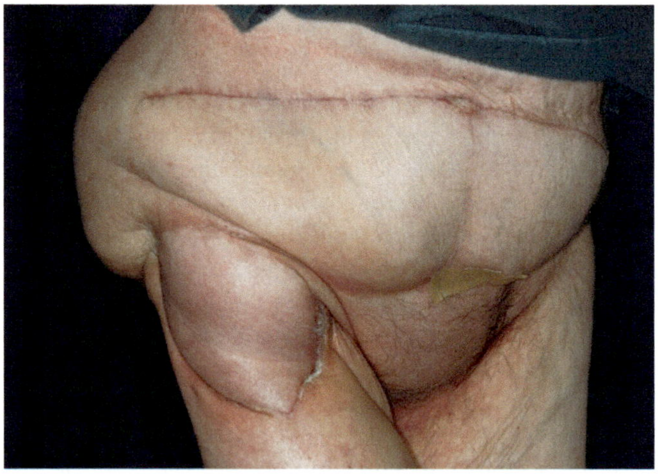

The wound remains healed. A small 1–2 mm rim medially of what might be eschar can be visualized.

Case-Based Conference

Case 2: Exposure of Vascular Reconstruction

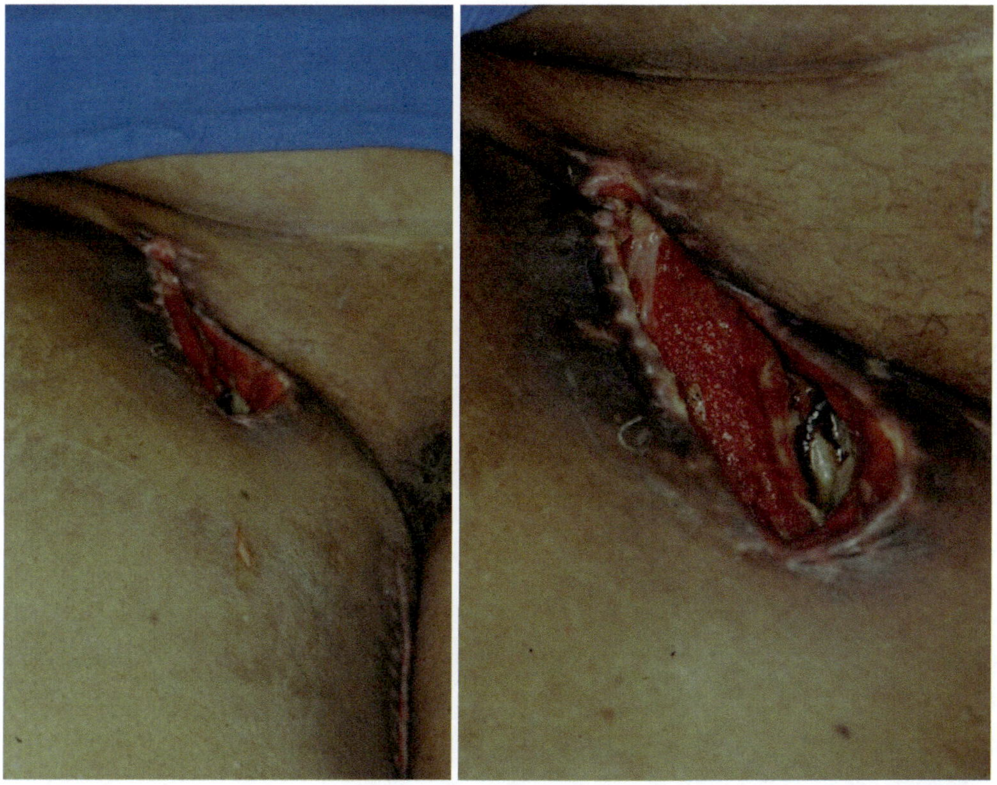

A 52-year-old diabetic who had vascular reconstruction 1 month ago and incision and drainage of the groin wound 10 days ago. Leg is viable.

1. Describe the photo(s) and add a *pertinent* history and P.E.
   (a) Any tests indicated? Additional information?
2. What is the pathology? Include a brief description of predisposing factors, a classification system, and summarize the clinical scenario and challenge.
3. List a menu of options for treatment and select the optimal plan and describe in detail.

Case-Based Conference: Discussion

Case 2: Exposure of Vascular Reconstruction

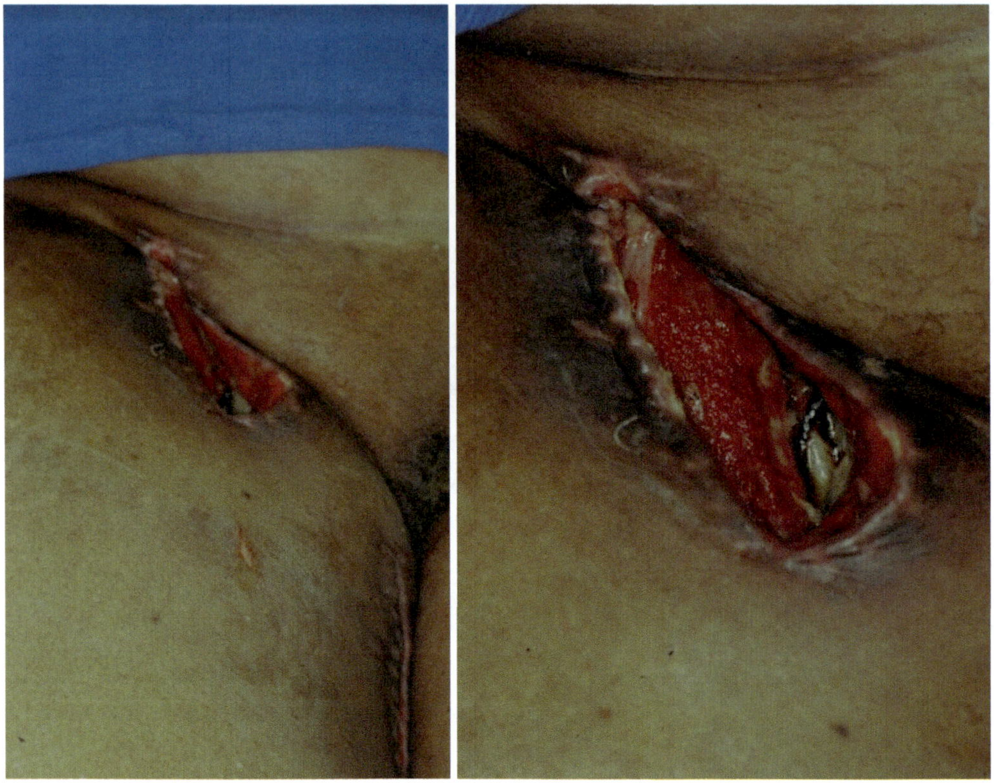

A 52-year-old diabetic who had vascular reconstruction 1 month ago and incision and drainage of the groin wound 10 days ago. Leg is viable.

1. Describe the photo(s) and add a *pertinent* history and P.E. (Two photos are provided. The first includes the right lower quadrant of the abdomen and anterior mid-thigh. Several findings are evident but the most pre-eminent feature is an open wound of a vertical or longitudinal distribution from the level of the inguinal crease extending in a slightly medial direction for 6–7 cm. The wound configuration is teardrop-shaped with an inferior width of approximately 4–5 cm. In the depths of the wound medially is a white tubular structure, consistent in appearance with a prosthetic vascular graft. The graft is exposed for a distance of 2 cm, but the characteristics of the wound are depicted more clearly in the closeup photo. Other findings include in the most medial thigh a healed incision, recent, that extends longitudinally inferior to and beyond the limits of the photo. A suggestion of a mature transverse scar exists in the lower abdominal crease. The closeup photo is dominated mostly by the wound. The lateral half is filled with a muscle, covered by early granulation tissue. The most superior aspect of the muscle contains some thin fibrinous exudate. The medial inferior portion of the wound contains, again, the exposed prosthetic vascular graft but also, not evident in the prior photo, is an additional 2 cm area of the superior graft covered in old clotted blood. No gross purulence or wound erythema is evident.

   The history would begin with questions that confirm the clinical course of events as outlined in the preamble with additional details, followed by some questions about wound management. Important to the treatment plan would be responses to questions about bleeding and, more particularly, the severity ranking from some spots on the dressings to oozing to necessity for intervention with wound packing. The urgency of the prior vascular operation should be determined as well as other past vascular procedures. The past medical history will document the severity of the diabetes, other comorbidities, and current medications. The social history includes tobacco and substance abuse, if any, and vocation. The physical exam would ascertain any limb edema, if any, inspect potential donor sites, and may include a gentle and careful wound inspection although perhaps that element of the examination could be deferred until the setting is within the operating room.)

(a) Any tests indicated? Additional information? (Other than assurance that the patient has been optimized nutritionally, diabetes is stable, and routine lab work, no, assuming any other comorbidities have been thoroughly assessed and managed.

Some critical additional information would be gleaned from review of the preoperative and, if performed, intraoperative angiogram. A conversation with the vascular surgeon would be crucial to provide details about the bypass, prior vascular procedures, nature of the circumstances that dictated return to the operating room postoperatively for incision and drainage, and subsequent wound management.)

2. What is the pathology? Include a brief description of predisposing factors, a classification system, and summarize the clinical scenario and challenge. (The predisposing factors besides diabetes include obesity and prior groin vascular surgery. Intraoperative factors include duration of operation which is probably a surrogate for level of operative difficulty. The postoperative factors are wound hematoma or lymphocele/fistula.

The simplest and established classification of infected arterial grafts is the Szilagi of Grade 1—superficial infection of skin only; Grade 2—an infection that extends into subcutaneous tissue but not to the graft and; Grade 3 infection involving the graft. Further modification divides Grade 3 into Stage I, no additional complications other than the infection; Stage II "minor complications" such as trickle bleeding; Stage III "major complications" of systemic sepsis, recurrent and/or massive bleeding, and thrombosis of the graft. Clearly, overlap exists particularly in Stage II and III. Also, the classification is of infected grafts but could include exposed prostheses because of wound dehiscence.

The clinical scenario and challenges are an open wound that contains an exposed vascular prosthesis. A small amount of clotted blood on the graft is of concern and if attended by episodes of bloody ooze, the specter of herald bleeding, bleeding that is a forerunner of massive hemorrhage. Dressings that are frequently soaked not with blood but fluid may signal the presence of lymph drainage, a lymph fistula. The challenge is to obtain definitive wound closure with vascularized tissue on an urgent basis.)

3. List a menu of options for treatment and select the optimal plan and describe in detail. (A number of options are available for treatment of this scenario. To some degree the selection of an option will hinge on the severity of the infection. Regardless, the most radical option is excision of the graft and extra-anatomic bypass. Graft preservation can be accomplished with incision, debridement, and utilization of negative wound pressure therapy, NWPT, with periodic VAC changes. The third option is incision, debridement, and rotation of a muscle flap with or without split-thickness skin graft for wound closure. Of course, any number of variations and combinations exist with these options.

As mentioned above, the institution of NWPT by VAC is an option in this scenario. Aggressive debridement, IV antibiotics, and close observation are prerequisites. Contraindications would be late, >30 days postoperative, graft infections or Grade 3 with bleeding. The late or chronic presentation of infected groin wounds with a draining sinus probably represents a graft infection that would be a poor candidate for management by VAC alone as is infection with pseudomonas. The optimal setting would be an early postoperative wound infection, particularly without graft exposure. The risk, particularly with prolonged therapy, is significant, perhaps even torrential hemorrhage from a ruptured arterial graft. The blended approach is debridement, application of a wound VAC as a bridge to definitive closure with a muscle flap.

The use of muscle flaps have emerged as the pre-eminent treatment option in management of complex groin wounds from the complications of vascular surgery. The benefits include bulk to address dead space concerns as well as well-vascularized tissue rotated into perhaps an inherently ischemic wound. Ample evidence exists from the classic studies of Mathes that muscle, if well-vascularized, has intrinsic bactericidal properties. The liabilities relate to the additional operative site and the functional loss, if any, from sacrifice of the donor muscle. The three regional muscles that have been utilized are the sartorius, rectus femoris, and gracilis. The possible fourth is the rectus abdominis, although probably should be considered a last resort option because of the arterial supply, the deep inferior epigastric, is a branch of the external iliac that may be involved by peripheral vascular disease and the rotation point is at a distance from the groin. The sartorius is easily accessible but has two significant disadvantages: one, a segmental blood supply and two, a blood supply derived from the superficial femoral artery which is usually occluded by peripheral vascular disease. The sartorius has been principally utilized as a prophylactic muscle flap in high-risk groin surgery. The gracilis is perfused by the medial circumflex femoral, a branch of the profunda, almost always patent. The disadvantages are insufficient bulk in some instances and the necessity to undermine medial thigh skin to rotate the flap into the groin which can result in delayed healing and skin necrosis. The rectus femoris is perfused by the lateral circumflex femoral, also a branch of the profunda with a dominant proximal pedicle readily visualized and has bulk as a component of the quadriceps. Harvest and rotation is easily accomplished either with a subcutaneous tunnel or an extension of the donor incision. The disadvantage is loss of 10–15° of terminal extension of the knee. At the level of the suprapatellar tendon and above, two to three sutures of 2° Prolene should be utilized to suture the medial and lateral vastus together.)

Postoperative (4 Months)

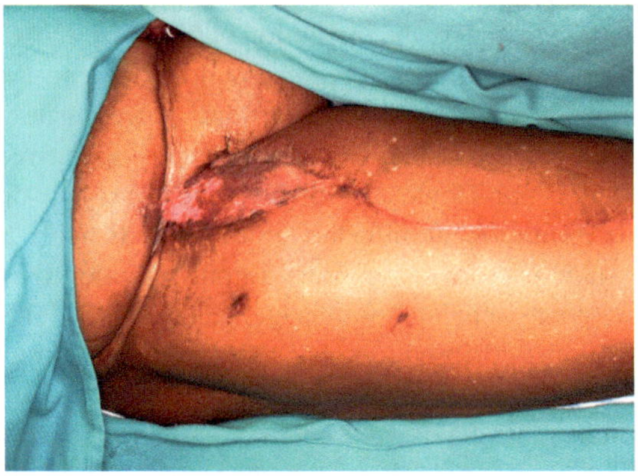

The single photo includes the same area as preoperative: suprapubic, right lower quadrant of the abdomen, groin, and mid thigh. A well-healed skin graft with some edge depigmentation is in place. A well-healed surgical incision courses inferiorly, probably reflective of access for harvest of the rectus femoris muscle flap.

Case-Based Conference

Case 3: Swollen Extremity

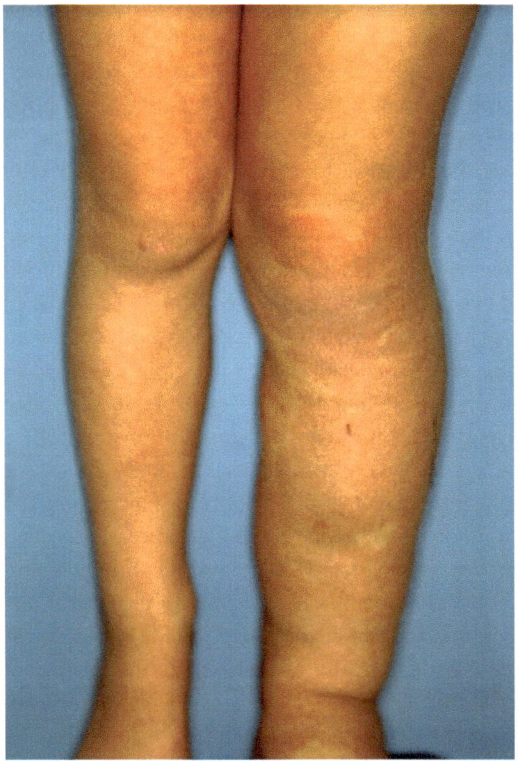

A 35 year old who had a regional lymph node dissection performed 18 months ago for a malignant melanoma. Swelling of the extremity began 6 weeks postoperatively.

1. Describe the slide(s) and add a focused clinical examination.
   (a) Tests indicated? Justify and explain.
2. Describe the pathophysiology of this condition. Give a classification of the severity based on your clinical examination.
3. List a menu of options available for treatment, select your treatment plan and describe.

Case-Based Conference: Discussion

Case 3: Swollen Extremity

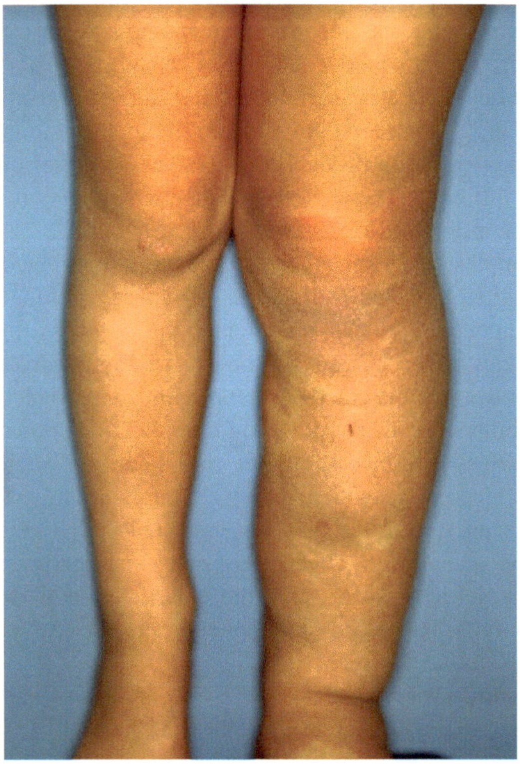

A 35 year old who had a regional lymph node dissection performed 18 months ago for a malignant melanoma. Swelling of the extremity began 6 weeks postoperatively.

1. Describe the slide(s) and add a focused clinical examination. (A single slide is a view of lower extremities with uniform swelling and asymmetry of the left leg that includes the ankle, leg, and thigh. The skin appears normal without color changes or lesions such as an excrescences or warty skin. The right leg appears completely normal. The oncologic history would entail the pathologic status of the nodes from the regional lymph node dissection, whether a superficial alone or superficial and deep iliac nodes were dissected and if postoperative radiotherapy was administered although unlikely. Also, the most recent oncologic assessment should be obtained.

Additional information of value would include treatment, if any, of the lymphedema and some assessment of the patient's burden by medical therapy. Additional history that helps establish the severity would be if the edema resolves in the morning and reoccurs during the day. Physical exam of the lymph node basin and primary site for any evidence of recurrence should be performed. Next, the severity of the lymphedema is assessed by circumference measurements with comparison to the opposite normal extremity, determination of the characteristics of the edema, pitting or non-pitting, and degree of firmness or fibrosis. The classification hinges on the physical exam finding, so for example, the presence of soft, pitting edema would indicate a Stage I or an ISL-1B.)

(a) Tests indicated? Justify and explain. (Although the clinical picture is compatible with secondary lymphedema, the possible diagnosis of deep venous thrombosis can be eliminated with an ultrasound evaluation of the deep venous system, the deep femoral vein. Assuming the diagnosis of secondary lymphedema, the nature of the obstruction and lymph flow can be evaluated with an MRI of the lower extremity lymphatic system and/or the use of indocyanine green laser-assisted imaging. ICG imaging consists of the injection into the venous system of the dye and then subsequent real-time imaging with a laser-assisted handheld probe. Initial circumference measurements at a fixed point above and below the knee is also important documentation.)

2. Describe the pathophysiology of this condition. Give a classification of the severity based on your clinical examination. (The pathophysiology of secondary lymphedema begins with the insult. Although worldwide the most common etiology is filariasis, a parasitic infection of the groin lymphatics, the common cause in developed countries is oncologic, lymphedema induced by a lymph node dissection of either the axillary or inguinal lymph nodes, in this instance for melanoma or more commonly, axillary lymph node dissection in patients with breast cancer. The subsequent fibrosis as the lymph node basins heal postoperatively produce an obstruction of the collecting lymphatics, a complication of which the probability of occurrence rises substantially with the administration of postoperative radiotherapy, the vast majority of axillary dissections for breast cancer. Obstruction increases the intraluminal pressure, upsets the normal homeostatic balance of the Starling's equation, and results in accumulation of excess lymphatic fluid in the interstitial space. What follows is fat deposition and further increase in circumference of the extremity, marked by the clinical findings of soft, pitting edema that partially improves overnight with elevation of the extremity. With time, the soft tissues become fibrotic, probably as a result of chronic edema, a common body reaction to the deposition of protein-rich interstitial fluid. The clinical picture is now firm, non-pitting edema with either pressure or elevation.

Treatment plans hinge on the stage of disease. Early stage may be addressed with decongestive non-surgical therapy that consist of frequent wrapping and elevation of the extremity. This treatment can be administered in a lymphedema clinic and those visits are required on a four to five times weekly. Maintenance of the program is necessary to avoid recurrence of the edema and only partial resolution is obtained.)

3. List a menu of options available for treatment, select your treatment plan and describe. (The excisional techniques or "non-physiologic" consist of the Charles procedure, excision of lymphedematous soft tissues to the deep fascia, and application of split-thickness skin grafts. Excisional procedures, uncommonly employed today, are restricted to end stage, Stage III lymphedema complicated by elephantiasis or extensive skin changes of exophytic, warty excrescences. Long-term, the split-thickness skin grafts undergo similar deterioration and changes. The other "non-physiologic" procedure is liposuction. Liposuction has been utilized in the early stages of lymphedema to reduce the total bulk of the extremity. The principal drawback is the disruption of the remaining lymphatics and the necessity of long-term postoperative compression therapy.

Two "physiologic" procedures are vascularized lymph node transfer and lymphaticovenous anastomosis. Vascularized lymph node transfer is performed by the harvest of a lymph node-bearing basin usually with the aid of lymphoscintigraphy. The donor sites are superficial inguinal, chest wall, and supraclavicular and require the incorporation of a named vessel, the superficial circumflex iliac, thoracodorsal, or supraclavicular, respectively, for a microvascular anastomosis. Careful consideration should be given to the harvest of the inguinal nodes that the nodes harvested are lateral and perhaps superior to the femoral vessels since the principal lymphatic draining lymph nodes for the lower extremity lie medial to the femoral vessels. The physiologic mechanisms consist of one or both of two explanations: one is that the transferred lymph nodes act as a sump for excess fluid and the other is the possibility of lymphangiogenesis stimulated by the presence of VEGF or vascular endothelial growth factor as a result of the transfer. Lymphaticovenous anastomosis is a super microsurgery technique since the lymphatic vessels and vein are quite small (0.3–0.8 mm). A distally injected dye, usually ICG, is utilized with infrared fluorescence to identify functioning lymphatic channels. A small vein with no backflow is utilized for the recipient vessels. Usually multiple anastomoses are performed and the short-term success in the hands of investigators has been quite good with significant reduction of limb circumference. Some concerns exist about the long-term patency of these anastomoses. Overall, additional investigations are necessary to firmly establish the efficacy of these procedures, either solely or in combination. The evidence to date is substantially encouraging.)

In-Service Examination

1. The principal disadvantages of the use of the sartorius muscle flap for coverage of an exposed arterial bypass graft in the groin include the following **EXCEPT:**
   (a) The sartorius is a Type II flap
   (b) The proximal sartorius is often involved in the inflammatory process
   (c) The blood supply is segmental rather than a major proximal pedicle
   (d) The blood supply is from the superficial femoral artery
2. Milroy's disease is:
   (a) Lymphedema and multiple enchondromatosis
   (b) Acquired lymphedema
   (c) Congenital lymphedema with onset in infancy
   (d) Lymphedema with onset in adolescence
3. A patient presents with lymphedema that has only partially responded to compression and elevation therapy. On exam the edema is non-pitting. The stage is:
   (a) I
   (b) II
   (c) III
   (d) IV

54 Vaginal, Perineum

Bibliography

Yavagal S, De Farias TF, Medlina CA, Takacs P, "Normal vulvovaginal, perineal, and pelvic anatomy with reconstructive considerations", *Seminars in Plastic Surgery*, (2011); 25(2):**121–124 ONLY**

Laufer MR, "Congenital absence of the vagina: In search of the perfect solution. When, and by what technique, should a vagina be created?", *Adult and Pediatric Gynecology*, (2002); 14:**441–444.**

"Committee Opinion: Nonsurgical diagnosis and management of vaginal agenesis", *Obstetrics and Gynecology*, (2002); 100:**213–216.**

Bialowas C, Nguyen B, Patel A, "Best Solutions for Perineal and Pressure Sore Reconstruction", *Plast Reconstr Surg.*, (2021);148:**1026e–30e, Videos 1 & 2 ONLY (Junior Residents Only)**

Jazayeri L., Pusic A.L., Cordeiro P.G., Chapter 15: "Reconstruction of Acquired Vaginal Defects", Neligan PC, Plastic Surgery, Elsevier 5th Edition, (2023), Volume 4: **pg. 452.**

Nelson RA and Butler CE, "Surgical outcomes of VRAM versus thigh flaps for immediate reconstruction of pelvic and perineal cancer resection defects", *Plast. Reconstr. Surg.*, (2009); 123(1):**175–183. (INTRODUCTION AND DISCUSSION ONLY)**

Wong S, Garvey P, Skibber J, Yu P, "Reconstruction of pelvic exenteration defects with anterolateral thigh—Vastus lateralis muscle flaps", *Plast. Reconstr. Surg.*, (2009); 124(4):**1177–1185.**

Kim JT, Ho SY, Hwang JH, et al., "Perineal perforator—based island flaps: The next frontier in perineal reconstruction", *Plast. Reconstr. Surg.*, (2014); 133(5):**683e–687e and Supplemental Digital Content 1–3.**

Hashimoto I, Abe Y, Nakanishi H, "The internal pudendal artery perforator flap: Free style pedicle perforator flaps for vulva, vagina, and buttock reconstruction", *Plast. Reconstr. Surg.*, (2014); 133(4):**924–933.**

Lannon DA, et al, "Versatility of the proximally pedicled anterolateral thigh flap and its use in complex abdominal and pelvic reconstruction", *Plast. Reconstr. Surg.*, (2011); 127(2):**677–688. Fig. 10 and Discussion ONLY**

Mericli AF, Martin JP, Campbell CA. "An Algorithmic Anatomical Subunit Approach to Pelvic Wound Reconstruction", *Plast. Reconstr. Surg.*, (2016); 137(3):**1004–1017. Figs. 1 and 2 ONLY.**

Faculty Discussion and Study Guide

Congenital Deformities of the Vagina, Vaginal Agenesis

1. A 16-year-old girl is brought to your office because the parents understand that you are a plastic surgeon who can handle almost anything, and they state that their daughter "doesn't have a vagina, and has not had any periods." On exam, the girl is of normal height and weight, has well-developed secondary sex characteristics (breasts, pubic and axillary hair) and no vagina with a normal urethra. What is the preliminary diagnosis and what is the treatment? (MRH Syndrome or Mayer–Rokitansky–Hauser syndrome. Basic workup would consist of an ultrasound or CT scan of the abdomen and pelvis and treatment is either non-surgical or surgical creation of a vagina. IVP may be indicated to workup urinary tract abnormalities. Another possible diagnosis is gonadal dysgenesis but not likely with the scenario given above.)
   - (a) The physical examination would reveal labia, yes or no? (Yes. The picture is one of Mullerian agenesis and the labia majora and minora are formed embryologically from the labiogenital folds which are not affected.)
   - (b) What rules out the diagnosis of gonadal dysgenesis? (The presence of pubic and axillary hair. Breast development can still occur with gonadal dysgenesis because of the peripheral conversion of circulating

E. Luce, *A Curriculum for Plastic Surgery*, https://doi.org/10.1007/978-3-031-62087-4_54

androgens to estrogen. Abdominal ultrasound can determine the presence of normal ovaries and a definitive diagnosis can be established by an elevated serum testosterone.)

2. Assume the patient has MRH Syndrome. What would be the results of the following: karyotyping, 17 testosterone levels, ultrasound of the pelvis (46XX, normal testosterone, and estradiol blood levels, absence of a uterus and fallopian tubes and the presence of normal ovaries on ultrasound. Patients with vaginal agenesis have normal cyclic ovarian function but of course are amenorrheic since the uterus is absent or rudimentary.)
3. What are the surgical methods of vaginal reconstruction in vaginal agenesis? (Use of loop of bowel, flaps, skin grafts.)
   (a) Critique each. (Neovagina created from bowel tends to be much less susceptible to problems of stenosis and stricture but is subject to heavy discharge and foul odor; skin flaps require donor site defects and the resultant scars externally and have a certain incidence of failure; skin grafts do not produce external scars other than the donor site but are more subject to stenosis and obliteration. The use of a fasciocutaneous flap, the pudendal or Singapore flap, is an effort to import sensation by incorporation of the perineal nerve.)
4. Describe the method and postoperative care for the McIndoe procedure (McIndoe technique is dissection of a space in the perineum between the bladder and the rectum and lining the space with a thick split-thickness skin graft. The skin graft is stented in the early postoperative period. Long-term care requires periodic dilation and is subject to stricture.)
5. The readings suggest reconstruction with a full-thickness skin graft. Critique. (Clearly, considerably less contracture will occur with a full-thickness skin graft than a split-thickness skin graft. Graft taken can be less with full thickness than split thickness. Equally as important, large grafts are necessary to accomplish a vagina of sufficient caliber and length. For example, a vagina of 12 cm. in length and 5 cm. in caliber would require 5 cm × 3.14 divided by 2, or two sheets of full-thickness skin, each measuring approximately 12 × 8 cm. in size, a very substantial sized donor site defect.)
6. Discuss the timing of vaginal reconstruction in vaginal agenesis as in the scenario above. (Surgical reconstruction of the vagina is probably best deferred into the early or mid teens because of the necessity for postoperative dilation which requires patient compliance. Parents may be uncomfortable with dilation of a preadolescent and a patient would not be able to perform self-dilatation. Deferral should be accomplished until late adolescence which permits the patient to arrive at the decision for surgery. The reconstruction is purely elective and can be deferred to the onset of intercourse.)
7. What is a non-surgical approach to reconstruction of the vagina in vaginal agenesis and how is such accomplished? (The use of pressure dilators made of glass or more recently laparoscopically placed internal–external devices.)
   (a) Critique. (The method is non-surgical and can be done in early adolescence. Considerable amount of time is necessary, possibly years, and perseverance and diligence is equally necessary. Nevertheless, if the commitment is present on the part of parents and the patient, the method does not burn any bridges.)

Acquired Vaginal Defects

1. Briefly describe the impetus for primary reconstruction of pelvic/perineal defects. (The reconstruction of a defect created by an oncologic resection may be dictated by the necessity of wound closure as in post-vulvectomy or a post-abdominoperineal resection, particularly in an irradiated field. Attempted primary closure of such defects is complicated by dehiscence and wound infection. The reconstruction may be directed toward function as well in the address of vaginectomy defects. The third objective in instances of anterior, posterior, and total exenteration is to fill the dead space created by the resection within the rigid peripelvic walls to prevent prolapse of small bowel into the inferior pelvis.)
2. Describe the pertinent vascular anatomy for perineal reconstruction with local flaps. (The pertinent branch of the common femoral is the external or superficial pudendal artery that provides vascular supply to the scrotum and labia majora. The third branch of the internal iliac, after superior and inferior gluteal, the internal pudendal in conjunction with the external pudendal provides blood supply to the same structures via the posterior labial and transverse perineal arteries. The former also has branches of the perineal nerve.)
3. Give a classification system for acquired vaginal defects. (See Figs. 54.1 and 54.2.) (IA. Anterior and/or lateral wall, usually urologic cancer surgery. IB. Posterior wall, usually colorectal cancer resections. IIA. Circumferential upper 2/3 vagina. IIB. Circumferential total vagina usually from radical hysterectomy total pelvic exenteration.) (Table 54.1) (Fig. 54.1)
4. Discuss the use of the VRAM for vaginal reconstruction including vascular supply, location of the pedicle, and design. (The VRAM flap is vascularized by the deep inferior epigastric, a medial branch of the external iliac artery, located on the lateral pelvic wall that enters the rectus laterally 6–8 cm above the pubis. The design is a

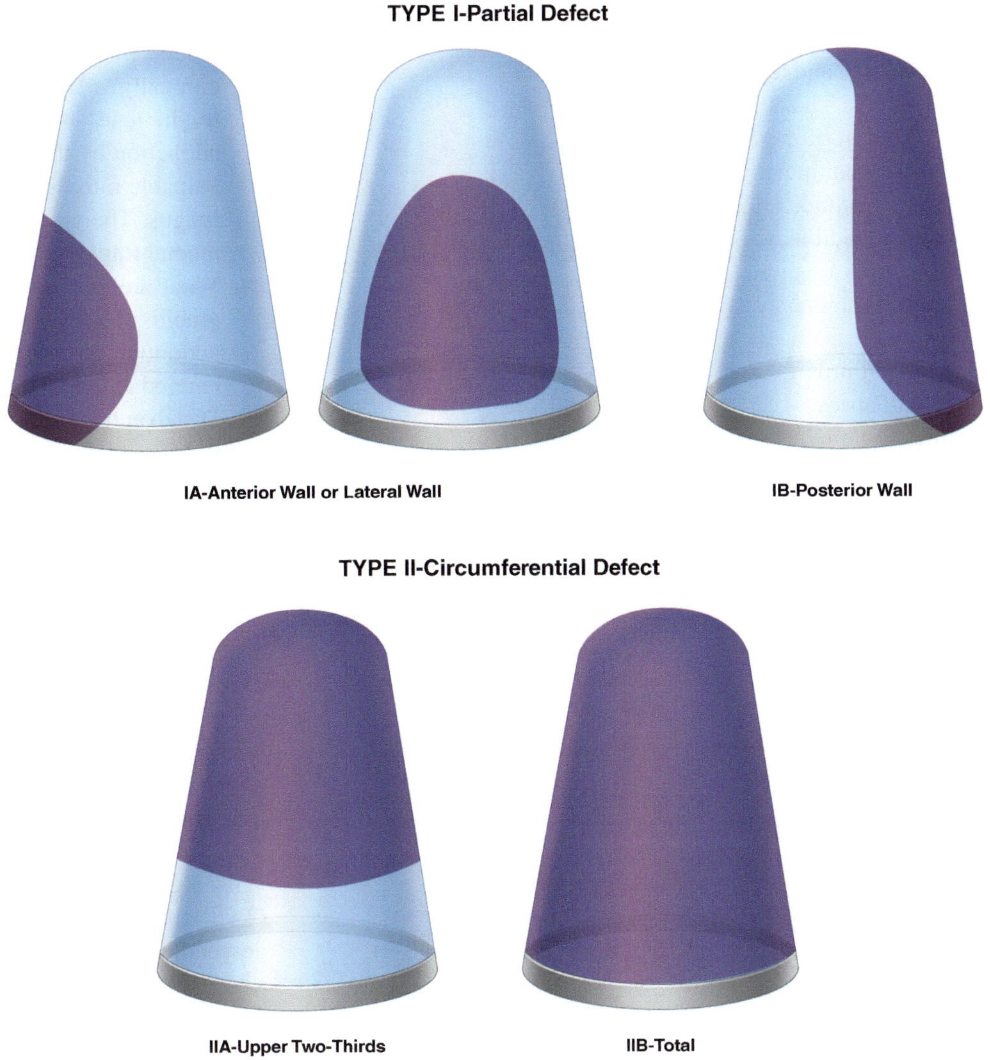

Fig. 54.1 Classification of vaginal defects

vertically oriented skin island over the rectus muscle with the elliptical skin island of 6–8 cm in width and a length of 12–15 cm and the inferior tip of skin island located at or slightly below the level of the umbilicus.)

(a) Discuss the advantages and disadvantages of the VRAM flap. (The advantage is that of a well-vascularized flap with a low incidence of necrosis with the necessary muscle bulk to fill the pelvic dead space. The principal disadvantage is sacrifice of anterior rectus sheath and the possibility of incisional hernia. In obese patients, the bulk may be quite considerable and difficult to place into the pelvis.)

(b) What is the principal limitation for total reconstruction of the vagina? (The flap size must be considerable in width to reconstruct a vagina of a 4 cm diameter caliber implying a 12 cm wide flap, creating a substantial difficulty in closure of the vertical soft tissue donor site in the upper abdomen. Folding the flap vertically can compensate with a more narrow dimension but at the expense of shortening the overall length.)

5. What are some of the technical aspects of the use of the VRAM for perineal reconstruction with respect to stoma placement and the umbilicus? (If an ileal loop and stoma is planned, placement of the laparotomy incision should be to the left of the umbilicus. If dual stomas would be necessary, the right side is still preferential for the ileal loop and placement of the colostomy can be done more laterally through the external oblique of the abdominal wall. This procedure still requires placement of the incision to the *left* of the umbilicus. If a colostomy only is planned, the right rectus is used for the VRAM.)
6. The oncologic surgeon plans a robotic abdominoperineal resection, APR. How does that resection plan affect your reconstruction? (A robotic resection precludes an open laparotomy unless performed solely for the harvest of a VRAM flap, an option that appears to cancel the purported advantages of a minimally invasive resection. Robotic harvest of the rectus abdominis muscle has been

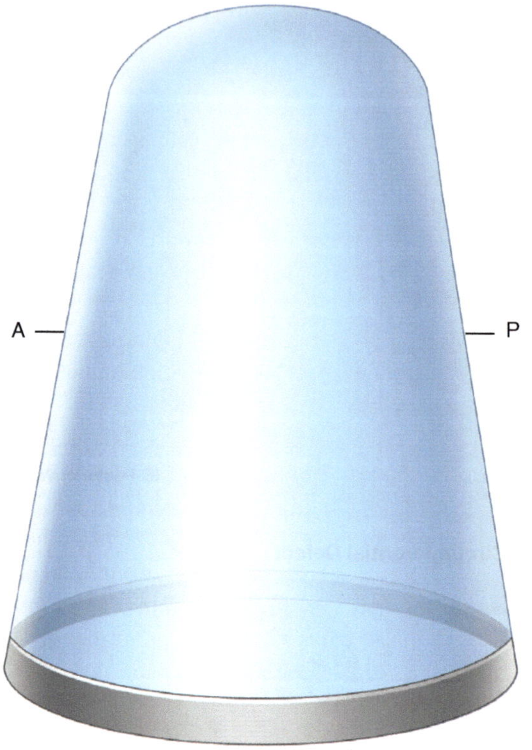

Fig. 54.2 Flap options

Table 54.1 Flap options for vaginal reconstruction

Defect type	Flap option
IA	Singapore flaps (aka pudendal fasciocutaneous flaps)
IB	Pedicled rectus myocutaneous flaps Pedicled rectus musculocutaneous flap Muscle-sparing rectus myocutaneous flap
IIA/B	Vertical rectus abdominis myocutaneous Gracilis Singapore flaps Pedicled jejunum Sigmoid colon

described but is limited to the muscle alone without skin island and requires experience with robotic instrumentation. On balance, the use of posterior thigh or pudendal perforator flaps would be an alternative approach. Both have some limitations and neither provides an address of the intrapelvic dead space with bulk as the VRAM flap.)

7. Discuss the use of gracilis flaps for vaginal reconstruction. Begin with the vascular supply, location of the vascular pedicle, and design. (The gracilis myocutaneous flap is vascularized by the medial femoral circumflex artery, which is located 8–10 cm inferior to the pubis and enters the muscle deep or lateral between adductor longus and magnus. The design is a vertical skin ellipse in line with the axis of the medial thigh, 6–8 cm. wide and 10–15 cm length.)
   (a) Describe the location of the gracilis muscle in the medial thigh and how can the muscle be identified clinically? (The gracilis muscle, an adductor of the thigh, can be identified by voluntary forced adduction by the patient against resistance. Readily palpable muscle in the medial thigh is the adductor longus. The gracilis is just posterior in the superior medial thigh.)
   (b) What are the advantages and disadvantages of the gracilis flap? (Advantages are the use of extra abdominal tissue particularly if the abdomen is not entered and a relatively thin flap in slender patients. Disadvantages are a significant incidence of skin flap necrosis estimated at 10–15% and probably higher, a relatively distal fixed point for pedicle rotation for vaginal reconstruction, and thick flaps in heavier patients.)
8. Readings are provided that perform a comparison between VRAM and thigh-based flaps for major perineal reconstruction. What was the outcome? (A significant difference in *recipient* site complications including an incidence of one-third pelvic abscess and 20% major wound dehiscence in thigh-based reconstruction. No difference was determined in donor site complications, an indication that abdominal wall morbidity is not increased with the use of abdominal-based flaps.)
9. What are the reconstructive options for perianal defects? (Two options: a posterior thigh flap based on the descending branch of the inferior gluteal artery, used as a rotation flap. The second option is bilateral V-Y gluteal advancement flaps, based on either perforators of the superior gluteal or the inferior gluteal artery. A criticism of the posterior thigh flap when rotated on the descending branch is the variability in the existence of this vessel.)
10. Describe the blood supply of the Singapore flap. (The posterior labial arteries which are in turn are a terminal branch of the superficial perineal artery, a branch of the internal pudendal artery of the internal iliac.)
    (a) Anastomoses with what other system and how? (Deep/superficial external pudendal as branches of the common femoral.)
    (b) Sensation? (Posterior labial branches of the pudendal nerve and perineal branches of the posterior cutaneous nerve of the thigh.)
11. Describe the design, dimensions, as well as the pros and cons of the Singapore flap. (The flap is posteriorly based with the harvest of medial posterior thigh skin and the immediately adjacent or lateral to the labia majora; common dimensions are 15 × 5 cm, which allows primary closure of the donor site. Since the flap contains some sensory nerve branches in the base, some sensation may

be present as well. Since the reconstruction is a flap and not a skin graft, the incidence of stenosis, if the flap survives, should be less. The principal shortcoming is that the blood supply may be damaged by either pelvic exenteration surgery and/or prior irradiation.)

(a) Why might this option not be desirable in some acquired vaginal defects? (The blood supply may be sacrificed with resection. For example, pelvic exenteration can sacrifice the major branches of the internal iliac including the internal pudendal artery.)

(b) Additional considerations? (If the labia are intact, the flap must be tunneled beneath the labia and distortion is a distinct possibility. From the oncologic standpoint, carcinoma of the vulva can involve the groin nodes and some consideration should be given to the necessity of groin dissection if Singapore flaps are under consideration.)

12. Since the Singapore flap is a posterior thigh-based flap, describe the application of the perforator concept to the design and development of a posterior thigh flap for perineal reconstruction. (The perforator concept requires identification of a specific cutaneous perforator, usually with a Doppler, and orientation of the flap, dependent on the soft-tissue defect requirements, in either a "propeller" or V-Y design. The former is a rotation flap, the latter usually an advancement technique. Regardless, the blood supply is the same as other posterior thigh-based flap such as the Singapore, namely the terminal branches including the posterior labial of the internal pudendal artery through the superficial or transverse perineal. These perforators arise in the ischio-rectal fossa.)

(a) Outline geometrically this location of the vascular perforators. (A triangle of which the base is formed by a vertical line drawn from the midline of the posterior vaginal introitus to the coccyx. The anterior limb is a line drawn from the coccyx to the ischium. A third line drawn from ischium to posterior vaginal fourchette completes the triangle.)

13. What are the anatomical limitations in the application of the perforator concept of flap dissection to use of the internal pudendal artery perforator flap for perineal reconstruction? ("Free-style" perforator flaps are raised and dissected into the base and feeding vessel incorporating the perforator including dissection of the perforator and feeding vessel for the necessary distance to allow tension-free rotation. Application of this principle is not possible in internal perforator pudendal artery-based flaps because the perforators arise from the ischiorectal fossa deep within the fat of the fossa. Deep dissection into the fat would be unnecessary and hazardous and the deep fascia is not readily accessible.)

14. What are the options for reconstruction of radical vulvectomy defects? Critique each. (The options are skin grafts, Singapore and gracilis flaps. Skin grafts can certainly be used in a skinning superficial vulvectomy done for carcinoma-in-situ or CIS. If so, the graft should be relatively thick to prevent secondary contracture. Singapore flaps are an excellent option for vulvectomy reconstruction if the pedicle, the posterior labial arteries, is intact. Gracilis flaps can be quite bulky for vulvectomy defects but certainly are an option as well.)

(a) What circumstance or set of circumstances would dictate flap reconstruction of vulvar defects? (Prior irradiation and/or a radical vulvectomy defect that includes labia minora and vaginal introitus to avoid contracture resulting from a skin graft.)

15. Describe the principal indications for the following flaps:

(a) Singapore flaps: (Anterior and lateral vaginal wall defects; radical vulvectomy defect, although vaginectomy alone defects will require a division of an intact vulva.)

(b) Gracilis flaps: (Radical vulvectomy defects; possibly vaginal reconstruction although the flaps are somewhat unreliable and as the readings indicated abdominal-based flaps such as the VRAM have an improved outcome.)

(c) VRAM: (Total vaginal reconstruction; obliteration of dead space created by anterior or posterior exenteration.)

(d) Intestinal segments: (Probably of historical interest only because of the heavy amount of secretions and unpleasant odors.)

16. What are the indications for the use of the anterolateral thigh flap for reconstruction of perineal defects? (Although some surgeons preferentially select the ALT flap, probably the principal indications would be a patient with mature stomas through both abdominal recti muscles, obviating the use of a VRAM flap or a perineal defect without intra-abdominal access such as oncologic resection by robotic technology. See Fig. 54.3.)

(a) What is the principal blood supply and methods of identification of the perforators? (The blood supply is the descending branch of the lateral femoral circumflex, usually musculocutaneous perforators, located at a midpoint of a line drawn from the anterior superior iliac spine to the lateral aspect of the patella. A circle with a radius of 3 cm contains the perforators, most commonly in the inferolateral quadrant.)

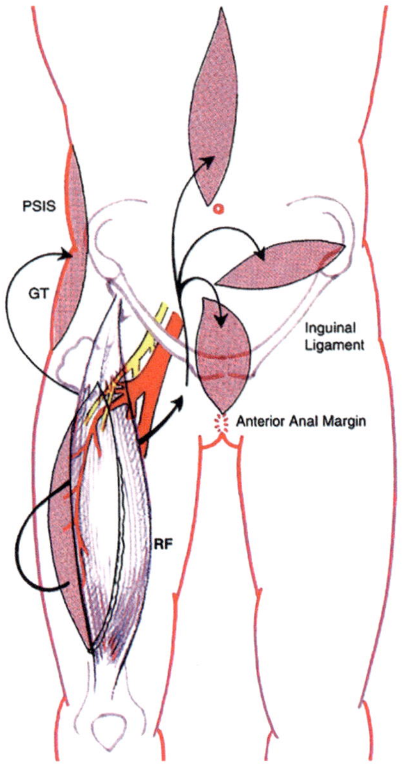

Fig. 54.3 Use of the pedicled anterolateral thigh flap for perineal and truncal defects. (Lannon DA, et al., "Versatility of the Proximally Pedicled Anterolateral Thigh Flap and Its Use in Complex Abdominal and Pelvic Reconstruction", *PRS*, (2011); 127(2):684. (Reprinted with Permission))

The pedicled anterolateral thigh flap pivot points, its arcs of rotation, and how they are affected by the rectus femoris muscle can be appreciated from this illustration. The illustration shows the femoral artery giving off the profunda, which then gives off the lateral circumflex femoral artery. The lateral circumflex femoral artery is very short in this illustration as it trifurcates almost immediately. The descending branch of the lateral circumflex femoral artery then gives off the pedicle to the rectus femoris and continues inferiorly, giving off musculocutaneous and septocutaneous perforators. The flap can be pivoted at the point of branching of the main pedicle to the rectus femoris muscle or more proximally if rectus femoris muscle viability is not compromised by ligation of this pedicle. More proximal pivot points can be at the origin of the descending branch of the lateral circumflex femoral artery, or just proximal to the trifurcation of this artery at the junction of the lateral circumflex femoral artery with the profunda femoris (or the femoral artery if it branches directly from it). As these vessels all travel posterior to the rectus femoris muscle, tunneling of the flap underneath the muscle is required for maximum reach in any superior or medial arc. Care should be taken to preserve the motor innervation to the rectus femoris during tunneling. The flap will reach the costal margin, the posterior superior iliac spine/greater trochanter, the anterior anal margin, and the contralateral iliac fossa. PSIS, posterior superior iliac spine; GT, greater trochanter; RF, rectus femoris; arcs of rotation are illustrated by dark arrows.

17. In the use of the pedicled antero-lateral thigh flap for reconstruction of perineal or lower abdominal defects, what operative maneuver will be necessary? (Once the flap is designed and raised, as discussed above, tunneling beneath the rectus femoris is necessary, a maneuver in which the motor nerve to the rectus and vastus lateralis must be carefully identified and preserved. If the flap is used for an intrapelvic defect, in addition to tunneling under the rectus femoris, division of the inguinal ligament will be necessary to pass the flap within the pelvis. If a concomitant perineal defect is present, the pedicle may be too short to prevent reconstruction of both.)
    (a) What patient population will present difficulties? (Obese patients with bulky ALT flaps may present a substantial difficulty in tunneling beneath the rectus femoris and the pedicle may be at risk.)

Case-Based Conference

Case 1: Persistent Perineal Sinus

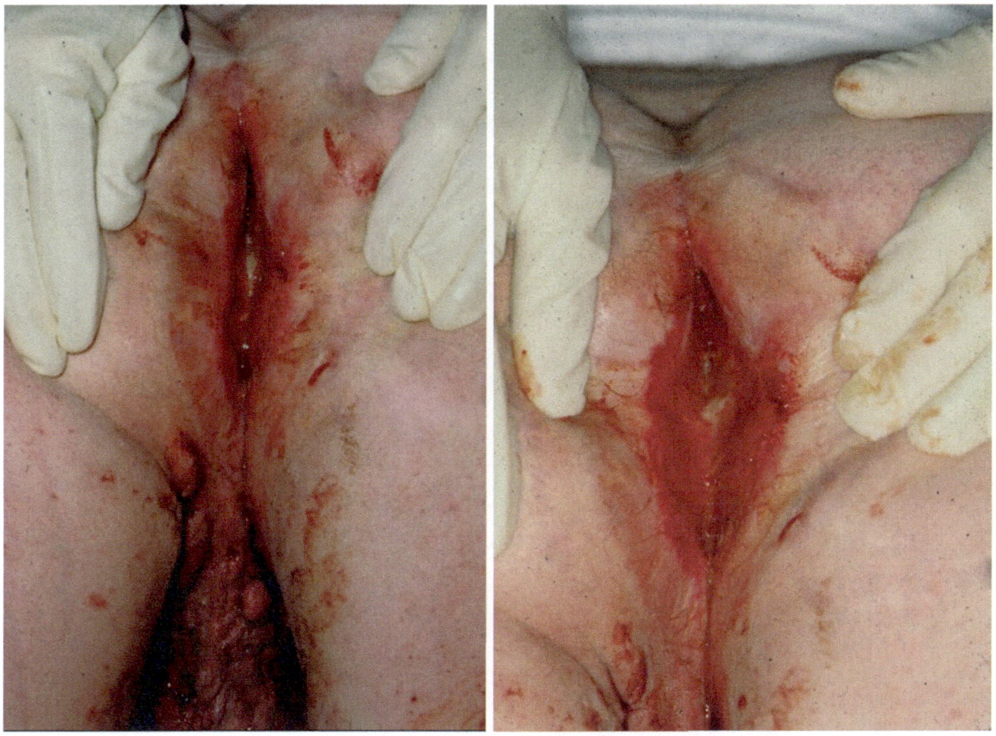

A 44-year-old man with persistent perineal wound 1 year after abdomino-perineal resection for inflammatory disease of the colon.

1. Describe the slide(s). Add a focused clinical examination.
   (a) Any test or imaging indicated?
2. What is the pathological anatomy of this problem?
3. Describe a treatment plan. Begin with options with the pros and cons, select yours, and describe.

Case-Based Conference: Discussion

Case 1: Persistent Perineal Sinus

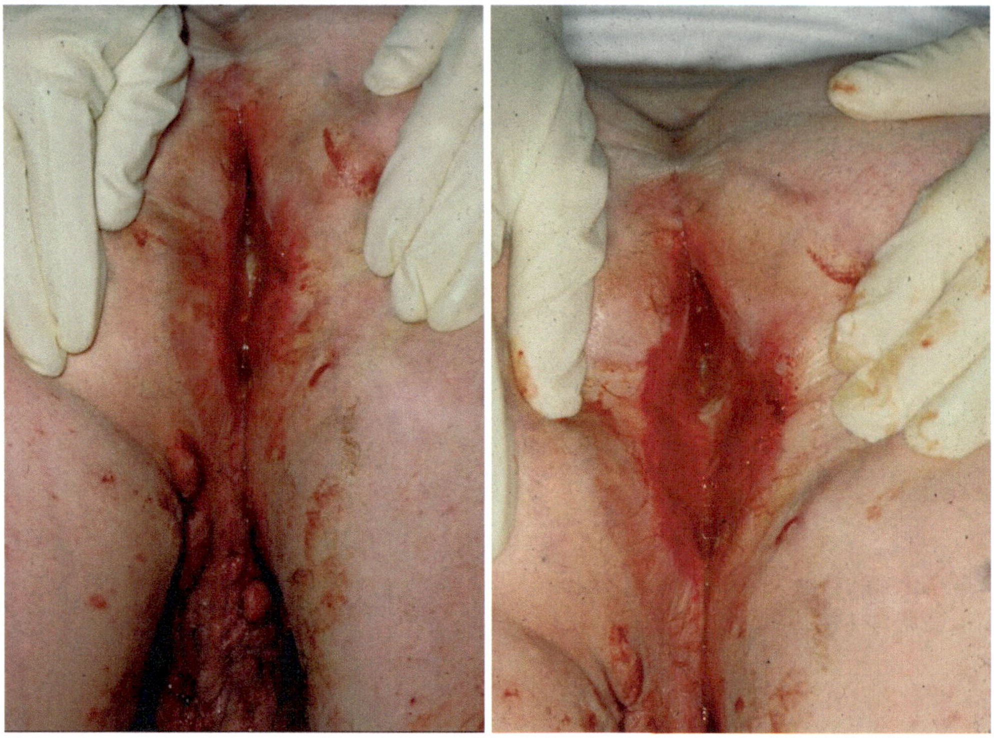

A 44-year-old man with persistent perineal wound 1 year after abdomino-perineal resection for inflammatory disease of the colon.

1. Describe the slide(s). Add a focused clinical examination. (Two slides are provided, both slightly different views of the posterior perineum. In the first, a view with a portion of the posterior scrotum visible, and a long, narrow, and apparently deep midline wound is evident between the inferior buttocks which are spread by the examiner's hands. The posterior depth of the wound cannot be ascertained because the walls are not clearly visible. The adjacent skin has a narrow zone of scarring but no erythema indicative of active infection. The scrotum has a small, smooth 1 cm nodule. The remainder of the thigh and perineum is unscarred. In the second slide, a modestly more close-up view, the wound is more readily visualized, perhaps because of more traction on the buttocks and the anterior one-half of the wound appears more shallow than the posterior. No additional information is provided by the second slide and the posterior depth cannot be readily visualized.

   Several elements of the history would be important to help shape the treatment plan. The nature, duration, and severity of the inflammatory bowel disease as well as the medical treatment and complications that may have occurred. In all likelihood the diagnosis is Crohn's disease, given the perineal component but perhaps the patient did not heal from a proctocolectomy for ulcerative colitis. If Crohn's disease was the diagnosis, was small bowel involved? Have the medications for the bowel disease, particularly immunosuppressants and or steroids been continued? The history should elicit information about primary healing of the perineal component of the anterior–posterior resection or was the wound allowed to heal secondarily? Has the perineal wound ever been healed? The past medical history would focus on the presence, if any, of co-morbidities and general performance status as well as tobacco use. Physical exam should assess overall nutritional status and then more clearly define the wound limits. If so, the wound should be probed for any evidence of tracts that may dictate the performance of a fistulagram. A thorough examination of the wound may not be feasible because of patient pain and may require a general anesthetic. See below. Potential flap donor sites are examined.)

   (a) Any test or imaging indicated? (The decision to image, CT, would hinge on the presence, if any, of characteristics of the wound suspicious for neoplasm. Similarly, the same rationale would exist for biopsy, particularly if a general anesthetic was deemed necessary for examination. Laboratory assessment of nutritional status is probably advisable.)

2. What is the pathological anatomy of this problem? (A clinical exam including the history would probably delineate the underlying cause, most likely the soft tissue perianal component, fistulae, of Crohn's disease. Since the patient required a proctocolectomy, in all likelihood an aggressive form of anorectal disease was present. If the anorectal element of the operation was performed with a narrow resection, residual disease may have remained, setting the stage for a deep and unhealed wound. Regardless, the chronicity either with or without an associated inflammatory component will dictate a similar treatment plan.)
3. Describe a treatment plan. Begin with options with the pros and cons, select yours, and describe. (Any medical or non-surgical approach to this complication is highly unlikely to be successful. The operative approach should incorporate excision/resection and address the resultant deep space with well-vascularized tissue transfer. The resection if done entirely from a posterior perineal approach establishes a risk of injury to the small bowel since post-abdominoperineal resection, APR, the bowel usually prolapses into the pelvic cavity. That risk can be minimized with a combined intra-abdominal and perineal approach that would provide mobilization of the bowel out of the pelvis followed by resection of the ulcer from the posterior route. Exposure from the supine lithotomy will require some modification of the patient positioning for both the resection and reconstruction.

   The rationale for flap transfer hinges on the necessity to provide soft tissue bulk to obliterate dead space and well-vascularized tissue to facilitate healing. The abdominal-based flap is the vertical rectus abdominal muscle, VRAM, flap, a choice that is contingent upon the decision to utilize a laparotomy. A number of perineal flap options are available in the absence of a history of irradiation. Those options include posterior-based thigh flaps, perfused by the terminal branches of the internal pudendal including the transverse perineal, often termed the Singapore or pudendal flap. The vessels emanating from the ischiorectal fossa should be detected with a Doppler. A considerable portion of the flap will need to be de-epithelized to fill the dead space and those requirements may dictate bilateral flaps. The other option is a single or bilateral gracilis muscle only flap, pedicled on the medial circumflex femoral artery. A final and probably secondary option is a rotational flap, also de-epithelized, based superiorly and perfused by the descending branch of the inferior gluteal artery, an occasionally absent vessel.)

Intraoperative

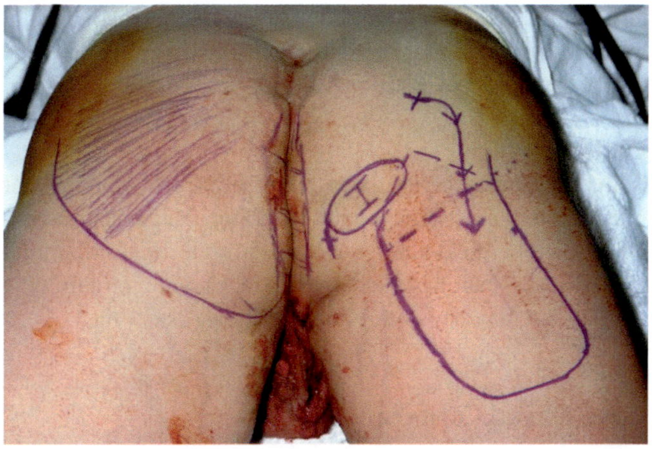

The patient is prone in a jackknife position. Outlined on the left buttock is a superior gluteal, possibly a VY advancement flap. Outlined on the right posterior thigh is a wide, encompassing half of the posterior thigh, a superiorly oriented flap with the base at the level of the ischium. An "X" on the right buttock is the location of the inferior gluteal artery and a line is drawn that represents the course of the descending branch. The plan is resection of the sinus, de-epithelialization of the flap, and rotation by tunneling into the perineal defect.

Postoperative (1 Year)

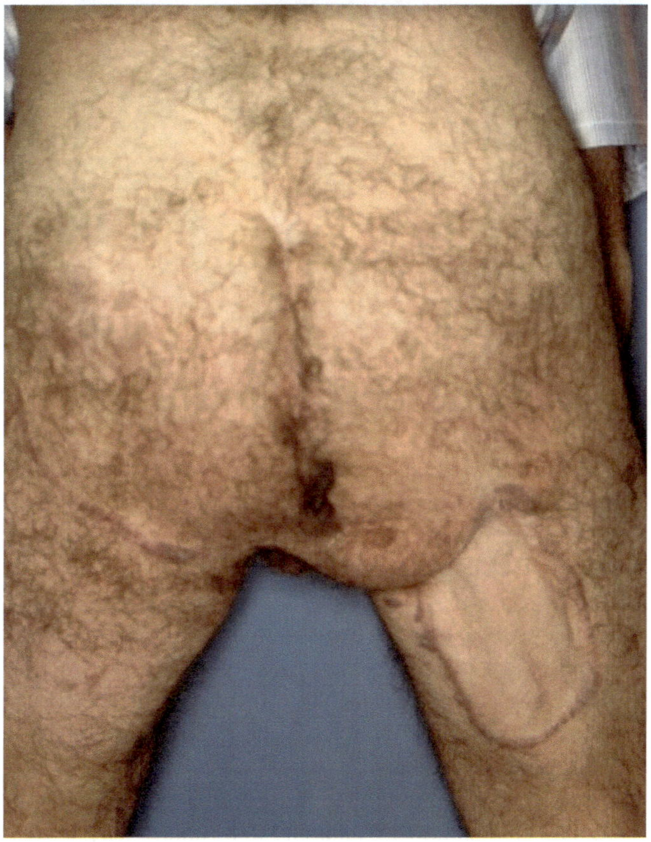

View from posterior—no evidence of recurrence. A well-healed split-thickness skin graft is in place on the right posterior thigh. Some minor redundancy of the medial right buttock is present that raises the question if a second-stage flap retrieval was ever accomplished.

Critique

Some variability of the descending branch of the inferior gluteal artery exists and a hand-held Doppler exam is advisable. Also, perineal sinuses from gastrointestinal inflammatory disease can have extensive tracks and a radiologic fistulagram may be helpful in preoperative planning.

Case-Based Conference

Case 2: Perineal Reconstruction

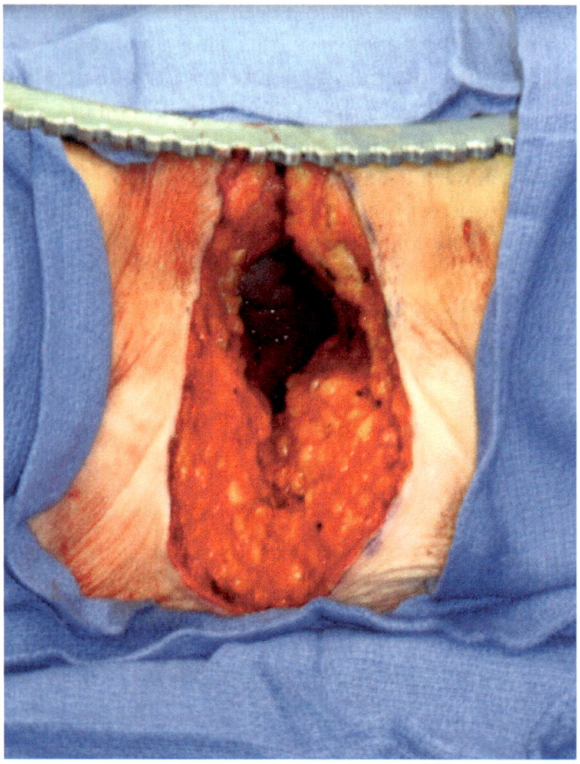

A 60-year-old woman was seen by you in preoperative consultation for reconstruction of a planned total pelvic exenteration. The patient has had prior pelvic irradiation. An intraoperative slide is provided.

1. Begin with a clinical examination and consultation. A pelvic exam is not necessary.
   (a) How would your discussion with the oncologic surgeon proceed? What issues need to be addressed?
   (b) Any tests indicated?
2. Describe and interpret the intraoperative photo.
3. What is the pathologic anatomy to be addressed?
4. Outline your treatment plan including timing and sequencing with the oncologic surgeon.
5. Complications?

Case-Based Conference: Discussion

Case 2: Perineal Reconstruction

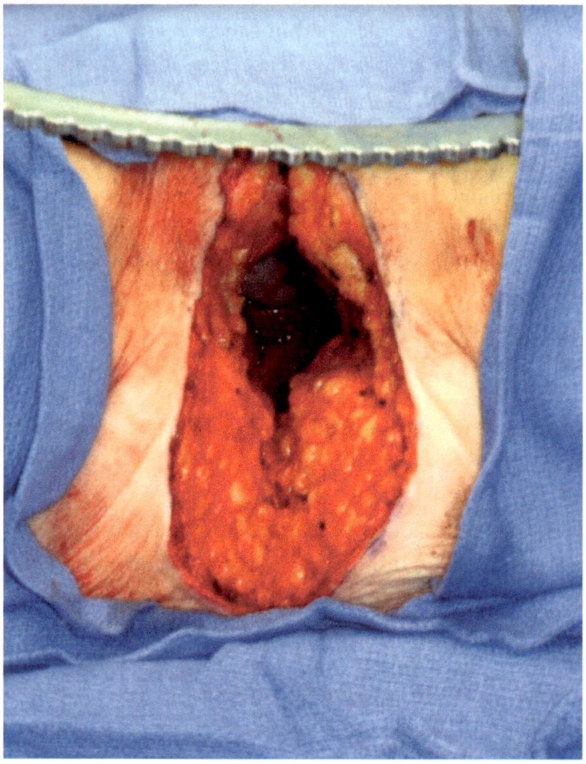

A 60-year-old woman was seen by you in preoperative consultation for reconstruction of a planned total pelvic exenteration. The patient has had prior pelvic irradiation. An intraoperative slide is provided.

1. Begin with a clinical examination and consultation. A pelvic exam is not necessary. (The historical data that can be gleaned from the patient would include the onset of the present illness, past operations, the amount of irradiation, and current symptoms. To elicit current symptoms aids in the establishment of some element of rapport with the patient. The amount of radiation can be roughly estimated if administered once daily and the duration in the number of weeks. An attempt to ascertain functional and nutritional status can be gained by questions about activities of daily living and weight loss. The past medical history is reviewed including medications and the social history of tobacco or other substance abuse, if any. The physical exam component includes inspection of the abdomen for incisional scars, the magnitude of central obesity, and hernias. Both lower extremities are examined for the presence of lymphedema.)

(a) How would your discussion with the oncologic surgeon proceed? What issues need to be addressed? (The discussion with the oncologist is crucial. The preamble states a "total" exenteration which implies cystectomy, hysterectomy and adnexa, and abdominal perineal resection. If so, the patient will require two abdominal stomas, one for the ileal loop and the other an end colostomy. In all likelihood, the right rectus will be desired for the ileal loop to enable an intramuscular placement, the colostomy must be located lateral to the left rectus, *if* a left vertical rectus abdominis muscle flap is selected for reconstruction. The location of the laparotomy incision and the sequencing of the procedural steps are also an important element of the discussion. Given the harvest of the left VRAM, the laparotomy incision optimally is periumbilical on the left. Sequencing is discussed below.)

(b) Any tests indicated? (Routine lab work, pre- and albumin levels. The gynecologist would have obtained the necessary imaging to rule out metastatic disease.)

2. Describe and interpret the intraoperative photo. (Pictured is the anticipated defect of the perineum that includes the labia, adjacent skin and soft tissue, some element of both perianal skin and soft tissue, and the visible portion of the intrapelvic defect. Obliteration of the resultant pelvic dead space, closure of the perineum with non-irradiated soft-tissue and skin; vaginal reconstruction, if performed.)
3. What is the pathologic anatomy to be addressed? (The pathologic anatomy includes a substantial perineal defect within an irradiated field as well as a considerable intrapelvic dead space which postoperatively will be filled in part by small bowel. The defect can be classified as a Corderio IIB.)
4. Outline your treatment plan including timing and sequencing with the oncologic surgeon. (Two most commonly employed options are the gracilis, probably bilateral, or a vertical rectus abdominis muscle flap, VRAM. The gracilis flap is based on the medial femoral circumflex artery and is innervated by the obturator nerve. In absence of labia, certainly the gracilis is an option. The liability is the more distal portion of the skin island that will be necessary for the more proximal or superior portion of the posterior vaginal reconstruction and the skin island is somewhat, 10–15% at least, unreliable. Recent evidence would indicate that a VRAM flap yields improved outcomes as compared to gracilis flaps and provides more muscle bulk to obliterate dead space.

   Other less commonly reconstructive options utilized in this scenario include the pudendal fasciocutaneous and, more recently, the posterior thigh flap. The former is perfused by the terminal branches of the superficial perineal, posterior labial and transverse perineal. The superficial perineal is a continuation of the internal pudendal, a part of the internal iliac system which can be sacrificed in the performance of a pelvic exenteration. However, a rich anastomosis and a collateral circulation with the external pudendal, a branch of the common femoral, probably ensures viability. The potential for sensation is because of inclusion of the perineal nerve, although no evidence exists that the flaps are sensate. The posterior thigh is perfused by the descending branch of the inferior gluteal and sensation is theoretically possible by including the posterior femoral cutaneous nerve. Because of a relatively short pedicle, application of this flap is restricted to superficial posterior perineal defects.

   The planning and execution of a VRAM flap needs to be carefully orchestrated with the extirpative surgeon. The laparotomy is *optimally,* in this case, is accomplished through a left paramedian or midline upper abdominal incision continuing circumumbilical to the pubis and the midline. That entry incision can be accomplished either by the extirpative or reconstructive surgeon. In this instance, a total exenteration, the VRAM will be harvested from the upper *left* abdomen.

   The reconstructive surgeon rejoins the operation after construction of the ileal loop, stapling of the sigmoid but *before* performance of the colostomy. The vertical RAM flap either with or without a superior transverse extension is then harvested with the necessary amount of anterior fascia and in this case with reconstruction of the perineal defect alone, approximately 5–6 cm of skin. The whole width of the rectus is harvested for bulk. The flap, based on the deep inferior epigastric artery and vein, is then tunneled into the pelvic defect with the superior end of the skin flap sutured posteriorly at the posterior perineum. The rectus muscle can be left attached to the pubis if not an undue amount of tension is present which in turn will protect against stress on the vascular pedicle. More frequently, the muscle is divided inferiorly.

   To return to the discussion of the gracilis, the criticism about reliability is discussed above. In addition, the distal portion of the flap frequently must be extended onto the distal thigh to obtain sufficient superior rotation into the depth of the proximal vagina. Finally, some variation of the blood supply may exist with the gracilis flap such that the medial femoral circumflex origin on the profunda femoral artery can be as far as 15 cm inferior to the pubis, thus shortening the pedicle substantially. The performance of the extirpative component of the operation endoscopically or robotically negates the option of abdominal-based flaps. Bilateral gracilis flaps are an acceptable alternative.)
5. Complications? (Acutely, hematoma, small bowel obstruction, perineal wound breakdown with heavily radiated skin. Long-term success can be judged by the absence of vaginal stenosis and the ability to have vaginal intercourse in those instances of vaginal reconstruction.)

Intraoperative

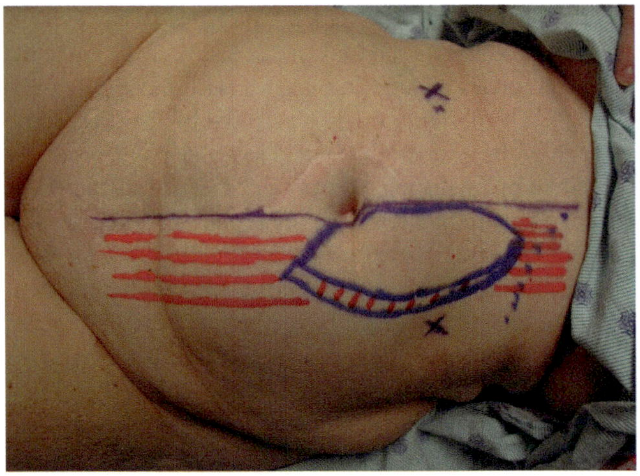

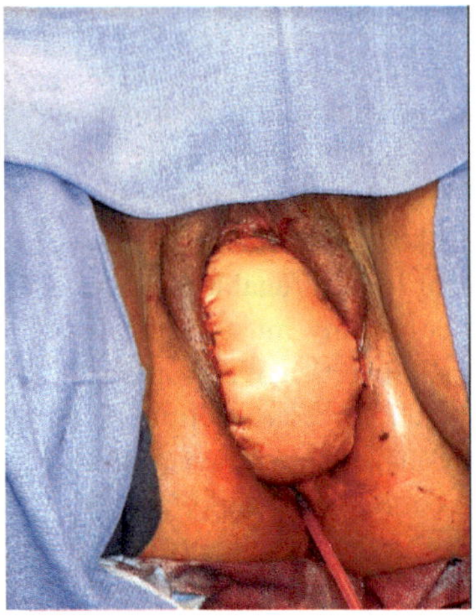

Illustrated and drawn on the anterior abdomen, a different patient, is a left-sided VRAM, based on the deep inferior epigastric vessels. The superior limit of the flap is the epigastrium where the rectus muscle is teased from the underlying rib and posterior fascia.

In the subsequent photo, the VRAM flap is sutured into the defect. The anticipated fullness is present.

Postoperative (3 Weeks)

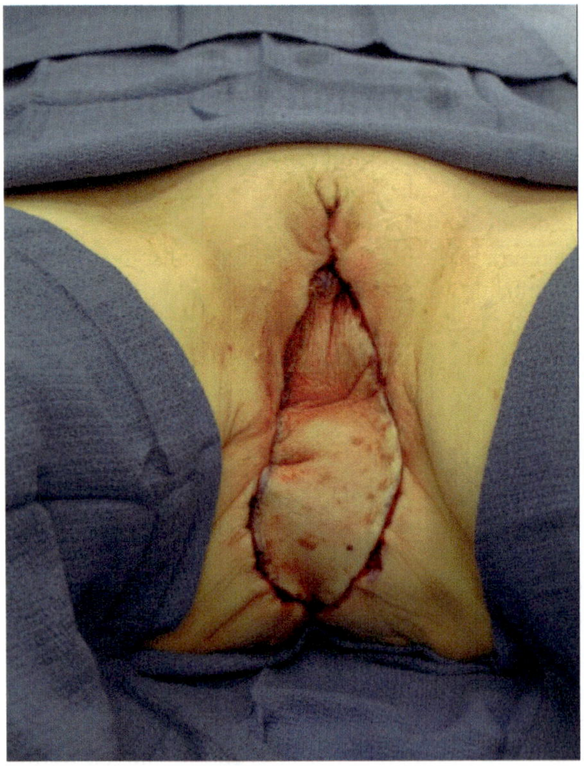

The edema has resolved and the wound is healing satisfactorily. The provision of well-vascularized tissue within an irradiated field will benefit the healing process considerably.

In-Service Examination

1. A 16-year-old girl presents with amenorrhea and on physical examination has well-developed secondary sex characteristics but no vagina. What is the initial step or treatment plan?
   (a) Chromosomal analysis
   (b) Laboratory determination of progesterone and estrogen levels
   (c) CT scan of the abdomen and pelvis
   (d) Urology consult
2. In the performance of a pelvic exenteration, all major branches of the internal iliac are ligated. The blood supply to which of the following flaps for perineal reconstruction would be compromised?
   (a) VRAM
   (b) Singapore
   (c) Gracilis
   (d) Groin
3. The pedicle to the gracilis flap can be located between:
   (a) Adductor magnus and sartorius
   (b) Adductor longus and sartorius
   (c) Vastus medialis and sartorius
   (d) Adductor magnus and adductor longus

55 Decubiti and Miscellaneous

Bibliography

Khansa I., Janis J.E., Chapter 16: "Pressure Sores", Neligan PC, Plastic Surgery, Elsevier 5th Edition, (2023), Volume 4: **pgs. 462**.

Ricci JA, Bayer LR, and Orgill DP. "Evidence-Based Medicine: The Evaluation and Treatment of Pressure Injuries", *Plast Reconstr Surg.*, (2017); 139(1):**275e–284e**.

Rubayi S and Chandrasekhar BS, "Trunk, Abdomen, and Pressure Sore Reconstruction", *Plast Reconstr Surg.*, (2011); 128(3):**205e-215e ONLY, and Video 2**.

Rubin, J.A., Whetzel, T.P., Stevenson, T.R., "The Posterior Thigh Fasciocutaneous Flap: Vascular Anatomy and Clinical Application", *Plast Reconstr Surg.*, (1995); 95:**1228–1239**.

Ahmadzadeh R, Bergeron L, Tang M, Morris SF, "The Superior and Inferior Gluteal Artery Perforator Flaps", *Plast Reconstr Surg.*, (2007);120(6):**1551–1556 ONLY**.

Faculty Discussion and Study Guide

Editorial comment: Decubitus wound care—wound care including dressings is discussed in the wound healing module, basic principles in Chap. 3.

General Principles

1. In terms of pressure distribution in the supine and seated positions, the points of greatest pressure are: (Sacrum about 60 mm Hg, ischium when seated 80–100 mm Hg).
   (a) In essence, what are the areas in the supine position that are at greatest risk for ulceration? (Sacrum, occiput, heel.)
2. What is the data about tissue perfusion and external pressure? (Essentially, if external pressure is greater than end-capillary pressure, 30 mm Hg, then diminished tissue perfusion occurs which can then lead to necrosis, particularly if the external pressure is two times capillary pressure for more than 2 h. This finding is the basis for turning supine comatose patients q 2 h.)
   (a) Besides pressure, what are the risk factors for the development of decubiti? (Friction, shear, moisture, malnutrition.)
3. The prevention of decubiti in hospitalized patients is best accomplished by: (Risk assessment with a risk assessment tool such as a Braden scale; appropriate skin care by avoidance of shearing/moisture and frequent turning, every 2 h.)
   (a) What is the Braden scale? (An assessment tool for the risk of development of decubiti or pressure sores with a 1–4 rating with 1 as worst and 4 as least. The parameters evaluated are sensation, potential for moisture, nutrition, mobility, as well as shear and fiction. The Braden scale is utilized by the nursing staff to determine if a particular inpatient or nursing home patient is at increased risk for the development of decubitus. No evidence exists that the Braden scale actually diminishes the incidence of inpatient-acquired decubiti.)
4. You evaluate a paraplegic with a newly discovered full-thickness eschar over the ischium that measures 3 cm in diameter. Is the underlying soft-tissue including muscle damage less than, equal to, or greater than the 3 cm? (Considerably greater. The cross-section of a decubitus is that of a cone with the tip of the cone the skin with increasing dimensions through fat, muscle with the eventual base lying over the bony prominence, the ischium.)
5. Give the characteristics of stage I–IV decubitus: (I—erythema without blanching on pressure; II—blistering and abrasion with presumed partial-thickness injury; III—full thickness into fat but not through fascia; IV—exposure and necrosis of muscle/tendon/joint/bone.)
6. A reading was provided that demonstrates a collaborative approach to the perioperative management of decubitus

E. Luce, *A Curriculum for Plastic Surgery*, https://doi.org/10.1007/978-3-031-62087-4_55

in an effort to reduce recurrence. Outline the particulars of that collaborative approach.

(a) Preoperative. (Nutritional status, wheelchair and mechanical device maintenance, and determination of the appropriateness of surgical therapy. The patients are admitted preoperatively to the rehabilitation service.)

(b) Postoperative. (All patients are maintained on Clinitron® or KinAire® beds for a 2-week period of time with initiation of physical therapy. Patient education centers on pressure-release maneuvers as well as education of participating family members. Once mobilization is initiated, the patients participate in a community reintegration program throughout the remainder of their hospitalization.)

Evaluation, Preoperative Assessment

1. What are the principal factors in preoperative global assessment of a decubitus patient? (One should assess the wound healing risk factors, nutrition, presence or absence of spasticity as well as the associated pulmonary and urologic complications. In the past, the principal eventual cause of mortality was urinary tract infections and urosepsis. Cessation of smoking is mandatory and some assessment of the patient's social situation for long-term maintenance of skin integrity is also important.)
   (a) What is the essential laboratory assessment of the decubitus patient? (Albumin, prealbumin, ESR, and if indicated imaging, preferable MRI, for osteomyelitis.)
2. What is the drug of choice for treatment of spasticity? (Baclofen; secondary drug is dantrolene. Gabapentin has been utilized as well.)
3. Discuss measures to offload pressure in paraplegic or patients who are unable to move. (Low air loss and air-fluidized beds both can decrease pressure points to less than 25 mm Hg and maintain a dry skin environment. Frequent patient repositioning or turning, q. 2 h, will decrease the occurrence of decubiti. Cost is a significant determinant and little evidence exists for the superiority of low air loss over static foam mattresses.)
4. Discuss the use of off-loading beds in the postoperative period. (The two types of off-loading beds that are available are low air loss and air fluidized beds. These types of beds or mattresses are of use also in prophylaxis in patients in whom a Braden's scale assessment would appear to be at high risk for the development of decubitus. Air-fluidized beds circulate warm air through fine ceramic beads within the mattress and have a drying effect similar to low air loss beds or mattresses. Air-fluidized beds tend to be more expensive and are certainly heavier than a low air loss mattress.)
   (a) Name other low-pressure devices. (A number of simple devices are available such as silicone, foam, and sheepskin. Alternative pressure devices vary the pressure to avoid prolonged pressure at a single anatomic point.)
5. What are the measures and usefulness of evaluation of osteomyelitis in decubiti? (Bone scan and CT are of little value since periostitis will light up on bone scan and CT is misleading unless advanced bone changes are present. MRI certainly can diagnose osteomyelitis but does not have the sensitivity and specificity of bone biopsy which remains the gold standard for the diagnosis.)
6. Outline a protocol for the management of the bone. (Since a bony prominence is the base for all decubiti, the bone is at least superficially colonized. More likely, some element of osteomyelitis exists, the magnitude dependent on a number of factors including the acuity and the size of the decubitus. One of the readings recommended a prior bone biopsy to establish osteomyelitis. An alternate treatment protocol is excision of all soft tissue involved as well as the osteomyelitic bone, the excision guided by the presence of bleeding non-infected bone. That protocol permits immediate soft tissue closure vs. bone biopsy, IV antibiotics for 6 weeks, and then ostectomy and delayed flap reconstruction. Regardless, the keystone is adequate debridement of bone.)
7. What is the advisability of ischiectomy for ischial decubitus? (As outlined in the prior question, adequate excision of the osteomyelitic bone is of paramount importance. In the past, an ischiectomy has been recommended but the outcome is the development of a decubitus on the opposite side because of the excessive load.)
8. What is the role of negative pressure wound therapy, NPWT, in the management of decubitus? (Similar to the management of other problematic wounds, NWPT can be used as a bridge if the patient situation merits delay. NWPT has the capability to permit downscaling of the wound in magnitude and perhaps for a less-extensive resection and flap closure.)
9. List the general principles in surgical therapy of decubiti. (Resect the ulcer and bursa; remove osteomyelitic bone; provide soft tissue cover usually with a flap; design flap so as not to burn bridges for possible future occurrence of decubiti.)
   (a) What are the theoretical and practical advantages of the use of musculocutaneous or muscle flaps in closure of decubiti? (The theoretical advantage is that well-vascularized musculocutaneous or muscle flaps have an innate ability to suppress and perhaps eradicate low bacterial colonization. The practical advantage is a dead space fill and a soft tissue buffer over the underlying bone.)

Specific Flaps

1. List and describe the vascular territory to the gluteal or buttock area. (Although not the thrust of the question, the area of the lumbar back just superior to the buttock is perfused by the lumbar and deep circumflex iliac arteries. The superior portion of the buttock is vascularized via the gluteus maximus by the superior gluteal and the inferior portion of the buttock by the superior gluteal and inferior gluteal arteries, respectively. The medial inferior area is perfused by the internal pudendal, a branch of the inferior gluteal artery. The lateral inferior region of the buttock is supplied by terminal branches of the lateral circumflex femoral. The immediately adjacent posterior thigh is vascularized by branches of the profunda femoris, the basis of the posterior thigh fasciocutaneous flap—see below.)
2. With respect to the gluteal flaps, describe the skin markings for "limits" of same. (Essentially, is the watershed area perfused by the superior and inferior gluteal arteries. The glut. Max. arises from the lateral edge of the sacrum and the posterior medial portion of the iliac crest and inserts on the greater trochanter and adjacent proximal posterior femur. Both rotational and advancement flap designs can be done.)
   (a) Where is the superior gluteal artery? (A branch of the internal iliac that emerges on a line drawn from the posterior superior iliac spine to the posterior superior trochanter, at a point approximately at the junction of the posterior and middle one-third of said line. The branch of interest is the superior branch. The perforators, 2–3 in number, are located on the same line but in the middle one-third.)
   (b) Describe the technique of a *rotational* gluteal flap. (The design consists of a large skin-muscle island based inferiorly with possible discrete identification of the superior gluteal artery pedicle as well as a back cut laterally and inferiorly on the gluteus muscle. In this writer's experience neither of those maneuvers are necessary and could be harmful. The flap can be designed as a fasciocutaneous flap.)
   (c) Describe bilateral v-y gluteal flaps. (The base of the v or triangle is the sacral defect and the tip points directly laterally at the greater trochanter. A large flap that consists of skin, fat, and gluteus muscle can be raised that will allow readvancement if additional decubiti occur in the future. Incision of the fascia and not the muscle is usually all that is necessary superiorly and laterally and then the muscle can be released from its attachments to the greater trochanter, also if necessary, to allow for greater advancement. Bilateral flaps are possible and advanced into the defect with closure of the donor site in a direct or V-Y fashion.)
3. In elevation of an inferior gluteus maximus island flap based on the inferior gluteal artery what muscle separates the superior gluteal from the inferior gluteal pedicle? (Pyriformis.)
   (a) A posterior thigh flap can be based on the descending branch of the inferior gluteal artery. What nerve accompanies the artery and what is the principal limitation? (The posterior femoral cutaneous nerve. The artery is absent in a significant percentage of cases.)
4. Describe the design of a posterior thigh fasciocutaneous flap not based on the inferior gluteal artery for closure of ischial defects. (For many plastic surgeons the posterior thigh v-y design has become the workhorse for closure of ischial decubitus. The design consists of a v with the base centered on the defect but an "open" area that is the base of the flap from the decubitus obliquely laterally and inferior toward a point 10 cm inferior to the greater trochanter. The tip of the flap is located at least and perhaps more than 10 cm from the popliteal fossa. The flap rotates superomedially into the defect with closure in a v-y fashion inferiorly. See Fig. 55.1.)
   (a) What is the blood supply to the posterior thigh flap? (The key is the cruciate anastomosis between the branches of the medial femoral circumflex artery and

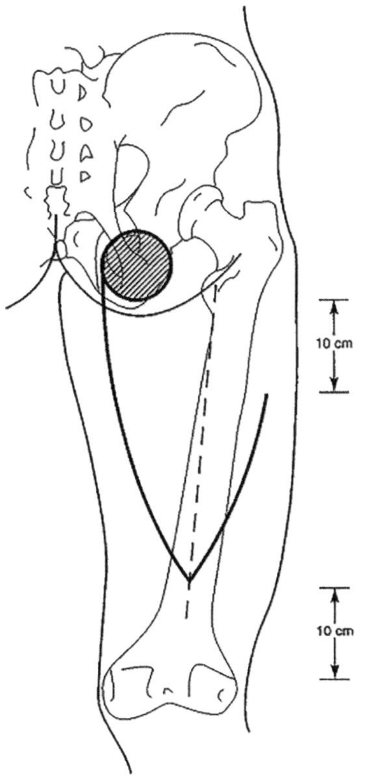

Fig. 55.1 Design of laterally based posterior thigh fasciocutaneous flap to reconstruct ischial defect. (Rubin, J.A., Whetzel, T.P., Stevenson, T.R., "The Posterior Thigh Fasciocutaneous Flap: Vascular Anatomy and Clinical Application." *PRS*, (1995); 95:1228–1239. (Reprinted with Permission))

the profunda perforator branches, principally the first though the third. The contribution of the terminal or descending branch of the inferior gluteal artery is probably overrated.)
   (b) Where are the first and second profunda perforators located? (The first is 2–4 cm and the second 4–6 cm inferior to the ischial tuberosity.)
5. Describe the design including blood supply of the gracilis flap. (The use of the gracilis flap is also covered in the perineum reconstruction section. A line is drawn between the pubic tubercle and the medial condyle of the femur with the gracilis muscle located about 2–3 cm posterior to that line. The adductor longus is palpated easily with the thigh in abduction. The gracilis is 2–3 cm posterior. The adductor magnus muscle is posterior to the gracilis. The skin island should be centered over the proximal third of the muscle, the location of most of the perforators, but can be extended over the middle third but is less reliable if extended. The pedicle is the ascending branch of the medial circumflex femoral artery located approximately 10 cm inferior to the pubic tubercle although variation exists.)
6. Describe the blood supply, design, and use of a tensor fascia lata flap. (Line drawn from the anterior superior iliac spine to the patella is the anterior extent of a tensor fascia lata flap, the muscle is located on the lateral and posterior iliac crest. The blood supply is the transverse or ascending branches of the lateral circumflex femoral artery that enter 10–12 cm below the anterior superior iliac spine. The flap is consistent for a length of the proximal one-half of the thigh but becomes progressively inconsistent with further distal extension. Incorporation of the underlying fascia lata is important in terms of vascularization. Larger, chimeric flaps can be harvested with incorporation of the anterolateral thigh flap by inclusion of the descending and transverse branches of the lateral femoral circumflex artery. Incorporation of the lateral femoral cutaneous nerve, a T_{10-12} branch, enables a sensate flap *if* the level of paraplegia is lower.)
7. A "total thigh flap" actually is designed and contains what? (Total thigh flap is an amputation of the lower extremity just above the popliteal fascia and a subperiosteal dissection along the femur. The actual skin component used is a composite flap of the total quadriceps musculature with the overlying anterior and lateral skin. The femur is discarded.)
8. What is the girdlestone procedure and when is that operation employed in the management of decubitus? (The girdlestone procedure consists of resection of the femoral head in instances of extensive decubiti with hip joint involvement. A substantial-size dead space results even when a portion of the acetabular portion is excised as well. The use of NWPT can assist in wound closure. Frequently, a muscle flap must be developed to close the dead space.)
9. What patient demographics set the stage for a significant incidence of recurrence? (The young, post-traumatic, paraplegic, or the demented elderly patient. Other significant factors include social situations such as lack of home support or substance abuse.)

Case-Based Conference

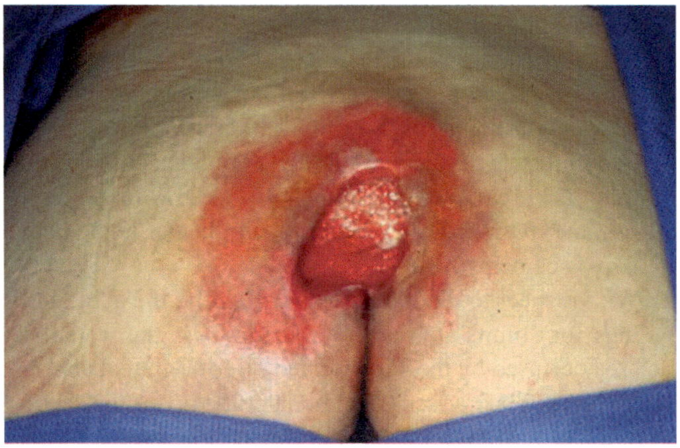

Case 1—Sacral Decubitus

The patient is a 42 year old paraplegic.

1. Describe the slide. Obtain a pertinent history and physical examination.
   (a) Any imaging necessary? Diagnostic testing?
2. Outline the pathophysiology of decubitus ulcer.
   (a) How do you integrate this knowledge of the pathophysiology into the treatment plan?
3. What are the goals of your treatment plan?
4. Outline the plan including perioperative care. If an operation is a component of the plan, list options, select yours, and draw the proposed wound closure.

Case-Based Conference: Discussion

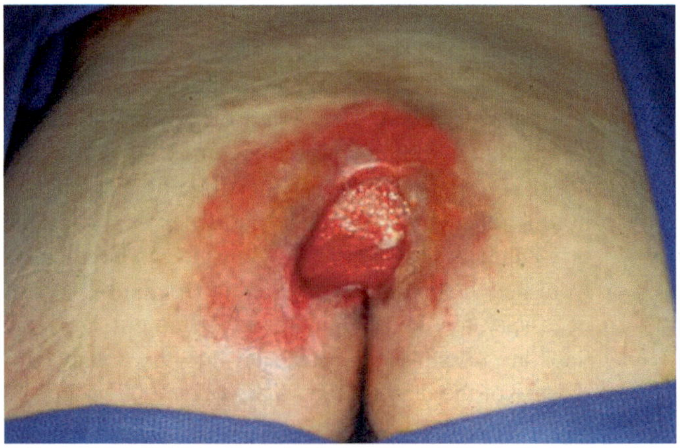

Case 1—Sacral Decubitus

The patient is a 42-year-old paraplegic.

1. Describe the slide. Obtain a pertinent history and physical examination. (A large sacral decubitus is depicted with a large area of circumferential adjacent reddened skin questionably more consistent in the appearance of irritation rather than cellulitis or pressure. The base of the decubitus has granulation tissue. No incisional or other scars are evident.

   Paraplegics with decubiti are subject to a number of associated complications including urinary tract infection leading to chronic renal failure, malnutrition, spasticity of the lower extremities, and, particularly with more proximal lesions, pulmonary insufficiency. More globally, an assessment of their social environment is important as well as tobacco and drug abuse. The physical exam in general is directed towards the physical findings of inanition, spasticity, and also direct probing of the decubitus for the magnitude of undermining. The anatomic level and the duration of injury should be established as well as any history of past decubiti.)

   (a) Any imaging necessary? Diagnostic testing? (Imaging can be done to detect osteomyelitis but CT scan, MRI, and bone scans are all non-specific. Erythrocyte sedimentation rate/WBC will be elevated and are not of value. The test of most diagnostic value in the detection of osteomyelitis is a bone biopsy. Objective nutritional assessment should be done with determination of levels of albumin and prealbumin. Social work and rehabilitation medicine input will be important in postoperative management.)

2. Outline the pathophysiology of decubitus ulcer. (The pathogenesis of decubiti stems from the descriptive term "pressure ulcer." The principal factor is unrelieved, sustained pressure greater than capillary pressure, 15–20 mm Hg, particularly if the external pressure is two times capillary pressure for greater than 2 h. The weight of the body part, for example in the sitting position, places pressure on underlying bony prominences, the ischium, and will produce necrosis of all overlying soft tissue including skin. The magnitude of soft-tissue necrosis is greater in progression from skin to bone, so viewed in cross section, the zone of tissue necrosis resembles an inverted cone, the tip at the skin. This pathologic anatomy has implications for debridement and closure.)

   (a) How do you integrate this knowledge of the pathophysiology into the treatment plan? (The understanding that the culprit in etiology of decubitus is the unrelenting pressure establishes the foundation for the postoperative management plan. The patient will need to be placed into a specialized bed, a number of models are available. A protocol is provided to the nursing staff for periodic repositioning of the patients. Arrangements are also established prospectively for subsequent intermediate care in a rehabilitation facility.)

3. What are the goals of your treatment plan? (Optimize nutrition, treat co-morbidities, involve social work, wound toilet, and wound closure. Establish a postoperative plan to ensure proper positioning with short- and long-term considerations to address predisposing factors for recurrence.)

4. Outline the plan including perioperative care. If an operation is a component of the plan, list options, select yours, and draw the proposed wound closure. (The redness of the surrounding skin may be secondary to the use of the VAC. Discontinuance of the VAC for 3–4 days may be of value. Nutrition is optimized and smoking cessation is mandated. The general principles in surgical therapy are resection of the ulcer and bursa, excision of osteomyelitic bone as judged by appearance at operation, and provide soft tissue cover and design flaps so as not to burn bridges for the possible occurrence of future decubiti.)

   Once those objectives are attained, intraoperative excision is followed by closure and reconstruction in a single stage. Excision of the bursa including the floor over the bony sacrum will expose the bone and excision of at least the superficial cortex will determine the depth, if any, of osteomyelitic bone, uncommon in the sacrum. Bilateral gluteal fasciocutaneous flaps with a V-Y design may be the option for wound closure. Gluteal flaps are perfused by the superior and inferior gluteal arteries. A V-Y design would include the superior gluteal artery, a branch of the internal iliac, located at a point 5 cm inferior to the posterior superior iliac spine and 5 cm lateral on a line drawn from the spine to the greater trochanter. The base of the triangle of a V-Y flap is the sacral defect, the tip just medial to the greater trochanter. Incision of the fascia and not the muscle, the gluteus maximus, is all that is necessary as well as the release of the attachments to the greater trochanter to allow for bilateral advancement. The lateral donor site can be closed in a V to Y fashion.

   A number of postoperative protocols exists, a common element to all is off-loading pressure through the use of specialized beds, physical therapy, and patient education.

   Finally, all plastic surgeons should be aware of the importance of nursing plans to prevent decubiti in hospitalized patients that includes risk assessment with a tool such as the Braden scale, appropriate skin care by the avoidance of shearing/moisture, frequent turning, and the use of air-loss beds in the high-risk patient.

Postoperative (Intraoperative)

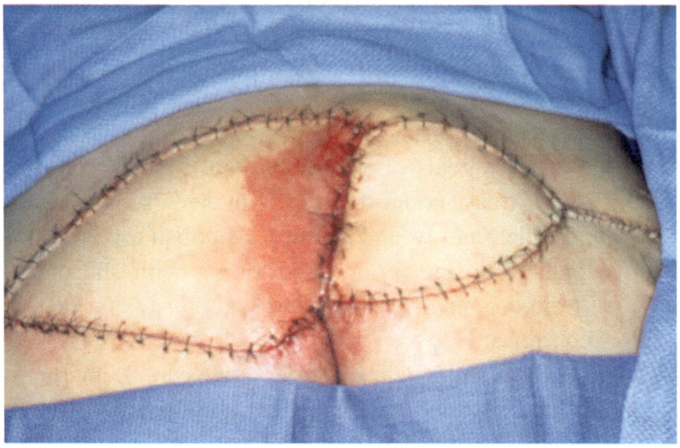

A single immediate postoperative photo illustrates excision and wound closure with asymmetric V-Y gluteal advancement flaps, the right considerably smaller than the left. Curiously, all of the adjacent area of irritation on the right medial buttock has been excised but residual on the left. Perhaps with discontinuance of the VAC, the right side responded.

In-Service Examination

1. The Braden scale is:
   (a) A classification lass of severity of decubiti
   (b) A classification of the size of an abdominal wall defect
   (c) Assessment tool for risk of decubitus
   (d) The bone height in an alveolar cleft
2. The blood supply to the rotational posterior thigh flap is:
   (a) Lateral femoral circumflex
   (b) Inferior gluteal
   (c) Internal pudendal
   (d) Profunda perforators
3. A decubitus complicated by osteomyelitis is optimally diagnosed by:
   (a) Technetium bone scan
   (b) Bone biopsy
   (c) Plane X-ray films
   (d) CT scan

56 Myelomeningocele, Complex Back Wound

Bibliography

Casas, L and Lewis VL, and Lewis Jr VL, "A Reliable Approach to the Closure of Large Acquired Midline Defects of the Back," *Plast. Reconstr. Surg.*, (1989);84:**634–641. (Overview)**

Mathes DW, Thornton JF, and Rohrich RJ, "Management of Posterior Trunk Defects." *Plast. Reconstr. Surg.;* (2006); 118:**73e–83e.**

Daly LT, Ortiz R, Shin JH, et al., "Reconstruction of Lumbar Spinal Defects: Case Series, Literature Review, and Treatment Algorithm", *Plast. Reconstr. Surg. Glob. Open*, (2019); 7:**Fig. 3, 4–6 ONLY.**

Garvey PB, Rhines LD, Dong W, and Chang DW, "Immediate soft-tissue reconstruction for complex defects of the spine following surgery for spinal neoplasm", *Plast. Reconstr. Surg.*, (2010); 125(5):**1463–65. (Discussion Only)**

Wilhelmi BJ, Snyder N, Colquhoun T, et al., "Bipedicle paraspinous muscle flaps for spinal wound closure: An anatomic and clinical study", *Plast. Reconstr. Surg.*, (2000); 106(6):**1305–1311.**

Devulapalli C., Broyles JM., Ricardo B. et al., "Soft-Tissue Reconstruction of Large Spinal Defects: A 12-Year Institutional Experience", *Plast Reconstr Surg.*, (2017) 140:**806, 810–813 ONLY.**

Sadigh PL, Chang LR, Hsieh CH, et al., "The trapezius perforator flap: An underused but versatile option in the reconstruction of local and distant soft-tissue defects", *Plast. Reconstr. Surg.*, (2014); 134(3):**449e–456e.**

Lynch JR, Hansen JE, Chaffoo R, et al. "The Lower Trapezius Musculocutaneous Flap Revisited: Versatile Coverage for Complicated Wounds to the Posterior Cervical and Occipital Regions Based on the Deep Branch of the Transverse Cervical Artery", *Plast. Reconstr. Surg.*, (2002); 109(2):**444–450.**

Luce EA, Discussion of "A New Technique for Closure of Large Meningomyelocele Defects." *Annals of Plastic Surgery,* (2007); 59:**544–545.**

Blanco-Dávila F, Luce EA, "Current Considerations for Myelomeningocele Repair", *The Journal of Craniofacial Surgery,* (2000); 11(5): **500–507.**

Faculty Discussion and Study Guide

Complex Back Wound—Anatomy

1. Describe the blood supply of the paraspinal muscles. (The vascular supply is from branches of the intercostal arteries in the lower one-half of the thoracic area and the lumbar region and from branches of the superior gluteal artery in the sacral region.)
   (a) Describe the configuration of the blood supply to any single intercostal segment. (Both a medial and lateral branch exit from the same intercostal trunk. The lateral branch is larger than the medial. The location of the medial is 3 cm, lateral 5 cm, from the main intercostal perforator, the source of these branches is usually located approximately 5 cm to the midline. To reiterate, the intercostal perforator, the source of these branches, is usually located approximately 5 cm from the midline.)
2. Group and name the posterior trunk muscles into a deep and superficial group. (The superficial or extrinsic group consists of the trapezius, latissimus dorsi, and possibly the gluteus maximus as well as the rhomboids medial to the scapula. The deep group consists of the intrinsics in the neck including the splenius and semispinalis capitis and cervicalis; the longissimus with cervical and thoracic component; iliocostalis with thoracic and lumbar components.)
3. Describe the essential anatomy of the scapular and parascapular flaps including the vascular supply. (The vascular supply of the scapular flap is the horizontal branch of the circumflex scapular artery and vein, the latter a major branch of the subscapular axis. The blood supply of the

E. Luce, *A Curriculum for Plastic Surgery*, https://doi.org/10.1007/978-3-031-62087-4_56

parascapular flap is the parascapular descending branch of the circumflex. The circumflex accesses the back via the triangular space formed by the teres major inferiorly, teres minor superiorly, and the long head of the triceps laterally.)

4. Describe the essential anatomy of the trapezius including function, origin and insertion, innervation, and blood supply. (The muscle is distributed as a "hood" over the posterior superior shoulders, the posterior cervical, and upper thoracic region arising from the nuchal line of the vertebrae and inserting on the scapular spine and lateral clavicle. Innervation is through the spinal accessory and C_{3-4} and the blood supply is the branches of the transverse cervical artery, derived from the thyrocervical trunk. The function is elevation or shrugging of the shoulder and lateral rotation of the scapula.)
5. Describe the essential anatomy of the latissimus dorsi including function, origin and insertion, innervation, and vascular supply. (Latissimus is a broad flat posterior trunk muscle that originates from the thoracolumbar fascia, posterior iliac crest, and T_{7-12} vertebra. Insertions on the proximal humerus, posterior-medially and functions to adduct, draw posteriorly, and medially rotate the humerus. Innervation and vascular supply is via the thoracodorsal nerve and artery, respectively.)
6. Describe the essential anatomy of the gluteal flaps including function, origin and insertion, innervation, and vascular supply. (The gluteal muscles, principally the maximus, are parallelogram-shaped muscle of the buttock originating from the lateral sacrum and the posterior superior iliac spine and inserting onto the greater trochanter and adjacent iliotibial tract. The function is extension and stabilization of the hip, innervation is by the inferior gluteal nerve, and perfusion by the superior and inferior gluteal arteries. The superior gluteal artery can be located at a distance of one-third to one-half on a line drawn from the posterior superior iliac spine to the superior aspect of the greater trochanter and the perforators are mostly within the middle third of that line. The inferior gluteal artery is at a point one-half to two-thirds on a line drawn from the posterior superior iliac spine to the lateral ischium. The perforators are located in the middle one-third of that line.)

Editorial note: Gluteal flaps are also included in Chap. 55.

Complex Back Wound—General

1. What is the general gestalt that outlines the difficulty in these particular types of truncal defects, namely an oncologic etiology referred to plastic surgery? (Large, irradiated, frequently infected, and/or multiple attempts at closure, presence of hardware.)
2. What are some general principles in determination of the method of reconstruction for difficult back wounds? (The particular zone of the back, namely cervical, thoracic, lumbar, lumbosacral; presence of irradiation; extent of previous surgery. All of these factors sum up to the fact that local flaps are not available; two-layer closure is frequently necessary; muscle flaps also may be necessary in the presence of contaminated and colonized wounds.)
3. What are the elements of optimization of the wounds and the patient? (Nutritional status, appropriate antibiotics, complete wound debridement.)
4. In what wound circumstances, would the paraspinal muscle flaps be perhaps most useful? (In deep defects that require two-layer muscle closure with the use of the paraspinal muscle flaps for the deep portions of the wound and a trapezius or latissimus flap for the next and more superficial layer.

   In the prophylactic or immediate reconstruction setting, elevation and advancement of the paraspinal muscles alone may suffice.)

   (a) Under what circumstances would the paraspinal muscle flaps be of limited usefulness? (With more lateral extension of either the previous wounds or operations such the more extensive lateral debridements have created loss of the intercostal arteries at the intercostal spaces.)
5. Describe two methods of use of the paraspinal muscles for wound closure. (Either as a "turnover" flap based principally on the medial branch and advancement flaps based more on the lateral branch. The former, turnover flaps, require mobilization by division of the thoracolumbar fascia and blunt dissection from the underlying bony skeleton. Medial advancement requires dissection deep to the transverse processes of the vertebral bodies, overlapping closure. Care must be directed towards not transecting, other than the medial branch, intercostal perforators emerging at 5 cm lateral.)
6. What are the landmarks for determination of the extent of the lateral or peripheral skin flap dissection? (Whether one plans to use turnover or sliding paraspinous muscle, the skin flaps should be elevated along the convex or posterior aspect of the muscle until the lateral groove is encountered, signaling the lateral extent of the paraspinous muscles and the location of the segmental blood supply. Although not explicitly discussed in the readings, simply release of the fascia lateral to the paraspinous muscles may not permit sufficient mobility for medial advancement and closure. In that instance, medial mobilization by dissection both medial and deep to the muscle mass may be necessary and perhaps liga-

tion of the medial perforators such that the muscles are pedicled on the lateral perforators alone.

   (a) The amount of bulk or muscle mass is more likely to be available in the lumbar or cervical region? (The paraspinous muscles become considerably thinner and less bulky in the more superior portions of the spine.)

7. Outline a possible role of the VAC in management of difficult and complex back wounds. (The VAC should not be used as a definitive modality in these complex cases. Rather the VAC, as used in other circumstances elsewhere, should be used as a bridge to definitive reconstructive closure.)
8. The trapezius can be utilized in closure of the back and neck wounds. Describe the vascular supply for each of those methods. (Direct elevation and bilateral advancement of the trapezius muscle based on the branches of the transverse cervical artery can be performed. A myocutaneous option consists of the inferior portion of the muscle and overlying skin based on the descending branch of the transverse cervical artery, rotated and/or advanced into a more superior wound as a myocutaneous flap.

   The trapezius perforator flap, based on the dorsal scapular artery is a second option, harvested from the posterior trapezius. As described above, the posterior trapezius myocutaneous flap is harvested as a skin and muscle island, based on the descending branch of the transverse cervical. The perforator flap, in contrast, harvests skin–soft tissue only by identification of a distal perforator at a point approximately 8–9 cm lateral to the midline and 6–8 cm inferior to the scapular spine. The perforators are located with a Doppler and retrograde intramuscular dissection is performed to isolate the flap on the dorsal scapular artery, a branch of either the subclavian or the transverse cervical artery. The pedicle may be short.)
9. Discuss the use of the scapular or periscapular flaps for back reconstruction. (Since the vascular leash for both flaps enters laterally and the subscapular axis is an axillary structure, only lateral and superior back wounds can be addressed, not midline. Also, both are fasciocutaneous flaps without the bulk that muscles provide for deep wounds.)
10. What are some different methods by which the latissimus dorsi can be utilized in closure? Describe the vascular supply for each of those methods. (Direct advancement flaps either with or without the overlying skin performed bilaterally enables closure of distal thoracic and proximal lumbar wounds, based on the dominant vascular pedicle, the thoraco-dorsal artery. The minor pedicle arises from posterior intercostal arteries and forms the basis for a "reverse" or turnover latissimus flap.)
    (a) Where is the minor vascular pedicle located and the potential inherent difficulty with a "reverse" latissimus dorsi flap? (The perforators are located consistently 5 cm from the midline, at the 9, 10, 11th intercostal space but may be damaged as a result of prior operations.)
11. Describe the use of a gluteal flap for an appropriate defect of the posterior trunk. (Probably the most commonly utilized option in gluteal flaps would be bilateral V-Y advancements based on a complete release of the gluteus maximus and laterally by division of the insertion on the greater trochanter and the sacro-tuberous ligaments and advancement into the midline.)
    (a) What perforator flaps are available? (A superior gluteal artery perforator based on the superior gluteal artery. See below.)
12. Free flaps are listed as an option for back reconstruction. Comment on some pros and cons of the following recipient vessels:
    (a) Intercostals (Resection may have sacrificed those vessels; also possible sacrifice of the nutrient vessels to the spinal cord at the level of T10.)
    (b) Lumbar perforators (The lumbar artery perforator is also an option, based on a segmental lumbar artery. The vessels are 5–8 cm off the midline and the pedicle is quite short. Dissection in an effort to lengthen the pedicle can place the dorsal spinal nerve at risk.)
    (c) Superior gluteal (The superior gluteal artery perforator is a possibility for low sacral defects. The intramuscular dissection is tedious and the pedicle also can be short.)
    (d) Thoracodorsal (Necessity for long vein grafts.)
13. What is another option besides the ones discussed above namely, trapezius, latissimus, paraspinal, and gluteal flaps that might be used uncommonly for closure of complex back wounds? (Probably the remaining option is the use of the omentum tunneled into the back. Clearly, this option would be one of last resort since utilization would require a laparotomy, position change and dissection of a tunnel into the back, and creation of a posterior hernia.)
14. Discuss closure of the following:
    (a) Large 8 × 10 cm defect of T2-T5 (Trapezius plus bilateral latissimus dorsi flaps.)
    (b) Similar size defect of L1-L5 (Turnover paraspinous muscle flaps plus thoraco-lumbar fascia as indicated; bilateral latissimus composite flaps with fasciocutaneous extension over gluteal region, probable STSG for skin closure.)
    (c) Moderate, 5 × 5 cm, size defect of the sacrum. (The first option is rotation of gluteal flap or flaps, based on the superior gluteal artery. The next line option is a lumbar artery perforator flap, based on a lumbar artery, usually more inferior as L_{4-5}.)

15. What is the argument for immediate versus delayed reconstruction of complex back wounds? (By definition the term "immediate reconstruction" implies other than primary closure. Since the operation is prophylactic or preventive of complications, the probability of occurrence of the same has to be sufficiently high to justify the risk and that proportion of the patients that will derive no benefit should be low since they are not destined to sustain a wound complication. To further refine the at-risk group, consideration for immediate reconstruction would include prior radiotherapy and/or operations, smoker, significant comorbidities as diabetes, perhaps also if extensive instrumentation will be required.)

Myelomeningocele

1. You and neurosurgery are consulted by the neonatologist for a newborn with a myelomeningocele of the thoracolumbar area. The neurosurgeon has never seen a myelomeningocele.
   (a) Comment on the appropriateness and urgency of treatment. (The use of past criteria of watchful waiting is not currently acceptable, so you must treat urgently.)
   (b) What is the overarching determination of the infant outcome both from the diagnosis and treatment perspectives? (Hydrocephalus and the treatment necessity of placement of a shunt.)
2. Discuss the dichotomy or dilemma in treatment of myelomeningocele for the neonate. (The neonate is inherently physiologically unstable, easily becomes hypothermic, and will not tolerate blood loss since the blood volume is small. The plastic surgeon must sail between the "rock" of adequate, consistent, and reliable closure of the defect vs. the "hard place" of the inherent physiologic instability of the neonate that limits the extent of the operation.)
3. Outline an option for closure of the following defects.
   (a) 6 × 6 cm thoracolumbar myelomeningocele (Advancement of compound latissimus–skin muscle flaps with lateral release if necessary.)
   (b) 4 × 4 cm sacral myelomeningocele (Sacral defects are quite difficult to obtain primary closure but, if possible, bilateral advancement gluteal flaps might suffice. In addition, these children are usually intact neurologically and ambulatory. Split-thickness skin graft is an option.)
   (c) 9 × 9 cm lumbosacral myelomeningocele (STSG and return at age 12–18 months and excise the skin graft and close with fasciocutaneous or musculocutaneous, gluteal V-Y advancement flaps.)
4. Associated anomalies of the CNS and significance? (Arnold–Chiari with hydrocephalus. These anomalies may result in an increase in CSF pressure, hydrocephalus, and bulging of the spinal dural closure. As such, a shunt may be necessary, in some instances even prophylactically.)
5. Discuss the role of prenatal prophylaxis as well as prenatal surgery. (The advent in widespread application of prenatal folic acid supplementation has dramatically reduced the incidence as well as the occurrence of large myelomeningocele.

   An exciting development in specialized centers has been the introduction of intrautero repair, capitalizing on the beneficial aspects of fetal wound healing.)
6. Parents present a 2 year-old male with a large "lipoma" of the buttock referred by the pediatrician, which has been present since birth. Your exam and management. (Look for long tract signs, such as delayed or atypical ambulation, and a history of increasing size. Suspect intraspinal involvement and will need a workup; refer to a neurosurgeon or neurologist.)
   (a) Other possible physical and possible CT findings? (Dermal sinus, hemangioma, hirsutism, or a patch of hair. Intraspinal lipoma, spina bifida occulta.)

Case-Based Conference

Case 1—Complex Back Wound

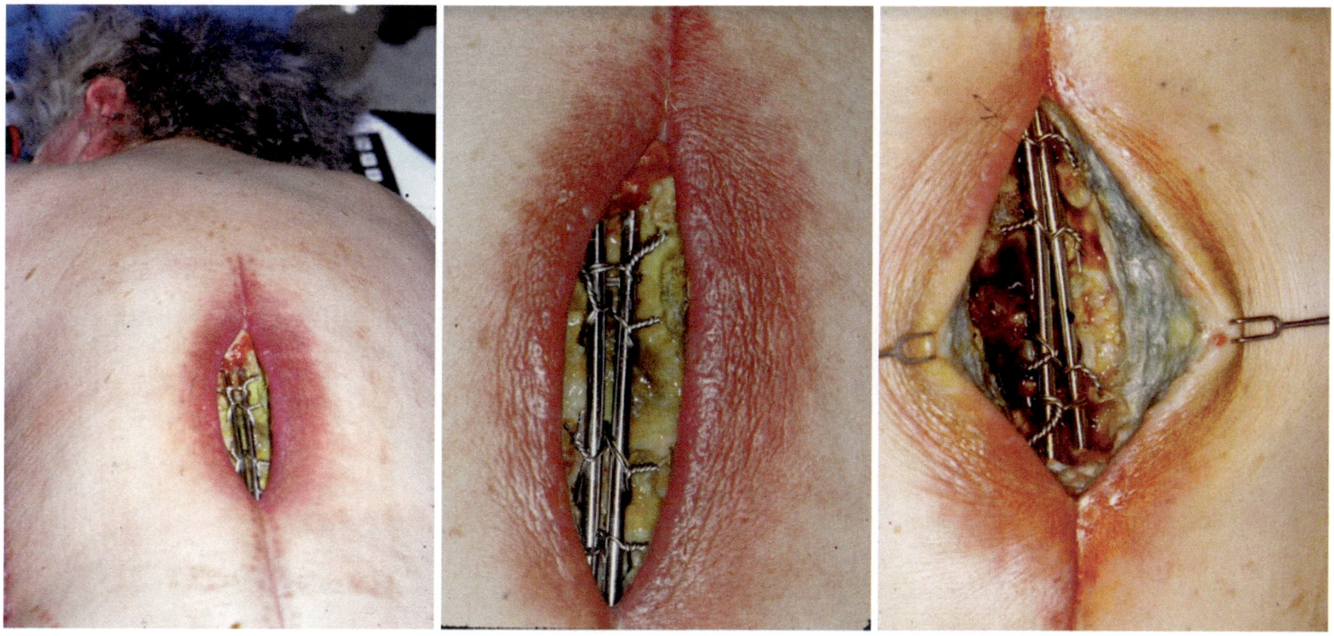

A 68-year-old woman who has received radiotherapy followed by instrumentation for a pathological fracture of the thoracic spine, complicated by wound breakdown 1 month postoperatively.

1. Describe the first two slide(s). Be specific about what the slides demonstrate. Add a focused clinical examination. Although the patient has metastatic disease, the oncologist advises you that the metastases are "stable."
2. Describe in detail the pathology of this patient's wound.
3. Outline a treatment plan. Assume the third slide represents adequate debridement.

Case-Based Conference: Discussion

Case 1—Complex Back Wound

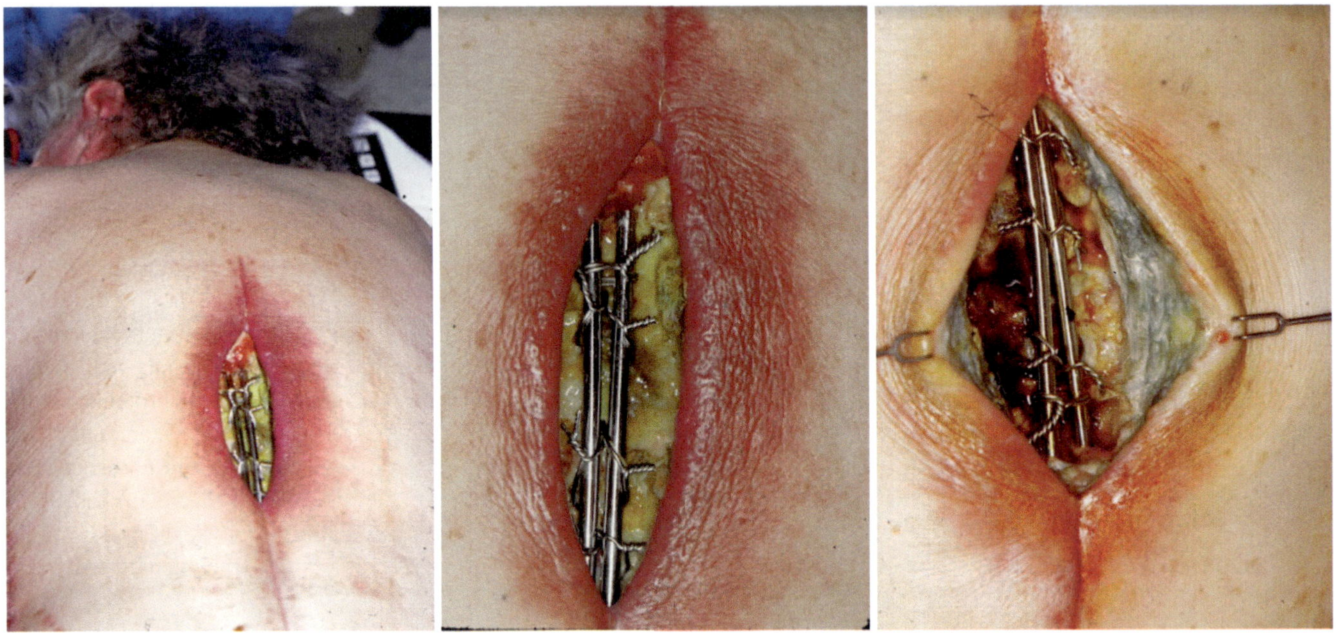

A 68-year-old woman who has received radiotherapy followed by instrumentation for a pathological fracture of the thoracic spine, complicated by wound breakdown 1 month postoperatively.

1. Describe the slide(s). Be specific about what the slides demonstrate. (A patient in prone position with the remarkable finding of a large, approximately 10 × 5 cm, wound in the midline of the low thoracic region. Exposed hardware consisting of large securing wires and rods is obvious. The surrounding skin for several centimeters on either side is red–purple in discoloration. A healed midline incision of recent duration is evident superior and inferior to the open wound. No other scars are evident. The first close-up view depicts all the visible wound soft tissue as necrotic and/or infected. The second close-up photo with retraction by double hooks demonstrates probable adjacent necrotic fascia throughout the length of the wound. Seen on the left side of the wound is some dark, liquid-appearing material, the bone is not readily visible.

   Add a focused clinical examination. Although the patient has metastatic disease, the oncologist advises you that the metastases are "stable." (The primary thrust of the history is assessment of the oncologic status. The oncologist has advised that metastases are "stable," but what is the extent of metastatic disease elsewhere, particularly pulmonary and hepatic. If the patient is currently on chemotherapy, that fact needs to be established as well as any comorbidities that exist. Ascertainment of the timing and dosage of the radiotherapy, neurologic function pre- and postoperative, as well as nutritional and functional status would all be important. Available information from the spine surgeon would include the quality of bone with placement of the transosseous wires as well as an impression whether the wound simply dehisced or was primarily infected, drained, and then dehisced. Physical exam would also evaluate neurologic status, particularly evidence of loss of some motor function in the lower extremities and assess as much as feasible the depth and extent of the wound, but thorough exploration will await the operating room. Overall functional status should be estimated.)

   (a) Any tests indicated? (Patient probably has had recent imaging, although at this early point postoperative, imaging would be of limited value. Routine lab work including albumin and prealbumin for evaluation of nutritional status.)

2. Describe in detail the pathology of this patient's wound. (Primary healing was not obtained in this postoperative wound for several reasons: the area was previously irradiated, substantial soft tissue dissection was necessary for exposure and implantation of the hardware, and the patient was probably in a catabolic state secondary to the metastatic cancer. The presenting problem now is exposed of recently implanted and essential spinal hardware in the depths of what appears to be a necrotic and infected wound. The status of the bone is somewhat uncertain but clearly has been irradiated.)

3. Outline a treatment plan and give your rationale. (The first of the steps to definitive wound closure is wound toilet by debridement. Debridement will require excision of the necrotic fascia, visible in the third photo, infected necrotic soft tissue, and irradiated skin. At the debridement setting, evaluation of the hardware with respect to tightness of the wires and the stability of the rods should be performed by the orthopedics service. A limited bone debridement is performed as well. Any request for removal and replacement of the hardware to orthopedics will, in all likelihood, encounter strong objection and, regardless, is not necessary at 1 month since established osteomyelitis is highly unlikely. The decision process, once the wound is thoroughly debrided, is the timing of definitive closure. If debridement consisted solely of excision of necrotic tissue and irradiated skin, strong consideration should be given to closure as a single-stage procedure, probably not likely in this particular scenario. If the specter of infection looms either because of purulence unroofed at debridement and/or a history of same, then the prudent decision would be an interval of wound management either with dressings or with negative wound pressure therapy, the wound VAC, assuming dura exposure with CSF leakage is not present.

The wound closure option needs to provide well-vascularized tissue for reconstruction as well as sufficient bulk to fill the inevitable dead space. Paraspinous muscles, as one component of the reconstructive plan, can fill a majority of the dead space as well as provide muscle for suppression of bacterial growth. The paraspinous muscles, relatively small in the cervical and lumbosacral region, are larger in the thoracic and thoraco-lumbar region. The muscles are perfused by the medial and lateral branches of the segmental intercostal perforators, both derived from the same trunk and can be utilized either as bilateral advancement or turnover flaps, sutured over the hardware and into the dead space. The lateral branch is larger than the medial. The location of the medial is 3 cm, lateral 5 cm, and main intercostal perforator, the source of these branches is usually located approximately 5–7 cm from the midline. The design of a "turnover" flap based principally on the medial branch or the advancement flap based more on the lateral branch. The former, turnover flaps, require mobilization by division of the thoraco-lumbar fascia and blunt dissection over the underlying bony skeleton. Medial advancement requires dissection deep to the transverse processes of the vertebral bodies, overlapping closure. Care must be directed with advancement towards not transecting the main intercostal perforators other than the medial branch, if necessary. In all likelihood, neither option is available in this case, as evident from the photo post-debridement. Exploration and debridement will provide the information for an intraoperative decision.

Provision of skin closure is accomplished by wide undermining deep to the latissimus on the chest wall, a process initiated by the undermining to expose the lateral aspect of the paraspinous muscles. The two latissimus muscles are opposed over the paraspinous closure, if accomplished, as a composite muscle and skin flap. Rarely, a longitudinal lateral release of skin and soft tissue may be necessary to advance the flaps. Drains are placed deep to the latissimus suture line and in each chest wall donor site. More distal wound locations than the scenario depicted will require bilateral gluteal V-Y advancement or lumbar perforator flaps.

Editorial note: Discussion of the technical highlights of the performance of gluteal fasciocutaneous V-Y flaps is included in Chap. 55, Case 1.

More superior defects, cervical and upper thoracic, require a similar approach with utilization of the trapezius muscles, again mobilized as a composite muscle and skin flap. (Dissection is performed in a plane deep to the trapezius but superficial to the rhomboids, scapula, and underlying supra- and infraspinatus muscles.)

Intraoperative

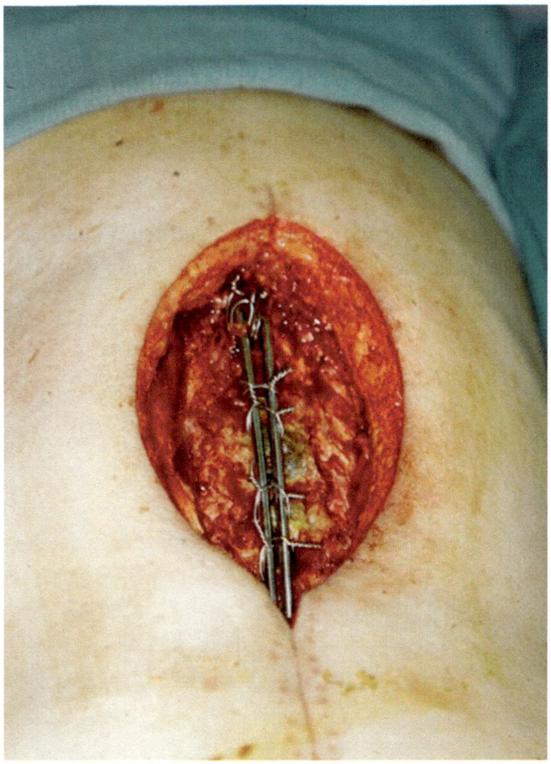

A debridement has excised necrotic and presumably contaminated or infected fascia, muscle, and skin. The resultant defect was closed with bilateral advancement composite flaps of latissimus, soft tissue, and skin.

Case-Based Conference

Case 2A—Myelomeningocele

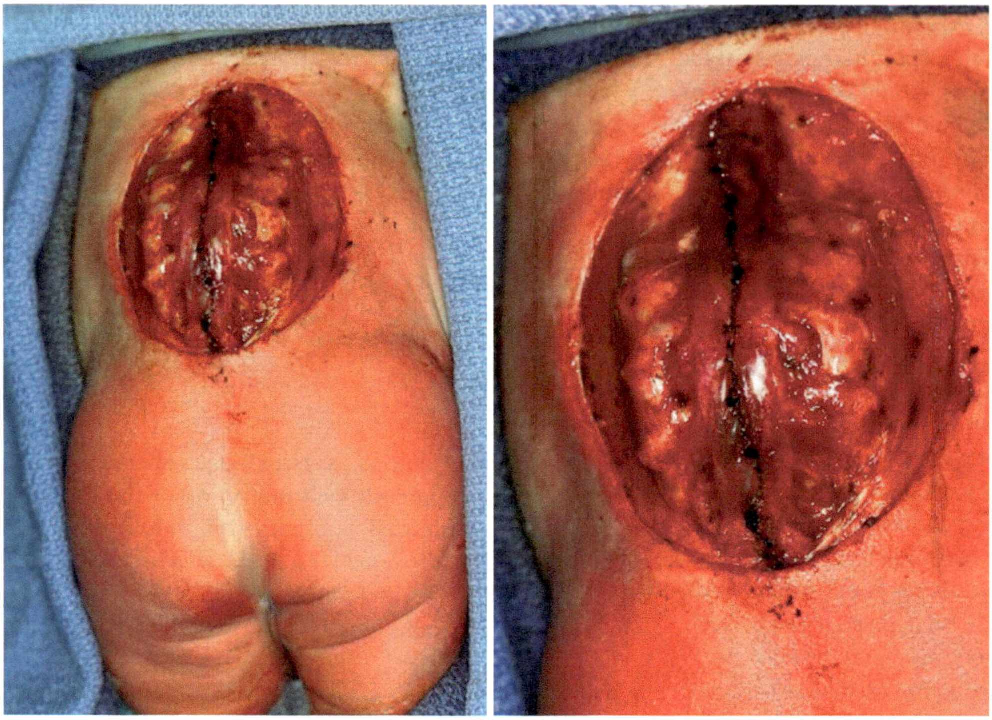

You are called to the OR by neurosurgery who has just completed dural repair of a large myelomeningocoele in a 18-h-old, 3000-gram infant. The defect measures 12 × 10 cm.

1. Describe the slides.
2. What additional information do you need from neurosurgery and anesthesia? What are the overarching concerns at this juncture?
3. Use the pathologic anatomy and natural history of myelomeningocele to help you formulate your treatment plan. What are the treatment objectives?
4. List a menu of options with pros and cons, select your treatment plan, and describe.
5. Short- and long-term follow-up including potential complications.

Case 2B—Myelomeningocele

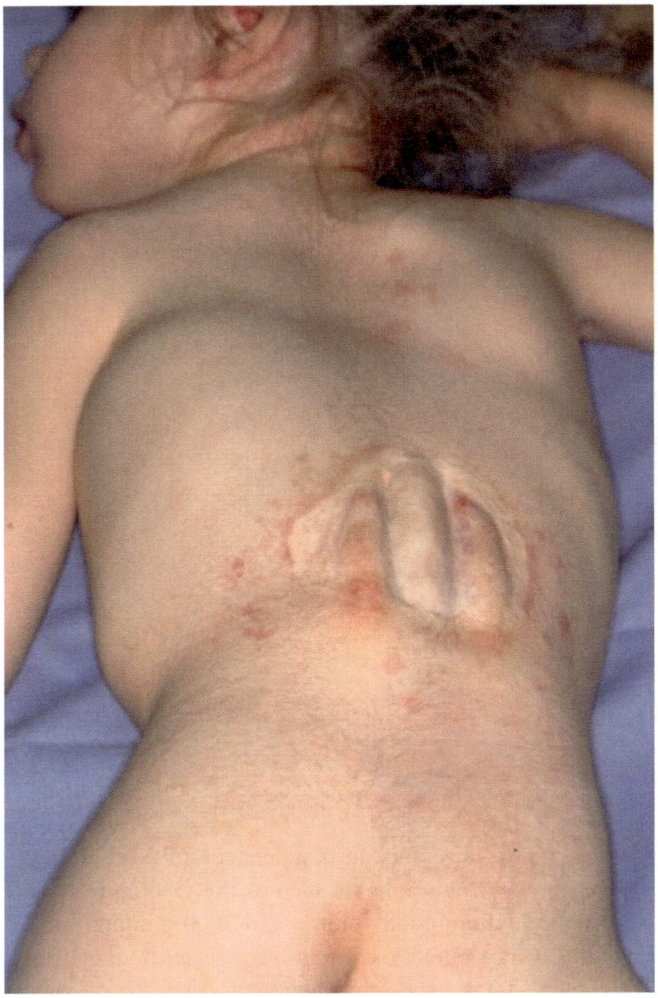

The child is now 3 years old. Orthopedics plans correction of kyphoscoliosis and desires "coverage."

1. Describe the slides, add a clinical exam.
   (a) Any tests?
2. What is the pathology and what is the underlying cause?
3. What will be required to provide "coverage" for ortho? Outline a treatment plan, including incisions, steps, and sequence.

Case-Based Conference: Discussion

Case 2A—Myelomeningocele

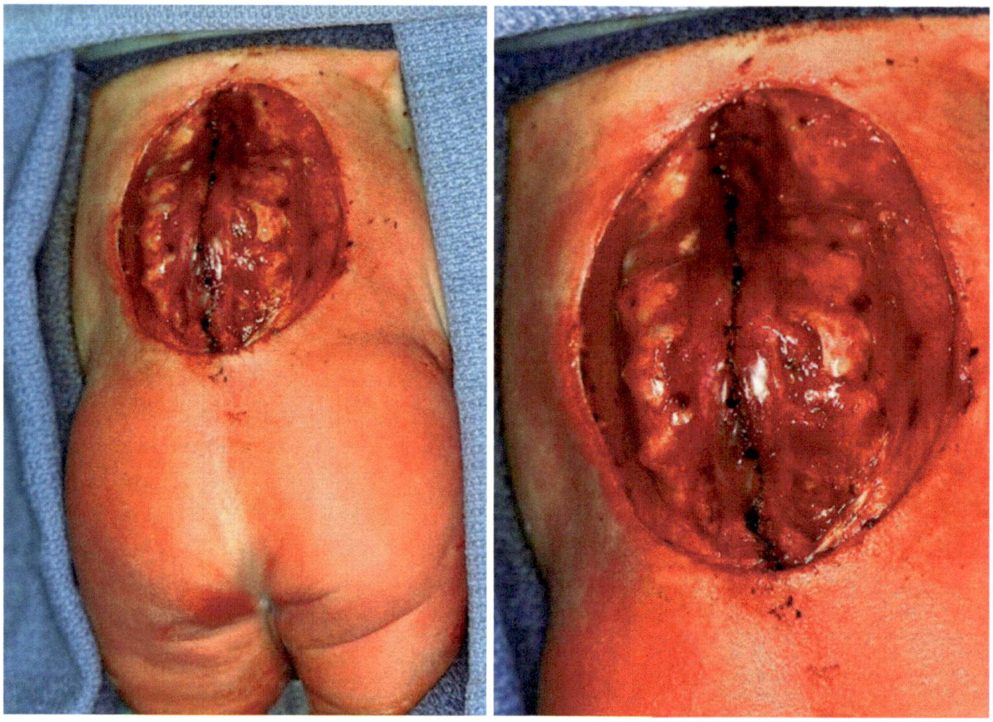

You are called to the OR by neurosurgery who has just completed dural repair of a large myelomeningocoele in a 18-h-old, 3000-gram infant. The defect measures 12 × 10 cm.

1. Describe the slides. (Two slides are provided of the infant in a prone position and include in the first a view from the proximal thigh to the upper back region. A large open wound consistent in size with the description of a 12 × 10 cm myelomeningocele is depicted. The defect extends from a point just superior to the buttock fold to the upper thoracic region. The myelomeningocele sac and placode has been excised and the dura closed with a suture line that courses throughout the length of the defect. The splayed vertebral bodies are evident on the right and left and lateral to the dural sac.)
2. What additional information do you need from neurosurgery and anesthesia? What are the overarching concerns at this juncture? (The stability of the infant. Information about duration of the procedure, blood loss, and core temperature changes are all crucial. Given the high incidence of hydrocephalus and elevated CSF and intraspinal pressure from a number of attendant malformations including Arnold–Chiari, does the neurosurgeon plan a shunt at this setting, preferable, or in the very near future?

   The overarching concern at this juncture is the inherent physiologic instability of the neonate, including most importantly, difficulty in maintenance of core temperature in cool environments such as the Operating Room. The circulating blood volume of a 3000 g infant implies that a 100 cc blood loss equates to greater than one-third of the total, the threshold of hypotonic shock. Intraoperative measures of controlled room temperature, heat lamps, and judicious administration of IV fluids provide the setting for safe surgery on a neonate, but these liabilities are the concerns that dominate this clinical setting.)
3. Use the pathologic anatomy and natural history of myelomeningocele to help you formulate your treatment plan. What are the treatment objectives? (The principal pathologic anatomy is a dysraphism or separation of the dorsal aspect of the involved soft tissue and bony vertebrae, exposing the involved spinal cord. As a result, the bony, muscular, and skin components are displaced laterally with exposure of the open neural tube. The covering of the meninges and placode is inadequate so the first priority is closure of the neural tube and the next is to obtain reliable skin coverage.

   The other particular is the necessity to optimize a functional outcome by early closure to prevent further loss of neural tissue. The open neural structures, leaking CSF fluid, exposes the infant to meningitis and sepsis. In the past, a policy of "watchful waiting" was adopted in large meningomyeloceles to permit secondary healing, a policy that has no contemporary application. In fact, some degree of urgency exists since the exposed cord or filaments are subject to desiccation, progressive neuronal loss, and sepsis as mentioned above.)

4. List a menu of options with pros and cons, select your treatment plan, and describe. (The list of options for closure of a myelomeningocele defect of this magnitude are few. Any type of transposition or rotation flap is destined for necrosis with the unacceptable sequelae described above. One option is advancement of large bilateral composite muscle–skin flaps bipedicled on the angiosomes of the thoracodorsal artery superiorly and the gluteal vessels inferiorly. To do so requires dissection deep to the latissimus over the chest wall superiorly and the lumbar fascia inferiorly. If the dissection continues laterally over the convexity of the trunk and advancement proves insufficient, a lateral release of skin–soft tissue has been described but probably not advisable in a neonate. This method will provide closure of most thoracolumbar myelomeningoceles but probably not for a lesion of these proportions.

   If so, and only a partial closure is obtained, the final resort is a split-thickness skin graft. Harvest of the skin graft from the buttock is associated with some blood loss even with tumescence and rather than bolstered, should be managed postoperatively with saline dressings, maintained constantly wet. Because the closure of the myelo defect with skin graft predisposes to gibbus formation and late ulceration, the treatment plan should include a deferral to age 18–24 months for excision of the graft, a tedious proposition, and definitive closure.
5. Short- and long-term follow-up including potential complications. (These patients are subject to a myriad of adverse consequences of their disability that span the specialty of plastic surgery, orthopedics, urology, and rehabilitation medicine and dictate long-term follow-up in a multidisciplinary clinic.)

Postoperative (8 Months)

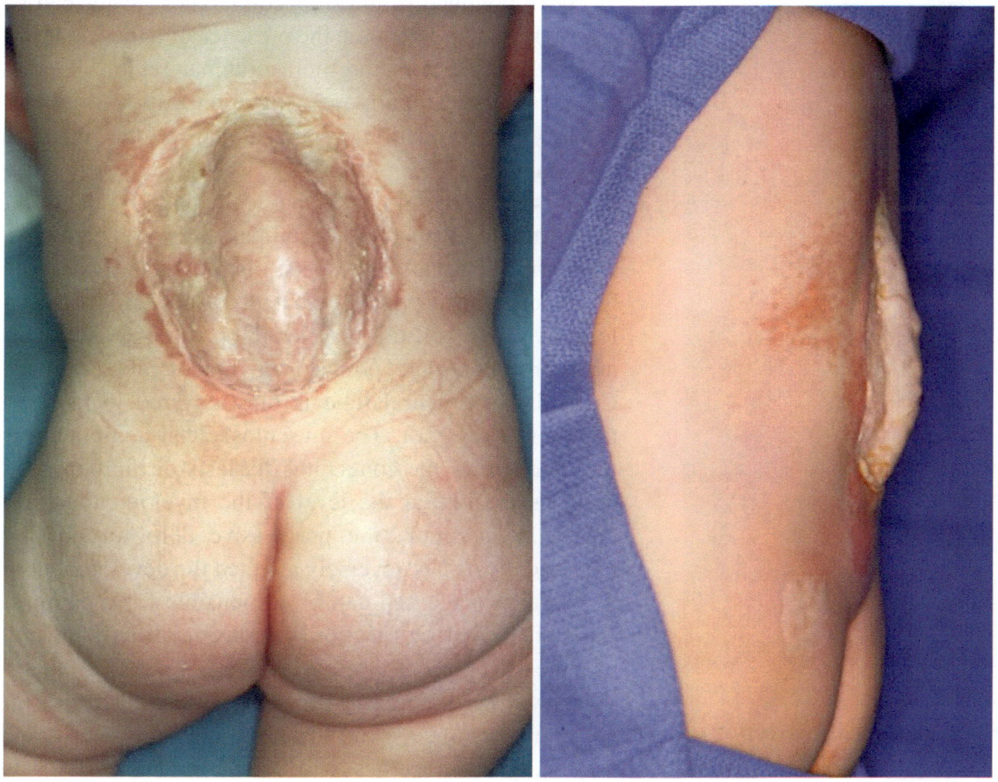

In two photos, posterior and lateral, the skin graft has fully healed and is reflective of the size of the original myelomeningocele. The skin-grafted defect incorporates a defect from midthoracic to mid sacral and demonstrates some secondary contraction of the original size. The central one-half is occupied by the bulging neural tube confirmed on the lateral view.

Critique

A split-thickness skin graft might have been the only option in this infant, particularly if somewhat unstable at birth. Nevertheless, progressive gibbus deformity can occur and at age 18–24 months, consideration should be given to excision of the skin graft. If so, a preliminary placement of bilateral tissue expanders beneath elevated compound latissimus muscle and skin flaps may assist considerably in utilization of those flaps for subsequent closure of the defect.

Case 2B—Myelomeningocele

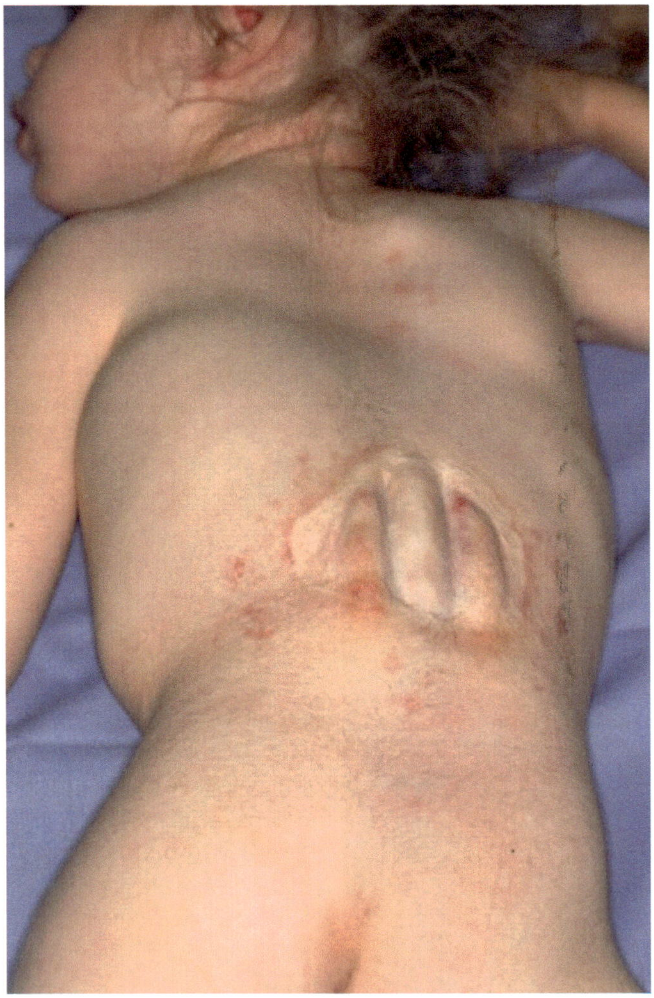

The child is now 3 years old. Orthopedics plans correction of kyphoscoliosis and desires "coverage."

1. Describe the slides, add a clinical exam. (The single photo is of the child in a prone position and encompasses the entire trunk and a portion of the buttocks. Several findings are evident including the skin-grafted defect of the thoracolumbar region. The defect is of substantial size, perhaps 10 × 10 cm. The central area is occupied by a fusiform and smooth structure, the neural tube. On the right and left lateral aspect of the neural tube are also two longitudinal raised prominences that course the length of the defect from cephalad to caudad. These prominences probably represent the splayed vertebrae. No ulcerations nor decubiti are evident. The appearance of the posterior thoracic rib cage is distinctly abnormal. The entire left side both posterior and lateral bulges outward from the tip of the scapula to or in proximity to the posterior iliac crest. The child's torso seems inclined to the left. A gibbus deformity is not evident in the photo.

   The clinical examination should establish the social support and multidisciplinary management of the attendant problems of the myelomeningocele patient. Of particular interest to the reconstructive surgeon is the pulmonary and nutritional status, since both can impact the management plan. The determination of ambulatory status should also be accomplished. The physical examination should assess the quality and pliability of the adjacent intact skin and soft tissue and, if possible, the presence of a functioning latissimus.)
   (a) Any tests? (In all likelihood, a CT scan or scans have been obtained from orthopedics. Those scans can be reviewed to determine the presence of a muscle layer, the latissimus in the thoracolumbar region. As discussed above, pulmonary function tests and laboratory determination of nutritional profile may be beneficial.)
2. What is the pathology and what is the underlying cause? (The pathologic anatomy encompasses several elements. First, the skin graft represents, obviously, is inadequate for the orthopedic procedure but also is not sufficient long term as stable soft tissue to avoid breakdown and ulceration from pressure points from braces and orthotics. Critically, the neural tube is only covered by a split-thickness skin graft. The musculoskeletal component is the outcome of the congenital diastasis of the bony and soft tissue spine at the level of the myelomeningocele defect. In addition, the progressive deformity of the kyphoscoliosis has adversely affected the development of the thoracic cage and can be responsible for a compromise of respiratory function—a consideration in general anesthesia for a protracted operation.)
3. What will be required to provide "coverage" for ortho? Outline a treatment plan, including incisions, steps, and sequence. (Orthopedics will resect bone and will do instrumentation and placement of hardware at several vertebral levels in a somewhat lengthy operation. The provision of the necessary full-thickness coverage can be accomplished simultaneously after completion of the orthopedics portion, but in all likelihood the available skin and soft tissue will not be adequate, enhanced by the mandate that ischemia, "epidermolysis," or wound heal-

ing problems cannot occur. The summary of the reconstructive requirements dictate some form of tissue transfer is necessary, in this instance tissue expansion. A prior placement of tissue expanders, bilaterally, in the plane beneath or deep to the latissimus muscle can recruit the additional tissue for the use of a compound muscle and skin flap. Two options exist: one, placement of the expanders, complete expansion, followed by a second procedure of removal of the expanders, excision of the skin graft, and closure. To do so will ensure a stable wound but deferral of the orthopedic spine surgery to a third operation. The other option is preliminary expansion, excision of the skin graft, completion of the orthopedic procedure followed by advancement of the expanded flaps for definitive closure. Two operations is the benefit of that option but dissection of the skin graft from the dura is a tedious procedure and is fraught with the hazard of a dural tear and resultant CSF leak—a complication more suitably addressed at a separate setting than the orthopedic intervention.)

Intra- and Postoperative (5 Days)

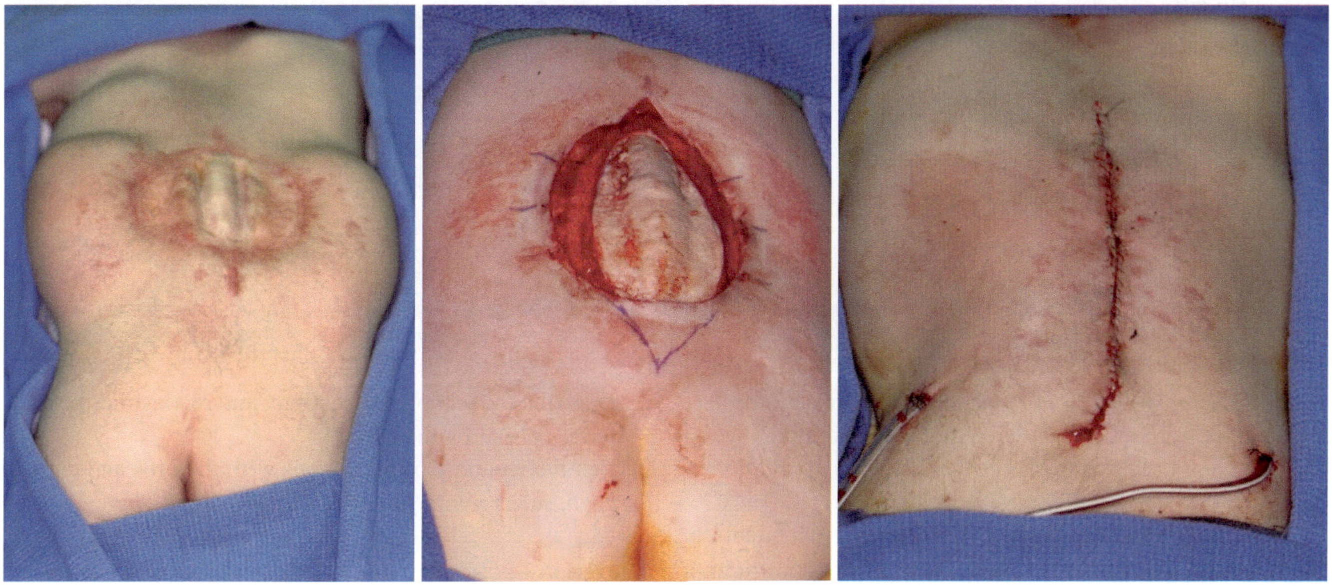

Bilateral submuscular rectangular tissue expanders were placed, expanded, and then the patient returned to the OR. The second operative procedure sequence consisted of excision of skin graft by plastic surgeon, then orthopedic spine surgery, and wound closure by plastic surgery.

The wound at an early point postoperatively demonstrates viable flaps and intact closure. The patient healed uneventfully.

Case-Based Conference

Case 3—Back Wound

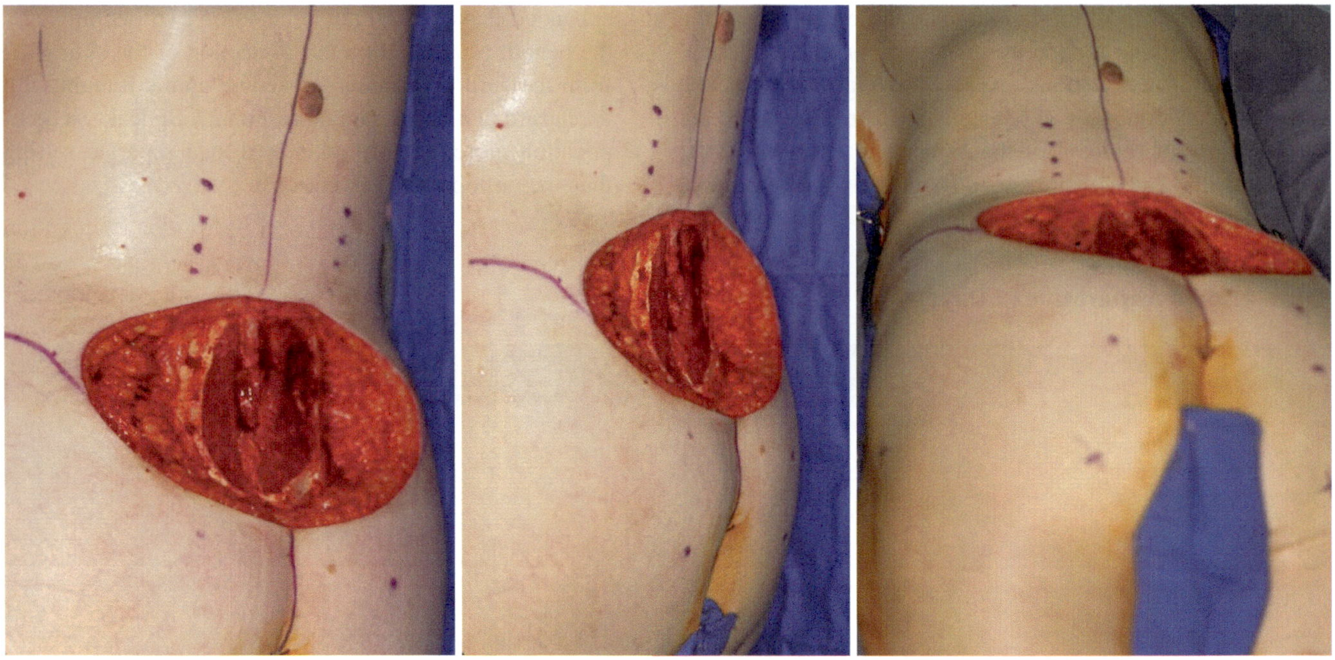

A lumbosacral wound after resection of a fibrosarcoma that included the spinous processes of the vertebrae in a 30 year-old. Adjuvant radiotherapy is planned.

1. Describe the slides and add a clinical examination. Assume the patient was seen in consultation preoperatively.
   (a) Any tests indicated? Assume imaging has been obtained by the surgical oncologist.
2. Describe the pathologic anatomy and reconstructive challenges posed by the defect.
3. List the wound closure options with the pros and cons of each, select yours, and describe and draw.

Case-Based Conference: Discussion

Case 3—Back Wound

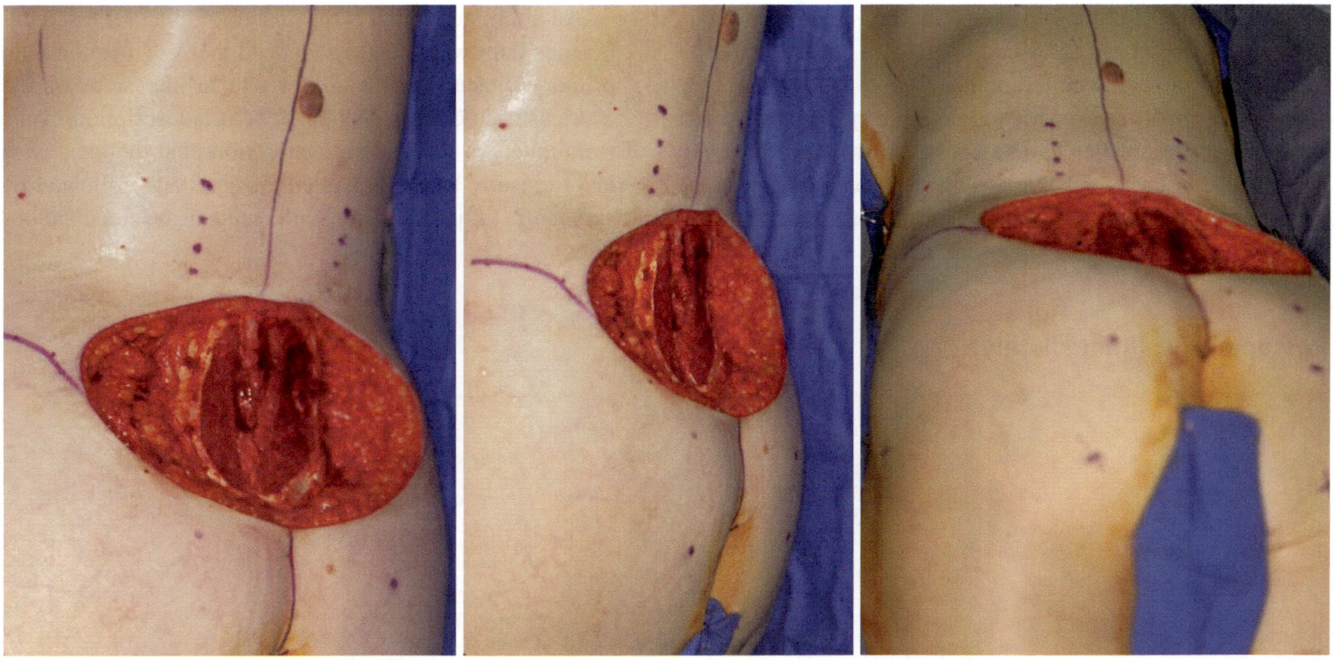

A lumbosacral wound after resection of a fibrosarcoma that included the spinous processes of the vertebrae in a 30 year-old. Adjuvant radiotherapy is planned.

1. Describe the slides and add a clinical examination. Assume the patient was seen in consultation preoperatively. (The first of these photos depict the posterior trunk of the patient in the prone position. The view is from the buttocks to mid thoracic. A large, fresh wound is present in the lumbosacral region, extending from the apex of the buttocks cleft to perhaps Lumbar 1 or 2. A line or surgical marking is visible on the left that appears to correspond to the iliac crest. The lateral extent of the wound is nearly to this line on the posterior iliac crest. Estimates of the size would be 15–18 cm wide by 12–15 cm. The characteristics of the defect include extensive exposure of the paraspinal muscles, absence of the investing fascia, except the far lateral extent. The most central or midline appears to consist of exposed bone. Other findings include surgical markings on the buttock and lumbar area in the paramedian line, dots only that perhaps mark the location of the superior gluteal artery in the former and intercostal perforators in the latter.

   The clinical examination is mostly to ensure as much as feasible that no significant comorbidities or bleeding diathesis exist. The consultation is also an opportunity to examine potential donor sites.)

   (a) Any tests indicated? Assume imaging has been obtained by the surgical oncologist. (Probably not. A discussion with the surgical oncologist re the resection plan would be important.)
2. Describe the pathologic anatomy and reconstructive challenges posed by the defect. (Soft-tissue defects of the lumbosacral area present a reconstructive challenge because of the paucity of options. In addition, the size of the wound is substantial and bone is exposed.)
3. List the wound closure options with the pros and cons of each, select yours, and describe and draw. (As described above, the reconstructive options in the lumbosacral area are limited and include skin grafts, lumbar and gluteal flaps. The application of split-thickness skin grafts to this particular defect would not be appropriate given the exposed bone in the central portion. One approach with utilization of local tissue is the use of the paraspinal muscles either bilaterally as turnover or advancement flaps. Once accomplished, the entire wound could be grafted. The cons of this choice is the absence of soft tissue padding and the issue of durability.

   The lumbar perforator flap has been described and utilized as a free flap for breast reconstruction. The flap is based on the posterior segmental arteries in the lumbar region, termed the lumbar arteries, and can be pedicled as a propeller flap. However, the dominant perforators lie at the level of L_{3-4} located approximately 7 cm at the midline, and undoubtedly sacrificed with the tumor resection. Perhaps a similar-style flap could be designed more superiorly, pivoted off one of the more proximal perforators. The difficulties to surmount, though, are the relatively small caliber of those vessels in the superior lumbar region, a drawback enhanced by the size and the anterior extent of the flap required in this case.

In contrast, the superior gluteal artery remains intact and a perforator flap can be harvested from the superior buttock. A unilateral flap would be prohibitively large, extended beyond the limits of the perfused angiosome, and precludes primary closure of the donor site. To address these liabilities, the employment of bilateral flaps would require the sometimes lengthy and tedious dissection to the source vessels times two and the donor site still may not permit primary closure.

An alternate choice is the design of bilateral fasciocutaneous flaps rotated and advanced in a V-Y fashion with primary closure of the donor site as the stem of the Y. Please see Case 1—Chap. 55. for a description of the technique. An optimal reconstruction plan then is a two-layer closure, local paraspinal muscle flaps, followed by skin–soft tissue closure with gluteal fasciocutaneous flaps.)

Postoperative (Immediately)

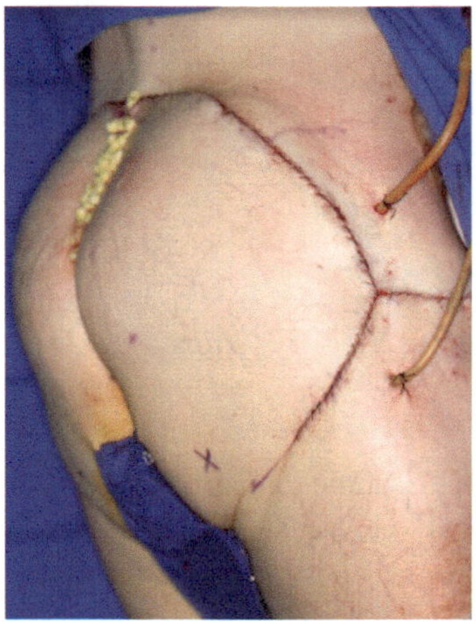

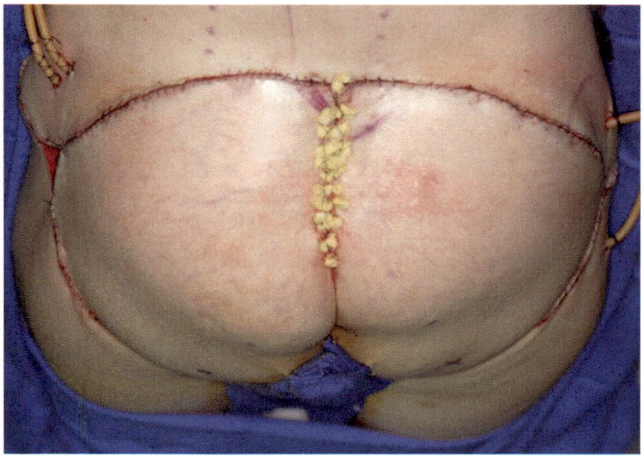

The two photos are of the patient still in the prone position. The defect has been closed by bilateral V-Y gluteal flaps that encompass the entire buttock. Direct closure of the flap donor defect laterally has been performed to create the V-Y configuration.

Case-Based Conference

Case 4—Difficult Wound

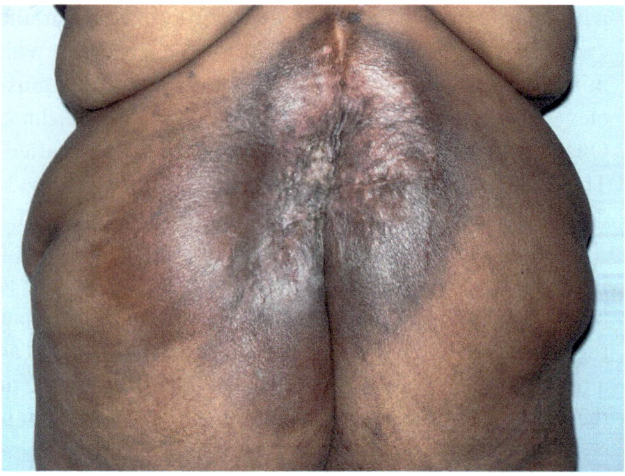

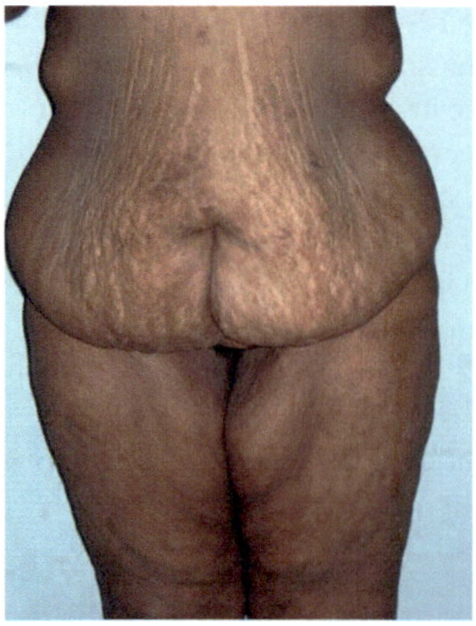

A 42-year-old non-insulin-dependent patient with a history of lumbosacral lesion for 2 to 3 years with gradual enlargement. Spontaneous drainage of pus for the past 6 months and incision and drainage and skin biopsy was performed 6 weeks ago. The skin biopsy was nondiagnostic.

1. Describe the slides and add a focused clinical examination.
   (a) Any tests indicated? Justify.
2. Outline a differential diagnosis. Explain how the clinical exam would narrow the list.
3. Describe a treatment plan that would address the new narrowed list of possible diagnoses. Any operation incorporated into the plan should also be outlined including drawing the excision, if so planned.

Case-Based Conference: Discussion

Case 4—Difficult Wound

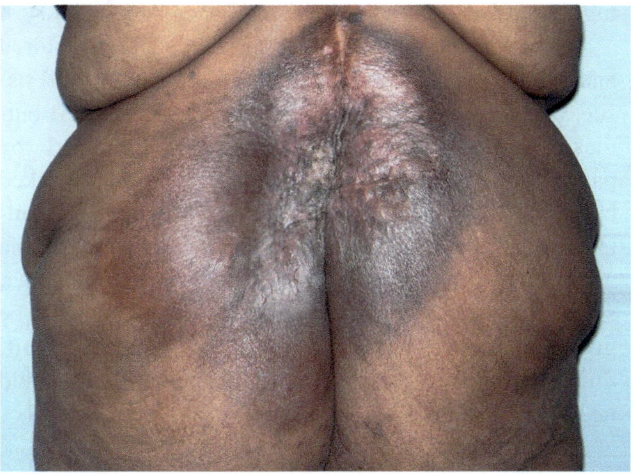

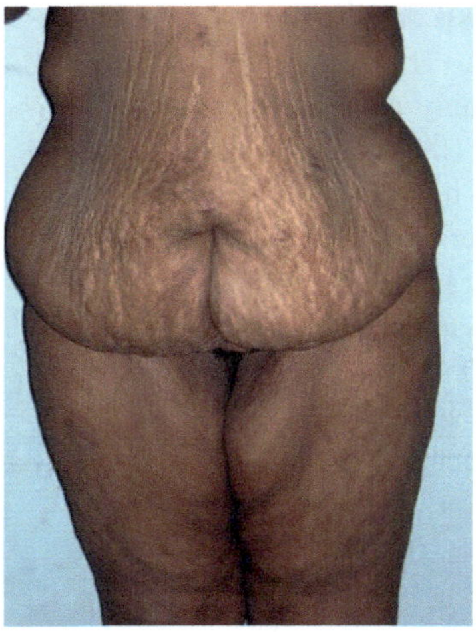

A 42-year-old non-insulin-dependent patient with a history of lumbosacral lesion for 2 to 3 years with gradual enlargement. Spontaneous drainage of pus for the past 6 months and incision and drainage and skin biopsy was performed 6 weeks ago. The skin biopsy was nondiagnostic.

1. Describe the slides and add a focused clinical examination. (Two photos of a Black obese patient, one limited to the posterior trunk from proximal or midthigh to lower thoracic region. Transverse rolls of skin and soft tissue are present at the junction of the hips and back. The other photo is of the anterior trunk also from midthoracic to knees. The most pertinent finding is a large central lesion that extends from the lumbar area to the midportion of the gluteal cleft. Laterally, more so on the left than the right, the lesion fans out into the buttock as well as the sacral and lumbar region. No ulceration or exophytic changes are evident but the skin has been altered markedly with darkening and plaque-like changes centrally and patchy lightening of skin superiorly as well as corrugation of the skin surface. The edges of the lesion are indistinct. On the left a triangular area, the tip pointed laterally, of lighter discoloration extends almost to the lateral edge of the buttock. Not including this latter area, the size of the central lesion is 15–18 cm in length and 10–12 cm in width. No other lesions are evident. The abdomen is marked by a substantially sized panniculus, redundant over the pubis onto the proximal thigh.

   The outcome of the clinical examination is crucial to the formulation of a treatment plan. The details of the history should be elucidated including initial appearance if known, the rate of growth over the past 6 months, and the nature of any past treatments. The subsequent questions would focus on associated symptoms including pain, factors that precipitate pain, nature and severity of the pain, and any dysfunction of the lower extremities. Any complaint of dysesthesia or paresthesia should be pursued for details. The presence of any systemic symptoms of malaise and/or any easily fatigability as well as comorbidities, in particular inflammatory bowel or autoimmune disease, is pursued. A social and family history and current medications will complete the history. The physical exam should ascertain the character of the lesion including palpation of firmness, mobility if any, and the nature and character of the soft tissue of the adjacent discolored skin of the buttocks for induration and firmness. A careful neurologic examination of the lower extremity including function and strength of the adductors of the thigh is also performed.)

(a) Any tests indicated? Justify. (Past medical records, if available, should be obtained including the pathology reading of the skin biopsy. Imaging of the lesion is mandatory, a CT scan initially. The composition of the soft tissue, the extent of the lesion, and any erosion and/or invasion of the underlying bone, the sacrum and lumbar vertebrae, should be observed. Additional tests would be triggered by a history suggestive of the presence of autoimmune disease or other comorbidities. Pathological examination of a repeat skin biopsy may be indicated.)

2. Outline a differential diagnosis. Explain how the clinical exam would narrow the list. (The preamble history and appearance of the lesion imply an inflammatory rather than a neoplastic etiology. The results of the CT scan would be helpful to establish the extent of the disease and a tentative diagnosis. Several possibilities exist that include necrobiosis lipoidica diabeticorum, pyoderma granulosum, calciphylaxis, and vasculitis. Necrobiosis lipoidica diabeticorum, NLD, has been described in diabetics but typically presents as red or yellow plaques on the lower extremity. The scenario illustrated would be a distinctly unusual presentation. Pyoderma granulosum is almost invariably ulcerated with undermined borders, also in association with a number of systemic disorders. Calciphylaxis occurs in renal failure patients and demonstrates calcium deposits in the small blood vessels. Vasculitis would be strongly suggested by inflammation and infiltrate of the dermal arterioles, although not necessarily universal, and would mandate the appropriate consultations for medical workup.)
3. Describe a treatment plan that would address the new narrowed list of possible diagnoses. Any operation incorporated into the plan should also be outlined including drawing the excision, if so planned. (Barring any additional diagnostic or medical information more than that provided by the case preamble and photos, excision by resection is the treatment of choice. Given the duration of the process and appearance of the lesion, a neoplasm is highly unlikely, confirmation by CT scan is mandatory.

   Resection should encompass all the deeply discolored and plaque-like lesion and neighboring indurated soft tissue, but in all probability spare the most lateral left buttock. Until a definitive diagnosis is obtained by pathological examination of the specimen, skin marked by a light discoloration would not be excised. The resultant defect would be substantial and in selection of the appropriate rung or option on the reconstructive ladder, skin graft, local or regional flaps, consideration should be given to the site of the defect, a weight-bearing area. Full-thickness coverage including fat to absorb pressure would be the optimal choice.)

Intraoperative

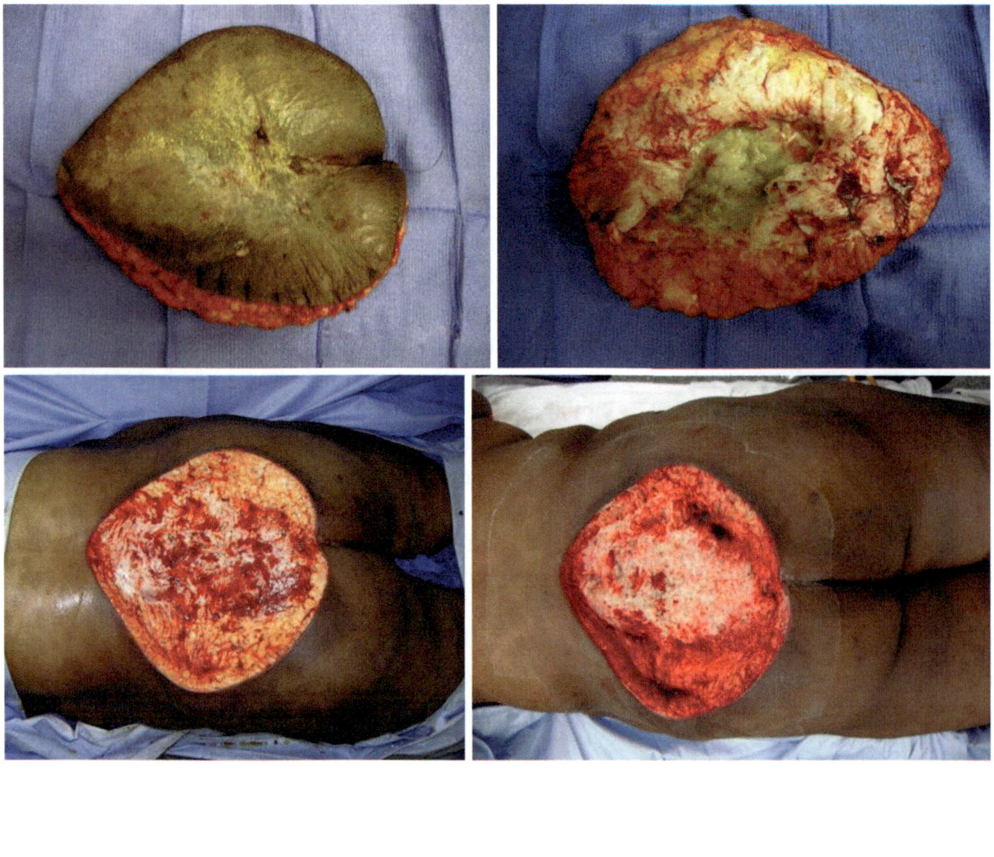

Two photos are of the skin side and deep aspect of the specimen. The thickness of the subcutaneous fat is substantial, probably 3 to 4 cm, but on the deep aspect of the specimen is a deep purulent crater with complete loss of fat.

The post-resection defect is also depicted. The excision involved the entire lesion and a portion of the discolored skin–soft tissue of the left buttock. The peripheral one-half of the bed consists of subcutaneous fat. The bed of the central portion appears to be lumbosacral fascia, although the photo is somewhat indistinct.

The patient was treated with negative wound pressure therapy for 6 days and then returned to the OR for definitive closure. A comprehensive pathological examination of the specimen failed to yield a definitive diagnosis.

Intraoperative (Post Closure)

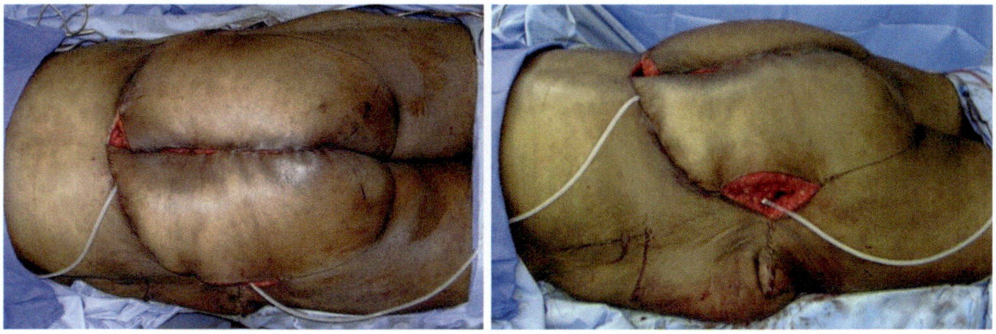

Intraoperative photos include the reconstruction after flap rotation and prior to definitive skin closure. Reconstruction has been accomplished by rotation of bilateral, large, inferiorly based buttock, sacral, and lumbar flaps with V to Y transverse closure of the lateral donor site.

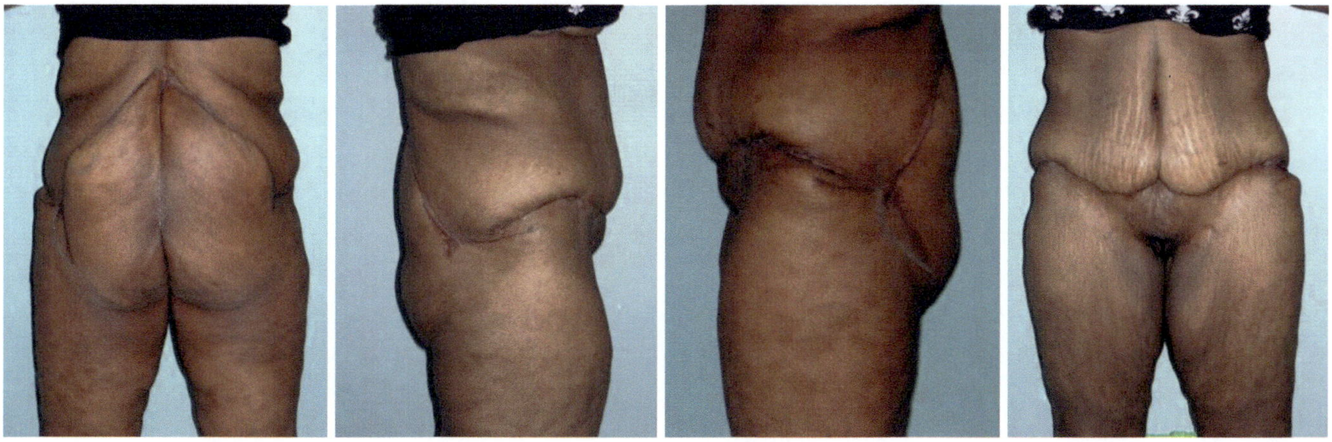

A subsequent series of photos obtained at 6 months demonstrate a healed wound without evidence of recurrence. At this juncture, the patient requested a panniculectomy.

The panniculectomy has healed as well.

Critique

The CT scan yielded important information of a large abscess located superficial to the deep fascia. A more conservative excision could have been performed but in all likelihood would have entailed an additional excision. The flaps were perfused by the superior and inferior gluteal vessels which should be identified with a pencil Doppler prior to flap elevation.

In-Service Examination

1. The intercostal perforators emerge at what distance from the midline?
   (a) 1 cm
   (b) 3 cm
   (c) 5 cm
   (d) 7 cm
2. The blood supply to the scapular flap:
   (a) Dorsal scapular
   (b) Circumflex scapular
   (c) Ascending branch of the parascapular
   (d) Posterior branch of the thoracodorsal
3. A 2-year-old presents with a sacral hemangioma with dark hair for possible excision. What is the next step in management?
   (a) Proceed with excision
   (b) Delay excision until age 5–7
   (c) Manage with Ng-switched laser
   (d) CT scan

57 Abdominal Wall

Bibliography

Everybody

Patel NG, Ratanshi I, Buchel EW. "The Best of Abdominal Wall Reconstruction", *Plast. Reconstr. Surg.*, (2018); 141(1): **113–31e, and Videos 1, 3.**

DeFranzo AJ, Pitzer K, Molnar JA, et al. "Vacuum-Assisted Closure for Defects of the Abdominal Wall.", *Plast. Reconstr. Surg.*, (2008); 121:**833, 836–839 (Discussion Only).**

Junior Residents (PGY 1, 2) Only

Ghazi B and Losken A, "Chapter 1: Abdominal Wall Anatomy", Losken A and Janis JE, Advances in Abdominal Wall Reconstruction, Quality Medical Publishing, (2012); **pgs. 8–10, 12–13 ONLY.**

Grevious MA, Cohen M, Jean-Pierre F, et al. "The Use of Prosthetics in Abdominal Wall Reconstruction", *Clinics in Plastic Surgery*, Saunders Elsevier Co., (2006); 33:**181–193**.

Nahabedian MY, Sosin M, Bhanot P. "A Current Review of Biologic Meshes in Abdominal Wall Reconstruction", *Plast. Reconstr. Surg.*, (2018); 142(3S): **74S–81S.**

Garvey PB. "Discussion: A Current Review of Biologic Meshes in Abdominal Wall Reconstruction", *Plast. Reconstr. Surg.*, (2018); 142(3S): **82S–3S.**

Middle (PGY 3, 4) and Senior (PGY 5, 6) Level Residents Only

Pauli EM and Rosen MJ, "Open ventral hernia repair with component separation", *Surg. Clin. N. Am.*, (2013); 93:**1111–1126.**

Butler CE. "Discussion: Anterior versus Posterior Compartment Separation: Which Is Better?" *Plast. Reconstr. Surg.*, (2018); 142(3S): **54S–55S.**

Novitsky YW, Belyansky I. "Discussion: Anterior versus Posterior Compartment Separation: Which Is Better?" *Plast. Reconstr. Surg.*, (2018); 142(3S): **56S–57S.**

Khansa I, Janis JE, "Complex Open Abdominal Wall Reconstruction: Management of the Skin and Subcutaneous Tissue", *Plast. Reconstr. Surg.*, (2018); 142(3S):**125S–129S ONLY and Videos 4 and 5 ONLY.**

Mericli AF, Baumann DP, Butler CE. "Reconstruction of the Abdominal Wall after Oncologic Reconstruction: Defect Classification and Management Strategies", *Plast. Reconstr. Surg.*, (2018); 142(3S): **187S–96S.**

Faculty Discussion and Study Guide

Anatomy, Function, and Assessment

1. In one method of abdominoplasty, the plane of dissection is performed superficial to the fascial system. What is the proper name for that system? (Scarpa's fascia.)
2. For breast reconstruction, you have raised a TRAM flap and are prepared to transect the rectus inferiorly just above the pubis when you note a muscle *superficial* to the rectus, arising from the linea alba. What is the muscle? (Pyramidalis.)
3. Outline the origin and insertion of the external and internal oblique. (The external oblique arises from the lower ribs and costal cartilage and runs inferior-medially to insert on the pubis, the semilunar line, and contributes to the inguinal ligament. The internal oblique in contrast arises from the anterior portion of the iliac crest and the thoraco-lumbar fascia, the inguinal ligament and inserts on the lower four ribs by coursing superior-laterally but still medial to the external oblique.)
   (a) What is, are, the structure or structures deep to the obliques? (Transversus muscle, transversalis fascia.)

E. Luce, *A Curriculum for Plastic Surgery*, https://doi.org/10.1007/978-3-031-62087-4_57

4. What are the principal components of the anterior rectus fascia at the level of the umbilicus? (The aponeurosis of the anterior and posterior fascia of the external oblique and the anterior fascia of the internal oblique.) Posterior rectus fascia? (Posterior fascia of the internal oblique, the transversus muscle, and transversalis fascia.)
   (a) What are the principal components of the anterior rectus fascia halfway between the umbilicus and the pubis or just below the arcuate line? (The aponeurosis of the anterior and posterior fascia of the external oblique and both the anterior and posterior fascia of the internal oblique as well as the transversus muscle.)
   (b) Posterior rectus fascia? (Transversalis fascia only.)
5. What is the relationship in cross section of the major blood supply of the inferior portion of the abdominal wall, the deep inferior epigastric artery, DIEA, and the superficial inferior epigastric artery, SIEA? (The SIEA is superficial to Scarpa's fascia and supplies subcutaneous fat and skin. The DIEA is deep to the rectus and is the principal blood supply to the perforators of the rectus muscle.)
6. The motor innervation of the rectus is a segmental pattern accompanying the vessels, entering the rectus at what point in cross section? (Posterior or deep at the junction of the lateral and middle one-third of the muscle.)
   (a) The neurovascular bundle travels from posterior to anterior in what layer? (Deep to the inferior oblique and superficial to the transversus. See below for the anatomy of components of separation.)
7. Describe Huger's classification of a blood supply to the anterior abdominal wall and the source vessels of the same. (Huger's zone I is essentially the upper and mid abdomen centrally oriented vertically and is supplied primarily by the perforators of the deep inferior and superior epigastric artery and arcade. The inferior portion of Zone I overlaps the central portion of Zone II. Zone II is the lower central abdomen oriented transversely and defined superiorly by a line drawn from the anterior superior iliac spines and inferiorly by the pubis and inguinal ligaments. Zone II is supplied by multiple vessels including the DIEA from the external iliac, and branches of the femoral artery including the SIEA, superficial circumflex iliac, and superficial external pudendal, although the last is a relatively minor contribution. Zone III is the flank and lateral abdomen and the principal blood supply is from the segmental lower thoracic and first lumbar intercostal vessels.)
   (a) What is the watershed or collateral point between the DIEA and the SIEA? (Halfway between the umbilicus and the subcostal angle.)
   (b) Describe the perfusion and distribution of the periumbilical perforators. (The periumbilical perforators consist of a medial and lateral row and are fed principally by the deep inferior epigastric arteries. The medial row may provide a greater perfusion across the midline and the lateral row the adjacent tissue lateral to the rectus. This subject is discussed in the breast reconstruction submodule, Chap. 88.)

Editor's note: One of the readings stated incorrectly that the "collateralization" occurred at the umbilicus.

8. Give a classification of ventral hernias based on risk of complications and/or recurrence. (See Table 57.1.)
9. List the risk factors for ventral hernia recurrence. (Smoking, obesity, diabetes, steroids, size, wound contamination.)
10. Although the thrust of this module is not toward early management of the open abdomen, what are two options and balance each? (The most widely utilized option, by general surgery, is application of Vicryl® or other absorbable mesh to hold the intraabdominal contents in place and management of the open wound with wet dressings. Once granulation occurs over the bowel, split-thickness skin grafts are applied and, eventually at 12–18 months, the skin grafts are removed and the abdomen reconstructed. The other option is application of the VAC either coincident with the Vicryl® mesh or as a primary modality as outlined in one of the readings.)
11. When should negative wound pressure therapy, NWPT, be employed in abdominal wall defects and why? (In the setting of wound infection, inflammation, and edema. NWPT decreases edema and bacteria colonization, increases local perfusion, promotes granulation tissue, and decreases the size of the defect.)
12. What are the two or three essential elements of the overall assessment of the patient besides the defect? (Pulmonary, nutritional, functional status. So possibly pulmonary function test, A1c levels, prealbumin and albumin, questions about activities of daily living.)
13. What are the essential elements of the assessment of the defect of the anterior abdominal wall? (In addition to the presence of a hernia, abdominal wall loss as necrotizing fasciitis, significant traumatic or oncologic loss of skin–soft tissue, history of radiotherapy, or presence of enterocutaneous fistulas.)
14. Describe the physical exam of an anterior abdominal wall defect. (Presence or absence of intact skin, pliability of the skin graft if present, exam in standing and supine position for the magnitude or size of the defect and degree of loss of abdominal domain, intact rectus or not, location on the abdominal wall such as central or lateral, upper or lower.)

Table 57.1 Ventral Hernia Working Group grading system for risk of complications at the surgical site with recommendation for each grade

Grade	Description
1	The healthy patient with no contamination and no history of wound infection; the VHWG recommends the use of prosthetic material to reinforce the repair of all incisional ventral hernias, regardless of whether or not the midline fascia can be closed
2	The patient who does not have wound contamination or infection but has one or more comorbidities that increase the risk of infection; the VHWG suggests that bioprosthetic material might have an advantage over synthetic material in these cases
3	The patient who has violation of bowel or the presence of nearby stoma or infection; synthetic mesh is not recommended*; bioprosthetic mesh maybe a good option
4	The patient with infected synthetic mesh or septic dehiscence; no repair material should be used in the setting of gross uncontrolled contamination; the surgeon may consider a delayed repair

VHWG Ventral Hernia Working Group
Breuing K, Butter CE, Ferzoco S. et al. Incisional ventral hernias: Review of the literature and recommendations regarding the grading and technique of repair. *Surgery* 2010;148:544–558
Althubaiti G and Butler CE, "Abdominal wall and chest wall reconstruction", *PRS*, (2014); 133:688e–710e. Reprinted with Permission

15. What is the role, if any, in imaging and assessment? (CT scan and contrast will assess size, location, and status of the remaining intact fascia.)

Separation of Components

1. Outline the anatomy that permits separation of anterior components closure of abdominal wall defects. (The neurovascular supply is at the level of the internal oblique/transversus muscles laterally; the linea semilunaris is conjoint of anterior and posterior fascia of the external and internal oblique; the transversus continues medial to the semilunar line as does transversalis fascia. Division of the external oblique just lateral to the semilunar line permits medial advancement of the remaining components of the abdominal wall.)
   (a) Describe the nature of innervation. (The innervation is segmental arising from T7 through T12 as well as branches of L1 that enter on the deep aspect of the rectus muscles. The internal and external oblique are innervated considerably further lateral to the semilunar line. As described above, the component of the intercostal nerves courses beneath the internal oblique and on top of or superficial to the transversus muscle.)
2. Describe the three or four essential steps in the procedure. (Identification of the edge of the fascia defect medially, wide lateral skin–soft tissue undermining, division of external oblique fascia 2–3 cm. lateral to the linea semilunaris, develop a plane between the external oblique and internal oblique to the level of the mid axillary line, plus or minus dissection of the rectus muscle off the posterior rectus fascia.)
   (a) How much uni*lateral* movement is possible at epigastrium, the umbilicus, and the suprapubic region? (3–4 cm at the epigastrium, 10 cm at the umbilicus, and 2–3 cm at the suprapubic region. Those numbers may include posterior rectus fascia release.)
   (b) Limitations? (Epigastric and suprapubic regions are difficult with limited mobility; wide skin undermining and the potential for devascularization secondary to separation of skin–soft tissue from the rectus and division of the perforators can lead to wound necrosis and dehiscence.)
   (c) Methods to address skin problem(s)? (Perform limited lateral skin incisions only to the point of exposure of the fascial defect to preserve medial blood supply from the periumbilical perforators, or endoscopic release. In reality, all of these techniques are technically difficult to perform.)
3. Briefly describe posterior components release. (The posterior rectus fascia is incised several millimeters off the medial edge and dissection is performed between the posterior rectus fascia and the posterior aspect of the rectus muscle. That dissection is continued to the semilunar line for identification of the transversus muscle lying immediately anterior or superficial to the transversalis fascia. At that point the muscle, the transversus, is incised longitudinally and further dissection laterally is performed deep or posterior to the transversus muscle, maintaining an intact transversalis fascia and peritoneum. Usually, a large sheet of prosthetic mesh is placed into the space and secured with interrupted deep sutures placed 4–6 cm from the edge of the defect.)
4. What are the advantages and disadvantages in release and/or division in the posterior rectus fascia? (Actually, the procedure was a part of the original description of separation of components technique. The advantage may be an additional 1–2 cm of advancement but the disadvantages are compromise of the anterior fascia closure if the posterior fascia is dissected separately as well as the potential exposure of intraperitoneal contents to raw soft tissue if the transversalis fascia is disrupted. The potential also exists for damage to the deep epigastric vessels on the posterior aspect of the rectus muscle as well as injury to the segmental intercostal neurovascular bundles located just anterior to the transversus muscle. Nevertheless, the technique has rapidly been incorporated into ventral hernia repair as a stand-alone operation independent of anterior component of separation.)
5. What is the underlying philosophy in the placement of prosthetic mesh in a retromuscular prefascial location

with several cm of overlap also known as the Stoppa technique? (The principal location of recurrent hernias with mesh is at the interface between the fascial tissue and the prosthetic mesh with an edge to edge inset technique. A considerable overlap of the fascia by mesh and placement of the sutures 4–6 cm from the medial fascial edge hopefully minimizes a cause for recurrence.)

6. List the relative and possible contraindications to separation of components method alone for closure of defects. (Defects with substantial soft tissue loss such as a shotgun wound or necrotizing fasciitis, lateral defects and particularly defects far superior or inferior in the area of the linea semilunaris where medial advancement is more limited, and an acute inflammatory setting.)
7. What are acute and long-term complications of separation of components technique for closure of central hernias? (Infection estimated as high as 15–20% particularly in the presence of enteral stomas; necrosis of the skin as noted above; inadvertent enterotomies. Late complications include recurrence, a lateral or Spigelian hernia resulting from inadvertent dissection deep to the inferior oblique with a resultant injury to the neurovascular pedicle, denervation of the rectus muscles, and loss of fascial continuity.)
   (a) After closure by components of separation, the anesthesiologist complains of an increased peak airway pressure and decrease in blood pressure. What is the problem, how diagnosed, and the solution? (The diagnosis is that of abdominal compartment syndrome, confirmed by a rise in bladder pressures as measured through the Foley catheter.

   The address of the problem is release of the closure accomplished by components of separation and placement of bridging mesh or bioprosthetics into the defect, ordinarily not desirable but the option in this scenario.)
   (b) What early postoperative complications should be anticipated? (Ileus and possible respiratory compromise as discussed.)

Use of Prosthetics and Bioprosthetics in Abdominal Wall Reconstruction

1. True or false: the most important factor in assessing any one of the various prosthetics in success or failure in repair of incisional or ventral hernias of the abdominal wall is the intrinsic tensile strength of the material (False—all have more than sufficient tensile strength for intra-abdominal wall pressure. Failure occurs at the mesh–tissue suture line.)
2. Classify and subclassify prosthetics used in abdominal wall reconstruction. (The first broad classification is absorbable vs. non-absorbable. Types of absorbable prosthetics are Vicryl® and Dexon® mesh. Non-absorbable mesh can be divided into bioprosthetic and synthetic. A number of bioprosthetic meshes exist including those of human origin, human acellular dermis, and animals including bovine and porcine. Synthetic meshes can be divided into macro and microporous. Macroporous can be further divided into monofilament and polyfilament.)
3. What is the role of porosity or pore size in the biologic behavior of various prosthetics? (Small pores, less than 70 micrometers, have a minimal cellular response and infiltration only while a larger pore size permits tissue ingrowth in the form of angiogenesis, fibroblasts, and collagen deposition.)
   (a) Could this difference play a role in infection? (Absolutely. Bacterial infiltration can occur in any pore size, yet only larger pores allow the infiltration of native tissue for host response. Also as described, larger pores allow collagen ingrowth.)
4. What is the role of the type of fibers, monofilament versus multifilament? (Bacterial infiltration can occur in interstices of multifilament fibers and yet the interstices are too small, 10 microns, to allow access for the local defense infiltrate of PMNs and macrophages.)
5. The readings discuss the use of prosthetics in fascial repair and list three considerations in choice of the same: (Contact with bowel, ability to be incorporated into surrounding tissue, and quality of soft tissue coverage. See Table 57.2.)
   (a) What are the options in terms of location with the use of prosthetics in abdominal wall reconstruction? Describe efficacy. (Essentially three. As an overlay, placed anteriorly to reinforce fascial repair; as an underlay, placed in retromuscular position; and, thirdly, to bridge a defect from fascial edge to fascial edge. Little evidence exists that the use of mesh in an overlay position provides a lower recurrence rate. Underlay references placement of the mesh poste-

Table 57.2 Methods of mesh placement in ventral hernia repair

Method	Description
Overlay	The mesh material is sutured ventral to the primary repair of fascial edges, with no contact with viscera
Underlay	The mesh material is sutured dorsal to the primary repair of fascial edges; less risk of mesh exposure if skin wound dehiscence occurs; mesh can be placed in the intraperitoneal, preperitoneal, or retrorectus plane
Interpositional	The mesh material is sutured to the fascial edges (bridging) with minimal overlap; not generally recommended because of high hernia recurrence rate

Althubaiti G and Butler CE, “Abdominal wall and chest wall reconstruction,” *Plas. Reconstr. Surg.*, (2014); 133: 688e–710e. Reprinted with Permission rior to the fascial closure but, most commonly currently, is placed in a retromuscular position posterior to the rectus and transversus muscles and is usually utilized as an element of posterior component release. The mesh is excluded from the peritoneal cavity by retention of the transversalis fascia posterior to the retromuscular mesh. The use of mesh to bridge a fascial defect is attended by a substantial and perhaps prohibitive incidence of recurrence of the hernia.)

(b) Evaluate the onlay technique of mesh placement from a physics standpoint (If you had a hole in a dike, would you put the plaster on the water side or the land side?)

(c) Give the pros and cons of the following: polypropylene, Prolene®, or Marlex®, expanded TFE or Gore-Tex®. (Marlex—allows tissue ingrowth and has a substantially good tensile strength. The disadvantage is if contact with bowel allows tissue ingrowth from the serosa and possibly bacterial translocation with the potential formation of fistulas as well as infection of the mesh. Prolene is monofilament and perhaps less likely to be infected, but still has the same issue with tissue ingrowth from the bowel and resultant infection and/or fistula. Once colonized, all mesh must be removed. Gore-Tex® does not allow tissue ingrowth and is not subject to the difficulties described above but has a high incidence of recurrent hernias at the junction of the mesh and native tissue as well as a propensity for the formation of seromas because of the lack of tissue ingrowth.)

(d) Explain biologically why Gore-Tex has a high incidence of recurrent hernias? (The nature of the material with the small pore size does not permit sufficient cellular infiltration to allow collagen deposition and good healing.)

6. Composite prosthetics have been advocated to address the problem of adhesions. Describe the composition of such composite meshes and the potential disadvantages. (The combination is the use of a polypropylene mesh as an outer layer and an inner layer composed most commonly of ePTFE or an absorbable mesh which theoretically avoids bowel adhesions against the Gore-tex or absorbable mesh and maintains the tissue ingrowth and strength capabilities of the Prolene. One example is Composix®. Unfortunately, the use of such composite mesh is complicated by high incidence of seroma formation as well as bowel adhesions where sutures are placed through the abdominal wall for the inset and composite mesh is quite expensive.)
7. Do a cost analysis by hierarchy from least to most expensive of the following: Prolene, Gore-tex, Composix, Alloderm. (As listed.)
8. How does a bioprosthetic differ from a synthetic prosthetic? (Retains sufficient structural integrity during a degradation/replacement process in order to substitute and replace the missing tissue reconstructed. By definition, bioprosthetics regardless of origin, are acellular but have retained key cytokines. A more comprehensible discussion is in **I. Basic Principles G. Biomaterials**.)
   (a) Although not specifically discussed in the readings, what are the three possible biological processes that can occur with insertion of a bioprosthetic in the body? (Encapsulation such as breast prostheses, inflammation, and degradation such as Vicryl® mesh, and regeneration, presumably the process that occurs with Integra or acellular human dermis.)
9. According to the readings, what are the advantages of Alloderm®? (Has little adhesion with good tissue ingrowth/replacement and so can be used in defects too large for autogenous reconstruction and/or contaminated wounds.)
   (a) Disadvantages of the use of acellular dermis? (Seroma formation, excessive extensibility with time, more marked in some than others.)
10. What are the available options for closure of fascial defects in heavily contaminated wounds, Grade III, with the advantages and disadvantages of each? (Vicryl® mesh; the advantage is temporary closure of the abdomen which entails a delayed reconstruction. Usually employed early in "damage control" situations. The disadvantage is absorption. Bioprosthetics such as human acellular dermis; disadvantage as discussed above is seroma formation and probable elasticity and stretching with time. As a result, bioprosthetics of xenograft origin have been developed to address this reconstructive need.)
11. The readings outline two non-human or porcine bioprosthetics, Surgisis and Permacol, one of which is pig small intestine submucosa, Surgisis, and pig dermis, Permacol. Discuss the advantages and disadvantages of each. (Surgisis consists of multiple layers, 4–8, of processed submucosa and has the advantages of unlimited availability and disadvantages of perhaps not regeneration but rather replacement by scar and/or encapsulation which raises concerns about use in a contaminated field. Although porcine dermis is a single layer, similar concerns have arisen about the use of Permacol. Those comments can perhaps be extended to the use of other xenograft types of bioprosthetics.)

Editorial note: Some of the initial enthusiasm for bioprosthetics in hernia repair has waned because of the inherent elasticity and loss of structural integrity or tensile strength over time. Perhaps the clinical scenario for the appropriate use needs to be defined.

Algorithm for Abdominal Wall Reconstruction

1. Describe the use of and indications for tissue expansion in abdominal wall reconstruction. (If the skin deficit is substantial, estimated by the readings anywhere between 10–20 cm in width, preliminary placement of tissue expanders for recruitment of additional skin/soft tissue is necessary. Some discussion exists about whether those expanders should be placed supra- or subfascial, namely beneath the external oblique. The latter may be subject to attenuation of the fascia and probably a suprafascial, subcutaneous placement is more appropriate and certainly simpler.)
   (a) Problems? (The incidence of exposure and loss is quite high, estimated at 20–25%. Also, expansion is difficult without an underlying non-yielding surface such as the rib cage.)
2. Give a classification system for post-extirpative defects of the abdominal wall. (See Fig. 57.1.)

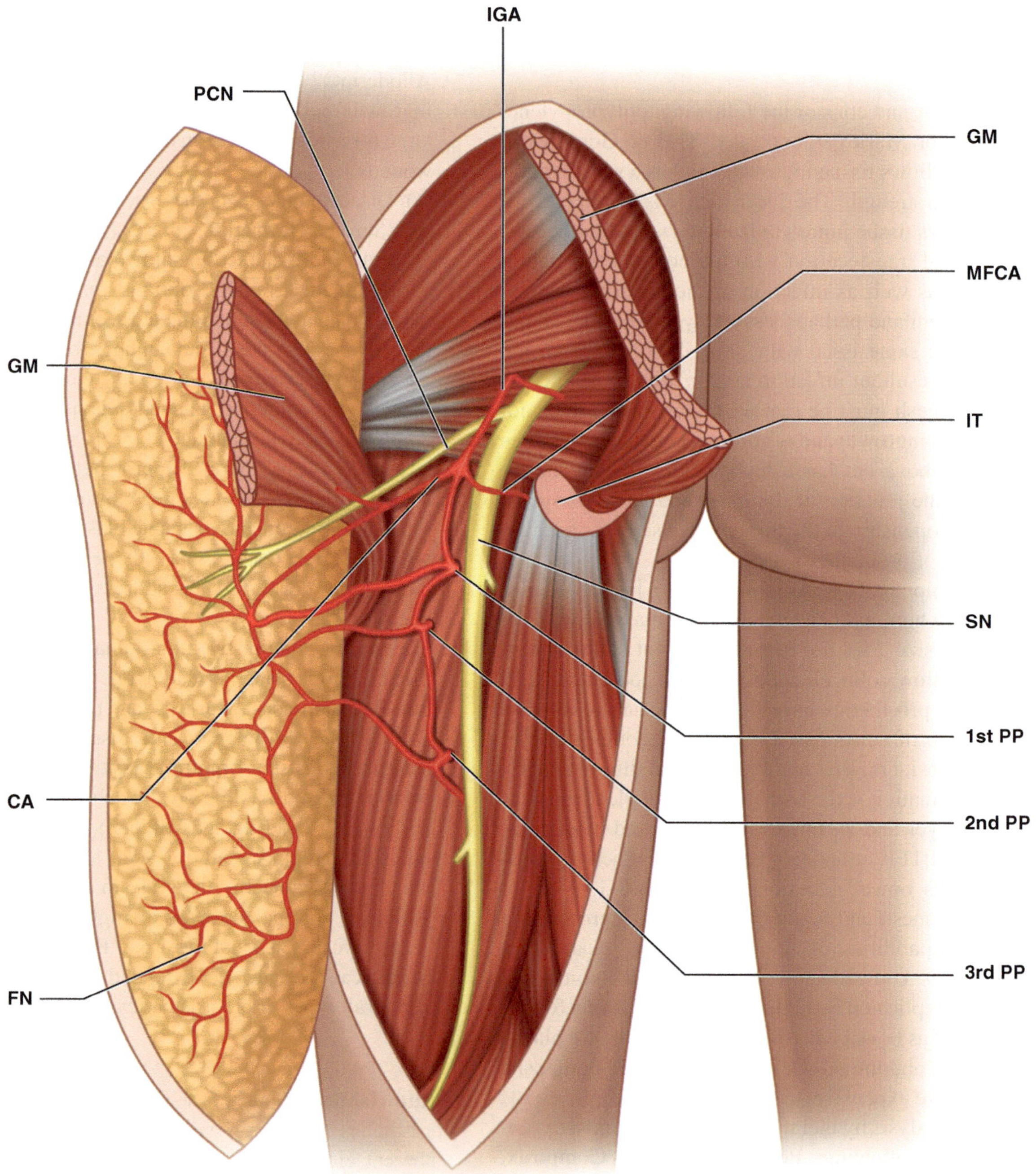

Fig. 57.1 Classification of oncologic defects of the abdominal wall. (Mericli AF, Baumann DP, Butler CE. "Reconstruction of the Abdominal Wall after Oncologic Reconstruction: Defect Classification and Management Strategies," *Plast. Reconstr. Surg.* (2018); 142 (3S): Fig. 1. 190S. (Reprinted with Permission))

3. Assuming a full-thickness defect of the abdominal wall including skin and soft tissue, describe the options for reconstruction in the areas outlined in the above question. (Central defects, Type I, if within limits of anterior component separation are best addressed with this approach, perhaps reinforced with an underlay retrorectus mesh. Smaller central superior or inferior defects as Type III or IV can also be addressed with components of separation. Larger defects, particularly Type II or lateral to the semilunar line of fascial fusion will probably require regional flap transfer. Superior lateral defects can be reconstructed with latissimus dorsi, inferior central, and lateral defects with thigh-based flaps as the anterolateral thigh and rectus femoris. A previously delayed tensor fascia lata flap can provide substantial fasciocutaneous closure particularly for lateral inferior defects. All thigh-based flaps usually require split-thickness skin graft of the donor site.)
4. With some difficulty, you have been successful with closure of a substantial-sized abdominal wall fascial defect and are preparing to excise excess skin and close when the anesthesiologist states the airway pressures have elevated considerably and the endotracheal tube and airway are clear of a possible causative role. What is the likely pathophysiology? (Abdominal compartment syndrome—the clinical picture of increased airway pressures and decreased blood pressure as a result of an increased pressure within the abdominal cavity. The pressure on the diaphragm and the diminished venous return by compression of the inferior vena cava. The inciting event in this instance is probably the return of intra-abdominal contents into the abdominal cavity that has some loss of domain. The increase in intra-abdominal compartment pressure compresses the inferior vena cava with a diminished venous return and cardiac filling volume. The only pliable structure of the four walls is the muscular diaphragm that is compressed and displaced superiorly.

   The intra-abdominal pressure is the crucial measurement and criterion. A modified intravesical catheter is capable of determination of bladder pressures, a surrogate for intraabdominal pressure. Intra-abdominal pressures of greater than 16 mmHg is considered Grade II hypertension and may require address. If pressure elevation is borderline, the patient may require maintenance of the endotracheal airway as a temporary measure until a later assessment. For more invasive measures include release with bridging mesh, accepting that the prohibitively high recurrence rate mandates a secondary operation.)
5. Outline a treatment plan for each of the following case scenarios.
   - Case #1: General surgery requests your assistance in the elective repair of an incisional hernia from a prior colon resection 1 year ago with a postoperative wound infection and dehiscence. On exam, the hernia is central and measures 8x8 cm. (Separation of components, probably anterior. The addition of a mesh overlay as reinforcement would be appropriate.)
   - Case #2: A 50-year-old healthy male has a 6x6 cm. sarcoma of the abdominal wall in the right upper quadrant. Surgical Oncology anticipates a full-thickness resection (Anticipate a 12x12 cm. defect. Use bioprosthetic plus latissimus dorsi.)
   - Case #3: A 50-year-old female has a 7x7 cm. radiation ulcer in the midline central lower abdomen. The surrounding skin has evidence of radiation changes and damage. (Keep posterior fascia or possibly the rectus intact. Use a tensor fascia lata flap, probably delayed; the second option is a rectus femoris or an anterolateral thigh flap but the donor deficit is greater. If sufficient skin laxity exists, use a VRAM if the deep inferior epigastric artery is intact on CT angiogram. Given the presence of a radiation ulcer, the adjacent skin, although intact, may be severely damaged by radiation changes.)
   - Case #4: A 12 × 12 cm. central abdominal incisional hernia? (Separation of components, then a composite mesh consisting of Gore-tex® and polypropylene into the residual deficit sutured by Stoppa technique or retro muscular, if possible, pre-posterior fascia with permanent sutures. The other option is the use of bioprosthetics.)

Case-Based Conference

Case 1—Abdominal Wall Reconstruction

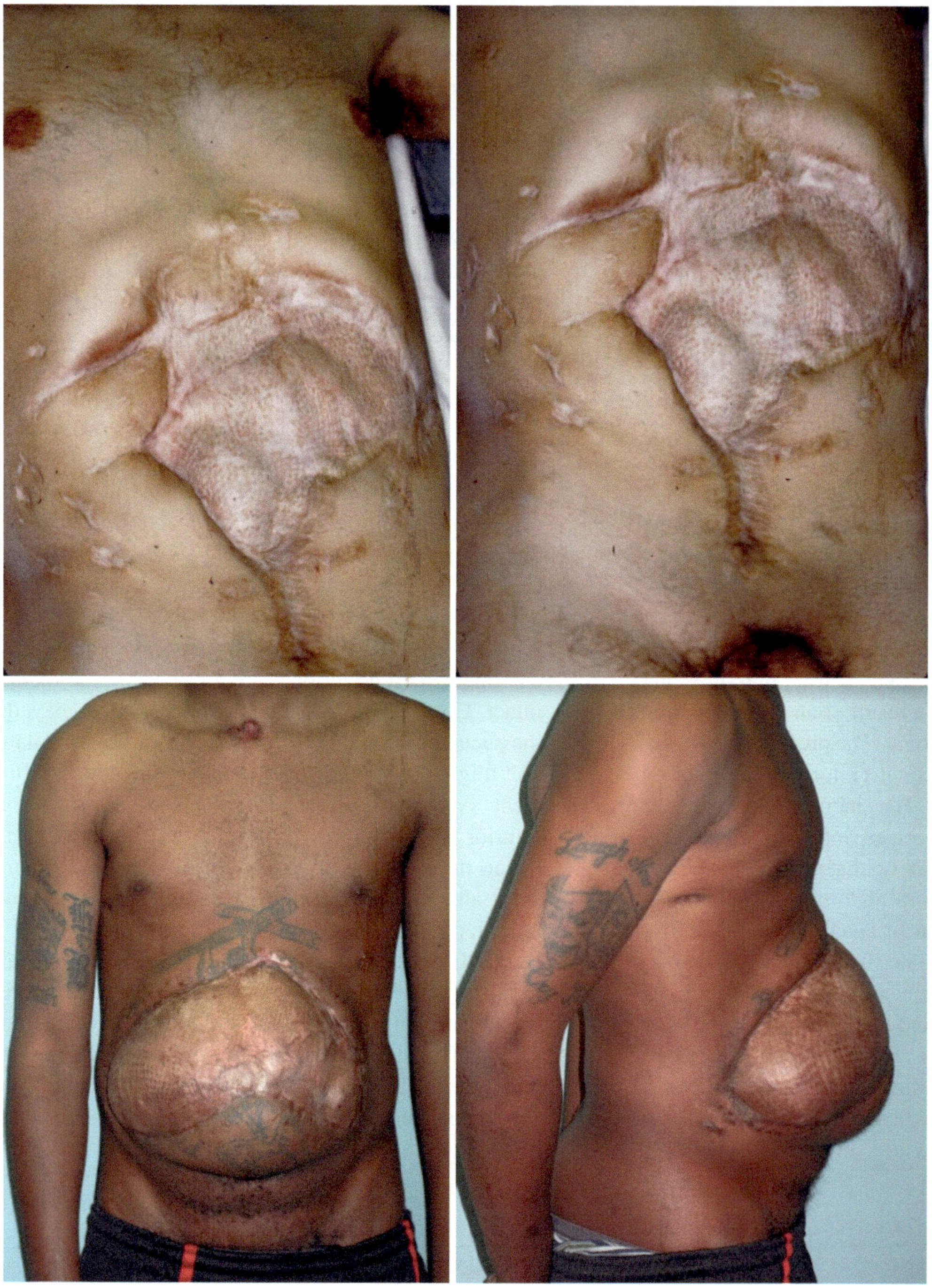

A 28-year-old who is 1 year after acute pancreatitis and necrotizing fasciitis requiring multiple washouts and skin grafts. The patient had Vicyrl mesh initially only. The patient is now fully healed without fistula and desires reconstruction of his abdominal wall.

The second set of photos are a patient who had an emergency laparotomy, open abdomen, and split-thickness skin graft.

1. After describing what you see in the slide, add a physical examination. The patient is supine.
   (a) Any additional diagnostic tests necessary?
2. In discussions with the patient what would you outline as the outcome if he ultimately decides not to reconstitute his anterior abdominal wall?

3. This patient on the second set of photos had an emergent transverse laparotomy for a stab wound and was treated with an open abdomen, absorbable mesh, and split-thickness skin graft. How does your case differ in complexity from this case? Or does it?

4. Outline a reconstructive plan and begin by summarizing the reconstructive needs. Include specifics regarding incisions, steps, and sequence.

Case-Based Conference: Discussion

Case 1—Abdominal Wall Reconstruction

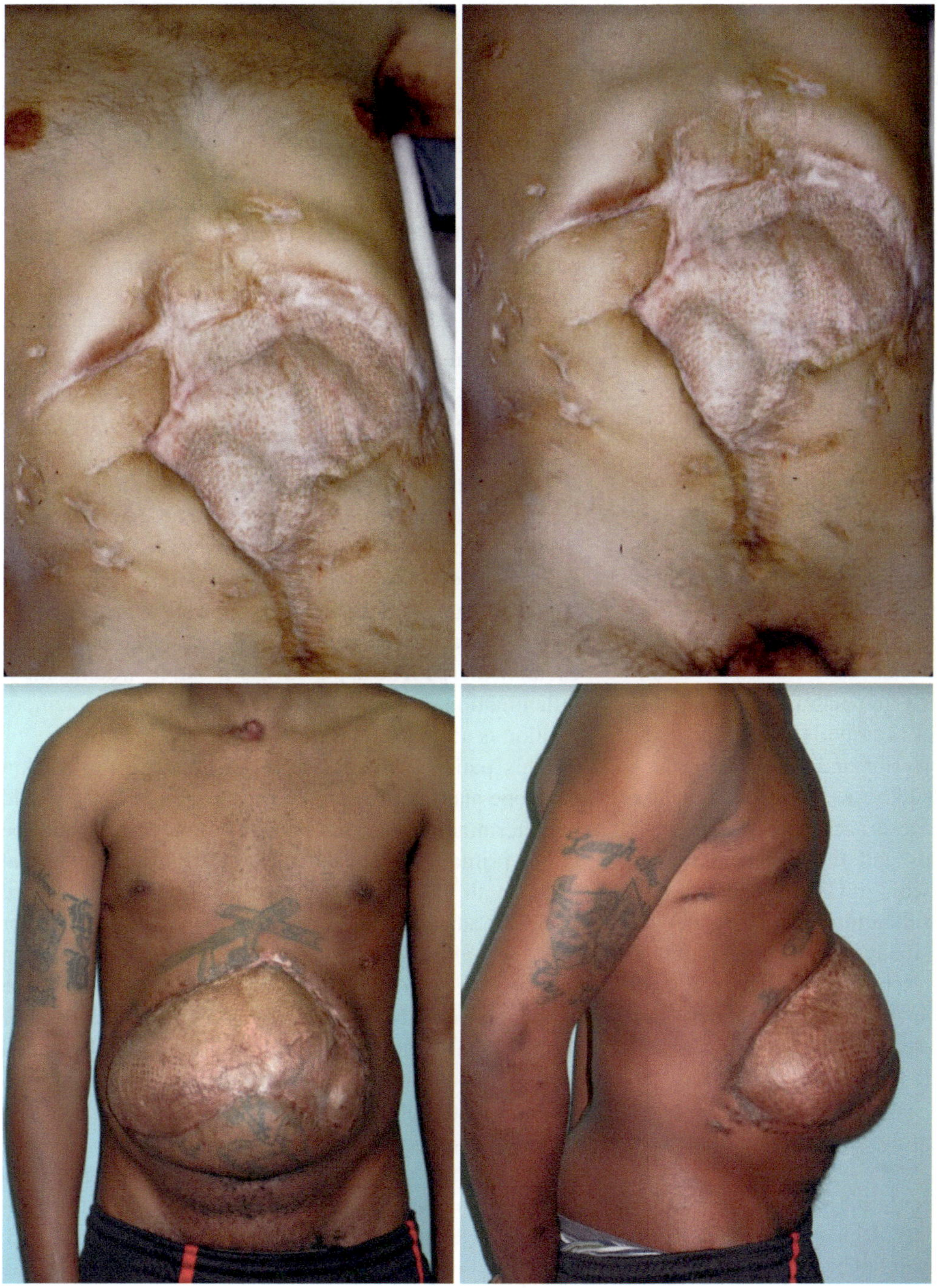

A 28-year-old who is 1 year after acute pancreatitis and necrotizing fasciitis requiring multiple washouts and skin grafts. The patient had Vicyrl mesh initially only. The patient is now fully healed without fistula and desires reconstruction of his abdominal wall.

1. After describing what you see in the slide, add a physical examination. The patient is supine. (Male in a supine position with a large central abdominal defect that extends from approximately 8–10 cm above the pubis to the xiphoid, left costal angle to the junction of the left upper and lower quadrant and measures approximately 20 by 25 cm. On the patient's right, a similar extent except some anterior flank and lateral abdominal wall is retained. The overall configuration of the defect is irregular in shape. The intact abdominal wall skin has a number of small scars consistent with past drain sites. In addition, extending from the central abdominal defect and the epigastrium along the right subcostal angle is a long, perhaps 10 cm in length, incisional scar. As stated, the patient is supine and as such a significant loss of intra-abdominal domain has probably not occurred. A mature meshed skin graft covers the defect. In the clinical examination, the pertinent medical information should be obtained and in particular: etiology of the pancreatitis and, if alcoholic, alcohol, a smoking history, diabetes secondary to the pancreatitis, current gastrointestinal function and performance status. Also, the old operative notes, if available, should be reviewed. The physical exam would focus on palpation of the fascial edges of the defect in the supine position and the degree of loss of domain in the standing position. A judgment about the maturity of the skin graft hinges on the finding of a pliable, non-adherent, and non-erythematous skin graft. Ascertainment of the magnitude of the skin–soft tissue defect is important for planning purposes. Examination of anterior and lateral thigh for potential flap donor sites should be accomplished.
    (a) Any additional diagnostic tests necessary? (Assuming no current GI difficulties and that a recent intra-abdominal assessment with a CT scan has been accomplished, some consideration should be given to pulmonary function tests if any suggestion of pulmonary compromise exists. Return of the intraabdominal contents solely within the abdominal cavity by abdominal wall reconstruction has the potential by elevation and pressure on the diaphragm for further pulmonary compromise. Of course, routine laboratory assessment of electrolytes and renal function should be obtained.)
2. In discussions with the patient, what would you outline as the outcome if he ultimately decides not to reconstitute his anterior abdominal wall? (The natural history of an unrepaired ventral hernia, particular hernias as a result of split-thickness skin graft closure of an abdominal wall defect, is one of progressive loss of domain as the intra-abdominal pressure gradually pushes the intestines anteriorly and out of the abdominal cavity. Large hernias as the one depicted are highly unlikely to incarcerate.)
3. This patient on the second set of photos had an emergent transverse laparotomy for a stab wound and was treated with an open abdomen, absorbable mesh, and split-thickness skin graft. How does your case differ in complexity from this case? Or does it? (The two photos are with the patient standing and demonstrate a large ventral hernia, the result of inability to definitively close the abdomen. Whether he has a loss of domain can be better assessed supine, but the important difference is that the patient has not suffered an absolute abdominal wall loss. Nevertheless, with lateral retraction of the musculofascial units, operative repair may entail advancement by component separation, either anterior or posterior, an underlay mesh reinforcement.)
4. Outline a reconstructive plan and begin by summarizing the reconstructive needs. Include specifics regarding incisions, steps, and sequence. (The assessment begins with consideration of reconstruction of the two components of the abdominal wall, the skin–soft tissue, and musculofascial elements. The pliability of the intact abdominal wall skin and soft tissue and the presence and extent of scars are important determinants, particularly if the lateral flaps will advance with digital pressure. As mentioned in the physical exam, some evaluation of the absolute size of the fascial defect will guide surgical decision-making. Clearly, the patient depicted has a stable wound but if inflammation or an unhealed wound bed persists, temporization is advisable.

    This patient will require reconstitution of both skin envelope and myofascial integrity. The initial step would be determination of what portion of the defect could be closed primarily by advancement of soft tissue and fascial flaps. In all likelihood, the lower one-fourth to one-third could be advanced and closed. Tethered by the inferior thoracic wall, little if any closure could be anticipated in the superior portion of the defect. Simultaneously, tissue expanders could be placed strategically, particularly over the rib cage and probably in the right lateral abdominal wall. Less skin will be recruited from tissue expanders situated in the abdomen because of the lack of a firm underlying structure as exists over the ribs.

    The second stage is removal of the skin graft and intraabdominal access for lysis of the adhesions is necessary to access the remnants of the intact abdominal wall, prosthetic repair of the abdominal wall defect, and advancement of skin coverage. At times, distant tissue may need to be imported from the thigh if tissue expansion is inadequate for provision of sufficient skin envelope for closure. The most common thigh-based pedicle flaps are tensor fascia lata, rectus femoris, and anterolateral thigh. Reconstruction of abdominal defects superior to the umbilicus with pedicled flaps from the thigh are difficult and unlikely.

The other element of reconstruction of the abdominal wall is reconstitution of the fascial envelope. As described above, some of the peripheral defect, inferior and lateral, can be closed primarily at the time of tissue expander placement. At the second stage, if possible, separation of components should be performed. On the patient's left, most if not all of the rectus appears to be absent, although a lateral remnant may still persist, so separation of components on the left appears unlikely. On the right, some anterior separation of components may be possible. Anterior separation of contents is accomplished by exposure of the semilunar line by the necessary skin undermining, followed by longitudinal incision of the external oblique 2–3 cm lateral to the semilunar line. The rectus abdominis and internal oblique unit is advanced medially. The abdomen with an intact, or relatively intact, rectus and obliques, the advancement available is 10 cm centrally, 4 cm in the epigastrium, and a similar amount above the pubis. The alternative option is a posterior compartment release performed by dissection of the posterior rectus fascia and lateral release of the transversus muscle with placement of retrorectus mesh. Inner position or bridging mesh is attended by a significant recurrence and should be avoided but underlay mesh placed retrorectus with a wide overlap is a beneficial reinforcement of the repair.

The choice in prosthetic repair is between alloplastic and bioprosthetic. Given the size of the defect and the potential tenuous nature of the skin coverage, certainly bioprosthetic would be appropriate. Also, use of a macroporous mesh Marlex® or Prolene® permits ingrowth of tissue, a characteristic that when adjacent to intestinal serosa can lead to infected mesh and/or intestinal fistula. Microporous mesh, pores less than 70 microns such as Gortex®, do not allow tissue ingrowth but can provoke seroma formation and a high incidence of hernia recurrence. Given the patient's history, omentum is probably not likely available for a barrier between mesh and the intra-abdominal contents. Mesh of a composite character composed of both elements, Gore Tex® next to the intra-abdominal components and other synthetic mesh superficial to Gortex® could be utilized. Probably an optimal choice is placement of such a mesh or a bioprosthetic as Strattice®, human acellular dermis, or Surgisis, porcine intestinal submucosa, to bridge any residual defect after separation of components advancement, placed in a retrorectus location but superficial to the posterior fascia. Use of a bioprosthetic also carries an increased risk of seroma.

Due consideration should be given to the possibility of precipitation of an abdominal compartment syndrome. Monitoring of intra-abdominal pressures via a Foley catheter and peak and plateau airway pressures is crucial. Maintenance of the endotracheal tube and ICU observation may be required.)

Postoperative (Intermediate Stage)

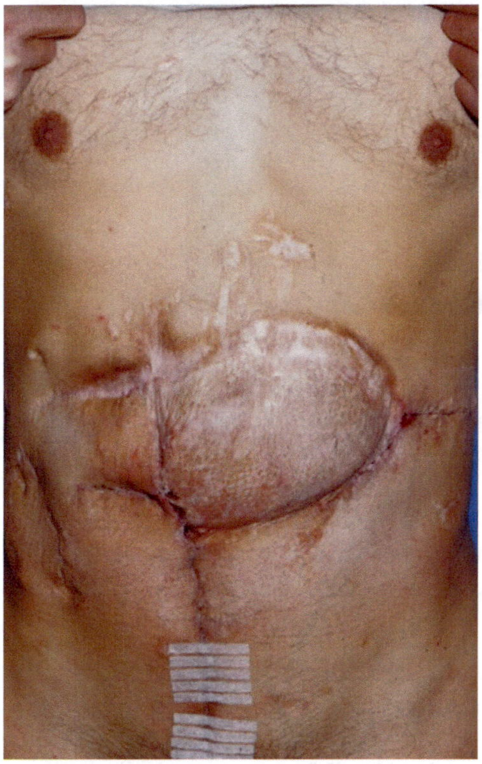

As described above, the first operation consisted of laparotomy and mobilization of the right abdominal wall and the remnant of the left lower quadrant wall. No tissue expander was placed concomitantly although that procedure could have been performed at the same setting prior to wound closure. Whether inserted at the time of laparotomy or subsequently, two large rectangular tissue expanders with remote ports, one placed over the left rib cage and the other in the left lower quadrant. Access incisions would be located at the scar and native skin interface and thus dictates a careful, secure two-layer closure with minimal initial fill line.

Postoperative (6 Months)

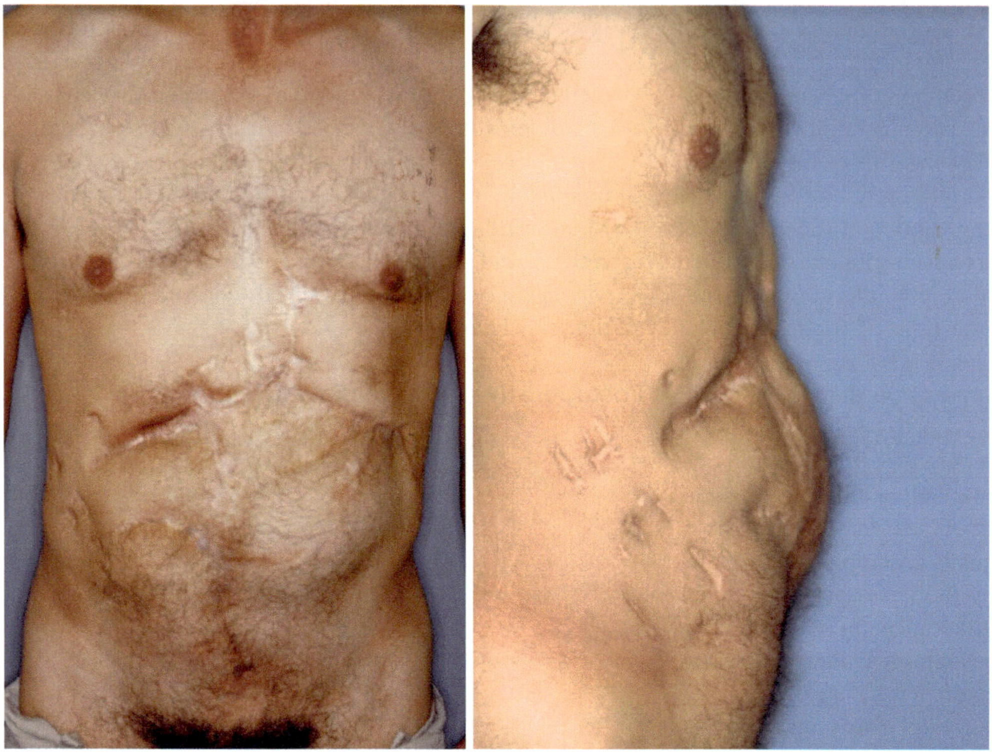

Closure has been obtained with a bioprosthetic for reconstitution of the fascia and the use of expanded skin and soft tissue for coverage.

Critique

Unless a contraindication existed, tissue expander insertion is optimally accomplished coincident with the initial partial abdominal wall closure. On the final result at 6 months, some element of bulge is apparent, probably secondary to some postoperative stretch of the bioprosthetic.

Case-Based Conference

Case 2—Abdominal Wall Reconstruction

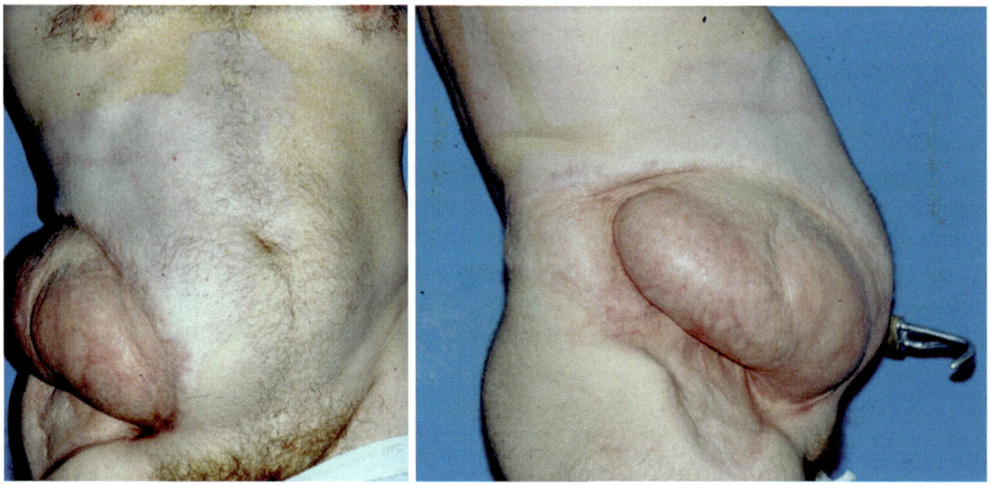

A 32 year old who is 9 months after an electrical burn to the abdominal wall. The patient had Vicryl mesh followed by split-thickness skin graft. The patient presents for reconstruction of his abdominal wall.

1. After describing what you see in the photos, add a physical examination.
   (a) Any additional diagnostic tests necessary?
2. In discussions with the patient, what would you outline as the outcome if he ultimately decides not to reconstitute his anterior abdominal wall?
3. What is the pathologic anatomy?
4. Outline a reconstructive plan and draw the plan.

Case-Based Conference: Discussion

Case 2—Abdominal Wall Reconstruction

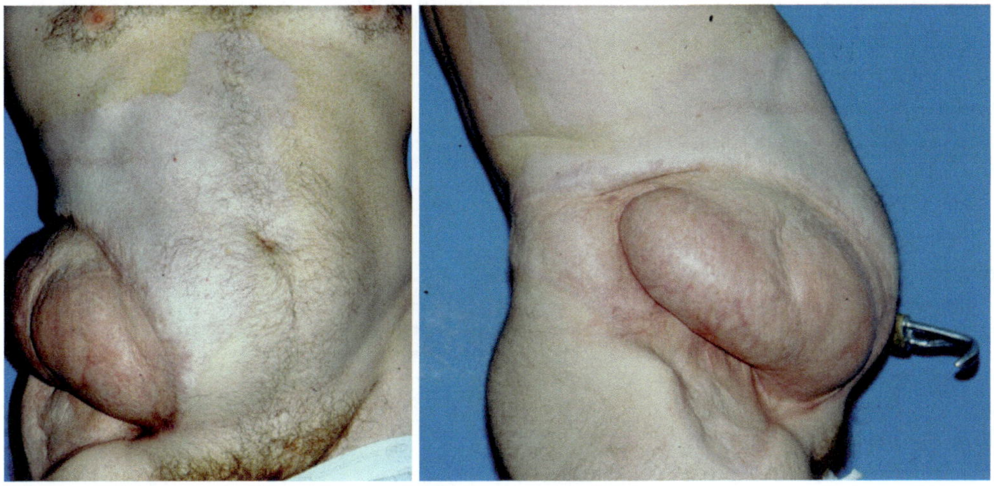

A 32 year old who is 9 months after an electrical burn to the abdominal wall. The patient had Vicryl mesh followed by split-thickness skin graft. The patient presents for reconstruction of his abdominal wall.

1. After describing what you see in the photos, add a physical examination. (Two photos illustrate a large hernia of the abdomen and flank. The first is a view of the anterior trunk from the nipples to the pubis. The remarkable finding is a large bulge of the right lateral abdominal wall, extending from the lateral superpubic region to the lateral and inferior edge of the rib cage. The posterior extent cannot be ascertained on this photo. Intra-abdominal contents are protruding well beyond the limits of the defect and are covered, apparently by split-thickness skin graft. An additional large skin grafted area is present, immediately adjacent, inferior, and posterior to the defect. This area, in contrast to the hernia, is somewhat sunken and depressed. The remainder of the abdomen and lower chest wall are without any scars, defects, or deformities but as suggested on both photos some asymmetrical protuberance and laxity of the right lower abdomen is present. The patient is neither obese nor asthenic. The second photo is a true lateral and does illustrate the posterior extent, well lateral into the flank. The approximate size of the defect is 30 × 20 cm. In addition, the adjacent area of skin graft is more clearly depicted and appears to extend beyond the hernia into the posterior flank. An incidental finding in the lateral view is the terminal end of an upper extremity prosthesis.

   The history portion of the clinical examination is of some importance. Given the prosthesis of the left upper extremity and the magnitude of the truncal defect, the patient apparently sustained a high-tension electrical injury. Other possible concomitant injuries include cardiac, pulmonary, and intra-abdominal. No evidence of laparotomy incisions is present, so questions would focus on if long-term cardiac or pulmonary complications have occurred and some information about current performance status. The patient should be queried about any gastrointestinal symptoms. Current medications and social history including alcohol and tobacco use would complete the history. The physical exam would ascertain the reduction of the intraabdominal contents in a supine position and palpation of the edges of the facial defect. Potential donor sites are examined.)

(a) Any additional diagnostic tests necessary? (CT angiogram may be advisable to determine available vascular supply to the planned reconstructive options, particularly in the setting of high-tension electrical injury. Some estimation of renal function should also be accomplished, also because of the nature of the original injury.)

2. In discussions with the patient, what would you outline as the outcome if he ultimately decides not to reconstitute his anterior abdominal wall? (The natural history of an unrepaired ventral hernia, particular hernias as a result of split-thickness skin graft closure of an abdominal wall defect, is one of progressive loss of domain as the intra-abdominal pressure gradually pushes the intestines anteriorly and out of the abdominal cavity. Large hernias as the one depicted are highly unlikely to incarcerate.)
3. What is the pathologic anatomy? (The pathologic anatomy is a large abdominal and flank hernia with an absolute, not relative, deficit of the abdominal wall and adjacent flank. The other component is the possible loss of integrity of the innervation. The principal muscles of abdominal wall, the rectus and obliques, are provided motor innervation by the intercostal branches of thoracic seven through twelve and lumbar one through four. The defect would appear to encompass a loss of a portion of the obliques laterally, but since the intercostal branches course medially from superior to inferior or obliquely, the segmental innervation of the lower rectus may have been lost.)
4. Outline a reconstructive plan and draw the plan. (The reconstruction of this patient's abdominal wall and correction of the large hernia presents a substantial challenge. Presumably, the original injury resulted in an element of absolute tissue loss of full thickness of the abdominal wall. As such, the reconstructive plan must include reconstitution of the fascia as well as skin–soft tissue coverage. Available regional options include thigh-based flaps and use of the remainder of the abdominal wall. The dominant factor in the decision process is the magnitude of the defect, since any flap harvested from the thigh will be inadequate. The remaining intact abdomen is an enticing choice but also will probably be insufficient to close the entire defect, particularly posterior. To utilize that choice will require incorporation of the entire right and left upper abdominal wall pedicled on the right deep inferior epigastric artery. The remainder of the defect posteriorly could be closed with a thigh-based flap, probably the tensor fascia lata, since the residual defect would be posterior and more amenable to a flap oriented from the lateral thigh. Excision of the old skin graft must be accomplished. If the skin graft is not adherent to the underlying bowel, a plane can be developed directly beneath the graft that will facilitate the dissection. The medial edges of the musculofascial defect can be identified, advanced, and secured to the bone laterally.

To improve perfusion and minimize the probability of ischemia, a preliminary delay of the tensor fascia lata would be advisable. If so, the design would be division of collateral supply with the delay and the distal portion of the flap. Reconstitution of the fascial defect could be accomplished with a bioprosthetic or a composite synthetic mesh. The other options are discussed in this chapter, Case 1.)

Intraoperative

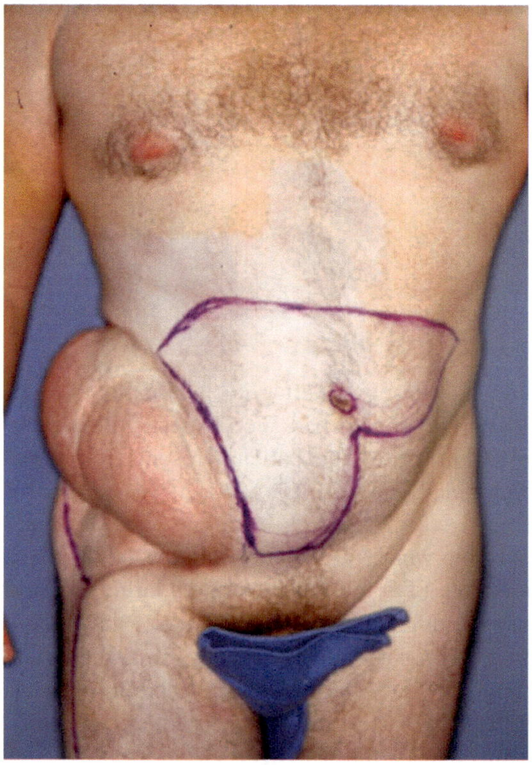

The photo illustrates the operative plan: mobilization of the entire remaining right abdominal and left upper quadrant. Surgical markings on the right anterolateral thigh illustrate the inclusion of a thigh-based flap in the reconstructive plan.

Postoperative (3 Months)

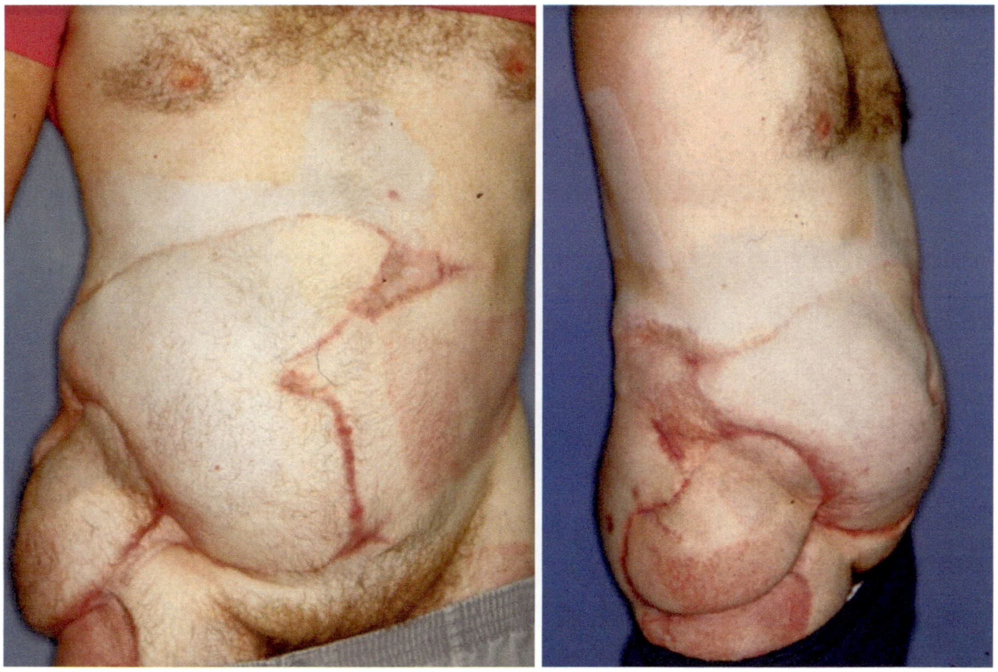

The two photos, anterior and lateral, demonstrate the healed reconstruction including the use of the tensor fascia lata flap inset into the more posterior and inferior portion of the defect.

In-Service Examination

1. The Ventral Hernia classification or staging of the risk of complications include the following variables **EXCEPT:**
   (a) Wound contamination
   (b) Comorbidities
   (c) Prior repair
   (d) Presence of a stoma in the vicinity
2. The technique of anterior separation of components repair of a ventral hernia entails dissection beneath what plane?
   (a) Subcutaneous and external oblique
   (b) Subcutaneous and rectus
   (c) Subcutaneous and external and internal oblique
   (d) Internal oblique, transversus, and rectus abdominis
3. A patient undergoes a pedicled TRAM for breast reconstruction. What structures remain in the flap donor site inferior to the arcuate line?
   (a) Parietal peritoneum only
   (b) Peritoneum and transversalis fascia
   (c) Parietal peritoneum, transversalis fascia, and transversus abdominis
   (d) Parietal peritoneum and internal oblique posterior aponeurosis

Chest Wall

58

Bibliography

Hever P., Singh P., Eiben I., Eiben P., Nikkhah D., "The Management of Deep Sternal Wound Infection: Literature Review and Reconstructive Algorithm", *JPRAS Open*, (2021); 28:77, **Table 1 ONLY.**

Agarwal J.P., Ogilvie M., Wu L.C., Lohman R.F., Gottlieb L.J., Franczyk M., Song D.H., "Vacuum-assisted closure for sternal wounds: a first-line therapeutic management approach", *Plast Reconstr Surg.*, (2005);116(4):**1035–40 ONLY.**

Hamaguchi R, Shekar PS, Johnson JA, et al., "Current Management of Sternal Wounds", *Plast. Reconstr. Surg.*, (2021); 148(6):**1012e-1022e ONLY and Videos 1–3.**

Ascherman M.D., J. A., et al., "Management of Sternal Wounds with Bilateral Pectoralis Major Myocutaneous Advancement Flaps in 114 Consecutively Treated Patients: Refinements in Technique and Outcomes Analysis," *Plast. Reconstr. Surg.*, (2004) 114:**Discussion 680–83 ONLY.**

Clemens, M. W., et al., "Introduction to Chest Wall Reconstruction: Anatomy and Physiology of the Chest and Indications for Chest Wall Reconstruction", *Seminars in Plastic Surgery*, (2011), 25(1):**5–13.**

Althubaiti G and Butler CE, "Abdominal wall and chest wall reconstruction", *Plast. Reconstr. Surg.*, (2014); 133(5):**694e-698e. (Overview)**

Losken A, Thourani VH, Carlson GW, et al., "A reconstructive algorithm for plastic surgery following extensive chest wall resection", *Br. J. Plast. Surg.*, Elsevier Ltd. (2004); 57:**Discussion 297–302 ONLY.**

Isaac KV, Elzinga K, Buchel EW, "The Best of Chest Wall Reconstruction: Principles and Clinical Application for Complex Oncologic and Sternal Defects", *Plast Reconstr Surg.*, (2022); 149(3):**547e, 552–558e ONLY (A different perspective).**

Ferraro P, Cugno S, Liberman M, et al., "Principles of Chest Wall Resection and Reconstruction", *Thorac. Surg. Clin.* (2010); 20: 465–73. **For Junior Residents ONLY.**

Asaad, M., Van Handel, A., Akhavan, A.A., et al., "Muscle Flap Transposition for the Management of Intrathoracic Fistulas", *Plast Reconstr Surg*, (2020); 145(4):**829e-830e and 833e-837e ONLY.**

Fix RJ and Vasconez LO, "Use of the Omentum in Chest-Wall Reconstruction", *The Surgical Clinics of North America*, (1989); 69(5):**1029 Figure 1, 7 ONLY.**

Botianu P.V.H., "Current Indications for the Intrathoracic Transposition of the Omentum", *J Cardiothoracic Surg.*, (2019);14:**Table 1 ONLY**.

Faculty Discussion and Study Guide

Chest Wall

1. Explain the role of the thoracic or chest wall musculoskeletal framework in respiratory physiology. (The skeletal framework consists of the ribs anchored anteriorly by the sternum and posteriorly by the vertebral column. Expansion of the thoracic cavity occurs with contracture and descent of the diaphragm as well as contraction of the intercostal muscles that compress the ribs and lift the thoracic skeletal cage. That expansion of the musculoskeletal system creates a negative intrathoracic pressure and an expansion of the lungs. During inspiration, the abdominal wall muscles relax. Expiration is created by a passive recoil of the lung, abdominal wall contracture by the rectus and oblique muscles, and relaxation and ascent of the diaphragm.)
   (a) How does the configuration, i.e., topography of the ribs facilitate respiration? (The structure of the thoracic cavity including the direction of the ribs anteriorly and posteriorly as well as the rigid anchor points of the sternum and the vertebral column, all create an accordion action with respiration. The inferior portion of the sternum lifts in a "pump-handle" action under the influence of the lifting action of the sternocleidomastoid and scalenes.)

E. Luce, *A Curriculum for Plastic Surgery*, https://doi.org/10.1007/978-3-031-62087-4_58

   (b) Explain the pathophysiology of a loss of the portion of the thoracic wall. (Without stabilization of the musculoskeletal framework, the segment of chest wall will collapse during inspiration under the influence of the negative intrathoracic pressure. The reverse will occur with expiration, the segment will expand. This phenomenon is known as a flail chest or paradoxical respiration.)
2. Discuss reconstructive goals of the chest wall, in particular the musculoskeletal framework. What is the complication of failure to do so? (The more anterior the defect, size for size, the more implications in terms of adverse effect on respiration. In general, defects of less than 5 cm in diameter do not require reconstruction whereas many three rib and most four and five rib resections, particularly if anterior or lateral, do require reconstruction. Elective sternectomy or resection of the manubrium will also require reconstruction of the skeletal framework in most instances.)
3. In preoperative assessment of a patient for determination of ability to tolerate a chest wall resection what pulmonary function tests, PFTs, should be ordered? (Forced expiratory volume or FEV_1 as well as functional vital capacity, and FEV_1/FVC ratio are the essential PFTs. The normal ratio is 0.8.)
4. What are some materials that are available for reconstitution of the musculoskeletal wall; disregard the soft tissue requirements. (A popular method has been the use of a methylmethacrylate sandwich that consists of an outer and inner layer of polypropylene mesh with a middle layer of methyl methacrylate or the use of mesh alone. The use of either will require stable and healthy soft tissue coverage. The advent of bioprosthetics has enabled the combination of a bioprosthetic as a deep layer in contact with lung and alloplastic mesh as the outer layer for chest wall stabilization.)
5. Give a general framework of indications for use of a particular material for restoration of chest wall stability and the benefits and liability of each. (Synthetics of polypropylene, such as Prolene® and Marlex®, provide strength and because of the large pore size permit tissue ingrowth but unfortunately also include lung and cannot be used in circumstances of wound contamination. Gore Tex® allows minimal tissue ingrowth with relatively small pore size, but does not heal to the edges of the defect. Bioprosthetics can be utilized in wound contamination circumstances but may lack sufficient rigidity for the thoracic skeleton. Methyl methacrylate does have rigidity but is subject to fracture and extrusion and remains a less than optimal choice.)
6. What are the factors to consider in addressing a chest wall resection defect? (Four factors: the size of the defect, location on the chest wall, the presence or not of wound contamination, and if prior radiation has been administered.)
7. What is the hierarchy or classification of types of reconstructive problems presented by thoracic post-resection infections? (Empyema alone without bronco-pleural fistula, empyema in the presence of bronco-pleural fistula with available muscle flaps; and, empyema, bronco-pleural fistula, and available muscle flaps that either have been utilized or divided at the time of prior operations.)
   (a) Define and briefly describe the following: Clagett procedure, Eloesser procedure, thoracoplasty. (The Clagett procedure consists of creation of an open cavity by resection of a rib or two to allow active drainage. The name Clagett procedure is also associated with drainage, debridement, followed by installation of antibiotic solution and a primary delayed closure. Eloesser procedure consists of an open thoracostomy by creation of an inferiorly based skin flap that is led into the thoracic cavity to control drainage and exteriorize a bronchopleural fistula. The procedure is utilized principally in debilitated patients. Thoracoplasty is resection of multiple ribs with collapse of the soft tissue. The Clagett and Eloesser procedures are both associated with a considerable amount of morbidity and even mortality and the healing process is usually lengthy. Thoracoplasty is quite deforming.)
8. Thoracic surgeons ordinarily manage postpneumonectomy empyema. When most commonly is a plastic surgeon's consultation requested? (Management is usually requested after tube thoracentesis, followed by VATS with decortication followed by perhaps a Clagett procedure and all have failed.)
9. Give a treatment plan for management of a bronchopleural fistula after pneumonectomy. (Surgical debridement must be accomplished including nonviable chest wall and intrathoracic tissue. Second, the site of the fistula from the bronchus must be identified and debrided to viable and healthy tissue. Third, the bronchial end of the fistula must be closed with healthy tissue, namely, muscle transposition to cover the closure of the fistula suture line is essential.)
   (a) What is the success rate with the above treatment plan based on published experience? (About 2/3 of the patients remained healed.)
   (b) What pedicled flaps are most useful? (The most commonly employed muscle for closure over the bronchial stump is serratus anterior, pedicled on the thoracodorsal artery. More anterior and proximal problems such as fistula arising from the tracheoesophageal fistulas, the pectoralis major, can be utilized. Resection of ribs two and three are necessary to move the pectoralis into the thoracic cavity, a lateral rib resection may be necessary to utilize the serratus

anterior. The importance of avoidance of compression of the pedicle is paramount in both instances. The latissimus muscle is commonly divided with thoracotomy and may not have sufficient length to meet reconstructive needs. The omentum is available but requires a laparotomy with a potential for introduction of sepsis into the abdominal cavity and hernia.)

Sternum

1. Outline a classification of sternal wound dehiscence both in space and in time. (I a, b; superficial either with or without exposure of the fascia and sternal periosteum and usually an aseptic sternal dehiscence secondary to poor technical closure; II a, b; infected exposed bone either stable or unstable sternum; III a, b; exposed necrotic and unstable bone, exposure of the mediastinal structures either with or without sepsis. The CDC has defined deep sternal wound infection as one of the following: a positive mediastinal culture, gross or biopsy evidence of mediastinitis, sternal instability, and pleural mediastinal drainage. Classification in time: acute, subacute, and chronic. Although a bright line does not exist between the three time components of acute, subacute, and chronic. Ordinarily, acute is less than 2 weeks and chronic is a matter of months. The acute problems are heavily weighted toward a sternal dehiscence that may not have been infectious but rather ischemic in etiology. The etiology of chronic infections are most commonly a period of osteomyelitis or chondritis.)
   (a) Hierarchy of frequency of occurrence? (II > III > I.)
2. Give several risk factors for the development of mediastinal osteomyelitis, mediastinitis, sternal dehiscence. Separate into preoperative and intraoperative. (Preoperative risk factors are obesity, diabetes, smoking, COPD, renal failure, chronic steroid use, and immunosuppression. Intraoperative include off-line sternotomy, bilateral internal mammary artery, IMA, harvest, transverse fracture of the sternum, and bypass greater than 2 h. Postoperative risk factors include the necessity for prolonged ventilator support. The evolution and advancement of percutaneous coronary artery stenting has probably contributed to a higher proportion of CABG patients with risk factors.)
   (a) Is harvest of the left internal mammary artery, LIMA, a risk factor? (Probably not.)
   (b) What is the approximate overall incidence of sternal dehiscence? (1–2%.)
3. Comment on the following imaging modalities for sternal wound infection. Chest x-ray, CT scan, nuclear scan. (Chest x-ray is of value to determine the presence of broken wires only. CT scan before 21 days will be of little value. Nuclear scans are almost always positive, perhaps falsely so, if the sternum has been exposed for any length of time. CT scan after 3 weeks postoperatively may be of value to detect an intra-mediastinal fluid collection.)
4. Readings were distributed to provide information about other methods of sternal fixation at the time of the primary procedure. What was the essence of the points made? (Since early or noninfectious sternal dehiscence is distinctly uncommon and may be technique-based, repair by some method such as Robicsek or other parasternal cerclage closures is preferable to a single wire transternal closure. Rigid fixation with plates and screws can be selectively employed in high-risk patients, particularly in repeat sternotomy. The readings and video from the REC illustrate the use of rigid fixation with 2.4 mm locking reconstruction plates instead of wires. The use of the technique as a secondary procedure would require careful judgment. An aseptic, early postoperative sternal dehiscence could be satisfactorily plated instead of rewired. Advanced osteomyelitis that requires debridement and subtotal sternectomy is optimally managed with conventional therapy.)
5. Comment on the use of closed irrigation and drainage-suction in the management of sternal wound infections. (A method of closed irrigation- and drainage-suction was instituted by cardiothoracic surgeons 50 years ago and was the mainstay of treatment until the development of muscle flap closure in the late 70 s, early 80 s. A number of studies have established that the morbidity and mortality of closed irrigation-suction is higher than a more aggressive approach of debridement and flap closure.)
6. Readings were provided about the role of the VAC in management of these problems. What is the bottom line message from these readings? (Agarwal and coauthors established the role of the VAC as "first line management" but the mortality rate was 20% and 2/3 of the patients actually had reconstructive closure after an average of 11 days of the use of the VAC. Other publications have defined the potentially adverse effect of prolonged use of the VAC for more than 21 days. The bottom line message is that the VAC could be an excellent bridge particularly in unstable patients between debridement and definitive closure but the duration of the VAC therapy should be limited to perhaps 2 weeks or less.)
7. With the information from several of the distributed papers, comment on staged vs. single-stage repair of sternal dehiscence/osteomyelitis. (Staged repair with multiple debridements, development of a granulating surface, and a closure has some traditional value. The readings indicate that a single-stage debridement and

reconstruction is possible with good results. Nevertheless, with the availability of the VAC, stabilization of the patient, and assurance of culture-specific antibiotic coverage, a two-stage approach is more prudent. Type III or chronic sternal infections with established osteomyelitis would lend themselves to a staged approach of debridement, application of a VAC, and definitive closure. As discussed above, a two-stage approach with short-term use of the VAC is an acceptable option.)

8. Describe methods of utilization of the pectoralis for closure of mediastinal defects. (Turnover pectoralis muscle flaps inherently devascularize the overlying pectoral skin because of the division of the thoracoacromial trunk and the necessity for elevation of the soft tissue and skin off the muscle in order to turnover a muscle flap. Any muscle splitting will be bloody. Turnover flaps have some traditional value but have been discarded by many for pectoralis advancement flaps. Two other methods of the use of the pectoralis consist of dissection of the pectoralis alone and advancement. To do so, devascularize the overlying skin and may set the stage for skin necrosis and wound dehiscence. The third method is advancement as a compound skin and muscle flap. See the next question.)
9. Describe the technique of bilateral pectoralis advancement flaps. (The chest wall skin and pectoralis muscle are raised as a single unit with a dissection beneath the pectoralis muscle after ligation of the internal mammary perforators. The flaps are advanced bilaterally with elevation of the superior portion of the anterior rectus fascia. Closure is accomplished over drains.)
   (a) Comment on the following: management of the humeral insertion, necessity of mediastinal "fill," principal blood supply to the flaps, duration of drains (The blood supply is the thoracoacromial and the principal point is to maintain drains until dry with an average duration of 22 days. Most frequently, the humeral insertion is not divided, the mediastinum does not necessarily have to be "filled" but should have drains deep and superficial to the muscular closure as well as both donor sites.)
   (b) Although low, a certain percentage of patients may sustain skin edge necrosis. Why? (Elevation of the flaps require division of the perforators from the internal mammary artery. Perfusion of the thoracic skin is then entirely from the thoracoacromial and the lateral thoracic arteries.)
10. What would be the role, benefit, and limitations of the use of a rectus muscle flap in these wounds? (If compound pectoralis skin and muscle flaps are utilized in an advancement fashion, the weakest portion of the closure is the distal one-fourth. That space could be filled with a superiorly based rectus muscle flap, although not commonly incorporated with bilateral pectoralis skin and muscle flap advancement for the reasons listed below.)
    (a) Why not combine bilateral advancement pectoral flaps with a rectus flap as described? (Probably the incidence of wound dehiscence would be increased considerably since the blood supply for the entire side of the trunk, not just the chest, would be deprived by division of the perforators from the deep superior and inferior epigastric and dependent on the thoracoacromial superiorly and secondary branches from the common femoral inferiorly.)
11. What difficulty can occur in treatment outcomes in type III or late osteomyelitis? (Necessity for reoperation can be as high as one-third, some of whom will require additional flaps. The reason for the significant recurrence rate is not clear but may be related to inadequate debridement of the associated costochondritis and underlines that the management of late sternal osteomyelitis has a significant recurrence and reoperation rate.)
12. The use of the omentum has been advocated as a tertiary solution to sternal dehiscence/mediastinitis. The vascular supply of the omentum is derived from a branch of the celiac axis. What vessels give off the left and right gastroepiploic arteries? (The left is derived from the splenic artery, the right the gastroduodenal artery.)
    (a) What is the name and consistency of the occurrence of the principal connecting vessel? (The marginal artery of Barkow; 85–90%.)
13. What are the indications for a tertiary use of the omentum in chest wall reconstruction? (The irradiated defect with possibly failed muscle reconstruction; a large sternal defect particularly inferior in location +/− use of muscle flaps that have failed.)
14. Briefly describe a technique for a right-sided pedicled omental flap. (Identification as high as possible on the lesser curvature of the stomach of the left gastroepiploic artery and ligation at that point. Care must be taken not to injure the spleen. The short gastric vessels derived from the superior marginal connection between the left and right gastroepiploic arteries must be individually ligated to pedicle the omentum completely on the right gastroepiploic artery. Of course, dissection of the omentum off the transverse colon is necessary regardless of how the omentum is pedicled.)
    (a) What is the method of entry for an omental flap into a sternal defect? (A small aperture is made in the anterior central portion of the diaphragm.)

15. What are the principal disadvantages in use of the omentum for either sternum or chest wall reconstruction? How to minimize? (The principal disadvantages are the necessity to enter the abdomen and harvest the omentum and the possible spread of wound sepsis into the abdominal cavity. An additional concern is the possible occurrence of hernia through the diaphragmatic aperture. Endoscopic harvest can minimize the possibility of both. Since a skin graft will be applied to the omentum, an inherent defect will exist without the presence of muscle and, obviously, bone.)

Videos

Hamaguchi R, Shekar PS, Johnson JA, et al., "Current Management of Sternal Wounds", *Plast. Reconstr. Surg.*, (2021); 148(6):1012e.

Video 1

Orgill is interviewed.

1. Lauded the role of VAC to convert to a semi-elective procedure; "limited" advancement by preservation of the perforators (probably not advisable).

Video 2

CT surgeons perspective.

1. Changed the method of wiring but does not utilize plates. Does use nasal mupirocin in patients with a positive nasopharyngeal culture.
2. Changed preoperative antibiotics to bank.

Case-Based Conference

Case 1—Chest Wall Ulcer

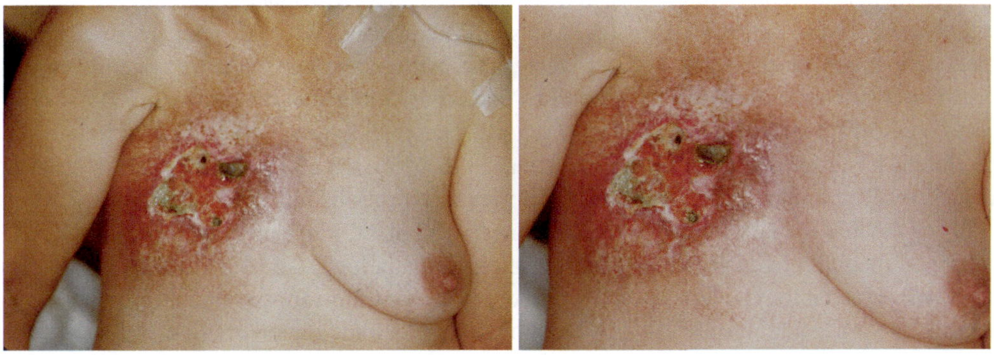

A 44 year old 2 years after radical mastectomy for a large Ca of the breast and 18 months after completion of radiation therapy.

1. Describe the slides and add a focused clinical examination.
   (a) Any studies indicated? Why?
2. What is the pathologic anatomy? How does the pathologic anatomy dictate your treatment plan?
3. Outline your treatment plan. If operative, draw your incisions.

Case-Based Conference: Discussion

Case 1—Chest Wall Ulcer

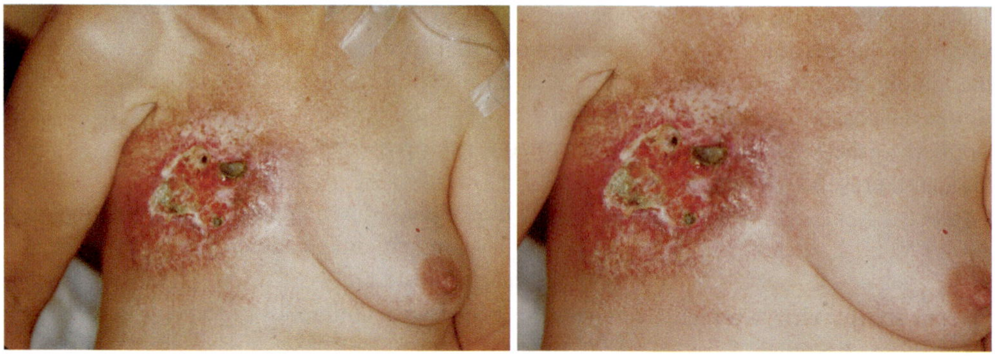

A 44 year old 2 years after radical mastectomy for a large Ca of the breast and 18 months after completion of radiation therapy.

1. Describe the slides and add a focused clinical examination. (Two photos of the patient's anterior chest from shoulders to epigastrium and a close-up view illustrates the salient finding, a large ulcerative lesion on the right chest wall with an absent breast. The characteristics of the ulcer include irregular edges and measures 7 x 8 cm. The surrounding skin has marked telangiectasia for a zone of 2–3 cm, more so inferior and superior. The medial extent is to the parasternal line, laterally to the mid axillary line. Within the ulceration superiorly and medially is an area of 2 cm of exposed rib which appears nonviable. The left breast is present and unremarkable. No other findings are depicted. In summary, the ulcer and telangiectatic skin occupy a substantial portion, probably greater than 50% of the right anterior chest wall.

   The history portion of the clinical exam would attempt to ascertain the size of the breast primary tumor, if regional lymph nodes were positive, and the duration and frequency of the radiotherapy administered postoperatively. In reality, that information will need to be supplemented by a review of the medical records including pathology and operative reports that would indicate the performance of an axillary lymph node dissection and if the pectoralis was sacrificed. Additional questions would focus on systemic symptoms such as shortness of breath, chest pain, limited exercise tolerance as well as easy fatigability, weight loss, and bone pain. The social history would be also reviewed that would include smoking, alcohol, or other substance abuse as well as the activities of daily living. The physical exam should include palpation of the axilla and supraclavicular fossa for evidence of axillary or scalene recurrence as well as the opposite breast and axilla. The abdomen is inspected for scars and the ipsilateral latissimus palpated with the shoulder in active adduction against resistance.)

   (a) Any studies indicated? Why? (If not performed previously, an oncologic workup to detect systemic metastases that would include at the minimum, CT scan of the head, chest, abdomen, and pelvis. Although not critical in the decision about the extent of resection, MRI may be more sensitive in the detection of osteoradionecrosis but a CT scan may be more sensitive to intrathoracic pathology. On balance, a PET/CT scan would probably suffice for the imaging components of the workup. In anticipation of chest wall resection, pulmonary function tests may be of value. Nutritional assessment includes, besides a history of weight loss, is a determination of albumin and prealbumin levels.)

2. What is the pathologic anatomy? How does the pathologic anatomy dictate your treatment plan? (Either neoplastic or radiation necrosis or both are present in this area of extensive ulceration and by implication, osteoradionecrosis of the ribs. The summary of those factors in the pathologic anatomy is the magnitude of chest wall involvement. The anterior and anterolateral skeletal chest wall play a crucial role in respiratory physiology. The ability to produce negative intrathoracic pressures to assist in expansion of the lung during inspiration is achieved by both downward movement of the diaphragm and expansion of the chest wall accomplished by the intercostals and secondary muscles of respiration.

Removal of ribs anteriorly and anterolaterally, but not posteriorly because of the splinting effect of the scapular and paraspinal muscles, can result in chest wall instability. If the resection is of sufficient magnitude, the stage may be set for paradoxical respiration, characterized by inward, rather than outward, collapse of the chest wall on inspiration and outward, rather than contraction, of the chest wall on expiration. The result is a decrease in tidal volume and loss of ability to clear small airways of mucus. Radiation fibrosis will, to some degree, impart some fixation of the chest wall by loss of pliability. Nevertheless, prior radiotherapy does not significantly alter the equation of determination of the magnitude of chest wall resection. Additional pathology includes the radiated skin and soft tissue and possibly the underlying lung parenchyma as well. The common thread, regardless of the end target, in radiation-induced injury is a progressive ischemia from an obliterative endarteritis of the small vessels.)

3. Outline your treatment plan. If operative, draw your incisions. (The overarching consideration is the patient's life expectancy. If the chest wall ulceration is a presentation of local recurrence, the probability of systemic metastases, even if not evident, is quite high. The point is somewhat moot, because the pathology will be unknown until a resection is completed and submitted as a specimen. If metastases are present, some estimation of the life expectancy would be helpful and should be balanced against the impact of the wound on the patient's quality of life. In this scenario, the short interval between initial diagnosis and the current situation would indicate that in the presence of demonstrable systemic metastases, a very careful and balanced decision process is necessary with extensive patient involvement.

   If resection is the plan, then one must consider that the ulcer and the adjacent irradiated skin and soft tissue will require resection. The principal challenge for reconstruction will be stabilization and wound closure of the thoracic cavity to prevent/minimize an unstable chest wall and provision of soft tissue coverage. The extent of the chest wall resection will dictate the necessity for chest wall stabilization. In general, resection of four and certainly five or greater ribs with the overlying soft tissue will mandate the address by reconstruction of the defect of the chest wall. An alternative yardstick is 5 cm or 25 cm^2. Prosthetic materials are utilized, most commonly polypropylene mesh either alone or as a "sandwich" incorporating methyl methacrylate as the central layer. The criticism of this method of chest wall reconstruction, the incorporation of methyl methacrylate, is twofold: one, the long-term infection and extrusion rate is not insignificant, perhaps secondary to lack of tissue ingrowth incorporation of the methyl methacrylate; second, from the standpoint of dynamic respiratory physiology, a rigid chest wall may not be desirable. More recently, description of the use of biologics such as acellular human dermis has emerged, the advantage is if a small area is exposed, not an infrequent occurrence, infection and loss of the mesh is not the inevitable outcome. Further experience with biologics is needed but one conceptual concern would be the elasticity and stretch in situ with time that would subsequently result in loss of a stable chest wall. Bioprosthetics may have an optimal application in the circumstances of infection or a contaminated wound. A compromise between rigidity, methyl methacrylate sandwich, and elasticity, bioprosthetics may be a composite mesh. One example includes polytetrafluoroethylene, Gore Tex ®, or a bioprosthetic as the layer against the lung and polypropylene, Prolene ® or Marlex ® exposed to the superficial or underside of the flap provided for coverage.

   The second reconstructive consideration is the full-thickness skin–soft tissue wound closure. The post-resection wound in this scenario will be large and the flap dimension requirements are substantial since closure of an open chest wound must by definition be complete. The adjacent latissimus dorsi with overlying skin is one choice in this setting but, because of the size of the defect, either will require skin grafting of the donor site or preoperative expansion to yield a sufficiently sized flap for primary closure. Other options to supply the requisite volume of tissue include a pedicled TRAM or a DIEP free flap. The former would benefit from a prior, 1 week, delay, the latter a consideration of the fate of the right internal mammary with the resection.

   The perioperative considerations are the possible prolonged period of postoperative ventilation and weaning particularly in those instances of massive resections that include chest wall and sternum. Although the incidence of long-term adverse laryngeal sequelae are the same for prolonged oral vs. nasal intubation, patient comfort is enhanced by nasal intubation at the time of resection.)

Intraoperative

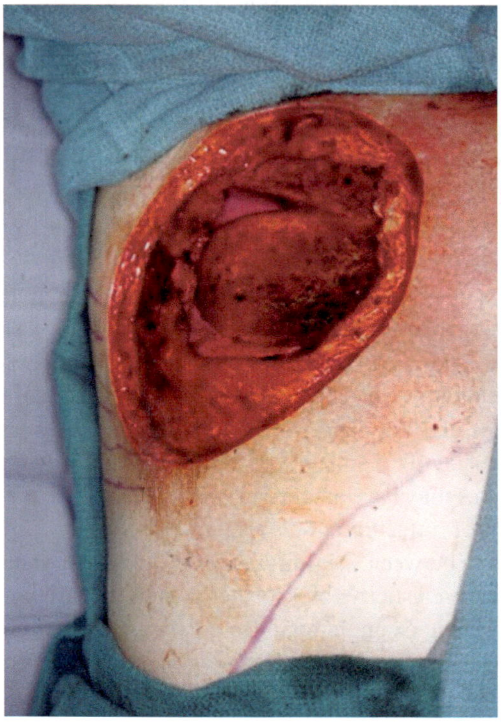

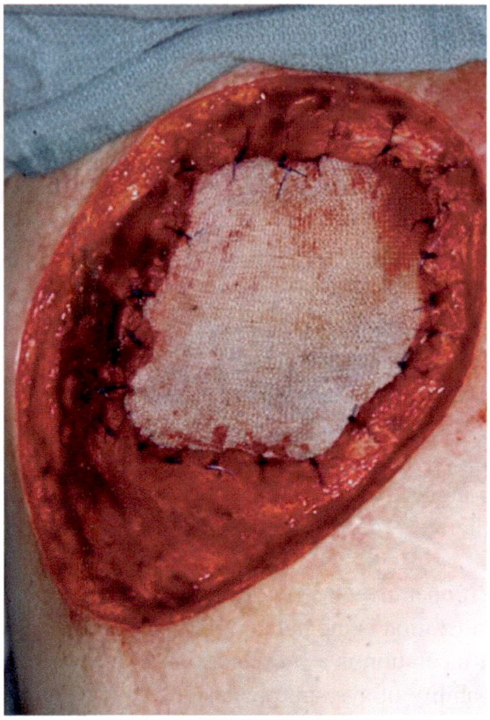

Two intraoperative photos illustrate the post-resection defect and repair. The first demonstrates a probable four rib resection with an unexpanded lung and pleural cavity visible. A blue mark curves obliquely across the lower margin of the surgical field that outlines the subcostal angle. In the second photo a close-up view, a prosthetic mesh has been sewn into the defect with large interrupted sutures.

Postoperative (3 Months)

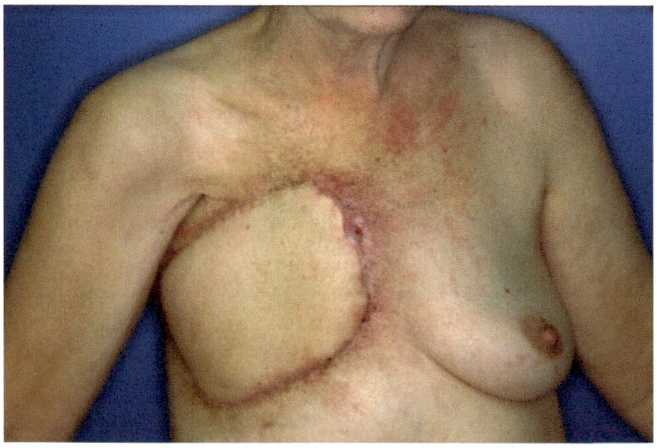

In a single view of the chest from shoulders to epigastrium, the defect has been reconstructed with a large, rectangular-shaped latissimus flap with a skin island. A small rim of 1–2 cm of irradiated skin persists medially. The peripheral incisions of the flap inset have healed.

Case-Based Conference

Case 2—Open Chest Wound

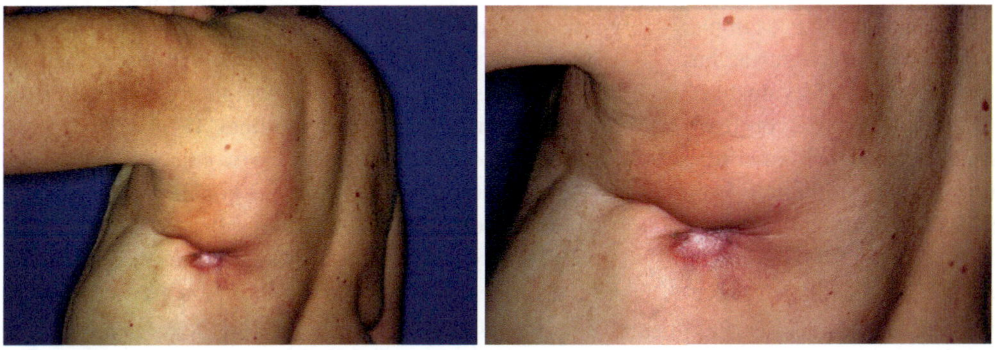

Patient is 51 year old and 6 months after upper lobectomy. The patient developed a bronchopleural fistula despite conservative treatment with chest tube and suction. Currently, the patient bubbles actively through the skin wound and the lower lobe remains only partially expanded.

1. Describe what you see on the slide and add a pertinent history and physical examination.
   (a) Any imaging studies or diagnostic tests indicated? Justify.
2. What is the pathologic anatomy and physiology of this problem?
3. In essence, what are the treatment goals? Outline a treatment management plan including steps and sequence.

Case-Based Conference: Discussion

Case 2—Open Chest Wound

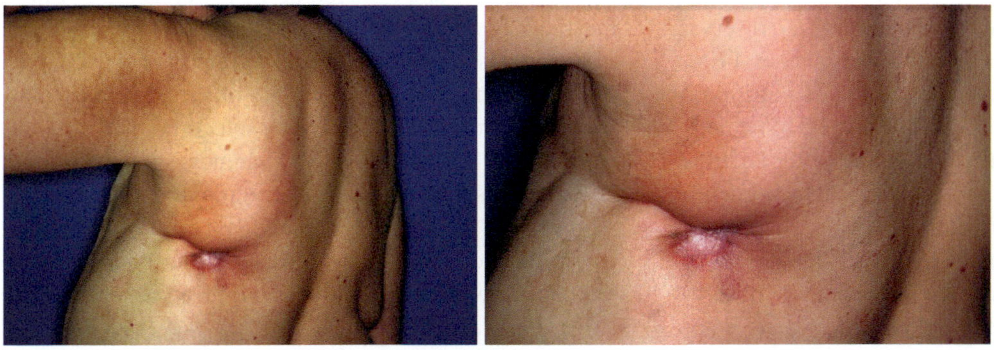

Patient is 51 years old and 6 months after upper lobectomy. The patient developed a bronchopleural fistula despite conservative treatment with chest tube and suction. Currently, the patient bubbles actively through the skin wound and the lower lobe remains only partially expanded.

1. Describe what you see on the slide and add a pertinent history and physical examination. (The two slides provide only a lateral view of the thorax, shoulder, and back of the patient. Apparent in the mid-posterior lateral thorax is a 6–7 cm area of transverse retracted skin and soft-tissue with an immediate adjacent round 2 cm of either ulceration or scar. No active drainage is evident. No incisional scar is apparent posterior, the anterior thorax cannot be visualized. The surrounding skin is not erythematous. The remaining portion of the trunk of the patient appears to be normal or even a moderately obese habitus. The second slide is a close-up view and does not provide additional information.

The principal function of the clinical examination will be to provide the necessary information about the treatment of the present illness to date. That history would begin with the initial diagnosis: malignant such as a neoplasm of the bronchus versus benign as, for example, lobar bronchiectasis. If neoplasm was the diagnosis, has the patient had a recent oncologic follow-up evaluation? The next tier of history questions would focus on treatment of his current complication, in particular, other than a thoracostomy, have other treatment modalities been implemented? For example, has an effort to close the bronchopleural fistula endoscopically been attempted? Does the fistula represent the outcome of a Clagett procedure, directed toward control of the fistula by creation of a skin–soft tissue flap? If the diagnosis was neoplasm, was postoperative irradiation administered? The following set of historical questions would focus on the patient's overall functional status. Judged by the activities of daily living, how compromised is the patient by his/her reduced respiratory status? The final set of questions would ascertain the presence, if any, of significant comorbidities, medications, tobacco and alcohol use, and pertinent social history.

The physical exam would be directed toward the wound, although little could be ascertained not already evident in the preamble. Other aspects of the exam, in addition to ascertainment of the overall nutritional status, would be evaluation of potential donor sites. See below.)

(a) Any imaging studies or diagnostic tests indicated? Justify. (In all probability, the patient has had multiple chest x-rays and multiple CT scans and those imaging studies should be reviewed. The other assessment is the patient's functional respiratory reserve. Pulmonary functional tests would consist of FEV_1 and FEV_1/FVC. If concerns exist about nutritional status, albumin and pre-albumin would be of value.)

2. What is the pathologic anatomy and physiology of this problem? (The occurrence of a postoperative bronchopleural fistula following a lobectomy is distinctly uncommon, perhaps more frequent in those instances of resection for infectious complications such as postobstructive disease. Regardless, the presence of a bronchopleural fistula 6 months postoperative implies a chronic inflammatory state and low probability of resolution with conservative measures alone. The bronchopleural fistula and attendant air leak signals inadequate expansion of the remaining lower lobe and ongoing respiratory insufficiency. The increase in work of respiration can deplete metabolic reserves and result in weight loss and inanition. The bronchial stump and confines of the fistula are incased in a chronic inflammatory wound.)
3. In essence, what are the treatment goals? Outline a treatment management plan including steps and sequence. (A goal of the patient's treatment plan is successful closure of the bronchial stump and obliteration of the fistulous tract. To do so will require the transfer of well-vascularized tissue, namely, a pedicled flap, preferably muscle. The three muscle options are the pectoralis major, latissimus dorsi, and serratus anterior. Although no posterior extension of the thoracotomy is present on the slides, the thoracic surgeon and operative note would need to be queried for possible division of the latissimus dorsi with the initial procedure. Use of the pectoralis is a distinct possibility since the bronchus under consideration is the left upper lobe. The third possibility is the serratus anterior, the workhorse for management of postoperative bronchopleural fistulas, usually post-pneumonectomy. The muscle can be harvested and pedicled on the branch of the thoracodorsal artery. Harvest of the serratus more than just the inferior 2–3 slips, necessary in this instance, often leads to a winged scapula. Access into the chest is provided by a rib resection, although a formal thoracotomy is necessary anyway to accomplish a decortication of the remaining lobe and excision of the fistulous tract. A non-muscular option is the use of the omentum, perhaps harvested endoscopically and tunneled into the chest. Given the consistency and the reliability of the muscle options, omentum is considered a tertiary selection.

The final consideration is awareness of the resultant skin–soft tissue defect with excision of the chronic chest wound and tract, since some degree of contraction occurred over the lengthy postoperative course. In all likelihood, wide undermining and advancement will be sufficient to address that deficit.)

Case-Based Conference

Case 3—GSW of Shoulder–Neck

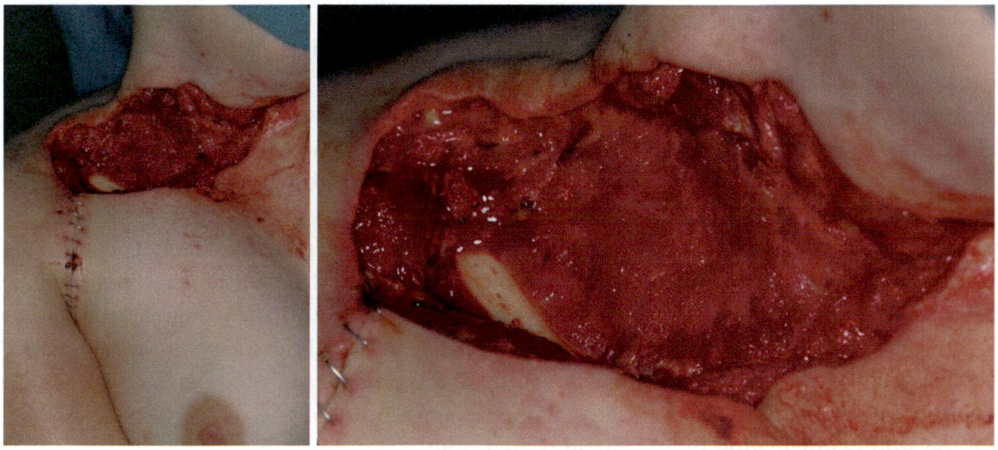

A 24-year-old-female shot at close range with a high-velocity rifle. The patient has been managed by the trauma service yesterday with wound exploration, debridement, and vascular repair of the subclavian artery with a saphenous vein graft which is palpable in the depths of the wound.

1. Describe the findings on the slide(s) and add a focused clinical examination.
   (a) Any test indicated?
2. Describe the pathologic anatomy. Outline the treatment goals.
3. Give your treatment plan.

Case-Based Conference: Discussion

Case 3—GSW of Shoulder–Neck

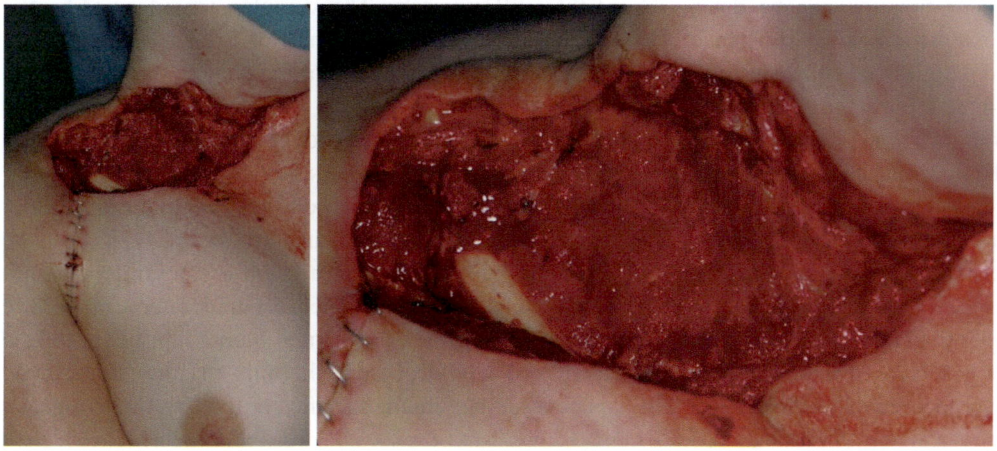

A 24-year-old-female shot at close range with a high-velocity rifle. The patient has been managed by the trauma service yesterday with wound exploration, debridement, and vascular repair of the subclavian artery with a saphenous vein graft which is palpable in the depths of the wound.

1. Describe the findings on the slide(s) and add a focused clinical examination. (The slides represent a limited view of the right shoulder, upper arm, and breast of the patient. The principal finding is a large acute wound that occupies most of the supraclavicular area, extends into the base of the anterolateral neck, and impinges on the infraclavicular area but not to the tip of the shoulder. The posterior shoulder appears intact. A stapled incision crosses obliquely from the inferior lateral edge of the wound into the axilla, the distal extent not visualized. The wound appears to have some element of depth and several centimeters of exposed bone, presumably the clavicle, is visible in the most lateral aspect. The surrounding skin appears quite viable. No active bleeding as depicted by clotted blood is evident.

   The initial history would quickly eliminate or establish the presence of any co-morbidities, doubtful in this young patient, and then move toward documentation of associated injuries. Presumably, the trauma service has ruled out concomitant injuries elsewhere including the chest and neck. A review with the operating surgeon about the extent of injury evident in the OR including the brachial plexus and the subclavian vein would be of value and in particular the location of the proximal anastomosis on the subclavian artery.

   Pertinent questions to the patient about pain, numbness, and upper extremity function should be folded into the physical exam. To limit patient discomfort, the neurovascular exam could be centered on the hand. Ulnar, radial, and median nerve motor and sensory function can provide valuable information about the status of the brachial plexus trunks. The upper and middle, more superiorly located, would have a higher probability of injury and those trunks contribute to the radial and median nerves. The radial nerve motor function can be determined by finger and wrist extension against resistance, the median assessed by flexor digitorum sublimis function. The wrist pulses are palpated. Further delineation of the presence of and extent of the brachial plexus injury by examination of deltoid and latissimus function will be limited by pain. Attention directed toward the wound would consist of a gentle palpation and determination of the location and degree of exposure of the saphenous vein graft.)

   (a) Any tests indicated? (Other than reviewing recent lab values, the principal test is review of the angiogram particularly if performed preoperatively as well as the on-table angiogram performed at the time of the subclavian artery repair. Determination of the status of the branches that perfuse the tissues that could potentially serve as a reconstructive option would be essential in treatment planning. A review of x-ray for determination of any clavicle fractures needs to be done as well.)

2. Describe the pathologic anatomy. Outline the treatment plan. (The wound has been inflicted by a high-velocity missile that imparts a substantial amount of kinetic energy, the end result a loss of skin, soft tissue, and injury to underlying neurovascular structures. Because of the high energy, the full extent of the damage may not be evident initially. Apparently, by the wound appearance in the photos, an aggressive debridement was accomplished at the setting of the vascular repair but an additional operative wound examination and possible additional debridement is advisable.

   Given the extent and depths of the wound and the presence of the saphenous vein graft and exposed clavicle, a full-thickness flap would be necessary to address the wound reconstructive requirements. Regional musculocutaneous flaps available include trapezius, latissimus, pectoralis, and possibly the scapular each with benefits and liabilities. The first step in consideration is the location of the perfusing vessels. The superior portion of the trapezius is vascularized by the transverse cervical artery, a branch of the thyrocervical trunk, the most proximal branch, arising from the first portion of the subclavian artery. An extension of the trapezius myocutaneous is the supraclavicular flap, perfused by the supraclavicular artery, a branch of the transverse cervical. The pectoralis major is vascularized by the thoracoacromial artery branching from the first or second part of the axillary artery. The scapular, vascularized by the circumflex scapular, a branch of the subscapular axis, would require a dissection of the pedicle through the triangular space and the flap must follow, a substantially tight fit. As such, some doubt about sufficient length would be present. The latissimus is perfused by the thoracodorsal artery, a branch of the subscapular axis, arising from the third part of the axillary artery. Use of the pectoralis will inflict a significant aesthetic deficit onto this patient and the thoracoacromial artery may have been damaged. The latissimus blood supply should be intact and would provide the bulk to address the dead space issue but entails sacrifice of the latissimus muscle.

Variants of the latissimus as the thoracodorsal artery perforator, TAP, flap would spare the latissimus muscle, a consideration since the extent of the brachial plexus injury is not clear, including the ultimate necessity for muscle transfer. The TAP flap, though, may or may not be sufficient in closing the dead space. The remaining consideration is rotation of a trapezius-based musculocutaneous or fasciocutaneous flap. The photos would appear to depict a wound that involves loss of a portion of the trapezius and, possibly, injury to the transverse cervical artery but not likely the thyrocervical trunk. Again, review of the angiograms would be key to determining the suitability of a transverse cervical artery flap perfused by most particularly the supraclavicular artery. Regardless, rotation of a flap will require a split skin graft to the donor site, perhaps excised later with the aid of tissue expansion. Certainly, one option to avoid a skin graft of the flap donor site, is something of a bilobed design. The primary option to fill the defect would be the supraclavicular flap in closure of the donor site with a flap, harvested from the adjacent back angiosome, perfused by the circumflex scapular. The tip of the supraclavicular flap must be designed to limit the length at the tip of the shoulder. Further extension into the arm encroaches on the posterior humeral reflex angiosome.

No consideration should be given to a primary repair of a brachial plexus injury, if present, since the circumstance of the wound are those of high energy, rendering the determination of the degree of nerve injury extremely difficult.)

Intraoperative

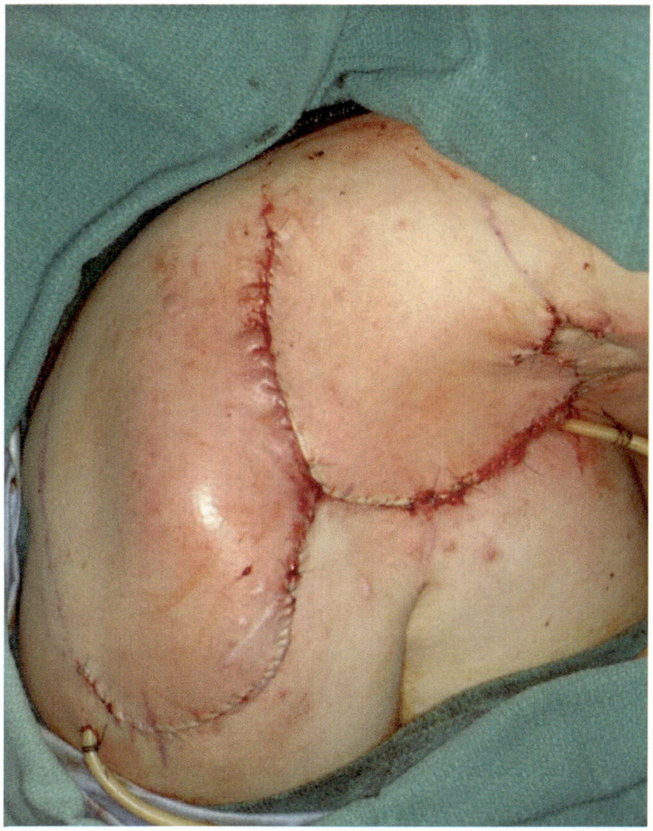

As described above, a bilobed design of two flaps were utilized.

Postoperative (4 Months)

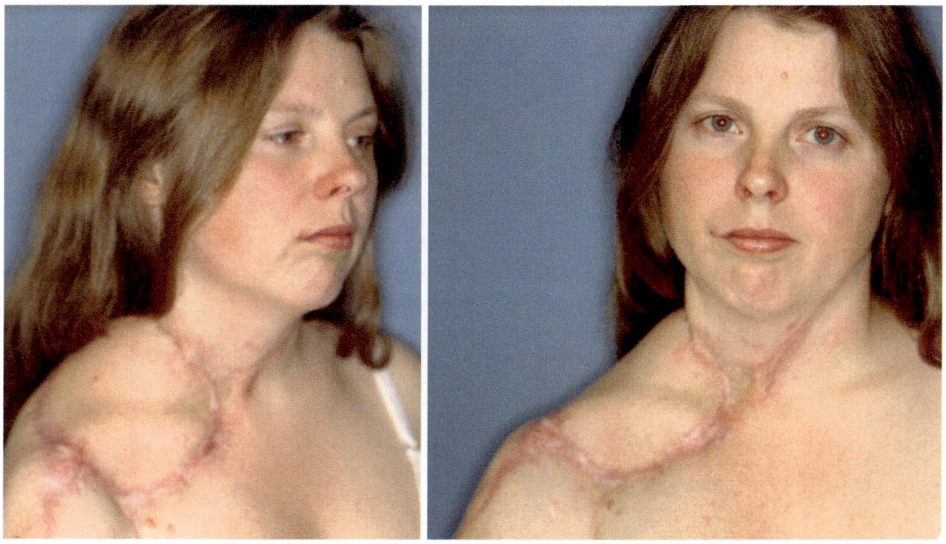

In the two views, frontal and oblique, the wound is fully healed. The right shoulder has a slump posture that would seem to reflect loss of deltoid and possibly some trapezius muscle function. The scars are somewhat hypertrophic, consistent with the patient's red hair and Fitzpatrick 1–2 complexion.

Case-Based Conference

Case 4—Sternal Dehiscence

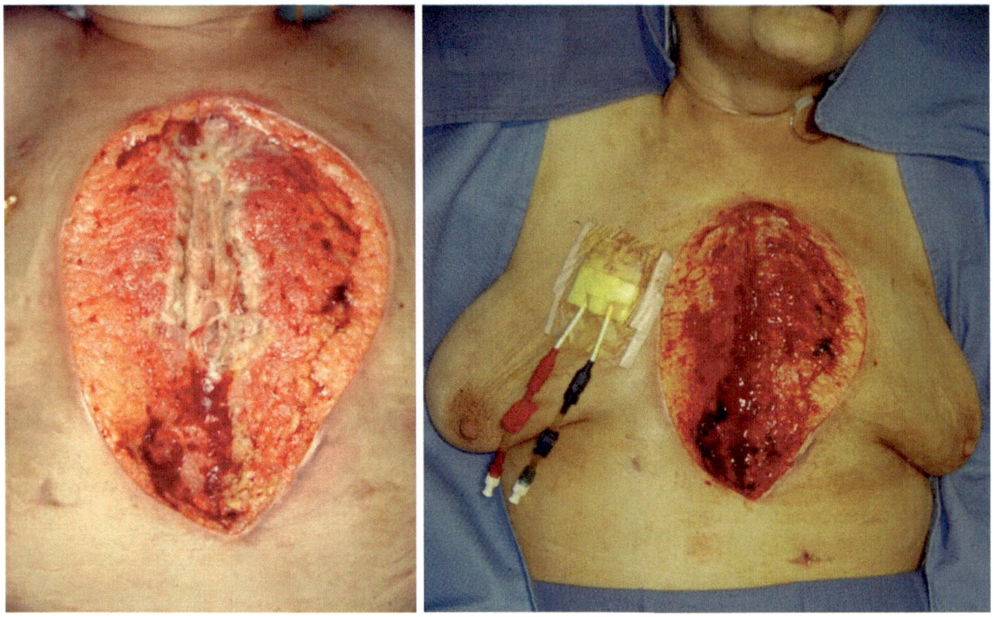

A 66-year-old diabetic 3 weeks post-CABG. The wound was opened, drained, and soft tissue debrided on the floor. The first photo is immediate after debridement, the second 3–4 days later. The patient is stable, not on the ventilator, and remains in the ICU.

1. Describe the slide; add any additional history that may be of value as well as a physical examination.
   (a) Any tests indicated? If so, why?
2. What may have been the risk factors operative in this patient's complication and how might those factors be minimized?
   (a) What is the pathological process? Describe in the framework of duration of onset postoperative.
3. Outline a menu of treatment options from your most acceptable to least acceptable. Give your rationale for your choices.
   (a) Is the hierarchy of procedures described in the preamble the same as yours?

Case-Based Conference: Discussion

Case 4—Sternal Dehiscence

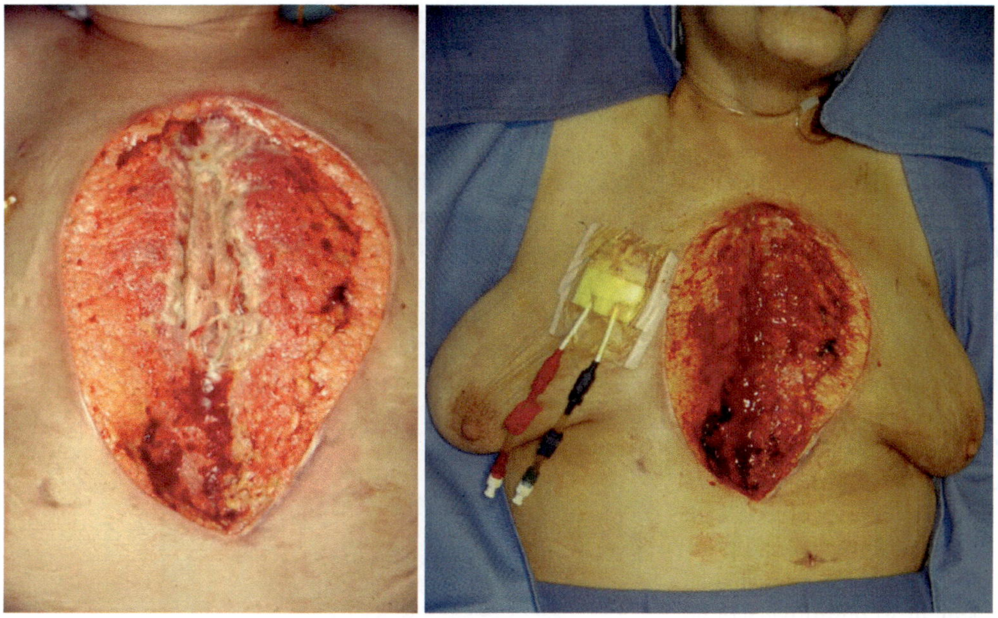

A 66-year-old diabetic 3 weeks post-CABG. The wound was opened, drained, and soft tissue debrided on the floor. The first photo is immediate after debridement, the second 3–4 days later. The patient is stable, not on the ventilator, and remains in the ICU.

1. Describe the slide; add any additional history that may be of value as well as a physical examination. (Two slides are provided, one at the time of skin–soft tissue debridement, the second 3–4 days later. The first depicts an extensive skin–soft tissue wound that involves the central chest area, medial left breast, and right parasternal region. Recently clotted blood is visible centrally. The fat at the wound edges appears viable and no necrotic skin is present. The second slide is a much wider view of the entire chest and breast and several things are evident. The external ports for two intracardiac catheters are evident through the upper pole of the right breast. The wound itself has a small amount of freshly clotted blood and appears to be adequately debrided. The patient also is moderately obese and the breasts are of moderate size. No upper abdominal scars are evident.

   Historical information of value, in addition to what is provided in the preamble, is the type of CABG performed and the donor vessels, particularly harvest of the LIMA or left internal mammary artery, the urgency of the procedure as an index of the severity of the disease as well as preoperative information with respect to cardiac performance. The presentation of the current complication as well as the appearance of the wound prior to debridement if another service performed, the debridement is also information of value. Current postoperative medications complete the history. The physical exam assesses the wound and status of the sternum, particularly the mobility of the two leaves of the bone. The wound is also examined for visibility of the parasternal wires and the abdomen is examined for extra scars.)

   (a) Any tests indicated? If so, why? (A CT scan may be of value to detect mediastinal fluid collection. CT scans performed prior to 3 weeks postoperatively have a high incidence of false positives. CT scans may also indicate the presence of osteomyelitis in late sternal infections, not likely detected though on imaging this acutely postoperative. The scan can also detect residual sternal wires, if any. If not already performed, a laboratory assessment of the patient's nutritional status and perhaps a dietary consult would be advisable.)

2. What may have been the risk factors operative in this patient's complication and how might those factors be minimized? (The risk factors for patients who undergo sternotomy are numerous and include obesity, diabetes, smoking, COPD, renal failure, steroids, bilateral IMA harvest, use of the aortic pump, and reoperation. Clearly, some are modifiable such as avoidance of bilateral IMA harvest, use of Vitamin A to offset steroid use and

optimization of renal status and diabetes. High-risk patients can be prophylactically addressed with compression plates and screws instead of sternal wiring, a measure that reduces the incidence of sternal complications.)

(a) What is the pathological process? Describe in the framework of duration of onset postoperative. (Early, within the first 2 weeks, is termed acute and presents as a soft-tissue wound infection. The underlying causation may be sternal instability or dehiscence secondary to broken wires or poor closure technique. These patients are managed with wound drainage and antibiotics if the sternum is stable. If the sternum is unstable and in the absence of gross purulence, rewiring with either the Robicsek circumsternal wires or plates and screws is an option. The second group, subacute, presents 2–6 weeks postoperatively and are associated with purulence and sternal dehiscence and are the most common. This group of patients require an aggressive approach of bone debridement, sternectomy, and costal cartilage excision if involved. With the advent of the wound VAC, negative wound pressure therapy, the patient can be bridged and managed from drainage and debridement to definitive wound closure. Mediastinal abscess, although rare, should be detected on CT scan. The management of late osteomyelitis is beyond the scope of the discussion of this case.)

3. Outline a menu of treatment options from your most acceptable to least acceptable. Give your rationale for your choices. (The workhorse for wound closure and reconstruction is advancement of pectoralis muscle and skin–soft tissue, based on the thoracoacromial and lateral thoracic vessels. The plane of wide dissection is directly upon the chest wall, ligating the medial intercostal perforators. Dissection continues inferiorly and inferior lateral where the plane transitions subcutaneously. The deep layer, muscle, is opposed with large caliber sutures over a drain. If tension is ascertained, a complementary maneuver is release of the insertion of the pectoralis on the humerus which necessitates a separate incision in the deltopectoral groove. Although once commonly employed, this release is rarely necessary. The skin is closed in layers also over a drain and an incisional VAC may assist in healing. The drains should remain in place for 3 weeks. Other options include turnover flaps of the pectoralis based on the internal mammary perforators, right side only if the LIMA has been harvested, rectus muscle pedicled on the deep superior epigastric artery, and omentum. Each have specific disadvantages including devascularization of the chest wall skin with pectoralis major turnover flaps, the potentially unreliable distal tip of the rectus, and the necessity of intraabdominal harvest of the omentum. The morbidity of the last option, omentum, can be minimized with an endoscopic approach and may be indicated in large wounds as in this particular patient.)

(a) Is the hierarchy of procedures described in the preamble the same as yours? (No. A preferable management plan if the patient's condition permits, would have been operative drainage and debridement of soft-tissue and bone and application of NWPT accomplished with the first stage, followed by definitive closure with the second operation.)

Intraoperative

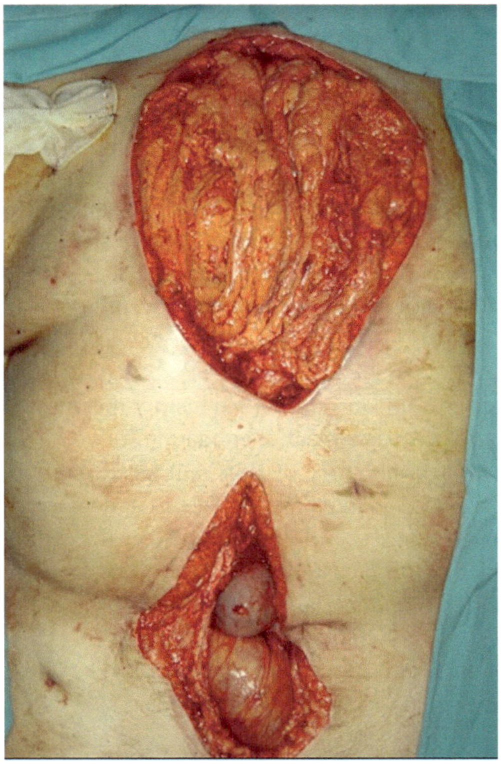

The intraoperative use of the omentum was selected for closure, harvested initially endoscopically. Difficulties were encountered and upper abdominal laparotomy was necessary.

Postoperative (4 Months)

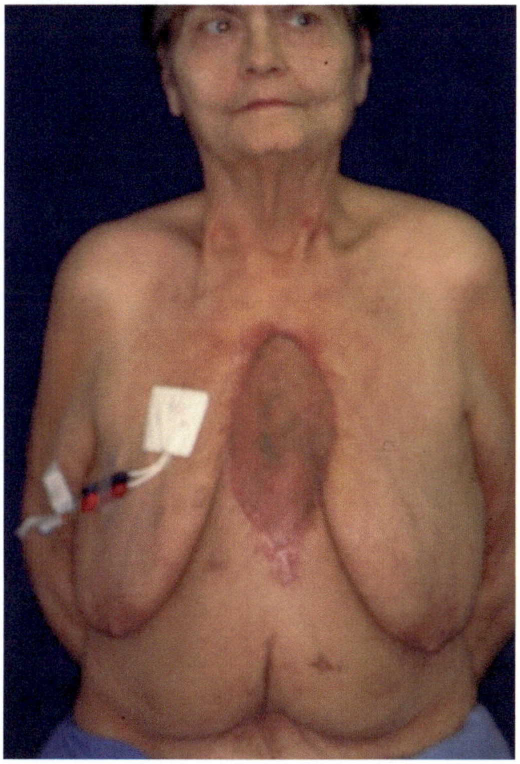

The patient was successfully skin-grafted. Over time, a secondary contracture of the graft has decreased the size of the defect considerably. The intracardiac catheters remain.

In-Service Examination

1. A patient presents with a 4 cm ulcer of the left anterior chest wall with exposed nonviable ribs 3 years after mastectomy and postoperative radiotherapy. Multiple biopsies reveal granulation tissue and inflammation only. The appropriate management is:
   (a) Dressing changes and HBO therapy
   (b) VAC and HBO treatment
   (c) Debridement of the ulcer, VAC, and flap coverage
   (d) Resection of full-thickness chest wall and radiated soft tissue plus flap closure
2. A 45-year-old patient developed a sternal infection and dehiscence 1 month after LIMA and CABG managed with bilateral pectoralis major advancement flaps. Partial necrosis and complete dehiscence occurs with a 10 mm wide defect. The appropriate option is:
   (a) VAC plus split-thickness skin graft
   (b) Omentum plus split-thickness skin graft
   (c) Left rectus plus split-thickness skin graft
   (d) Right rectus plus split-thickness skin graft
3. The most likely cause of persistent infection following reconstruction of the dehisced sternum is:
   (a) Immunosuppressed host
   (b) Presence of MRSA and/or VRSA
   (c) Inadequate debridement
   (d) Poorly vascularized pectoralis

Part VII

Burns, Difficult Soft Tissue Infections

59 Pathophysiology, Resuscitation, and Pulmonary Complications

Bibliography

Zuo K.J., Medina A, Tredget EE. "Important Developments in Burn Care", *Plast. Reconstr. Surg.*, (2017); 139(1):**120e–25e (Overview).**

Yowler C.J. and Fratianne RB, Editor—Luce, EA, "Current Status of Burn Resuscitation", *Clinics in Plastic Surgery: Burn Care and Management*. (2000), 27(1):**1–10. (Junior Level Residents).**

Cartotto R., "Fluid Resuscitation of the Thermally Injured Patient." Cartotto, R., *Clinics in Plastic Surgery*. Elsevier Inc. (2009), 36(4):**569–579.**

Deutsch C.J., Tan A., Smailes S., Dziewulski P., "The Diagnosis and Management of Inhalation Injury: An Evidence Based Approach", *Burns*, (2018);44(5):**1041–1049.**

Butts C.C., Holmes JH, Carter JE, "Surgical Escharotomy and Decompressive Therapies in Burns", J. Burn Care Res., (2020); 41(2):**1–13 ONLY.**

Faculty Discussion and Study Guide

Resuscitation

1. The most important determinants of burn patient survival are: (Burn size, age, proportion of burn of full-thickness injury, presence or not of inhalation injury.)
2. Differentiation between partial and full-thickness burns can be estimated clinically but ascertainment of those burns that will heal spontaneously can be difficult. Describe an objective technique or technology. (The use of a laser Doppler performed in the early, 2–5 days, post-burn has been the most frequent application of a technology. Standardization and determination of efficacy of the readings await further experience.)
3. In a patient with a large, 50% burn from the waist upward, what explains the edema formation in the lower extremities during resuscitation? (A tremendous increase in permeability, particularly in the venules, occurs with loss of venule and capillary integrity that allows transudation of fluid and small molecular weight proteins from the intravascular system into the interstitial space. This shift creates diminished intravascular volume and increase in interstitial fluid volume that results clinically in the appearance of edema.)
   (a) What are some possible explanations for this loss of integrity? (The exact mechanism is not known but the culprits appear to be histamine release from mast cells, activation of the proteolytic cascade including kinins, and vasoactive products as prostaglandins—all of which can create not only an increase in vascular permeability but also an increase in relative intravascular hydrostatic pressure in the microcirculation.)
4. Explain the role of the alteration of Starling's forces in the production of burn edema. (The Starling equation states that in normal circumstances, fluid moves from the intravascular space across the capillary membrane and into the interstitial space but that fluid is equally removed by the lymphatic system so that edema does not occur. The fluid shift in that direction is driven by the intravascular hydrostatic pressure which is greater than the interstitial hydrostatic pressure. Yet, a positive gradient exists in the opposite direction, interstitial to intravascular space by the difference between plasma colloid osmotic pressure, higher than interstitial colloid osmotic pressure, so that difference is driven by a higher concentration of protein within the intravascular rather than the interstitial space. As a result of the burn injury, the capillary and venule membranes become permeable to plasma proteins including albumin which then "leak" into the interstitial space thus negating, in fact, even reversing the normal difference in colloid osmotic pressure. Of course, the same dramatic increase in permeability allows fluid as well to move easily from the vascular into the interstitial space.)

E. Luce, *A Curriculum for Plastic Surgery*, https://doi.org/10.1007/978-3-031-62087-4_59

(a) What impact do these pathophysiologic changes have on the fluid resuscitation regime? (The tremendous loss of vascular volume in large burns requires a large volume of administered intravascular fluids to maintain cardiac filling pressures—see below. Also, the loss of capillary integrity to the passage of intravascular proteins would also imply that colloid or protein administration in the first 24 h would be counterproductive—as well as expensive.)

5. What would be the hemodynamics of a 30-year-old burn patient with a 50% body surface area burn *prior* to resuscitation in terms of the following: intravascular volume, red cell mass, total body water, cardiac output? (Intravascular volume would be markedly diminished because of the mechanisms outlined in question 1, red cell mass would be only slightly diminished secondary to direct red cell damage by the burn, total body water would be essentially the same as preburn except for a minimal loss due to direct burn damage, cardiac output would be markedly diminished.)
   (a) What is the mechanism(s) for the above? (The loss of intravascular volume is explained by the loss of vascular system integrity and the transudation of fluid and protein into the interstitial space; cardiac output is markedly diminished in the burn patient due to not only diminished intravascular volume but also perhaps a direct negative cardiac inotropic effect of some circulating agent as a result of the burn injury.)

6. How was the Parkland or Baxter formulas *initially* derived? (The Parkland formula, 4 ml/kg/% body surface area burn with one-half administered in the first 8 h post-burn, was developed by Baxter and Shires at Parkland hospital. The formula was derived as a result of both experimental and clinical or retrospective review of successful vs. unsuccessful resuscitated patients vs. the volume in fluids given.)
   (a) Recommended urine output? (0.5–1.0 cc/kg/hr. in adults.)
   (b) What is the role of colloid in the Parkland formula? Why? (Colloid was given *after* the first 24 h post-burn usually as albumin and at a volume of approximately 0.5 cc of colloid/kg/% body surface area burn administered with D5w to maintain urine output. Restoration of capillary membrane integrity is necessary such that administered colloid remains intravascular, an event that may be incomplete at 24 h post-burn.)
   (c) What are the current thoughts about the role of colloid in resuscitation? (Three principal schools of thought exist on the use of colloid in burn resuscitation: One that incorporates colloid from the initiation of resuscitation, another that avoids colloid altogether and administers crystalloid throughout the whole resuscitation period, and a third group that utilizes colloid on a selective basis after the first 24 h.)

7. What is "fluid creep" and what are the adverse effects of fluid creep? (Fluid creep is the term applied to a relatively recently described phenomenon that references administration of resuscitation fluids considerably greater than those predicted by a formula such as the Parkland formula. The adverse effects of fluid creep are those of abdominal compartment syndrome, the necessity for more frequent escharotomies, and possibly an increased incidence of pulmonary complications.)
   (a) How can the diagnosis of abdominal compartment syndrome be established and what are some of the clinical signs? (Increase in bladder pressure greater than 20 mm Hg, the appearance of impaired ventilation with high peak airway pressures, worsening metabolic acidosis, and hemodynamic instability. Also, discussed in the escharotomy section.)

8. What clinical scenarios may require greater than predicted fluid resuscitation volume? (Delay in initiation of therapy, inhalation injury, which may appear counter intuitive, electrical injury, perhaps advancing age.)

9. What particular challenges does the pediatric patient represent for resuscitation and how are the burn resuscitation formulas modified for the pediatric age group? (Characteristically, pediatric patients require greater volumes of fluid for resuscitation than the various formulas would calculate. Also, free water, D_5W, should be added because of increased free water requirements and the necessity to avoid hypernatremia.)

10. Discuss the use of pulmonary artery catheters for monitoring. (The results of the use of central pressure monitoring through a Swan–Ganz catheter are inconclusive and mixed. Much of the information has been derived from the use of pulmonary artery catheters in trauma patients for monitoring pulmonary wedge pressure, cardiac output, and O_2 consumption. Although these indices correlate more closely with the actual physiologic state than urine output, the widespread use of pulmonary artery catheters have not led to an increased survival in the burn patient. An optimal application would be in the elderly patients with preexisting cardiovascular disease and patients who are not adequately resuscitated and more information is needed to direct further resuscitation.)
    (a) What would be the Swan–Ganz readings in an early (4 h post-burn) large burn inadequately resuscitated? (Pulmonary wedge pressure would be extremely low as well as cardiac index. The systemic vascular resistance would be quite high.)

11. Discuss the following:
    Swan–Ganz reading in a 25 year old 20 h post-burn, 50% BSA with a pulse of 96, normal BP, urine output of 50–60 cc/hour: PAP 30/15, PCWP of 2, C.O. 3.5 L per m^2. (The patient is adequately resuscitated.)
12. Discuss the pros and cons of the use of hypertonic saline in burn resuscitation. (The theory underlying the use of hypertonic saline is the administration of the required amount of sodium ion yet much smaller volumes of fluid. The proposed benefits were those of decreased tissue edema, less necessity for escharotomies, and fewer pulmonary complications. The potential problems include hypernatremia and hyperosmolarity with possible CNS and renal complications and is probably of historical interest only.)
13. What are the two objections to the use of Dextran as a resuscitation vehicle? (Dextran has a number of potential problems including coagulopathy, allergic reaction, and can interfere with blood typing.)

Inhalation Injury

1. In general terms, describe the impact of inhalation injury in burn patients, i.e., frequency, correlation with burn surface area, effect on mortality. (The occurrence of inhalation injury has a positive correlation with body surface area burn and has an additive effect on mortality. As outlined below, the frequency of occurrence hinges on the circumstances surrounding the burn injury.)
   (a) Discuss the three clinical stages of inhalation injury. (The first phase within 24 h consists of carbon monoxide poisoning, hypoxemia, and bronchospasm, all which can result in acute pulmonary insufficiency. The second phase consists of pulmonary edema, atelectasis, and tracheobronchitis with respiratory failure. The third stage is bronchial pneumonia, characteristically occurring after 3–4 days post injury.)
2. Briefly discuss the toxic components of smoke and the effect on the respiratory tract. (The toxic components are secondary to a chemical injury induced by the products of incomplete combustion. In some circumstances, hydrogen cyanide may be a culprit.)
   (a) Describe the effects of this pathophysiologic process. (The resultant chemical or irritative tracheobronchitis can result in mechanical plugging of the distal bronchial airway. The combination of the irritative damage to the larynx and the edema induced by the resuscitation phase can produce acute complete upper airway obstruction.)
   (b) Briefly and succinctly, what is the pathophysiology of lower airway injury in inhalation injury? (The damage to the terminal bronchioles can produce premature airway closure during the respiratory cycle with focal atelectasis. These areas of atelectasis produce ventilation/perfusion mismatches and functional shunting. The systemic response to burn injury of increased capillary permeability occurs within the lungs as well with transudation of fluid into the alveoli, further exacerbating the deleterious effects of inhalation injury.)
3. What is the pathology of airway injury that sets the stage for the onset of infectious complications, tracheobronchitis, and pneumonia? (The stage for the development of the third phase of inhalation injury, bronchial pneumonia, is set by mucosal damage of the tracheobronchial tree with bronchorrhea and slough, the increase in pulmonary secretions and diminished ciliary response and bacterial colonization by intubation of the airway or from the burn wound.)
4. Diagnostic findings to establish inhalation injury? (A careful history may be one of the most important diagnostic findings, namely, a history of burn injury sustained in a closed space such as a house fire and a prolonged extraction from the scene. Other important physical findings are singed nasal hair, intraoral soot, or sooty sputum, none are diagnostic but suggest a heightened awareness. The presence of hoarseness may indicate damage to the larynx and, of course, stridor would indicate impending upper airway obstruction.)
5. Discuss the laboratory diagnosis of the inhalation injury, including a critique of each modality. (Although not considered a laboratory study, chest x-ray at the early stage is normal as well as arterial blood gasses. Other laboratory methods that have been utilized are Xe 133 nuclear scans and pulmonary function tests, both of which are not logistically feasible and have not been incorporated routinely into the diagnosis of inhalation injury.)
   (a) Expand on the role of fiberoptic bronchoscopy. (Early fiberoptic bronchoscopy can play an important diagnostic and therapeutic role. The findings of soot and inflamed mucosa within the trachea and large bronchi is indicative of a significant inhalation injury. As the inhalation injury unfolds with secondary small airway edema and airway plugging, bronchoscopy can perform pulmonary toilet directly administer bronchodilators, and obtain cultures for culture-specific antibiotic therapy.)
6. What is the pathophysiology of carbon monoxide (CO) poisoning? (Exposure to carbon monoxide results in a stable intracellular compound within the red blood cell that is preferential and will replace oxygen. The carbon monoxide thus shifts the hemoglobin–oxygen curve to the left that will impair oxygen diffusion at the level of the tissues. Carbon monoxide cannot be measured by

Table 59.1 Clinical presentation for different levels of carbon monoxide

% Levels	Carbon monoxide intoxication
CO Hgb	Symptoms
0–5	Normal value
15–20	Headache—Confusion
20–40	Disorientation, fatigue, nausea, visual changes
40–60	Hallucination, combativeness, coma, shock state
60 or above	Cardiopulmonary arrest

arterial blood gasses since laboratory measurement of blood gasses is dependent on the partial pressure within the plasma, not the hemoglobin or carboxyhemoglobin content. The level of carboxyhemoglobin is measured by spectrophotometry.)

(a) Outline levels and a comparable clinical picture. (See Table 59.1.)

(b) Discuss the management of carbon monoxide poisoning and give the half-life of carbon monoxide with different treatment modalities. (The treatment of carbon monoxide toxicity involves the displacement of the carbon monoxide moiety from the intracellular hemoglobin by the administration of oxygen. The half-life of carboxyhemoglobin on 100% oxygen is reduced from 180 minutes to about 30 minutes. Hyperbaric oxygen can result in even a shorter half-life but the logistical difficulty is the placement of a patient into a hyperbaric oxygen atmosphere, i.e., chamber, during the resuscitation period, a period marked by hemodynamic instability. The efficacy of HBO in the prevention of delayed neurocognitive deficits is unproven.)

7. True or false: The optimal management of the airway in the burn patients dictates endotracheal intubation only with appearance in the post-burn period of dyspnea and stridor? (False. Once the clinical signs of upper airway obstruction and stridor are apparent, the patient may require tracheostomy instead of endotracheal intubation, attended by increased morbidity and even mortality.)
   (a) What are some clinical characteristics that may point toward early or "prophylactic" intubation? (Head and neck burns, large >50% body burn, full-thickness circumferential burns of the trunk, high clinical suspicion of inhalation injury.)
8. In an intubated patient with circumferential third degree burns of the trunk, what are some reliable indications of the necessity for escharotomies? (The mechanics of respiration can be restricted significantly by a circumferential truncal eschar. As a result the airway pressures will rise to produce the same tidal volume, the chest wall component of dynamic compliance will decrease if calculated, P_{CO2} increases and shunting or a widened A-a DO_2 will be apparent on 100% oxygen. To summarize:
   - Rising P_{CO2} on arterial blood gasses
   - A widened A-a DO_2 on 100% O_2
   - Decrease in dynamic compliance
   - Increase in airway pressures for the same tidal volume.)
9. Discuss the efficacy of the following: systemic steroids, prophylactic antibiotics, the use of PEEP, and the use of extracorporeal membrane oxygenation. (Although steroids would seem indicated to diminish the inflammatory response and antibiotics to forestall infection, both have been proven to have no beneficial effect on inhalation injury and may be detrimental in addition. PEEP or positive end expiratory pressure may be of benefit to address the V-Q mismatch of ventilation and perfusion by addressing the problem with premature airway closure in the terminal bronchioles and focal atelectatic changes. The use of ECMO requires pulmonary bypass capability and cardiothoracic anesthesia. Efficacy in terms of improved outcomes has not been established.)

Escharotomy

1. Indications for chest wall escharotomy is discussed above. What are the indications in the extremities? (The indications may be more subtle if the patient is intubated and sedated which is likely the case in those circumstances of burn severity that produce massive edema. If the patient is responsive, one can use the measures of sensation in the hands, for example, but often the hands are burned as well. If not, decreased capillary filling of the fingernails or loss of digital pulse on doppler exam may heighten suspicion. The most important objective finding is an elevated compartment pressure as measured in the volar forearm, greater than 30 mm Hg as worrisome and greater than 40 mm Hg an absolute indication for escharotomy.)
2. Briefly describe the technique of escharotomy of the upper extremity. (Parallel incisions on the radial and ulnar aspect of the forearm, extending above the elbow into the arm if necessary. Escharotomies should only be performed, as the name implies, through eschar and not violate the deep fascia. Repeated tissue pressure measurements should decline. In the absence of electrical injury, fasciotomies are uncommonly indicated.

   No substantial evidence exists of the efficacy of the performance of escharotomies of the digits.)
3. What is the analogous situation in the abdomen? (Hemodynamic instability, oliguria, intracompartmental pressure of greater than 20–25 mm Hg as measured through a Foley catheter.)

Case-Based Conference

Case 1—Acute Burn

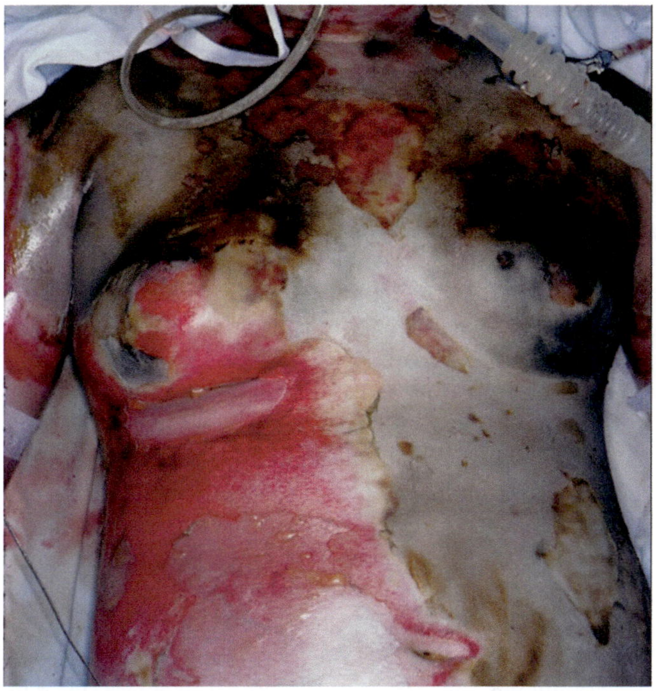

A 50-year-old woman sustained burns in a house fire and was intubated at the scene and is 2 h post-burn. She has circumferential burns of the thorax and both of her extremities.

1. Describe the slide and your initial assessment.
   (a) What initial tests are indicated, if any, besides routine blood work and chest x-ray?
   (b) What are the major management priorities for this particular patient for the next 12 h?
2. What individual factors will play a significant role in the determination of the patient's fluid needs? What is the physiologic explanation?
3. Address the following scenarios:
   (a) Two hours after admission despite your fluid regimen and a fluid bolus, urine output has fallen to 15 cc./hour. Explain your treatment plan in terms of the pathophysiology involved.
   (b) At 8 h, the patient has developed rising airway pressures and a falling Po2 on a FIO2 of 100%. What is (are) the possible explanation(s) and your management?
   (c) One consideration in the patient with massive burns including the extremity is the necessity for escharotomy. Describe the indications and technique.
4. Outline a management plan for administration of fluids in the second 24 h.

Case-Based Conference: Discussion

Case 1—Acute Burn

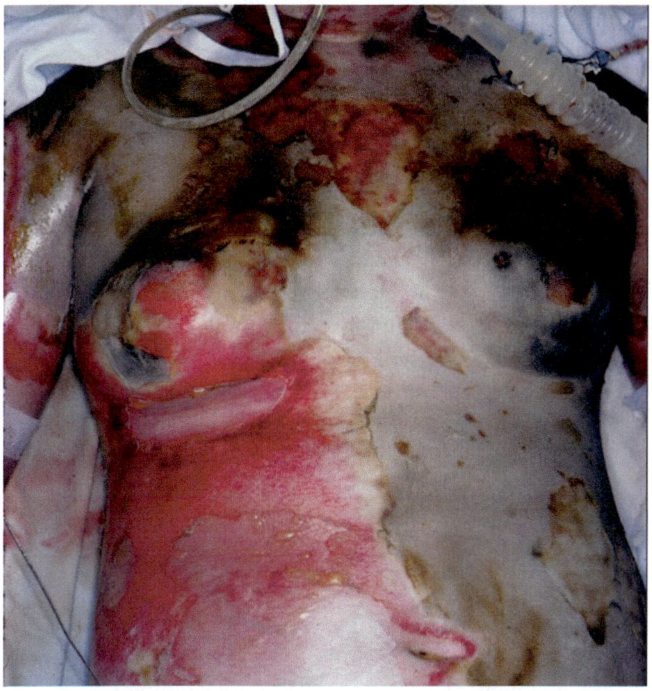

A 50-year-old woman sustained burns in a house fire and was intubated at the scene and is 2 h post-burn. She has circumferential burns of the thorax and both of her extremities.

1. Describe the slide and your initial assessment. (The single slide depicts the anterior trunk of a severely burned woman. The superior limit of the photo is the neck and inferiorly approximately the umbilicus. Visible are the connections for presumably an endotracheal tube. Also visible is a nasogastric tube and perhaps on the left shoulder a percutaneous deep venous access or "deep line." The entire upper chest, left breast, and visible left abdomen is occupied by a leathery and in some areas blackened skin. The right breast and right abdomen is a bright pink. The neck may be unburned. Some substantial edema is evident.

   Since the patient is intubated, the initial history will need to be obtained from the EMTs or others. That history would focus on indications for the on-scene intubation as loss of consciousness, for example, and location of the patient when rescued, if applicable. The circumstances of the fire, for example, a bedroom fire, may be of value. Patient's past medical history is obtained to establish co-morbidities as well as tobacco and alcohol use. The physical exam is an initial trauma survey. Although the patient in question has been intubated, if not, the probability of inhalation injury and potential for upper airway obstruction should be ascertained. A history of burns sustained in a closed space, the presence of head and neck burns, and the expectoration of or the presence of sooty sputum in the endotracheal suction all signal a high likelihood of an inhalation injury. The perfusion of the extremities, in this instance, the upper extremities by assessment of color and doppler exam will set the baseline for future observations.)

(a) What initial tests are indicated, if any, besides routine blood work and chest x-ray? (The stem provides for a chest x-ray which would be probably normal. The lab tests should include carbon monoxide levels, and, possibly, myoglobin. An initial bladder pressure obtained via the Foley catheter will also establish a baseline. Whenever feasible during the resuscitation period, the airway is examined by flexible bronchoscopy for the detection of the presence of soot in the tracheobronchial tree, highly diagnostic of the presence of inhalation injury. The indications for other test or imaging would be driven by the individual patient findings.)

(b) What are the major management priorities for this particular patient for the next 12 h? (The initial management of this patient assuming intubation, placement of nasogastric tube, and Foley catheter is fluid resuscitation, ventilatory support, and observation for the acute complications of oliguria, respiratory failure, and extremity compartment syndrome. If not intubated on arrival, since the patient has sustained greater than a 50% body surface area of probably full-thickness burns in a house fire, prophylactic intubation would be advisable rather than an emergent effort to secure the airway in an obstructed patient.)

2. What individual factors will play a significant role in the determination of the patient's fluid needs? What is the physiologic explanation? (The loss of intravascular volume is explained by the loss of vascular system integrity and the transudation of fluid and small molecular weight protein into the interstitial space. Cardiac output is markedly decreased in the burn patient due to not only diminished intravascular volume but also a direct negative cardiac inotropic effect of some circulating agent as a result of the burn injury. The fluid requirements to resuscitate a burn patient can be calculated from a number of formulas but all use percentage body surface area burn and pre-burn body weight. The most widely utilized is the Parkland formula that dictates a requirement of 4 ccs/kg/percent body surface area as measured on a Lund–Browder chart to a maximum of 50% BSA in some practitioners' opinion. One-half is given the first 8 post-burn and the remainder in the next 16 h. Larger volumes are dictated by the presence of inhalation injury, delay in initiation of resuscitation, and electrical injury. Modification may be necessary in the elderly and/or the presence of heart disease. See below.)

3. Address the following scenarios:

(a) Two hours after admission despite your fluid regimen and a fluid bolus, urine output has fallen to 15 cc./hour. Explain your treatment plan in terms of the pathophysiology involved. (The patient was oliguric and, if a sufficient bolus was administered without response, cardiovascular hemodynamics should probably be assessed with central pressures. Other indications for central pressure measurements via a Swan–Ganz catheter is an elderly and/or patient with pre-existing cardiac disease. A low end-capillary wedge pressure and a concomitant high systemic vascular resistance, signals hypovolemia. Some practitioners would administer colloid, in the form of 5% or 20% albumin, but many would not, theorizing that administered colloid would not be retained in the intravascular system. A low cardiac output might mandate the administration of inotropic agents. In summary, the most likely explanation for the scenario is hypovolemia secondary to inadequate resuscitation and dictates an urgent increase in fluid administration.)

(b) At 8 h, the patient has developed rising airway pressures and a falling pO2 on a FIO2 of 50%. What (are) the possible explanation(s) and your management? (Mechanical causes of the picture such as a partially obstructed endotracheal tube from secretions or a pneumothorax should be eliminated first. In this patient a loss of chest wall compliance from a circumferential restricting eschar is a likely culprit since the mechanics of respiration can be restricted significantly by circumferential eschar. As a result the airway pressures will rise to produce the same tidal volume, the chest wall component of dynamic compliance will decrease if calculated, Pco2 increases and shunting or a widened A-aDO2 will be apparent on 100% oxygen. Release will require escharotomies in both transverse and vertical planes, accomplished with a "tic-tac-toe" distribution. The airway pressure should decrease promptly.)

(c) One consideration in the patient with massive burns including the extremity is the necessity for escharotomy. Describe the indications and technique. (The indications may be more subtle if the patient is intubated and sedated which is likely the case in those circumstances of burn severity that produce massive edema. If the patient is responsive, one can use the measures of sensation in the hands, for example. If not, decreased capillary filling of the fingernails or loss of digital pulse on doppler exam may heighten suspicion. The most important objective finding is an elevated compartment pressure, greater than 30 mm Hg as worrisome and greater than 40 mm Hg an absolute indication for escharotomy.

Parallel incisions on the radial and ulnar aspect of the forearm, extending above the elbow into the arm if necessary. Escharotomies should only be performed, as the name implies, through eschar and not violate the deep fascia. Repeated tissue pressure measurements should decline. In the absence of electrical injury fasciotomies are uncommonly indicated. No substantial evidence exists for performing escharotomies of the digits.)

4. Outline a management plan for administration of fluids in the second 24 h. (Resuscitation may need to be continued in the second 24 h, particularly in larger burns. The diuretic phase may not have an onset until after 48 h in some patients, including large pediatric burns. One estimate that includes maintenance and evaporative loss is roughly one-half of the volume that was required in the first 24 h for a satisfactory resuscitation. A role for colloid infusion, 5% albumin, in addition to crystalloid is a component of some burn resuscitation formulas.)

In-Service Examination

1. The hemodynamics in body composition of a 30-year-old patient 2 h post 50% BSA burn and prior to resuscitation is:
   (a) Increase in RBC mass
   (b) Total body water markedly diminished
   (c) Cardiac output markedly diminished
   (d) Intravascular volume slightly diminished
2. A 30-year-old 70 kg patient sustains a BSA burn, admitted 2 h after injury. What are the initial resuscitation orders?
   (a) 875 cc/hour of Ringer's lactate
   (b) 437 cc/hour of Ringer's lactate
   (c) 1170 cc/hour of Ringer's lactate
   (d) 220 cc/hour of 5% albumin
3. A patient who sustained burns of heads and neck, thorax and upper extremities in a house fire is coughing up sooty sputum and has stridor. After IV access, the next treatment step is:
   (a) Chest X-ray and arterial blood gasses
   (b) Intubation
   (c) Intracompartmental pressure readings of volar forearms
   (d) Application of burn dressings after cleaning of burn wounds

60 Wound Care and Coverage

Bibliography

Lang T.C., Zhao R., Kim A., Wijewardena A., et al., "A Critical Update of the Assessment and Acute Management of Patients with Severe Burns", *Advances in Wound Care*, (2019);8:**607, 618–625 (For Junior Residents for Overview).**

Davis B.N., Xu H., Gottlieb L.J., Vrouwe S.Q., "Acute Burn Care", *Plastic and Reconstructive Surgery*, (2024);153(4): **804e, 812e-820e ONLY.**

Pruitt Jr. BA and Wolf SE, "An Historical Perspective on Advances in Burn Care Over the Past 100 Years." Cartotto, R., *Clinics in Plastic Surgery*. Elsevier Inc. (2009), 36(4):**533–37 ONLY**.

Zuo KJ, Medina A, Tredget EE. "Important Developments in Burn Care", *Plast. Reconstr. Surg.*, (2017); 139(1): **125e-131e ONLY. (Overview)**

Greenhalgh DG, "Topical Antimicrobial Agents for Burn Wounds", *Clinics in Plastic Surgery*, (Oct. 2009); 36(4):**597–606.**

Isilali M.E., et al., Chapter 12: "Operative Wound Management", Total Burn Care, 5th edition, Elsevier (2018); **pgs. 114–130.**

Mosier MJ and Gibran NS, "Surgical excision of the burn wound", *Clinics in Plastic Surgery*, (2009); **617–622.**

Saffle JR, "Closure of the Excised Burn Wound: Temporary Skin Substitutes", *Clinics in Plastic Surgery*, (Oct. 2009); 36(4):**627–638 ONLY.**

Sheridan R, "Closure of the Excised Burn Wound: Autografts, Semipermanent Skin Substitutes, and Permanent Skin Substitutes", *Clinics in Plastic Surgery*, (Oct. 2009); 36(4):**643–651.**

Hill DM, Sinclair SE, Hickerson WL, "Rational Selection and Use of Antimicrobials in Patients with Burn Injuries", *Clin Plastic Surg.*, (2017); 44:**521–529 ONLY.**

Faculty Discussion and Study Guide

Topical Microbial Agents/Burn Wound Infection

1. *Briefly* describe the natural progression of the disease process of burn wound infection. (Initially, the burn wound is relatively sterile except for some bacteria in the skin appendages and hair follicles, most commonly S. aureus. If not prevented or minimized, bacterial colonization will initially occur in a more superficial portion of the burn wound and then gradually penetrate into the deeper eschar. The next phase is proliferation of the bacteria at the interface between nonviable tissue, the eschar, and the deeper viable tissue. Once that proliferation reaches a critical mass or concentration, the microorganisms then are capable of invasion of the adjacent viable, undamaged soft tissue.)
2. Define "burn wound sepsis." (Bacterial growth reaching a level of much greater than 10^5 organisms per gram of tissue with invasion of viable subcutaneous tissues and blood vessels. The diagnosis is made by a full-thickness wound biopsy.)
3. Differentiate clinically and laboratory between burn wound cellulitis and burn wound infection. (Cellulitis, as the name implies, demonstrates erythema and edema of adjacent unburned skin/soft tissue and may be the precursor to burn wound infection. Burn wound infection implies an active invasion of unexcised eschar as well as adjacent viable tissue. Ordinarily, this development means that the bacterial colonization has proliferated to the point of 10^7 or 10^8 and is accompanied by or closely followed by systemic sepsis. Diagnosis can be established by histologic examination of viable tissue. Clinical diagnosis is suggested by profound changes in

E. Luce, *A Curriculum for Plastic Surgery*, https://doi.org/10.1007/978-3-031-62087-4_60

the appearance of the burn wound and eschar such as hemorrhagic or color changes. These changes can also occur in already-excised burn wounds.)

   (a) What is the specific and cardinal histologic sign of burn wound infection? (The presence of microorganisms in unburned tissue.)

4. Outline a staging or grading system for the histologic assessment of the burn wound colonization or invasion and why that system is consistent with burn wound pathophysiology. (A system dividing burn wound infection into that of colonization or invasion parallels what occurs with burn wound infection evolving into burn sepsis. Superficial penetrating colonization is reflective of the process of bacterial colonization within the eschar up to the point of proliferation of the bacteria in the subeschar space. Staging of the invasive process is similar, namely, the early presence of bacteria in the viable tissue immediately beneath the subeschar space and then progressive invasion of that bacteria into normal tissue with invasion of small blood vessels and lymphatics.)
5. Burn wound sepsis and pneumonia are the two most common infections in burn patients. What is the most common mechanism by which these patients contract pneumonia? (Most commonly by aerosolization of bacteria emanating from the wound surface during manipulation of the patient. This is also the reason why topical antimicrobials decrease the incidence of pneumonia.)
6. What is the basic philosophy underlying conservative management of burns with topical agents? (The philosophy is to treat superficial partial-thickness burn wounds with an agent capable of suppressing bacterial colonization until re-epithelialization occurs, hopefully, prior to hypertrophic scarring, normally 2–3 weeks. Extension of that same philosophy to deeper burns requires the application of a topical antimicrobial agent to minimize infection while the eschar spontaneously separates and granulation tissue develops capable of supporting a split-thickness skin graft. Separation of the eschar occurs as a result of subeschar proliferation and invasion of bacteria. Those bacteria then lyse the nonviable tissue that allows the eschar to separate, a prolonged process. As discussed in the next session, unless extenuating circumstances exist, the contemporary management of deeper burns is excision and coverage.)
   (a) What is the evolution over time of the type of microorganism that colonizes the burn wound? (Initially, gram-positive cocci such as S. aureus are the predominant organisms, replaced in time by gram-negative organisms such as Pseudomonas. With even additional time fungi, yeast such as Candida and drug-resistant organisms become dominant.)
   (b) Name two contemporary organisms of concern? (MRSA and acinetobacter.)
7. What is the basic issue with antimicrobial ointments, as different from creams discussed below, such as Bacitracin, Neosporin, etc.? (The agents rapidly produce secondary involvement with fungus and molds and some have a significant, 10%, incidence of hypersensitivity reactions.)
8. Discuss the possible concerns in complications in the use of silver sulfadiazine. (In large body burns in the early post-burn period, leukopenia and thrombocytopenia occurs, an effect that is usually transient. The cream cannot be used in patients with a sulfa allergy and should not be used on the face because of potential for eye irritation or injury. Probably the most significant historical concern has been the probable impairment of re-epithelization.)
   (a) What are the two principal components? (As the name implies silver and a sulfa compound, sulfadiazine.)
   (b) What is the ability of silver sulfadiazine to penetrate the eschar? (Does penetrate the eschar but to a limited degree—see below.)
9. Discuss the principal concerns and complications in the use of mafenide acetate in treatment of burns. (Mafenide acetate or Sulfamylon has an excellent eschar penetration ability. The agent also seems quite effective against Pseudomonas but appears to have little activity against fungi or yeast. Sulfamylon can be quite painful in partial thickness burns and cannot be used in patients with sulfa allergies. The principal complication, particularly in large burns, is the development of a metabolic acidosis as a result of the inhibition of carbonic anhydrase characteristic. Metabolic acidosis can also lead to potassium loss and an increase in respiratory rate.)
10. Briefly, discuss the solutions of silver nitrate, Dakin's, and acetic acid. (Silver nitrate solution as a primary agent for the treatment of large body burns is probably of historical interest only. The agent does not penetrate the eschar and can produce hyponatremia and requires close monitoring of electrolytes in large surface burns. Dakin's solution is dilute bleach and has toxicity to tissue cells. Dilute acetic acid can be effective against Pseudomonas but is relatively infrequently used.)
11. Discuss the mechanism of action of silver as an antimicrobial agent and the practical clinical applications. (Silver is a heavy metal and as such is toxic to bacteria but has an additional antimicrobial dimension that is not clearly understood. To be active, silver must be soluble in solution since the silver ion binds to proteins in the serum and/or tissues, so silver concentrations must be maintained at least at a minimal level. The metallic form is inert and must become ionized to become reactive and thus bind to proteins in cell membranes. Whether the silver is applied in solution, silver nitrate, or as a cream, silver sulfadiazine, application must be done two to three times daily.)

(a) To avoid the necessity of frequent application, discuss silver-eluting agents. (Dressings have been developed that incorporate nanocrystalline silver that elutes the active silver ion in an uncharged form when exposed to water/fluid and are changed every 3 days. Examples include Acticoat, Aquacell, and Mepilex.)
(b) Discuss potential problems with the use of silver-impregnated dressings. (The principal problem is staining of the adjacent unburned skin as well as the care keeper's clothing, dressings etc., the possibility of argyria from systemic absorption of the silver, and the potential problem of retardation of wound healing.)

12. What is the role of intravenous antibiotics in treatment of burn patients? (Prophylactic intravenous antibiotic use is discouraged. Systemic antibiotics are indicated for those patients that demonstrate sepsis. Burn patients have altered binding and metabolism of antibiotics and serum levels must be frequently monitored.)
13. What explains why adequate serum levels of some antibiotics may require more frequent dosing than normal? (The hyperdynamic and hypermetabolic state of the burn patient results in a shortened half-life for most pharmaceutical agents.)
14. Give some clinical and laboratory evidence for the establishment of the diagnosis of burn wound infection. (Probably the most important clinical finding indicative of burn wound infection is an alteration in the appearance of the burn including color. A transformation to a more dark or violaceous eschar can be indicative of the evolution into burn wound infection. Probably the most important laboratory indication, outside of systemic signs of sepsis, is a quantitative wound biopsy with a result of $>10^5$ bacteria colonies.)
15. What is the treatment for suspected invasive burn wound infection? (Treatment of the systemic sepsis, of course, but also the application of a eschar-penetrating agent such as sulfamylon on a 2–3 times per 24 h basis. The keystone of the treatment is surgical excision of the infected tissue with application of topical antimicrobial agents in solution.)
    (a) From an infection point of view, what is the logic of early excision of eschar? (Removal of necrotic eschar appears to reverse many immunologic abnormalities and defects that are seen in the burn patient. Second, the longer burn wounds remain open, the longer they are at risk for infection. Timely closure minimizes risk.)
16. What are the most likely non-bacteria organisms to produce burn wound infection? (Candida, fungi such as Aspergillus and herpes simplex virus.)

Burn Wound Excision and Closure

The readings that have been included provide both enthusiastic endorsement of burn wound excision as well as perhaps a more balanced perspective.

1. Describe the three zones of burn wound injury. (The theoretical basis for tangential excision is the three zones of injury. The deepest or central zone is the nonviable eschar, the surrounding zone is the zone of stasis or possible microvascular compromise of blood flow and potentially reversible injury, and finally, the least-injured zone of hyperemia or increased blood flow.)
2. What are the principal advantages of burn wound excision? (Early burn wound excision has the potential for reduction of mortality, shortening of hospital stay, and not subjecting the patients to prolonged daily wound debridement. Early burn wound excision of deep partial thickness burns may also avoid hypertrophic scars.)
    (a) Disadvantages? (Increased blood loss, potential for excision of a burn that will heal spontaneously without hypertrophic scarring. Shortening of hospital length of stay in large burns has not been definitively proven.)
3. In those studies that have demonstrated improved survival, that improvement has been limited to what group? (Patients 16–30 years of age without inhalation injury and 40–60% body surface area burn.)
4. Although discussed in more depth in the next module, metabolism and nutrition, what is the basis for the abnormal metabolic response to the burn injury? (The burned tissue, skin and subcutaneous fat, promotes an inflammatory response at the junction of the eschar and the underlying viable tissue. Bacterial proliferation can attract PMN's that in turn are responsible for the release of inflammatory mediators. The systemic response to these inflammatory mediators is increased metabolism and energy expenditure, weight loss, and immunodepression.)
5. Discuss the technique and the perspective of tangential excision of partial-thickness burns of less than 20–25% total body surface area. (Tangential excision is the use of large knives to remove sequential slices of burn tissue followed by the application of split-thickness skin grafts. The sequential excision of burn tissue is continued until a pattern of dermal bleeding, indicative of viable tissue, is encountered. The papillary dermis will have a diffuse and pinpoint pattern of bleeding rather than coarse as seen in the reticular dermis. One perspective is that the blood loss is substantial: approximately 100 cc's for every 1% body surface area excised, the wounds may heal without hypertrophic scarring without excision, and the demonstration of improved functional or cosmetic result is unproven. Immediate application of skin grafts, either auto- or allo-,

are mandated to preserve their residual dermis. Some shortening of hospital stay may occur, but at the expense of general anesthesia and blood transfusions.)

6. What are two different concepts, not techniques, of burn wound excision? (Early or acute total excision of the burned wound and staged excision and grafting with the extent of excision guided by available donor sites.)
   (a) In those units that have adopted early primary excision of the burn wound, in general, what is the approach in very large, greater than 60% TBSA burn? (In general, fascial rather than tangential excision and the treatment plan is completion of the excision by the fifth day postburn and coverage with very thin widely meshed skin grafts ± bilaminar skin substitute.)
7. Describe in detail the techniques of tangential excision, fascial excision, and methods to control blood loss. (Tangential excision, as described above, consists of sequential excision of deeper layers of burned eschar until a viable layer is reached, whether deep dermis or subcutaneous fat. Fascial excision in contrast, excises burned and unburned tissue to the level of the deep fascia. The pros and cons of each is that fascial excision results in less blood loss but can create a substantial aesthetic contour defect. Tangential excision results in substantially greater blood loss but limits excision to burned tissue only. Some methods that can control blood loss include the use of tourniquets in extremity excision as well as pharmacologic products such as fibrin spray, epinephrine/thrombin soaks, etc. The use of tumescence solution, dilute epinephrine solutions in Ringer's lactate or saline, also have the capability to reduce blood loss.)
8. Describe the essentials of the operative management of a large body burn. (Methods need to be provided to prevent hypothermia which consist of a warm operative room and perhaps warming lamps, expectant blood loss with early replacement including methods to minimize blood loss such as the use of tourniquets and compressive dressings.)

Coverage of the Excised Burn Wound

Excision of specific anatomical areas, e.g., hands, will be addressed in the Burn Reconstruction module (Chap. 63). A more detailed discussion of skin substitutes is also included in the biomaterials (Chap. 11).

1. What is the essential difference between a synthetic dressing as Biobrane® and allograft when applied to a wound? (A synthetic dressing may *adhere* to the wound as a result of fibrin deposition but will not become *incorporated*. At 24–48 h the allograft skin will begin to vascularize as the capillaries migrate from the wound bed into the graft and the graft begins to "take," duplicating the sequence seen in autografts.)
   (a) Advantage of the allograft? (Both materials in the early period, 24–48 h, can reduce evaporative loss and perhaps even adhere to the wound as the result of fibrin deposition. As the allograft becomes vascularized, the capability to decrease bacterial count is enhanced. Synthetic dressings require frequent dressing changes in order to decrease bacterial count.)
   (b) What wound characteristics must be present to allow allograft take? (Exactly the same as autograft, namely free of infection and a well-vascularized bed.)
2. Differentiate the ultimate fate of the epidermis vs. the dermis components of an allograft placed on an open wound. (Even with vascularization, if not provided with sufficient diffusion of oxygen and nutrients the epidermis may be lost. The epidermis has the Langerhans cells which contain the histocompatibility antigens and as such will be the stimulus for rejection. Rejection consists of loss of the epidermis although the dermis may survive and persist for an extended period of time because of the diminished patient antigenicity in very large burns. Rejection followed by secondary infection, particularly in the adnexal structures within the dermis, frequently results in lysis of the entire autograft. Unfortunately, the process of rejection of the epidermis often leads to sufficient inflammation and infection that the remaining dermis is lyzed as well and the quality of the wound may regress.)
3. Discuss methods of preparation of allograft including the pros and cons of each. (The behavior of refrigerated or fresh allograft is the same as stored autograft, namely after 5 days tends to lose viability precipitously. Cryopreserved allograft is frozen and retains some viability for a prolonged period of time. Although treated, frozen allograft loses substantial viability in comparison to fresh allograft. The benefit is obviously prolonged shelf life in comparison to fresh allografts. As such, commercially available allograft is almost always frozen.)
4. Summarize the overall risk and clinical usefulness of each. (Fresh allograft is excellent protection and coverage for excised burned wounds and is also a good test for the suitability of wounds for autografting. The cost and limited availability are the principal limitations. The risks include the possibility of viral disease transmission, although that occurrence is extremely rare. Frozen allografts are good, although not as excellent as fresh allograft, for coverage of excised burns and are a more practical use as a test of the suitability of a wound for autografting. Frozen allograft shares the same risk of disease transmission as fresh allograft.)

5. Describe how allograft could be utilized to determine the suitability of autografting and wound closure of a chronic granulating wound. (Allografts are not viewed as “foreign” for the first few days after transplantation before the type II hypersensitivity reaction is stimulated. As such, the allograft simulates autografting and if infection supervenes, the wound is too heavily colonized.)
6. Describe the use of combined auto- and allografts in large burns. Comment on pros and cons. (The effort in very large burns is to mesh the autograft widely, perhaps even at a 9:1 ratio. To do so, creates a large amount of open wound because of the wide mesh. Allograft is placed over the autograft in effort to close, temporarily, the open wounds. The difficulty is the allograft will be recognized as foreign and undergo rejection with the secondary effect of lysis, infection, etc., described above with loss of both auto- and allograft.)
7. What are CEAs or cultured epithelial autografts? (CEAs are developed from a skin biopsy taken from the patient and then cultured, eventually yielding a preparation of sheets of epithelial cells about 6–12 cells thick.)
    (a) Describe the performance and limitations. (The culture process requires about 3 weeks. The end product lacks long-term durability and the overall take or engraftment rate is quite low. The expense is high. The lack of durability stems from the absence of dermis and delayed breakdown with blistering and open wounds are not infrequent.)
8. Are porcine xenografts vascularized by the host? (No. Adherence as well as **sealing** the wound against evaporative fluid loss are an advantage of xenografts, but they do not vascularize.)
9. Although dermal analogs are discussed in the biomaterials module, briefly describe the composition and use of the following: Integra® and human acellular dermis. (Integra® is bovine collagen fibers immersed in shark ground substance or a glycosaminoglycan and an outer layer of a silicone polymer. Integra® is intended to provide dermal wound coverage until incorporation into the host is manifested by a thin layer of vascularized tissue beneath the silicone, ordinarily at about 2 or 3 weeks. Thin autografts can then be applied. Integra® is expensive and a contaminated wound may become infected.

    Human acellular dermis is a commercially available dermal substitute and is cryopreserved cadaver acellular dermis. Although used widely in breast and abdominal reconstruction, Alloderm has had a limited application in burns.)
10. Discuss the composition of as well as the benefits and limitations of Biobrane®. (Biobrane® can seal the wound and prevent evaporative loss and bacterial contamination. The principal limitations are the accumulation of fluid and susceptibility to infection as a synthetic material. Biobrane® has no inherent bacteriostatic capability and is a synthetic bilaminar substitute composed of nylon and silicone. The Biobrane® can be easily dislodged by patient movement.)

Case-Based Conference

Case 1: Acute Burn

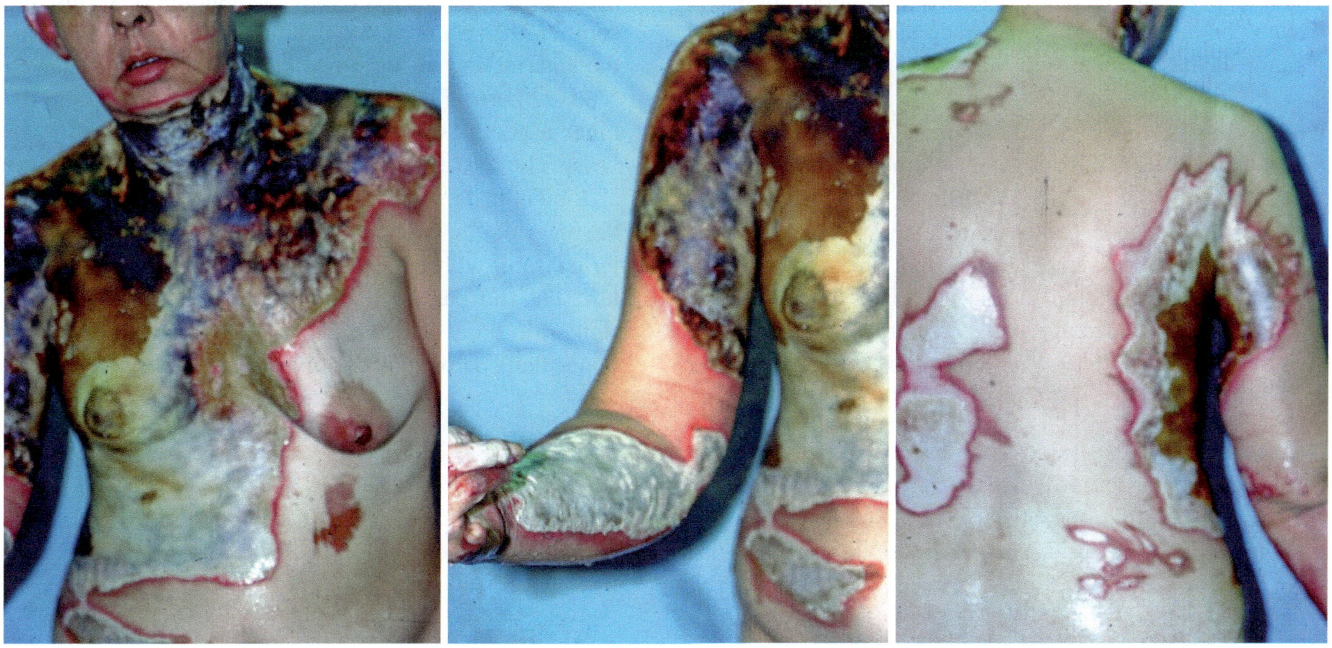

A 50-year-old woman transferred to a community hospital 72+ h post-burn from a house fire. Had application of a "cream" on admission but none since that time She had transferred because she has become "febrile and confused."

1. Describe the slides and add a clinical exam.
   (a) Besides the routine lab studies, any specific tests indicated? Justify.
2. What is your tentative clinical diagnosis and the pathophysiology of your diagnosis?
3. Outline a treatment plan including short term (on admission), intermediate (24+ h), and definitive (after 24+ h).

Case-Based Conference: Discussion

Case 1: Acute Burn

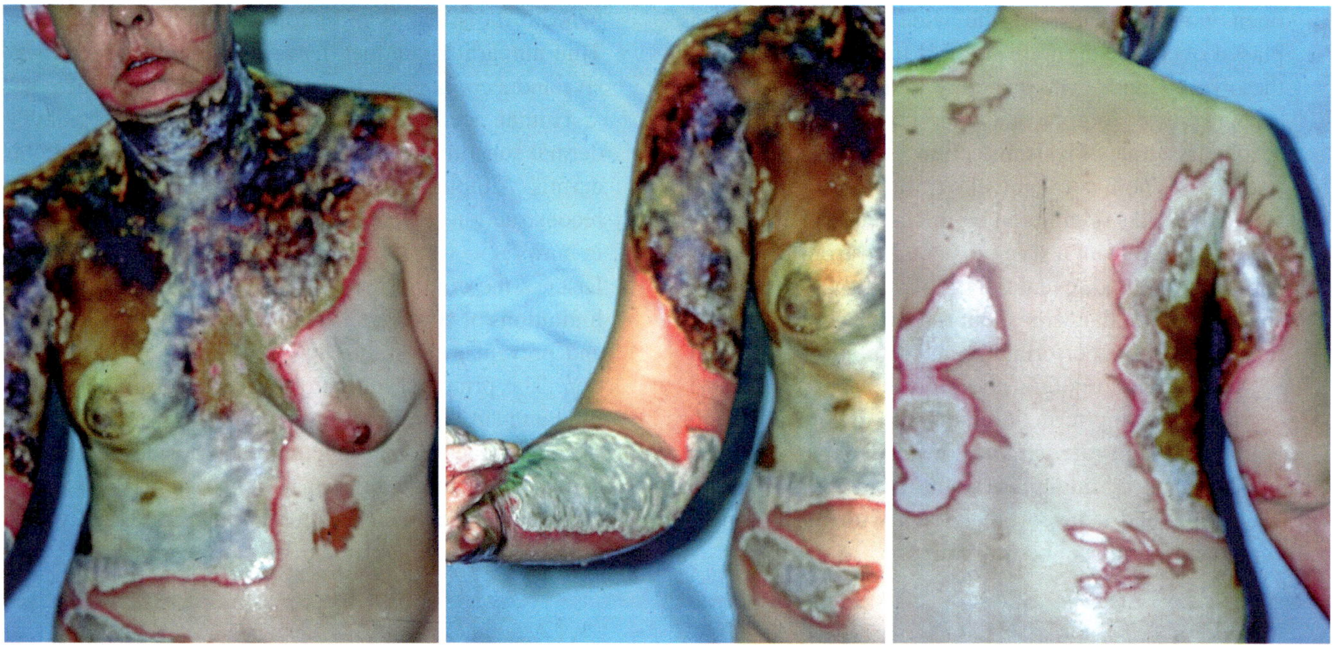

A 50-year-old woman transferred from a community hospital 72+ h post-burn from a house fire. Had application of a "cream" on admission but none since that time. Transferred because she has become "febrile and confused."

1. Describe the slides and add a clinical exam. (Three photos depict a frontal, back, and right upper extremity and adjacent truncal views. The frontal view provides the photo of a female patient with extensive burns of the entire visible neck, upper chest, right breast, right upper abdomen, and right upper arm. Although only the lower one-half is included, the face is unburned. The burns are a thick, diffusely blackened eschar except for the upper abdomen which is a silver gray in appearance. The patient is not intubated and appears to be standing or sitting, not supine. The second photo demonstrates a burn eschar of the anterior and medial two-thirds of the right arm and a separate burn of the entire volar forearm, tailing into the ulnar aspect of the elbow and terminating at the volar wrist. The forearm eschar is similar in appearance to the abdomen, the arm eschar is blackened in color similar to the anterior chest. The third photo, the length of the posterior trunk with the exception of a small portion of the left side and buttock, demonstrates an extension of the right side burn onto the lateral aspect of the chest and upper flank as well as the upper extremity burn into the

axilla and posterior and superior arm. A separate patch of burn is evident to the left of the midline that measures 15 × 4 cm. None of the three photos depict any evidence of erythema of the adjacent unburned skin. The history portion of the clinical exam would establish the circumstances of injury, the initial treatment and particular timing of intervention, the necessity of intubation or not, resumption of oral alimentation, and wound management. Pursuit of past medical history would document the presence of comorbidities, if any, to assist in the determination of the particulars of the current treatment plan. The physical exam would essentially establish the degree of critical illness including vital signs. Since the patient was transferred with "confusion," some aspect of the physical exam should establish mental status. The other aspects of the exam of the wound are outlined in the photo description.)

(a) Besides the routine lab studies, any specific tests indicated? Justify. (Clearly, the initial lab profile should include blood cultures as well as CBC and a basic metabolic panel. If indicated and dictated by the degree of septic state, arterial blood gasses should be drawn. Although quantitative wound cultures may be of assistance in directing antibiotic therapy, the operative treatment plan, see below, is of precedence.)

2. What is your tentative clinical diagnosis and the pathophysiology of your diagnosis? (The scenario is one of 50-year-old patient who has sustained substantial body burns. The photos portray an estimated 22–23% body surface area, BSA, full-thickness burn. In addition, the history of inadequately treated, a single application of a topical burn wound creme, and a recent onset of fever and confusion as well as the appearance of the eschar all point toward a diagnosis of incipient wound sepsis. The judgment of the dimension of the degree of the critical illness hinges on admission of vital signs, namely the presence of hypotension, tachycardia, tachypnea, fever, and mental status. Regardless, despite the benign overall appearance on the photos, the patient is probably on the cusp of systemic sepsis.)

3. Outline a treatment plan including short term (on admission), intermediate (24+ h), and definitive (after 24+ h). (Dependent on the patient's clinical picture on presentation a secure venous access is mandatory. If tachypnic, tachycardic, and/or hypotensive endotracheal intubation would be indicated and some element of fluid resuscitation would be initiated. Systemic antibiotics also should be initiated with venous access since the patient has essentially an acute, 72 h, untreated full-thickness burn wound. The high likelihood of burn wound infection is by colonization of Staphylococcus, MRSA, given the probability of hospital-acquired Staphylococcus infection. The antibiotic of choice would be vancomycin, a profile modified by subsequent wound cultures obtained operatively. Presuming eschar colonization and subeschar proliferation of the infecting organism, the initial choice of burn wound creme is mafenide acetate or sulfamylon®. Sulfamylon® has excellent capability to penetrate the eschar with efficacy against Staphylococcus. Because of the rapid absorption, Sulfamylon® should be applied q. 6 h, at least for the first 48 h. The patient should be carefully monitored for the detection of metabolic acidosis, the outcome of inhibition of carbonic anhydrase activity. Once stable, probably after 24 h of resuscitation and antibiotics, operative excision of the eschar should be accomplished. Given the presence of full-thickness burns, the most expeditious, rapid, and definitive excision is at the level of the fascia. Since wound closure of the resultant defect involves the investment of a substantial magnitude of split-thickness autograft, the application of allograft to ensure a receptive wound bed is a prudent temporizing measure. Assuming adherence of the allograft, the absence of purulence and an afebrile patient a return to the operative room at 72 h for autografting definitive wound closure should be accomplished. Given the degree of skin grafts necessary, one can anticipate the necessity for release of burn contractures at some juncture, particularly the neck and axilla.)

Postoperative (2 Months)

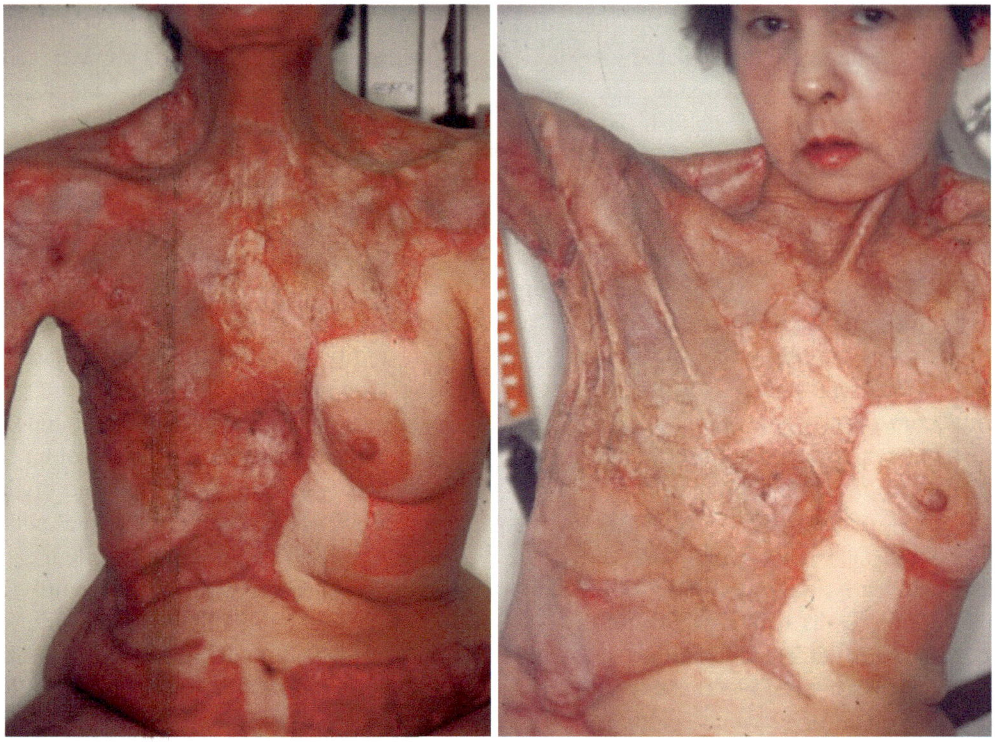

Two photos illustrate a closed wound, an absent right breast, and some hypertrophic scars of the most inferior right anterior abdomen. Besides the axilla, the entire right upper extremity is not included in either photo. In the second photo, the right shoulder is in near full abduction and some mild banding is present anteriorly. Although the neck is in a neutral position, no anterior cervical contracture is present. The band in the second photo is the sternal left sternocleidomastoid.

Critique

This outcome is probably the optimal result, given the clinical scenario.

In-Service Examination

1. The clinical onset of systemic sepsis occurs when what pathological event occurs?
   (a) Bacterial colonization occurs in the burn eschar
   (b) Invasion of viable tissue by bacteria
   (c) The predominant organism in the burn wound is staphylococcus aureus
   (d) Proliferation of bacteria in the interface of eschar and undamaged soft tissue
2. What is the complication and the application of silver sulfadiazine in burn wounds?
   (a) Metabolic acidosis
   (b) Metabolic alkalosis
   (c) Neutropenia
   (d) Hyponatremia
3. Patient admitted with untreated burns of 25–30% of 48 h duration and is in the early stage of systemic burn wound sepsis. In addition to resuscitation and systemic antibiotics what is the initial management?
   (a) Emergent excision in the OR
   (b) Application of mafenide acetate to the burn wound
   (c) Application of silver sulfadiazine to the burn wound
   (d) Application of silver nitrate to the burn wound

Metabolism, Nutritional Support, Electrical and Chemical Burns

61

Bibliography

Pruitt Jr. BA and Wolf SE, "An Historical Perspective on Advances in Burn Care Over the Past 100 Years." Cartotto, R., *Clinics in Plastic Surgery*. Elsevier Inc. (2009), 36(4):**537–42 ONLY**.

Williams FN, Herndon DN, "Metabolic and Endocrine Considerations After Burn Injury", *Clin Plastic Surg*. Elsevier Inc., (2017); 44:**541–45.**

Rollins C, Huettner F, Neumeister MW, "Clinician's Guide to Nutritional Therapy Following Major Burn Injury", *Clin Plastic Surg*., Elsevier Inc., (2017); 44:**555–66.**

Friedstat J, Brown DA, Levi B, "Chemical, Electrical, and Radiation Injuries", *Clin Plastic Surg*., Elsevier Inc., (2017); 44:**657–61.**

Demling RH, Chapter 5: "Electrical Injury", Thermal Injury, ACS Curriculum (1995); pgs. **3–10.**

CDROM PowerPoint presentation, "Electrical Burns", (2007); from Hoopes curriculum, **Slides 1–56.**

Luce EA, "Electrical burns", *Clinics in Plastic Surgery*, Elsevier Inc., (2000); 27(1):**133–143.**

Faculty Discussion and Study Guide

Nutrition and Metabolic Support

1. The primary mediators of the large burn hypermetabolic response are? What are the effects of the same? (The catabolic hormones of catecholamines, particularly epinephrine, cortisol, and glucagon, all of which can lead to proteolysis, gluconeogenesis, as well as an increase in production of endogenous corticosteroids, decreased protein, and lipid synthesis.)
   (a) Since muscle protein catabolism leads to a decrease in lean body mass, what are the negative consequences of importance to the burn patient? (Diminished capacity for wound healing, increased predisposition to sepsis, diminished immune response.)
2. What are the outcomes of the unaddressed hypermetabolic response in the major burn injury? (Increased resting energy expenditures, increased cardiac work and O_2 consumption, muscle wasting, hepatic dysfunction.)
   (a) What is the magnitude of the hypermetabolism? (For burns greater than 40% BSA and dependent on the opinion of which of the readings distributed, from 50–100% greater than the basal metabolic rate.)
   (b) What is the broad index of this response? (Increased nitrogen excretion in the urine reflects the protein breakdown as a result of the burn hypermetabolic response.)
   (c) True or false: Wound closure returns the basal metabolic rate to normal. (False—even with healing and wound closure, basal metabolic rate, BMR, is in the range of 130% and even at 1 year resting energy expenditure is 110–120%.)
3. Rank the following pathologic states in terms of magnitude of protein breakdown as reflected by increased nitrogen excretion: Starvation, 40% + burn injury, severe sepsis, multiple skeletal trauma. (40% + burn injury, multiple skeletal trauma, severe sepsis, starvation. See Fig. 61.1.)
   (a) What is the estimated maximal weight loss in a 40% + body burn without routine nutritional support? (25%) When? (2–3 months post burn. See Fig. 61.2.)
4. What is the primary method to modulate the burn hypermetabolic response? (The single most effective method is early excision and grafting of the burn, namely wound closure. One of the readings suggest in the first 72 h or perhaps the first week. Other measures are discussed below.)
5. Describe the role of ambient temperature control and non-operative methods and the physiologic basis for the same to assist in modulation of the hypermetabolic response. (Burn patients sustain a tremendous increase in water and heat loss through the burn wounds, both of

E. Luce, *A Curriculum for Plastic Surgery*, https://doi.org/10.1007/978-3-031-62087-4_61

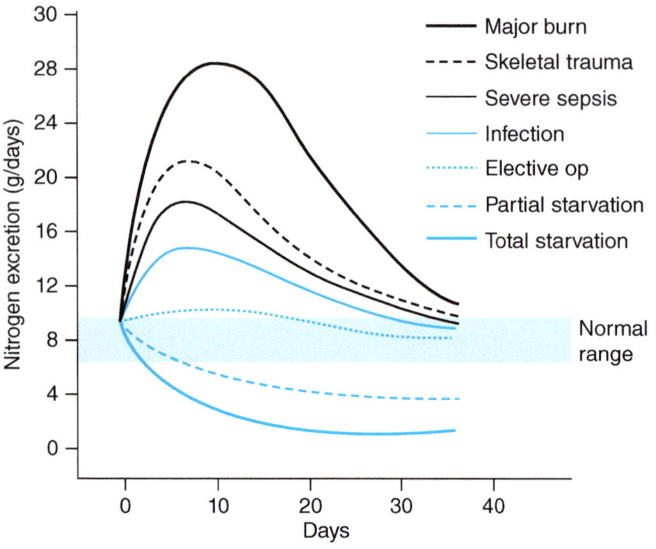

Fig. 61.1 Magnitude of catabolism with a variety of clinical scenarios. (Saffle JR, Graves C, and Cochran A. Chapter 29: Nutritional support of the burned patient. Herndon DN. Total burn care. Saunders; 2012. p. 333–353. (Reprinted with Permission))

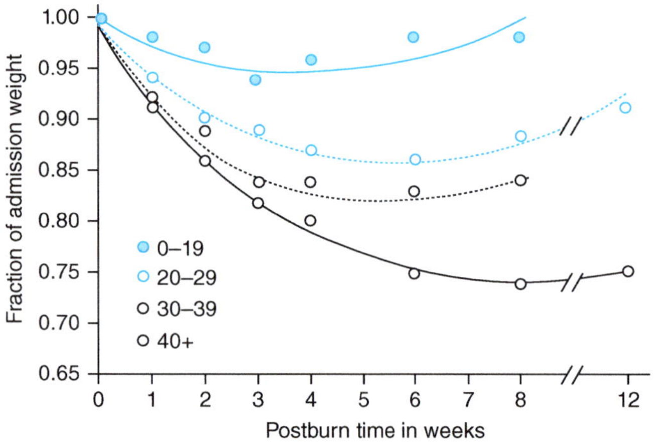

Fig. 61.2 Weight loss vs. burn body surface area in absence of nutritional support. (Saffle JR, Graves C, and Cochran A, Chapter 29: "Nutritional support of the burned patient", Herndon, D. N., Total Burn Care, Saunders. 2012. p. 333–353. (Reprinted with Permission))

which result in energy loss and expenditure. Increase in the ambient temperature in the patient's environment, hospital room, and OR, to 28–33 °C, attenuates this component of the hypermetabolic response.)

6. Describe the efficacy of the following in attenuation of the post-burn systemic inflammatory response: anti-inflammatory agents such as ibuprofen, glucocorticoids, and monoclonal antibodies. (Essentially, none of those modalities have proven to be efficacious in treatment of the systemic inflammatory response.)
   (a) If the above modalities are ineffective, what are the essential elements of address of the same? (The obvious: adequate fluid resuscitation, use of vasoactive agents as necessary, excision of the burns, enteral support, prompt diagnosis, and treatment of burn wound sepsis.)
7. What is indirect calorimetry? (Measurements of volume of expired gas and the concentration of oxygen, O_2, and carbon dioxide, CO_2.)
   (a) What is the respiratory quotient? (Ratio of CO_2 produced/O_2 consumed or VCO_2/VO_2.)
   (b) What is the role of bedside indirect calorimetry? (Calculate resting energy expenditure.)
8. Discuss address of the nutritional needs of the burn patient. (The measurement, as described above, of the resting energy requirements by beside indirect calorimetry can establish nutritional needs. These needs can be delivered most optimally by enteral feedings. Parenteral feeding by the intravenous route has significant drawbacks including bacterial intestinal translocation, loss of gut motility, and impaired immune response.)
   (a) What are some methods of monitoring nutritional status and support? (Because of wide fluctuations with infections, ventilator support, and fluid balance, body weight is notoriously unreliable but easily obtained. Nitrogen balance performed 1–2×/per week with 24 h urine collection will provide an estimation of nitrogen losses. Serum markers as prealbumin may provide a rough estimate if performed serially.)
9. Give a formula for calculating caloric needs. (The most widely used states 25 cal/Lg body weight + 40 cal/% BSA burned. Formulas tend to overestimate caloric needs. Another estimate is 1.4 × the resting energy expenditure.)
10. The major energy source for burn patients is? (Carbohydrates.)
    (a) Why? (Essentially, the fuel for healing wounds and the metabolic pathways is carbohydrates.)
    (b) The paradox is that despite increased demands and production of glucose, utilization is hampered by what? (The presence of insulin resistance resulting in hyperglycemia which also mandates for strict blood glucose control with exogenous insulin.)
11. Give an estimate of the needs of carbohydrate, fat, and protein, expressed in per kg for a large body burn. (7 g of carbohydrate, 1 g of fat, and 2 g of protein or 28 + 9 + 10 calories or a total of 47–50 calories per kg; less so in smaller burns perhaps more so in larger burns.)
12. Overfeeding can result in what? (Overfeeding, particularly of carbohydrates, can result in an increase in fat synthesis with fatty filtration of the liver. Overfeeding can further intensify the hyperglycemic characteristic of the major burn inflammatory response, rendering glucose control more difficult. Careful calculation of nutritional needs is imperative.)

Chemical Burns

1. What is the chemical property that differs the extent of acid vs. alkali burns? (Acids cause coagulation necrosis with precipitation of protein that will limit the depth-extent of the injury by neutralization of the agent. An exception may be hydrofluoric acid. See below. Alkalis create liquefaction necrosis by dissolution of the tissue protein and continuation of the extent and depth of injury.)
   (a) What is the keystone and implications of treatment? (Copious irrigation with water. Irrigation of alkali burns may be necessary initially for a prolonged, 1–2 h, and repeated every 4–6 h for 24 h. Achievement of a neutral skin pH as measured by litmus paper is the treatment goal.)
2. Hydrofluoric acid is a commonly used agent in industry. Besides the acidic component of the injury by exposure, what are the principal electrolyte disorders? (The fluoride ion combines with tissue calcium and magnesium resulting in hypocalcemia and hypomagnesaemia. Calcium and magnesium are essential elements of cellular function and lethal cardiac arrhythmias can occur. Hydrofluoric acid may also result in liquefative necrosis secondary to the free fluoride.)
   (a) Give a general classification of concentration of hydrofluoric acid exposure vs. injury. (Concentrations greater than 50% cause immediate tissue destruction and pain; 20–50% the injury may be apparent within several hours; concentrations less than 20% may take up to 24 h to become apparent.)
   (b) For significant exposures, what agent can be used to assist in neutralization of the hydrofluoric acid? (Application of a topical gel of 2.5% calcium gluconate as well as calcium gluconate injections of 5–10% concentration into the subcutaneous tissue of the wound.)
3. Phosphorus is an incendiary compound used in military armaments as well as some agricultural fertilizers. What is the method for identification of soft tissue particles and the treatment of the same? (Use of a Wood's light will assist in identification of embedded particles by ultraviolet light. Injection of a solution of 0.5% copper sulfate will assist in neutralization as well as identification of particles. The copper agent has its own potential for toxicity and renal injury and lacking availability, irrigating with water may be equally as efficacious.)

Electrical Burns

1. What is the essential equation that estimates the degree of tissue damage by an electrical injury? (Ohm's Law, $I = V/R$, or the intensity of the current in amperage.)
   (a) In fact, only one factor in the equation, voltage, is known. So, how can that number be useful? (Electrical injuries are classified as high vs. low based on the magnitude of the voltage. High-voltage injuries are considered greater than 1000 volts, low voltage less than 1000, although as the readings explain the tissue resistance can be important as well. See below.)
   (b) How does Joule's Law enter the picture in terms of tissue damage? (Adds the element of time, so the duration of heat or energy transfer to the tissues is considered.)
2. Discuss the element of resistance and how that factor can vary widely. (The skin resistance of a moist palm is much less than that of a heavily calloused hand. A hierarchy of resistance exists in the different tissues.)
   (a) List the hierarchy of the specific tissue resistance from low to high. (Nerve, blood vessels, muscle, skin, bone, and tendon. Bone and tendon are relatively avascular and acellular compared to the other tissues on the list.)
3. Differentiate the types of electric burns that occur from a high-voltage source. (Three types of electrical burns can occur and include contact, arc, and flash. The first two are considered "true" electrical injuries or burns. The contact burn occurs from either the entrance into or exit from the body of the current source. An arc burn occurs when the current from a high-voltage source is transmitted and conducted by air from source to the contact point on the body. Characteristically, the generation of heat by the arcing process can be 2000–3000°. A "flash" burn is when clothes are ignited and skin burns occur that are not essentially different from thermal burns.)
   (a) Give some characteristics of arc and contact electrical burns. (The contact points will sustain full-thickness skin injury but the extent of the skin injury will not reflect the magnitude of underlying tissue damage. The readings discuss the more extensive nature of the underlying muscle injury and the implications for treatment. In addition to the arc component of the contact injury, arc burns also may occur, dependent on the voltage, on flexion creases of the extremities; wrist, antecubital fossa, and axilla as well as popliteal fossa and the groin area. The skin burns at these skip areas conceal a much larger area of muscle and soft tissue injury as a result of the high temperatures generated by the arc phenomenon.)
4. Outline the principle, beyond ATLS, of the initial, 24 h care of the electrical burn patient. Begin with assessment. (The history needs to center on the circumstances surrounding the injury, namely if a fall occurred or momentary loss of consciousness occurred. If the voltage of the current source can be determined that number should be ascertained. The physical exam centers on the contact

points of the head, chest, abdomen, and extremities because of the implications of each.)
   (a) Give the implications of the specific body region of the contact points. (Contact points on the head may have reconstructive needs for exposed damaged skulls. The depth of injury may be limited to the skin but can also involve the cranial bone. Early debridement and even coverage of non-viable bone with well-vascularized tissue can permit reossification, if the bone is not colonized. Patients with scalp contact points are at risk for the late recurrence of gait disturbances and balance as well as other CNS sequelae including seizures. Contact points of the chest may have resulted in direct cardiac or pulmonary injury. An entrance or exit point on the abdomen may conceal underlying visceral injury. The same principles apply to contact injury of the extremities, concealed deep tissue injury beneath essentially intact skin.)
5. What are the three principal treatment needs or considerations for the first 24 h? (EKG monitoring for cardiac arrhythmias, fluid resuscitation, the necessity for extremity decompression. Cardiac monitoring in the presence of direct chest contact injury may require monitoring beyond 24 h. The volume of fluid resuscitation hinges on the degree of muscle injury. The presence of macroscopic or visible myoglobinuria mandates fluid administration beyond that of body surface area burned in order to achieve urine output of 1 + cc/kg/h and urine clear of pigment. A rough guideline is 9 cc/% BSA/kg.

   Extremities should be monitored clinically and with compartment pressures for the possible necessity of decompression by fasciotomies. Unlike thermal injury burns, the restrictive structure is the deep muscular fascia. Most high ultra voltage contact points on the hand, presumably entrance, will require early fasciotomies of the forearm. Two adjuncts to IV fluids advocated by some are mannitol and bicarbonate, given intravenously; mannitol to induce diuresis by volume expansion and bicarbonate to alkalize the urine, since myoglobin is more soluble in an alkaline medium. High-volume lactated Ringer's induces an alkaline urine and administration of mannitol seems somewhat counterintuitive.)
6. What are the essential elements in wound care of the electrical burn? (Serial debridement every 24–48 h, temporizing wound coverage with allograft, awareness of possibility of deep muscle damage, early definitive wound coverage, and/or amputation.)

Case-Based Conference

Case 1: Deep Burn of Scalp

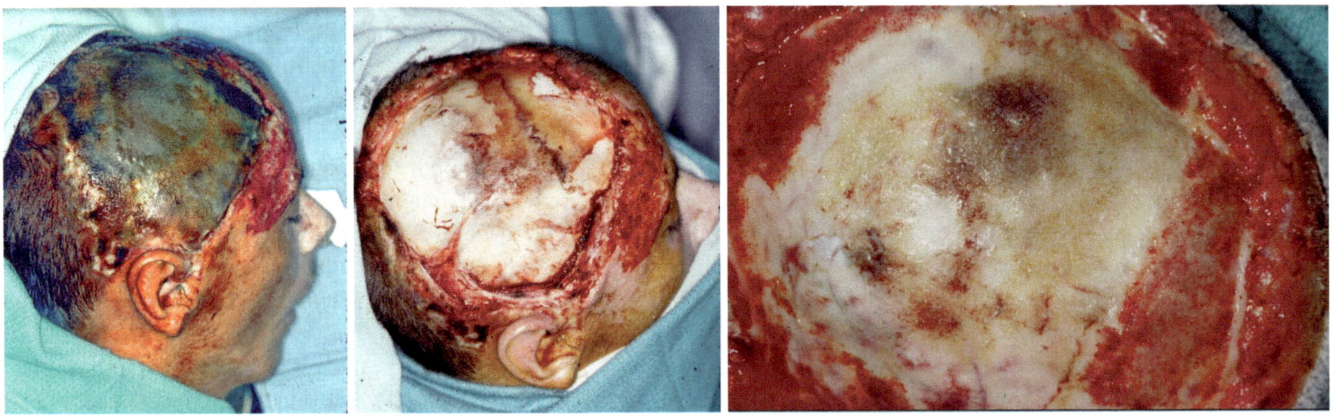

A 26 year old, 2 weeks ago sustained a contact high-tension electric contact burn as well as hepatic and splenic lacerations sustained in a fall, acute care elsewhere was rendered, and has been transferred to you. He has no other burns and has recovered from his other injuries.

1. Describe the photo(s). Add a focused clinical examination.
   (a) Tests or imaging indicated? Why?
2. What is the pathologic anatomy or possible scenarios?
3. Outline a treatment plan that hinges on your response to question 2.

Case-Based Conference: Discussion

Case 1: Deep Burn of Scalp

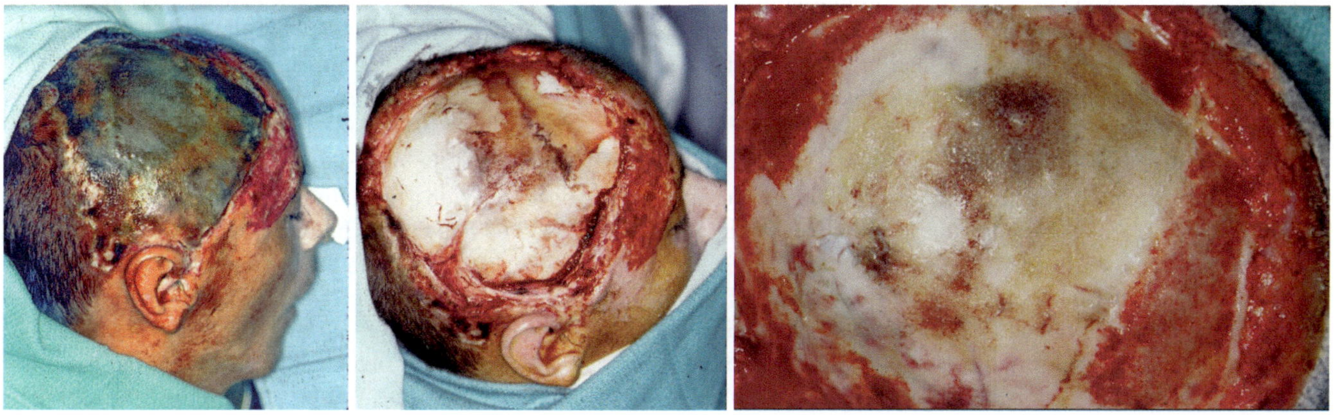

A 26 year old, 2 weeks ago sustained a contact high-tension electric contact burn as well hepatic and splenic lacerations sustained in a fall, acute care elsewhere was rendered, and has been transferred to you. He has no other burns and has recovered from his other injuries.

1. Describe the photo(s). Add a focused clinical examination. (The set of photos depict an extensive burn of the scalp and skull. The first photo is a lateral view and pictures a large eschar that occupies nearly the entire temporal and parietal scalp. The eschar is of variegated color. An additional extension of the wound is evident over the remaining temple and adjacent forehead. The subsequent photo, also accomplished from the lateral perspective, was apparently after debridement and demonstrates a bare skull devoid of periosteum with some apparent discoloration of bone. The last photo is a close-up of the bone and illustrates an area of grayish discoloration of the cranium with surrounding bone more normal in appearance and color.

   The history would center on the circumstances of injury, the duration of contact if known, and the approximate voltage, if available. The prior management of the hepatic and splenic lacerations would be of value as well as his clinical course over the subsequent 2 weeks prior to transfer. Additional history would assess the overall status as eating, ambulating, and functional capacity and exertion tolerance. In addition, given the location of the wounds, the history would attempt to establish the presence of CNS symptoms as seizures, episodes of confusion or ataxia. Although the preamble stated no other burns, a full-body examination is mandatory as well as an assessment of the scalp wound. That assessment performed when eschar is still intact would include adherence, the presence or not of expressible purulence, and the presence or not of adjacent cellulitis.)

   (a) Tests or imaging indicated? Why? (Assuming the patient has good renal function, an assessment of the contiguous skull by imaging would be appropriate. The objective is a determination of the viability of the involved skull and in particular the status of the inner cortex. The choice between MRI or CT would tilt toward MRI in the capability to ascertain intact bone. Of course, given the other injuries, the necessary lab tests of CBC and basic metabolic panel should be performed.)
2. What is the pathologic anatomy or possible scenarios? (The principal pathology is electrical injury to bone, in this instance calvarial bone. Bone of all the body tissues has the highest inherent resistance so the passage of high voltage, presumed in this case, generates tremendous heat as dictated by Joule's Law: Power or heat is a product of current squared times the resistance. Since the current also passes or traverses the vascular channels within cortical and cancellous bone, the bone is rendered non-viable if the heat generated is significant. If the non-viable bone remains undebrided, colonization is inevitable and eventually infected, or the outcome of osteomyelitis. A burn of scalp and skull may vary in severity to skin only to one of full thickness of soft-tissue including periosteum. Bone involvement can also be either partial thickness of the outer cortex only or full thickness of diploe or inner cortex and even in rare instances dural injury. From the perspective of pathophysiology does the lower resistance and hence the less heat generated by the diploe cavity lessen the possibility of full thickness injury?)
3. Outline a treatment plan that hinges on your response to question 2. (If possible, the depth of injury should be ascertained with imaging either CT or MRI. Since the preamble states that the patient has fully recovered from his intra-abdominal injuries, his wound closure/recon-

struction is accomplished with either a single or multi-staged approach. Operative debridement of the eschar is the first step toward the determination of the depth of injury. If the periosteum is intact, the wound is immediately skin-grafted. If in contrast, the periosteum is lost and the bone is involved as is evident in the case under discussion, the depth of injury must be determined by the removal of the outer cortex by burring with copious irrigation. If bleeding diploe cavity is encountered with viable cancellous bone, the preferable course of action is delayed skin grafting. One drawback of the placement of the split-thickness skin grafts directly on granulating calvarial bone in this manner is lack of durability and the frequent occurrence of late ulceration with minor trauma of the activities of daily living. This disadvantage can be minimized with the application of a dermal template, Integra®, use of negative wound pressure therapy, and delayed split-thickness skin grafts.

If full-thickness bony injury is encountered, a difficult treatment decision looms. A craniectomy signals a neurosurgical procedure and complex late reconstruction. An option is retention of the non-viable bone and coverage with a well-vascularized flap, in this case a large free flap. The probability of success of that option lies on the degree, if any, of colonization of the bone. If the hiatus between injury and definitive debridement is relatively short, 2 weeks in this case, and the inner cortical bone is not infected or even significantly colonized, then after debridement of the outer cortex and curettage of the diploe, coverage with a free latissimus flap provides definitive closure. The flap can be muscle only, covered with split-thickness skin graft. With time and atrophy of the muscle, the contour will improve. The final option for discussion is the placement of the flap over the intact skull without removal of even the outer cortex, avoiding the necessity of bone debridement. The potential and disastrous outcome is camouflaged infection underneath the flap, osteomyelitis, and eventually epidural abscess. Perhaps a bone sample of the central area for culture may assist the decision process.)

Postoperative

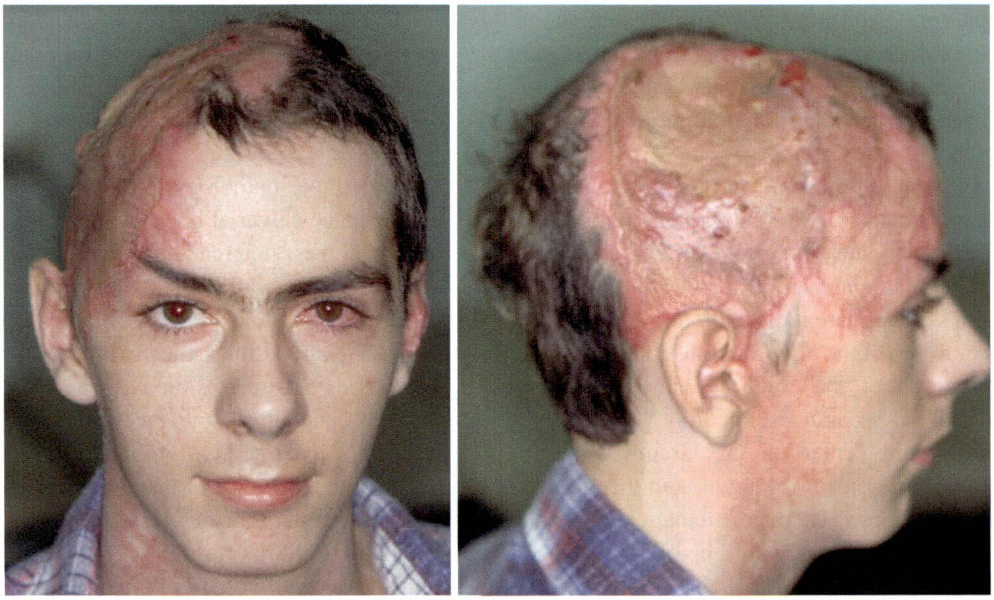

The two postoperative photos demonstrate a healed wound with some perceptible contour deformity secondary to loss of the outer cortex.

Case-Based Conference

Case 2: Electrical Burn

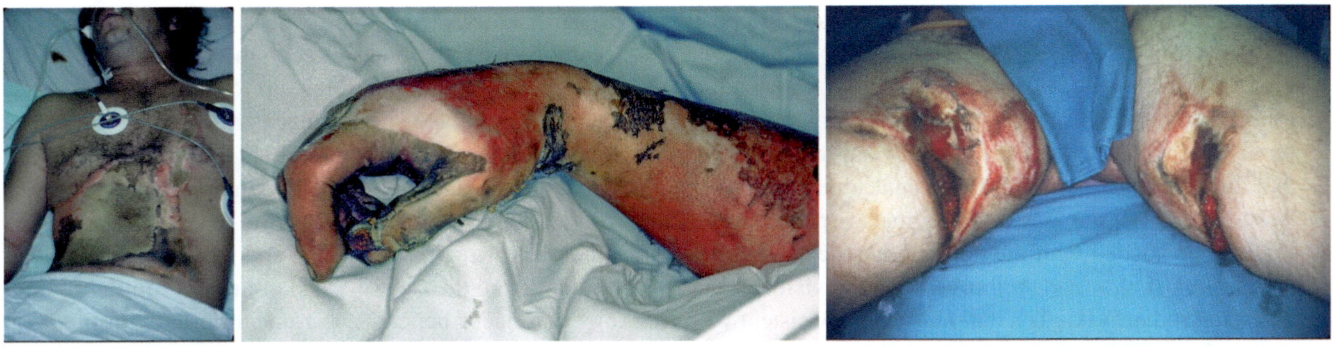

A 30-year-old lineman sustained injury 1 h ago. Conscious and responsive. Vital signs blood pressure 110/70, pulse 112. The patient has had an IV and nasogastric tube inserted as well as blood drawn. The trauma team has completed assessment including a screening CT scan of the head, chest, and abdomen.

1. Describe the findings in the photo(s). Add a focused clinical examination.
   (a) What tests, if any besides blood work and CT scan are indicated? Justify.
2. What is the pathophysiology involved in the patient's injury?
3. Based on the response to question 2, outline a treatment plan. Do so in the sequence of priority.
4. Complications?

Case-Based Conference: Discussion

Case 2: Electrical Burn

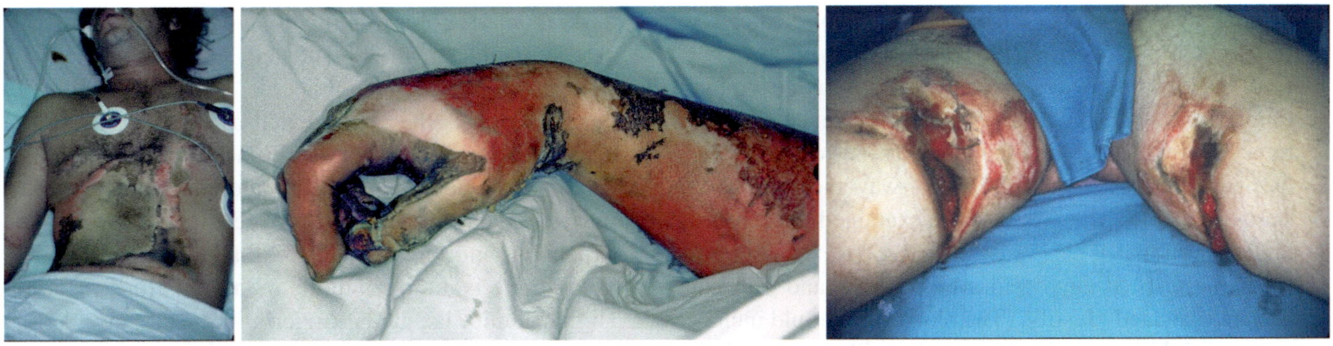

A 30-year-old lineman sustained injury 1 h ago. Conscious and responsive. Vital signs blood pressure 110/70, pulse 112. The patient has had an IV and nasogastric tube inserted as well as blood drawn. The trauma team has completed assessment including a screening CT scan of the head, chest, and abdomen.

1. Describe the findings in the photo(s). Add a focused clinical examination. (The first photo is the recumbent patient, anterior chest and upper abdomen and most of the head and neck is included. EKG leads are in place, IV access in the neck, as well as a nasogastric tube. The patient is not intubated. The most impressive finding depicted is a large

burn of the left chest and upper abdomen. The burn extends from the right parasternal line to beyond the lateral chest and from the left nipple-areola to the left midabdomen. Neither upper extremity is visible except for the upper right arm. Nearly the entire burn has the appearance of a third degree injury, depressed in contour and grayish in color with only a small zone of surrounding pink-white burn. No other burns are evident. The second photo is limited to an upper extremity and includes hand and forearm from just distal to the antecubital fossa. The wrist is in a flexed posture, the metacarpophalangeal joints are extended with the digital joints flexed. Burned and peeling skin is evident throughout. The visible radial and ulnar forearm skin is a dull red-white consistent with a deep burn. The radial and dorsal skin of the hand is snow white distally and similar to the forearm reddish hue more proximal. The volar aspect of the wrist and palmar skin is not discernible. The third photo is limited to an inclusion of only both medial thighs. In the central mid-third of the left thigh is a burn wound with darkened skin and, more posterior, an open transversely oriented elliptical-shaped open wound. The burn wound of the right thigh is more extensive and involves the medial one-half of the thigh as well as extension onto a considerable portion of the anterior thigh. A similar open wound of similar shape is also present. The burns are a mixture of pink and white with sharp demarcation from the surrounding skin.

The clinical examination gleans important information about the circumstances of the injury including was a fall involved, any loss of consciousness, duration of contact, and current complaints including shortness of breath. The line voltage at the moment of injury will be available from the electric power company. The physical examination beyond vital signs establishes the presence of respiratory distress, if any, although the presence of the IV and nasogastric access would suggest airway and respiratory status is stable. The wounds are examined. See below under question 3.)

(a) What tests, if any besides blood work and CT scan are indicated? Justify. (The blood work could include myoglobin levels but the results will not materially affect the treatment plan.)

2. What is the pathophysiology involved in the patient's injury? (The principles underlying electrical injury is Ohm's law or I = V/R that states the energy intensity, I, is the magnitude of the voltage modified by the degree of resistance. The burn is the result of heat generated, since Joule's Law dictates that power, or heat, is I^2 x R or resistance. The body tissues have a hierarchy of resistance to the passage of electrical current, from least to highest as nerve, blood vessels, muscle, skin, and bone. As a result, the same current or voltage will generate substantially more heat in contact with bone than with blood vessels. The other element of the pathophysiology is the arcing of electrical current. Arcing refers to the passage of high-voltage electrical current through air for short distances from one contact point to another, for example, from the line source to the victim. In doing so, extremely high temperatures, up to 2–3000°, are generated. High-voltage circumstances can create arc burns at flexion creases of the extremities as wrist, antecubital fossa, axilla, and the groin. The importance of both the contact points and the arc burns is these areas conceal a much larger region of muscle and soft tissue injury, not evident from the size of the skin burn. A similar pathology can occur beneath the truncal burns with injury to the underlying viscera.

The systemic consequences of electrical injury are those of hypovolemia and direct renal tubular damage from myoglobin. The degree of fluid loss from the intravascular volume into the interstitial space is greater than the body surface area burn, reflective of injury to the deeper tissues. Those tissues include skeletal muscle that once damaged, releases myoglobin into the circulation which in turn is excreted by the kidneys. Once precipitated, myoglobin inflicts a direct injury into the renal tubules which if not adequately addressed results in acute tubular necrosis and acute renal failure.)

3. Based on the response to question 2, outline a treatment plan. Do so in the sequence of priority. (The first priority is to address hypovolemia and hemoglobinuria. Administration of high-volume lactated Ringer's solution is the keystone of the resuscitation. If the urine is dark, indicative of a significant myoglobin load, aggressive IV management is mandated, readily tolerated in a young patient such as in this case. Urine output of 1 cc/kg or greater is the goal as well as the clearing of the urine of gross pigment. Two adjuncts to IV fluids advocated by some are mannitol and bicarbonate, given intravenously, mannitol to induce diuresis by volume expansion and bicarbonate to alkalize the urine, since myoglobin is more soluble in an alkaline medium. High-volume lactated Ringer's induces an alkaline urine in administration of mannitol seems somewhat counterintuitive.

Continuous ECG monitoring is critical not just for this patient with a chest burn but all electrical burn patients for the first 24–48 h. In addition, this patient with a contact burn of the chest from a high-tension source is at risk for ARDS, acute respiratory distress syndrome, secondary to a pulmonary injury. As such, monitoring with pulse oximetry is essential.

After resuscitation, the next priority is fasciotomy of the involved upper extremity. Forearm fasciotomies should be performed in the OR and should be considered a procedure to determine the extent of the underlying injury to forearm muscle. In fact, the operative setting is the opportunity to perform exploration and aggressive debridement of all wounds. To do so may lessen the load of myoglobin as well as other noxious byproducts of the injury. If indicated by the extent of injury, as apparent in the photo of the hand and forearm, early amputation should be accomplished. The implication from the standpoint of systemic stability is that prior to the OR, the patient's resuscitation is well underway, urine output is 1 cc/kg and clearing of pigment, vital signs are stable, and no EKG changes are evident. Wound coverage is temporalized with allograft and plans are established for serial debridements every 24–48 h in preparation for early definitive coverage.)

4. Complications? (A myriad of early and late complications can occur following a high-tension electrical injury. Acute renal failure may result from inadequate fluid resuscitation and myoglobinuria. Visceral injury, intra-abdominal or cardiopulmonary, are the potential consequences of contact points on the trunk. As indicated in this case, limb amputation is not uncommon.

Patients who sustained contact injury of the skull are at risk for late CNS complications.)

Intraoperative

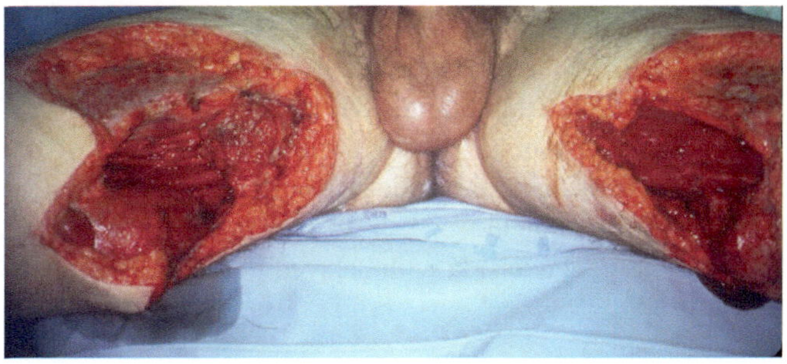

In the single photo, an extensive debridement of both thighs has been accomplished with a resultant large open wound. On the left, skin, subcutaneous fat, and deep fascia has been excised, revealing an intact adductor. On the right, though, both a proximal and distal muscle stump can be discerned at either extreme of the wound, indicative that the underlying muscle has been excised.

Postoperative (3 and 6 Months)

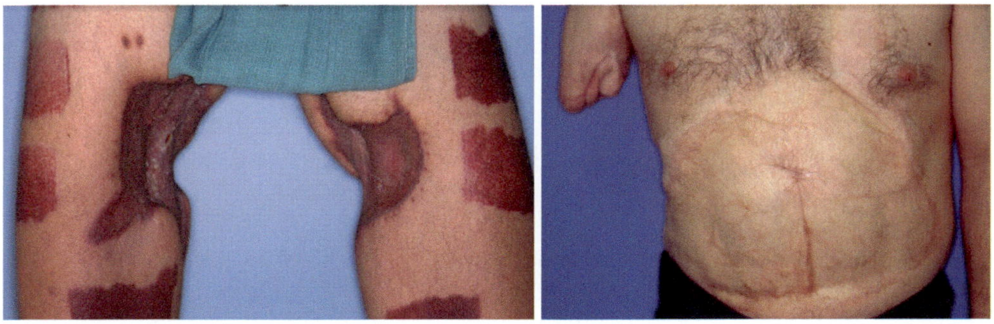

In the first photo, limited to the thighs the consequence of the extent of the debridement necessary is apparent. On the left the outline of the intact muscle is evident within a contour defect, secondary to loss of skin and subcutaneous fat. On the right the defect is substantially deeper. All wounds are skin-grafted and closed.

The six-month photo includes most of the anterior trunk and right upper arm. The face has been excluded. The area of the chest and abdomen has been skin-grafted. A transhumeral amputation of the right arm is present with a well-healed stump.

In-Service Examination

1. The hierarchy of magnitude of catabolism in protein breakdown in a 40% BSA burn is:
   (a) Total starvation, 40% burn
   (b) Systemic sepsis, 40% burn
   (c) 40% burn, major skeletal trauma
   (d) Major skeletal trauma, 40% burn
2. A patient sustains a 10% hydrofluoric acid burn of the torso in an industrial accident. Appropriate management of the wounds include:
   (a) Emergent excision with delayed grafting
   (b) Irrigation of the wounds, application of calcium gluconate gel
   (c) Irrigation of the wounds, application of mafenide acetate
   (d) Irrigation of the wounds, application of silver nitrate
3. An acute electrical injury is taken to OR for fasciotomy. What agents are absolutely contraindicated?
   (a) Isoflurane
   (b) Vancomycin
   (c) Succinylcholine
   (d) Propofol
   (e) Nitrous oxide

62 Reconstruction (Eyelids, Ears, Nose, Cheek, Face, Neck)

Bibliography

Donelan M.B., Bojovic B., "Reconstruction of the Head and Neck", Total Burn Care, 5th edition, Elsevier (2018); **pgs. 532–554.**

Dougherty, W. R. and Spence, R. J., Chapter 14 "Reconstruction of the burned face/cheek: acute and delayed." Sood, R., Burn Surgery: Reconstruction and Rehabilitation. Saunders Elsevier (2006), **pp 238–244 ONLY**.

Spence, R. J., "An Algorithm for Facial Reconstruction Using an Expanded Transposition Flap." *Plast. Reconstr. Surg.*, (2008); 121:**795–805.**

Achauer MD, B. M. and Adair MD, S. R., "Acute and Reconstructive Management of the Burned Eyelid." *Clinics in Plastic Surgery*. (January 2000), **pp 87–96.**

Bernard MD, S. L., "Reconstruction of the burned nose and ear." *Clinics in Plastic Surgery*. (January 2000), **pp 97–112 ONLY.**

Hickerson, W and Rives, J. M., Chapter 15 *Reconstruction of the burned neck*. Sood, R., Burn Surgery: Reconstruction and Rehabilitation. Saunders Elsevier (2006), **pp 254–263.**

Zuccaro J, Ziolkowski N, and Fish J. "A Systematic Review of the Effectiveness of Laser Therapy for Hypertrophic Burn Scars", *Clin. Plast. Surg.*, (2017); 44:**767, 769, 776–9 ONLY.**

Faculty Discussion and Study Guide

Editor's Note: Burn reconstruction of the nose and ear is similar to reconstruction in skin cancer (Chaps. 29 and 31).

General

1. The readings establish the dilemma in treatment of acute facial burns. Outline the dilemma. (If burns are sufficiently deep, healing will be principally by contracture and the production of hypertrophic scars. If that outcome can be predicted, then early excision and skin grafting will provide a more desirable outcome. Yet, the excision of a superficial burn that would otherwise spontaneously re-epithelialize will result in an inappropriately grafted face. The readings offer 3 weeks as the watershed point to permit healing if depth of burn cannot be ascertained.)
2. Give a classification system of facial burn scarring. (Essentially two classes. A normal-appearing facies without deformity but diffuse hypertrophic scars. The other is scarring, contracture, and distortion of facial features.)
3. What are the specific stigmata of facial burn scars? (The stigmata of facial burn scars consist of lower lid ectropion, a shortened nose with inadequate soft tissue coverage and skeletonization, alar flaring, and a short retruded upper lip. Eversion of the lower lip occurs because of scar contracture with inferior displacement. Overall, the facial features are flat with loss of jawline definition.)
4. What are some nonoperative modalities employed to treat hypertrophic scarring? (The use of prefabricated, custom-made, silicone-lined compression masks, and/or compression garments are conventional and traditional methods to address facial burn scars.)
5. What lasers have been principally utilized for the treatment of hypertrophic burn scars? (Either ablative, the CO_2 laser, or 585 nm pulsed dye laser. Although a wide variety of lasers can be employed, the only other laser reported is the intense pulsed light.)
   (a) What measures or assessment instruments can be utilized? (The two tools are modified Vancouver Scar Scale and patient observer assessment scale or POAS.)

E. Luce, *A Curriculum for Plastic Surgery*, https://doi.org/10.1007/978-3-031-62087-4_62

6. Give a perspective on the use of laser therapy in the management of burns. (Although laser therapy, particularly the pulsed dye laser, has been described and advocated in the early and late management of burn scars, the readings offer a note of caution. A systematic review of past contributions revealed low-quality studies and methodology such that no clear evidence of efficacy could be established.)

Eyelids

1. Discuss the examination of the eye in burn patients. (Vision, conjunctival burn, pupillary reaction and extraocular muscles, clarity of cornea and anterior chamber, corneal staining with fluorescein strip, measurement of intraocular pressure.)
2. Discuss the management of alkali burns of the eye. (Alkali burns tend to cause more penetration injuries than acid, and emergency treatment with irrigation is the cornerstone. A litmus test can document that neutral pH has been reached in the cul-de-sac. Intraocular pressure should be followed and the patient started on 1% atropine drops. Complications are symblepharon and ulceration.)
3. What are the methods available to protect the cornea in instances of severe lid loss? (A saran-wrap moisture chamber, scleral lens, or a Gunderson conjunctival flap and even simply antibiotic ointment alone in less severe cases. The use of ointment during the early days post-burn is sufficient. If more aggressive procedures are necessary, a Gunderson flap that consists of mobilization of conjunctiva to place over the cornea may be necessary. Early consideration should be given if persistent staining of the cornea indicates exposure. Full-thickness graft release may be necessary with the recognition that additional release later in the post-burn period will also be necessary.)
4. Other than contracture and exposure, what other mechanism that is an outcome of burned eyelids can predispose to corneal ulceration? (Destruction of the Meibomian glands on the lash margin will result in loss of the lipid component of tears. The lipid component in addition to the aqueous and mucin components provides protection and helps to minimize the evaporation of the tears.)
5. What were the recommendations and thoughts about temporary tarsorrhaphy for protection? (The readings were of the opinion that temporary tarsorrhaphy has less of a role than in the past because they are not effective and often dehisce and break down. They recommended early skin grafting even on granulation tissue if necessary.)
6. Briefly describe the technique of permanent tarsorrhaphy. (An intermarginal tarsorrhaphy is the most straightforward and is accomplished by excision of a strip of conjunctiva over the superior, the upper eyelid, and the inferior, the lower eyelid, margin of the tarsus to create a raw surface, placed at the most lateral aspect of the lids. Two horizontal sutures of a 5° prolene are placed with the use of small silastic catheter tubing to prevent lid skin erosion by the sutures.)
7. Describe the masquerade procedure. (Probably an extremely uncommon operation. Consists of suturing the upper and lower eyelid tarsal or lid conjunctiva to each other and application of a skin graft over the raw surface of the conjunctiva. Second stage consists of division of the skin graft. Clearly, a number of shortcomings exist in this procedure.)
8. Define symblepharon. (Adhesion of the eyelid to the underlying globe with loss and obliteration of the conjunctival-lined sulci. Address would require release and the liberal use of mucosal graft.)
9. Discuss the management of burn ectropion, including early vs. late, upper vs. lower eyelid, flaps vs. types of skin grafts. (The indications for early ectropion release are corneal exposure, irritation, and risk of ulceration. If possible, release should be deferred as long as feasible to permit maturation of the burn scar. The release should be oriented transversely and extend to and beyond each canthus, with the incision reasonably close to the lid margin in the lower eyelid and palpebral fold in the upper lid. The readings state that flaps have no role in release of eyelid contractions and advocate full-thickness skin grafts for the lower eyelids and thick split grafts for the upper lids. What the readings did not discuss was the "third dimension" release of burn ectropion, namely the importance of complete release of skin, orbicularis, and septum to accomplish a complete release. An oversized bolster should be applied to the graft which will essentially push the lash margin upward and serve as a tarsorrhaphy. A Frost suture can be utilized for upward traction during the release but is not necessary postoperative.)
10. Describe a technique for release-reconstruction of epicanthal folds. (A variety of procedures exist, most of which center on the use of a multiple Z-plasty concept. The jumping man is the use of several advancement flaps to address the contracture as represented by the straight line of the trunk.)
11. What methods are available for eyebrow reconstruction? (Free scalp grafts, either single or multiple strips, as well as punch grafts, an island flap on the superficial temporal vessels, and scalp flap.)
12. Discuss the pros and cons of grafts vs. flap approach to eyebrow reconstruction. (The authors quote the Pensler

study that determined that actually partial loss and misalignment was less common in free grafts than in the vascularized flaps. Probably gender, status of the other brow, and the degree of scarring on the recipient side all should be considered in the choice of reconstruction.)

Ear

Editor's Note: Partial and total ear and nose reconstruction are both addressed in Chaps. 29 and 31. (Skin Tumors)

1. What is the principal concern with acute deep burns of the ear? (Secondary infection of the cartilage, the development of chondritis.)
   (a) What is the primary treatment to minimize the development of burn chondritis? (Application of Sulfamylon as well as avoidance of compression of the ear.)
   (b) What are the findings in acute burn chondritis? (Red, tender, swollen ear with obliteration of the normal anatomical landmark.)
   (c) Treatment of choice for burn chondritis. (Systemic antibiotics as well as bivalving and debridement of the clearly necrotic cartilage. The outcome is frequently, even usually, a significant deformity.)
2. Give one classification of ear deformity secondary to burns. (Subtotal absence of the helical rim, total absence of the helical rim, ear lobule deformity, and meatal stenosis.)
   (a) What is the most common? (Loss of the superior helical rim.)
3. Outline the pros and cons of excision of burned ear tissue and skin grafting. (The obvious pro is that the burned skin can be excised and replaced with either thin full-thickness or split-thickness grafts with preservation of the underlying cartilaginous framework. The disadvantages or cons are at least two: one, the ear, could heal satisfactorily without deformity; second, most commonly, when the skin has sustained a full-thickness burn because of the absence of any significant tissue between skin and perichondrium, the perichondrium is damaged as well. Clearly, large areas of auricular cartilage without perichondrium will not sustain a skin graft.)
   (a) What is an alternative for coverage? (Probably the most popular is a temporoparietal fascial flap covered by skin graft. Although this technique has been utilized in post-traumatic as well as congenital ear loss, in severe burns the ear cartilage is significantly damaged and will often result in a deformed ear without discernible normal landmarks.)
4. Describe the use of an alloplastic or synthetic ear reconstruction. (As mentioned in the readings, silastic framework has fallen out of favor as an alternative to the use of autogenous cartilage because of high exposure and extrusion rates. A more recent development is the use of porous polyethylene or Medpor as a framework, an extension of the experience with congenital microtia, covered with a temporoparietal fascial flap. Little experience with the use of Medpor in total burn reconstruction has been published to date but results are promising.)
5. The readings describe the use of tissue expansion with small expanders for ear reconstruction. What do you believe would be the principal limitation(s)? (Quite frequently the tissue in the preauricular area is scarred from the burn injury. The use of an expanded scalp is quite problematic because of the hair follicles.)
6. Describe the use of prosthetic ear reconstruction with the use of osteo-integration. (The essential principle of osteo-integration is the placement of titanium implants that allow for some element of tissue/bone ingrowth and a second- or third-stage placement of the prosthetic ear portion of the implant. The soft tissue cover must be thin and minimally scarred, however.)

Face/Cheek

1. Discuss and describe the regional aesthetic units of the face in burn reconstruction. (The seams of any flap or skin graft reconstruction should be placed along a border between the units to accomplish optimal camouflage. This concept would imply seams below the lower border of the body of the mandible, the periorbital region and an interface between the temple and cheek. See Fig. 62.1.)
   (a) What is the "gold standard" in facial burn reconstruction? (The use of full-thickness skin grafts.)
   (b) What are some time guidelines re: excision "and grafting of facial burns? (As the readings outline, burns that have not healed by 3 weeks will heal by contracture and secondary epithelialization with resultant hypertrophic burn contractures and scars.)
   (c) Discuss primary excision and skin grafting versus grafting onto a granulating surface. (Split-thickness skin grafts placed on granulation tissue are prone to substantially more contracture than skin grafts placed on a freshly excised wound. The same principle of a hiatus of 2–3 weeks post-burn to allow for possible complete healing by re-epithelialization. So, primary excision of the burn combined with an application of a thick skin-graft is preferable.)

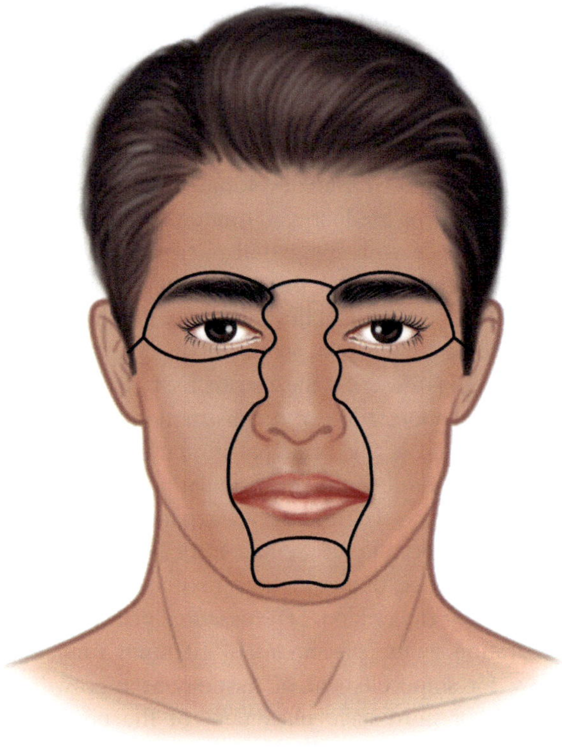

Fig. 62.1 Aesthetics of the face

2. What is the hierarchy of correction of burn scars/contractures in the face? What are the treatment implications? (The eyelids, the lower lip/chin unit, the upper lip, cheeks, and finally the nose. The readings classify facial burn reconstruction into two categories: one, no facial distortion but diffuse burn scarring without contractures and; second, facial burn contracture and deformities. The division would appear to be somewhat simplistic even though a facial deformity as eyelid or ectropion or nasal loss may not be present, diffuse scarring may still dictate the necessity for a reconstructive plan. The point established by the readings is that perhaps limited Z-plasties, local excisions, etc., may suffice. Perhaps the division into peripheral and central has more concise reconstructive implications. See question below.)
3. Contrast the reconstructive needs of the peripheral aesthetic units of the forehead, temple, and cheeks with the central units. (In general, the featureless flat, peripheral facial reconstructive units can be addressed with full-thickness skin grafts and are preferred over flaps, particularly the forehead and temple. The cheek, as the readings describe, may require the use of expanded transposition flaps harvested from the shoulder to provide a more full and round appearance. The central units are the nose and lips. Release, in the instance of the lower lip, or resurfacing, in the instances of the upper lip and the nose, may optimally be addressed with full-thickness skin grafts harvested from the "blush" area. The "blush" area refers to skin above the clavicles and provides an optimal color match and texture. (Reconstruction of the nose is covered in the Chap. 29. Nose Reconstruction.)
4. What is the advisability of a rotational-transposition flap from the neck to address the cheek? (Probably not advisable because of the downward traction from gravity and the secondary occurrence of lower lid ectropion unless the area is small and can be addressed with a cervicofacial flap. Similarly, expanded neck flaps rotated rather than advanced are at a less risk for the same complication.)
5. Give a general category of methods of burn reconstruction of the face/cheek with pros and cons of each. (A broad classification would be full-thickness skin grafts, either direct or harvested from expanded skin, split-thickness skin grafts, flaps, flaps either expanded or not expanded, and synthetics such as Integra. One of the readings provides an algorithm for the use of each. Expanded neck and adjacent supra-clavicular shoulder skin if available provides an elegant one unit reconstruction. Full-thickness skin graft if harvested from expanded supra-clavicular skin is also extremely useful as a large sheet-type skin replacement, but neither may be available. The use of Integra as a two-stage approach with application of a thin split-thickness skin graft after vascularization of the Integra is an option but recontracture and reoperation may be an attendant complication.)

Neck

1. What measures can be used in the burn unit to minimize neck contracture occurrence? (Efforts to avoid patient positioning that flexes the cervical spine/neck.)
2. A patient has a severe anterior cervical burn contracture and you plan release of the same. What are the anesthesia considerations? (The principal complication is the airway. An awake nasotracheal intubation and/or fiber-optic intubation is the contemporary management. More traditional techniques are the release of the contracture under local anesthesia and then routine intubation, not often employed today.)
3. Discuss the technical points and release of neck scar contractures. (Transverse release should be placed, as in other joint scar releases, from mid axial to mid axial point which would imply the mid cervical lateral line. Less severe contractures would not require that extent of an incision. With respect to depth, platysma is almost always incised and released and the head/neck progressively extended as the contracture release is accomplished. Not infrequently, the cervical fascia beneath the platysma needs release as well. Vertical lateral incisions, if scar

excision is accomplished, should be designed as a z or an s to minimize contracture.)

4. Discuss the use of Integra and release of neck burn contractures. (Placement of Integra, a dermal substitute, is done after contracture release and overlaps 2–3 mm onto native skin. Either a bolster or VAC is employed for the next 2 weeks in combination with a splint, fabricated by occupational therapy. After 2 weeks the silicon layer is removed and a thin split-thickness skin graft placed over the Integra. The advantage is, if a dermal template is not utilized, a thick split-thickness graft, 14+/1000 inches in thickness, will be necessary. Regardless of technique, postoperative splinting for 4–6 months is necessary to prevent recontracture.)

Case-Based Conference

Case 1A: Acute Burn of the Eyelids

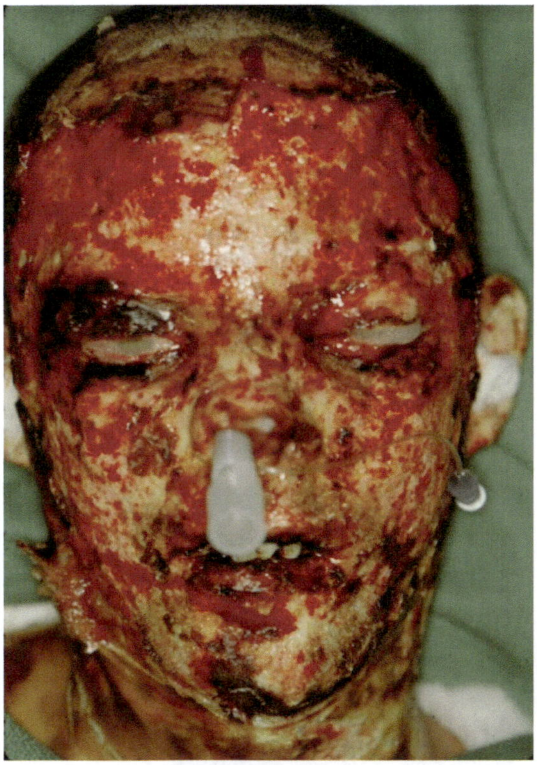

A 38 year old who sustained facial and trunk burns as well as severe inhalation injury. Patient is 2 weeks post-burn with improving pulmonary status but increasing corneal exposure.

1. Describe the slide. What is the pertinent clinical information that you need at this juncture to determine a plan of management?
2. Describe your plan.

Case 1B: Late Burn of the Eyelids

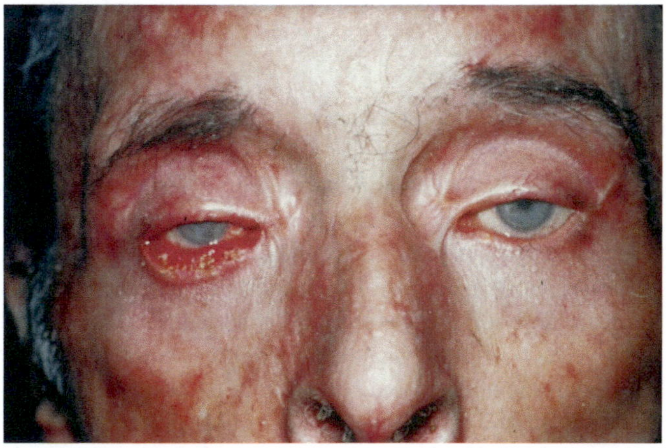

The patient is 2½ months post-burn and your acute management is successful; now the patient is seen as an outpatient.

1. Describe the slide, add a focused clinical exam.
2. Describe the pathologic anatomy in detail.
3. Give an operative plan, if indicated, and draw the same.

Case-Based Conference: Discussion

Case 1A: Acute Burn of the Eyelids

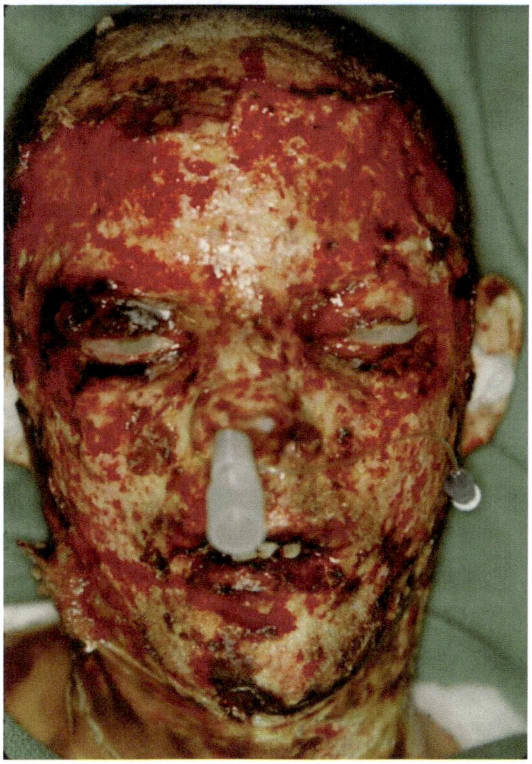

A 38 year old who sustained facial and limited trunk burns as well as severe inhalation injury. Patient is 2 weeks post-burn with improving pulmonary status but increasing corneal exposure.

1. Describe the slides. (Patient with total facial burn of indeterminate depth but appears to be at least deep dermal and perhaps full-thickness in nature with a nasotracheal tube in place. The patient has a considerable amount of ointment in the eyes and no comment can be made from the slides about the status of the underlying globe or corneas because both are covered by ointment. At this point 2 weeks post-burn, what is needed is an assessment of the magnitude of the cornea exposure, i.e., fluorescein staining and estimation of the degree of bulbar and tarsal conjunctivitis. If, in conjunction with ophthalmologic consult, intervention beyond the use of eye lubricant such as Lacrilube®, then two limbs of the decision tree exist. One, if the patient's systemic status is unstable or a massive burn exists, as in a different scenario, or the clinical situation suggests that further temporizing may culminate in insufficient healing and risk of corneal ulceration and perforation, then cornea protection with a moisture chamber and/or a Gunderson conjunctival flap may suffice at this stage. The other option, if more aggressive intervention appears indicated and donor sites exist, then excision/release with wound closure by split-thickness or full-thickness skin grafts will provide definitive corneal protection, although further release and grafting, particularly if split-thickness skin grafts are utilized, may be necessary later in the facial healing/contracture process. Since this patient has approximately a 45% body surface area burn, limited full-thickness or split-thickness skin graft donor sites may be available, although the size needs are not great. Full-thickness skin grafts are the highly preferable option.

   A temporary tarsorrhaphy may be tempting as another temporizing procedure but, in fact, frequently fails. The contracture process overpowers the sutures of the tarsorrhaphy and the tarsorrhaphy breaks down and dehisces. If tarsorrhaphy is indicated, an intermarginal tarsorrhaphy may be accomplished. That operation consists of an excision of a strip of conjunctiva over the upper eyelid as well as the inferior or lower eyelid margin of the tarsus to create two raw surfaces, placed at the most lateral aspect of the lids. Two horizontal sutures of a 5° prolene are placed with the use of a small silastic catheter tubing to prevent skin erosion from the sutures. A tarsorrhaphy coincident with contracture release and grafting may be advantageous.)

Postoperative (Immediate and 1 Year)

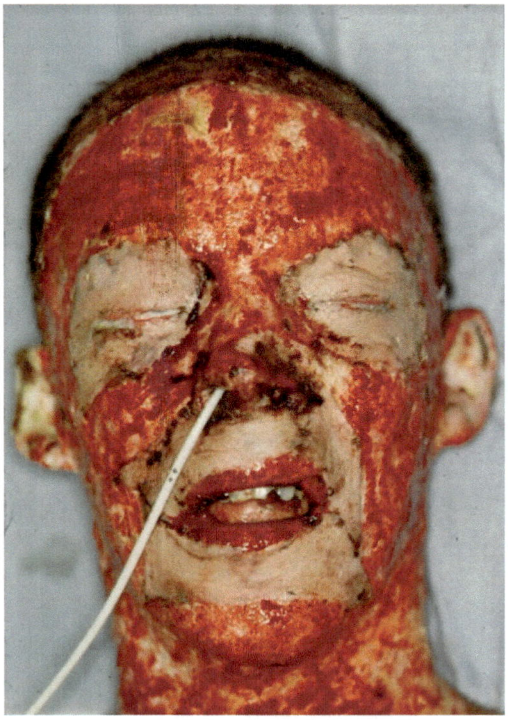

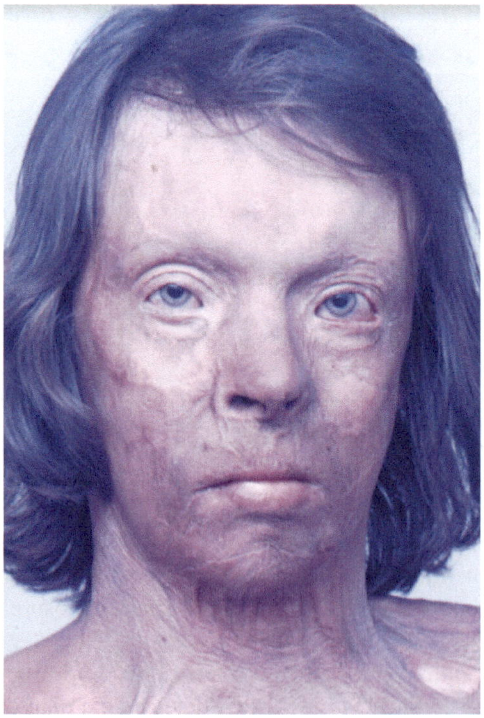

The patient has had early, 3 weeks post-burn, excision and full-thickness skin grafts of the periorbital and perioral regions. At 1 year (photo provided by patient) some laxity of the left lateral eyelid is evident.

Critique

The difficult decision in this case is intervention in the early post-burn period. Unhealed burns of the eyelids at the 3-week milestone are likely to culminate in ectropion. Release at this juncture, dependent on the urgency, may be through immature scar.

Case 1B: Late Burn of the Eyelids

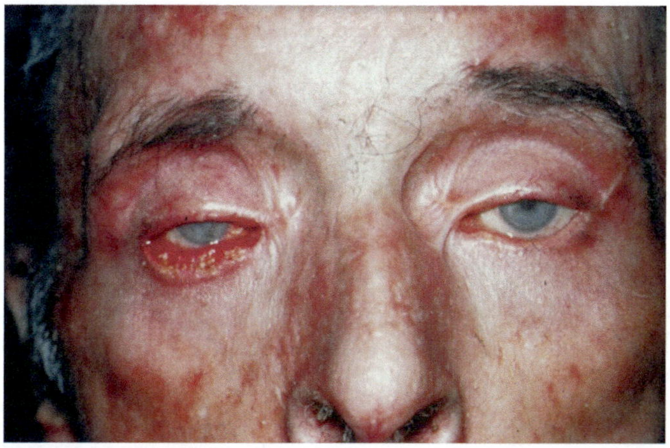

The patient is 2½ months post-burn and the patient is seen as an outpatient.

1. Describe the slide, add a focused clinical exam. (The patient has healed facial burns with the photos restricted to the lower forehead, periorbital, nose, and upper cheek region. Bilateral epicanthal folds are present left greater than right. Pertinent clinical findings are those of a significant cicatricial ectropion of the right lower eyelid with exposed, inflamed tarsal or lid conjunctiva. The bulbar conjunctiva is moderately inflamed as well. The palpebral fold of the upper eyelid is superiorly retracted bilaterally. Patient has bilateral ptosis of the upper eyelids right greater than left. The ptosis of the right eye is severe, 4–5 mm, and the left moderate 2–3 mm. No hollowing of the sulcus is evident and, in fact, the sulcus is somewhat shallow. A significant epicanthal fold is present on the left, less so on the right side. The folds may either exacerbate or be responsible for the ptosis. Evidence against that conclusion is that the ptosis of the right is severe, yet the epicanthal contracture is relatively mild. In contrast on the opposite side, the ptosis is moderate yet the epicanthal contracture is considerably more significant. The clinical exam should consist of fluorescein staining to detect early corneal damage, examine for the presence of a Bell's phenomenon, and estimate the degree of soft tissue deficiency.)
2. Describe the pathologic anatomy in detail. (The ectropion is the end result of healing of a full-thickness wound by contracture. The fixed unit of the lower lid is orbital soft tissue/skin at the level of the infraorbital rim or the lid/cheek interface and the mobile component is the lid margin. The cicatricial ectropion exposes tarsal, lid, conjunctiva and prevents lid closure and proper corneal coverage. An active Bell's phenomenon, upward and outward rotation of the globe with attempted lid closure, may provide sufficient corneal protection, particularly in the case of this patient who has some element of upper lid ptosis. Nevertheless, ectropion release is indicated.)
3. Give an operative plan, if indicated, and draw the same. (Optimal operative planning mandates an understanding of a role of the "third dimension" in the scarring process. With contracture of skin and the attached underlying orbicularis muscle or the anterior lamella, a parallel contractile process also occurs in the middle lamella, the orbital septum. The posterior lamella, tarsus, conjunctiva, and capsulopalpebral fascia are unaffected or, if anything, lengthened. Again, the indications for surgery is corneal exposure sufficiently severe that ulceration is a risk.

   Operative release should be oriented transversely and extend to and perhaps beyond both the lateral and the medial canthus, with the incision reasonably close to the lid margin in the lower eyelid or at the inferior tarsal border. The importance is recognition of the necessity of complete release of skin, orbicularis, and septum. The release should extend into the epicanthal area to release that contracture as well. Once lid and epicanthus have been released, a consideration could be given to repair of the levator in the same setting. Yet, assessment of levator status will be difficult under general anesthesia and simultaneous repair is a dynamic in opposition to the contracture release. Perhaps the issue of evaluation and possible treatment of levator dysfunction should await a secondary procedure. The resultant skin and soft tissue defect will be sizable in this patient extending essentially from the infraorbital rim to the lid margin. To avoid the necessity for repeated grafting, wound closure with a full-thickness skin graft is optimal. Because of the probable horizontal laxity of the tarsus, a lateral canthopexy or canthoplasty may be necessary.)

Intraoperative

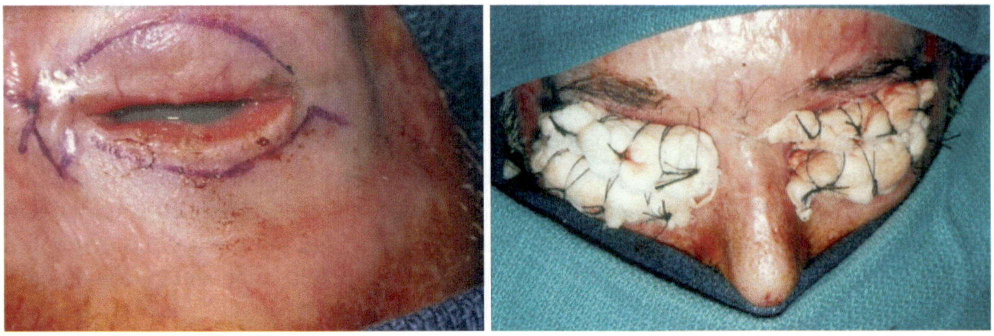

Proposed incisions for release. The intraoperative photo demonstrates the necessity for quite large bolsters to ensure a complete take.

Postoperative (1 Week, 3 Months)

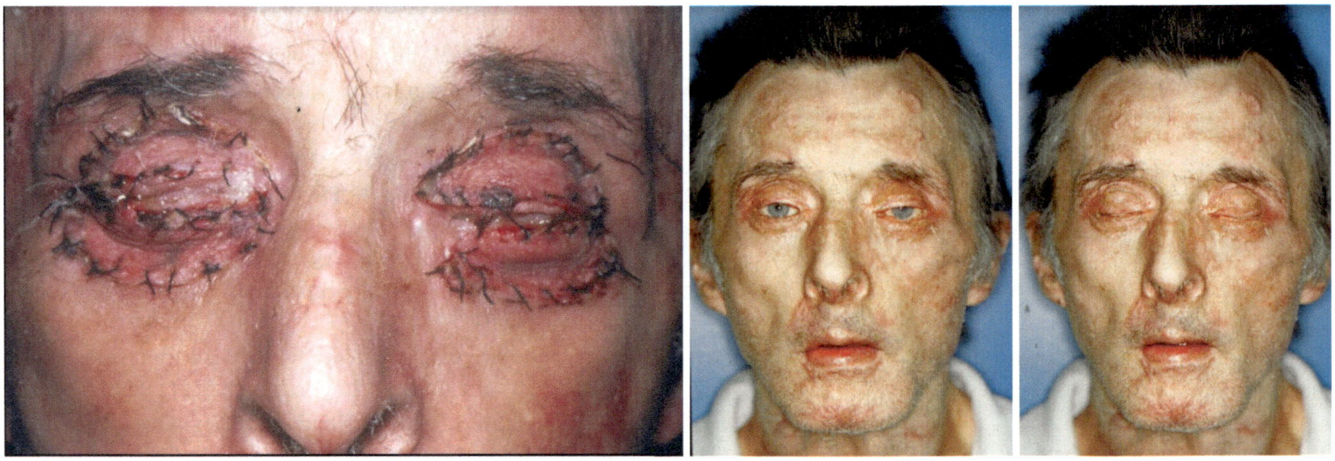

The patient, two and a half months post-burn has been addressed with ectropion release of both lower lids and contracture or lagophthalmos release with full-thickness skin grafts.

In the postoperative views, a satisfactory and complete release of his lower lid ectropion has been accomplished as well as the upper lids. However, residual ptosis is still present of 1–2 mm in the right and 3–4 mm in the left eye. Clearly, a secondary correction of levator attenuation and an advancement procedure will be necessary.

Case-Based Conference

Case 2: Head/Neck Burn Reconstruction

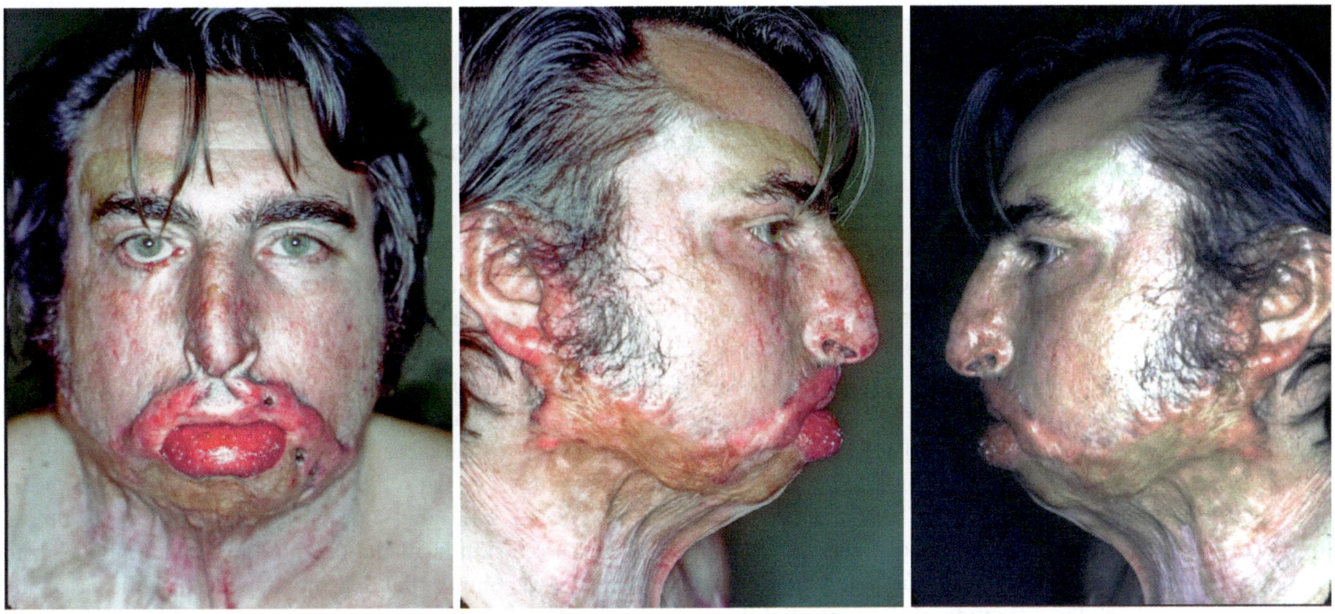

A 38-year-old man who sustained head/neck burns from an industrial explosion 18 months ago. He had some grafting performed at the time of the acute injury. He is otherwise in good health. His chief complaints are tearing and irritation of the right eye, "tightness" of the neck, and some element of oral incompetence.

1. Describe what you see on the slides. Add a pertinent clinical examination including additional information or questions not available from the slides.
2. Outline a hierarchy of his reconstructive needs.
3. Design a plan to include the address of his complaints, stages (if any), and anticipate his outcome.

Case-Based Conference: Discussion

Case 2: Head/Neck Burn Reconstruction

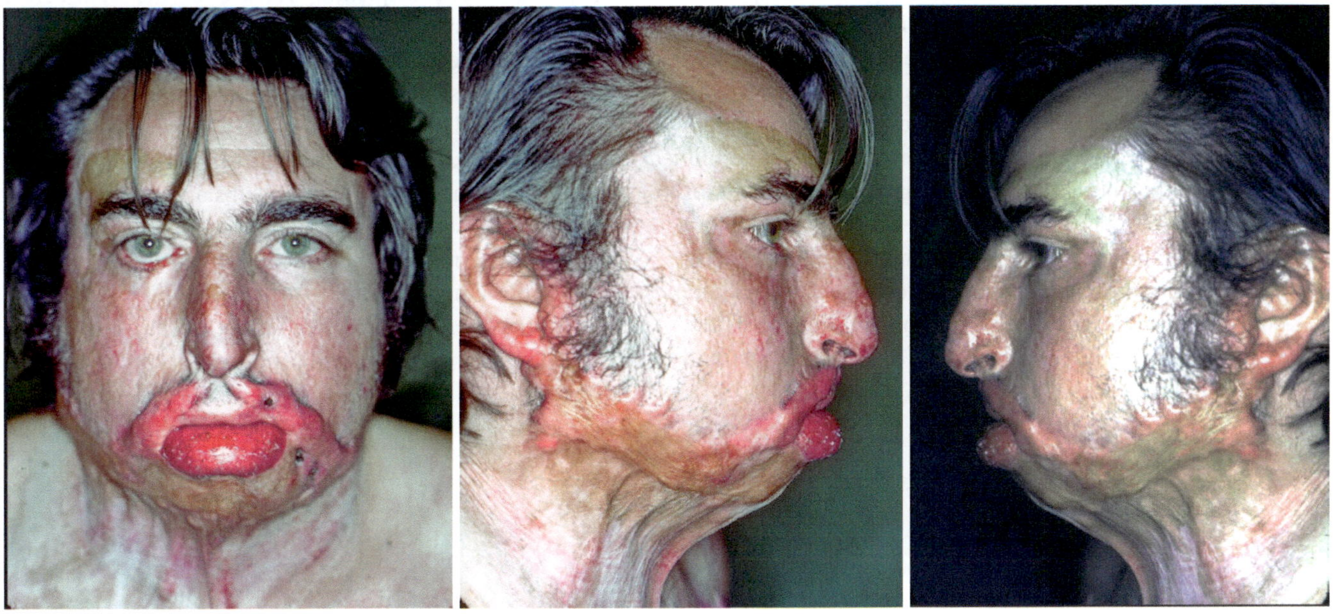

A 38-year-old man who sustained head/neck burns from an industrial explosion 18 months ago. He had some grafting performed at the time of the acute injury. He is otherwise in good health. His chief complaints are tearing and irritation of the right eye, "tightness" of the neck, and some element of oral incompetence.

1. Describe what you see on the slides. Add a pertinent clinical examination including additional information or questions not available from the slides. (Three photos: a frontal and full right and left lateral include the head and neck of the patient. Several late sequelae or outcomes of facial burns are depicted. These findings include on the frontal view healed but not hypertrophic or contracted forehead and cheek skin. The nose, in contrast, has an intact osteocartilaginous framework but the skin and soft tissue envelope has shrunk narrowing the nostrils and obliterating the alar groove and nasolabial fold. The right lower eyelid has a moderate ectropion with eversion of the lash margin and 2 mm of scleral show. Although two areas, each less than a millimeter, of tarsal conjunctiva are reddened, no evidence of exposure keratoconjunctivitis is present. With the exception of the central philtrum, the upper lip cutaneous component has been replaced by thickened, hypertrophic scar. The mucosa portion of the philtrum is intact but otherwise more laterally is obscured by scar. The lower lip is deformed by a significant protuberance and severe eversion of the mucosa. The normal proportions of the face have been distorted by a significant reduction in the lower one-third, the mandible. Although somewhat out of focus, the anterior cervical region appears to have contractions centrally as well as on the right and to a lesser degree on the left. An area of brownish discolored skin is pictured on the inferior aspect of the mandible centrally and extending onto the visible right side. Three small, 1-2 mm crusting areas are present in the hypertrophic scar on the left side.

   The lateral photo provides some additional information. The most remarkable finding is the complete loss of cutaneous lower lip and contracture of the remaining chin skin without a discernible bony mention of the mandible. In fact, the profile is severely retrognathic with perhaps an element of microgenia as well. The remaining chin skin blends into the contracted anterior cervical skin without a discernible submental or cervico-hyoid angle. Additional findings include a 2 cm wide strip of tan, wrinkled skin paralleling the body of the mandible and terminating in a hypertrophic scar at the lobule of the ear. The appearance is consistent with a contracted skin graft, harvested from a donor site remote from the head and neck "blush" area. The preauricular and lobular skin have been replaced by hypertrophic scar. The nasal tip lacks projection and the nostril rims are retracted with a resultant columellar show. The third photo, left lateral, is quite similar in appearance to the right.)
2. Outline a hierarchy of his reconstructive needs. (As illustrated in the above description, any number of objective reconstructive needs are present, but the hierarchy is dictated by the wishes of the patient. One could anticipate the lip deformities, occupying the central third of the face would be of the highest priority on the part of the patient.)
3. Design a plan to include the address of his complaints, stages (if any), and anticipate his outcome. (With the assumption that the patient wants to proceed, excision of the hypertrophic scar of the upper lip and release of the lower lip eversion will require full-thickness skin grafts harvested from the supraclavicular blush areas unless unscarred skin is available from the neck, although from the lateral photos that does not appear to be the case. The graft needs for the upper lip can be anticipated by direct measurement, but the lower lip deficit requirement will be substantial and should be anticipated. Although the mouth is closed in the photo, the patient does not seem to have microstomia but a mucosal advancement flap will be necessary to recreate visible mucosa of the right and left lateral upper lip. A transverse wedge excision of lower lip mucosa should be deferred to a secondary setting.

   Release of the right lid ectropion could be accomplished at the same setting and full-thickness skin graft utilized to close the defect. See Chap. 61, Case 1.

   The next priority may well be release of the cervical contracture. The sequential release of the contracture through a transverse incision should extend, as in all burn contracture release, from mid axial to mid axial points. A thorough release encompasses skin, contracted platysma, and superficial fascia. The defect can be reconstructed with split-thickness skin graft but, similar to the chin the amount of skin required will be substantial. One modification is the use of an intermediate stage of placement of Integra®, a dermal template, use of the VAC for 2 weeks, and the placement of a split-thickness skin graft. Address of the other, perhaps more secondary, needs as the hypertrophic scar of the ears would follow as desired.)

Postoperative

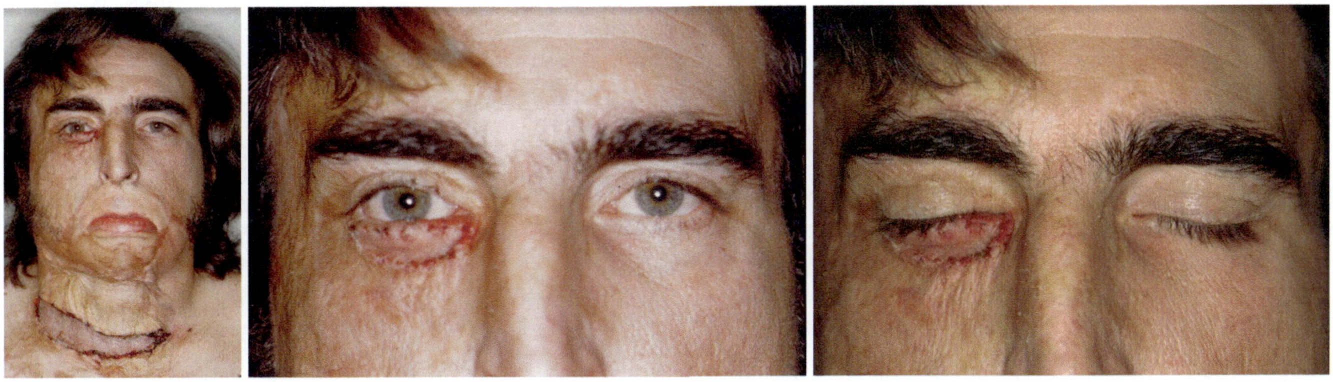

In the photos, the patient has had prior reconstruction of both upper and lower lip with excision of hypertrophic scar and full-thickness skin graft of the upper lip and release and full-thickness grafting of the lower lip. More recently, release of both the right ectropion and cervical contracture has been accomplished with a full-thickness skin graft of the former and non-meshed split-thickness skin graft of the latter. The lower lid is in a normal position with good correction.

Critique

The lower lip is somewhat everted despite release and full-thickness skin graft of the cutaneous component. An additional correction component would consist of a transverse wedge excision of mucosa.

In-Service Examination

1. The structures of the lower lid released in correction of burn ectropion are:
   (a) Skin only
   (b) Skin and orbicularis
   (c) Skin orbicularis and orbital septum
   (d) Skin orbicularis, orbital septum, and capsulopalpebral fascia
2. The burned ear is optimally managed with:
   (a) Saline dressings
   (b) Neosporin® ointment
   (c) Mafenide ointment
   (d) Silver sulfadiazine ointment

63 Reconstruction (Hand, Upper Extremities, Axilla, Breast, Foot, Splinting)

Bibliography

Luce EA, "The acute and subacute management of the burned hand", Luce EA, ed., *Clinics in Plastic Surgery*, (January 2000); 27(1):**49–63.**

Achauer BM, Chapter 10: "Burns of the upper extremity", Burn Reconstruction, Thieme New York, New York, (1991); **pp. 100–109**.

Kreymerman PA, Andres LA, Lucas HD, et al. "Reconstruction of the burned hand", *Plast. Reconstr. Surg.*, (2011); 127(2):**752–759.**

Jordan RB, Daher J, and Wasil K, "Splints and scar management for the acute and reconstructive burn care", Luce EA, ed., *Clinics in Plastic Surgery*, (January 2000); 27(1):**71–85.**

Duncan SF and Smith AA, Chapter 18 "Treatment of the burned axilla", Sood R, Burn Surgery: Reconstruction and Rehabilitation, Saunders Elsevier, (2006); **pp 282–298.**

Goldberg DP, "Reconstruction of the burned foot", Luce EA, ed., *Clinics in Plastic Surgery*, (January 2000); 27(1):**145–161.**

MacLeannan SE, Wells MD, and Neale HW, "Reconstruction of the burned breast", Luce EA, ed., *Clinics in Plastic Surgery*, (January 2000); 27(1):**113–119.**

Neale HW and Kurtzman LC, "Discussion: Postburn breast reconstruction: Tissue expansion prior to contracture release", *Plast. Reconstr. Surg.*, (1992); 90(4): **672–674.**

Supplemental Reading

- Palao R, Gomez P, and Huguet P, "Burned breast reconstructive surgery with Integra dermal regeneration template", *Br. J. Plast. Surg.*, (2003); **252–259.**

Faculty Discussion and Study Guide

Splints and Scar Management

1. Discuss the correct positioning for application of splints to the elbow and the wrist. (The elbow should be splinted in full extension minus 5–10°; the wrist splinted with slight extension 15–20° with neutral radial–ulnar deviation and in neutral pronation–supination.)
   (a) To splint the wrist, the splint should be how far distally? The distal palmar crease, the proximal palmar crease, or the proximal carpal row? (The distal aspect of the proximal carpal row. If the splint is to mid palm or more distal, MCP joint flexion cannot be obtained because of the blocking action of the splint. See Chap. 65 for further discussion of hand splinting. See Table 63.1.)
2. What element of the splinting regimen may need to be added during the proliferative phase of healing? (Some type of progressive motion such as the use of a rubber band traction to improve MP joint function, levered against a static wrist splint. The protocol is a combination of splinting and exercise.)
3. What is a method to conservatively address a PIP joint contracture with splinting? (A "joint-jack" or wire spring PIP extension splint as pictured in one of the readings.)
   (a) A similar approach to elbow contracture? (If less than 30°, serial splinting may regain nearly full extension. A commercial dynamic elbow splint is also available.)
4. What is a common sequela of chin and anterior cervical burns in addition to neck contracture? (Lower lip eversion with loss of oral competence and exposure of the mandibular dentition.)
   (a) The principal objective in splinting of perioral burns is? (Prevention of microstomia.)

E. Luce, *A Curriculum for Plastic Surgery*, https://doi.org/10.1007/978-3-031-62087-4_63

Table 63.1 Positioning for acute burns

Region/joint	Position of function	Splints	Accessory devices
Neck	Neutral or slight extension Neutral rotation	Neck conformer splint Triple component neck splint	No pillows under hand Small pillow under neck
Shoulders	Neutral rotation/elevation	Figure-of-eight soft splint	Soft vertical roll between scapulae
Axilla	Abduction: 70–80° Horizontal adduction: 15–20°	Airplane splint	Arm through Bedside table Abduction wedge
Elbow	Extension: −5° to −10 Forearm: Neutral to supinated	Volar-based extension splint	
Wrist	Neutral to slight extension Neutral radial/ulnar deviation	Intrinsic-plus splint Wrist cock-up	
Hand	Dorsal/circumferential burn MCP joints 50–70° of flexion IP joints in extension Palmar burns MCP and IP joints in extension Thumb in full flexion Digits abducted	Intrinsic-plus splint C-bar for thumb Hand extension splint Halo or horseshoe splint	K-wire fixation Webspace inserts

5. What is the common thread or element of the use of garments to treat hypertrophic burn scars? (Pressure.)
   (a) The physiologic basis? (The mechanism is not truly understood but what occurs is reorientation of the collagen bundles, diminished levels of ground substance including chondroitin and hyaluronic acid. Whether these effects are due to decreased fibroblast proliferation and thus unopposed collagenase activity or some other molecular mechanism is not known.)
6. Describe some methods for both early and late compression. (Early compression can be done with elastic bandages, Coban, etc., to reduce tissue edema. Late compression can be provided by custom-measured and fitted garments that can provide even uniform pressure to burn scars. Commercially available garments are manufactured by Jobst.)
7. Describe the use of facial masks in burn scars. (Usually composed of a transparent mask manufactured after a plaster mold is made. Such masks are almost always of a single unit. A variety of inserts can be placed within the mask itself.)

Hand/Upper Extremity

1. Describe the position of the burn claw hand deformity. (Wrist flexed, MP joints extended, PIP joints flexed with boutonniere deformity with early DIP joint flexion and later extension. Thumb adducted with contracted first webspace shortened with recurvatum deformity of the MP joint.)
2. What are the three processes responsible for burn wound edema, and how does that edema have a detrimental effect on hand function? (The three processes are direct burn injury, "leaky" capillaries due to a circulating vasoactive kinin, and a change in oncotic pressure due to leakage of protein from an intravascular to an extravascular or interstitial site. Dorsal edema of the hand limits skin flexibility and so decreases MP joint flexion; the fluid is protein rich with matrix metalloproteinases that set the stage for inflammation and scarring.)
3. In what position should the MP joints be splinted and why? PIP joints? The thumb? (MP joints should be splinted in flexion, 80°, because the collateral ligaments are stretched in that position; the PIP joints in extension to prevent contracture and adherence of the volar plate and check-rein ligaments, and the thumb in abduction with some opposition. This posture is the position of function.)
4. What is the role of wrist splinting in management of the burned hand? (The wrist in extension will utilize the tenodesis effect that is secondary to the stretched long finger flexors that possibly will facilitate splinting of the MP joint in flexion.)
5. Failure to properly splint the thumb can lead to what? (First webspace adductor contracture; hyperextension deformity of the MP joint.)
6. What is the anatomical explanation for the susceptibility of the little finger MCP joint to a hyperextension deformity? (The unique mobility of the carpometacarpal joint, as well as the loss of the normal transverse palmar arch because of soft tissue contracture.)
   (a) What can be the consequent effect on the PIP joint? (If sufficient hyperextension deformity of the MCP joint occurs, a zigzag deformity results in a PIP joint contracture or pseudo-boutonniere.)

7. Describe the indications and the technique of an upper extremity escharotomy? (Radial and ulnar incisions from just above the elbow to the level of the wrist.)
   (a) What is the technique for digital escharotomy and intrinsic fasciotomy? (Mid-axial incisions for release of digits and two dorsal hand incisions for release of the intrinsics; both of these procedures are controversial whether they have a beneficial role.)
8. What is the consequence of full-thickness palmar burns? (Cupping deformity of the hand that pulls the radial and ulnar components centrally with loss of full abduction of the thumb and conversion of the palmar mild concave curve to a severe or cup deformity.)
9. What is the underlying or consequent problem related to failure to splint the PIP joint in extension in digital burns? (If the middle phalanx is in flexion, the volar plate and check-rein ligaments are slack or relaxed which can lead to contracture of the same. The base of the proximal phalanx may also place pressure on the central slip particularly with burn loss of the overlying thin skin with the result of attenuation, exposure, and ultimate loss of the central slip. Loss of the central slip can lead to a boutonniere deformity; contracture of the volar plate and check-rein ligaments can lead to flexion contracture of the PIP joint.)
10. What is a maneuver that will determine severity of PIP joint contractures in burned hands? (If the flexion contracture can be relieved by flexion of MP joint and extension of PIP joint, complete extension with that maneuver is type I, incomplete is type II, and fixed PIP joint position regardless of MP joint position is type III.)
11. Discuss the management plan of the burned hand in the subacute period including pros and cons. (Only prompt application of compression hand dressings and elevation prior to the onset of burn wound edema of the hands allows proper splinting. This position, described in a prior question, is maintained for 4 or 5 days with the use of tissue pressure monitoring if necessary. Depending upon the patient's general condition, extubated and has diuresed the excess fluid, removal of the dressings at 5 days permits inspection of the burn wound and initiation of a program of therapy. The patient is replaced in bulky dressings for a day or two and then nighttime and daytime splints when not in therapy with burn wound dressing changes. If still intubated with little ability to cooperate, reapplication of the bulky dressing for an additional 2 days is advisable. Because of the risk of burn sepsis beneath a closed dressing after 7 days, a switched burn wound dressing should be accomplished. A decision about burn wound excision needs to be made if the burns are clearly third degree. If not, that decision is deferred until some point 15–20 days post burn, if healing has not taken place substantially or almost completely by that juncture. This plan should be aborted at any point that the patient fails to continue to progress with evident decrease in ROM and participation in daily therapy.)
12. Discuss the potential benefits and limitations of tangential excision of hand burns. (Tangential excision defines the depth of burn, but commits to grafting, which may lead to unnecessary excision and grafting of wounds that would otherwise heal satisfactorily.)
13. What is the underlying or consequent problem related to failure to splint the PIP joint in extension in digital burns? (If the middle phalanx is in flexion, the volar plate and check-rein ligaments are slack or relaxed which can lead to contracture of same. The base of the proximal phalanx may also place pressure on the central slip particularly with burn loss of the overlying thin skin with the result of attenuation, exposure, and ultimate loss of the central slip. Loss of the central slip can lead to a boutonniere deformity because of the progressive volar displacement of the lateral bands; contracture of the volar plate and check-rein ligaments can lead to flexion contracture of the PIP joint. The risk of burn dressing sepsis after 7 days, a switched burn wound dressing should be accomplished.)
14. A number of procedures have been described for the release of burn syndactyly. What is the problem and what is the common thread throughout those procedure options? (Secondary contracture of the webspace and distal migration of the dorsal, and occasionally palmar, skin components of varying severity from mild to severe, namely obliteration of the webspace, occasionally as far distal as the PIP joint. Release of quite mild forms can be done with local flaps such as multiple Z-plasties but severe forms require split- or full-thickness skin grafting. The common component of most options is release of the contracture and use of the dorsal skin to suture to the palmar skin release to define the cleft and then placement of skin grafts in the resultant donor site defect. The use of multiple smaller flaps are at risk for ischemic necrosis and secondary healing with the final result an incomplete release of the syndactyly.)
15. Discuss the prevention of and address of first webspace contracture. (As outlined earlier, proper positioning of the thumb into a posture of abduction–opposition is important to prevent secondary contracture of skin, adductor, and first dorsal interosseous muscles. Once established, release of quite minor contractures can be accomplished with four-flap Z-plasties but much more commonly will require at the minimum split-thickness skin grafts after release. Since the adductor and first dorsal interosseous are both adductor muscles of the thumb, more severe contractures will require release of the adductor fascia or in more extreme cases the muscle itself. If so, closure of the wound with a flap may be necessary.)

Axilla

1. What is the appropriate position to splint the shoulder to minimize axillary contractures? (Abduction and external rotation.)
2. What is the argument and a specific anatomical explanation for early release of axillary contractures? (Although some may advocate to allow maturation of the burn contracture since skin contracture recurrence rate is lower with release of a mature rather than an immature contracture, some specific anatomical reasons exist for early release. These include foreshortening of the principal adductors of the shoulder, the pectoralis, and to lesser degree the latissimus. Also, shoulder joint capsule contracture can occur.)
   (a) What are the components of the anterior and posterior axillary folds? (The principal muscular components of the anterior axillary fold are the pectoralis major and minor; the components of the posterior axillary fold are the latissimus and the teres major.)
3. Give a classification of axillary burn contractures. (Type I anterior and/or posterior axillary fold only which usually can be released with some type of Z-plasty or V-Y plasty. Type II is involvement of both the anterior and posterior axillary folds and usually split-thickness skin grafts are necessary after release. Type III involves the entire axilla except for apex or cupola and flaps may be necessary. Type IV includes severe scarring of the axilla and adjacent areas with loss of shoulder joint motion.)
4. Give the pros and cons of the following coverage methods after axillary contracture release: Z-plasties, thick split-thickness skin grafts, fasciocutaneous flaps. (Z-plasties can be useful for very mild axillary contractures but involve the use of transposition of burn skin and are subject to necrosis of the tips and recontracture. Split-thickness skin grafts are a reliable method, yet require long-term splinting of the axilla, and occasionally re-release and re-grafting. Fasciocutaneous flaps provide full-thickness coverage and are not likely to recontract but often are not available because of burn involvement of the adjacent soft-tissue and also the donor site cannot be closed primarily.)
5. What principle should be followed with release of axillary contractures? (First, the principle that joint release usually involves skin/soft-tissue release from mid axial point to mid axial point of the joint; second, adequate release of both the superficial and, rarely, deep fascia.)
6. The readings describe the use of thoracodorsal artery perforator flap. What have we learned about the TAP flap? (In only about 60–65% of patients is a true thoracodorsal perforator present, the implication is the absolute necessity for a Doppler identification of such perforator as with all perforator flaps.)
7. The vessel that supplies the scapular flap and parascapular flap arises from the triangular space. Name the vessel and define the three sides of the triangular space. (The vessels are the circumflex scapular and the triangular space is bounded by the long head of the triceps on the lateral aspect, the teres minor superiorly, and the teres major inferiorly. This anatomy is also discussed in the Head/Neck Tumor reconstruction Chap. 38.)
   (a) What is the parascapular flap? (A flap based just on the descending or vertical branch of the circumflex scapular vessels. The drawings on the reference included, Duncan and Smith, on two successive pages illustrate the parascapular flap only. The vascular supply to the scapular flap is the transverse branch.)
8. An alternative option for the treatment of axillary contractures is use of Integra. Describe the same. (The protocol is much the same as the use of Integra elsewhere, namely the complete release of the contracture, placement of the Integra with or without a VAC, followed 2–3 weeks later by application of thin split-thickness skin grafts. In all likelihood, prolonged splinting would be necessary in this scenario as well.)

Breast

1. Essentially, what are the three reconstructive problems in the burned breast? (One, full-thickness burns in prepubescent girls can destroy all or a portion of the breast bud and have an effect on ultimate breast growth. Two, extensive involvement of the skin envelope of the breast may result in unyielding contracted soft tissues that do not permit proper breast development in adolescence. Third, the nipple areola complex may be destroyed and may require reconstruction.)
2. Discuss timing and technique of release of a constricted breast mound. (The timing is best accomplished when the opposite breast, if present, has begun development. The inframammary crease is mapped out on the contracted breast and a 180° release is accomplished through scar tissue and down to the deep fascia. To create a natural cleavage plane, thick, 0.016″ split-thickness skin grafts are placed into the resultant defect both on the inferior pole of the breast and on the adjacent chest wall. Certainly, one alternate option to split-thickness skin grafts is the use of Integra, a 2–3 week hiatus and then followed by secondary skin grafts. The combination of scar contracture release, placement of a tissue expander, and Integra is probably not recommended as a combined procedure since inevitably the inferior portion of the tissue expander will be beneath the Integra with prolonged and incomplete vascularization of the Integra as a consequence.)

(a) Superior pole restriction. (Basically the same principle, although more commonly some scar excision in addition may be accomplished. Pressure garments are worn in the extended postoperative period as well as custom-made silicone molds.)

3. What was the sequence advocated by the readings? (The readings cite very substantial experience with burn breast reconstruction and advocates release when the retardation of breast development by the burn scar is detected, proposed excision of scar contracture of the superior portion of the breast, and a deep incisional release to the chest wall to create a natural cleavage plane. A thick split-thickness skin graft is placed into the defect. One year later the expander is placed and ultimately an implant. Secondary subpectoral breast implants with or without prior tissue expansion may assist in achievement of symmetry and an adequate breast mound.)
4. Why not place a tissue expander as a first aid, followed by an inframammary release and skin grafts? (Thickened fibrotic skin will expand poorly. Incision/excision of scarred skin–soft tissue will set the stage for successful expansion. See the following questions.)
5. If tissue expansion is employed, what is the timing and the purpose? (*After* adequate release of the breast mound has been accomplished with split-thickness skin grafting *and* the estimation is that implants alone will not overall provide balance, then a tissue expander can be placed in the subpectoral plane and exchanged with a second-stage breast implant.)
6. What options exist for reconstruction, not release, of the breast mound? (The usual options in breast reconstruction. A valuable alternative to, for example, the standard latissimus flap is the thoracodorsal perforator flap, if the lateral chest wall skin and soft tissues are not badly damaged and if a perforator can be identified.)
7. What are the options in nipple reconstruction? (Not many. The burned skin will obviate the use of standard techniques such as the skate flap, etc., that rely upon dermal circulation. A composite graft of toe pulp may be an option as well as the use of alloderm stuffed into the burned skin envelope or a circular release and purse-string suture to mimic a nipple, followed by full-thickness skin graft and perhaps tattoo to reconstruct areola.)

Foot

The readings established the importance of burn injuries to the feet since foot burns are one of the indications for a referral to a burn center.

1. What are the important factors to be included in the assessment of a burn of the foot? (Some are fairly obvious such as depth of burn. Others deserve emphasis such as weight bearing vs. non-weight bearing components of the foot as well as associated circumferential burn injury of the lower extremity.)
2. Discuss stance and swing phases and weight loading during gait. (60% of the duration of the gait is spent in the stance phase which is initiated once heel strike occurs and terminates with the push off of the forefoot. During the stance phase, the weight load is split between the metatarsal heads and the heel. Of the metatarsals, the first supports 1/3 of the load with the remaining distributed over the full remaining metatarsals although the fifth may share more compared to the other three. Once the load is shifted from heel to the forefoot, some of that increase in load is shifted to the second metatarsal head. Discussed also in Chap. 52.)
3. What is the role of the plantar fascia? (Prevents longitudinal collapse of the arch of the foot, provides a platform to support body weight. The fascia is the principal stabilizing structure of the foot.)
4. Define the "rocker-bottom" foot deformity and its treatment. (The terminology refers to soft–tissue contracture of the dorsum of the foot as well as extensor tendon shortening and plantar subluxation of the phalanges and a complete reversal of the normal convex–concave plantar arch. Treatment requires release of the contracture often including tenotomy of the extensors and application of thick skin grafts. The toes may need to be K-wired into extension.)
5. Describe the following: medial plantar flap, flexor digitorum brevis flap, abductor hallucis flap. (Medial plantar artery is a major pedal branch of the posterior tibial artery and a flap consisting of the instep glabrous skin can be fashioned on this artery; the muscle bellies of the short flexors of the toes can be rotated posteriorly to cover small heel defects as can the principal abductor of the big toe, the abductor hallucis.)
6. Describe the principal limitations of free tissue transfer for foot defects. (The use of free muscle transfer with overlying skin graft provides less shear and more durability than myocutaneous flaps. The problem is the use of insensate tissue for the weight-bearing portion of the sole of the foot.)
   (a) Would the provision of neurotized flaps be of benefit in this situation? (Theoretically, yes; practically, the results are no different than non-neurotized flaps.)

Case-Based Conference

Case 1: Hand Burn

A 34-year-old woman who has sustained burns, of a total BSA of 60% head and neck, upper extremities, and a portion of the trunk.

Case 1: Hand Burn A

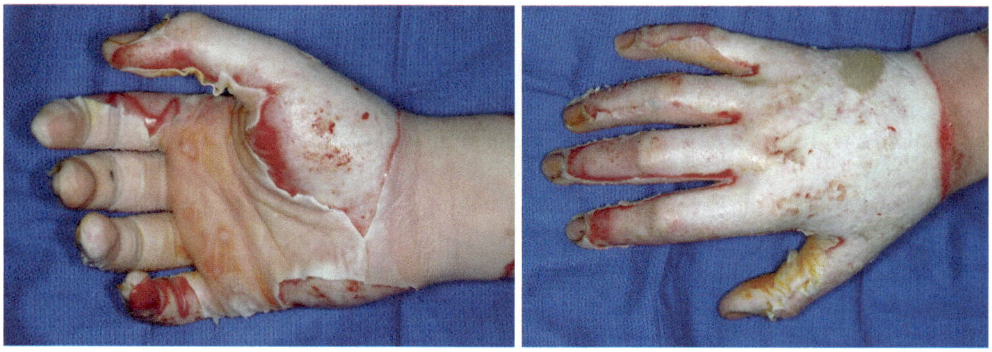

The photos depict the patient 1 h post-burn. The patient is intubated and resuscitation has been initiated.

1. Describe the photos. Add a focused clinical examination.
   (a) Any tests indicated?
2. What is the pathophysiology of this injury and based on that understanding, outline an acute (first several days) and a subacute (2–3 weeks) treatment plan.

Case 1: Hand Burn B

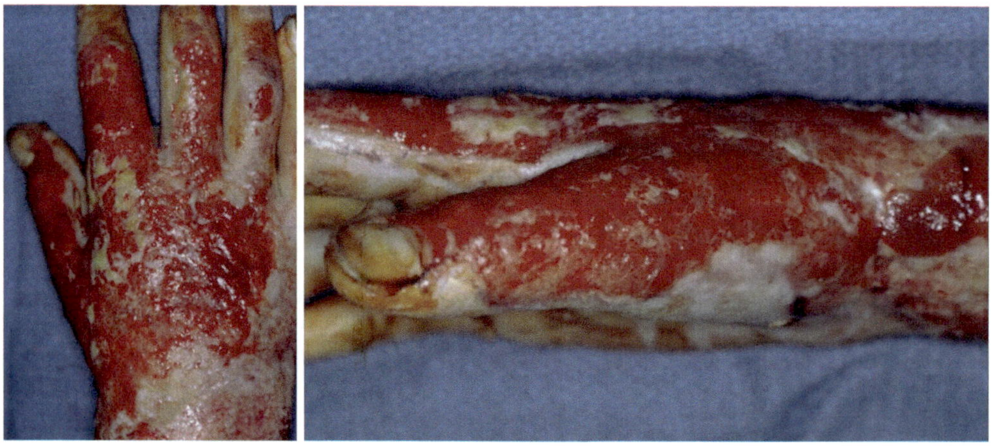

The patient is now extubated and stable at 2.5 weeks post-burn.

1. Describe the photos. Add a focused clinical examination.
2. What is the underlying pathophysiologic mechanism in this instance?
3. Outline a treatment plan.

Case 1: Hand Burn C

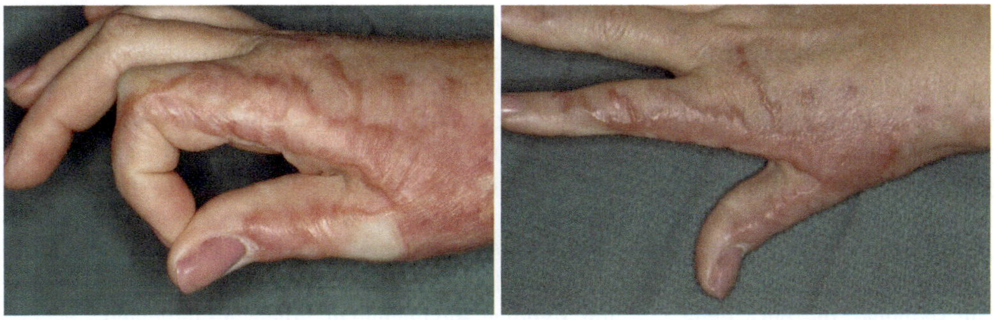

The patient's opposite hand at 3 months post-burn. The patient's chief complaint is inability to grasp larger objects. The second picture depicts an attempt at full thumb abduction.

1. Describe the photos. Add a focused clinical examination.
2. Explain in terms of functional anatomy the problem presented.
3. Outline a treatment plan.

Case-Based Conference: Discussion

Case 1: Hand Burn

A 34-year-old woman who has sustained burns, rib fractures, and possible intra-abdominal injury in a MVA. Her total BSA is 60% head and neck, upper extremities, and a portion of the trunk.

Case 1: Hand Burn A

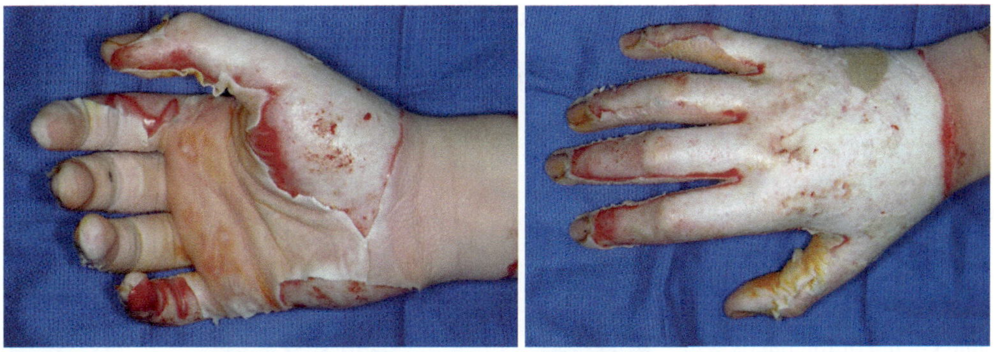

The photos depict the patient 1 h post-burn. The patient is intubated and resuscitation has been initiated.

1. Describe the photos. Add a focused clinical examination. (The two photos offer a palmar and dorsal view of a burn of the entire hand and wrist. The palm has sustained burns of the little and index finger, the ring and long appear spared. All of the visible palmar and radial aspect of the thumb has sustained burns. The skin is pale white and apparently blistered skin has been removed since the edges of the prior blister are visible. A rim of skin at the distal thenar eminence appears pink rather than pale. The posture of the hand is the normal flexion cascade and little edema is evident. The dorsal view demonstrates a burn uniform in appearance of the entire dorsum including all of the digits and the thumb. Although the entire dorsum of the fingers have been burned, a sharp demarcation between burned and unburned skin can be seen along the radial and ulnar aspect of each digit. Also, a transverse demarcation between burned and normal skin is present at the wrist. The overall appearance of the burn is a pale white-gray similar to the volar aspect of the thumb.

   The clinical exam would focus on a succinct history from a provider about the circumstances of the accident, including if possible, the duration of exposure. A general assessment by the trauma service would be helpful as well. The physical exam is centered on the hands. If the patient is intubated and sedated, the examination would be extremely limited and essentially would establish the adequacy of perfusion and sensate or insensate status of the burns.)

   (a) Any tests indicated? (If any doubt exists about the necessity of escharotomy, unlikely at the first hour post-burn, tissue pressures can be measured in the forearm.)

2. What is the pathophysiology of this injury and based on that understanding, outline an acute, first several days, and a subacute, 2–3 weeks, treatment plan. (An understanding of the pathophysiology that must be successfully addressed begins with the late sequelae, the burn claw deformity. The burn claw deformity consists of wrist flexion, hyperextension of the metacarpophalangeal, MP, joints, the proximal interphalangeal, PIP, joints in flexion with an associated boutonniere deformity and early distal interphalangeal, DIP, joint flexion and the later development of hyperextension. The burn deformity also includes the thumb. The thumb is adducted with a contracted first webspace and a recurvatum deformity of the MP joint.

   The initial treatment to avoid the occurrence of these sequelae begins immediately post-burn. The three processes that are responsible for generalized burn wound edema also occur in the hand. The three processes are direct burn injury, "leaky" capillaries or loss of integrity of the endothelial basement membrane due to a circulating vasoactive kinin, and a change in oncotic pressure due to leakage of protein from the intravascular to extravascular or interstitial space. Dorsal edema of the hand limits skin flexibility and so decreases MP joint flexion. The fluid is protein rich with matrix metalloproteinases that set the stage for inflammation and scarring. To offset these processes requires the application of bulky compressive dressing in the immediate post-burn period with a bacteriostatic gauze over the burn wounds. Only prompt application of compression hand dressings and elevation *prior* to the onset of burn wound edema of the hands will permit proper splinting. This position is the opposite of the burn claw deformity and consists of moderate, 25–30°, extension of the wrist that by a tenodesis effect will assist in MP joint flexion. The MP joints are flexed to 70–80° and the PIP joints maintained in full extension. Since this patient has a large body burn and is intubated, she will not be able to participate actively in physical therapy. The dressings are maintained with elevation for 4–5 days with the use of tissue pressure monitoring by an indwelling catheter, if necessary. If the patient's general condition permits extubation and by diuresis has excreted the excess fluid, the removal of the dressings at 5 days permits inspection of the burn wound and then initiation of a program of therapy. A principal consideration is the close monitoring of perfusion that might signal the necessity of escharotomy. The prompt application of bulky dressings and elevation has diminished the necessity for escharotomy to a minimum but an indwelling tissue pressure catheter can assist in the observation. Because of concern about the duration of bacteriostasis of the original dressing, removal and change at 5 days are indicated.

   The subacute management consists of perhaps a reinitiation of another bulky dressing for an additional day or so but then removal for application of nighttime and daytime splints when not in therapy with burn wound dressing changes. That treatment plan continues into either spontaneous healing has occurred or the next treatment intersection point is reached at 2½ weeks.

   The other possible treatment approach is early tangential excision. Tangential excision can define the depth of burn but commits to the immediate application of skin grafts which may lead to an unnecessary excision and skin grafts to wounds that would otherwise have healed satisfactorily.)

Intraoperative

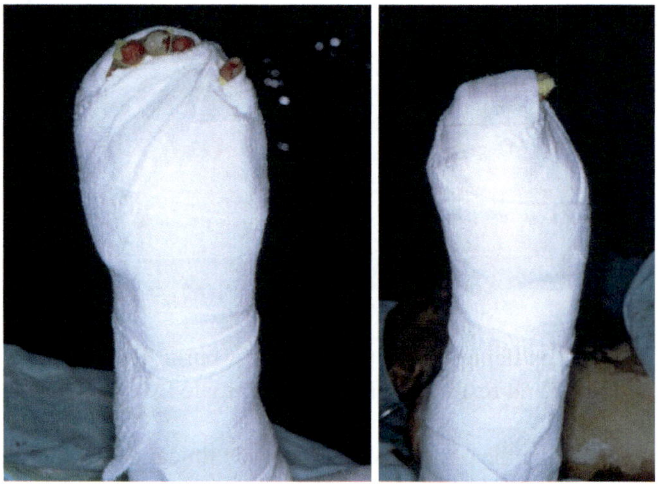

Pictured is a bulky compressive dressing incorporating a volar splint with elevation of the extremity. The fingertips are visible and the hand and fingers are in a position of function.

Postoperative (5 Days)

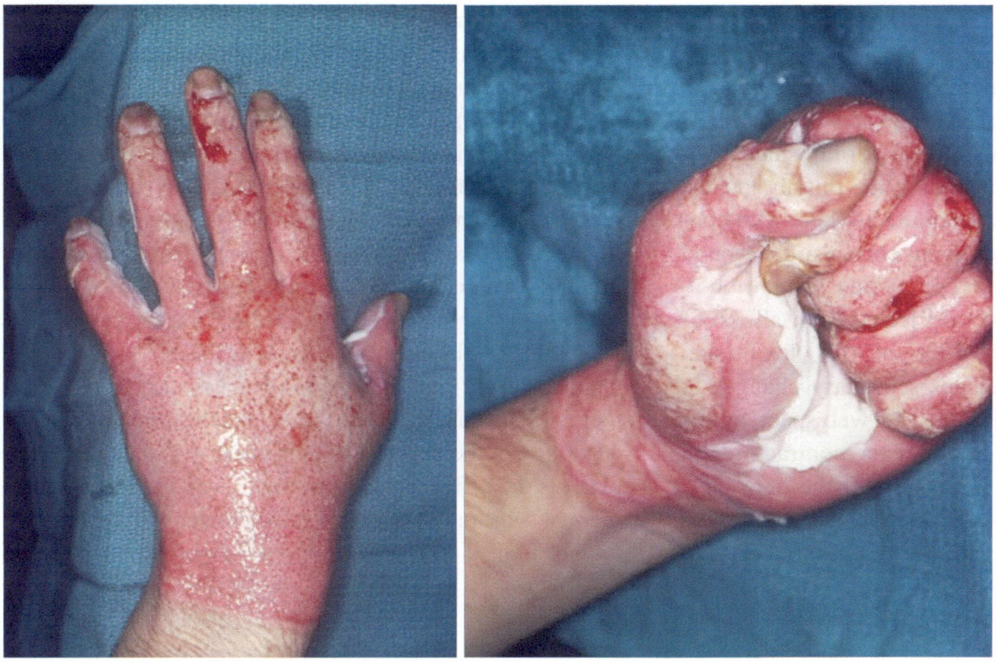

The hand is mildly edematous but with full digital flexion.

Case 1: Hand Burn B

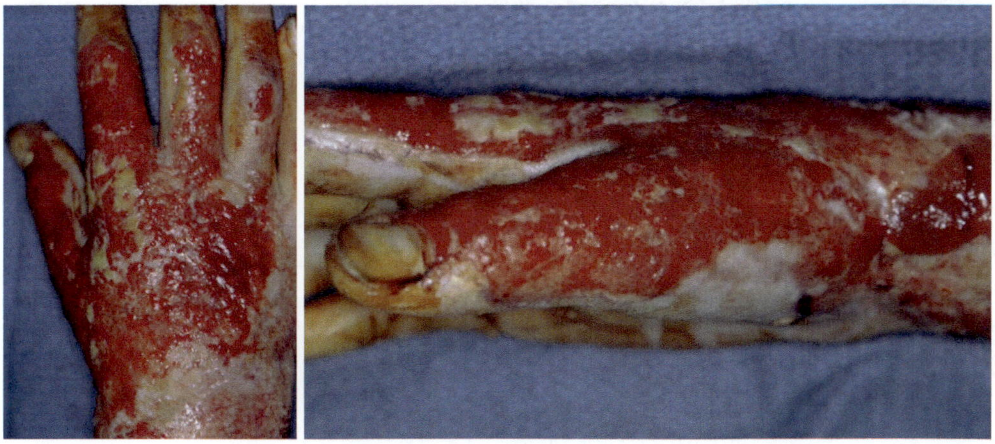

The patient is now extubated and stable at 2.5 weeks post-burn.

1. Describe the photos. Add a focused clinical examination. (Two views are provided, a dorsal view that includes most of the dorsum of the hand, wrist, and the thumb, the most ulnar aspect of the hand and little finger are not included. The hand is in the posture of a full pronation. A granulating surface is evident over most of the dorsal wrist and dorsum of the hand except the most ulnar aspect that appears unburned or healed. The granulation tissue extends over the index and long fingers to the PIP joint and is evident on the entire dorsum and ulnar surface of the thumb to the level of the nail. A small one cm area is also present on the dorsum of the proximal phalanx of the ring digit. All fingers are in extension. The second photo is a lateral view of the radial aspect and includes the thumb, index finger, and dorsum of the first webspace. An area of unburned palmar skin is evident over the most radial portion of the thenar eminence and palmar index but the remainder of the visible hand skin is occupied by granulation tissue.

   The clinical exam would assess the degree of function, in particular the range of motion. Sequentially, the wrist, metacarpophalangeal, and digital joints are examined for active, and if limitation of motion is present, gentle passive flexion and extension. The thumb is also evaluated for full abduction and extension. Potential donor sites are determined.)

(a) Any tests indicated? (No.)

2. What is the underlying pathophysiologic mechanism in this instance? (The clinical scenario is now one of a partially healed burn but most of the dorsum of the hand consists of granulation tissue, including the thumb and the dorsum of the radial digits. If permitted to heal with conservative management and dressing changes, the wound healing process will consist of contraction in addition to re-epithelialization. The cost or price paid, in all likelihood, will be some element of loss of MPJ flexion and PIP joint extension with perhaps secondary changes in the joint structures. Healing of the first web space by the same process will lead to an adductor contracture. In sum, these changes are the foundation of the burn claw deformity. That outcome cannot be prevented with physical therapy since the forces of wound contracture are relentless and greater than those generated by intermittent physical therapy.)
3. Outline a treatment plan. (As a result of the above pathologic process, a decision for operative management at this junction will interrupt the wound contraction process. The operation is excision of the burn wound and application of skin grafts. The excision is performed deep to the superficial fascia but retains the thin filmy layer including paratenon over the extensor tendons. Excision should be designed with multiple darts to avoid straight-line contracture and includes minimal, a mm., of normal skin. Coverage can be accomplished with one of two options, either a thick split-thickness skin graft or placement of a sheet of Integra® and delayed application of thin skin grafts after vascularization of the dermal substitute. The disadvantage of the former is the consumption of the donor sites by harvest of thicker grafts, the latter is the 2–3 week delay to permit vascularization of the dermal substitute, a period in which finger and hand motion will be limited and perhaps ultimately more stiff.)

Intraoperative

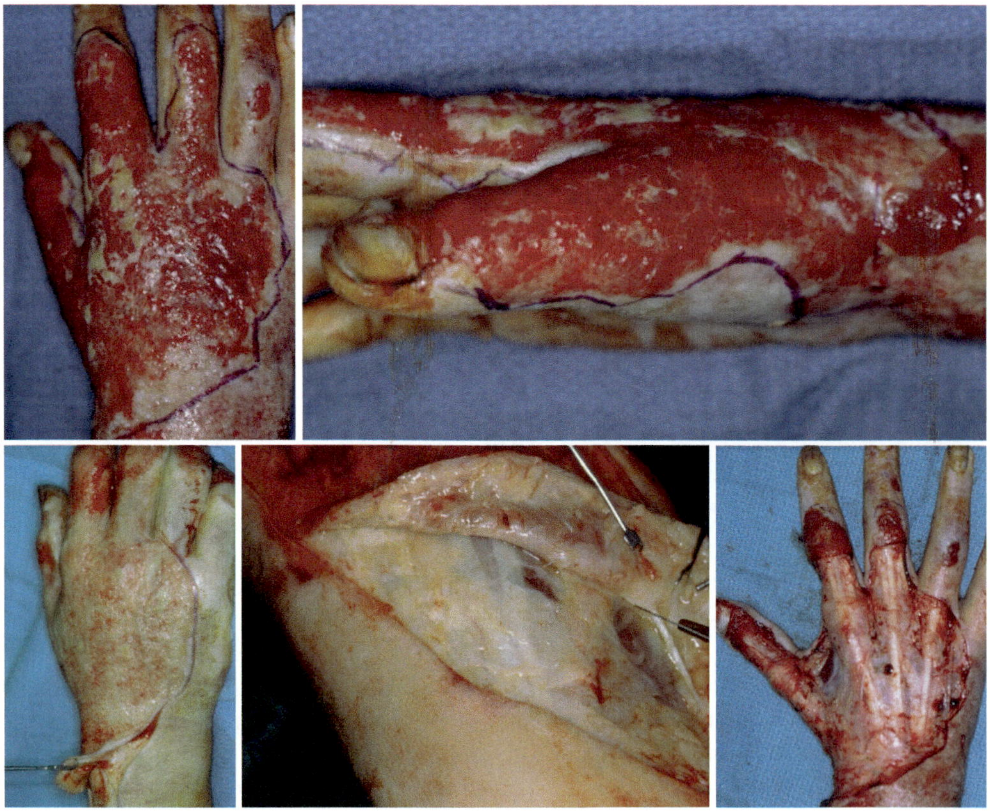

Sharp excision of the entire granulating surface is accomplished at the level of the deep fascia, retaining paratenon over the extensor tendons. Granulation tissue over the PIP joints is abraded clean rather than excised to avoid loss of the dorsal joint capsule.

Postoperative (10 Days)

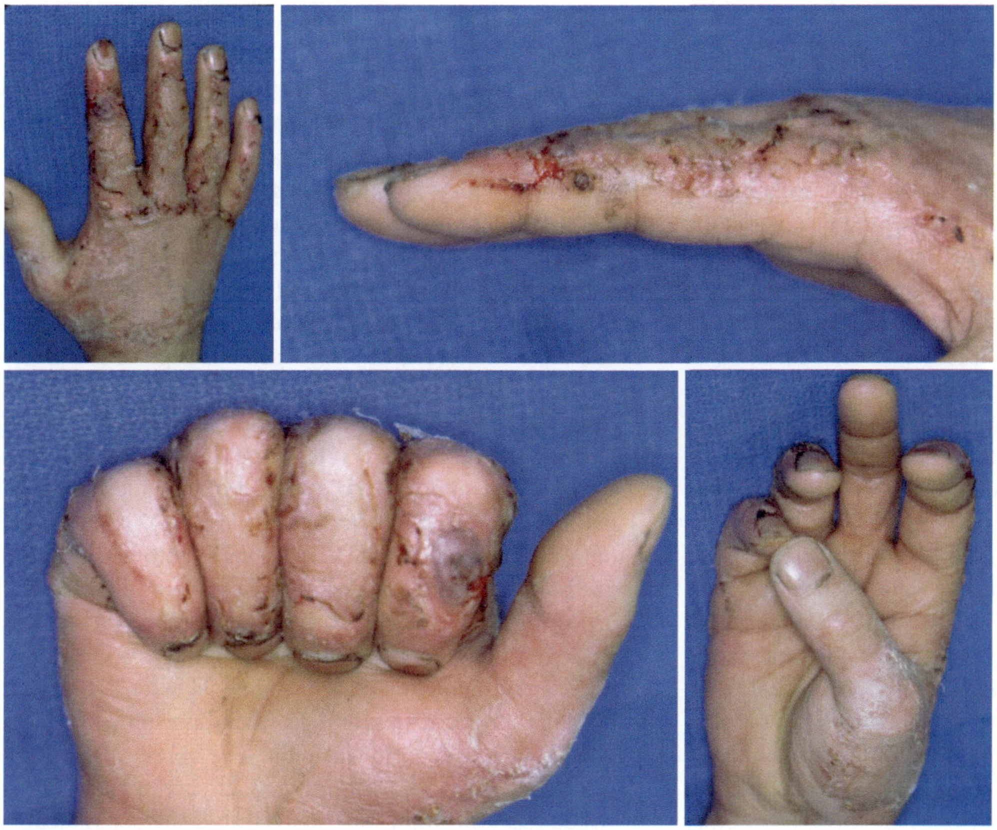

A full range of motion of flexion, extension, and opposition is demonstrated.

Case 1: Hand Burn C

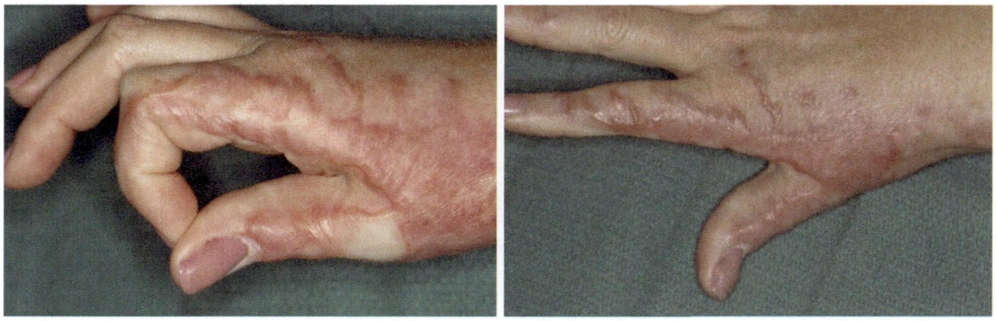

The patient's opposite hand at 3 months post-burn. The patient's chief complaint is inability to grasp larger objects. The second picture depicts an attempt at full thumb abduction.

1. Describe the photos. Add a focused clinical examination. (Two photos are provided. The first demonstrates the thumb in pulp-to-pulp pinch with the interphalangeal joint in hyperextension and the metacarpophalangeal joint in neutral. The thumb is in a sharply adducted position. The radial and dorsal aspect of the proximal phalanx contains a thickened hypertrophic scar that continues proximal onto the dorsum overlying the thumb metacarpal. A similar hypertrophic scar is present on the dorsal aspect of the thumb. The second photo which the preamble describes as an attempt at full abduction, depicts the thumb at approximately 45° of abduction and again a hyperextended posture of the interphalangeal joint. The thickened band of hypertrophic scar visible on the radial aspect of the proximal portion of the index finger contin-

ues across the dorsal aspect of the first webspace to approximately to the metacarpophalangeal joint or dorsal aspect of the thumb metacarpal.)

2. Explain in terms of functional anatomy the problem presented. (The pertinent pathologic anatomy is a scar contracture of the first webspace. That contracture restricts a full, 90°, abduction of the thumb from the index metacarpal. Full abduction is dependent on adequate pliability of the skin of the first webspace. Shortening or contracture of that skin will limit the ability of the thumb to abduct. In this instance, the contracture is secondary to delayed healing of burn wounds of the dorsum of thumb, first web space, and index finger. As a result of the limitation of motion from the skin contraction, additional pathology may occur in the underlying musculoskeletal structures including secondary contracture of the adductor mechanism, composed of the adductor pollicis and first dorsal interosseous. The adductor pollicis with the two heads, oblique arising from the volar aspect of the capitate and base of the third metacarpal as well as the transverse head, arising from the palmar aspect of the long finger metacarpal both insert on the ulnar sesamoid and extensor apparatus of the thumb metacarpophalangeal joint. Shortening of muscle and fascia aponeurosis can occur in instances of first webspace contracture. The other muscle, the first dorsal interosseous, also serves as an adductor, a consequence of the head that originates from the ulnar aspect of the thumb metacarpal and unites with the second head, originating from the radial aspect of the index metacarpal, to contribute to the extensor mechanism of the thumb metacarpophalangeal joint. The final component in the most severe adductor contracture are the secondary changes in the thumb carpal–metacarpal joint proper.)
3. Outline a treatment plan. (The treatment plan is dictated by the severity of the first web space contracture. Mild contractures with modest limitation of abduction can be addressed with a simple Z-plasty or perhaps a four flap Z-plasty after release of the skin contracture. More severe contractures may dictate a more extensive release of skin and fascia of the adductor pollicis. The resultant defect will require grafting, preferably with a thick split-thickness skin graft. One approach is design of a Z-plasty but the proximal flap is based radially and proximal and inset into the more distal and palmar limb of the Z-plasty which also serves as a release of the contracture. The resultant defect on the radial aspect of the index metacarpal is skin grafted. This option places full-thickness skin onto the palm and volar base of the thumb and the skin graft in contrast, onto the soft tissues overlying the radial aspect of the index metacarpal. This design is known as the stiletto flap.

   Severe contractures will mandate an extensive release of skin, adductor muscle, and fascia as well as the first dorsal interosseous by incision. The release is accomplished sequentially, judging at each step what residual structures still limit full abduction. Characteristically, these extensive defects require flap closure, a reverse radial forearm as a pedicled option or the lateral arm as a free flap choice.)

Intraoperative

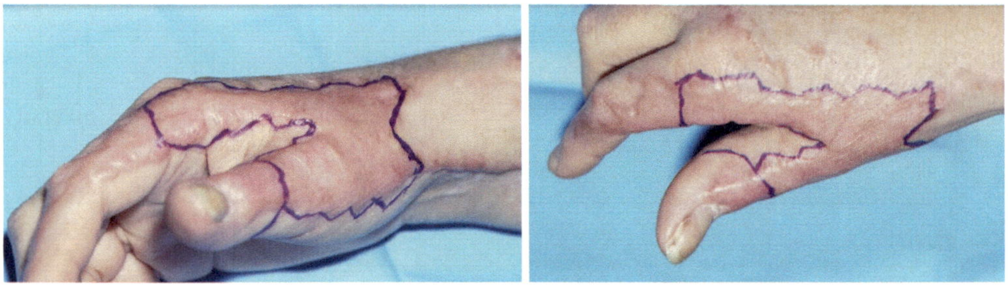

Excision of the entire area of hypertrophic burn scar has been outlined with a design that incorporates multiple small darts into unburned skin to avoid straight-line contracture in the healing process.

Postoperative

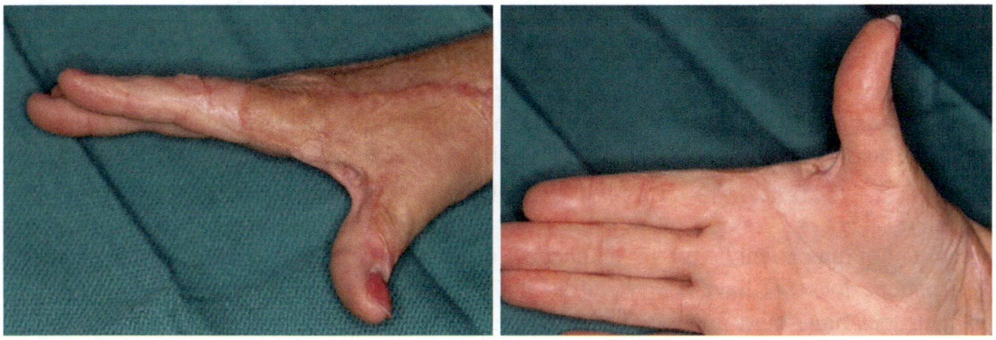

A dorsal and palmar view demonstrates a full thumb abduction of 90°.

Case-Based Conference

Case 2: Burn Contracture of the Trunk in Adolescent Female

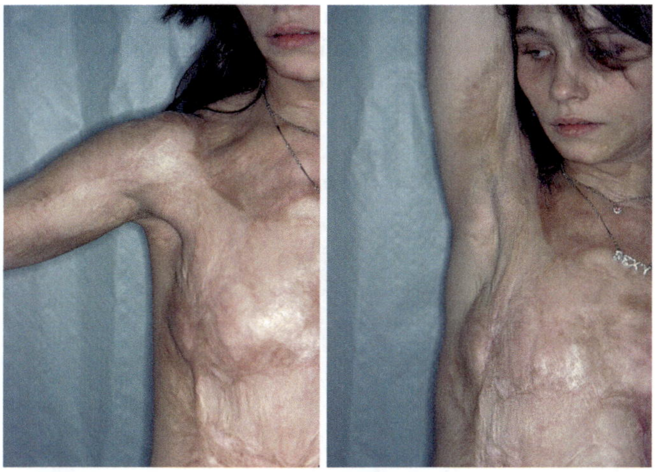

A 13 year old presents with history of burns of the trunk with skin-grafting performed acutely at age 2. Patient and family has concerns about the "breasts."

1. Describe the photo(s). The opposite side of the chest is similar in appearance to that depicted. Add a clinical examination.
   (a) Any tests indicated? Justify.
2. What are the indications for treatment of the patient? Are those indications present?
3. What is the pathologic process that explains the response to question two?
4. Outline a treatment plan. If an operation or operations are a component, explain your rationale and draw incisions.

Case-Based Conference: Discussion

Case 2: Burn Contracture of the Trunk in Adolescent Female

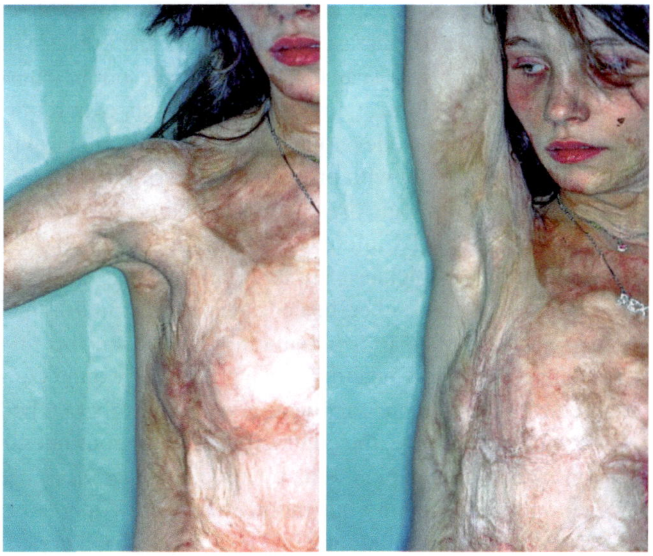

A 13 year old presents with history of burns of the trunk with skin-grafting performed acutely at age 2. Patient and family have concerns about the "breasts."

1. Describe the photo(s). The opposite side of the chest is similar in appearance to that depicted. Add a clinical examination. (The first view is of the right side of the upper trunk with diffuse and dense burn scarring of the visible upper arm, and upper and lower chest. The scarring appears to be mature. The second view is with the arm fully extended and elevated and a vertical scar contracture is visible on the lateral chest wall from the lateral breast to the anterior axilla and superiorly to the proximal medial arm. Axillary hair is present indicative of onset of

puberty. The pertinent history would be questions about the onset of menarche and functional complaints related to the shoulder although the shoulder does not seem to be limited significantly. The physical exam would focus on the degree of development present on the opposite breast, particularly if unburned, range of motion of the shoulder and limitation of motion if present, and availability of donor sites.)

(a) Any tests indicated? Justify. (No.)

2. What are the indications for treatment of the patient? Are those indications present? (The patient does not have a significant axillary contracture but does have burn contracture of the visible right breast, the severity of which is difficult to judge from the photo(s). Regardless, a release of said contracture is essential to remove as much as possible any restriction or constriction to normal breast development. The indication is the presence of a chest wall contracture involving the breast, because if unaddressed, as development occurs throughout adolescence, the deformity will increase either because the breast will be "pancaked" by a scarring involving the entire chest wall or if areas of intact, unburned skin exists over a portion of the breast, development and enlargement will occur preferentially with progressive deformity.)
3. What is the pathologic process that explains the response to question two? (By inference, the patient sustained deep dermal and full-thickness burns. Again, judging from the photos the burns either healed secondarily and/or had skin grafts applied to a granulating surface. In the first instance, secondary healing is by a process of wound contracture. In the second, application of skin grafts to a bed of granulation tissue, the contraction process continues.)
4. Outline a treatment plan. If an operation or operations are a component, explain your rationale and draw incisions. (A release of the contracture and a skin graft to the resultant defect will be required. The release is optimally accomplished by an incision placed in the inframammary crease, the extent of which is a semicircle or 180°, even into unburned skin if necessary. The result and defect will be sizable and should be closed with a thick split-thickness skin graft, bolstered for a complete take. The graft will encompass both the inferior pole of the breast superiorly and the inferior chest wall and may be quite extensive in size. A conformer may be useful to mold breast development after release of the constriction but the keystone of treatment is contracture release and grafting. An equally efficacious method is a similar release, application of the dermal substitute, Integra®, use of NWPT for 2 weeks, followed by closure with a thin split-thickness skin graft. The advantage is the harvest of a thin skin graft with more rapid healing of the donor site, disadvantage is the delay and two-stage approach.

The graft subsequently should be allowed to mature and soften. The next step has three options. One, if contracture release and grafting is sufficient, distinctly uncommon, nothing further is indicated. If not, an implant alone would suffice as a single-stage reconstruction, a minority of the instances. If also not possible, the third option, the majority of instances, is insertion of a tissue expander through an inframammary crease incision within the mature soft tissue skin graft, followed by a second-stage implant once the expansion process is complete.

Nipple-areola reconstruction can be a challenge since little dermis may exist beneath burn scars and previously placed grafts. As such, dermal-based flaps as the c-v and skate designs will not be successful nor will be areolar tattooing. The resemblance of a nipple bud may be constructed by tenting up a burn scar with multiple radial incisions, embedding a plug of Alloderm®, and encircling the newly constructed nipple with a full-thickness skin graft.

Finally, if complete breast reconstruction is necessary, then autogenous tissue transfer is the appropriate option but probably should be deferred until adulthood. The full menu of autologous tissue donor sites can be considered, for example, the use of bilateral free DIEP flaps.)

Postoperative (1 Year, 3 Years)

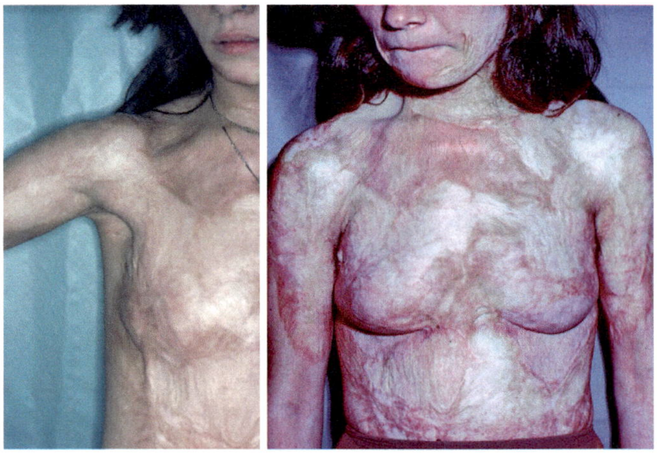

Some breast development is apparent 1 year after bilateral split-thickness skin graft release. The second photo is following staged tissue expansion and implants. The postoperative view following staged split-thickness skin grafts, tissue expansion, and implants depicts small breasts with an absent nipple-areola complex.

Critique

Some asymmetry of the inframammary crease, left lower than right, is present. As a result, the left implant is positioned lower on the chest wall. Revision would consist of elevation as well as increased definition of the inframammary crease with a superior capsulotomy and perhaps a larger implant. The patient is still in early adolescence and after a hiatus, 2 or 3 years, additional tissue expansion and implants could be accomplished.

Case-Based Conference

Case 3: Burn Contracture of Upper Extremity

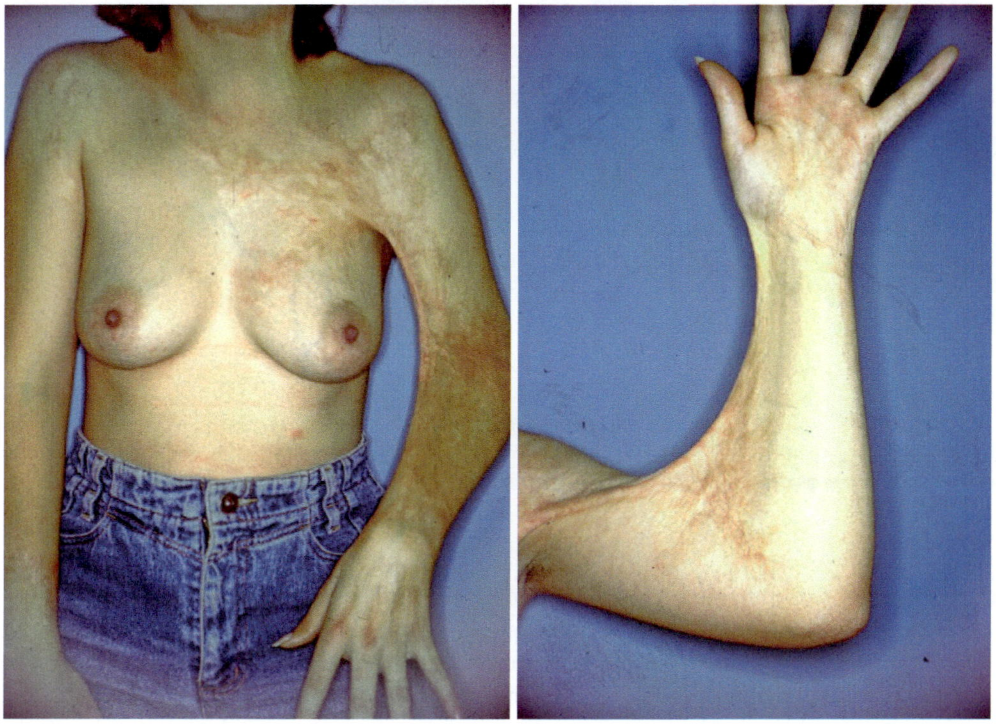

A 25 year old sustained burns of the left upper extremity and head injury 2 years ago in a MVA. Now fully recovered.

1. Describe the photo(s), add a focused clinical exam.
   (a) Any tests indicated? Why?
2. Describe the pathologic process that explains the findings depicted on the photo(s) as well as the pathologic anatomy.
   (a) How will the findings on clinical exam perhaps influence your treatment plan?
3. Outline a treatment plan including perioperative care.
4. Draw your incisions.

Case-Based Conference: Discussion

Case 3: Burn Contracture of Upper Extremity

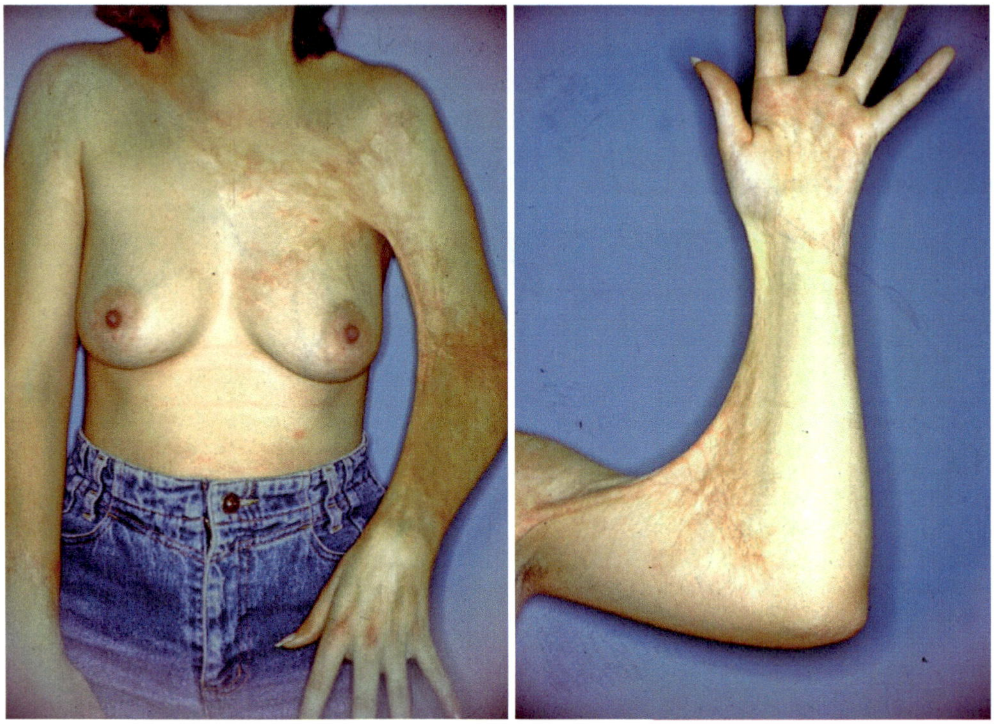

A 25 year old sustained burns of the left upper extremity and head injury 2 years ago in a MVA. Now fully recovered.

1. Describe the photos(s), add a focused clinical exam. (Two slides are provided, the first a frontal half trunk view. The slide depicts a young woman with the obvious findings of a band-like contracture and web extending from the area of the anterior axillary fold and adjacent lateral anterior chest wall. The contracture band continues on the medial aspect of the arm distally and the length of the radial portion of the forearm. A confluent scar is also present over the superior portion of the left anterior chest extending onto the superior pole of the breast. Most of the breast is unscarred and similar in shape and size to the opposite breast which is unscarred as is the opposite chest and the visible upper abdomen. The contracture of the upper extremity appears taut despite the shoulder and arm in a posture of adduction and a carrying angle of an incomplete extension of the elbow to a full 180°. Some light burn scars are visible on the posterior–lateral arm and the dorsum of the forearm. The hand is normal in appearance and unscarred. The second view is restricted to the volar aspect upper extremity from the hand to the axilla. The elbow is flexed to 90°, the hand and forearm are pronated. The extent of the contracture is evident, beginning at the anterior axilla and adjacent chest wall, coursing obliquely across the arm toward the antecubital fossa, but spanning the elbow as a large web and into the radial aspect of the forearm and wrist, ending at the base of the thumb. In doing so, the contracture has created a dense web of skin and soft tissue the apex of which appears several centimeters anterior to the antecubital fossa. The hand posture is one of the digits fully extended and no burn scars are evident of the palm, thumb, or fingers. The described web consists of burn scar.

   The clinical exam would elicit pertinent details regarding treatment at the time of injury and any residual sequelae although the preamble states, "Fully recovered." The appearance of the burn scar is what leads to the conclusion that no grafting was attempted, a conclusion to be confirmed by history. The physical exam would also establish normal function of the hand and wrist with the exception of the ability to deviate ulnarly. The elbow joint range of motion from full flexion to the limitation of full extension is also examined.)

(a) Any tests indicated? Why? (Plain x-rays are necessary to determine the presence, if any, of joint pathology including heterotopic ossification.) Why? (Burn patients are at risk for the development of periarticular heterotopic ossification, particularly at the elbow joint.)

2. Describe the pathologic process that explains the findings depicted on the photo(s) as well as the pathologic anatomy. (The process that culminated in the finding of an extensive contracture was the end result of burn wound healing by secondary intention. Assuming the area of scarring of the anterior chest, arm, and forearm represented full-thickness or deep partial thickness burns, the healing process must have consisted of eschar separation, granulation tissue formation, and eventual healing by wound contracture at the expense of the axilla and elbow range of motion. The pathology may include secondary scarring of the elbow joint capsule as well as certainly the possibility of heterotopic ossification of the periarticular structures of the elbow. Loss of full extension can occur in long-standing flexion deformities of the elbow as a result of skin and soft tissue scarring, secondary to intrinsic shortening of the principle flexors of the elbow, the biceps, brachioradialis, and brachialis.)

(a) How will the findings on the clinical exam perhaps influence your treatment plan? (Unlike the hand, isolation of the components of joint limitation of motion secondary to skin alone vs. intrinsic joint changes by flexion of the more proximal joint is not readily accomplished in the elbow. The exam can be facilitated by flexion and adduction of the shoulder and then attempted extension of the elbow. Given the severity of the skin contracture and all likelihood, the examination of the elbow joint will be incomplete. Regardless, if joint changes and muscle shortening are suspected, thought must be given to the same in management and development of the postoperative treatment plan.)

3. Outline a treatment plan including perioperative care. (Two decisions need to be made in the development of the treatment plan. The first is scar incision or scar excision. One of the determinants of that decision will be the pliability or thickness of the scar, a thickened scar would perhaps indicate excision. In severe burn contractures, the scar will usually soften with release and, in general, incision-release is preferred. The other treatment decision is management of any residual inability to fully extend the elbow after skin contracture release because of the presence of musculoskeletal alterations described above, a presence that probably won't be manifest until intraoperative and post skin release. Three options will then exist with mostly different implications. One is release of the principal flexors of the elbow, the biceps, and brachioradialis. To do so will require an incision of the lacertus fibrosus and tendon lengthening of those two muscles. The vital structures of the antecubital fossa, the brachial artery, and median and radial nerves will, by virtue of the operative approach, be exposed. Exposure of those structures mandates coverage by placement of a dermal substitute with implicit risks and delayed application of skin grafts. The other possibility is wound closure by full-thickness flap, pedicled or free. Other than perhaps a reverse lateral arm flap or a proximally based radial forearm, neither of which is preferable in these instances, no pedicled options are available. A variety of free flaps are available. In summary, operative release of the joint at this juncture is probably not advisable.

A second approach is operative release, placement of a temporary dressing of allograft, insertion of pins, and the use of postoperative traction to passively stretch the joint. Unfortunately, the neurovascular structures have shortened as well and postoperative traction will be extremely painful and of limited success.

A third option is immediate closure with a thick split-thickness skin graft after contracture release and then initiation of postoperative physical therapy after the wound is healed. Given the youth of the patient and the 2 year duration of the contracture, that option may be most appropriate.)

4. Draw your incisions. (The proposed incisions should be designed as in all contracture release to extend from axis to axis of the joint in a U-shaped fashion. To do so will also create a short flap that will retract a substantial distance proximal in order to create the resultant soft-tissue defect. The design of the transverse contracture release component of that incision should be done to permit the flap to slide proximal into and coverage of the antecubital fossa.)

Postoperative (2 Weeks)

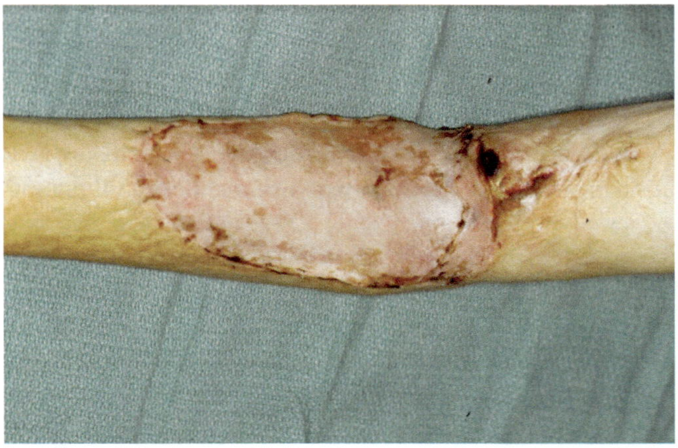

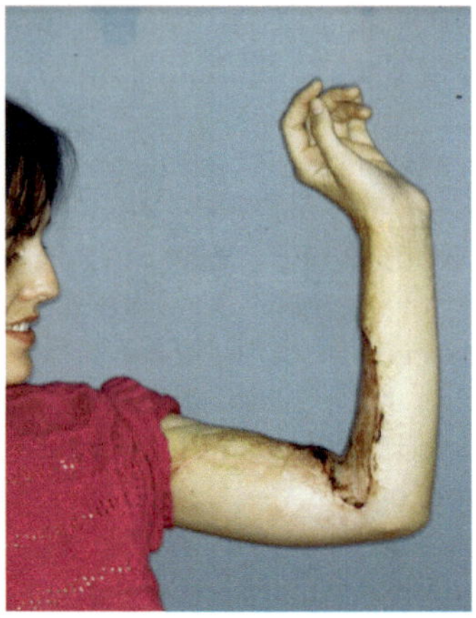

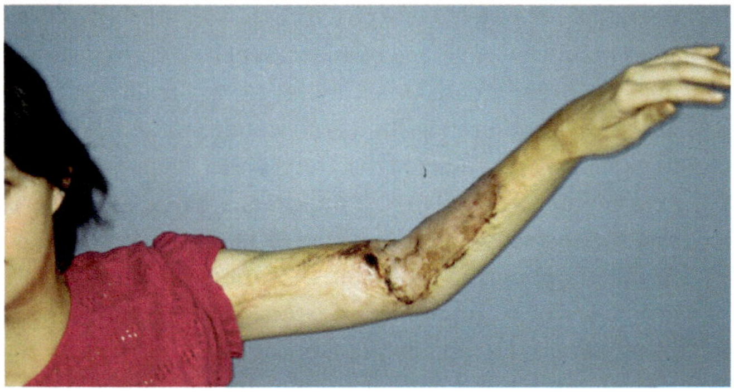

The three photos depict immediate, 2 week, postoperative results. A large defect extending from the antecubital fossa for one-half of the volar forearm has been closed successfully with a non-meshed split-thickness skin graft. The patient demonstrates elbow flexion to 90° and residual incomplete extension.

Critique

The patient will need prompt and aggressive physical therapy to achieve additional elbow extension. To avoid periarticular bleeding and inflammation, therapy should be primarily active. If necessary, serial splinting can be added later.

In-Service Examination

1. The appropriate immediate post-burn splinting in a patient of 60% BSA burns of head and neck, upper extremity, and torso consist of the following **EXCEPT:**
   (a) Head and neck at 0°.
   (b) Hands in intrinsic minus.
   (c) Elbows at 180°.
   (d) Shoulders at 90° abduction and externally rotated.
2. A 10-year-old female 2 years after sustaining partial thickness burns of the right chest has reached menarche and has constriction and lack of development of the right breast. What is the appropriate management?
   (a) Observation and treatment after full breast development.
   (b) Insertion of a tissue expander beneath the right breast bud.
   (c) Release of contracture with application of Integra® and delayed skin grafting.
   (d) Release of contracture with application of Integra® and delayed skin grafting; small augmentation implant, plans for later larger implant.
3. The classic position of the untreated burn claw deformity is:
   (a) Wrist flexed, MP joints flexed, PIP joints flexed.
   (b) Wrist flexed, MP joints extended, PIP joints flexed.
   (c) Wrist extended, MP joints flexed, PIP joints extended.
   (d) Wrist extended, MP joints extended, PIP joints flexed.

64 Soft Tissue Infections, Bites, Frostbite

Bibliography

Thompson S. and Townsend R., "Pharmacological agents for soft tissue and bone infected with MRSA: Which agent and for how long?", *Injury, Int. J. Care Injured*, (2011); 42:**S7-S10.**

Bonne SL, Kadri SS., "Evaluation and Management of Necrotizing Soft Tissue Infections", *Infect. Dis. Clin. N. Am.*, (2017); **497–507 ONLY.**

Fagan S, Chai J, Spies M, et al., Chapter 43: "Exfoliative disease of the integument and soft tissue necrotizing infections", Herndon, D. N., Total Burn Care, Saunders, (2012); **pgs. 471–81.**

Stevens DL, Bryant AE, "Necrotizing Soft-Tissue Infections", *N Engl J Med.*, (2017); 377:**Figure 2 ONLY.**

Taylor EM, Hamaguchi R, Kramer KM, et al., "Plastic Surgical Management of Hidradenitis Suppurativa", *Plast. Reconstr. Surg.*, (2021); 147(3):**479e-491e.**

Anz AW, Schweppe M, Halvorson J, et al., "Management of Venomous Snakebite Injury to the Extremities", *J. Am. Acad. of Orthopedic Surgeons*, (2010); 18(12):**752–59 ONLY.**

Swanson DL and Vetter RS, "Bites of brown recluse spiders and suspected necrotic arachnidism", *New England Journal of Medicine*, (2005); 352(7):**700–7.**

Mohr WJ, Jenabzadeh K, Ahrenholz DH., "Cold Injury", *Hand Clin*, (2009); **481–93 ONLY.**

Gottlieb M, Long B, Koyfman A., "The evaluation and management of toxic shock syndrome in the emergency department: A review of the literature" *Journal of Emergency Medicine*, (2017); 54(6): **807-11.**

Noonburg GE, "Management of extremity trauma and related infections occurring in the aquatic nvironment", *J Am Acad Orthop Surg*, (2005); 13(4): **243–49 ONLY.**

For Supplemental Reading Only

Dryden M. S., "Complicated skin and soft tissue infection", *J. Antimicrob. Chemother.*, (2010); 65 Suppl. 3:iii35–44.

Faculty Discussion and Study Guide

Editor's Note: Chronic wounds are discussed in Chap. 3.

Complex Soft Tissue Infections

1. The readings divided complicated soft tissue infections into necrotizing and non-necrotizing. How do these two differ microbially? (The pathogen in non-necrotizing complex soft tissue infections is quite frequently staphylococcus aureus and of course methicillin-resistant or MRSA is quite common. In contrast, streptococcus is perhaps the most common microbe in single organism necrotizing fasciitis although polymicrobial infections are the most frequent necrotizing fasciitis.)
2. You are asked to consult on an ICU patient with a forearm abscess and cellulitis secondary to a radial artery puncture. You plan incision and drainage and your antibiotic of choice should be a cephalosporin. True or false? (False. The patient in all likelihood has hospital acquired MRSA, HA-MRSA, and the agent of choice is vancomycin or linezolid.)
3. You are asked to consult on the medicine service for an otherwise healthy patient who has been admitted with acute lower leg cellulitis without sepsis. The most likely organism and the antibiotic of choice? (ß-hemolytic streptococcus, group A, is the most likely culprit and leg elevation, warmth, and any Gram-positive antibiotic such as cefazolin or even high dose of penicillin added to the treatment regime. Failure to respond may represent a community-acquired MRSA or a polymicrobial infection and are indications for change in antibiotic therapy such as the initiation of vancomycin, possibly combined with Zosyn.)
4. Describe the two types of necrotizing fasciitis and their differentiating characteristics. (Type I is a polymicrobial

E. Luce, *A Curriculum for Plastic Surgery*, https://doi.org/10.1007/978-3-031-62087-4_64

infection with usually an anaerobic species in combination with another organism usually a streptococcus β-hemolytic or an enteric bacteria. The anatomical location is usually the trunk or the perineum or a postoperative wound. The patients are more likely to have comorbidity or morbidities than Type II. Type II is a monomicrobial infection usually group A strep or perhaps Aeromonas from a fresh water infection. The microbe is much more likely a single organism such as group A ß-hemolytic Streptococcus or perhaps MRSA and much more commonly located in the extremities in a patient who is otherwise healthy and immunocompetent. MRSA has become increasingly prevalent as the principal organism in type II necrotizing fasciitis infections.)
   (a) Describe a third type, associated with infections from a salt water source. (Fulminant infections from bites or shellfish injuries resulting from Vibrio organisms that are characteristically an extremely virulent course with a very significant mortality, particularly in the immunocompromised patient.)
5. Although, as described in an above question, streptococcus is the most common organism, what is the general microbial composition of necrotizing soft tissue infections? (Polymicrobial with frequent contributions from gram-negative rods as well.)
6. The estimated overall mortality in necrotizing soft tissue infections is approximately: (20%.)
   (a) What is the most significant determinant of prognosis/mortality? (Early diagnosis, initiation of antibiotic therapy, and aggressive surgical debridement.)
7. What are the common comorbidities present in a patient who presents with necrotizing fasciitis? (Perirectal infection, IV drug abuse, diabetes, an undetected retroperitoneal infectious process such as perforated distal sigmoid diverticulitis.)
8. What are some clinical and test methods of establishing a diagnosis of necrotizing fasciitis? (The clinical picture may be indistinct but includes skin bullae and ecchymosis, edema, erythema, as well as a patient who is systemically septic. Severe pain including myalgia may be an important clinical sign. A CT or MRI may detect fluid or even gas in fascial planes and obliteration of facial definition. Laboratory evidence of hyponatremia and elevated BUN and WBC and perhaps coagulopathy are nonspecific laboratory parameters.)
   (a) What pathologic feature explains the progressive nature of necrotizing fasciitis? (Thrombosis of small blood vessels as well as a toxin capable of lysing tissue barriers.)
9. What is the antibiotic protocol for a diagnosis of necrotizing fasciitis? (The necessity to consider the high likelihood of polymicrobial infection implies the use of a combination of antibiotics. One such combination could be linezolid and minocycline or as described above, Vancomycin and Zosyn. See below.)
10. What are some general principles in surgical management of necrotizing fasciitis? (Early, less than 8 h after admission/diagnosis, excision of full-thickness skin, subcutaneous fat, and fascial involvement. Careful inspection of the periphery of the excision margin for evidence of further disease, examination of the muscle for viability, and a return to the operating room on a every 24 h basis for further inspection and debridement. A diverting colostomy may be necessary in perineal infections as well.)
    (a) Operative findings? (Grey necrotic fascia, thrombosed superficial veins, watery and foul smelling drainage, a relatively easy blunt dissection of skin/subcutaneous tissue from the deep fascia and little resistance to subfascial finger dissection.)
11. Fournier's gangrene refers to? (A necrotizing fasciitis with polymicrobial infection; almost always a gram-negative rod component in a compromised patient such as diabetes, cirrhosis, or renal insufficiency with the process usually limited to the scrotum/perineum.)
12. What is at least hypothetically an advantage of clindamycin in treatment of MRSA infections? (Capable of direct action on exotoxin to reduce concentration of the same.)
    (a) Disadvantages? (15–20% of MRSA resistance as tested by "double D" dimer test. Potential for C. difficile enteritis/colitis.)
    (b) Another oral agent? (Doxycycline, a tetracycline derivative; linezolid but is expensive.)
13. A previously healthy young adult sustains a life-threatening rapidly progressive necrotizing fasciitis from a water skiing soft tissue injury. What is the most likely organism and the explanation? (Aeromonas hydrophila is an organism in contaminated fresh water that is capable of producing exotoxins that contribute significantly to the pathogenicity.)
    (a) Other organisms that may produce a similar virulent clinical picture? (Group A, ß-hemolytic streptococcus, community-acquired MRSA, and clostridium species. A vibrio infection from contaminated salt water with the picture of overwhelming sepsis may or may not be attended by a necrotizing soft tissue infection and more commonly occurs in immunocompromised patients.)

Other Complex Soft Tissue Infections

1. Your mammaplasty patient, 24 h postoperatively presents to the ER with hypotension, hepatic and renal failure, coagulopathy, and acute respiratory distress syndrome, ARDS. A rash is present over much of the anterior trunk and the dressings have a small amount of serosanguineous drainage. Your diagnosis? (Toxic shock syndrome probably group A strep but toxic shock from staph has also been reported. The treatment is immediate removal of the implants even prior to resuscitation and initiation of antibiotics.)
2. Toxic epidermal necrolysis, TENS, Stevens–Johnson syndrome, linked to what etiology? (The current etiology of TENS or Stevens–Johnson syndrome is almost invariably linked to oral medications including antibiotics, anticonvulsants, and analgesics including NSAIDS in perhaps susceptible individuals.)
   (a) What is the pathology? (Dermal–epidermal separation with a normal reticular dermis but damaged papillary dermis. The postoperative setting strongly suggests staphylococcus most likely MRSA and initiation of Vancomycin is appropriate.)
3. Outline the clinical picture. (The onset is preceded by a prodromal phase of 2–3 days of low-grade fever, malaise perhaps closely followed by the development of mucosal lesions, then the occurrence of multiple bullae with desquamation of the epidermis.)
4. Outline the essential management? (Transfer to burn unit is indicated with initial fluid resuscitation, although considerably less than for a similar size burn, wound care to permit re-epithelialization, and nutritional support.)
   (a) What is one important consultation? (Ophthalmologic because of the associated involvement of the conjunctiva with possible secondary complications. Gastroenterology consultation if evidence of intestinal involvement.)
5. Give an estimate of outcomes and mortality. (Mortality, particularly in the elderly or immunocompromised can be above 50%. If wound infection can be prevented and spontaneous healing occurs, the mortality is reduced substantially.)
6. Differentiate the staphylococcal scalded syndrome, SSS, from TENS. (Staphylococcal syndrome is as the name implies a soft tissue infection produced by staphylococcus and differs from TENS in that the cleavage point and loss of the skin layer is intraepidermal while TENS occurs at the epidermal–dermal junction. Another differentiation is the absence of mucosal lesions. A skin biopsy can help with diagnosis and the clinical course is usually benign with spontaneous healing within a week or two of onset but TENS in contrast may require longer duration to heal and most commonly occurs in immunocompromised patients. SSS occurs predominantly at the pediatric age group.)

Hidradenitis Suppurativa

1. What is epidemiology of hidradenitis suppurativa, HS? (Female preponderance, a ratio of 3:1, onset in early adulthood and waning in middle age, higher incidence in smokers and the obese, and a probable genetic predisposition in some.)
2. Pathology? (Infection of the apocrine sweat glands that secrete primarily via an excretory duct into the hair follicle. Occlusion of the latter by keratinization may lead to rupture with spilling of keratin into the dermis, a material that induces an intense inflammatory response and secondary bacterial contamination. Abscesses and sinus tracts then occur.)
   (a) Hereditary component? (Yes, possibly autosomal dominant with a variable penetrance. Yet, HS is regarded as a complex disorder with multiple environmental factors that may trigger the disease.)
   (b) Exacerbating factors? (Obesity, tobacco use.)
3. Outline the Hurley classification of severity. (Not particularly useful since usually only the severely afflicted patients are referred for surgical management. Three stages: stage I consists of isolated abscesses; stage II is recurrent disease, abscess, and sinus tracts but with expanses of uninvolved skin; stage III is diffuse involvement. A number of other classifications have been described, the use primarily limited to research studies.)
4. Differential diagnosis? (Acne conglobata; folliculitis of the scalp or capitans, both of which may be related.)
5. Antibiotic therapy? (As the readings imply, the microbiology is not well defined. One preferable choice is clindamycin and/or doxycycline but recurrence after cessation of therapy is common and prolonged administration of clindamycin is not recommended because of the potential occurrence of c.difficile, enterocolitis.)
6. Outline the elements and efficacy of medical treatment. (Weight loss, tobacco cessation, topical clindamycin, anti-androgen therapy. Non-surgical management of HS has limited efficacy and only in mild or early disease, Hurley I.)

7. What are some adjunctive measures in addition to surgery? (Use of isotretinoin perioperatively and perhaps finasteride, an antiandrogen agent, as a short course preoperatively but efficacy has not been demonstrated.)
8. What is the principal surgical treatment of hidradenitis? (Wide excision of not only the pathologically involved skin but the area of apocrine sweat glands in addition as delineated by the extent of the hair-bearing skin, for example in the axilla. Wound management can be by primary closure, delayed closure with use of negative wound pressure therapy followed by skin grafting and/or secondary healing. Although the use of rotational flaps for both the axilla and the perineum have been described, the prerequisite is an assurance that excision is complete and the probability of recurrence is an absolute minimum.)
9. Comment on the possible role of biologic therapy. (Some work has been performed with use of immunomodulators such as Humira® with some positive benefits in control of the disease. Those benefits need to be weighed against the significant side effects and possible complications as well as the difficulty in acquisition of insurance coverage. Humira® is the only FDA-approved biologic for HS.)

Snake, Spider Bites

1. A stat consultation is requested in the ER of a patient who has sustained a snake bite, perhaps copperhead. What are the important aspects of the clinical examination? (Time of injury, associated comorbidities, location of the bite, presence of two puncture marks consistent with a pit viper bite. Patient questioning re: degree of pain and any associated paresthesia, weakness or CNS symptoms. An exam would focus on the presence of edema and ecchymosis if an extremity is involved.)
   (a) Laboratory studies? (Coagulation profile including PT, PTT, fibrinogen, and platelet count if coagulopathy is suspected.)
   (b) What is the overall gestalt in copperhead bites? (Local swelling and injury to the extremity but less likely systemic effects.)
2. What are the significance of the local effects of the venom? (Venom is a complex mixture of multiple cytotoxins and proteolytic enzymes that are capable of inducing loss of vascular permeability with extravasation of fluid into the interstitial space and a rising compartmental pressure as a result. The implications are that the careful monitoring of clinical status is paramount in extremity pit viper bites. The timelines are that edema begins to occur quite promptly within the first 6 h post-injury and reaches a peak 12–18 h after envenomation.)
   (a) Modality to monitor? (Tissue compartment pressures for the presence of compartment syndrome as indicated by pressures greater than 30 mm Hg.)
3. Discuss the pros and cons of administration of contemporary antivenin. (CroFab® is a preparation of antibodies harvested from sheep immunized with pit viper venom. The potential problem with antivenin is either acute or delayed hypersensitivity reactions with an approximate incidence of 15% each. The delayed hypersensitivity reaction is serum sickness characterized by fever, rash, and arthralgia with a low but worrisome incidence of long-term morbidity. Antivenin should probably not be given prophylactically unless massive envenomation is suspected. Therapeutic or symptomatic antivenin is given to the patient who has evidence of systemic manifestations of cardiac, coagulopathy, or rhabdomyolysis.)
4. The role of fasciotomy as mentioned above should be performed in the presence of signs, symptoms, and pressures indicative of compartment syndrome. The use of fasciotomy has diminished dramatically over the past several decades (Table 64.1).
5. What was the thrust of the readings with respect to diagnosis of brown recluse spider bites? (The thrust was that the diagnosis should be suspect if the contact is outside of the normal geographic home of the brown recluse which is the southeast except the coastal region, Texas, Missouri, Kansas. The stated implication was that most soft tissue infections even within that geographic area are probably not the result of spider bite.)
6. What is the overarching principle in the management of brown recluse bites? (In the absence of the offending spider, the treatment is conservative. First, as mentioned above, the diagnosis may be suspect. Second, the wound is usually self-limited and commonly heals without intervention.)
   (a) What are the available modalities with the benefits and liabilities? (Dapsone is an agent that *may* limit the degree of skin necrosis. Dapsone does induce some element of hemolysis in most patients as the result of the sulfone moiety. Glucose 6-phosphate dehydrogenase levels should be obtained as well as liver function tests. Primary excision has fallen heavily out of favor and is reserved only for well-demarcated necrotic lesions.)

Table 64.1 Classification of snakebite severity and recommended intervention

Degree of envenomation	Clinical manifestation	Extremity treatment	Antivenin
0	Mild pain at bite site	Local wound care	None
I	Local edema, ecchymosis	Local wound care, strict elevation	Copperhead or cottonmouth bite and normal blood panel: None Rattlesnake bite or abnormal blood tests: 5 vials
II	Edema extending proximally from the bite site, mild coagulopathy, mild change in renal/liver profile, nausea, vomiting	Local wound care, strict elevation, evaluation for signs and symptoms of compartment syndrome every 2–4 h	5–15 vials
III	Swelling of entire extremity, intense pain, severe systemic signs, moderate abnormality in blood tests	Strict elevation, hourly evaluation for signs and symptoms of compartment syndrome	15–20 vials
IV	Hypotension, obtundation, cardiac arrhythmia, severe abnormality in blood tests (e.g., platelet count <20,000/mm^3)	Strict elevation, evaluation for signs and symptoms of compartment syndrome, consider measuring compartment pressure	≥20 vials

Frostbite

1. What is the pathophysiology of frostbite or cold-induced injury? (The formation of extracellular ice crystals with the resultant fluid shift from intra-extracellular and cellular dehydration. Intracellular ice crystals can form subsequently or, if freezing is rapid. Those changes at the cellular level may even be overshadowed by the pathology at the microvascular level. Vasoconstriction of arterioles and venules perhaps induced by increased levels of free radicals, similar to the changes of the no-reflow phenomenon in ischemic flaps, that then culminates in microthrombosis.)
2. Compare frostbite and frostnip. (Frostnip is a reversible cold-induced injury that will not result in tissue loss. The numbness and pallor of exposed skin, particularly the tip of the nose and ears, cheek, penis, tips of fingers and toes, can be seen in both. Frostbite is a worsening of severity as exemplified by the subsequent appearance of blebs or blisters.)
   (a) What is the pathognomonic appearance immediately in both rewarming? (Flushing, hyperemia.)
   (b) What may differentiate the two? (Severe pain with rewarming in frostbite as well as the formation of blebs in 12–24 h.)
3. What is a classification of frostbite? (First degree is no blebs but with pallor that develops erythema and edema on rewarming. The overlap between frostnip and first degree frostbite is quite substantial. Second degree frostbite has blebs with light colored fluid that will result in just superficial epidermal loss and spontaneous healing. In third degree frostbite, the blebs and bullae are filled with dark hemorrhagic fluid that over a period of 10–14 days will become firm black eschar. Fourth degree is involvement of bone and tendon and inevitably results in amputation.)
4. A role for imaging and frostbite? (CT/MRI is no better than triple-phase bone scan done early, as early as 2–3 days post-injury but clinical assessment is usually sufficient.)
5. Outline management of the frostbite injury. (Initial rapid rewarming in a tub with circulating water set at 40 °C (104–108° F) with concomitant administration of the necessary narcotics followed by application of aloe vera cream plus silver-impregnated gauze. Adjunctive measures consist of ibuprofen, Trental or pentoxifylline, and narcotics as necessary. If the core temperature is less than normal, the entire patient, not just the extremity should be placed in the tub.)
6. Other measures? (The readings describe the use by several centers of intra-arterial thrombolytic therapy with tPA. Although the administration of a thrombolytic is appealing and perhaps appropriate from a pathophysiology perspective, the benefits need to be weighed against the known complications of angioplasty.)
7. What is the role of surgical intervention? (The overarching theme in frostbite is conservative management with deferred debridement until amputation is evident and obvious. The phrase "frostbite in January, amputate in July" is an exaggeration but the underlying theme is correct.)

Case-Based Conference

Case 1: Severe Infection of the Axillae

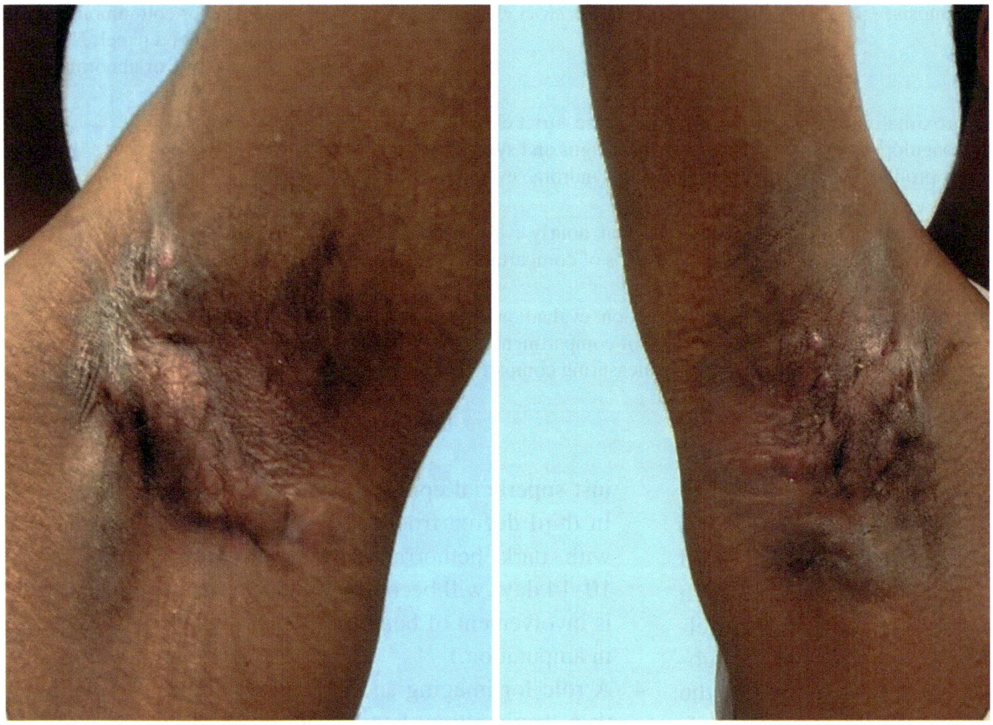

A 40-year-old man with a 12–18 month history of multiple drawing sinuses and abscesses of both axillae who had multiple courses of antibiotics.

1. Describe the photos and add a clinical examination.
   (a) Any tests indicated? Justify.
2. What is the pathophysiology of this disorder? How does the pathophysiology impact the treatment plan?
3. Outline a treatment plan. Include a commentary on conservative management. If surgery is a component of the treatment plan, describe and include perioperative care.

Case-Based Conference: Discussion

Case 1: Severe Infection of the Axillae

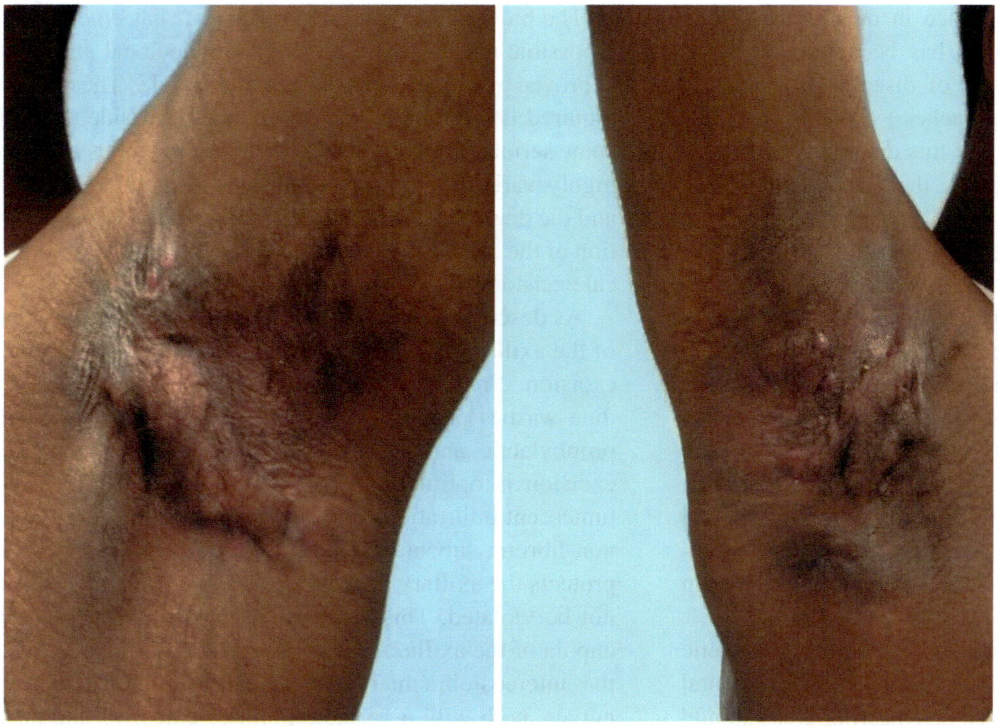

A 40-year-old man with a 12–18 month history of multiple drawing sinuses and abscesses of both axillae. Has had multiple courses of antibiotics.

1. Describe the photos and add a clinical examination. (Two photos are available of the left and right axillae. In both the arms are extended and include the proximal one third of the medial arm and the immediately adjacent inferior and lateral chest wall. The most conspicuous finding in both axillae is an inflammatory process marked by multiple pustules, more so on the right than the left, and large nodules of raised and contracted skin, more apparent on the left than the right. The involved areas on the left extend to the borders of the axilla. The process on the right has some pustules for 1–2 cm of the medial arm and inferiorly for a short distance of 2–3 cm onto the superior chest wall skin. The patient is a Fitzpatrick 6 skin coloration. The clinical exam would document the time of onset, the subsequent course, past treatments both medical and incision and drainage, and other areas in the body currently afflicted. The presence of comorbidities as diabetes or immunocompromised state as lupus erythematosus is documented. Some associated diseases include inflammatory bowel disease and pyoderma granulosum. Social history of tobacco or drug abuse is important since both are risk factors for the probable diagnosis in this case, hidradenitis suppurativa, HS. Since a genetic component may exist, a family history is equally important. The physical exam would focus on possible extent of disease beyond what is evident on observation including acute inflammation as signaled by erythema of adjacent, apparently uninvolved skin. Other possible body areas involved by history as breast and perineum are examined. The BMI is calculated.)

(a) Any tests indicated? Justify. (Although any number of biomarkers are increased in HS, none are of treatment or predictive value. Because of the polymicrobial nature of the secondary bacterial infection, cultures are not of assistance in development of a treatment plan. Ultrasound has been utilized as an effort to define the extent of disease but has little impact on excisional approaches.)

2. What is the pathophysiology of this disorder? How does the pathophysiology impact the treatment plan? (Occlusion of the sebaceous gland, an apocrine gland that secretes sebum into the base of the hair follicle, results in rupture of the gland and spillage of keratin and sebum into the soft tissue including the dermis. Both are highly provocative agents of an inflammatory response. Secondary bacterial colonization follows with the inevitable development of abscesses and multiple sinus tracts. The primary etiologic event, occlusion of the duct of the follicular sebaceous gland, is of interest. The pathological process is keratinization of the duct. What the actual pathogenetic mechanism of the process remains undefined although causative cytokine agents have been identified.

   The involvement of the pilosebaceous unit by a genetic predisposition and unknown individual environmental factors implies that uninvolved hair-bearing areas should be incorporated in any treatment plan that includes excision.)

3. Outline a treatment plan. Include a commentary on conservative management. If surgery is a component of the treatment plan, describe and include perioperative care. (The patient depicted is burdened with Hurley's stage III disease, the most severe of the Hurley classification and success of a medical protocol is highly improbable. Conservative measures include weight loss, patient education re personal hygiene, and topical and systemic antibiotics. Other modalities utilized include finasteride such as antiandrogen therapy and keratolytic drugs. Tobacco cessation is important and should be implemented regardless of the treatment plan. All of the above measures may have some efficacy in the early stages of the disease process, Hurley I and II, but not in advanced disease as pictured in the scenario. In addition, prolonged antibiotic administration may not be advisable. The agents utilized include clindamycin, rapamycin, and doxycycline and all can have substantial complications with long-term administration. Severe HS inflicts a substantial emotional burden as the disease negatively impacts the patient's quality of life on a daily basis. The rationale for a definitive surgical solution is excision.

   The biologic adalimumab or Humira® has emerged as a possible agent. Adalimumab is a monoclonal antibody approved by the FDA for the treatment of HS. The dosage required is substantial and the incidence of side effects, some serious, is considerable. In addition, the response is highly variable, complete remission distinctly unusual, and the degree of efficacy is inversely related to the duration of the disease. The role as adjunct therapy with surgical excision has not been defined.

   As described above, the uninvolved hair-bearing area of the axilla is at risk and should be encompassed in the excision. Preoperative preparation includes chlorhexidine washes prior to the day of surgery and the usual prophylactic antibiotic immediately preoperative. The excision is optimally accomplished with a knife after tumescent infiltration. The plane of dissection is normal, non-fibrotic subcutaneous fat. The deep brachial fascia protects the axillary neurovascular structures and should not be violated. This risk is the greatest at the apex or cupola of the axilla. Additional structures at risk include the intercostobrachial and medial brachial cutaneous nerves, both with a variable point of exit from the brachial fascia into the subcutaneous space. Although both can be identified and preserved, patients should be counseled about the possibility of diminished sensation of the upper medial arm.

   A variety of closure methods are available, the choice selection hinging to a large degree on the extent of the excision. In the clinical case presented, primary closure over drains with sling and circumferential swath dressing is a likely option. The useful adjunct recently employed is a primary closure, followed postoperatively by application of a portable negative wound pressure therapy. In bilateral disease, a staged approach will respect the patient's personal hygiene and other daily life needs. Larger defects will require more conservative closure options such as negative wound pressure followed by delayed closure with a skin graft. In the use of local rotational flaps including thoracodorsal artery perforator flaps, the prerequisite is the assurance that an excision is complete, probability of recurrence is an absolute minimum, and the longer operative times are justifiable.)

Case-Based Conference

Case 2: Difficult Wound

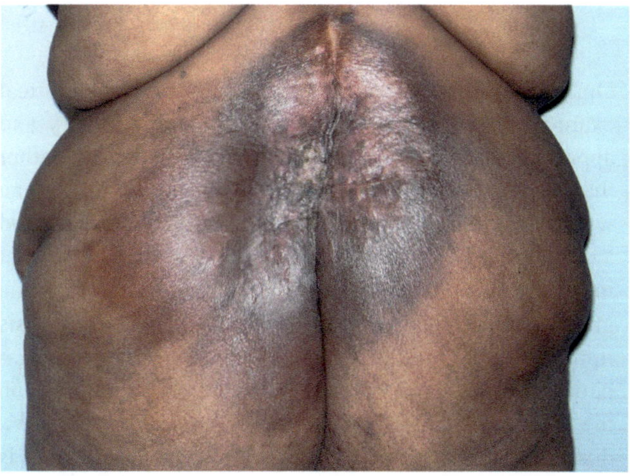
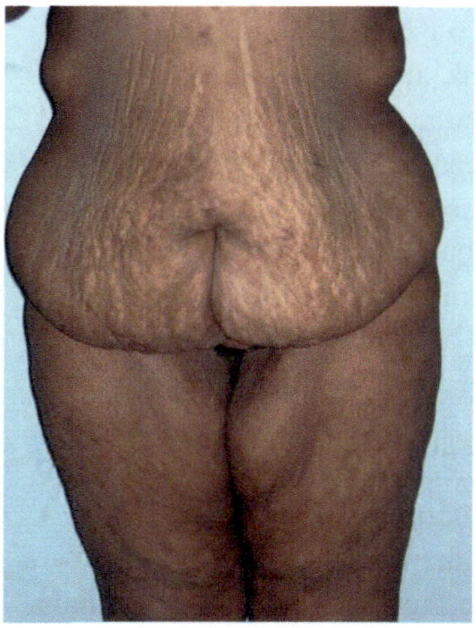

A 42-year-old non-insulin dependent patient with a history of lumbosacral lesion for 2–3 years with gradual enlargement. Spontaneous drainage of pus for the past 6 months and incision and drainage and skin biopsy was performed 6 weeks ago. The skin biopsy was nondiagnostic.

1. Describe the slides and add a focused clinical examination.
   (a) Any tests indicated? Justify.
2. Outline a differential diagnosis. Explain how the clinical exam would narrow the list.
3. Describe a treatment plan that would address the new narrowed list of possible diagnoses. Any operation incorporated into the plan should also be outlined including drawing the excision, if so planned.

Case-Based Conference: Discussion

Case 2: Difficult Wound

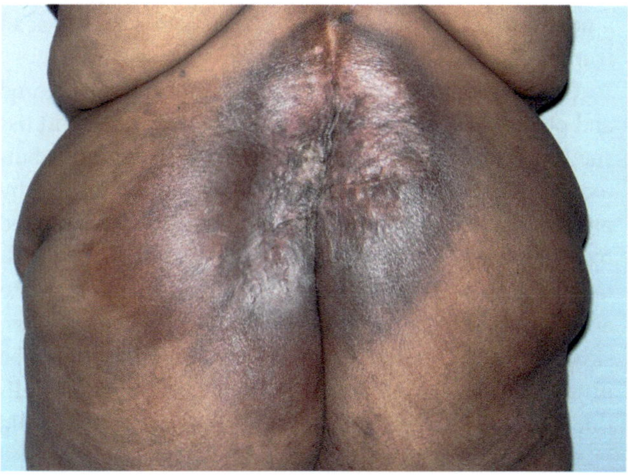
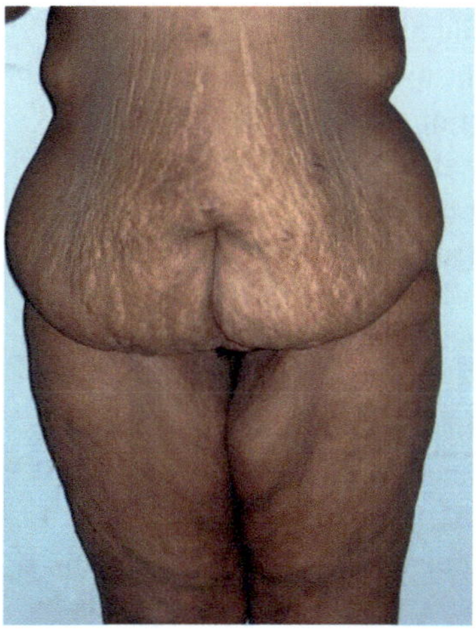

A 42-year-old non-insulin dependent patient with a history of lumbosacral lesion for 2–3 years with gradual enlargement. Spontaneous drainage of pus for the past 6 months and incision and drainage and skin biopsy was performed 6 weeks ago. The skin biopsy was nondiagnostic.

1. Describe the slides and add a focused clinical examination. (Two photos of a Black obese patient, one limited to the posterior trunk from proximal or mid-thigh to lower thoracic region. Transverse rolls of skin and soft tissue are present at the junction of the hips and back. The other photo is of the anterior trunk also from midthoracic to knees. The most pertinent finding is a large central lesion that extends from the lumbar area to the midportion of the gluteal cleft. Laterally, more so on the left than the right, the lesion fans out into the buttock as well as the sacral and lumbar region. No ulceration or exophytic changes are evident but the skin has been altered markedly with darkening and plaque-like changes centrally and patchy lightening of skin superiorly as well as corrugation of the skin surface. The edges of the lesion are indistinct. On the left a triangular area, the tip pointed laterally, of lighter discoloration extends almost to the lateral edge of the buttock. Not including this latter area, the size of the central lesion is 15–18 cm in length and 10–12 cm in width. No other lesions are evident. The abdomen is marked by a substantially sized panniculus, redundant over the pubis onto the proximal thigh.

   The outcome of the clinical examination is crucial to the formulation of a treatment plan. The details of the history should be elucidated including initial appearance if known, the rate of growth over the past 5 months, and the nature of any past treatments. The subsequent questions would focus on associated symptoms including pain, factors that precipitate pain, nature and severity of the pain, and any dysfunction of the lower extremities. Any complaint of dysesthesia or paresthesia should be pursued for details. The presence of any systemic symptoms of malaise and/or any easily fatigability as well as comorbidities, in particular inflammatory bowel or autoimmune disease, is pursued. A social and family history and current medications will complete the history. The physical exam should ascertain the character of the lesion including palpation of firmness, mobility if any, and the nature and character of the soft tissue of the adjacent discolored skin of the buttocks for induration and firmness. A careful neurologic examination of the lower extremity including function and strength of the adductors of the thigh is also performed.)

   (a) Any tests indicated? Justify. (Past medical records, if available, should be obtained including the pathology reading of the skin biopsy. Imaging of the lesion is mandatory, a CT scan initially. The composition of the soft tissue, the extent of the lesion, and any erosion and/or invasion of the underlying bone, the sacrum and lumbar vertebrae, should be observed. Additional tests would be triggered by a history suggestive of the presence of autoimmune disease or other comorbidities. Pathological examination of a repeat skin biopsy may be indicated.)

2. Outline a differential diagnosis. Explain how the clinical exam would narrow the list. (The preamble history and appearance of the lesion imply an inflammatory rather than a neoplastic etiology. The results of the CT scan would be helpful to establish the extent of the disease and a tentative diagnosis. Several possibilities exist that include necrobiosis lipoidica diabeticorum, pyoderma granulosum, calciphylaxis, and vasculitis. Necrobiosis lipoidica diabeticorum, NLD, has been described in diabetics but typically presents as red or yellow plaques on the lower extremity. The scenario illustrated would be a distinctly unusual presentation. Pyoderma granulosum is almost invariably ulcerated with undermined borders, also in association with a number of systemic disorders. Calciphylaxis occurs in renal failure patients and demonstrates calcium deposits in the small blood vessels. Vasculitis would be strongly suggested by inflammation and infiltrate of the dermal arterioles, although not necessarily universal, and would mandate the appropriate consultations for medical workup.)

3. Describe a treatment plan that would address the new narrowed list of possible diagnoses. Any operation incorporated into the plan should also be outlined including drawing the excision, if so planned. (Barring any additional diagnostic or medical information more than that provided by the case preamble and photos, excision by resection is the treatment of choice. Given the duration of the process and appearance of the lesion, a neoplasm is highly unlikely, confirmation by CT scan is mandatory.

   Resection should encompass all the deeply discolored and plaque-like lesion and neighboring indurated soft tissue, but in all probability spare the most lateral left buttock. Until a definitive diagnosis is obtained by pathological examination of the specimen, skin marked by a light discoloration would not be excised. The resultant defect would be substantial and in selection of the appropriate rung or option on the reconstructive ladder, skin graft, local or regional flaps, consideration should be given to the site of the defect, a weight-bearing area. Full-thickness coverage including fat to absorb pressure would be the optimal choice.)

Intraoperative

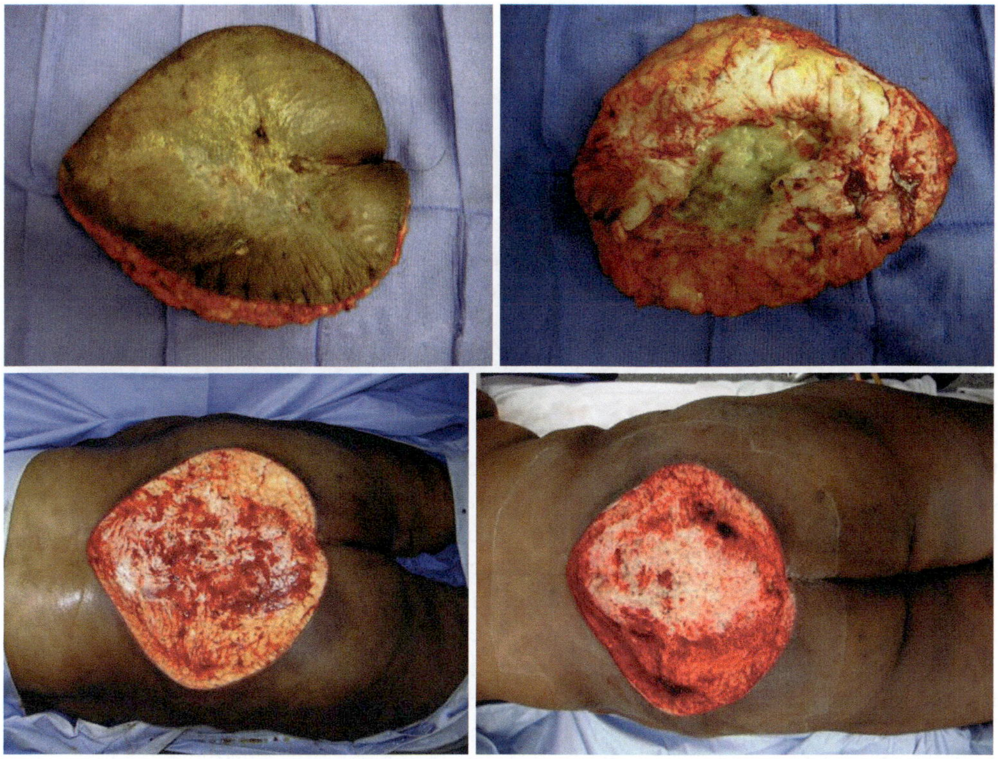

Two photos are of the skin side and deep aspect of the specimen. The thickness of the subcutaneous fat is substantial, probably 3–4 cm, but on the deep aspect of the specimen is a deep purulent crater with complete loss of fat.

The post-resection defect is also depicted. The excision involved the entire lesion and a portion of the discolored skin–soft tissue of the left buttock. The peripheral one-half of the bed consists of subcutaneous fat. The bed of the central portion appears to be lumbosacral fascia, although the photo is somewhat indistinct.

The patient was treated with negative wound pressure therapy for 6 days and then returned to the OR for definitive closure. A comprehensive pathological examination of the specimen failed to yield a definitive diagnosis.

Intraoperative (Post Closure)

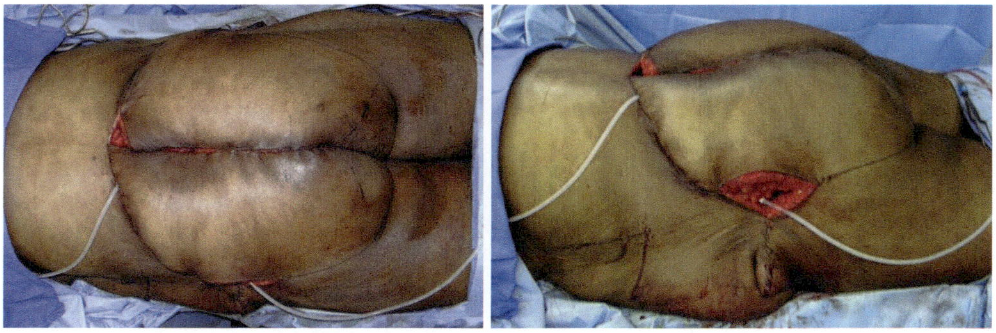

Intraoperative photos include the reconstruction after flap rotation and prior to definitive skin closure. Reconstruction has been accomplished by rotation of bilateral, large, inferiorly based buttock, sacral, and lumbar flaps with V to Y transverse closure of the lateral donor site.

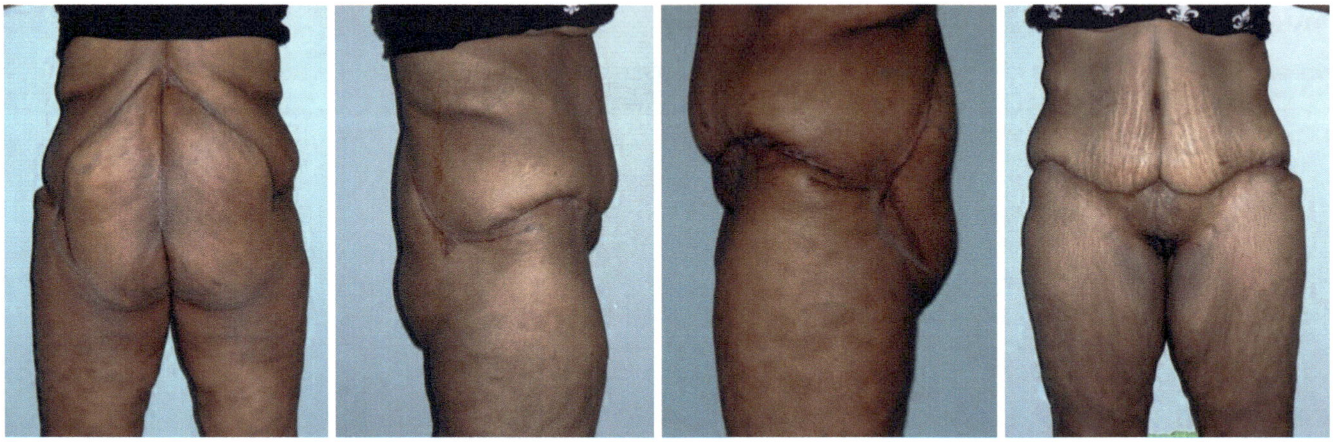

A subsequent series of photos obtained at 6 months demonstrate a healed wound without evidence of recurrence. At this juncture, the patient requested a panniculectomy.

The panniculectomy has healed as well.

Critique

The CT scan yielded important information of a large abscess located superficial to the deep fascia. A more conservative excision could have been performed but in all likelihood would have entailed an additional excision. The flaps were perfused by the superior and inferior gluteal vessels which should be identified with a pencil Doppler prior to flap elevation.

In-Service Examination

1. A patient on an immunomodulator for ulcerative colitis sustained a hand laceration from cleaning lobster 24 h ago and is admitted with sepsis. The most probable organism is:
   (a) MRSA
   (b) Streptococcus beta-hemolytic
   (c) Clostridia
   (d) Vibrio vulnificus
   (e) Mycobacterium marinum
2. The principal culprit in hidradenitis is occlusion of the:
   (a) Apocrine sweat glands
   (b) Eccrine sweat glands
   (c) Apocrine sebaceous glands
   (d) Eccrine sebaceous glands
3. Dapsone is an agent for treatment of brown recluse spider bites and is contraindicated in which of the following?
   (a) Renal compromise
   (b) Elevated liver function test
   (c) 6-phosphate dehydrogenase deficiency
   (d) Congestive heart failure

GPSR Compliance

The European Union's (EU) General Product Safety Regulation (GPSR) is a set of rules that requires consumer products to be safe and our obligations to ensure this.

If you have any concerns about our products, you can contact us on ProductSafety@springernature.com

In case Publisher is established outside the EU, the EU authorized representative is:

Springer Nature Customer Service Center GmbH
Europaplatz 3
69115 Heidelberg, Germany

Batch number: 10731665

Printed by Printforce, the Netherlands